THE WASHINGTON MANUAL®
OF MEDICAL THERAPEUTICS

34th Edition

Department of Medicine
Washington University
School of Medicine
St. Louis, Missouri

Editors

Hemant Godara, MD

Angela Hirbe, MD

Michael Nassif, MD

Hannah Otepka, MD

Aron Rosenstock, MD

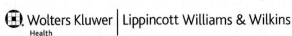
Wolters Kluwer | Lippincott Williams & Wilkins
Health
Philadelphia • Baltimore • New York • London
Buenos Aires • Hong Kong • Sydney • Tokyo

Executive Editor: Rebecca S. Gaertner
Senior Product Manager: Kristina Oberle
Production Manager: David Saltzberg
Manufacturing Manager: Beth Welsh
Senior Marketing Manager: Kimberly Schonberger
Design Coordinator: Teresa Mallon
Production Service: Absolute Service, Inc.
Editorial Coordinator: Katie Sharp

34th Edition

Printed in China

Adhesive binding:
ISBN: 978-1-4511-8851-6
ISBN: 1-4511-8851-X

The Washington Manual® is an intent-to-use mark belonging to Washington University in St. Louis to which international legal protection applies. The mark is used in this publication by LWW under license from Washington University.

Care has been taken to confirm the accuracy of the information presented and to describe generally accepted practices. However, the authors, editors, and publisher are not responsible for errors or omissions or for any consequences from application of the information in this book and make no warranty, expressed or implied, with respect to the currency, completeness, or accuracy of the contents of the publication. Application of the information in a particular situation remains the professional responsibility of the practitioner.

The authors, editors, and publisher have exerted every effort to ensure that drug selection and dosage set forth in this text are in accordance with current recommendations and practice at the time of publication. However, in view of ongoing research, changes in government regulations, and the constant flow of information relating to drug therapy and drug reactions, the reader is urged to check the package insert for each drug for any change in indications and dosage and for added warnings and precautions. This is particularly important when the recommended agent is a new or infrequently employed drug.

Some drugs and medical devices presented in the publication have Food and Drug Administration (FDA) clearance for limited use in restricted research settings. It is the responsibility of the health care provider to ascertain the FDA status of each drug or device planned for use in their clinical practice.

To purchase additional copies of this book, call our customer service department at (800) 638-3030 or fax orders to (301) 223-2320. International customers should call (301) 223-2300.

Visit Lippincott Williams & Wilkins on the Internet: at LWW.com. Lippincott Williams & Wilkins customer service representatives are available from 8:30 am to 6:00 pm, EST.

We dedicate this manual to the outstanding medicine house staff at Washington University and Barnes-Jewish Hospital—their wisdom, dedication, and compassion continue to inspire us each and every day.

Contents

1 Patient Care in Internal Medicine   1

Mark Thoelke, John Cras, Nathan Martin, and Amy Sheldahl

21 Hematologic Disorders and Transfusion Therapy   760

Ronald Jackups, Kristen Sanfilippo, Tzu-Fei Wang, and Morey Blinder

22 Medical Management of Malignant Disease   796

Saiama N. Waqar, Janakiraman Subramanian, George Ansstas, and Ramaswamy Govindan

28 Toxicology 1002
S. Eliza Halcomb, Evan Schwarz, and Michael E. Mullins

Overdoses 1002

Appendix A Immunizations and Postexposure Therapies 1070

Carlos A. Q. Santos and Victoria J. Fraser

Appendix B Infection Control and Isolation Recommendations 1088

Carlos A. Q. Santos and Victoria J. Fraser

Appendix C Advanced Cardiac Life Support Algorithms 1094

Contributors

Zarmeena Ali, MD
Instructor of Medicine Division of Rheumatology

Beau Ances, MD, PhD, MS
Assistant Professor Division of Neurology

George Ansstas, MD
Instructor of Medicine Hospitalist-BMT

Jeffrey J. Atkinson, MD
Assistant Professor of Medicine Division of Pulmonary Medicine

Rachel Bardowell, MD
Instructor in Medicine Hospitalist Service

Rebecca Bavolek, MD
Instructor in Emergency Medicine Division of Emergency Medicine

Morey Blinder, MD
Associate Professor of Medicine Division of Hematology

Anthony Boyer, MD
Clinical Fellow Division of Pulmonary Medicine

Ben P. Bradenham, Jr., MD
Resident Department of Medicine

Angela L. Brown, MD
Assistant Professor of Medicine Division of Cardiology

Robert C. Bucelli, MD, PhD
Assistant Professor Department of Neurology

Bernard C. Camins, MD
Assistant Professor of Medicine Division of Infectious Diseases

Mario Castro, MD
Professor of Medicine Division of Pulmonary and Critical Care

Murali Chakinala, MD
Associate Professor of Medicine Division of Pulmonary and Critical Care

Alexander Chen, MD
Assistant Professor of Medicine Division of Pulmonary and Critical Care

Steven Cheng, MD
Assistant Professor of Medicine Division of Renal Diseases

William E. Clutter, MD
Associate Professor of Medicine Division of Medical Education

Daniel H. Cooper, MD
Assistant Professor of Medicine Division of Cardiovascular Medicine

Daniel Coyne, MD
Professor of Medicine Division of Renal Diseases

John Cras, MD
Assistant Professor of Medicine Hospitalist Service

Sara L. Cross, MD
Clinical Fellow Division of Infectious Diseases

Charles Eby, MD
Professor Department of Pathology & Immunology

Gregory A. Ewald, MD
Associate Professor of Medicine Division of Cardiovascular Medicine

Mitchell N. Faddis, MD, PhD
Associate Professor of Medicine Division of Cardiovascular Medicine

Timothy J. Fendler, MD
Resident Department of Medicine

Victoria J. Fraser, MD
Adolphus Busch Professor of Medicine and Chairman Department of Medicine

Brian F. Gage, MD
Professor of Medicine Division of General Medical Sciences

Anne C. Goldberg, MD
Associate Professor of Medicine Division of Endocrinology and Metabolism

Seth Goldberg, MD
Assistant Professor of Medicine Division of Nephrology

Ramaswamy Govindan, MD
Professor of Medicine Division of Medical Oncology

C. Prakash Gyawali, MD
Professor of Medicine Division of Gastroenterology

S. Eliza Halcomb, MD
Assistant Professor Department of Emergency Medicine

Ronald Jackups, MD
Assistant Professor of Pathology and Immunology Laboratory and Genomic Medicine

Judy L. Jang, MD
Assistant Professor of Medicine Division of Renal Diseases

Susan M. Joseph, MD
Assistant Professor of Medicine Division of Cardiovascular Medicine

Andrew L. Kau, MD
Clinical Fellow Division of Allergy and Immunology

Thomas Kerr, MD
Assistant Professor of Medicine Division of Gastroenterology

Nigar Kirmani, MD
Professor of Medicine Division of Infectious Diseases

Mohammad Kizilbash, MD
Assistant Professor of Medicine Division of Cardiovascular Medicine

Christina L. Klein, MD
Assistant Professor of Medicine Division of Renal Diseases

Marin H. Kollef, MD
Professor of Medicine Division of Pulmonary & Critical Care

Shane J. LaRue, MD
Clinical Fellow Division of Cardiovascular Medicine

Stephen Y. Liang, MD
Instructor in Medicine Division of Infectious Diseases

Brian R. Lindman, MD
Assistant Professor of Medicine Division of Cardiovascular Medicine

Mauricio Lisker-Melman, MD
Professor of Medicine Division of Gastroenterology

Nathan Martin, MD
Instructor in Medicine Hospitalist Service

Colleen McEvoy, MD
Clinical Fellow Division of Pulmonary and Critical Care

Janet B. McGill, MD
Professor of Medicine Division of Endocrinology

Jason D. Meyers, MD
Clinical Fellow Division of Cardiovascular Medicine

Scott T. Micek, PharmD, BCPS
Department of Pharmacy Barnes-Jewish Hospital

Brent W. Miller, MD
Associate Professor of Medicine Division of Nephrology

Hector Molina, MD
Associate Professor of Medicine Division of Rheumatology

Michael E. Mullins, MD
Associate Professor of Emergency Medicine Department of Medicine

E. Turner Overton, MD
Adjunct Assistant Professor of Medicine Division of Infectious Diseases

Jeffrey R. Parker, MD
Instructor in Medicine Division of Hospitalist Medicine

Amit Patel, MD
Resident Department of Medicine

Dominic Reeds, MD
Assistant Professor in Medicine Director, Clinical Nutrition Support Service

David J. Ritchie, PharmD
Clinical Pharmacist Division of Infectious Diseases

Daniel B. Rosenbluth, MD
Professor of Medicine and Pediatrics Division of Pulmonary and Critical Care

M. Katherine Rude, MD
Clinical Fellow Division of Gastroenterology

Tonya D. Russell, MD
Associate Professor of Medicine Division of Pulmonary and Critical Care

Christopher Sampson, MD
Assistant Professor of Emergency Medicine Division of Emergency Medicine

Kristen Sanfilippo, MD
Clinical Fellow Division of Medical Oncology

Carlos A. Q. Santos, MD
Assistant Professor of Medicine Division of Infectious Diseases

Muhammad A. Sarwar, MD
Research Fellow Division of Cardiovascular Medicine

Sarena Sawlani, MD
Clinical Fellow Division of Allergy and Immunology

Evan Schwarz, MD
Assistant Professor of Emergency Medicine Division of Emergency Medicine

Robert M. Senior, MD
D & H Moog Professor of Pulmonary Diseases Division of Pulmonary and Critical Care

Jay Shah, MD
Instructor in Medicine Division of Cardiovascular Medicine

Shivak Sharma, MD
Clinical Fellow Division of Cardiovascular Medicine

Amy Sheldahl, MD
Instructor in Medicine Hospitalist Service

Ajay Sheshadri, MD
Clinical Fellow Division of Pulmonary and Critical Care

Janakiraman Subramanian, MD
Instructor in Medicine Division of Medical Oncology

Mark Thoelke, MD
Associate Professor Division of Hospital Medicine

Jason Wagner, MD
Assistant Professor of Emergency Medicine Division of Emergency Medicine

Tzu-Fei Wang, MD
Clinical Fellow Division of Medical Oncology

Saiama N. Waqar, MD
Instructor in Medicine Division of Medical Oncology

Jennifer M. Welch, MD
Clinical Fellow Division of Immunology

Roger Yusen, MD, MPH
Associate Professor of Medicine Division of Pulmonary and Critical Care

Chairman's Note

The rate of increase of medical knowledge places an enormous burden on physicians to keep up with recent advances, particularly in novel therapies that will improve patient outcomes. The *Washington Manual*® *of Medical Therapeutics* provides an easily accessible source of current information that covers a practical clinical approach to the diagnosis, investigation, and treatment of common medical conditions that internists encounter on a regular basis. The pocketbook size of the *Manual* ensures that it will continue to be of enormous assistance to interns, residents, medical students, and other practitioners in need of readily accessible practical clinical information. It meets an important unmet need in an era of information overload.

I acknowledge the authors, who include house officers, fellows, and attendings, at Washington University/Barnes-Jewish Hospital. Their efforts and outstanding skill are evident in the quality of the final product. In particular, I am proud of our editors—Hemant Godara, Angela Hirbe, Michael Nassif, Hannah Otepka, and Aron Rosenstock—and the series editors—Tom De Fer and Katherine Henderson—who have worked tirelessly to produce another outstanding edition of the *Manual*. I also recognize Melvin Blanchard, MD, Chief of the Division of Medical Education in the Department of Medicine at Washington University, for his guidance and advice. I am confident that this *Manual* will meet its desired goal of providing practical knowledge that can be directly applied to improving patient care.

Victoria J. Fraser, MD
Adolphus Busch Professor of Medicine
Chairman, Department of Medicine
Washington University School of Medicine
St. Louis, Missouri

Preface

We have the pleasure of introducing the 34th edition of *The Washington Manual of Medical Therapeutics*. "The Manual," as it has been labeled here at Washington University, has a proud tradition of being edited by the Internal Medicine Chief Residents. It was initially intended for use by local medical students and house staff but has now grown to be the best-selling medical text in the world. Beyond the increase in production, the *Manual* has grown in size and complexity, mirroring the practice of medicine. Wayland MacFarlane served as the initial editor in 1943, and numerous revisions have occurred in its 70 years of existence, moving from a short textbook to a portable reference. Today, we hope to continue that evolution in providing the rich text in both written and electronic form with availability on portable electronic devices.

We continue the virtues that made the work a success: a concise discussion of pathophysiology, an evidence-based presentation of current therapies, and a sensible format. Additionally, we have diligently updated the content to reflect ever-changing advances in medicine.

The Washington Manual of Medical Therapeutics has established a tradition of excellence that we aspire to preserve. Throughout this year, the medicine house staff, fellows, medical students, and attendings have inspired us. Their brilliance, commitment, and compassion are truly remarkable. We are honored that they turn to the *Manual* for guidance. We are deeply indebted for the substantial support and direction that Tom De Fer, the series editor, provided in the creation of this edition of the *Manual*. We also thank Katie Sharp and the editorial staff at Lippincott Williams & Wilkins for their assistance and patience with our busy schedules.

We have had the honor and pleasure of serving as Chief Residents of Shatz-Strauss, Karl-Flance, Kipnis-Daughaday, North Campus firms, and The Primary Care Medicine Clinic in the Barnes-Jewish Center for Outpatient Health. Our Firm Chiefs, Megan Wren, William Clutter, Geoffrey Cislo, and E-P Barrette, have been instrumental over the course of the year, serving as mentors and role models. Our program director, Melvin Blanchard, has been a great help in the production of the *Manual*. Our Chairman of Medicine, Vicky Fraser, provided guidance and support in the creation of this text. We thank our families for their support and inspiration. To Ram Kumar, Malka, and Robbie; Patrick and Carla, TJ and Gabriel; Edward, Cecelia, and Karla; Steve, Karen, and Arun; Julio, Katty, and Jessi ... our gratitude is beyond measure.

Hemant Godara, MD
Angela Hirbe, MD, PhD
Michael Nassif, MD
Hannah Otepka, MD
Aron Rosenstock, MD

1

Patient Care in Internal Medicine

Mark Thoelke, John Cras, Nathan Martin, and Amy Sheldahl

General Care of the Hospitalized Patient

GENERAL PRINCIPLES

- Although a general approach to common problems can be outlined, **therapy must be individualized**. All diagnostic and therapeutic procedures should be explained carefully to the patient, including the potential risks, benefits, and alternatives. This explanation minimizes anxiety and provides the patient and the physician with appropriate expectations.
- The period of hospitalization represents a complex interplay of multiple caregivers that subjects the patient to potential harm by **medical errors and iatrogenic complications**. Every effort must be made to minimize these risks. Basic measures include:
  - Use of standardized abbreviations and dose designations
  - Excellent communication between physicians and other caregivers
  - Institution of appropriate prophylactic precautions
  - Prevention of nosocomial infections, including attention to hygiene and discontinuation of unnecessary catheters
  - Medicine reconciliation at all transfers of care
- **Hospital orders**
  - **Admission orders** should be written promptly after evaluation of a patient. Each set of orders should bear the **date and time** of writing and the legible signature of the physician. Consideration should be given to including a **printed signature** and a **contact number**. All orders should be clear, concise, organized, and legible. Computer order entry facilitates aspects of this process.
  - To ensure that no important therapeutic measures are overlooked, the content and organization of admission orders may follow the outline that follows (the **mnemonic ADC VANDISMAL**):
    - **A**dmitting service, location, and physician responsible for the patient
    - **D**iagnoses
    - **C**ondition of the patient
    - **V**ital signs with frequency
    - **A**ctivity limitations
    - **N**ursing instructions (e.g., Foley catheter to gravity drainage, wound care, daily weights)
    - **D**iet. Remember that "NPO" may preclude oral medications unless specified
    - **I**ntravenous (IV) fluids, including composition and rate
    - **S**edatives, analgesics, and other as needed (PRN) medications
    - **M**edications, including dose, frequency, route, and indication; state "first dose now" when appropriate

- Allergies, sensitivities, and previous drug reactions
- Laboratory tests and radiographic studies
○ Orders should be reevaluated frequently and altered as patient status dictates.
○ Daily rounds should include assessment for ongoing need of IV fluids, medications, telemetry, and supplemental oxygen.
• **Discharge**
  ○ **Discharge planning** begins at the time of admission. Assessment of the patient's social situation and potential discharge needs should be made at this time.
  ○ **Early coordination** with nursing, social work, and case coordinators/managers facilitates efficient discharge and a complete postdischarge plan.
  ○ **Patient education** should occur regarding changes in medications and other new therapies. Compliance with treatment is influenced by patient's understanding of that treatment.
  ○ **Prescriptions** should be written for all new medication, and the patient should be provided with a complete medication list including instructions and indications.
  ○ **Communication** with physicians who will be resuming care of the patient after discharge is important for optimal follow-up care.

PROPHYLACTIC MEASURES

Venous Thromboembolism Prophylaxis

GENERAL PRINCIPLES

Epidemiology
Venous thromboembolism (VTE) is among the most common preventable causes of death in hospitalized patients. Between 70% and 80% of fatal pulmonary emboli occur in nonsurgical patients (*Chest 2007;132:936*). Approximately 40% of medical inpatients are considered high risk for VTE by risk factors (≥4 points) described in the following and would therefore benefit from VTE prophylaxis (*J Thromb Haemost 2010;8:2450*).

Risk Factors
Weighted risk factors for VTE in hospitalized medical patients include:
• 3 points: active cancer, previous VTE (excluding superficial vein thrombosis), known thrombophilic condition, bed rest for at least 3 days
• 2 points: trauma or surgery <1 month ago
• 1 point: age over 70, obesity (body mass index [BMI] >30), heart and/or respiratory failure, acute myocardial infarction (MI), ischemic stroke, acute infection and/or rheumatologic disorder, ongoing hormonal treatment

Prevention
• **Pharmacologic prophylaxis results in a 50% decrease in VTE risk.**
• All able patients should be encouraged to ambulate several times a day.
• Acutely ill patients at high risk of VTE using risk factors described previously without active bleeding or high risk for bleeding should be initiated on **prophylactic dosing** of low-dose unfractionated heparin (UFH), 5,000 units SC q8h or q12, or low–molecular-weight heparin (LMWH), enoxaparin, 40 mg SC daily or dalteparin, 5,000 units SC daily, or fondaparinux, 2.5 mg SC daily. Aspirin alone is not sufficient for prophylaxis (*Chest 2012;141:e195S*).

- At-risk patients with contraindications to anticoagulation prophylaxis may receive mechanical prophylaxis with intermittent pneumatic compression or graded compression stockings, although evidence of benefit is lacking in medical patients (*Chest 2012;141:e195S*; *Ann Intern Med 2011;155:625*).

Decubitus Ulcers

GENERAL PRINCIPLES

Epidemiology

Decubitus ulcers typically occur within the first 2 weeks of hospitalization and can develop within 2 to 6 hours. Once they develop, decubitus ulcers are difficult to heal and have been associated with increased mortality (*J Gerontol A Biol Sci Med Sci 1997;52:M106*). Risk factors for the development of decubitus ulcers include, advanced age, paralysis, and severe illness (*Clin Dermatol 2010;28(5):527*).

Prevention

Prevention is the key to management of decubitus ulcers. While the majority of decubitus ulcers are preventable, evidence for best practices is lacking, and it is likely not all decubitus ulcers are avoidable). Measures include:

- **Risk factor assessment**, including immobility, limited activity, incontinence, impaired nutritional status, impaired circulation, and altered level of consciousness.
- **Skin care**, including daily inspection with particular attention to bony prominences, minimizing exposure to moisture from incontinence, perspiration, or wound drainage, and applying moisturizers to dry sacral skin.
- Nutritional supplements should be provided to patients at risk.
- Interventions aimed at **relieving or redistributing pressure**, including frequent repositioning (minimum of every 2 hours, or every 1 hour for wheelchair-bound patients), pillows or foam wedges between bony prominences, maintenance of the head of the bed at the lowest degree of elevation, and use of lifting devices when moving patients. **Pressure-reducing and relieving devices** (foam, dynamic air mattresses, low–air-loss and air-fluidized beds) can also be used (*JAMA 2006; 296:974*).

DIAGNOSIS

Clinical Presentation

National Pressure Ulcer Advisory Panel Staging:

- **Suspected deep tissue injury:** Purple or maroon localized area of discolored intact skin or blood-filled blister due to damage of underlying soft tissue from pressure and/or shear. The area may be preceded by tissue that is painful, firm, mushy, boggy, warmer, or cooler as compared to adjacent tissue.
- **Stage I:** Intact skin with nonblanchable redness of a localized area usually over a bony prominence. Darkly pigmented skin may not have visible blanching; its color may differ from the surrounding area.
- **Stage II:** Partial thickness loss of dermis presenting as a shallow open ulcer with a red pink wound bed without slough. May also present as an intact or open/ ruptured serum-filled blister.
- **Stage III:** Full thickness tissue loss. Subcutaneous fat may be visible but bone, tendon, or muscle are not exposed. Slough may be present but does not obscure the depth of tissue loss. May include undermining and tunneling.

- **Stage IV:** Full thickness tissue loss with exposed bone, tendon, or muscle. Slough or eschar may be present on some parts of the wound bed. Often include undermining and tunneling.
- **Unstageable:** Full thickness tissue loss in which the base of the ulcer is covered by slough (yellow, tan, gray, green, or brown) and/or eschar (tan, brown, or black) in the wound bed.

TREATMENT

- **Initial interventions** include use of pressure-relieving devices, pain control, normal saline for cleansing, avoidance of agents that delay healing (antiseptic agents [Dakin solution, hydrogen peroxide, chlorhexidine] and wet-to-dry gauze), and removal of necrotic debris. Moist wounds heal best, and **occlusive dressings** (such as hydrocolloid dressings) should be used to maintain a moist environment while controlling exudate. **Topical agents** can also be used (silver sulfadiazine [Silvadene], bacitracin, Neosporin, Polysporin) to optimizing healing or for minor slough debridement (Santyl, Xenaderm).
- **Adequate nutrition** is recommended, although there is insufficient data to recommend a specific supplement regimen (*Cochrane Database Syst Rev. 2003;(4): CD003216*).
- Infected decubitus ulcers with evidence of cellulitis or lymphangitis require systemic antibiotics, but there is no role for antibiotics to aid healing of a noninfected ulcer.
- **Other adjunctive therapies** for nonhealing ulcers include electrical stimulation, radiant heat, negative pressure therapy, and surgical intervention (*JAMA 2008; 300:2647*).

Other Precautions

GENERAL PRINCIPLES

- **Fall precautions** should be written for patients who have a history of falls or are at high risk of a fall (i.e., those with dementia, syncope, orthostatic hypotension). Falls are the most common accident in hospitalized patients, frequently leading to injury. Fall risk should not be equated with confinement to bed, which may lead to debilitation and higher risk of future falls.
- **Seizure precautions** should be considered for patients with a history of seizures or those at risk of seizing. Precautions include padded bed rails and an oral airway at the bedside.
- **Restraint orders** are written for patients who are at risk of injuring themselves or interfering with their treatment due to disruptive or dangerous behaviors. Restraint orders must be reviewed and renewed every 24 hours. Physical restraints may exacerbate agitation. Bed alarms or sitters are alternatives in appropriate settings.

ACUTE INPATIENT CARE

- New or recurrent symptoms that require evaluation and management frequently develop in hospitalized patients.
- Evaluation should generally include a directed history, including a complete description of the symptom (i.e., alleviating and precipitating factors, quality of the

symptom, associated symptoms, and the course of the symptom, including acuity of onset, severity, duration, and previous episodes), a directed physical examination, review of the medical problem list, review of medications with attention to recent medication changes, and consideration of recent procedures.
- Further evaluation should be directed by the initial assessment, the acuity and severity of the complaint, and the diagnostic possibilities.
- An approach to selected common complaints is presented in this section.

Chest Pain

GENERAL PRINCIPLES

Chest pain is a common complaint in the hospitalized patient, and the severity of chest discomfort does not always correlate with the gravity of its cause.

DIAGNOSIS

Clinical Presentation

History
History should be taken in the context of the patient's other medical conditions, particularly previous cardiac or vascular history, cardiac risk factors, and factors that would predispose the patient to a pulmonary embolus.

Physical Examination
Physical examination is ideally conducted during an episode of pain and includes vital signs (with bilateral blood pressure [BP] measurements if considering aortic dissection), a careful cardiopulmonary and abdominal examination, and inspection and palpation of the chest for possible trauma, rash, and reproducibility of the pain.

Differential Diagnosis

Causes of chest pain in the medical inpatient range from life-threatening causes such as MI, aortic dissection, and pulmonary embolism to other causes including esophageal reflux, peptic ulcer disease, pneumonia, costochondritis, shingles, trauma to chest wall, and anxiety.

Diagnostic Testing

Assessment of **oxygenation status, chest radiography, and electrocardiogram (ECG)** is appropriate in most patients. Serial cardiac enzymes should be obtained if there is suspicion of ischemia. Spiral computed tomography (CT) and ventilation/perfusion (VQ) scans are employed to diagnose pulmonary embolus.

TREATMENT

- If **cardiac ischemia** is a concern, initial therapy should include supplemental oxygen, aspirin, and administration of nitroglycerin, 0.4 mg SL, or morphine sulfate, 1 to 2 mg IV, or both. (See Chapter 4, Ischemic Heart Disease.)
- If a **gastrointestinal (GI) source** of chest pain is suspected, a combination of Maalox and diphenhydramine (30 mL of each in a 1:1 mix) can be administered.

- **Musculoskeletal pain** typically responds to acetaminophen or nonsteroidal anti-inflammatory drug (NSAID) therapy.
- **Prompt empiric anticoagulation** while awaiting testing should be considered if there is high suspicion for MI or pulmonary embolism (barring contraindication).

Dyspnea

GENERAL PRINCIPLES

Dyspnea is most commonly caused by a cardiopulmonary abnormality, such as congestive heart failure (CHF), cardiac ischemia, bronchospasm, pulmonary embolus, infection, mucus plugging, and aspiration. Dyspnea must be promptly and carefully evaluated.

DIAGNOSIS

Clinical Presentation

History
Initial evaluation should include a review of the medical history for underlying pulmonary or cardiovascular disease and a directed history.

Physical Examination
A detailed cardiopulmonary examination should take place, including vital signs with comparison of current findings to those documented earlier. Auscultation of the heart and lungs are vital to the exam in patients with dyspnea.

Diagnostic Testing
- Oxygen assessment should take place promptly. Arterial blood gas measurement provides more information than pulse oximetry. Chest radiography is useful in most patients.
- Other diagnostic and therapeutic measures should be directed by the findings in the initial evaluation and the severity of the suspected diagnosis.

TREATMENT

Therapeutic measures should be directed by the findings in the initial evaluation and the severity of the suspected diagnoses. If the patient is hypoxic, oxygen administration should be delivered in a prompt fashion.

Acute Hypertensive Episodes

GENERAL PRINCIPLES

- Acute hypertensive episodes in the hospital are most often caused by inadequately treated essential hypertension.
- Volume overload and pain may exacerbate hypertension and should be recognized appropriately and treated.
- Hypertension associated with withdrawal syndromes (e.g., alcohol, cocaine) and rebound hypertension associated with sudden withdrawal of antihypertensive medi-

cations (i.e., clonidine, α-adrenergic antagonists) should be considered. These entities should be treated as discussed in Chapter 3, Preventive Cardiology.

TREATMENT

Treatment decisions should consider baseline BP, presence of symptoms (e.g., chest pain or shortness of breath), and current and baseline antihypertensive medications. **Overtreatment with IV medications should be avoided.**

Fever

GENERAL PRINCIPLES

Fever accompanies many illnesses and is a valuable marker of disease activity.

DIAGNOSIS

Clinical Presentation
History
History should include chronology of the fever and associated symptoms, medications, potential exposures, and a complete social and travel history.

Physical Examination
• Physical examination should include **oral or rectal temperature** monitoring from a consistent site. In the hospitalized patient, special attention should be paid to any rash, new murmur, abnormal fluid accumulation, IV lines, and indwelling devices such as gastric tubes or Foley catheters.
• In the **neutropenic patient**, the skin, oral cavity, and perineal area should be examined carefully for breaches of mucosal integrity. For management of neutropenic fever, see Chapter 22, Medical Management of Malignant Disease.

Differential Diagnosis
• Infection is a primary concern. Drug reaction, malignancy, VTE, vasculitis, central fever, and tissue infarction are other possibilities but are diagnoses of exclusion.
• The pace and complexity of the workup depends on the diagnostic considerations taken in the context of the clinical stability and immune status of the patient.

Diagnostic Testing
• Testing includes culture of blood and urine, complete blood count (CBC) with differential, serum chemistries with liver function tests, and urinalysis.
• Diagnostic evaluation generally includes chest radiography.
• Cultures of abnormal fluid collections, sputum, cerebrospinal fluid, and stool should be sent if clinically indicated. Cultures are ideally obtained prior to initiation of antibiotics; however, antibiotics should not be delayed if serious infection is suspected.

TREATMENT

• Not all fevers require treatment. **Antipyretic drugs** may be given to decrease associated discomfort. Aspirin, 325 mg, and acetaminophen, 325 to 650 mg PO or per rectum q4h, are the drugs of choice. **Aspirin should be avoided in adolescents** with possible viral infections because this combination has been associated with Reye syndrome.

- **Tepid water baths** are effective in treating hyperpyrexia. Use of hypothermic (cooling) blankets and ice packs are uncomfortable and should generally be discouraged.
- **Empiric antibiotics** should be considered in hemodynamically unstable patients in whom infection is a primary concern, as well as in neutropenic and asplenic patients.
- **Heat stroke and malignant hyperthermia** are medical emergencies that require prompt recognition and treatment (see Chapter 27, Medical Emergencies).

Pain

GENERAL PRINCIPLES

Definition

Pain is subjective, and therapy must be individualized. Chronic pain may not be associated with any objective physical findings. **Pain scales** should be employed for quantitation.

Classification

- Acute pain usually requires only temporary therapy.
- For chronic pain, a combination of basal pain medication with bolus as needed doses may be needed.
- Anticonvulsants and antidepressants, such as gabapentin and tricyclic antidepressants (TCAs), are useful adjuncts for neuropathic pain. If pain is refractory to conventional therapy, then nonpharmacologic modalities, such as nerve blocks, sympathectomy, and cognitive behavioral therapy, may be appropriate.

TREATMENT

Medications

- **Acetaminophen**
  - **Effects:** Antipyretic and analgesic actions but no anti-inflammatory or antiplatelet properties.
  - **Preparations and dosage:** Acetaminophen, 325 to 1,000 mg q4–6h (maximum dose, 4 g/d), is available in tablet, caplet, liquid, intravenous, and rectal suppository form. It should be used at low doses in patients with liver disease (less than 2 g/d).
  - **Adverse effects**
    - The principal advantage of acetaminophen is its lack of gastric toxicity.
    - **Hepatic toxicity** may be serious, and acute overdose with 10 to 15 g can cause fatal hepatic necrosis (see Chapter 19, Liver Diseases, and Chapter 27, Medical Emergencies).
- **Aspirin**
  - **Effects:** Aspirin has analgesic, antipyretic, anti-inflammatory, and antiplatelet effects.
  - **Preparations and dosages**
    - 325 to 650 mg PO q4h PRN (maximum dose, 4 g/d).

- Rectal suppositories, 300 to 600 mg q3–4h may be irritating to the mucosa and have variable absorption.
  - Enteric-coated tablets may cause less injury to the gastric mucosa than buffered or plain aspirin.
  ○ **Adverse effects**
    - Dose-related side effects include tinnitus, dizziness, and hearing loss.
    - Dyspepsia and GI bleeding can develop and may be severe.
    - Hypersensitivity reactions, including bronchospasm, laryngeal edema, and urticaria, are uncommon, but patients with asthma and nasal polyps are more susceptible.
    - **Patients with allergic or bronchospastic reactions to aspirin should not be given NSAIDs.**
    - Chronic excessive use can result in interstitial nephritis and papillary necrosis.
    - Aspirin should be used with caution in patients with hepatic or renal disease, bleeding disorders, pregnancy, and those who are receiving anticoagulation therapy.
    - **Antiplatelet effects** may last for up to 1 week after a single dose.
- **NSAIDs**
  ○ **Effects:** NSAIDs have analgesic, antipyretic, and anti-inflammatory properties mediated by inhibition of cyclooxygenase. All NSAIDs have similar efficacy and toxicities, with a side-effect profile similar to that of aspirin.
  ○ **Adverse effects**
    - NSAIDs may blunt the cardioprotective effects of aspirin.
    - **NSAIDs should be used with caution in patients with impaired renal or hepatic function** (see Chapter 25, Arthritis and Rheumatologic Diseases).
    - The U.S. Food and Drug Administration (FDA) has issued a boxed warning that all NSAIDs (including cyclooxygenase-2 [COX-2] inhibitors) are associated with an increased risk of adverse cardiovascular thrombotic events, including MI and stroke. NSAIDs are contraindicated immediately postoperative from coronary artery bypass surgery.
- **Ketorolac** is an NSAID analgesic that can be given intramuscularly (IM) or IV, 15 to 30 mg q8h, and is often used postoperatively; however, parenteral therapy should not exceed 5 days. Nephrotoxicity is more pronounced with IM than with PO administration.
- **Cyclooxygenase-2 (COX-2) inhibitors**
  ○ **Effects:** COX-2 inhibitors act primarily on COX-2, an inducible form of cyclooxygenase and an important mediator of pain and inflammation. COX-2 inhibitors have little significant effect on the gastric mucosa. COX-2 inhibitors offer no analgesic advantage over other NSAIDs.
  ○ **Preparations and dosages:** The currently available selective COX-2 inhibitor is **celecoxib**. **Meloxicam** is also available but is less selective for COX-2.
  ○ **Adverse effects**
    - Chronic, high-dose COX-2 inhibitor increased the risk of adverse cardiovascular events in one study, but a subsequent meta-analysis of randomized controlled trials showed no increased risk of adverse cardiovascular outcomes, although most patients in these studies received only a short course of celecoxib (*N Engl J Med 2006;355:873*; *Am J Cardiol 2007;99:91*). While pharmacologic data suggest celecoxib has no effects on the platelet inhibitory effects of aspirin or Plavix, there is some concern for increased thrombotic risk when celecoxib is

used after cardiac stenting (*J Clin Pharmacology 2002;42:1027; Korean Circ J 2010; 40(7):321; Eur Heart J 2012 Mar 8. [Epub ahead of print]*).

- COX-2 inhibitors should not be used in patients who have allergic or bronchospastic reactions to aspirin or other NSAIDs.
- Celecoxib is contraindicated in patients with allergic-type **reactions to sulfonamides**.
- **Opioid analgesics**
  - **Effects:** Opioid analgesics are pharmacologically similar to opium or morphine and are the drugs of choice when analgesia without antipyretic action is desired.
  - **Preparations and dosages:** Table 1-1 lists equianalgesic dosages.
  - **Constant pain**
    - Constant pain requires continuous (basal) analgesia with supplementary, PRN doses for breakthrough pain at doses of roughly 5% to 15% of the daily basal dose. Medication dosages should be maintained at the lowest level that provides adequate analgesia. If frequent PRN doses are required, the maintenance dose should be increased, or the dosing interval should be decreased.
    - **If adequate analgesia** cannot be achieved at the maximum recommended dose of one narcotic or if the side effects are intolerable, the patient should be changed to another preparation beginning at one half of the equianalgesic dose to account for incomplete cross-tolerance.
    - **Oral medications** should be used when possible.
    - **Parenteral and transdermal administration** are useful in the setting of dysphagia, emesis, or decreased GI absorption.
    - **Continuous IV administration** provides steady blood levels and allows for rapid dose adjustment.
    - Agents with short half-lives, such as morphine, should be used. Narcotic-naïve patients should be started on the lowest possible doses, whereas patients with demonstrated tolerance will require higher doses.
    - **Patient-controlled analgesia** is often used to control pain in a postoperative or terminally ill patient.
    - Advantages of patient-controlled analgesia include enhancement in pain relief, and decrease in anxiety. Opioid-naïve patients should not have basal rates prescribed due to risk of overdose.

Table 1-1	Equipotent Doses of Opioid Analgesics			
Drug	**Onset (min)**	**Duration (hr)**	**IM/IV/SC (mg)**	**PO (mg)**
Fentanyl	7–8	1–2	0.1	NA
Levorphanol	30–90	4–6	2	4
Hydromorphone	15–30	2–4	1.5–2.0	7.5
Methadone	30–60	4–12	10	20
Morphine	15–30	2–4	10	30[a]
Oxycodone	15–30	3–4	NA	20
Codeine	15–30	4–6	120	200

Note: Equivalences are based on single-dose studies.
[a]An IM:PO ratio of 1:2 to 1:3 used for repetitive dosing.
NA, not applicable.

○ **Selected drugs**
- **Codeine** is usually given in combination with aspirin or acetaminophen. It is also an effective cough suppressant at a dosage of 10 to 15 mg PO q4–6h.
- **Oxycodone and hydrocodone** are also usually prescribed orally in combination with acetaminophen. Available tablets include oxycodone with acetaminophen, 5 mg/325 or 7.5 mg/325 PO q6h, and hydrocodone with acetaminophen, 5 mg/325, 5 mg/500, 7.5 mg/325, or 7.5 mg/500 PO q4–6h. Care should be taken to avoid acetaminophen overdose with these formulations. Oxycodone is available without acetaminophen and should be used for patients requiring higher opioid doses to avoid acetaminophen toxicity.
- **Immediate-release and sustained-release morphine sulfate** preparations (immediate-release, 5 to 30 mg PO q2–8h, sustained-release, 15 to 120 mg PO q12h or a rectal suppository) can be used. The liquid form can be useful in patients who have difficulty in swallowing pills. Larger doses of morphine may be necessary to control pain as tolerance develops. Morphine should be used with caution in renal insufficiency.
- **Meperidine** is no longer recommended for pain treatment due to limited efficacy and a very short duration of analgesia with significant euphoria.
- **Methadone** is very effective when administered orally and suppresses the symptoms of withdrawal from other opioids because of its extended half-life. Despite its long elimination half-life, its analgesic duration of action is much shorter.
- **Hydromorphone**, 2 to 4 mg PO q4–6h; 1 to 2 mg IM, IV, or SC q4–6h, is a potent morphine derivative. It is also available as a 3-mg rectal suppository.
- **Fentanyl** is available in a transdermal patch with sustained release over 72 hours. Initial onset of action is delayed. Respiratory depression may occur more frequently with fentanyl.
- **Mixed agonist–antagonist agents** (butorphanol, nalbuphine, oxymorphone, pentazocine) offer few advantages and produce more adverse effects than do the other agents.

○ **Precautions**
- **Opioids are relatively contraindicated** in acute disease states in which the pattern and degree of pain are important diagnostic signs (e.g., head injuries, abdominal pain). They may also increase intracranial pressure.
- **Opioids should be used with caution** in patients with hypothyroidism, Addison disease, hypopituitarism, anemia, respiratory disease (e.g., chronic obstructive pulmonary disease [COPD], asthma, kyphoscoliosis, severe obesity), severe malnutrition, debilitation, or chronic cor pulmonale.
- Opioid dosage should be adjusted for patients with impaired hepatic function.
- Drugs that potentiate the adverse effects of opioids include phenothiazines, antidepressants, benzodiazepines, and alcohol.
- **Tolerance** develops with chronic use and coincides with the development of physical dependence.
- **Physical dependence** is characterized by a withdrawal syndrome (anxiety, irritability, diaphoresis, tachycardia, GI distress, and temperature instability) when the drug is stopped abruptly. It may occur after only 2 weeks of therapy.
- Administration of an opioid antagonist may precipitate withdrawal after only 3 days of therapy. Withdrawal can be minimized by tapering the medication slowly over several days.

○ **Adverse and toxic effects**
  ▪ Although individuals may tolerate some preparations better than others, at equianalgesic doses, few differences in side effects exist.
  ▪ **Central nervous system (CNS) effects** include sedation, euphoria, and pupillary constriction.
  ▪ **Respiratory depression** is dose related and is especially pronounced after IV administration.
  ▪ **Cardiovascular effects** include peripheral vasodilation and hypotension, especially after IV administration.
  ▪ **GI effects** include constipation, nausea, and vomiting. Patients who are receiving opioid medications should be provided with stool softeners and laxatives. Benzodiazepines, dopamine antagonists (e.g., prochlorperazine, metoclopramide), and ondansetron can be used as antiemetics. Opioids may precipitate toxic megacolon in patients with inflammatory bowel disease.
  ▪ **Urinary retention** may be caused by increased bladder, ureter, and urethral sphincter tone.
  ▪ **Pruritus** occurs most commonly with spinal administration.
○ **Opioid overdose**
  ▪ **Naloxone**, an opioid antagonist, should be readily available for administration in the case of accidental or intentional overdose. For details of administration, see Chapter 27, Medical Emergencies.
  ▪ Side effects include hypertension or hypotension, irritability, anxiety, restlessness, tremulousness, nausea, and vomiting.
  ▪ Naloxone can also precipitate seizure activity and cardiac arrhythmias.
• **Alternative medications**
  ○ **Tramadol** is an opioid agonist, and a centrally acting nonopioid analgesic that acts on pain processing pathways.
    ▪ **Preparations and dosages:** Between 50 and 100 mg PO q4–6h can be used for acute pain. For elderly patients and those with renal or liver dysfunction, dosage reduction is recommended.
    ▪ **Adverse effects:** Because CNS effects include sedation, concomitant use of alcohol, sedatives, or narcotics should be avoided. Nausea, dizziness, constipation, and headache may also occur. Respiratory depression has not been described at prescribed dosages but may occur with overdose. **Tramadol should not be used in patients who are taking a monoamine oxidase inhibitor**, as it can contribute to serotonin syndrome.
  ○ **Anticonvulsants** (e.g., gabapentin, pregabalin, carbamazepine and oxcarbazepine), **tricyclic antidepressants** (e.g., amitriptyline), and **duloxetine** are PO agents that can be used to treat neuropathic pain.
  ○ **Topical anesthetics** (e.g., lidocaine) may provide analgesia to a localized region (e.g., postherpetic neuralgia).

Altered Mental Status

GENERAL PRINCIPLES

Mental status changes have a broad differential diagnosis that includes neurologic (e.g., stroke, seizure, delirium), metabolic (e.g., hypoxemia, hypoglycemia), toxic (e.g., drug effects, alcohol withdrawal), and other etiologies. Infection (e.g., urinary tract infections, pneumonia) is a common cause in the elderly and patients with underlying neurologic disease. **Sundown syndrome** refers to the appearance of worsening confusion in the evening and is associated with dementia, delirium, and unfamiliar environments.

DIAGNOSIS

Clinical Presentation

History
- Focus particularly on medications, underlying dementia, cognitive impairment, neurologic or psychiatric disorders, and a history of alcohol and drug use.
- Directed history should be obtained from the patient. Family and nursing personnel may be able to provide additional details.

Physical Examination
Physical examination generally includes vital signs, a search for sites of infection, a complete cardiopulmonary examination, and a detailed neurologic examination including mental status evaluation.

Diagnostic Testing

- Testing includes blood glucose, serum electrolytes, creatinine, CBC, urinalysis, oxygen assessment, and chest radiograph.
- Other evaluation, including culture, lumbar puncture, toxicology screen, thyroid function tests, and B_{12} levels, should be directed by initial findings and diagnostic possibilities.
- If indicated by initial findings and diagnostic possibilities, the following should be obtained:
  - CT of the head (initially, a noncontrast study is appropriate)
  - Electroencephalogram (EEG)
  - ECG

TREATMENT

Management of specific disorders is discussed in Chapter 26, Neurologic Disorders.

Medications

Agitation and psychosis may be features of a change in mental status. The antipsychotic, haloperidol, and the benzodiazepine, lorazepam, are commonly used in the **acute management** of these symptoms. Second-generation antipsychotics **(risperidone, olanzapine, quetiapine, clozapine, ziprasidone, aripiprazole, paliperidone)** are alternative agents that may lead to decreased incidence of extrapyramidal symptoms. All of these agents pose risks to elderly, demented patients if given for long term.
- **Haloperidol** is the initial drug of choice for acute management of agitation and psychosis. The initial dose of 0.5 to 5 mg (0.25 mg in **elderly patients**) PO and 2 to 10 mg IM or IV can be repeated every 30 to 60 minutes until the desired effect is achieved. Sedation is usually achieved with 10 to 20 mg PO or IM. **IV infusions** (1 to 40 mg/hr) can also be used as an alternative to bolus injections. Haloperidol has fewer active metabolites and fewer anticholinergic, sedative, and hypotensive effects than other antipsychotics but may have more extrapyramidal

side effects. In low dosages, haloperidol rarely causes hypotension, cardiovascular compromise, or excessive sedation.

- ○ **Prolongation of the QT interval** with development of torsades de pointes may be seen with high-dose IV therapy. In patients who are receiving IV therapy, QT_c and electrolytes (primarily potassium and magnesium) should be monitored. Use should be discontinued with prolongation of QT_c >450 milliseconds or 25% above baseline.
- ○ **Postural hypotension** may occasionally be acute and severe after IM administration. If significant hypotension occurs, administration of IV fluids with the patient in the Trendelenburg position is usually sufficient. If **vasopressors** are required, dopamine should be avoided, as it may exacerbate the psychotic state.
- ○ **Neuroleptic malignant syndrome** is an infrequent, potentially lethal complication of antipsychotic drug therapy. Clinical manifestations include rigidity, akinesia, altered sensorium, fever, tachycardia, and alteration in BP. Severe muscle rigidity can cause rhabdomyolysis and acute renal failure. **Laboratory abnormalities** include elevations in creatine kinase, liver function tests, and white blood cell count (see Chapter 26, Neurologic Disorders).
- **Lorazepam** is a benzodiazepine that is useful for agitation and psychosis in the setting of hepatic dysfunction and sedative or alcohol withdrawal, and in patients who are refractory to monotherapy with antipsychotics. The **initial dose** is 0.5 to 2.0 mg IV. The **key features** of lorazepam are its short duration of action and few active metabolites. The use of lorazepam, as with all benzodiazepines, is limited by excess sedation and respiratory depression. Caution is advised when using benzodiazepines in the elderly as they may paradoxically worsen agitation.

Nonpharmacologic Therapies

Patients with delirium of any etiology often respond to frequent reorientation, observance of the day–night light cycle, and maintenance of a familiar environment.

Insomnia and Anxiety

GENERAL PRINCIPLES

- Insomnia and anxiety may be attributed to a variety of underlying medical or psychiatric disorders, and symptoms may be exacerbated by hospitalization.
- Causes of **insomnia** include environmental disruptions, mood and anxiety disorders, substance abuse disorders, common medications (i.e., β-blockers, steroids, bronchodilators), sleep apnea, hyperthyroidism, and nocturnal myoclonus.
- **Anxiety** may be seen in anxiety disorder, depression, substance abuse disorders, hyperthyroidism, and complex partial seizures.

DIAGNOSIS

The diagnosis of insomnia and anxiety is a clinical one. No laboratory or imaging tests help in establishing the diagnosis; however, they can help to rule out other etiologies. A thorough history is essential.

TREATMENT

Selected medications for insomnia or anxiety or both:
- **Benzodiazepines** are frequently used in management of anxiety and insomnia. Table 1-2 provides a list of selected benzodiazepines and their common uses and dosages.
  - **Pharmacology:** Most benzodiazepines undergo oxidation to active metabolites in the liver. **Lorazepam, oxazepam, and temazepam** undergo glucuronidation to inactive metabolites; therefore, these agents may be particularly useful in the elderly and in those with liver disease. **Benzodiazepine toxicity** is heightened by malnutrition, advanced age, hepatic disease and concomitant use of alcohol, other CNS depressants, and CYP3A4 inhibitors. Benzodiazepines with long half-lives may accumulate substantially in the elderly, in whom the half-life may be increased manyfold.
  - **Dosages**
    - **Relief of anxiety and insomnia** is achieved at the doses outlined in Table 1-2. Therapy should be started at the lowest recommended dosage with intermittent dosing schedules.
    - **Side effects** include drowsiness, dizziness, fatigue, psychomotor impairment, and anterograde amnesia.
    - The elderly are more sensitive to these agents and may experience falls, paradoxical agitation, and delirium.
    - **IV administration of diazepam and midazolam** can be associated with hypotension, bradycardia, and respiratory or cardiac arrest.
    - **Respiratory depression** can occur even with oral administration in patients with respiratory compromise.
    - **Tolerance** to benzodiazepines can develop.
    - **Dependence** may develop after only 2 to 4 weeks of therapy.
    - **Seizures and delirium** may also occur with sudden discontinuation of benzodiazepines.
    - **A withdrawal syndrome** consisting of agitation, irritability, insomnia, tremor, palpitations, headache, GI distress, and perceptual disturbance begins 1 to 10 days after a rapid decrease in dosage or abrupt cessation of therapy and may last for several weeks. Although the severity and incidence of withdrawal symptoms appears to be related to dose and duration of treatment, withdrawal symptoms have been reported even after brief therapy at doses in the recommended range. Short-acting and intermediate-acting drugs should be decreased by 10% to 20% every 5 days, with a slower taper in the final few weeks. Long-acting preparations can be tapered more quickly.
  - **Overdose**
    - **Flumazenil**, a benzodiazepine antagonist, should be readily available in case of accidental or intentional overdose. For details of administration, see Chapter 27, Medical Emergencies. Common side effects include dizziness, nausea, and vomiting.
    - **Flumazenil should be used with caution in patients with a history of seizure disorder or if overdose with tricyclic antidepressants is suspected.**
- **Trazodone**
  - Trazodone is a serotonin receptor antagonist antidepressant that may be useful for the treatment of severe anxiety or insomnia. Common dosing is 50 to 100 mg at bedtime.

| Table 1-2 | | Characteristics of Selected Benzodiazepines | | |

Drug	Route	Common Uses	Usual Dosage	Half-life (hr)[a]
Alprazolam	PO	Anxiety disorders	0.75–4.0 mg/24 hr (in three doses)	12–15
Chlordiazepoxide	PO	Anxiety disorders, alcohol withdrawal	15–100 mg/24 hr (in divided doses)	5–30
Clonazepam	PO	Anxiety disorders, seizure disorders	0.5–4.0 mg/24 hr (in two doses)	18–28
Diazepam	PO	Anxiety disorders, seizure disorders, preanesthesia	6–40 mg/24 hr (in one to four doses)	20–50
	IV		2.5–20.0 mg (slow IV push)	20–50
Flurazepam	PO	Insomnia	15–30 mg at bedtime	50–100
Lorazepam[b]	PO	Anxiety disorders	1–10 mg/24 hr (in two to three doses)	10–20
	IV or IM	Preanesthetic medication	0.05 mg/kg (4 mg max)	10–20
Midazolam	IV	Preanesthetic and intraoperative medication	0.01–0.05 mg/kg	1–12
	IM		0.08 mg/kg	1–12
Oxazepam[b]	PO	Anxiety disorders	10–30 mg/24 hr (in three to four doses)	5–10
Temazepam[b]	PO	Insomnia	15–30 mg at bedtime	8–12
Triazolam	PO	Insomnia	0.125–0.250 mg at bedtime	2–5

[a]Half-life of active metabolites may differ.
[b]Metabolites are inactive.

○ **Side effects**
  ▪ Highly sedating, causes postural hypotension, and is rarely associated with priapism.
  ▪ Levels may be substantially increased when used with CYP3A4 inhibitors.
• **Nonbenzodiazepine hypnotics** appear to act on the benzodiazepine receptor. These agents have been shown to be safe and effective for initiating sleep. All should be used with caution in patients with impaired respiratory function. Zolpidem in high, chronic doses is rarely associated with withdrawal syndromes, rebound insomnia, and tolerance (*Drug Saf 2009;32(9):735*). Zaleplon and eszopiclone have not been shown to be associated with rebound insomnia or tolerance. All three agents are associated with abuse potential and are therefore Schedule IV drugs by the U.S. Drug Enforcement Administration (DEA).
○ **Zolpidem** is an imidazopyridine hypnotic agent that is useful for the treatment of insomnia. It has no withdrawal syndrome, rebound insomnia, or tolerance. Side effects include headache, daytime somnolence, and GI upset. The starting dose is 5 mg PO every night at bedtime for the elderly and 10 mg for other patients, titrating up to 20 mg as needed. Doses should be reduced in cirrhosis.
○ **Zaleplon** has a half-life of approximately 1 hour and has no active metabolites. Side effects include drowsiness, dizziness, and impaired coordination. Zaleplon should be used with caution in those with compromised respiratory function. The starting dose is 5 mg PO at bedtime for the elderly or patients with hepatic dysfunction and 10 to 20 mg PO at bedtime for other patients.
○ **Eszopiclone** offers a longer half-life compared to the previous agents. Side effects include headache, somnolence, and dizziness. Starting dose is 2 mg, with reduced dosing in the elderly, debilitated, and patients with liver disease.
○ **Ramelteon** is a melatonin analog with similar efficacy as the nonbenzodiazepine hypnotics. The usual dose is 8 mg PO at bedtime. There is no evidence for withdrawal, tolerance, rebound insomnia, or abuse potential, and it is therefore not a scheduled drug.
○ **Antihistamines:** Over-the-counter antihistamines can be used for insomnia and anxiety, particularly in patients with a history of drug dependence. Anticholinergic side effects limit the utility, especially in the elderly.

PERIOPERATIVE MEDICINE

Preoperative Cardiac Evaluation

GENERAL PRINCIPLES

• The role of the medical consultant is to estimate the level of cardiac risk associated with a given procedure. "Clearance" cannot be readily granted, as **there is always some level of risk**.
• Based on the estimated risk, the consultant should then determine the need for further evaluation and prescribe possible interventions to mitigate risk.
• Though preoperative consultations often focus on cardiac risk, it is essential to remember that poor outcomes can result from significant disease in other organ systems. **Evaluation of the entire patient is necessary to provide optimal perioperative care.**

Definition

Perioperative cardiac complications are generally defined as cardiac death, MIs (both ST and non-ST elevation), CHF, and clinically significant rhythm disturbances.

Epidemiology

- The incidence of perioperative cardiac complications varies markedly depending on the definitions employed and the population studied. Overall, an estimated 50,000 perioperative infarctions and 1 million other cardiovascular complications occur annually (*N Engl J Med 2001;345:1677*).
- Of those who have a perioperative MI, the risk of in-hospital mortality is estimated at 10% to 15% (*Chest 2006;130:584*).
- Perioperative MI (PMI) is believed to occur via two distinct mechanisms:
  - **Type I PMI** occurs via erosion or rupture of unstable atherosclerotic plaque, leading to coronary thrombosis, ischemia, and infarction.
  - **Type II PMI** results from an imbalance in myocardial oxygen supply/demand, leading to prolonged ischemia and ST-segment depression.
- Angiographic data suggest that existing stenoses may play a role with some perioperative events; however, a significant number of PMIs are "stress" related (Type II PMI) and not due to plaque rupture (*Am J Cardiol 1996;77:1126; J Cardiothorac Vasc Anesth 2003;17:90*).
- Autopsy data suggest fatal PMIs occur predominantly in patients with multivessel and especially left main disease, via the same mechanism as non-PMIs (*Int J Cardiol 1996;57:37*).

DIAGNOSIS

Clinical Presentation

History

- The focus of the history is to identify factors and comorbid conditions that will affect perioperative risk.
- Current guidelines focus on identification of active cardiac disease and known risk factors for perioperative events.
  - Evidence of **active** cardiac conditions for which the patient should undergo evaluation and treatment:
    - Unstable coronary syndromes
    - Unstable or severe angina
    - Recent MI (defined as more than 7 but less than 30 days)
    - Decompensated CHF (NY Heart Association [NYHA] class IV, worsening or new-onset heart failure [HF])
    - Significant arrhythmias
    - Severe valvular disease
  - Clinical **risk factors**
    - Preexisting, stable coronary artery disease (CAD)
    - Compensated or prior CHF
    - Diabetes mellitus
    - Prior cerebrovascular accident (CVA) or transient ischemic attack (TIA)
    - Renal insufficiency

- Other
  - Age >70 years has been identified in several studies as a significant risk factor (*JAMA 2001;285:1865*; *Eur Heart J 2008;29:394*). Not uniformly accepted as an independent risk factor.
  - Abnormal ECG (e.g., LVH, LBBB, ST-T wave abnormalities)
  - Nonsinus rhythm (rate controlled and stable)
  - Poorly controlled hypertension

Physical Examination
- A complete physical exam is essential.
- Specific attention should be paid to:
  - **Vital signs**, particularly evidence of **hypertension**.
    - Systolic blood pressure (SBP) <180 and diastolic blood pressure (DBP) <110 are generally considered acceptable.
    - The management of stage III hypertension (SBP >180 or DBP >110) is controversial. Postponing elective surgery to allow adequate BP control in this setting is acceptable, but this is poorly studied and how long to wait after treatment is instituted is unclear.
  - Evidence of **CHF** (elevated JVP, crackles, S3, etc.).
  - **Murmurs** suggestive of **significant valvular lesions**.
    - Symptomatic stenotic lesions such as **mitral** and **aortic stenosis (AS)** are thought to be associated with the greatest risk.
      - Severe **AS** (valve area <0.7 cm^2 or mean gradient ≥50 mm Hg) is associated with an approximate 30% incidence of cardiac morbidity with a mortality of approximately 10% (*Am J Med 2004;116:8*; *Am J Cardiol 1998;81:448*).
      - The risk of asymptomatic, moderate AS appears to be less, and surgery can be considered in this group with careful evaluation (*Chest 2005;128:2944*).
      - **Mitral stenosis** is not well studied in the perioperative setting. Percutaneous valvotomy should be considered with severe stenosis.
    - Symptomatic **regurgitant lesions** are generally tolerated perioperatively and can be managed medically as long as the patient is well compensated preoperatively.

Diagnostic Criteria

- **Risk Stratification**
  The 2007 American College of Cardiology/American Heart Association (ACC/ AHA) Guidelines on Perioperative Cardiovascular Evaluation and Care for Noncardiac Surgery offer a stepwise approach to preoperative evaluation (Figure 1-1).
- **Step 1: Establish the urgency of surgery.**
  Important to note that many surgeries, though not absolutely emergent, are urgent and are unlikely to allow for a time-consuming evaluation.
- **Step 2: Assess for active cardiac conditions** (see History section previously).
- **Step 3: Determine the surgery-specific risk.**
  - Though professional judgement is required, surgical risk can generally be divided as follows:
    - **Low-risk surgeries** (<1% expected risk of adverse cardiac events) include superficial procedures, cataract surgery, breast surgery, endoscopic procedures, and most procedures that can be performed in an ambulatory setting.
    - **Intermediate risk surgeries** (1% to 5% risk of adverse cardiac events) include carotid endarterectomy, intraperitoneal surgeries, intrathoracic surgeries, orthopedic surgeries, head and neck surgeries, and prostate surgery.

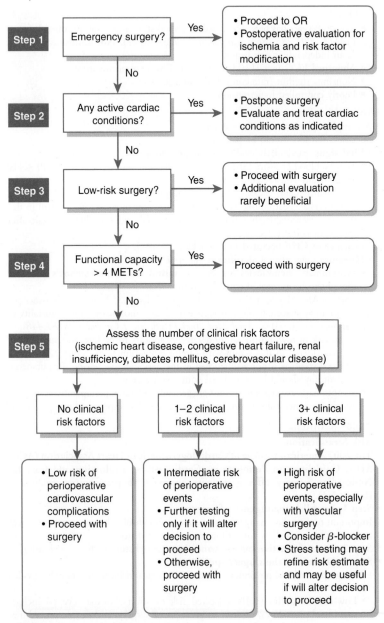

Figure 1-1. Cardiac evaluation algorithm for noncardiac surgery. (Adapted from the *2007 ACC/AHA guidelines on perioperative evaluation for noncardiac surgery. Circulation 2007; 116:e418.*)

- **Vascular surgery** involving extremity revascularization and aortic surgeries is generally found to carry the highest risk (>5% risk of adverse cardiac events).
- **Step 4: Assess the patient's functional capacity.**
  - Poor functional capacity (<4 metabolic equivalents [METs]) is associated with an increased risk of perioperative cardiac events (*Arch Intern Med 1999;159:2185*; *Chest 1999;116:355*).
  - Though exercise testing is the gold standard, functional capacity can be reliably estimated by patient self-report (*Am J Cardiol 1989;64:651*).
  - Examples of activities that suggest at least a moderate functional capacity (>4 METs) include:
    - Climbing one to two flights of stairs
    - Able to walk up a hill
    - Walk a block at a brisk pace
  - **Patients with a functional capacity of >4 METs without symptoms can proceed to surgery with relatively low risk.**
- **Step 5: Assess the patient's clinical risk factors**
  - The number of risk factors combined with the surgery-specific risk (intermediate vs. vascular) determines further management.
  - The clinical risk factors are adapted from the *Revised Cardiac Risk Index (RCRI)* (*Circulation 1999;100:1043*):
    - Ischemic heart disease
    - History of TIA or CVA
    - History of CHF
    - Renal insufficiency (Cr ≥ 2.0)
    - Diabetes mellitus, requiring insulin
  - Patients with **no clinical risk factors** are inherently **low risk** (<1% risk of cardiac events) and are unlikely to benefit from further intervention. They may proceed to surgery.
  - Patients with **one or two clinical risk factors** are generally at **intermediate risk** and may proceed to surgery.
    - Stress testing may provide a better estimate of cardiovascular risk, and so may be considered if knowledge of this increased risk would change management (*J Am Coll Cardiol 2006;48:964*).
    - It is important to note that revascularization is unlikely to improve upon this risk and is not recommended solely to reduce perioperative risk (see Revascularization section) (*N Engl J Med 2004;351:2795*).
  - Patients with **three or more clinical risk factors** are at **high risk** of adverse cardiac events, particularly when undergoing vascular surgery.
    - Stress testing can provide a better estimate of the degree of risk and can be considered if a more precise estimate of risk will alter the decision to proceed with the planned surgery.
    - Despite the increased risk, there is evidence that preoperative revascularization fails to improve perioperative cardiovascular outcomes in this population (see Revascularization section) (*N Engl J Med 2004;351:2795*; *J Am Coll Cardiol 2007;49:1763*).

Diagnostic Testing

- **12-Lead electrocardiogram**
  - The value of a routine ECG is controversial, and it is often unnecessary.

- ○ The current ACC/AHA guidelines recommend an ECG in:
  - Patients with 1+ risk factors undergoing vascular surgery and patients with peripheral vascular disease (PVD), CAD, or cerebrovascular disease (CVD) undergoing intermediate risk surgery (Class I recommendation).
  - Patients without risk factors undergoing vascular surgery and patients with other clinical risk factors undergoing intermediate risk surgery (Class II recommendation) (*Circulation 2007;116:e418*).
- **Resting echocardiogram**
  - ○ In general, the indications for echocardiographic evaluation in the preoperative setting are no different than in the nonoperative setting. **An echo is not routinely necessary.**
  - ○ Murmurs found on physical exam suggestive of significant underlying valvular disease should be evaluated by echocardiogram.
  - ○ An assessment of left ventricular function should be considered when there is clinical concern for underlying CHF not previously diagnosed or if there is concern for deterioration since the last exam.
- **Stress evaluation**
  - ○ The decision to pursue a stress evaluation should be guided by an assessment of preoperative risk as detailed previously.
  - ○ **Routine stress evaluation of all patients undergoing surgery is not warranted.**
  - ○ Even if revascularization is not warranted (see Revascularization section), a stress evaluation does add to the evaluation of the potentially high-risk patient. **A positive test indicates a substantially increased risk of a perioperative cardiac event, while a negative study suggests a lower risk than that predicted by clinical factors alone** (*JAMA 2001;285:1865*).
  - ○ For further details on stress testing see Chapter 4, Ischemic Heart Disease.

TREATMENT

Medications

- **β-Blockers**
  - ○ **Evidence**
    - Multiple studies have provided support for perioperative β-blockade in patients with or at risk for CAD undergoing noncardiac surgeries (*N Engl J Med 1996;335:1713*). The most pronounced benefit has been in high-risk patients undergoing vascular surgery where β-blocker dose was titrated to heart rate control (*J Am Coll Cardiol 2006;48:964; Circulation 2006;114(suppl):I344*).
    - In the trial, a relatively high dose of extended-release metoprolol beginning on the day of surgery led to decrease in cardiac events but an increase in overall mortality and stroke risk (*Lancet 2008;371:1839*).
  - ○ **Recommendations**
    - Per ACC/AHA guidelines, routine administration of **high-dose** β-blockers in the absence of dose titration is not recommended for patients undergoing intermediate risk surgery who are not already taking β-blockers (*Circulation 2009;54:13*).
    - For patients undergoing vascular surgery with known CAD or evidence of cardiac ischemia on preoperative testing, β-blockers **titrated to heart rate** (target pulse of 60 bpm) and blood pressure are recommended (*Anesth Analg 2008;106:1039*).
    - For patients undergoing vascular or intermediate risk with two or more clinical risk factors, β-blockers are reasonable.
    - Patients already taking β-blockers should be continued on their medication.

- **Statins**
  - **Evidence**
    - Statins are believed to improve cardiovascular outcomes by enhancing endothelial function, reducing vascular inflammation, and stabilizing atherosclerotic plaque, in addition to their lipid lowering effects.
    - Two trials have shown a decrease in perioperative cardiac events with statins in patients undergoing vascular surgery (*J Vasc Surg 2004;39:967*; *J Am Coll Cardiol 2008;52:2032*).
    - A recent meta-analysis of statin therapy in statin-naïve patients revealed statistically significant reductions in risk of perioperative atrial fibrillation and MI, as well as reduced mean length of stay. Notably, only 4 of the 15 studies included involved noncardiac surgery patients.
  - **Recommendations**
    - Patients currently taking statins should be maintained on therapy.
    - Patients undergoing vascular surgery, and those with risk factors undergoing intermediate surgery, may benefit from initiation of statin therapy perioperatively.
    - The dose, duration of therapy, and target low-density lipoprotein (LDL) levels for perioperative risk reduction are unclear.
- **α_2-Agonists**
  - **Evidence**
    Multiple studies of the perioperative cardiovascular benefit of α_2-agonists (e.g., clonidine) have been performed. These included a variety of agents and revealed α_2-agonists were able to decrease the incidence of perioperative ischemia in both cardiac and noncardiac surgeries (*Anesthesiology 2002;96:323*; *Anesthesiology 2004;101:284*).
  - **Recommendations**
    - It appears clonidine does have cardioprotective benefits, but the evidence is not conclusive.
    - The use of α_2-agonists as a risk-reduction strategy in patients at risk for adverse cardiac outcomes when β-blockers are contraindicated appears a reasonable consideration.
    - If given, no particular administration protocol is clearly superior. The protocol used in the study cited previously consisted of clonidine 0.2 mg orally on the evening prior with the concurrent placement of a 0.2 mg/d clonidine patch (one time only). An additional 0.2-mg dose of clonidine was given on the morning of surgery due to the expected lag in onset of action of the transdermal preparation. Hemodynamics need to be monitored closely.
- **Aspirin**
  For discussion, see Revascularization and Perioperative Anticoagulation and Antithrombotic Management sections.

Revascularization

The best available data on preoperative revascularization come from the CARP trial, a prospective study of patients scheduled to undergo vascular surgery (*N Engl J Med 2004;351:2795*):

- Patients with angiographically proven significant CAD were randomized to revascularization versus no revascularization. There was no difference between the groups in the occurrence of MI or death at 30 days or in mortality with long-term follow-up. Patients with three or more clinical risk factors and extensive ischemia on stress testing were evaluated in a separate small study (*J Am Coll Cardiol 2007;49:1763*).

High event rates were seen in both the revascularization and no revascularization arms, and there was no benefit seen with revascularization.

- Taken together, these studies suggest the risk of adverse cardiac events is not altered by attempts at preoperative revascularization, even in high-risk populations.
- A notable possible exception are patients with **left main disease**, who appeared to have benefited from preoperative revascularization in a subset analysis of the CARP trial data (*Am J Cardiol 2008;102:809*).
- Based on these cumulative results, **a strategy of routinely pursuing coronary revascularization as a method of decreasing perioperative cardiac risk cannot be recommended**.
- However, careful screening of patients is still essential to **identify those high-risk subsets** who may obtain a survival benefit from revascularization **independent of their need for noncardiac surgery**.
- **Patients with coronary stents:** see Perioperative Anticoagulation and Antithrombotic Management section.

SPECIAL CONSIDERATIONS

Risk Assessment in Orthopedic Trauma

- Multiple studies have reported a correlation between delayed repair of hip fracture and increased morbidity and mortality (*Br Med J (Clin Res Ed). 1986 Nov 8;293 (6556):1203; Clin Orthop 1984;(186):45*).
- For urgent surgical procedures (i.e., those that should be done within 48 hours of diagnosis) the value of additional testing is typically outweighed by the risk of worsened short- and long-term outcomes incurred with surgical delay.
- Unnecessary preoperative cardiac testing may be an independent risk factor for postoperative complications in hip fracture patients (*Am J Orthop 2008 Jan; 37(1):32*).
- In such cases, it is advisable to optimize the patient's medical status and modifiable risk factors and then proceed to the operating room.

MONITORING/FOLLOW-UP

Postoperative Infarction and Surveillance

- Most events will occur within 48 to 72 hours of surgery, with the majority in the first 24 hours (*Anesthesiology 1998;88:572; Arch Surg 2003;138:596; CMAJ 2005;173:779*).
- Most are not heralded by chest pain and may be **clinically asymptomatic** (*Anesthesiology 1990;72:153*).
- The current ACC/AHA guidelines recommend:
  - Obtaining ECGs postoperatively and on postoperative days 1 and 2 for patients with known or suspected CAD undergoing intermediate or high-risk surgeries.
  - **Troponin measurements** are only recommended in the setting of ECG changes or clinical symptoms.
  - There is no need to perform surveillance in low-risk surgeries. However, several studies suggest an increased risk of cardiac events and death in patients with abnormal troponins postoperatively (*Eur Heart J 2005;26:2448; Anaesthesia 2004;59:318; Ann Intern Med 2011;154:523*).

○ Aggressive medical management triggered by a finding of elevated troponins in the otherwise asymptomatic patient may, therefore, be warranted.

• Symptomatic infarctions should be addressed according to standard therapy of acute coronary syndromes (see Chapter 4, Ischemic Heart Disease). The major caveat is that bleeding risk with anticoagulants must be carefully considered.

Perioperative Anticoagulation and Antithrombotic Management

GENERAL PRINCIPLES

• Patients on chronic anticoagulation for atrial fibrillation, VTE, or mechanical heart valves often need to undergo procedures that pose risk of bleeding. Providing optimal anticoagulation treatment is challenging.

• The risk of thromboembolic events must be weighed against the risk of surgical bleeding. Patient preferences regarding the associated complications (e.g., increased risk of stroke vs. increased risk of reoperation to control hemorrhage) must be considered.

• The **perioperative risk of thromboembolism is greater than expected** from extrapolation of annual rates in otherwise stable patients, likely due to a rebound hypercoagulable state from cessation of anticoagulants and hypercoagulability due to surgical trauma.

• New oral anticoagulation agents with shorter half-lives may simplify this process in the future but presently have limited indications.

• Until better research is available, decisions regarding perioperative anticoagulation will have to be made by clinicians with the help of guidelines with relatively weak strength of evidence (*Chest 2012;141:326S*).

DIAGNOSIS

• It is essential to **determine the indication for any anticoagulant**.

• Any history of hypercoagulability and/or prior thromboembolism, including timing, should be sought.

• The details of the planned surgery will need to be reviewed, and the surgical team involved.

○ The surgeon's perspective on bleeding risk and the consequences of increased surgical bleeding will need to be determined.

○ The use of regional anesthesia (e.g., epidural) can be greatly impacted by the use of anticoagulant medications, and therefore, the anesthesiologist will need to be involved early in the care of patients who may need perioperative treatment with anticoagulants.

TREATMENT

• Recommended management varies according to the indication for anticoagulation, medication used, and surgical bleeding risk.

- **For patients being treated with oral anticoagulants/vitamin K antagonists (VKA):**
  - **Low bleeding risk** procedures permit continuation of **oral anticoagulation** through the perioperative period (e.g., minor dental and dermatologic procedures, cataract extraction, endoscopy without biopsy, arthrocentesis).
  - **Significant bleeding risk procedures** require the anticoagulation to be discontinued.
    - Though the international normalized ratio (INR) at which surgery can be safely performed is subjective, **an INR of <1.5 is typically a reasonable goal**.
    - The VKA (e.g., warfarin) will typically need to be stopped 5 days preoperatively.
    - The INR should be checked the day before surgery. If a level <1.5 is not obtained, a single 1-mg oral dose of vitamin K appears to be a safe and effective method of achieving an INR <1.5 on the anticipated day of surgery.
    - The VKA can generally be resumed 12 to 24 hours postoperatively if postoperative bleeding has been controlled (*Chest 2012;141:326S*).
  - **High bleeding risk procedures** (e.g., intracranial or spinal) with potential catastrophic outcomes due to bleeding will preclude any anticoagulation in the perioperative period. Other procedures with high bleeding risk (e.g., sessile polypectomy, bowel resection, kidney, liver, or spleen biopsy, extensive orthopedic or plastic surgery) should lead to a delay of at least 48 hours prior to resumption of anticoagulation.
- **Bridging therapy** refers to the administration of an alternative anticoagulation during the time the INR is anticipated to be below the therapeutic range. The benefit conferred by bridging in decreasing thrombosis must be weighed against the increased risk of bleeding.
- **High thrombotic risk patients** should typically be treated with bridging therapy. Examples include:
  - Mechanical mitral valve
  - Older generation mechanical valve (e.g., Starr–Edwards ball-in-cage valve) in aortic or mitral position
  - Any mechanical valve with a history of cardioembolism within the preceding 6 months
  - Nonvalvular atrial fibrillation with either a history of embolism in the last 3 months or $CHADS_2$ score ≥5 (*JAMA 2001;285:2921*) (see Chapter 7, Cardiac Arrhythmias).
  - Valvular atrial fibrillation
  - Recent VTE (<3 months)
  - Known thrombophilic state (e.g., protein C deficiency)
- For **moderate thrombotic risk patients**, treatment with bridging may be considered, although evidence is less compelling. Treatment with deep vein thrombosis (DVT) prophylaxis dosing of LMWH is considered an acceptable alternative. This includes patients with:
  - Mechanical aortic valve (bileaflet) with one or more associated risk factors for thromboembolism: atrial fibrillation (AF), CHF, hypertension, age ≥75, diabetes mellitus, and prior history of CVA or TIA
  - Atrial fibrillation with a $CHADS_2$ score of 3 or 4 or history of prior embolism with lower score
  - History of VTE within preceding 3 to 12 months
  - Non–high-risk thrombophilia (e.g., heterozygous factor V Leiden mutation)

- ○ History of recurrent VTE
- ○ Active malignancy
- **Low thrombotic risk** patients are **not** felt to require bridging therapy. Treatment with DVT prophylaxis doses of LMWH or UFH is an alternative. This group includes patients with:
  - ○ Mechanical aortic valve (bileaflet) without associated risk factors (as outlined previously).
  - ○ Nonvalvular atrial fibrillation with a CHADS$_2$ score ≤2 and no history of embolism.
  - ○ Prior VTE >12 months prior (without history of recurrent VTE or known hypercoagulable state).
- **Choices for bridging therapy** are generally the LMWHs and UFH. There is less experience in this setting with other agents (e.g., fondaparinux), and their use cannot be considered routine.
  - ○ **LMWHs** have the advantages of relatively predictable pharmacokinetics and ability to be administered subcutaneously. Monitoring of anticoagulant effect is typically not required. Renal dosing is available for patients not on dialysis.
  - ○ Subcutaneous administration allows for outpatient therapy in appropriate patients. This decreases the amount of time the patient must be hospitalized and also has economic advantages. For these reasons, LMWH is the agent of choice for bridging in anticoagulation, including patients with mechanical heart valves (*Chest 2012;141:326S; Circulation 2011;123:269*). The last dose should be given 24 hours prior to surgery. Also, if the medication is being given on a once-daily regimen, the dose should be 50% of the usual dose.
  - ○ **UFH** is the agent of choice for patients with end stage renal disease. It is typically administered IV and requires frequent monitoring of the aPTT. UFH should be stopped at least 4 hours prior to the planned surgical procedure to allow the anticoagulant effect to wane. Fixed dose subcutaneous UFH has been proven efficacious for treatment of VTE, and may be considered as an option (*JAMA 2006;295:1152*).
- **Patients being treated with antiplatelet agents.**
  - ○ Continuing antiplatelets agents perioperatively also carries a risk of bleeding, while discontinuation may increase cardiovascular events. Irreversible agents must be withheld for 5 to 7 days several days before effects fully abate. Clinicians are again left with little evidence and sometimes conflicting guidelines.
  - ○ **Low bleeding risk procedures** (e.g., minor dermatologic or dental procedures) allow continuation of aspirin (ASA) being given for secondary prevention of cardiovascular disease.
  - ○ **Noncardiac surgery patients** should generally have clopidogrel (or other thienopyridines) held 5 days preoperatively. Prompt reinitiation with a loading dose of 300 mg should take place postoperatively. Further stratification drives decisions regarding ASA:
    - ▪ **Moderate to high cardiac risk**, in which case ASA should be continued perioperatively
    - ▪ **Low cardiac risk**, in which case ASA should be held 7 days preoperatively
  - ○ **Coronary artery bypass graft** candidates should generally continue ASA perioperatively, and have clopidogrel held 5 days preoperatively.
  - ○ **Coronary stents** pose a particular risk of in-stent thrombosis and transmural infarction if dual antiplatelet therapy is prematurely withheld. Whenever possible,

surgery should be deferred until the minimum period of dual antiplatelet therapy is completed:
- Drug-eluting stents, 6 months
- Bare metal stents, 6 weeks
- Balloon angioplasty without stent, 14 days
- **Urgent surgeries** within the previous time frames should proceed with continued dual antiplatelet treatment, if possible. If the bleeding risk is felt to be prohibitive, ASA should be continued. Heparin bridging has not been shown to be of benefit. Bridging with IV glycoprotein IIb/IIIa antagonists, or reversible oral agents (e.g., ticagrelor) is controversial (*Chest 2012;141:326S*).

PERIOPERATIVE MANAGEMENT OF SPECIFIC CONDITIONS

Hypertension

GENERAL PRINCIPLES

- **Severe hypertension** (BP >180/110) preoperatively often results in wider fluctuations in intraoperative BP and has been associated with an increased rate of perioperative cardiac events (see Preoperative Cardiac Evaluation section previously).
- Antihypertensive agents that the patients are taking prior to admission for surgery may have an impact on the perioperative period.
  - When the patient is receiving β-blockers or clonidine chronically, withdrawal of these medications may result in tachycardia and rebound hypertension, respectively.
  - Evidence suggests that holding angiotensin-converting enzyme inhibitors and angiotensin II receptor blockers on the day of surgery may reduce perioperative hypotension. This is believed to be due to the effect of this class of medication in blunting the compensatory activation of the renin–angiotensin system perioperatively.

DIAGNOSIS

BP monitoring should be done as part of a patient's routine vital signs. A portable or wall blood pressure cuff should be used. In the setting of severe hypertension, BP should be checked in both arms and with two different types of BP cuffs in order to ensure accuracy.

TREATMENT

- Hypertension in the postoperative period is a common problem with multiple possible causes.
  - All **remediable causes of hypertension**, such as pain, agitation, hypercarbia, hypoxia, hypervolemia, and bladder distention, should be excluded or treated.

- o Poor control of essential hypertension secondary to discontinuation of medications the patient was previously taking in the immediate postoperative period is not uncommon. Reviewing the patient's home medication list is recommended.
- o A rare cause of perioperative hypertension is **pheochromocytoma**, particularly if its presence was unrecognized. Patients can develop an acute hypertensive crisis perioperatively. Treatment with **phentolamine** or **nitroprusside** is recommended in this situation. Preoperative treatment when the diagnosis is suspected to minimize this risk is recommended. This is classically accomplished by titration of **phenoxybenzamine** preoperatively.
- Many parenteral antihypertensive medications are available for patients who are unable to take medications orally. Transdermal clonidine is also an option, but the onset of action is delayed.

Pacemakers and Implantable Cardioverter Defibrillators (ICDs)

GENERAL PRINCIPLES

- The use of electrocautery intraoperatively can have adverse effects on the function of implanted cardiac devices.
- A variety of errors can occur from resetting of the device to inadvertent discharge of an ICD.
- Complications are rare but are more likely with abdominal and thoracic surgeries.

DIAGNOSIS

- The type of device (i.e., pacemaker or ICD) and manufacturer should be determined.
- The initial indication for placement and the patient's underlying rhythm should be determined. Ideally, this can be determined from the history and an ECG.
- When the device was last formally interrogated should be ascertained.
- The device should be interrogated within 3 to 6 months of a significant surgical procedure.

TREATMENT

If the patient is pacemaker dependent, the device should be reprogrammed to an asynchronous mode (e.g., VOO, DOO) for the surgery.
- The application of a magnet will cause most pacemakers to revert to an asynchronous pacing mode, but if this is the planned management, it should be tested preoperatively, especially in the pacemaker-dependent patient.
- It should be noted that the effect of a magnet on ICDs is typically different than the effect on pacemakers in that it affects the antitachycardia function but does not alter the pacing function of most models. If the pacing function of an ICD needs to be altered perioperatively, the device will need to be reprogrammed.
- The antitachycardia function of an ICD will typically need to be programmed off for surgical procedures where electrocautery may cause interference with device function, leading to the potential of unintentional discharge.

- ○ The effect of a magnet on this function is variable, so programming is the preferred management.
- ○ Continuous monitoring for arrhythmia during the period when this function is suspended is essential.
- Continuous ECG and pulse monitoring is recommended during surgery. Pulse monitoring should not be affected by electrocautery interference.
- Postoperative interrogation may be necessary, particularly if the device settings were changed perioperatively or if the patient is pacemaker dependent.
- **Consultation with an electrophysiologist** is strongly recommended if there is any uncertainty regarding the perioperative management of a device.

Pulmonary Disease and Preoperative Pulmonary Evaluation

GENERAL PRINCIPLES

Epidemiology

- **Clinically significant postoperative pulmonary complications are probably more common than cardiac complications**, and the occurrence of one may increase the chance of the other occurring (*Am J Respir Crit Care Med 2005;171:514*; *Am J Med 2003;115:515*).
- Though definitions vary, clinically significant pulmonary complications generally include pneumonia, respiratory failure, bronchospasm, atelectasis, and exacerbation of underlying chronic lung disease.
- Postoperative respiratory failure can be a life-threatening complication with a 30-day mortality rate as high as 26.5% (*J Am Coll Surg 2007;204:1188*).

Etiology

Both patient-dependent risk factors and surgery-specific risk factors combine to produce the level of risk. These are reviewed in detail in a 2006 guideline from the American College of Physicians (*Ann Intern Med 2006;144:575*).

Risk Factors

- **Procedure-related risk factors**
  - ○ The **surgical site** is generally considered the greatest determinant of risk, with **upper abdominal and thoracic surgeries** imparting the greatest risk (*N Engl J Med 1999;340:937*). Surgical procedures not involving the torso can also impart increased risk of pulmonary complications. Examples include neurosurgery and surgeries involving the mouth and palate (*Ann Surg 2000;232:242*; *J Am Coll Surg 2007;204:1188*).
  - ○ The **surgery duration** also imparts risk, with prolonged procedures increasing the risk of pulmonary complications (*Arch Intern Med 1992;152:967*).
  - ○ The **type of anesthesia** utilized appears to affect pulmonary risk as well. Though somewhat controversial, it appears neuraxial anesthesia carries less risk of pneumonia and respiratory failure (*BMJ 2000;321:1*; *Lancet 2002;359:1276*).
- **Patient-dependent risk factors**
  - ○ **Chronic lung disease**, particularly COPD, has reliably been found to be a risk factor for postoperative pulmonary complications. Unsurprisingly, patients with progressively more severe disease appear to be at increased risk for more serious

complications (*Chest 1993;104:1445*). However, even patients with advanced lung disease can safely undergo surgery if it is deemed necessary (*Br Med J 1975;3:670*). Thus, **there is no identified degree of COPD that precludes surgery**.

- Data on non-COPD chronic lung disease are not well studied.
  - **Asthma** that is compensated does not appear to be a significant risk factor.
  - **Interstitial lung disease** likely places patients at higher risk, but it is not well studied in patients undergoing general surgery (*Chest 2007;132:1637*). Restriction associated with **obesity** does not appear to be a significant risk factor (*Ann Intern Med 2006;144:575*).
  - **Pulmonary hypertension** is associated with significant morbidity in patients undergoing surgery (*J Am Coll Cardiol 2005;45:1691*; *Br J Anaesth 2007; 99:184*).
- **Poor general health status** is associated with increased perioperative pulmonary risk. Multiple measures of general health status have been correlated with poor pulmonary outcomes.
- **Advanced age** has also been identified as a predictor of postoperative pulmonary complications. The degree to which medical comorbidities confound this information is unclear, but multiple studies have found a significant association and it is included as a factor in risk prediction models, particularly age >60 years (*Ann Surg 2000;232:242*; *Ann Intern Med 2001;135:847*).
- **Smoking** is a risk factor for pulmonary complications. The degree of tobacco abuse correlates with the degree of risk (*Am J Respir Crit Care Med 2003;167:741*).
- **Obstructive sleep apnea** is increasingly being recognized as a risk factor for perioperative complications, both pulmonary and cardiac (*Chest 2008;133:1128*). The most frequent pulmonary complication appears to be hypoxemia (*Anesthesiology 2008;108:822*). Unrecognized sleep apnea may pose an even greater risk (*Mayo Clin Proc 2001;76:897*).

DIAGNOSIS

Clinical Presentation

History
- The preoperative pulmonary evaluation should focus on evaluating the presence and severity of patient-dependent risk factors.
  - Any history of chronic lung disease should be detailed. An effort should be made to determine the patient's baseline and whether there has been any recent deterioration, such as increased cough or sputum production.
  - Any symptoms of a current upper respiratory infection should be ascertained. Though not an absolute contraindication to surgery, it seems prudent to postpone purely elective procedures until such infections have resolved.
  - A full smoking history should be obtained.
- As noted, comorbid conditions impact the likelihood of pulmonary complications. Therefore, a complete medical history is necessary.

Physical Examination
- A complete physical examination should be part of any preoperative evaluation.
- Attention should be paid to evidence of chronic lung disease such as increased anteroposterior (AP) dimensions of the chest and the presence of adventitious lung sounds, particularly wheezing.

- The **maximum laryngeal height** should be determined. A value of <4 cm has been associated with pulmonary complications. Persistent coughing after a voluntary cough is also an indicator of increased risk (*Am J Respir Crit Care Med 2003;167:741*).

Diagnostic Criteria

- Unlike the situation for preoperative cardiac risk stratification, relatively few tools for quantifying preoperative pulmonary risk are available.
- In general, patients are deemed to be at an elevated risk of complications if they are undergoing high-risk procedures as noted previously and have one or more of the identified patient-dependent risk factors. To what degree their risk is elevated remains, by and large, a subjective assessment. It does appear that the risk of increasing numbers of risk factors is additive, such that patients with multiple risk factors are at increasingly high levels of risk.
- Risk indices for predicting postoperative respiratory failure and pneumonia have been developed (*Ann Surg 2000;232:242*; *Ann Intern Med 2001;135:847*). Though somewhat cumbersome, these represent the best available objective risk prediction tools. The former was refined in a more recent study, but it remains somewhat unwieldy for routine clinical use (*J Am Coll Surg 2007;204:1188*).

Diagnostic Testing

- **Pulmonary function tests (PFTs)**
  - The value of preoperative PFTs is unclear and controversial outside of lung resection surgery, where its role is better defined.
  - Though PFTs can clearly be used to define lung disease, in the setting of nonpulmonary surgery there is concern that they add little beyond what can be gathered clinically (*Chest 1997;111:1536*).
  - Firm recommendations for or against PFTs cannot be made. However, in patients with unexplained pulmonary symptoms and patients with lung disease and an unclear baseline, PFTs should be considered.
- **Arterial blood gas (ABG) analysis**
  - It is unclear that ABG results add to the estimate of preoperative pulmonary risk beyond other clinically derived variables.
  - In general, an ABG is not an integral part of the preoperative pulmonary evaluation.
  - An ABG should be obtained when otherwise clinically necessary, such as to determine if a patient's lung disease is compensated.
- **Chest radiography**
  - The value of a routine chest radiograph is variable.
  - Many findings deemed abnormal are chronic and do not affect management (*Can J Anesth 2005;52:568*).
  - In general, a chest radiograph is recommended only if otherwise clinically indicated.
- **Serum albumin**
  - A decreased serum albumin level has been shown to be a strong predictor of increased pulmonary risk, though a more recent large study found a lesser risk than suggested previously (*Ann Intern Med 2006;144:581*; *J Am Coll Surg 2007;204:1188*).
  - Though studies vary in definition, a level <3.5 mg/dL appears to be indicative of increased risk.

○ Despite the evidence identifying a decreased albumin level as a strong predictor of perioperative risk, there is at present no conclusive evidence that enteral or parenteral **nutritional supplementation** decreases risk (*Ann Intern Med 2006;144:596*).

TREATMENT

- **Modifiable patient-related risk factors**
  ○ The effect of preoperative **smoking cessation** on pulmonary complications has been largely described in cardiothoracic surgeries, where a benefit to smoking cessation **at least 2 months** prior to surgery has been shown (*Mayo Clin Proc 1989;64:609*). The effect on a general surgical population is less clear, as most of the benefit of smoking cessation has been related to improvements in nonpulmonary outcomes such as fewer wound complications (*Ann Surg 2008;248:739*). Nevertheless, given the long-term benefits of smoking cessation, all patients should be counseled to stop smoking even if <8 weeks from surgery. Previous concerns about a paradoxical increase in complications appear unwarranted (*Chest 2005;127:1977*).
  ○ **COPD therapy** should be optimized. Symptoms should be aggressively treated preoperatively. Although not all patients with COPD respond to corticosteroid therapy, a preoperative course of steroids is reasonable for symptomatic patients already receiving maximal bronchodilator therapy who are not at their best personal baseline level. Patients with recent sputum changes may benefit from a preoperative course of antibiotics.
- **Modifiable procedure-related risk factors**
  ○ Consideration of alternative procedures with the lowest possible pulmonary risk should be undertaken for high-risk patients.
  ○ **Laparoscopic procedures** may yield fewer pulmonary complications (*Br J Anaesth 1996;77:448*). Typically, though, the pulmonary benefits demonstrated with laparoscopic procedures have been in laboratory variables such as spirometry, and it is unclear if this will lead consistently to fewer clinical pulmonary complications.
  ○ Where possible, use of **neuraxial/regional anesthetic** methods may be preferable in higher risk patients.
- **Postoperative interventions**
  ○ **Lung expansion maneuvers**, such as incentive spirometry or deep breathing exercises, should be employed. Intensive preoperative training has been shown to reduce pulmonary complications in patients undergoing coronary artery bypass (*JAMA 2006;296:1851*). Whether the same would be true in a general surgical population or with less intensive training is not clear. However, the intervention is benign and is probably helpful.
  ○ **Noninvasive positive pressure ventilation (NPPV)** is an option for both the prevention and treatment of postoperative respiratory failure. Continuous positive airway pressure (CPAP) was shown in a recent review to decrease postoperative pulmonary complications in patients undergoing abdominal surgery and in those undergoing thoracoabdominal aortic surgery (*Ann Surg 2008;247:617; Chest 2005;128:821*). For patients who do develop postoperative respiratory failure, there is evidence to suggest NPPV will improve pulmonary outcomes (*JAMA 2005;293:589*). The best studied of the NPPV modalities is CPAP, but other modalities have also been used (*Chest 2005;128:2688*). The optimal modality

and delivery system is undefined. Because of the potential complications of its use, patients being treated with NPPV require intensive monitoring.

o **Appropriate analgesia** is essential to prevent splinting, but oversedation needs to be carefully avoided. There is some evidence to suggest that epidural analgesia can reduce postoperative pulmonary complications relative to other regimens (*Arch Surg 2008;143:990*).

o A strategy of **selective nasogastric tube placement** rather than routine use has also been shown to decrease the risk of pulmonary complications (*Cochrane Database Syst Rev 2007(3)*). Communication with the surgical team is important to determine if this is an appropriate consideration.

o Appropriate **DVT prophylaxis** is strongly encouraged.

Anemia and Transfusion Issues in Surgery

GENERAL PRINCIPLES

- Blood products represent a finite and costly resource.
- Transfusion of blood products is associated with substantial risks including transmission of bloodborne infections, transfusion-related acute lung injury (TRALI), transfusion reactions, and immunosuppressive effects.
- Preoperatively, anemia is present in 5% to 76% of patients, with the wide variance related to the definition of anemia and type of surgery studied (*Am J Med 2004;116(S):58S*). Regardless, it is a common clinical occurrence.

DIAGNOSIS

- Patients should be asked about a history of anemia or hematologic disease. Any history of a bleeding diathesis should be noted.
- Any clinical signs of anemia (e.g., pallor) or coagulopathy (e.g., petechiae) should be duly noted.
- Prior medical records and testing should be reviewed.
- In patients without findings from the initial evaluation to suggest a hematologic abnormality, the degree of testing is controversial.
  - o For **low-risk procedures**, it is not clear that otherwise asymptomatic individuals require any preoperative testing, and there is no evidence that routine testing before low-risk procedures increases safety (*N Engl J Med 2000;342:168*).
  - o For **higher risk procedures**, particularly those with a more substantial bleeding risk, a baseline CBC and coagulation profile is typically obtained. If recent results are available, repeating the tests is likely unnecessary.
  - o Further testing of patients found to have significant anemia or coagulopathy should be performed as clinically indicated.

TREATMENT

It is essential to remember that volume resuscitation and control of active bleeding is the initial therapy of anemia, particularly in the perioperative period when acute blood loss is a common occurrence.

- Anemia to a hemoglobin concentration of 5 gm/dL is reasonably well tolerated in euvolemic, otherwise healthy individuals under stable, experimental conditions (*Anesthesiology 2000;93:1004*).
- Data from patients who refused transfusion are consistent with this finding, as nearly all deaths attributed to anemia occurred at a hemoglobin concentration <5 gm/dL (*Transfusion 1994;34:396*).
- How this applies to patients undergoing surgery is less clear.
  - Preoperative hemoglobin levels <10 gm/dL are associated with an increase in morbidity/mortality risk. The risk increases steadily with decreasing hemoglobin levels, with a pronounced surge in risk at levels <6 gm/dL (*Lancet 1996; 348:1055*).
  - Postoperatively, in a cohort of patients who refused transfusion, no mortality was observed until the hemoglobin decreased below 7 gm/dL. A marked increase in risk was seen as hemoglobin levels dropped below the 5 gm/dL threshold (*Transfusion 2002;42:812*).
  - As these were observational studies, the degree to which the anemia was a causative factor rather than a marker of illness cannot be determined.
  - Increased surgical blood loss, as evidenced by the degree of decrease in hemoglobin from the preoperative to the postoperative values, was noted to be associated with increased morbidity and mortality.
  - The benefit of transfusion at physiologically tolerable levels of anemia is unclear.
    - A study of intensive care unit patients suggested that the classic transfusion threshold of a hemoglobin of 10 gm/dL was too liberal, as patients treated with a more "restrictive" strategy (with a trigger of 7 gm/dL) had outcomes that were at least equivalent and in some cases better (*N Engl J Med 1999;336:933*). The applicability of this study to the perioperative setting is uncertain, particularly as postcardiac surgery patients were excluded from the trial.
    - Other observational studies have suggested that transfusion may actually increase the risk of adverse outcomes (*Crit Care Med 2006;34:1608*; *J Surg Res 2002; 102:237*).
- It is generally agreed that transfusion is not required when the hemoglobin exceeds 10 gm/dL. Likewise, it is generally agreed that a hemoglobin <6 gm/dL necessitates transfusion (*Anesthesiology 2006;105:198*).
- The best strategy for patients with hemoglobin between 6 and 10 gm/dL is unclear.
  - Markers of intolerance of anemia (e.g., tachycardia) should be considered.
  - Evidence of end-organ dysfunction (e.g., myocardial ischemia) should prompt transfusion.
  - Preoperatively, consideration of the expected blood loss with the planned surgery may alter the threshold for transfusion.
  - **The presence of cardiovascular disease** may influence the decision to transfuse:
    - Concomitant cardiovascular disease appears to increase the risk of perioperative mortality for any given level of anemia (*Lancet 1996;348:1055*).
    - Two studies have demonstrated an increase in myocardial ischemia with a hematocrit <28%, though analysis of critically ill patients with cardiovascular disease showed no significant increase in adverse outcomes with a transfusion threshold of a hemoglobin of 7 gm/dL (*Transfusion 1998;38:924*; *Crit Care Med 1993;21:860*; *Crit Care Med 2001;29:227*). It is difficult to establish the effect of volume status on these results, particularly in the patients with anemia postoperatively.

▪ Thus, no firm recommendations can be made. It appears reasonable to **consider transfusion at a hemoglobin <9 gm/dL in this population**, though other groups have recommended tolerance of a lower hemoglobin, suggesting a threshold for transfusion of 8 gm/dL (*Br J Haematol 2001;113:24*).

Other Nonpharmacologic Therapies

Measures to **reduce the need for allergenic blood** should be utilized where feasible.

- Preoperative **autologous blood donation** should be considered for elective procedures where the anticipated need for transfusion is high.
- **Preoperative erythropoietin** can be considered in patients with decreased hemoglobin concentration (*N Engl J Med 1997;336:933*). Patients need to have adequate iron stores when this is utilized; supplemental iron therapy may be required. There are also concerns about increased risk for DVT in patients treated with erythropoietin preoperatively that have been included in an FDA-mandated "black box" warning that limit its use in this setting (*Med Lett Drugs Ther 2007;49:37*).
- **Intraoperative measures** include **normovolemic hemodilution** for surgeries with high expected blood loss. This approach has the advantage of requiring minimal preoperative preparation (*Arch Pathol Lab Med 2007;1331:695*). **Intraoperative blood salvage and autotransfusion and positional blood pooling** are the other options.
- Avoidance of perioperative hypothermia may also limit blood loss, and thereby decrease transfusion requirements (*Anesthesiology 2008;108:71*).

SPECIAL CONSIDERATIONS

Patients with **sickle cell anemia** should generally be transfused to a hemoglobin of 10 gm/dL preoperatively to decrease the incidence of complications.

Liver Disease

GENERAL PRINCIPLES

- Patients with hepatic dysfunction suffer from an increased risk of morbid outcomes when undergoing surgery.
- Patients with underlying liver disease are at substantial risk for acute hepatic decompensation postoperatively.
- The myriad systemic effects of liver dysfunction result in an increased frequency of other complications as well, such as bleeding and infection.

Classification

- The best validated measure of perioperative risk in patients with cirrhosis is the **Child–Pugh score**, reflecting increased risk with greater degrees of hepatic dysfunction (see Chapter 19, Liver Diseases).
  - A large review of patients undergoing a variety of surgical procedures clearly identified a demarcation between Child's class A (score <7) and those with more severe class B and C disease (*Anesthesiology 1999;90:42*).
    - ▪ Thirty-day mortality was 9.4% in the Child's class A group versus 16.7% in classes B and C group combined. Other complications were also significantly more common.

- Interestingly, the type of cirrhosis appears to have an impact as well, as **patients with primary biliary cirrhosis and primary sclerosing cholangitis appear to tolerate surgery better**.
  - Other studies have shown further that patients with Child's class C disease have extremely high operative risk, with perioperative mortality exceeding 80% with abdominal surgery in this group (*Surgery 1997;122:730*).
- The **MELD score** may also be an indicator of postoperative mortality in cirrhotics (see Chapter 19, Liver Diseases). One study of cholecystectomies found a MELD score ≥8 to be a marker of increased risk relative to the Child–Pugh score (*Clin Gastroenterol Hepatol 2004;2:1123*). However, other studies have found the Child–Pugh score to be superior (*Clin Gastroenterol Hepatol 2004;2:719*).

DIAGNOSIS

Clinical Presentation

History
- As part of the preoperative history and physical, evidence of liver disease should be sought.
- Historical details suggesting a risk for hepatic disease, such as alcohol or drug abuse and prior blood transfusion, should be sought.
- Other indicators of a risk for liver disease may be noted in the preoperative evaluation (e.g., family history of hemochromatosis).

Physical Examination
Physical examination evidence of liver dysfunction should be noted. Some should be obvious, such as icterus and abdominal distension with ascites, but other abnormalities such as spider nevi, palmar erythema, and testicular atrophy may be more subtle.

Diagnostic Testing
- Because of the low prevalence and because significant disease is usually clinically suspected, routine laboratory screening for hepatic dysfunction in patients presenting for surgery who are without clinically suspected or known liver disease is not recommended (*Med Clin N Am 2003;87:211*).
- Patients with known or suspected liver disease should undergo a thorough evaluation of liver function including **hepatic enzyme levels**, **albumin** and **bilirubin** measurements, and **evaluation for coagulopathy**.
- **Renal function**, including electrolytes, blood urea nitrogen (BUN), and creatinine measurements, should also be evaluated.

TREATMENT

- Patients with **acute viral or alcoholic hepatitis** tolerate surgery poorly, and delaying surgery until recovery is recommended if possible.
- Patients with **chronic hepatitis** without evidence of hepatic decompensation generally tolerate surgery well.
- Based on the high perioperative mortality rates in patients with **advanced cirrhosis**, nonoperative alternatives should be strongly considered.
- For patients who do require surgery, steps should be taken to **optimize the preoperative status**.

- **Coagulopathy** should be corrected.
  - Vitamin K should be administered if the INR is elevated. As the coagulopathy may well be refractory to this measure in the setting of liver disease, fresh frozen plasma and cryoprecipitate may be required.
  - **Thrombocytopenia** is a common occurrence and should generally be corrected if severe. The general recommendation for most surgical procedures is a minimum platelet count of 50,000. However, in the setting of liver disease, the coexistence of platelet dysfunction should be considered, particularly if there is clinical bleeding with an otherwise adequate platelet count.
- Renal and electrolyte abnormalities should be addressed.
  - Careful attention should be paid to **volume status**.
  - Nephrotoxic substances, such as NSAIDs and aminoglycosides, should be avoided.
  - Patients with cirrhosis often have **hypokalemia** and **alkalosis**. These conditions should be corrected preoperatively to minimize the risks of cardiac arrhythmias and to limit encephalopathy.
  - If **hyponatremia** occurs, free water restriction may be required.
- **Ascites** should be treated.
  - Ascites has been found to be an independent risk factor for postoperative pulmonary complications (*J Am Coll Surg 2007;204:1188*).
  - If time permits, **diuretic therapy** should be instituted.
  - **Paracentesis** should be considered preoperatively if diuretics are ineffective or if time constraints prevent their use.
- **Encephalopathy** should be treated.
  - **Lactulose** titrated to two to three soft bowel movements per day should be started in patients with encephalopathy.
  - Protein restriction has been recommended for individuals who respond poorly to lactulose but should be done cautiously, because excessive restriction may actually contribute to malnutrition.
  - **Sedatives and other narcotics** can precipitate or worsen encephalopathy. They should be used only cautiously and dose reductions should be considered.
  - **Hypokalemia** should be avoided.
- Adequate **nutrition** should be provided.

Diabetes Mellitus

GENERAL PRINCIPLES

- Medical and surgical patients with hyperglycemia are at increased risk for poor outcomes (*J Clin Endocrinol Metab 2002;87:978*).
- Poor preoperative glucose control, as indicated by elevated hemoglobin A1c levels, is associated with an increased risk of surgical infections (*Arch Surg 2006;141:375*). Hyperglycemia postoperatively also appears to be associated with an increased risk of postoperative infection (*JPEN J Parenter Enteral Nutr 1998;22:77*).
- There is some suggestion, particularly in patients undergoing cardiothoracic surgery, that more aggressive medical management of hyperglycemia mitigates the risk of infection and possibly mortality (*Ann Thorac Surg 1997;63:356; J Thorac Cardiovasc Surg 2003;125:1007*).
- The fact that hyperglycemia is a marker for poor outcomes appears to be relatively clear. However, whether aggressive management truly improves outcomes is uncertain. Trial results have been mixed.

- In a population of mostly surgical patients requiring critical care, impressive reductions in mortality were demonstrated in a single institution study (*N Engl J Med 2001;345:1359*). The results of this trial prompted widespread adoption of aggressive insulin protocols in surgical intensive care units.
- However, a recent larger multicenter trial of both surgical and medical critical care patients was unable to show improvements in outcome and actually found a slight increase in risk with aggressive treatment of hyperglycemia (*N Engl J Med 2009;360:1283*).
- Diabetics are at **increased risk for cardiovascular disease**. Appropriate risk stratification for cardiac complications of surgery is vital to the perioperative evaluation of these patients.

Classification

- Establishing the etiology of hyperglycemia has important implications for subsequent patient care.
  - **Stress hyperglycemia** can occur in the perioperative setting because of the body's response to surgery with the release of counterregulatory hormones and cytokines that impede glucose metabolism. These patients need adequate glucose control during the perioperative period but are unlikely to require such treatment later.
  - Type 2 diabetes is notoriously underdiagnosed, however, and the notation of perioperative hyperglycemia may be the first indication of its presence.
- It is also essential to distinguish between type 1 and type 2 diabetes mellitus.
  - **Type 1 diabetics** will require a continuous supply of insulin regardless of glucose level and oral intake.
  - The insulin requirement, if any, of **type 2 diabetics** during the perioperative period will vary.

DIAGNOSIS

- Most patients should have a **hemoglobin A1c** obtained.
  - This can assist in differentiating perioperative stress hyperglycemia from undiagnosed diabetes.
  - Knowledge of recent glycemic control in known diabetics is also helpful in determining what therapy is required.
- Evaluating **renal function** is also recommended given the increased prevalence of renal disease in diabetics.
- Cardiovascular risk stratification may require other evaluations (see Preoperative Cardiovascular Evaluation section previously).

TREATMENT

- Elective surgery in patients with uncontrolled diabetes mellitus should preferably be scheduled after acceptable glycemic control has been achieved.
- If possible, the operation should be scheduled for early morning to minimize prolonged fasting.
- Frequent monitoring of blood glucose levels is required in all situations.
- **Type 1 diabetes**
  - Some form of basal insulin is required at all times.
  - On the evening prior to surgery, the regularly scheduled basal insulin should be continued. If taken in the morning, it is still recommended to give the regularly

scheduled basal insulin without dose adjustment (*Diabetes Care 2004;27:553*). However, patients who are very tightly controlled may be at increased risk for hypoglycemia and will need to be monitored closely. A decrease in the last preoperative basal insulin dose may be considered in this circumstance.

○ Glucose infusions (e.g., D5-containing fluids) can be administered to avoid hypoglycemia while the patient is NPO and until tolerance of oral intake postoperatively is established.

○ For complex procedures and procedures requiring a prolonged NPO status, a continuous insulin infusion will likely be necessary.

○ **Caution should be exercised with the use of subcutaneous insulin** in the intraoperative and critical care settings, as alterations in tissue perfusion may result in variable absorption.

• **Type 2 diabetes**

○ Treatment of type 2 diabetics varies according to their preoperative requirements and the complexity of the planned procedure (*Med Clin N Am 2003;87:175*).

○ Consideration should be given to the efficacy of the patient's current regimen. If they are not well controlled at baseline, then an escalation in therapy may be required.

▪ **Diet-controlled type 2 diabetes** can generally be managed without insulin therapy. Glucose values should be checked regularly and elevated levels (>180 mg/dL) can be treated with intermittent doses of short-acting insulin.

▪ **Type 2 diabetes managed with oral therapy**

□ **Short-acting sulfonylureas** and **other oral agents** should be withheld on the operative day.

□ **Metformin** and **long-acting sulfonylureas** (e.g., chlorpropamide) should be withheld 1 day before planned surgical procedures. Metformin is generally held for 48 hours postoperatively. Renal function should be normal prior to resuming treatment. Other oral agents can be resumed when patients are tolerating their preprocedure diet.

□ Most patients can be managed without an insulin infusion.

□ Glucose values should be checked regularly and elevated levels (>180 mg/dL) can be treated with intermittent doses of short-acting insulin.

▪ **Type 2 diabetes managed with insulin**

□ If it is anticipated the patient will be able to eat postoperatively, basal insulin is still given on the morning of surgery.

□ If given as long-acting insulin (e.g., glargine insulin) and the patient usually takes the dose in the morning, 50% to 100% of the usual dose can be given.

□ If the patient utilizes intermediate-acting insulin (e.g., NPH), one half to two thirds of the usual morning dose is given to avoid periprocedural hyperglycemia.

□ Dextrose-containing IV fluids may be required to avoid hypoglycemia.

□ Patients undergoing major procedures will typically require an insulin drip perioperatively.

□ The usual insulin treatment can be reintroduced once oral intake is established postoperatively.

• **Target glucose levels**

○ There are no generally agreed upon target glucose levels applicable to the entire postsurgical population.

- Previous recommendations for aggressive glucose control in the critical care setting (*Diabetes Care 2008;31S:S12*) were published prior to the aforementioned NICE-SUGAR trial.
- In a general medical–surgical population, recurring glucose values >200 mg/dL were associated with a poor outcome (*J Clin Endocrinol Metab 2002;87:978*).
  - Pending further research, a goal of maintaining glucose levels <180 mg/d in the postoperative setting seems reasonable. It should be noted that this may still require intensive treatments such as insulin infusion.
  - In patients treated with sliding scale insulin, it is essential to monitor the response to therapy. Patients who are hyperglycemic consistently are unlikely to have adequate glucose control with intermittent treatment alone, and a basal/bolus regimen should be introduced if hyperglycemia is persistent (*Diabetes Care 2007;30:2181*).

Adrenal Insufficiency and Corticosteroid Management

GENERAL PRINCIPLES

- Surgery is a potent activator of the hypothalamic–pituitary axis, and patients with adrenal insufficiency may lack the ability to respond appropriately to surgical stress.
- Patients receiving corticosteroids as medical therapy for indications other than adrenal dysfunction may develop adrenal insufficiency. Case reports of presumed adrenal insufficiency from the 1950s led to the widespread use of perioperative "stress-dose" steroids in this population (*JAMA 1952;149:1542*; *Ann Intern Med 1953;39:116*).

Classification
- The subtype of adrenal insufficiency has implications on management.
  - **Tertiary adrenal insufficiency** due to exogenous corticosteroid administration is the most common adrenal problem encountered. These patients should have intact mineralocorticoid function and therefore, if treated, should require only glucocorticoid supplementation (*N Engl J Med 2003;348:727*).
  - Likewise, **secondary adrenal insufficiency** should not result in mineralocorticoid deficiency. The possibility of deficits in other hormones due to pituitary disease should be considered.
  - **Primary adrenal insufficiency** requires replacement of both mineralocorticoids and glucocorticoids.
- The dose and duration of exogenous corticosteroids required to produce clinically significant tertiary adrenal insufficiency is highly variable, but general principles can be outlined (*Med Clin N Am 2003;87:175*).
  - Daily therapy with **5 mg or less of prednisone** (or its equivalent), **alternate-day corticosteroid therapy**, and **any dose given for <3 weeks** should not result in clinically significant adrenal suppression.
  - Patients receiving **>20 mg/d of prednisone (or equivalent) for >3 weeks** and patients who are clinically "**cushingoid**" **in appearance** can be expected to have significant suppression of adrenal responsiveness.
- The function of the hypothalamic–pituitary axis cannot be readily predicted in **patients receiving doses of prednisone 5 to 20 mg for >3 weeks**.

DIAGNOSIS

Clinical Presentation

History

- The dose and duration of prior corticosteroid therapy should be clarified.
- The coexistence of diseases that suggest the possibility of primary adrenal insufficiency should be sought (e.g., autoimmune thyroid disease, malignant tumors that metastasize to the adrenal such as lung cancer).

Physical Examination

Physical exam findings suggestive of adrenal hypofunction such as hyperpigmentation should be noted. As previously, inspection for features of a "cushingoid" appearance should be performed (see Chapter 24, Endocrine Diseases).

Diagnostic Testing

- For patients in whom clinical prediction of adrenal function is difficult, a **cosyntropin stimulation test** can be performed to determine adrenal responsiveness.
- **Electrolyte abnormalities** should be sought in patients with primary adrenal insufficiency. Patients with other forms of adrenal insufficiency are unlikely to manifest the classic hyperkalemia and hyponatremia due to intact mineralocorticoid function.

TREATMENT

- **Patients expected to have an intact adrenal function** (as outlined previously) should take their regularly scheduled dose of corticosteroid. No further treatment is required.
- Whether patients should otherwise be treated depends on the type of adrenal insufficiency encountered and the anticipated surgical stress.
  - For **patients with primary disease of the hypothalamic–pituitary–adrenal (HPA) axis**, adrenal supplementation is generally recommended. These recommendations are based on extrapolation from small studies in the literature, expert opinion, and clinical experience (*JAMA 2002;287:236*).
    - **Minor surgical stress** (e.g., colonoscopy, cataract surgery): Administer 25 mg hydrocortisone or 5 mg methylprednisolone IV on the day of the procedure only.
    - **Moderate surgical stress** (e.g., cholecystectomy, hemicolectomy): Administer 50 to 75 mg hydrocortisone or 10 to 15 mg methylprednisolone IV on the day of the procedure and taper quickly over 1 to 2 days to the usual dose.
    - **Major surgical stress** (e.g., major cardiothoracic surgery, Whipple procedure): Administer 100 to 150 mg hydrocortisone or 20 to 30 mg methylprednisolone IV on the day of the procedure and taper to the usual dose over the next 1 to 2 days.
    - **Critically ill patients undergoing emergent surgery** (e.g., sepsis, hypotension): Administer 50 to 100 mg hydrocortisone IV every 6 to 8 hours or 0.18 mg/kg/hour as a continuous infusion plus 50 mg/d of fludrocortisone until the shock has resolved. Then gradually taper the dose, monitoring vital signs and serum sodium closely.
    - Additional **mineralocorticoid supplementation** for patients with primary adrenal insufficiency may or may not be necessary, depending on the dose and mineralocorticoid potency of the corticosteroid given.

- ○ For patients with adrenal insufficiency due to **exogenous steroid administration**, the necessity of further treatment is controversial.
  - ▪ Two trials of glucocorticoid supplementation in patients receiving exogenous steroids undergoing surgery found no evidence of adrenal crisis when the patient's baseline steroid dose was continued (*Surgery 1997;121:123*; *J Clin Periodontol 1999;26:577*).
  - ▪ Several other observational studies examined perioperative cessation of all steroids in this population and found clinical adrenal insufficiency to be a very rare occurrence (*Arch Surg 2008;143:1222*). Patients who did develop clinical symptoms of adrenal insufficiency all responded to treatment with supplemental steroids.
  - ▪ Based on this evidence, **continuation of the patient's baseline steroid dose without additional steroid treatment** is a reasonable treatment strategy. Patients should be monitored closely for signs/symptoms of adrenal insufficiency. Given the fact that oral medications are often held on the morning of surgery, it may be prudent to convert the steroid to intravenous form in the perioperative period.
  - ▪ Some still recommend supplemental steroid therapy in this population. If this management strategy is pursued, treatment as outlined previously for patients with primary disease of the HPA axis is reasonable.

Chronic Renal Insufficiency and End-Stage Renal Disease

GENERAL PRINCIPLES

- **Chronic renal insufficiency (CRI)** is an independent risk factor for **perioperative cardiac complications**, so all patients with renal disease need appropriate cardiac risk stratification (*JAMA 2001;285:1865*).
- **Patients with end-stage renal disease (ESRD)** have a substantial mortality risk when undergoing surgery (*Arch Intern Med 1994;154:1674*).
- Most general anesthetic agents have no appreciable nephrotoxicity or effect on renal function other than that mediated through hemodynamic changes (*Anesthesiol Clin 2006;24:523*).

TREATMENT

- **Volume status**
  - ○ Every effort should be made to **achieve euvolemia** preoperatively to reduce the incidence of volume-related complications intraoperatively and postoperatively (*Med Clin N Am 2003;87:193*).
  - ○ Though this typically entails removing volume, some patients may be hypovolemic and require hydration.
  - ○ Patients with CRI not receiving hemodialysis may require treatment with loop diuretics.
  - ○ Patients being treated with **hemodialysis** should undergo dialysis preoperatively.
    - ▪ This is commonly performed on the day prior to surgery.
    - ▪ Hemodialysis can be performed on the day of surgery as well, but the possibility that transient electrolyte abnormalities and hemodynamic changes postdialysis can occur should be considered.

- **Electrolyte abnormalities**
  - **Hyperkalemia** in the preoperative setting should be treated, particularly as tissue breakdown associated with surgery may elevate the potassium level further postoperatively.
    - For patients on dialysis, preoperative dialysis should be utilized.
    - For patients with CRI not undergoing dialysis, alternative methods of potassium excretion will be necessary.
      - **Loop diuretics** can be utilized, particularly if the patient is also hypervolemic.
      - **Sodium polystyrene sulfonate (SPS) resins** can also be utilized. The possibility that **intestinal necrosis** with SPS resins occurs more frequently in the perioperative setting has been suggested (*Am J Kidney Dis 1992;20:159*).
  - Although chronic **metabolic acidosis** has not been associated with elevated perioperative risk, some local anesthetics have reduced efficacy in acidotic patients. Preoperative metabolic acidosis should be corrected with sodium bicarbonate infusions or dialysis.
- **Bleeding diathesis**
  - **Platelet dysfunction** has long been associated with uremia.
    - The value of a preoperative bleeding time in predicting postoperative bleeding has been questioned (*Blood 1991;77:2547*). A preoperative bleeding time is, therefore, not recommended.
    - Patients with evidence of perioperative bleeding should, however, be treated.
      - **Dialysis** for patients with ESRD will improve platelet function.
      - **Desmopressin** (0.3 µg/kg IV or intranasally) can be utilized.
      - **Cryoprecipitate,** 10 U over 30 minutes IV, is an additional option.
      - In patients with coexisting anemia, **red blood cell transfusions** can improve uremic bleeding.
      - For patients **with a history of prior uremic bleeding**, preoperative desmopressin or **conjugated estrogens** (0.5 mg/kg/day IV for 5 days) should be considered.
  - **Heparin** given with dialysis can increase bleeding risk. Heparin-free dialysis should be discussed with the patient's nephrologist when surgery is planned.

Acute Renal Failure

GENERAL PRINCIPLES

Surgery has been associated with an increased risk of **acute renal failure (ARF)** (*Med Clin N Am 2003;87:193*).
- Patients with **CRI** are at increased risk of ARF.
- ARF among patients with normal preoperative renal function is a relatively rare event but is associated with increased mortality when it occurs (*Anesthesiology 2007;107:892*).

DIAGNOSIS

- The approach to ARF in the perioperative setting is not substantially different from that in the nonoperative setting (see Chapter 13, Renal Diseases).
- However, certain additional factors have to be considered when evaluating the cause in the perioperative setting:

- ○ **Intraoperative hemodynamic changes**, particularly hypotension, should be considered.
  - ■ Intraoperative factors associated with ARF postoperatively include vasopressor use and diuretic use (*Anesthesiology 2007;107:892*).
  - ■ A careful review of the operative record is advised.
- ○ Certain procedures can have an adverse effect on the renal function (e.g., aortic clamping procedures). Therefore, careful attention to the details of the procedure is necessary.
- ○ The possibility that bleeding is responsible for a prerenal state deserves special attention.

TREATMENT

For a detailed discussion regarding the management of acute renal failure, please refer to Chapter 13, Renal Diseases.

2 Nutrition Support

Dominic Reeds and Ben P. Bradenham, Jr.

Nutrient Requirements

GENERAL PRINCIPLES

- **Energy**
  - **Total daily energy expenditure** (TEE) is composed of resting energy expenditure (normally ~70% of TEE), the thermic effect of food (normally ~10% of TEE), and energy expenditure of physical activity (normally ~20% of TEE).
  - It is impossible to determine **daily energy requirements** precisely with predictive equations because of the complexity of factors that affect metabolic rate. Judicious use of predictive equations can provide a reasonable estimate that should be modified as needed based on the patient's clinical course.
  - **Malnutrition** and **hypocaloric feeding** may decrease resting energy expenditure to values 15% to 20% below those expected for actual body size, whereas metabolic stressors, such as inflammatory diseases or trauma, often increase energy requirements (usually by <50% of preillness values).
  - The **Harris–Benedict equation** provides a reasonable estimate of resting energy expenditure (in kilocalories per day) in healthy adults. The equation takes into account the effect of body size and lean tissue mass (which is influenced by gender and age) on energy requirements and can be used to estimate total daily energy needs in hospitalized patients:

$$\text{Men} = 66 + (13.7 \times W) + (5 \times H) - (6.8 \times A)$$
$$\text{Women} = 665 + (9.6 \times W) + (1.8 \times H) - (4.7 \times A)$$

  where W is the weight in kilograms, H the height in centimeters, and A is the age in years (*Publication No. 279. Carnegie Institute of Washington. Philadelphia: JB Lippincott, 1919:223*).

  - Energy requirements per kilogram of body weight are inversely related to body mass index (BMI) (Table 2-1). The lower range within each category should be considered in insulin-resistant, critically ill patients unless they are depleted in body fat.
  - **Ideal body weight** can be estimated based on height:
    - For men: 106 lb + 6 lb for each inch over 5 ft
    - For women, 100 lb + 5 lb for each inch over 5 ft
- **Protein**
  - Protein intake of 0.8 g/kg/d meets the requirements of 97% of the adult population.
  - Protein requirements are affected by several factors, such as the amount of nonprotein calories provided, overall energy requirements, protein quality, the patient's baseline nutritional status and the presence of metabolic stressors (Table 2-2).

Table 2-1	Estimated Energy Requirements for Hospitalized Patients Based on Body Mass Index

Body Mass Index (kg/m^2)	Energy Requirements (kcal/kg/d)
15	35–40
15–19	30–35
20–24	20–25
25–29	15–20
≥30	<15

Note: These values are recommended for critically ill patients and all obese patients; add 20% of total calories in estimating energy requirements in non–critically ill patients.

- ○ Inadequate amounts of any of the essential amino acids result in inefficient utilization.
- ○ Illness increases the efflux of amino acids from skeletal muscle; however, it should be noted that increasing protein intake to >1.2 g/kg/d of prehospitalization body weight in critically ill patients may not reduce the impact of illness on loss of lean body mass (*Crit Care Med 1998;26(9):1529*).
- **Essential fatty acids**
  - ○ The liver can synthesize most fatty acids, but humans lack the desaturase enzyme needed to produce the n-3 and n-6 fatty acid series. Therefore, linoleic acid should constitute at least 2% and linolenic acid at least 0.5% of the daily caloric intake to prevent the occurrence of essential fatty acid deficiency.
  - ○ The plasma pattern of increased triene-to-tetraene ratio (>0.4) can be used to detect essential fatty acid deficiency.
  - ○ Patients who are unable to receive intravenous (IV) or oral lipid solutions may receive a daily topical application of 1 Tbsp of safflower oil to provide essential fatty acids.

Table 2-2	Recommended Daily Protein Intake

Clinical Condition	Protein Requirements (g/kg IBW/d)[a]
Normal	0.8
Metabolic ªstress° (illness/injury)	1.0–1.5
Acute renal failure (undialyzed)	0.8–1.0
Hemodialysis	1.2–1.4
Peritoneal dialysis	1.3–1.5

[a]Additional protein intake may be needed to compensate for excess protein loss in specific patient populations such as those with burn injury, open wounds, and protein-losing enteropathy or nephropathy. Lower protein intake may be necessary in patients with chronic renal insufficiency who are not treated by dialysis and certain patients with hepatic encephalopathy.
IBW, ideal body weight.

- **Carbohydrates**
  Certain tissues, such as bone marrow, erythrocytes, leukocytes, renal medulla, eye tissues, and peripheral nerves, cannot metabolize fatty acids and require glucose (~40 g/d) as a fuel. Other tissues such as the brain prefer glucose (~120 g/d).
- **Major minerals**
  Major minerals are important for ionic equilibrium, water balance, and normal cell function.
- **Micronutrients (trace elements and vitamins)**
  Trace elements and vitamins are essential constituents of enzyme complexes. The recommended dietary intake for trace elements, fat-soluble vitamins, and water-soluble vitamins is set at two standard deviations above the estimated mean so that it will cover the needs of 97% of the healthy population. See Table 2-3 for specifics regarding the assessment of micronutrient nutritional states as well as signs and symptoms of micronutrient deficiency and toxicity.

SPECIAL CONSIDERATIONS

- Both the amount and location of prior gut resection influences nutrient needs. Patients with a reduced length of functional small bowel may require additional vitamins and minerals if they are not receiving parenteral nutrition. Table 2-4 provides guidelines for supplementation in these patients.
- Distal ileum inflammation, resection, inflammatory bowel disease (IBD), and bypass (ileojejunal bypass) can cause rapid development of B_{12} deficiency and bile salt loss. Diarrhea in this setting may be improved with oral cholestyramine given with the first meal of the day.
- Proximal gut resection (stomach or duodenum) via partial gastrectomy, Billroth I and II, duodenal switch/biliopancreatic diversion, Roux-en Y gastric bypass, pancreaticoduodenectomy (Whipple), and sleeve gastrectomy may impair absorption of divalent cations such as iron, calcium, and copper. Copper deficiency is extremely common in post–gastric bypass patients who do not receive routine supplementation (*Int J Obes (Lond) 2012;36(3):328*).
- Patients with excessive gastrointestinal (GI) tract losses require additional fluids and electrolytes. An assessment of fluid losses due to diarrhea, ostomy output, and fistula volume should be made to help determine fluid requirements. Knowledge of fluid losses is also useful in calculating intestinal mineral losses by multiplying the volume of fluid loss by an estimate of intestinal fluid electrolyte concentration (Table 2-5).

Assessment of Nutritional Status

GENERAL PRINCIPLES

- Patients should be assessed for protein-energy malnutrition as well as specific nutrient deficiencies.
- A thorough history and physical exam combined with appropriate laboratory studies is the best approach to evaluate nutritional status.

DIAGNOSIS

Clinical Presentation

History
- Assess for changes in diet pattern (size, number, and content of meals). If present, the reason for altered food intake should be investigated.

Table 2-3	Trace Minerals, Fat-Soluble Vitamins, and Water-Soluble Vitamins: Recommended Daily Intake, Deficiency, At Risk Populations, Toxicity, and Status Evaluation				
Nutrient	Recommended Daily Enteral[1] Intake/ Parenteral Intake[2]	Signs and Symptoms of Deficiency[4]	Populations At Risk for Deficiency[1,4]	Signs and Symptoms of Toxicity[4]	Status Evaluation[4,5]
Chromium (Cr^{3+})	30–35 mcg/ *10–15 mcg*	Glucose intolerance, peripheral neuropathy[A]	None[A,4]	PO: gastritis IV: skin irritation Cr^{-6+}: (steel, welding) lung carcinogen if inhaled	Chromium$_s$
Copper (Cu^{2+})	900 mcg/ *300–500 mcg*	Hypochromic normocytic or macrocytic anemia (rarely microcytic), neutropenia, thrombocytopenia, diarrhea, osteoporosis/ pathologic fractures[A] Intrinsic: Menkes' disease[18]	Chronic diarrhea, high zinc/low protein diets[7,8]	PO: gastritis, nausea, vomiting, coma, movement/neurologic abnormalities, hepatic necrosis Intrinsic: Wilson's Disease	Copper$_{s,u}$ Ceruloplasmin$_p$

(continued)

Table 2-3 Trace Minerals, Fat-Soluble Vitamins, and Water-Soluble Vitamins: Recommended Daily Intake, Deficiency, At Risk Populations, Toxicity, and Status Evaluation (Continued)

Nutrient	Recommended Daily Enteral[1] Intake/ Parenteral Intake[2]	Signs and Symptoms of Deficiency[4]	Populations At Risk for Deficiency[1,4]	Signs and Symptoms of Toxicity[4]	Status Evaluation[4,5]
Iodine (I⁻)	150 mcg/ **70–140 mcg** (*not routinely added*)	Thyroid hyperplasia (goiter) + functional hypothyroidism Intrinsic in utero: cretinism, poor CNS development, hypothyroidism	Those without access to fortified salt, grain, milk, or cooking oil[11]	Hypothyroidism blocks thyroxine synthesis OR hyperthyroidism Excess supplementation in severe deficiency	TSH_s, iodine$_u$ (24 hr intake or iodine: Cr ratio are more representative than a single sample) Thyroglobulin$_s$[13]
Iron (Fe²⁺,³⁺)	8 mg/ **1.0–1.5 mg** (*not routinely added*)	Fatigue, hypochromic microcytic anemia, glossitis, koilonychia	Reproductive age females, pregnant females, chronic anemias, hemoglobinopathies, post-gastric bypass/ duodenectomy, alcoholics	PO or IV: hemosiderosis, followed by deposition in liver, pancreas, heart and glands Intrinsic: Hereditary hemochromatosis	Ferritin$_s$, TIBC$_s$, % Transferrin saturation$_c$, iron$_s$
Manganese (Mn²⁺)	2.3 mg/ **60–100 mcg**	Hypercholesterolemia, dermatitis, dementia, weight loss[B]	Chronic liver disease, iron deficient populations	PO: None[B] Inhalation: Hallucination, Parkinsonian-type symptoms[9]	No reliable markers Manganese$_s$ does not reflect bodily stores, especially in the CNS

Element	RDA / Dose	Deficiency	Causes	Toxicity	Laboratory
Selenium (SeO_4^{2-})	55 mcg/ **20–60 mcg**	Myalgias, cardiomyopathy[A] Intrinsic: Keshan's disease (Chinese children), Kashin-Beck disease, myxedematous endemic cretinism	Endemic areas of low soil content include certain parts of China and New Zealand[13]	PO: Nausea, diarrhea, AMS, irritability, fatigue, peripheral neuropathy, hair loss, white splotchy nails, halitosis (garlic-like odor)	Selenium$_s$, glutathione peroxidase activity$_b$
Zinc (Zn^{2+})	11 mg/ **2.5–5.0 mg**	Poor wound healing, diarrhea (high fistula risk), dysgeusia, teratogenicity, hypogonadism, infertility, acro-orificial skin lesions (glossitis, alopecia), behavioral changes Intrinsic: Acrodermatitis enteropathica	Chronic diarrhea, cereal-based diets, alcoholics, chronic liver disease, sickle cell, HIV, pancreatic insufficiency/any intestinal malabsorptive states, fistulas/ostomies, nephrotic syndrome, diabetes, post-gastric bypass/duodenectomy, anorexia, pregnancy[12] Intrinsic: Acrodermatitis enteropathica	PO: Nausea, vomiting, gastritis, diarrhea, low HDL, gastric erosions, Competition with GI absorption can precipitate Cu^{2+} *deficiency* Inhaled: Hyperpnea, weakness, diaphoresis	Zinc$_{S,P}$, alkaline phosphatase$_s$ (good for those on TPN, but in general Zinc$_{S,P}$, hair, RBC, WBC levels can be misleading) Zinc radioisotope studies (most accurate tests at present; limited by cost and availability)[12]

(continued)

Table 2-3 Trace Minerals, Fat-Soluble Vitamins, and Water-Soluble Vitamins: Recommended Daily Intake, Deficiency, At Risk Populations, Toxicity, and Status Evaluation (*Continued*)

Nutrient	Recommended Daily Enteral Intake[1] / Parenteral Intake[2]	Signs and Symptoms of Deficiency[4]	Populations At Risk for Deficiency[1,4]	Signs and Symptoms of Toxicity[4]	Status Evaluation[4,5]
Molybdenum	45 mcg/**45 mcg**	CNS toxicity, hyperoxypurinemia, hypouricemia, low urinary sulfate excretion[A,10] (also reported with parenteral sulfite infusion) Intrinsic: Molybdenum cofactor deficiency, isolated sulfite oxidase deficiency	None[A]	PO or any exposure: Hyperuricemia + gout Inhaled: Pneumoconiosis (industrial exposure)	Molybdenum$_b$

Vitamin A *Retinol*	900 mcg/ ***3,300 IU***	Conjunctival xerosis, keratomalacia, follicular hyperkeratosis, night blindness, *Bitot spots*, corneal + retinal dysfunction	Any malabsorptive state involving proximal small bowel, vegetarians, chronic liver disease	Acute: Teratogenic, skin exfoliation, intracranial hypertension, hepatocellular necrosis Chronic: Alopecia, ataxia, cheilitis, dermatitis, conjunctivitis, pseudotumor cerebri, hyperlipidemia, hyperostosis	Retinol$_s$, retinol esters$_p$, electroretinogram, liver biopsy (diagnostic for toxicity), retinol binding protein (useful in ESRD, accurately assesses blood levels)[14]
Vitamin D *Ergocalciferol*	5–15 mcg/ ***200 IU***	Rickets/osteomalacia	Any malabsorptive state involving proximal small bowel, chronic liver disease Of note: Those with higher skin melanin content (i.e., darker skin) have low baseline 25-OH vitamin D levels; it is unclear whether this merits their inclusion as an "at risk" population[15]	Hypercalcemia, hyperphosphatemia, which can lead to CaPO$_4$ precipitation, systemic calcification +/− AMS +/− AKI	25-OH vitamin D$_s$ Of note: lively debate between IOM and Endocrine Society regarding definitions of deficiency, goal serum 25-OH levels, and at risk populations[15,16]

(continued)

Table 2-3 | Trace Minerals, Fat-Soluble Vitamins, and Water-Soluble Vitamins: Recommended Daily Intake, Deficiency, At Risk Populations, Toxicity, and Status Evaluation (*Continued*)

Nutrient	Recommended Daily Enteral Intake[1]/Parenteral Intake[2]	Signs and Symptoms of Deficiency[4]	Populations At Risk for Deficiency[1,4]	Signs and Symptoms of Toxicity[4]	Status Evaluation[4,5]
Vitamin E (α,γ)-*Tocopherol*	15 mg/*10 IU*	Hemolytic anemia, posterior column degeneration, ophthalmoplegia, peripheral neuropathy Seen in severe malabsorption, abetalipoproteinemia	Any malabsorptive state involving proximal small bowel, chronic liver disease	Possible increase risk in hemorrhagic CVA, functional inhibition of vitamin K–mediated procoagulants	Tocopherol Must account for cholesterol/triglyceride ratio: otherwise, higher cholesterol/triglyceride ratio overestimates vitamin E, lower cholesterol/triglyceride ratio underestimates vitamin E[2c]
Vitamin K *Phylloquinone*	120 mcg/*150 IU*	Hemorrhagic disease of newborn, coagulopathy	Any malabsorptive state involving proximal small bowel, chronic liver disease	In utero: Hemolytic anemia, hyperbilirubinemia, kernicterus IV: flushing, dyspnea, hypotension (possibly related to dispersal agent)	Prothrombin time_p

Vitamin		Deficiency	At-risk populations	Toxicity	Laboratory test
Vitamin B1	*Thiamine*	1.2 mg/**6 mg**	Irritability, fatigue, headache Wernicke's encephalopathy, Korsakoff psychosis, "Wet" beri-beri, "Dry" beri-beri	Alcoholics, severely malnourished	IV: Lethargy and ataxia	RBC transketolase activity[b], thiamine[b&u]
Vitamin B2	*Riboflavin*	1.3 mg/**3.6 mg**	Cheilosis, angular stomatitis, glossitis, seborrheic dermatitis, normocytic normochromic anemia	Alcoholics, severely malnourished	None[B]	RBC glutathione reductase activity[p]
Vitamin B3	*Niacin*	16 mg/**40 mg**	Pellagra dysesthesias, glossitis, stomatitis, vaginitis, vertigo Intrinsic: Hartnup disease	Alcoholics, malignant carcinoid syndrome, severely malnourished	Flushing, hyperglycemia, hyperuricemia, hepatocellular injury[B]	N-methyl-nicotinamide[u]
Vitamin B5	*Pantothenic acid*	5 mg/**15 mg**	Fatigue, abdominal pain, vomiting, insomnia, paresthesias[B]	Alcoholics[6]	PO: Diarrhea	Pantothenic acid[u]
Vitamin B6	*Pyridoxine*	1.3–1.7 mg/**6 mg**	Cheilosis, stomatitis, glossitis, irritability, depression, confusion, normochromic normocytic anemia	Alcoholics, diabetics, celiac sprue, chronic isoniazid or penicillamine use[6]	Peripheral neuropathy, photosensitivity	Pyridoxal phosphate[p]

(continued)

Table 2-3	Trace Minerals, Fat-Soluble Vitamins, and Water-Soluble Vitamins: Recommended Daily Intake, Deficiency, At Risk Populations, Toxicity, and Status Evaluation (Continued)				
Nutrient	Recommended Daily Enteral[1] Intake/ Parenteral Intake[2]	Signs and Symptoms of Deficiency[4]	Populations At Risk for Deficiency[1,4]	Signs and Symptoms of Toxicity[4]	Status Evaluation[4,5]
Vitamin B7 *Biotin*	30 mcg/**60 mcg**	Mental status changes, myalgias, hyperesthesias, anorexia[C,5] (excessive egg white consumption results in avidin-mediated biotin inactivation)	Alcoholics[6]	None[B,5]	$Biotin_p$, methyl-citrate$_u$, 3-methyl-crotonylglycine$_u$, 3-hydroxyisovalerate$_u$
Vitamin B9 *Folic acid*	400 mcg/ **600 mcg**	Bone marrow suppression, macrocytic megaloblastic anemia, glossitis, diarrhea Can be precipitated by Sulfasalazine + Phenytoin	Alcoholics, celiac or tropical sprue, chronic sulfasalazine use[6]	PO: May lower seizure threshold in those taking anticonvulsants	Folic acid$_s$, RBC folic acid$_p$

Vitamin B12 Cobalamin	2.4 mcg/**5 mcg**	Bone marrow suppression, macrocytic megaloblastic anemia, glossitis, diarrhea posterolateral column demyelination, AMS, depression, psychosis	Vegetarians, atrophic gastritis, pernicious anemia, celiac sprue, Crohn's disease, patients postgastrectomy or ileal resection	None[B]	Cobalamin (B12)[s], methylmalonic acid[s&p]
Vitamin C Ascorbic acid	90 mg/**200 mg**	Scurvy, ossification abnormalities Tobacco lowers plasma and WBC vitamin C[2] Sudden cessation of high dose vitamin C can precipitate scurvy	Fruit-deficient diet, smokers[1], ESRD[3].	Nausea, diarrhea, increased oxalate synthesis (theoretical nephrolithiasis risk)	Ascorbic acid[p], leukocyte ascorbic acid

AKI, acute kidney injury; AMS, altered mental status; CNS, central nervous system; CVA, cerebrovascular accident; ESRD, end-stage renal disease; IOM, Institute of Medicine; IV, intravenous; GI, gastrointestinal; HDL, high-density lipoprotein (cholesterol); TIBC, total iron bonding capacity; TPN, total parenteral nutrition.

Subscript: b, blood; c, calculated; p, plasma; s, serum; u, urine.

[A]Only reported in patients on long-term TPN.

[B]Never demonstrated in humans.

[C]Only able to induce under experimental conditions and/or only been able to induce in animals.

(continued)

Table 2-3	Trace Minerals, Fat-Soluble Vitamins, and Water-Soluble Vitamins: Recommended Daily Intake, Deficiency, At Risk Populations, Toxicity, and Status Evaluation (Continued)

[1]Trumbo P, Yates AA, Schlicker S, et al. Institute of Medicine, Food and Nutrition Board. Dietary reference intakes for vitamin A, vitamin K, arsenic, boron, chromium, copper, iodine, iron, manganese, molybdenum, nickel, silicon, vanadium, and zinc. *J Am Diet Assoc.* 2001;101(3):294–301.

[2]Mirtallo J, Canada T, Johnson D, et al. Safe practices for parenteral nutrition. *JPEN J Parenter Enteral Nutr.* 2004;28:S39–S74.

[3]Deicher R, Hörl WH Vitamin C in chronic kidney disease and hemodialysis patients. *Kidney Blood Press Res.* 2003;26:100–106.

[4]Office of Dietary Supplements: National Institutes of Health. Dietary supplement fact sheet: chromium. Office of Dietary Supplements: National Institutes of Health. http://ods.od.nih.gov/pdf/factsheets/Chromium-HealthProfessional.pdf. August 5, 2005. Accessed March 10–25, 2012.

Ibid. (June 24, 2011). Dietary supplement fact sheet: iodine. Office of Dietary Supplements: National Institutes of Health. http://ods.od.nih.gov/pdf/factsheets/Iodine-HealthProfessional.pdf. June 24, 2011. Accessed March 10–25, 2012.

Ibid. (August 24, 2007). Dietary supplement fact sheet: iron. Office of Dietary Supplements: National Institutes of Health. http://ods.od.nih.gov/factsheets/Iron-HealthProfessional/. August 24, 2007. Accessed March 10–25, 2012.

Ibid. (October 11,2011). Dietary supplement fact sheet: selenium. Office of Dietary Supplement: National Institutes of Health. Retrieved March 10–25, 2012, from http://ods.od.nih.gov/factsheets/Selenium-HealthProfessional/

Ibid. (April 23, 2006). Dietary supplement fact sheet: vitamin A. Office of Dietary Supplements: National Institutes of Health. Retrieved March 10–25, 2012, from http://ods.od.nih.gov/factsheets/VitaminA-HealthProfessional/

Ibid. (June 24, 2011). Dietary supplement fact sheet: vitamin B12. Office of Dietary Supplements: National Institutes of Health. Retrieved March 10–25, 2012, from http://ods.od.nih.gov/factsheets/VitaminB12-HealthProfessional/. June 24, 2011. Accessed March 10–25, 2012.

Ibid. (June 24, 2011). Dietary supplement fact sheet: vitamin C. Office of Dietary Supplements: National Institutes of Health. http://ods.od.nih.gov/factsheets/VitaminC-HealthProfessional/. June 24, 2011. Accessed March 10–25, 2012.

Ibid. (June 24, 2011). Dietary supplement fact sheet: vitamin D. Office of Dietary Supplements: National Institutes of Health. http://ods.od.nih.gov/factsheets/VitaminD-HealthProfessional/. June 24, 2011. Accessed March 10–25, 2012.

Ibid. (September 15, 2011). Dietary supplement fact sheet: vitamin B6. Office of Dietary Supplements: National Institutes of Health. http://ods.od.nih.gov/factsheets/VitaminB6-HealthProfessional/. September 15, 2011. Accessed March 10–25, 2012.

Ibid. (October 11, 2011). Dietary Supplement fact sheet: vitamin E. Office of Dietary Supplements: National Institutes of Health. http://ods.od.nih.gov/factsheets/VitaminE-HealthProfessional/. October 11, 2011. Accessed March 10–25, 2012.

Ibid. (September 20, 2011). Dietary Supplement fact sheet: zinc. Office of Dietary Supplements: National Institutes of Health. http://ods.od.nih.gov/factsheets/Zinc-HealthProfessional/. September 20, 2011. Accessed March 10–25, 2012.

[5]Feldman M, Friedman LS, Brandt LJ. Sleisenger and Fordtran's Gastrointestinal and Liver Disease, 9th ed. Philadelphia: Saunders Elsevier, 2010.

[6]Said HM. Intestinal absorption of water-soluble vitamins in health and disease. Biochem J. 2011;437:357–372.

[7]Stern BR. Essentiality and toxicity in copper health risk assessment: overview, update and regulatory considerations. J Toxicol Environ Health A. 2010;73:114–127.

[8]Abumrad NN, Schneider AJ, Steel D, et al. Amino acid intolerance during prolonged total parenteral nutrition reversed by molybdate therapy. Am J Clin Nutr. 1981;34(11):2551–2559.

[9]Santamaria AB, Sulsky, SI. Risk assessment of an essential element: manganese. J Toxicol Environ Health A. 2010;73:128–155.

[10]Linus Pauling Institute. http://lpi.oregonstate.edu/

Higdon J, Drake VL, Turnlund JR. Micronutrient information center: moylbdenum. Linus Pauling Institute, Micronutrient Research and Optimum Health. http://lpi.oregonstate.edu/infocenter/minerals/molybdenum/. Accessed March 10–25, 2012.

Higdon J, Drake VL, Mock D. Micronutrient information center: biotin. Linus Pauling Institute, Micronutrient Research and Optimum Health. http://lpi.oregonstate.edu/infocenter/vitamins/biotin/. Accessed March 10–25, 2012.

[11]Zimmermann MB. Iodine deficiency. Endocr Rev. 2009 Jun;30(4):376–408.

[12]Semrad C. Zinc and intestinal function. Curr Gastroenterol Rep. 1999;1:398–403.

[13]Fairweather-Tait SJ, Collings R, Hurst R. Selenium bioavailability: current knowledge and future research requirements. Am J Clin Nutr. 2010;91(suppl):1484S–1491S.

[14]Mahmood K, Samo AH, Lairamani KL, et al. Serum retinol binding protein as an indicator of vitamin A status in cirrhotic patients with night blindness. Saudi J Gastroenterol. 2008;14(1):7–11.

[15]Rosen CJ, Abrams SA, Aloia JF, et al. IOM committee members respond to Endocrine Society vitamin D guideline. J Clin Endocrinol Metab. 2012;97:1146–1152.

[16]Holick MF, Binkley NC, Bischoff-Ferrari HA, et al. Evaluation, treatment, and prevention of vitamin D deficiency: an Endocrine Society clinical practice guideline. J Clin Endocrinol Metab. 2001;96:1911–1930.

[17]Ford L, Farr J, Morris P, et al. The value of measuring serum cholesterol-adjusted vitamin E in routine practice. Ann Clin Biochem. 2006;43:130–134.

[18]Uauy R, Olivares O, Gonzales M. Essentiality of copper in humans. Am J Clin Nutr. 1998;67(suppl):952S–959S.

Table 2-4	Guidelines for Vitamin and Mineral Supplementation in Patients with Severe Malabsorption	
Supplement	**Dose**	**Route**
Prenatal multivitamin with minerals[a]	1 tablet daily	PO
Vitamin D[a]	50,000 U two to three times per week	PO
Calcium[a]	500 mg elemental calcium tid–qid	PO
Vitamin B$_{12}$[b]	1 mg daily	PO
100–500 mcg q1–2 mo		SC
Vitamin A[b]	10,000–50,000 U daily	PO
Vitamin K[b]	5 mg/d	PO
	5–10 mg/wk	SC
Vitamin E[b]	30 U/d	PO
Magnesium gluconate[b]	108–169 mg elemental magnesium qid	PO
Magnesium sulfate[b]	290 mg elemental magnesium one to three times per week	IM/IV
Zinc gluconate or zinc sulfate[b]	25 mg elemental zinc daily plus 100 mg elemental zinc per liter intestinal output	PO
Ferrous sulfate[b]	60 mg elemental iron tid	PO
Iron dextran[b]	Daily dose based on formula or table	IV

[a]Recommended routinely for all patients.
[b]Recommended for patients with documented nutrient deficiency or malabsorption.

- Unintentional weight loss of >10% body weight in the last 6 months is associated with a poor clinical outcome (*Am J Med 1980;69:491*).
- Look for evidence of **malabsorption** (diarrhea, weight loss).
- For symptoms of specific **nutrient deficiencies**, see Table 2-3.
- Consider factors that may increase metabolic stress (e.g., infection, inflammatory disease, malignancy).
- Assess patient's functional status (e.g., bedridden, suboptimally active, very active).

Table 2-5	Electrolyte Concentrations in Gastrointestinal Fluids			
Location	Na (mEq/L)	K (mEq/L)	Cl (mEq/L)	HCO$_3$ (mEq/L)
Stomach	65	10	100	–
Bile	150	4	100	35
Pancreas	150	7	80	75
Duodenum	90	15	90	15
Mid–small bowel	140	6	100	20
Terminal ileum	140	8	60	70
Rectum	40	90	15	30

Physical Examination
- By World Health Organization (WHO) criteria, patients can be classified by BMI as underweight (<18.5 kg/m^2), normal weight (18.5 to 24.9 kg/m^2), overweight (25.0 to 29.9 kg/m^2), class I obesity (30.0 to 34.9 kg/m^2), class II obesity (35.0 to 39.9 kg/m^2), or class III obesity (≥40.0 kg/m^2) (*Obes Res 1998;6(suppl 2):S53*).
- Patients who are **extremely underweight** (BMI <14 kg/m^2) or those **with rapid, severe weight loss** (even with supranormal BMI) have a high risk of death and should be considered for admission to the hospital for nutritional support.
- Look for **tissue depletion** (loss of body fat and skeletal muscle wasting).
- Assess **muscle function** (strength testing of individual muscle groups).
- **Fluid status:** Evaluate patients for dehydration (e.g., hypotension, tachycardia, mucosal xerosis) or excess body fluid (edema or ascites).
- Evaluate patient for sources of protein or nutrient losses: large wounds, burns, nephrotic syndrome, surgical drains, etc. Quantify the volume of drainage and the concentration of fat and protein content.

Diagnostic Testing
- Perform laboratory studies to determine specific nutrient deficiencies only when clinically indicated, as the plasma concentration of many nutrients may not reflect true body stores (Table 2-3).
- Plasma albumin and prealbumin concentration should not be used to assess patients for protein-calorie malnutrition or to monitor the adequacy of nutrition support. While levels of these plasma proteins correlate with clinical outcome, inflammation and injury can alter their synthesis and degradation, consequently limiting their utility in nutritional assessment (*Crit Care Med 1982;10:305*; *Gastroenterology 1990;99:1845*).
- Most hospitalized patients are vitamin D deficient, and caregivers should have a low threshold for checking plasma 25-OH vitamin D levels (*N Engl J Med 1998;338:777*).

Enteral Nutrition

GENERAL PRINCIPLES

Whenever possible, **oral/enteral** feeding (Figure 2-1) is preferred to parenteral **feeding** because it limits mucosal atrophy, maintains immunoglobulin A (IgA) secretion, and prevents cholelithiasis. Additionally, oral/enteral feeds are less expensive than parenteral nutrition.
- **Types of feedings**
  - **Hospital diets** include a regular diet and those modified in either nutrient content (amount of fiber, fat, protein, or sodium) or consistency (liquid, puréed, soft). There are ways that food intake can often be increased:
    - Encourage patients to eat.
    - Provide assistance at mealtime.
    - Allow some food to be supplied by relatives and friends.
    - Limit missed meals for medical tests and procedures.
    - Avoid unpalatable diets. Milk-based formulas (e.g., Carnation Instant Breakfast) contain milk as a source of protein and fat and tend to be more palatable than other defined formula diets.
    - Use of calorically dense supplements (e.g., Ensure, Boost).

1) Calculate the basics:
  - Calculate **BMI** (kg/m^2): You will need it to calculate total daily caloric requirements (TEE = surrogate).
  - Calculate **IBW**: You will need to calculate daily protein requirements.

2) Calculate both total caloric and total protein requirements:
  - There are many equations used to estimate energy requirements including:
    ○ Extrapolation of TEE from **Harris-Benedict**, which estimates REE (70% of TEE) (i.e., multiply calculated result by 1.3 for TEE estimate).
    ○ WHO guidelines for given calories per kilogram for a given BMI.[1]
    ○ Washington University equivalent to WHO guideline (Table 2-1).
  - Calculating daily protein requirements: *Calculate using ideal body weight*
    ○ Evaluate for presence of metabolic stressors (e.g., SIRS, burns, trauma, hemodialysis (see Table 2-2).

3) Estimate protein requirements (see Table 2-2) and calculate calories derived from protein
  - Protein delivered (g) $\times$ 4 (cal/g) = protein caloric requirement
  - Protein caloric requirement $\div$ total daily caloric requirement ($\times$ 100) = % total daily calorie requirement in protein

4) Choose the best product based both on special considerations and protein requirements.
  a) Renal failure? Low protein, K^+ and PO_4^{3-}
  b) Fluid restriction? High caloric concentration
  c) Pancreatic insufficiency? Enzyme replacement vs. oligomeric vs. elemental formula
  d) Severe COPD or sepsis? Consider low carbohydrate formula

  See Table 2-6 for examples of several currently available products.

5) Calculate rate of feeding:
  - Now that a product has been chosen, one needs to assess how much product is needed to meet total daily caloric requirements.
  - KEY: Attempting to meet protein needs is the FIRST priority. Meeting total daily caloric requirements is secondary in most hospitalized patients.
  - Total daily caloric requirement $\div$ (calories/mL of formula X) = mL formula.
  - See bolus vs. gravity vs. continuous feedings.

6) Calculate free H20 requirement:
  - Start at 30–50 mL q 4 hours. May initially need to supplement IV to meet requirements.

Figure 2-1. A step-by-step approach to enteral nutrition. BMI, body mass index; (*continued*)

Case scenario: 30-yo female with chronic pancreatitis, calorically dependent enteral nutrition via a jejunostomy tube, presents from home with fever and hypoxia found to be secondary to pneumonia. Below is one way to calculate her new caloric requirement.

1) She weighs 45 kg, and is 160 cm tall:
   a. BMI = 45 kg/1.6 m^2 = 17.6 kg/m^2
   b. IBW = 45.5 kg + 4.6 kg* = 50.1 kg
      *Rounded 160 cm to approximately 5 feet 2 inches

2) Estimate total caloric and protein requirements:
   a. Calories: From Table 2-1, she requires approximately 35 kcal/kg/d given her BMI of 17.6 kg/m^2.
      i. 35 kcal/kg/d × 45 kg = 1,575 kcal/d
   b. Taking into consideration her chronic pancreatitis and current pneumonia, an appropriate modification of her protein content would be 1.5 g/kg IBW/d (normal = 0.8 g/kg/d)
      i. 1.5 g/kg IBW/d × 50.1 kg IBW = approximately 75 g protein/d

3) Protein requirements in terms of total calories:
   a. 75 g protein/d × 4 kcal/g protein = 300 kcal/d
   b. 300 kcal/1,575 kcal = 19% of total calories should be in the form of protein

4) Taking into consideration her chronic pancreatitis and resulting malabsorption, Peptamen AF or Vivonex would both be reasonable formulas to consider. Vivonex, however, at 20% protein comes slightly closer to her estimated protein requirements.

5) Calculating rate of feeding with Vivonex:
   a. How many milliliters of product will be needed to account for total protein needs?
      i. 300 kcal protein/d/0.2 kcal protein/mL = 1,500 mL/d
   b. How many milliliters of product will be needed to account for total caloric needs?
      i. 1,575 kcal/d/1 kcal/mL = 1,575 mL
   c. Note: It is rare that the protein composition of a formula so closely approximates a patient's protein needs. In general, in a hospitalized population, if one must choose between two formulas, choose the formula with the higher protein content.
   d. Jejunal feeding: Continuous feeds at a goal of approximately 66.7 mL/hr is a reasonable initial option. Start at 10–25 mL/hr and uptitrate the rate as tolerated until goal is met.

Figure 2-1. (*Continued*). COPD, chronic obstructive pulmonary disease; IBW, ideal body weight; IV, intravenous; REE, resting energy expenditure; SIRS, systemic inflammatory response syndrome; TEE, total energy expenditure; WHO, World Health Organization. (Data from Feldman M, Friedman LS, Brandt LJ. *Sleisenger and Fordtran's Gastrointestinal and Liver Disease*. 9th ed. Philadelphia, PA: Saunders Elsevier; 2010.)

- **Defined liquid formulas**
  - **Polymeric formulas** (e.g., Osmolite, Jevity) are appropriate for most patients. They contain nitrogen in the form of whole proteins and include blenderized food, milk-based, and lactose-free formulas. Other formulas are available with modified nutritional content including high-nitrogen, high-calorie, fiber-enriched, and low-potassium/phosphorus/magnesium formulas.
  - **Semielemental *oligomeric* formulas** (e.g., Propeptide, Peptamen) contain hydrolyzed protein in the form of small peptides and free amino acids. While these formulas may have benefit in those with exocrine pancreatic insufficiency or short gut, pancreatic enzyme replacement is a less expensive, equally effective intervention in most of these patients.
  - **Elemental monomeric formulas** (e.g., Vivonex, Glutasorb) contain nitrogen in the form of free amino acids and small amounts of fat (<5% of total calories), and are hyperosmolar (550 to 650 mOsm/kg). These formulas are not palatable and therefore require either tube feeding or mixing with other foods or flavorings for oral ingestion. Free amino acids are poorly absorbed, and as a result, absorption of monomeric formulas is not clinically superior to that of oligomeric or polymeric formulas in patients with adequate pancreatic digestive function. These formulas may exacerbate osmotic diarrhea in patients with short gut.
  - **Oral rehydration solutions** stimulate sodium and water absorption by taking advantage of the sodium–glucose cotransporter present in the brush border of intestinal epithelium. Oral rehydration therapy (using 90 to 120 mEq/L solutions to avoid intestinal sodium secretion and negative sodium and water balance) can be especially useful in patients with short bowel syndrome (*Clin Ther 1990; 12(suppl A):129*). The characteristics of several oral rehydration solutions are listed in Table 2-6.
- **Tube feeding**
  - Tube feeding is useful in patients who have a **functional GI tract** but who cannot or will not ingest adequate nutrients.
  - The type of tube feeding approach selected (nasogastric, nasoduodenal, nasojejunal, gastrostomy, jejunostomy, pharyngostomy, and esophagostomy tubes) depends on physician experience, clinical prognosis, gut patency and motility, risk of aspirating gastric contents, patient preference, and anticipated duration of feeding.
  - Short-term (<6 weeks) tube feeding can be achieved by placement of a soft, small-bore nasogastric or nasoenteric feeding tube. Although nasogastric feeding is usually the most appropriate route, orogastric feeding may be needed in those who are intubated, or in patients with nasal injury or deformity. Nasoduodenal and nasojejunal feeding tubes can be placed at the bedside with a success rate approaching 90% when inserted by experienced personnel (*Nutr Clin Pract 2001;16:258*).
  - Long-term (>6 weeks) tube feeding usually requires a gastrostomy or jejunostomy tube that can be placed percutaneously by endoscopic (*PEG*) or radiographic assistance. Alternatively, they can be placed surgically, depending on the clinical situation and local expertise.
- **Feeding schedules:** Patients who have feeding tubes in the stomach can often tolerate intermittent bolus or gravity feedings, in which the total amount of daily formula is divided into four to six equal portions.
  - **Bolus feedings** are given by syringe as rapidly as tolerated.
  - **Gravity feedings** are infused over 30 to 60 minutes.

Table 2-6	Enteral Feeding Formulas: Comparing Composition						
Formula	kcal/mL	% Protein	% Lipid	% Carbohydrate	K⁺ mEq/L	PO4³⁻ mg/L	Purpose/Niche
Osmolite	1.0	16.7	29	54.3	40.2	760	Standard polymeric
Jevity	1.5	17	29	53.6	40.2	1,200	Standard polymeric
TwoCal HN	2	16.7	40.1	43.2	62.6	1,050	Volume restricted
Nepro with Carb Steady	1.8	18	48	34	27.2	700	ESRD
Glucerna	1.2	20	45	35	51.8	800	Glucose intolerance/ diabetes
Promote	1.0	25	23	52	50.8	1,200	High protein
Peptamen AF	1.2	25	39	36	41	800	Short gut, exocrine pancreatic insufficiency
Vivonex RTF	1.0	20	10	70	31	670	Fat malabsorption
Oxepa	1.5	16.7	55.2	28.1	50.1	1,060	SIRS, ARDS, sepsis

ARDS, acute respiratory distress syndrome; ESRD, end-stage renal disease; SIRS, systemic inflammatory response syndrome.
Table adapted from Barnes-Jewish Hospital Enteral Nutrition Formulary (8/2009).

- The patient's upper body should be elevated by 30 to 45 degrees during feeding and for at least 2 hours afterward. Tubes should be flushed with water after each feeding. Intermittent feedings are useful for patients who cannot be positioned with continuous head-of-the-bed elevation or who require greater freedom from feeding. Patients who experience nausea and early satiety with bolus gravity feedings may require continuous infusion at a slower rate.
- **Continuous feeding** can often be started at 20 to 30 mL/hr and advanced by 10 mL/hr every 6 hours until the feeding goal is reached. Patients who have gastroparesis often tolerate gastric tube feedings when they are started at a slow rate (e.g., 10 mL/hr) and advanced by small increments (e.g., 10 mL/hr every 8 to 12 hours). Patients with severe gastroparesis may require passage of the feeding tube tip past the ligament of Treitz. **Continuous feeding should always be used when feeding directly into the duodenum or jejunum to avoid distention, abdominal pain, and dumping syndrome.**
- **Jejunal feeding** may be possible in closely monitored patients with mild to moderate **acute pancreatitis** (*J Am Coll Nutr 1995;14(6):662*).
- **Contraindications:** The intestinal tract cannot be used effectively in some patients due to:
  - Persistent nausea or vomiting
  - Intolerable postprandial abdominal pain or diarrhea
  - Mechanical obstruction or severe hypomotility
  - Severe malabsorption
  - Presence of high-output fistula

COMPLICATIONS

- **Mechanical complications**
  - **Nasogastric feeding tube misplacement** occurs more commonly in unconscious patients. Intubation of the tracheobronchial tree has been reported in up to 15% of patients. Intracranial placement can occur in patients with skull fractures.
  - **Erosive tissue damage** can lead to nasopharyngeal erosions, pharyngitis, sinusitis, otitis media, pneumothorax, and GI tract perforation.
  - **Tube occlusion** is often caused by inspissated feedings or pulverized medications given through small-diameter (<#10 French) tubes. Frequent flushing of the tube with 30 to 60 mL of water and avoiding administration of pill fragments or "thick" medications help to prevent occlusion. Techniques used to unclog tubes include the use of a small-volume syringe (10 mL) to flush warm water or pancreatic enzymes (Viokase dissolved in water) through the tube.
- **Hyperglycemia**
  - The precise level at which glucose should be maintained in hospitalized patients remains controversial.
  - Subcutaneously administered insulin can usually maintain good glycemic control. IV insulin drip protocols may be used to control blood glucose in critically ill patients with anasarca or hemodynamic instability to ensure adequate insulin absorption.
  - Intermediate-duration insulin (e.g., NPH) can often be used safely once tube feedings reach 1,000 kcal/d. Long-duration insulin (e.g., detemir, glargine) should be used with caution in critically ill patients because changes in clinical status may affect pharmacokinetics and increase the risk of sustained hypoglycemia.

- Patients who are receiving bolus feeds should receive short-acting insulin at the time of the feed.
- Patients who are being given continuous (24 hours per day) feeding should receive intermediate- or long-duration insulin every 12 to 24 hours when clinically stable.

- **Pulmonary aspiration**
  - The etiology of **pulmonary aspiration** can be difficult to determine in tube-fed patients because aspiration can occur from refluxed tube feedings or oropharyngeal secretions that are unrelated to feedings.
  - Addition of food coloring to tube feeds **should not be used** for the diagnosis of aspiration. This method is insensitive for diagnosis, and several case reports suggest that food coloring can be absorbed by the GI tract in critically ill patients, which can lead to serious complications and death (*N Engl J Med 2000;343:1047*).
  - Gastric residuals are poorly predictive of aspiration risk.
  - Prevention of reflux: Decrease gastric acid secretion with pharmacologic therapy (H2 blocker, PPI), elevate head of bed during feeds, and avoid gastric feeding in high-risk patients (e.g., those with gastroparesis, frequent vomiting, gastric outlet obstruction).

- **GI complications**
  - Nausea, vomiting, and abdominal pain are common.
  - **Diarrhea** is often associated with antibiotic therapy (*JPEN J Parenter Enteral Nutr 1991;15:27*) and the use of liquid medications that contain nonabsorbable carbohydrates, such as sorbitol (*Am J Med 1990;88:91*). If diarrhea from tube feeding persists after proper evaluation of possible causes, a trial of antidiarrheal agents or fiber is justified. Diarrhea is common in patients who receive tube feeding and occurs in up to 50% of critically ill patients.
  - Diarrhea in patients with short gut, who do not have other causes such as *Clostridium difficile* infection, may be minimized by use of small, frequent meals that do not contain concentrated sweets (e.g., soda). Intestinal transit time should be maximized to allow nutrient absorption using tincture of opium, loperamide, or diphenoxylate. Low-dose clonidine (0.025 to 0.05 mg orally twice a day) may be used to reduce diarrhea in hemodynamically stable patients with short bowel syndrome (*JPEN J Parenter Enteral Nutr 2004;28(4):265*).
  - **Intestinal ischemia/necrosis** has been reported in patients receiving tube feeding. These cases have occurred predominantly in critically ill patients receiving vasopressors for blood pressure support in conjunction with enteral feeding. There are no reliable clinical signs for diagnosis, and the mortality rate is high. **Caution should be used when enterally feeding critically ill patients requiring vasopressors.**

Parenteral Nutrition

GENERAL PRINCIPLES

- Parenteral nutrition should be considered if energy intake has been or is anticipated to be inadequate (<50% of daily requirements) for more than 7 to 10 days and enteral feeding is not feasible. This guideline originates from two intensive care unit (ICU)-focused meta-analyses discussed in the 2009 A.S.P.E.N. (American Society for Parenteral and Enteral Nutrition) guidelines citing increased infectious complications, overall complications (*Am J Clin Nutr 2001;74:534*) and increased overall mortality (*JAMA 1998;280:2013*) in ICU patients receiving early parenteral nutrition (i.e., within 7 days of admission) (*JPEN J Parenter Enteral Nutr 2009;33(3):285*). Results from Casaer et al. corroborate these recommendations citing faster recovery, as well as fewer infectious and cholestatic complications in critically ill patients fed after day 8, compared to those in whom parenteral nutrition was begun on the first hospital day (*N Engl J Med 2011;365:506*).

- Routine use of immediate postoperative total parenteral nutrition (TPN) does not appear to improve outcomes in unselected patients (*Ann Surg 1993; 217(2):185*).
- **Recommendations**
  - **Central parenteral nutrition (CPN)**
    - The infusion of hyperosmolar (usually >1,500 mOsm/L) nutrient solutions requires a large-bore, high-flow vessel to minimize vessel irritation and damage.
    - Percutaneous subclavian vein **catheterization** and peripherally inserted central venous catheterization (PICC) are the most commonly used techniques for CPN access. The internal jugular, saphenous, and femoral veins are also used, although are less desirable due to decreased patient comfort and difficulty in maintaining sterility. Tunneled catheters are preferred in patients who are likely to receive >8 weeks of TPN to reduce the risk of mechanical failure.
    - PICCs (which reduce the risk of pneumothorax) are increasingly used to provide CPN in patients with adequate antecubital vein access. These catheters are not suitable for patients in whom CPN is anticipated to be necessary for an extended duration (>6 months).
  - **CPN macronutrient solutions**
    - Crystalline **amino acid solutions** containing 40% to 50% essential and 50% to 60% nonessential amino acids (usually with little or no glutamine, glutamate, aspartate, asparagine, tyrosine, and cysteine) are used to provide protein needs (Table 2-2). Infused amino acids are oxidized and should be included in the estimate of energy provided as part of the parenteral formulation.
    - Some amino acid solutions have been modified for specific disease states such as those enriched in branched-chain amino acids for use in patients who have hepatic encephalopathy and solutions that contain mostly essential amino acids for use in patients with renal insufficiency.
    - **Glucose** (dextrose) in IV solutions is hydrated; each gram of dextrose monohydrate provides 3.4 kcal. While there is no absolute requirement for glucose in most patients, providing >150 g glucose per day maximizes protein balance.
    - **Lipid emulsions** are available as a 10% (1.1 kcal/mL) or 20% (2.0 kcal/mL) solution and provide energy as well as a source of essential fatty acids. Emulsion particles are similar in size and structure to chylomicrons and are metabolized like nascent chylomicrons after acquiring apoproteins from contact with circulating endogenous high-density lipoprotein-cholesterol particles. Lipid emulsions are as effective as glucose in conserving body nitrogen economy once absolute tissue requirements for glucose are met. The optimal percentage of calories that should be infused as fat is not known, but 20% to 30% of total calories is reasonable for most patients. The rate of infusion should not exceed 1.0 kcal/kg/hr (0.11 g/kg/hr) because most complications associated with lipid infusions have been reported when providing more than this amount (*Curr Opin Gastroenterol 1991;7:306*). A rate of 0.03 to 0.05 g/kg/hr is adequate for most patients who

are receiving continuous CPN. Lipid emulsions should not be given to patients who have triglyceride concentrations of >400 mg/dL. Moreover, patients at risk for hypertriglyceridemia should have serum triglyceride concentrations checked at least once during lipid emulsion infusion to ensure adequate clearance. Underfeeding obese patients by the amount of lipid calories that would normally be given (e.g., 20% to 30% of calories) facilitates mobilization of endogenous fat stores for fuel and may improve insulin sensitivity. IV lipids should still be administered twice per week to these patients to provide essential fatty acids.

COMPLICATIONS

- **Mechanical complications**
  - Complications at time of line placement include pneumothorax, air embolism, arterial puncture, hemothorax, and brachial plexus injury.
  - Thrombosis and pulmonary embolus: Radiologically evident subclavian vein thrombosis occurs commonly; however, clinical manifestations (upper extremity edema, superior vena cava syndrome) are rare. Fatal microvascular pulmonary emboli can be caused by nonvisible precipitate in parenteral nutrition solutions. Inline filters should be used with all solutions to minimize the risk of these emboli.
- **Metabolic complications:** Usually caused by overzealous or inadequate nutrient administration:
  - Fluid overload
  - Hypertriglyceridemia
  - Hypercalcemia
  - Specific nutrient deficiencies. Consider providing supplemental **thiamine** (100 mg for 3 to 5 days) during initiation of CPN in patients at risk for thiamine deficiency (e.g., alcoholism).
  - Hypoglycemia
  - **Hyperglycemia.** For the past decade, tight blood glucose control (between 90 and 120 mg/dL) has been the standard dogma in ICU populations (*N Engl J Med 2001;345:1359*); however, this practice has been called into question in light of a 2009 randomized controlled trial (RCT) illustrating significantly higher overall mortality and incidence of critical hypoglycemia in patients whose blood glucose was being tightly controlled (*N Engl J Med 2009;360(13):1283*). Management of patients with hyperglycemia or type 2 diabetes (*Mayo Clin Proc 1996;71:587*) can be performed in the following way:
    - If blood glucose is >200 mg/dL, consider obtaining better control of blood glucose before starting CPN.
    - If CPN is started, (a) limit dextrose to <200 g/d, (b) add 0.1 U of regular insulin for each gram of dextrose in CPN solution (e.g., 15 U for 150 g), (c) discontinue other sources of IV dextrose, and (d) order routine, regular insulin with blood glucose monitoring by fingerstick every 4 to 6 hours or IV regular insulin infusion with blood glucose monitoring by fingerstick every 1 to 2 hours.
    - In outpatients who use insulin, an estimate of the reduction in blood sugar that will be caused by the administration of 1 U of insulin may be calculated by dividing 1,500 by the total daily insulin dose (e.g., for a patient receiving

50 U of insulin as an outpatient, 1 U of insulin may be predicted to reduce plasma glucose concentration by 1,500/50 = 30 mg/dL.

- If blood glucose remains >200 mg/dL and the patient has been requiring SC insulin, add 50% of the supplemental short-acting insulin given in the last 24 hours to the next day's CPN solution and double the amount of SC insulin sliding-scale dose for blood glucose values >200 mg/dL.
- The insulin-to-dextrose ratio in the CPN formulation should be maintained while the CPN dextrose content is changed.

- **Infectious complications**
  - Catheter-related sepsis is the most common life-threatening complication in patients who receive CPN and is most commonly caused by skin flora: *Staphylococcus epidermidis* and *Staphylococcus aureus*.
  - In **immunocompromised patients** and those with long-term (>2 weeks) CPN, *Enterococcus*, *Candida* species, *Escherichia coli*, *Pseudomonas*, *Klebsiella*, *Enterobacter*, *Acinetobacter*, *Proteus*, and *Xanthomonas* should be considered.
  - The principles of **evaluation and management** of suspected catheter-related infection are outlined in the Infectious Disease section.
  - Although antibiotics are often infused through the central line, the **antibiotic lock technique** has been used successfully to treat and prevent central catheter-related infections (*Nutrition 1998;14:466*; *Antimicrob Agents Chemother 1999;43:2200*). This technique involves local delivery of antibiotics in the catheter without systemic administration.

- **Hepatobiliary complications.** Although these abnormalities are usually benign and transient, more serious and progressive disease may develop in a small subset of patients, usually after 16 weeks of CPN therapy or in those with short bowel (*Diseases of the Liver. 7th ed. Philadelphia: JB Lippincott; 1993:1505*).
  - Biochemical: Elevated aminotransferases and alkaline phosphatase are commonly seen.
  - Histologic alterations: Steatosis, steatohepatitis, lipidosis, phospholipidosis, cholestasis, fibrosis, and cirrhosis have all been seen.
  - Biliary complications usually occur in patients who receive CPN for >3 weeks.
    - Acalculous cholecystitis
    - Gallbladder sludge
    - Cholelithiasis
    - Routine efforts to prevent hepatobiliary complications in all patients receiving long-term CPN include providing a portion (20% to 40%) of calories as fat, cycling CPN so that the glucose infusion is stopped for at least 8 to 10 hours per day, encouraging enteral intake to stimulate gallbladder contraction and maintain mucosal integrity, avoiding excessive calories, and preventing hyperglycemia.
    - If abnormal liver biochemistries or other evidence of liver damage occurs, evaluation for other possible causes of liver disease should be performed.
    - If mild hepatobiliary complications are noted parenteral nutrition does not need to be discontinued, but the same principles used in preventing hepatic complications can be applied therapeutically.
    - When cholestasis is present, copper and manganese should be deleted from the CPN formula to prevent accumulation in the liver and basal ganglia. A 4-week trial of metronidazole or ursodeoxycholic acid has been reported to be helpful in some patients.

- **Metabolic bone disease**
  - Metabolic bone disease has been observed in patients receiving long-term (>3 months) CPN.
  - Patients may be asymptomatic. Clinical manifestations include bone fractures and pain (*Annu Rev Nutr 1991;11:93*). Demineralization may be seen in radiologic studies. Osteopenia, osteomalacia, or both may be present.
  - The precise causes of metabolic bone disease are not known, but several mechanisms have been proposed, including aluminum toxicity, vitamin D toxicity, and negative calcium balance.
  - Several therapeutic options should be considered in patients who have evidence of bone abnormalities.
  - Remove vitamin D from the CPN formulation if the parathyroid hormone and 1,25-hydroxy vitamin D levels are low.
  - Reduce protein to <1.5 g/kg/d because amino acids cause hypercalciuria.
  - Maintain normal magnesium status because magnesium is necessary for normal parathormone action and renal conservation of calcium.
  - Provide oral calcium supplements of 1 to 2 g/d.
  - Consider bisphosphonate therapy to decrease bone resorption.
- **Peripheral parenteral nutrition**
  - Peripheral parenteral nutrition is often considered to have limited usefulness because of the high risk of thrombophlebitis.
  - Appropriate adjustments in the management of peripheral parenteral nutrition can increase the life of a single infusion site to >10 days. The following guidelines are recommended:
    - Provide at least 50% of total energy as a lipid emulsion piggybacked with the dextrose–amino acid solution.
    - Add 500 to 1,000 U heparin and 5 mg hydrocortisone per liter (to decrease phlebitis).
    - Place a fine-bore 22- or 23-gauge polyvinylpyrrolidone-coated polyurethane catheter in as large a vein as possible in the proximal forearm using sterile technique.
    - Place a 5-mg glycerol trinitrate ointment patch (or 0.25 in. of 2% nitroglycerin ointment) over the infusion site.
    - Infuse the solution with a volumetric pump.
    - Keep the total infused volume <3,500 mL/d.
    - Filter the solution with an inline 1.2-m filter (*Nutrition 1994;10:49*).
- **Long-term home parenteral nutrition**
  - Long-term home parenteral nutrition is usually given through a **tunneled catheter** or an implantable subcutaneous port inserted in the subclavian vein.
  - **Nutrient formulations** can be infused overnight to permit daytime activities in patients who are able to tolerate the fluid load. IV lipids may not be necessary in patients who are able to ingest and absorb adequate amounts of fat.
- **Monitoring nutrition support**
  - Adjustment of the nutrient formulation is often needed as medical therapy or clinical status changes.
  - When nutrition support is initiated, other sources of **glucose** (e.g., peripheral IV dextrose infusions) should be stopped and the volume of other IV fluids adjusted to account for CPN.
  - Vital signs should be checked every 8 hours.

○ In certain patients, body weight, fluid intake, and fluid output should be followed daily.

○ Serum electrolytes (including phosphorus) should be measured every 1 or 2 days after CPN is started until values are stable and then rechecked weekly.

○ Serum glucose should be checked up to every 4 to 6 hours by fingerstick until blood glucose concentrations are stable and then rechecked weekly.

○ If lipid emulsions are being given, **serum triglycerides** should be measured during lipid infusion in patients at risk for hypertriglyceridemia to demonstrate adequate clearance (triglyceride concentrations should be <400 mg/dL).

○ Careful attention to the catheter and catheter site can help to prevent **catheter-related infections**.

  ▪ Gauze dressings should be changed every 48 to 72 hours or when contaminated or wet, but transparent dressings can be changed weekly.

  ▪ Tubing that connects the parenteral solutions with the catheter should be changed every 24 hours.

  ▪ A 0.22-μm filter should be inserted between the IV tubing and the catheter when **lipid-free CPN** is infused and should be changed with the tubing.

  ▪ A 1.2-μm filter should be used when a total nutrient admixture containing a **lipid emulsion** is infused.

  ▪ When a **single-lumen** catheter is used to deliver CPN, the catheter should not be used to infuse other solutions or medications (with the exception of compatible antibiotics) and it should not be used to monitor central venous pressure.

  ▪ When a **triple-lumen** catheter is used, the distal port should be reserved solely for the administration of CPN.

Refeeding the Severely Malnourished Patient

COMPLICATIONS

Initiating nutritional therapy in patients who are severely malnourished and have had minimal nutrient intake can have adverse clinical consequences and precipitate the refeeding syndrome.

- **Hypophosphatemia, hypokalemia, and hypomagnesemia:** Rapid and marked decreases in these electrolytes occur during initial refeeding because of insulin-stimulated increases in cellular mineral uptake from extracellular fluid. For example, plasma phosphorus concentration can fall below 1 mg/dL and cause death within hours of initiating nutritional therapy if adequate phosphate is not given (*Am J Clin Nutr 1981;34:393*).

- **Fluid overload** and **congestive heart failure** are associated with decreased cardiac function and insulin-induced increased sodium and water reabsorption in conjunction with nutritional therapy containing water, glucose, and sodium. Renal mass may be reduced, limiting the ability to excrete salt or water loads.

- **Cardiac arrhythmias:** Patients who are severely malnourished often have bradycardia. Sudden death from ventricular tachyarrhythmias can occur during the first week of refeeding in severely malnourished patients and may be associated with a prolonged QT interval (*Ann Intern Med 1985;102:49*) or plasma electrolyte abnormalities. Patients with electrocardiogram (ECG) changes should be monitored on telemetry, possibly in an ICU.

- **Glucose intolerance:** Starvation causes insulin resistance such that refeeding with high-carbohydrate meals or large amounts of parenteral glucose can cause marked

Table 2-7	Major Mineral Daily Requirements, Deficiency, Toxicity, and Diagnostic Evaluation			
Mineral	Recommended Daily Enteral[1] Intake/ Parenteral[2] Intake	Signs and Symptoms of Deficiency	Signs and Symptoms of Toxicity	Diagnostic Evaluation
Sodium	1.2–1.5 g[3,5]/ **1–2 mEq/kg**	Encephalopathy, seizure, weakness, dehydration, cerebral edema	Encephalopathy, seizure	Sodium$_p$ (correct for hyperglycemia) Sodium$_u$ (will often only provide a rough estimate [i.e., too low, too high])
Potassium	4,700 mg[4,5]/ **1–2 mEq/kg**	Abdominal cramping; diarrhea, paresthesias, QT prolongation, weakness	QRS widening, QT shortening (sin wave morphology in extreme cases), peaked T waves	Potassium$_{w,b}$
Calcium	1,000–1,200 mg/ **10–15 mEq**	QRS widening, paresthesias (Trousseau's sign), tetany (Chvostek's sign), osteomalacia	Encephalopathy, headache, abdominal pain, nephrolithiasis, metastatic calcification	Calcium$_{w,b}$, 24-hour Calcium$_u$ (correct for albumin$_s$)

(continued)

Table 2-7   Major Mineral Daily Requirements, Deficiency, Toxicity, and Diagnostic Evaluation (Continued)

Mineral	Recommended Daily Enteral[1] Intake/ Parenteral[2] Intake	Signs and Symptoms of Deficiency	Signs and Symptoms of Toxicity	Diagnostic Evaluation
Magnesium	420 mg/ **8–20 mEq**	Tachyarrhythmia, weakness, muscle cramping, peripheral and central nervous system overstimulation (seizure, tetany)	Hyporeflexia, nausea, vomiting, weakness, encephalopathy, decreased respiratory drive, hypocalcemia, hyperkalemia, heart block	Magnesium$_s$, Magnesium$_u$
Phosphorus	700 mg/ **20–40 mMol**	Weakness, fatigue, increased cell membrane fragility (hemolytic anemias, leukocyte + platelet dysfunction), encephalopathy	Metastatic calcification, theoretic higher risk of nephrolithiasis, secondary hyperparathyroidism	Phosphorus$_p$

b, blood; p, plasma; s, serum; u, urine; w, whole blood.

[1]Trumbo P, Yates AA, Schlicker S, et al. Institute of Medicine, Food and Nutrition Board. Dietary reference intakes for vitamin A, vitamin K, arsenic, boron, chromium, copper, iodine, iron, manganese, molybdenum, nickel, silicon, vanadium, and zinc. *J Am Diet Assoc.* 2001;101(3):294–301.

[2]Mirtallo J, Canada T, Johnson D, et al. Safe practices for parenteral nutrition. *JPEN J Parenter Enteral Nutr.* 2004;28: S39–S74.

[3]Higdon J, Drake V, Obarzanek E. Micronutrient Information Center: sodium (chloride). Linus Pauling Institute: Micronutrient Research for Optimum Health. http://lpi.oregonstate.edu/infocenter/minerals/sodium/. Accessed March 10–27, 2012.

[4]Higdon J, Drake V, Pao-Hwa L. Micronutrient Information Center: potassium. Linus Pauling Institute: Micronutrient Research for Optimum Health. http://lpi.oregonstate.edu/infocenter/minerals/potassium/. Accessed March 10–27, 2012.

[5]*Note: Adequate daily intake.*

elevations in blood glucose concentration, glycosuria, dehydration, and hyperosmolar coma. In addition, carbohydrate refeeding in patients who are depleted in thiamine can precipitate Wernicke's encephalopathy.

- **Recommendations**
- Careful **evaluation** of cardiovascular function and plasma electrolytes (history, physical examination, ECG, and blood tests) and correction of abnormal plasma electrolytes are **important before initiation of feeding**.
- Refeeding by the oral or enteral route involves the frequent or continuous administration of small amounts of food or an isotonic liquid formula.
- Parenteral supplementation or complete parenteral nutrition may be necessary if the intestine cannot tolerate feeding.
- During initial refeeding, fluid intake should be limited to approximately 800 mL/d plus insensible losses. Adjustments in fluid and sodium intake are needed in patients who have evidence of fluid overload or dehydration.
- Changes in body weight provide a useful guide for evaluating the efficacy of fluid administration. Weight gain greater than 0.25 kg/d or 1.5 kg/wk probably represents fluid accumulation in excess of tissue repletion. Initially approximately 15 kcal/kg, containing approximately 100 g carbohydrate and 1.5 g protein per kilogram of actual body weight, should be given daily.
- The rate at which the caloric intake can be increased depends on the severity of the malnutrition and the tolerance to feeding. In general, increases of 2 to 4 kcal/kg every 24 to 48 hours are appropriate.
- Sodium should be restricted to approximately 60 mEq or 1.5 g/d, but liberal amounts of phosphorus, potassium, and magnesium should be given to patients who have normal renal function.
- All other nutrients should be given in amounts needed to meet the recommended dietary intake (Table 2-7).
- Body weight, fluid intake, urine output, plasma glucose, and electrolyte values should be **monitored daily** during early refeeding (first 3 to 7 days) so that nutritional therapy can be appropriately modified when necessary.

Preventive Cardiology

Angela L. Brown, Timothy J. Fendler, and
Anne C. Goldberg

Hypertension

GENERAL PRINCIPLES

Definition

Hypertension is defined as the presence of a blood pressure (BP) elevation to a level
that places patients at increased risk for target organ damage in several vascular beds
including the retina, brain, heart, kidneys, and large conduit arteries (Table 3-1).

Classification

- **Normal BP** is defined as systolic blood pressure (SBP) <120 mm Hg and diastolic
  blood pressure (DBP) <80 mm Hg; pharmacologic intervention is not indicated.
- **Prehypertension** is defined as SBP 120 to 139 mm Hg or DBP 80 to 89 mm Hg.
  These patients should engage in comprehensive lifestyle modifications to delay
  progression or prevent the development of hypertension. Pharmacologic therapy
  should be initiated in prehypertensive patients with evidence of target organ damage
  or diabetes.
- **In stage 1** (SBP 140 to 159 mm Hg or DBP 90 to 99 mm Hg) **and stage 2**
  (SBP >160 mm Hg or DBP >100 mm Hg) **hypertension**, pharmacologic therapy
  should be initiated in addition to lifestyle modification to lower BP below
  140/90 mm Hg in patients without diabetes or chronic kidney disease. In patients
  with diabetes or chronic kidney disease, BP should be lowered below 130/80 mm Hg.
  Patients with BP levels more than 20/10 mm Hg above their treatment target will
  often require more than one medication to achieve adequate control, and a two-
  drug regimen may be initiated as initial therapy. Patients with an average BP of
  200/120 mm Hg or greater require immediate therapy and, if symptomatic end-
  organ damage is present, hospitalization.
- **Hypertensive crisis** includes hypertensive emergencies and urgencies. It usually
  develops in patients with a previous history of elevated BP but may arise in those
  who were previously normotensive. The severity of a hypertensive crisis correlates
  not only with the absolute level of BP elevation but also with the rapidity of
  development because autoregulatory mechanisms have not had sufficient time
  to adapt.
- **Hypertensive urgencies** are defined as a substantial increase in BP, usually with
  a DBP >120 mm Hg, and occur in approximately 1% of hypertensive patients.
  Hypertensive urgencies (i.e., upper levels of stage 2 hypertension, hypertension
  with optic disk edema, progressive end-organ complications rather than damage,
  and severe perioperative hypertension) warrant BP reduction within several hours
  (*JAMA 2003;289:2560*).
- **Hypertensive emergencies** include **accelerated hypertension**, typically defined
  as an SBP >210 mm Hg and DBP >130 mm Hg presenting with headaches,

Table 3-1	Manifestations of Target Organ Disease
Organ System	**Manifestations**
Large vessels	Aneurysmal dilation Accelerated atherosclerosis Aortic dissection
Cardiac	
Acute	Pulmonary edema, myocardial infarction
Chronic	Clinical or ECG evidence of CAD; LVH by ECG or echocardiogram
Cerebrovascular	
Acute	Intracerebral bleeding, coma, seizures, mental status changes, TIA, stroke
Chronic	TIA, stroke
Renal	
Acute	Hematuria, azotemia
Chronic	Serum creatinine >1.5 mg/dL, proteinuria >1+ on dipstick
Retinopathy	
Acute	Papilledema, hemorrhages
Chronic	Hemorrhages, exudates, arterial nicking

CAD, coronary artery disease; ECG, electrocardiogram; LVH, left ventricular hypertrophy; TIA, transient ischemic attack.

blurred vision, or focal neurologic symptoms and **malignant hypertension** (which requires the presence of papilledema). Hypertensive emergencies require immediate BP reduction by 20% to 25% to prevent or minimize end-organ damage (i.e., hypertensive encephalopathy, intracranial hemorrhage, unstable angina [UA] pectoris, acute myocardial infarction [MI], acute left ventricular failure with pulmonary edema, dissecting aortic aneurysm, progressive renal failure, or eclampsia).

- **Isolated systolic hypertension**, defined as an SBP >140 mm Hg and normal DBP, occurs frequently in the elderly (beginning after the fifth decade and increasing with age). Nonpharmacologic therapy should be initiated with medications added as needed to lower SBP to <140 mm Hg. Patient tolerance of antihypertensive therapy should be assessed frequently.

Epidemiology

- The public health burden of hypertension is enormous, affecting an estimated 68 million American adults (*MMWR Feb 2011;60*). Indeed, for nonhypertensive individuals aged 55 to 65 years, the lifetime risk of developing hypertension is 90% (*JAMA 2002;287:1003*).
- Data derived from the Framingham study have shown that hypertensive patients have a fourfold increase in cerebrovascular accidents as well as a sixfold increase in congestive heart failure (CHF) when compared to normotensive control subjects.
- Disease-associated morbidity and mortality, including atherosclerotic cardiovascular disease, stroke, heart failure (HF), and renal insufficiency, increase with higher levels of SBP and DBP.

- Over the past three decades, aggressive treatment of hypertension has resulted in a substantial decrease in death rates from stroke and coronary heart disease (CHD). Unfortunately, rates of end-stage renal disease (ESRD) and hospitalization for CHF have continued to increase. BP control rates have improved but remain poor with only 50.1% of treated hypertensive patients below their goal BP level (*JAMA 2010;303:2043*).

Etiology

Of all hypertensive patients, more than 90% have primary or essential hypertension; the remainder have secondary hypertension due to causes such as renal parenchymal disease, renovascular disease, pheochromocytoma, Cushing's syndrome, primary hyperaldosteronism, coarctation of the aorta, obstructive sleep apnea, and uncommon autosomal dominant or autosomal recessive diseases of the adrenal–renal axis that result in salt retention.

Risk Factors

BP rises with age. Other contributing factors include overweight/obesity, increased dietary sodium intake, decreased physical activity, increased alcohol consumption, and lower dietary intake of fruits, vegetables, and potassium.

Prevention

Prevention should be focused on risk factor modification. Strategies must address cultural and social barriers related to health care delivery and behavioral modification.

DIAGNOSIS

Clinical Presentation

- BP elevation is usually discovered in asymptomatic individuals during routine health visits.
- Optimal detection and evaluation of hypertension requires accurate noninvasive BP measurement, which should be obtained in a seated patient with the arm resting level with the heart. A calibrated, appropriately fitting BP cuff (inflatable bladder encircling at least 80% of the arm) should be used because falsely high readings can be obtained if the cuff is too small.
- Two readings should be taken, separated by 2 minutes. SBP should be noted with the appearance of Korotkoff sounds (phase I) and DBP with the disappearance of sounds (phase V).
- In certain patients, the Korotkoff sounds do not disappear but are present to 0 mm Hg. In this case, the initial muffling of Korotkoff sounds (phase IV) should be taken as the DBP. One should be careful to avoid reporting spuriously low BP readings due to an auscultatory gap, which is caused by the disappearance and reappearance of Korotkoff sounds in hypertensive patients and may account for up to a 25-mm Hg gap between true and measured SBP. Hypertension should be confirmed in both arms, and the higher reading should be used.

History
- The history should seek to discover secondary causes of hypertension and note the presence of medications and supplements that can affect BP (e.g., decongestants, oral contraceptives, appetite suppressants, cyclosporine, nonsteroidal anti-

inflammatory agents, exogenous thyroid hormone, recent alcohol consumption, caffeine, anabolic steroids, ma huang, and illicit stimulants such as cocaine).
- A diagnosis of secondary hypertension should be considered in the following situations:
  - Age at onset younger than 30 or older than 60 years
  - Hypertension that is difficult to control after therapy has been initiated
  - Stable hypertension that becomes difficult to control
  - Clinical occurrence of a hypertensive crisis
  - The presence of signs or symptoms of a secondary cause such as hypokalemia or metabolic alkalosis that is not explained by diuretic therapy
- In patients who present with significant hypertension at a young age, a careful family history may give clues to forms of hypertension that follow simple Mendelian inheritance.

Physical Examination
The physical examination should include investigation for target organ damage or a secondary cause of hypertension by noting the presence of carotid bruits, an S_3 or S_4, cardiac murmurs, neurologic deficits, elevated jugular venous pressure, rales, retinopathy, unequal pulses, enlarged or small kidneys, cushingoid features, and abdominal bruits. Overweight/obesity should be assessed by measurement of height and weight and/or abdominal waist circumference.

Differential Diagnosis
- Hypertension may be part of several important syndromes of withdrawal from drugs, including alcohol, cocaine, and opioid analgesics. Rebound increases in BP also may be seen in patients who abruptly discontinue antihypertensive therapy, particularly β-adrenergic antagonists and central α_2-agonists (see Complications).
- Cocaine and other sympathomimetic drugs (e.g., amphetamines, phencyclidine hydrochloride) can produce hypertension in the setting of acute intoxication and when the agents are discontinued abruptly after chronic use. Hypertension is often complicated by other end-organ insults, such as ischemic heart disease, stroke, and seizures. Phentolamine is effective in acute management, and sodium nitroprusside or nitroglycerin can be used as an alternative (Table 3-2). β-Adrenergic antagonists should be avoided due to the risk of unopposed α-adrenergic activity, which can exacerbate hypertension.

Diagnostic Testing
Laboratories
Tests are needed to help identify patients with possible target organ damage, to help assess cardiovascular risk, and to provide a baseline for monitoring the adverse effects of therapy:
- Urinalysis
- Hematocrit
- Plasma glucose
- Serum potassium
- Serum creatinine
- Calcium
- Uric acid
- Fasting lipid levels
- Electrocardiogram (ECG)

Table 3-2	Commonly Used Antihypertensive Agents by Functional Class

Drugs by Class	Properties	Initial Dose	Usual Dosage Range (mg)
β-Adrenergic Antagonists			
Atenolol[a,b]	Selective	50 mg PO daily	25–100
Betaxolol	Selective	10 mg PO daily	5–40
Bisoprolol[a]	Selective	5 mg PO daily	2.5–20
Metoprolol	Selective	50 mg PO bid	50–450
Metoprolol XL	Selective	50–100 mg PO daily	50–400
Nebivolol	Selective with vasodilatory properties	5 mg PO daily	5–40
Nadolol[a]	Nonselective	40 mg PO daily	20–240
Propranolol[b]	Nonselective	40 mg PO bid	40–240
Propranolol LA	Nonselective	80 mg PO daily	60–240
Timolol[b]	Nonselective	10 mg PO bid	20–40
Carteolol[a]	ISA	2.5 mg PO daily	2.5–10
Penbutolol	ISA	20 mg PO daily	20–80
Pindolol	ISA	5 mg PO daily	10–60
Labetalol	α- and β-antagonist properties	100 mg PO bid	200–1,200
Carvedilol	α- and β-antagonist properties	6.25 mg PO bid	12.5–50
Acebutolol[a]	ISA, selective	200 mg PO bid, 400 mg PO daily	200–1,200
Calcium Channel Antagonists			
Amlodipine	DHP	5 mg PO daily	2.5–10
Diltiazem		30 mg PO qid	90–360
Diltiazem SR		60–120 mg PO bid	120–360
Diltiazem CD		180 mg PO bid	180–360
Diltiazem XR		80 mg daily	180–480
Isradipine	DHP	2.5 mg PO bid	2.5–10
Nicardipine[b]	DHP	20 mg PO tid	60–120
Nicardipine SR	DHP	30 mg PO bid	60–120
Nifedipine	DHP	10 mg PO tid	30–120
Nifedipine XL (or CC)	DHP	30 mg PO daily	30–90
Nisoldipine	DHP	20 mg PO daily	20–40
Verapamil[b]		80 mg PO tid	80–480
Verapamil COER		80 mg PO daily	180–480
Verapamil SR		120–140 mg PO daily	120–480

(continued)

Table 3-2	Commonly Used Antihypertensive Agents by Functional Class (*Continued*)

Drugs by Class	Properties	Initial Dose	Usual Dosage Range (mg)
Angiotensin-Converting Enzyme Inhibitors			
Benazepril[a]		10 mg PO bid	10–40
Captopril[a]		25 mg PO bid–tid	50–450
Enalapril[a]		5 mg PO daily	2.5–40
Fosinopril		10 mg PO daily	10–40
Lisinopril[a]		10 mg PO daily	5–40
Moexipril		7.5 mg PO daily	7.5–30
Quinapril[a]		10 mg PO daily	5–80
Ramipril[a]		2.5 mg PO daily	1.25–20
Trandolapril		1–2 mg PO daily	1–4
Angiotensin II Receptor Blocker			
Azilsartan		40 mg PO daily	40–80
Candesartan		8 mg PO daily	8–32
Eprosartan		600 mg PO daily	600–800
Irbesartan		150 mg PO daily	150–300
Olmesartan		20 mg PO daily	20–40
Losartan		50 mg PO daily	25–100
Telmisartan		40 mg PO daily	20–80
Valsartan		80 mg PO daily	80–320
Diuretics			
Bendroflumethiazide	Thiazide diuretic	5 mg PO daily	2.5–15
Benzthiazide	Thiazide diuretic	25 mg PO bid	50–100
Chlorothiazide	Thiazide diuretic	500 mg PO daily (or IV)	125–1,000
Chlorthalidone	Thiazide diuretic	25 mg PO daily	12.5–50
Hydrochlorothiazide	Thiazide diuretic	12.5 mg PO daily	12.5–50
Hydroflumethiazide	Thiazide diuretic	50 mg PO daily	50–100
Indapamide	Thiazide diuretic	1.25 mg PO daily	2.5–5.0
Methyclothiazide	Thiazide diuretic	2.5 mg PO daily	2.5–5.0
Metolazone	Thiazide diuretic	2.5 mg PO daily	1.25–5
Polythiazide	Thiazide diuretic	2.0 mg PO daily	1–4
Quinethazone	Thiazide diuretic	50 mg PO daily	25–100
Trichlormethiazide	Thiazide diuretic	2.0 mg PO daily	1–4
Bumetanide	Loop diuretic	0.5 mg PO daily (or IV)	0.5–5

(*continued*)

Table 3-2	Commonly Used Antihypertensive Agents by Functional Class (*Continued*)		

Drugs by Class	Properties	Initial Dose	Usual Dosage Range (mg)
Ethacrynic acid	Loop diuretic	50 mg PO daily (or IV)	25–100
Furosemide	Loop diuretic	20 mg PO daily (or IV)	20–320
Torsemide	Loop diuretic	5 mg PO daily (or IV)	5–10
Amiloride	Potassium-sparing diuretic	5 mg PO daily	5–10
Triamterene	Potassium-sparing diuretic	50 mg PO bid	50–200
Eplerenone	Aldosterone antagonist	25 mg PO daily	25–100
Spironolactone	Aldosterone antagonist	25 mg PO daily	25–100
α-Adrenergic Antagonists			
Doxazosin		1 mg PO daily	1–16
Prazosin		1 mg PO bid–tid	1–20
Terazosin		1 mg PO at bedtime	1–20
Centrally Acting Adrenergic Agents			
Clonidine[b]		0.1 mg PO bid	0.1–1.2
Clonidine patch		TTS 1/wk (equivalent to 0.1 mg/d release)	0.1–0.3
Guanfacine		1 mg PO daily	1–3
Guanabenz		4 mg PO bid	4–64
Methyldopa[b]		250 mg PO bid–tid	250–2,000
Direct-Acting Vasodilators			
Hydralazine		10 mg PO qid	50–300
Minoxidil		5 mg PO daily	2.5–100
Miscellaneous			
Reserpine[b]		0.5 mg PO daily	0.01–0.25

[a]Adjusted in renal failure.
[b]Available in generic form.
DHP, dihydropyridine; ISA, intrinsic sympathomimetic activity; IV, intravenous; TTS, transdermal therapeutic system.

- Chest radiography
- Echocardiography may be of value for certain patients to assess cardiac function or detection of left ventricular hypertrophy (LVH)

TREATMENT

Medications

- **Initial drug therapy.** Data from the ALLHAT trial have shown decreased cardiovascular and cerebrovascular morbidity and mortality with the use of thiazide diuretics (*JAMA 2002;288:2981*); thus, this class of drug is favored as first-line therapy unless there is a contraindication to their use or the characteristics of a patient's profile (concomitant disease, age, race) mandate the institution of a different agent. Calcium channel antagonists and angiotensin-converting enzyme (ACE) inhibitors have a low side-effect profile and have been shown to decrease BP to degrees similar to those observed with diuretics and β-adrenergic antagonists. In ALLHAT, reductions in morbidity and mortality were similar to diuretics, making them reasonable initial agents. In patients with stage 2 hypertension, therapy may be initiated with a two-drug combination, typically a thiazide diuretic plus a calcium antagonist, ACE inhibitor, angiotensin receptor blocker (ARB), or β-adrenergic antagonists. Initial drug choice may be affected by coexistent factors such as age, race, angina, HF, renal insufficiency, LVH, obesity, hyperlipidemia, gout, and bronchospasm. Cost and drug interactions should also be considered. The BP response is usually consistent within a given class of agents; therefore, if a drug fails to control BP, another agent from the same class is unlikely to be effective. At times, however, a change within drug class may be useful in reducing adverse effects. The lowest possible effective dosage should be used to control BP, adjusted every 1 to 2 months as needed.
- **Additional therapy.** When a second drug is needed, it should generally be chosen from among the other first-line agents. A diuretic should be added first, as doing so may enhance effectiveness of the first drug, yielding more than a simple additive effect.
- **Adjustments of a therapeutic regimen.** In considering a modification of therapy because of inadequate response to the current regimen, the physician should investigate other possible contributing factors. Poor patient compliance, use of antagonistic drugs (i.e., sympathomimetics, antidepressants, steroids, nonsteroidal anti-inflammatory drugs [NSAIDs], cyclosporine, caffeine, thyroid hormones, cocaine, erythropoietin), inappropriately high sodium intake, or increased alcohol consumption should be considered before antihypertensive drug therapy is modified. Secondary causes of hypertension must be considered when a previously effective regimen becomes inadequate and other confounding factors are absent.
- **Diuretics** (see Table 3-2) are effective agents in the therapy of hypertension, and data have accumulated to demonstrate their safety and benefit in reducing the incidence of stroke and cardiovascular events.
  - ○ **Several classes of diuretics** are available, generally categorized by their site of action in the kidney. Thiazide and thiazide-like diuretics (e.g., hydrochlorothiazide, chlorthalidone) block sodium reabsorption predominantly in the distal convoluted tubule by inhibition of the thiazide-sensitive Na/Cl cotransporter. Loop diuretics (e.g., furosemide, bumetanide, ethacrynic acid, and torsemide) block sodium reabsorption in the thick ascending loop of Henle through inhibi-

tion of the Na/K/2Cl cotransporter and are the most effective agents in patients with renal insufficiency (estimated glomerular filtration rate [eGFR] <35 mL/min/1.73 m²). Spironolactone and eplerenone, potassium-sparing agents, act by competitively inhibiting the actions of aldosterone on the kidney. Triamterene and amiloride are potassium-sparing drugs that inhibit the epithelial Na⁺ channel in the distal nephron to inhibit reabsorption of Na⁺ and secretion of potassium ions. Potassium-sparing diuretics are weak agents when used alone; thus, they are often combined with a thiazide for added potency. Aldosterone antagonists may have an additional benefit in improving myocardial function in HF; this effect may be independent of its effect on renal transport mechanisms.

○ **Side effects** of diuretics vary by class. Thiazide diuretics can produce weakness, muscle cramps, and impotence. Metabolic side effects include hypokalemia, hypomagnesemia, hyperlipidemia (with increases in low-density lipoproteins [LDLs] and triglyceride levels), hypercalcemia, hyperglycemia, hyperuricemia, hyponatremia, and rarely, azotemia. Thiazide-induced pancreatitis has also been reported. Metabolic side effects may be limited when thiazides are used in low doses (e.g., hydrochlorothiazide, 12.5 to 25.0 mg/d). Loop diuretics can cause electrolyte abnormalities such as hypomagnesemia, hypocalcemia, and hypokalemia and can also produce irreversible ototoxicity (usually dose related and more common with parenteral therapy). Spironolactone and eplerenone can produce hyperkalemia; however, the gynecomastia that may occur in men and breast tenderness in women are not seen with eplerenone. Triamterene (usually in combination with hydrochlorothiazide) can cause renal tubular damage and renal calculi. Unlike thiazides, potassium-sparing and loop diuretics do not cause adverse lipid effects.

• **β-Adrenergic antagonists** (see Table 3-2) are effective antihypertensive agents and are part of medical regimens that have been proven to decrease the incidence of stroke, MI, and HF.

○ The **mechanism of action** of β-adrenergic antagonists is competitive inhibition of the effects of catecholamines at β-adrenergic receptors, which decreases heart rate and cardiac output. These agents also decrease plasma renin and cause a resetting of baroreceptors to accept a lower level of BP. β-Adrenergic antagonists cause release of vasodilatory prostaglandins, decrease plasma volume, and may also have a central nervous system (CNS)–mediated antihypertensive effect.

○ **Classes of β-adrenergic antagonists** can be subdivided into those that are cardioselective, with primarily β₁-blocking effects, and those that are nonselective, with β₁- and β₂-blocking effects. At low doses, the cardioselective agents can be given with caution to patients with mild chronic obstructive pulmonary disease, diabetes mellitus (DM), or peripheral vascular disease. At higher doses, these agents lose their β₁ selectivity and may cause unwanted effects in these patients. β-Adrenergic antagonists can also be categorized according to the presence or absence of partial agonist or intrinsic sympathomimetic activity (ISA). β-Adrenergic antagonists with ISA cause less bradycardia than do those without it. In addition, there are agents with mixed properties having both α- and β-adrenergic antagonist actions (labetalol and carvedilol). Nebivolol is a highly selective β-adrenergic antagonist that is vasodilatory through an unclear mechanism.

○ **Side effects** include high-degree atrioventricular (AV) block, HF, Raynaud's phenomenon, and impotence. Lipophilic β-adrenergic antagonists, such as propranolol, have a higher incidence of CNS side effects including insomnia and depression. Propranolol can also cause nasal congestion. β-Adrenergic antagonists can cause adverse effects on the lipid profile; increased triglyceride and decreased high-density lipoprotein (HDL) levels occur mainly with nonselective β-adrenergic antagonists but generally do not occur when β-adrenergic antagonists with ISA are used. Pindolol, a selective β-adrenergic antagonist with ISA, may actually increase HDL and nominally increase triglycerides. Side effects of labetalol include hepatocellular damage, postural hypotension, a positive antinuclear antibody (ANA) test, a lupus-like syndrome, tremors, and potential hypotension in the setting of halothane anesthesia. Carvedilol appears to have a similar side-effect profile to other β-adrenergic antagonists. Both labetalol and carvedilol have negligible effects on lipids. Rarely, reflex tachycardia may occur because of the initial vasodilatory effect of labetalol and carvedilol. Because β-receptor density is increased with chronic antagonism, abrupt withdrawal of these agents can precipitate angina pectoris, increases in BP, and other effects attributable to an increase in adrenergic tone.

- **Selective α-adrenergic antagonists** such as prazosin, terazosin, and doxazosin have replaced nonselective α-adrenergic antagonists such as phenoxybenzamine (see Table 3-2) in the treatment of essential hypertension. Based on the ALLHAT trial, these drugs appear to be less efficacious than diuretics, calcium channel blockers, and ACE inhibitors in reducing primary end points of cardiovascular disease when used as monotherapy (*JAMA 2002;283:1967*; *JAMA 2002; 288:2981*).
  - **Side effects** of these agents include a "first-dose effect," which results from a greater decrease in BP with the first dose than with subsequent doses. Selective α_1-adrenergic antagonists can cause syncope, orthostatic hypotension, dizziness, headache, and drowsiness. In most cases, side effects are self-limited and do not recur with continued therapy. Selective α_1-adrenergic antagonists may improve lipid profiles by decreasing total cholesterol and triglyceride levels and increasing HDL levels. Additionally, these agents can improve the negative effects on lipids induced by thiazide diuretics and β-adrenergic antagonists. Doxazosin specifically may be less effective at lowering SBP than thiazide diuretics and may additionally be associated with a higher risk of cardiovascular disease, particularly HF and stroke in patients with hypertension, and at least one additional risk factor for coronary artery disease (CAD) (*JAMA 2002;283:1967*).
- **Centrally acting adrenergic agents** (see Table 3-2) are potent antihypertensive agents. In addition to its oral dosage forms, clonidine is available as a transdermal patch that is applied weekly.
  - **Side effects** may include bradycardia, drowsiness, dry mouth, orthostatic hypotension, galactorrhea, and sexual dysfunction. Transdermal clonidine causes a rash in up to 20% of patients. These agents can precipitate HF in patients with decreased left ventricular function, and abrupt cessation can precipitate an acute withdrawal syndrome (AWS) of elevated BP, tachycardia, and diaphoresis (see Complications). Methyldopa produces a positive direct antibody (Coombs) test in up to 25% of patients, but significant hemolytic anemia is much less common. If hemolytic anemia develops secondary to methyldopa, the drug should be withdrawn. Severe cases of hemolytic anemia may require treatment with glucocorticoids. Methyldopa also causes positive ANA test results in approximately 10% of patients and can cause an inflammatory reaction in the liver that is indistinguishable from viral hepatitis; fatal hepatitis has been reported. Guanabenz and guanfa-

cine decrease total cholesterol levels, and guanfacine can also decrease serum triglyceride levels.

- **Reserpine, guanethidine, and guanadrel** (see Table 3-2) were among the first effective antihypertensive agents available. Currently, these drugs are not regarded as first- or second-line therapy because of their significant side effects.
  - ○ **Side effects** of reserpine include severe depression in approximately 2% of patients. Sedation and nasal stuffiness also are potential side effects. Guanethidine can cause severe postural hypotension through a decrease in cardiac output, a decrease in peripheral resistance, and venous pooling in the extremities. Patients who are receiving guanethidine with orthostatic hypotension should be cautioned to arise slowly and to wear support hose. Guanethidine can also cause ejaculatory failure and diarrhea.
- **Calcium channel antagonists** (see Table 3-2) are effective agents in the treatment of hypertension. Generally, they have no significant CNS side effects and can be used to treat diseases, such as angina pectoris, that can coexist with hypertension. **Due to the concern that the use of short-acting dihydropyridine calcium channel antagonists may increase the number of ischemic cardiac events, they are not indicated for hypertension management** (*JAMA 1995;274:620*); long-acting agents are considered safe in the management of hypertension (*Am J Cardiol 1996;77:81*).
  - ○ **Classes of calcium channel antagonists** include diphenylalkylamines (e.g., verapamil), benzothiazepines (e.g., diltiazem), and dihydropyridines (e.g., nifedipine). The dihydropyridines include many newer second-generation drugs (e.g., amlodipine, felodipine, isradipine, and nicardipine), which are more vasoselective and have longer plasma half-lives than nifedipine. Verapamil and diltiazem have negative cardiac inotropic and chronotropic effects. Nifedipine also has a negative inotropic effect, but in clinical use, this effect is much less pronounced than that of verapamil or diltiazem because of peripheral vasodilation and reflex tachycardia. Less negative inotropic effects have been observed with the second-generation dihydropyridines. All calcium channel antagonists are metabolized in the liver; thus in patients with cirrhosis, the dosing interval should be adjusted accordingly. Some of these drugs also inhibit the metabolism of other hepatically cleared medications (e.g., cyclosporine). Verapamil and diltiazem should be used with caution in patients with cardiac conduction abnormalities as they can worsen HF in patients with decreased left ventricular function.
  - ○ **Side effects** of verapamil include constipation, nausea, headache, and orthostatic hypotension. Diltiazem can cause nausea, headache, and rash. Dihydropyridines can cause lower extremity edema, flushing, headache, and rash. Calcium channel antagonists have no significant effects on glucose tolerance, electrolytes, or lipid profiles. In general, calcium channel antagonists should not be initiated in patients immediately after MI because of increased mortality in all but the most stable patients without evidence of HF.
- **Inhibitors of the renin–angiotensin system** (see Table 3-2) are effective antihypertensive agents in a broad array of patients.
  - ○ **ACE inhibitors** may have beneficial effects in patients with concomitant HF or kidney disease. One study has also suggested that ACE inhibitors (ramipril) may significantly reduce the rate of death, MI, and stroke in patients without HF or low ejection fraction (*N Engl J Med 2000;342:145*). Additionally, they can reduce hypokalemia, hypercholesterolemia, hyperglycemia, and hyperuricemia

caused by diuretic therapy and are particularly effective in states of hypertension associated with a high renin state (e.g., scleroderma renal crisis).

○ **Side effects** associated with the use of ACE inhibitors are infrequent. They can cause a dry cough (up to 20% of patients), angioneurotic edema, and hypotension, but they do not cause levels of lipids, glucose, or uric acid to increase. ACE inhibitors that contain a sulfhydryl group (e.g., captopril) may cause taste disturbance, leukopenia, and a glomerulopathy with proteinuria. Because ACE inhibitors cause preferential vasodilation of the efferent arteriole in the kidney, worsening of renal function may occur in patients who have decreased renal perfusion or who have preexisting severe renal insufficiency. ACE inhibitors can cause hyperkalemia and should be used with caution in patients with a decreased GFR who are taking potassium supplements or who are receiving potassium-sparing diuretics.

- **ARBs** are a class of antihypertensive drugs that are effective in diverse patient populations (*N Engl J Med 1996;334:1649*). Several of these agents are now approved for the management of mild-to-moderate hypertension (see Table 3-2). Additionally, ARBs may be useful alternatives in patients with HF who are unable to tolerate ACE inhibitors (*N Engl J Med 2001;345:1667*). **Side effects** of ARBs occur rarely but include angioedema, allergic reaction, and rash.

- **Direct renin inhibitor (DRI)** class consists of one agent, aliskiren, that is indicated solely for the treatment of hypertension. It may be used in combination with other antihypertensive agents; however, combined use with ACE inhibitors or ARBs is contraindicated in patients with diabetes. (*FDA Drug Safety Communication, April 2012*).

- **Direct-acting vasodilators** are potent antihypertensive agents (see Table 3-2) now reserved for refractory hypertension or specific circumstances such as the use of hydralazine in pregnancy. Hydralazine in combination with nitrates is useful in treating patients with hypertension and HF (see Chapter 5, Heart Failure and Cardiomyopathy). **Side effects** of hydralazine therapy may include headache, nausea, emesis, tachycardia, and postural hypotension. Asymptomatic patients may have a positive ANA test result, and a hydralazine-induced systemic lupus-like syndrome may develop in approximately 10% of patients. Patients who may be at increased risk for this latter complication include those treated with excessive doses (e.g., >400 mg/d), those with impaired renal or cardiac function, and those with the slow acetylation phenotype. Hydralazine should be discontinued if clinical evidence of a lupus-like syndrome develops and a positive ANA test result is present. The syndrome usually resolves with discontinuation of the drug, leaving no adverse long-term effects. **Side effects** of minoxidil include weight gain, hypertrichosis, hirsutism, ECG abnormalities, and pericardial effusions.

- **Parenteral antihypertensive agents** are indicated for the immediate reduction of BP in patients with hypertensive emergencies. Judicious administration of these agents (Table 3-3) may also be appropriate in patients with hypertension complicated by HF or MI. These drugs are also indicated for individuals who have perioperative hypertensive urgency or are in need of emergency surgery. If possible, an accurate baseline BP should be determined before the initiation of therapy. In the setting of hypertensive emergency, the patient should be admitted to an intensive care unit (ICU) for close monitoring, and an intra-arterial monitor should be used when available. Although parenteral agents are indicated as a first line in hypertensive emergencies, oral agents may also be effective in this group; the choice of drug

Table 3-3 Parental Antihypertensive Drug Preparations

Drug	Administration	Onset	Duration of Action	Dosage	Adverse Effects and Comments
Fenoldopam	IV infusion	<5 min	30 min	0.1–0.3 mcg/kg/min	Tachycardia, nausea, vomiting
Sodium nitroprusside	IV infusion	Immediate	2–3 min	0.5–10 mcg/kg/min (initial dose, 0.25 mcg/kg/min for eclampsia and renal insufficiency)	Hypotension, nausea, vomiting, apprehension. Risk of thiocyanate and cyanide toxicity is increased in renal and hepatic insufficiency, respectively; levels should be monitored; must shield from light
Diazoxide	IV bolus	15 min	6–12 hr	50–100 mg q5–10min, up to 600 mg	Hypotension, tachycardia, nausea, vomiting, fluid retention, hyperglycemia; may exacerbate myocardial ischemia, heart failure, or aortic dissection
Labetalol	IV bolus	5–10 min	3–6 hr	20–80 mg q5–10min, up to 300 mg	Hypotension, heart block, heart failure, bronchospasm, nausea, vomiting, scalp tingling, paradoxical pressor response; may not be effective in patients receiving α- or β-antagonists
	IV infusion			0.5–2 mg/min	

Drug	Route	Onset	Duration	Dose	Adverse effects
Nitroglycerin	IV infusion	1–2 min	3–5 min	5–250 mcg/min	Headache, nausea, vomiting. Tolerance may develop with prolonged use.
Esmolol	IV bolus	1–5 min	10 min	500 mcg/kg/min for first 1 min / 50–300 mcg/kg/min	Hypotension, heart block, heart failure, bronchospasm
Phentolamine	IV infusion / IV bolus	1–2 min	3–10 min	5–10 mg q5–15min	Hypotension, tachycardia, headache, angina, paradoxical pressor response
Hydralazine (for treatment of eclampsia)	IV bolus	10–20 min	3–6 hr	10–20 mg q20min (if no effect after 20 mg, try another agent)	Hypotension, fetal distress, tachycardia, headache, nausea, vomiting, local thrombophlebitis. Infusion site should be changed after 12 hr
Methyldopa (for treatment of eclampsia)	IV bolus	30–60 min	10–16 hr	250–500 mg	Hypotension
Nicardipine	IV infusion	1–5 min	3–6 hr	5 mg/hr, increased by 1.0–2.5 mg/hr q15min, up to 15 mg/hr	Hypotension, headache, tachycardia, nausea, vomiting
Enalaprilat	IV bolus	5–15 min	1–6 hr	0.6255 mg q6h	Hypotension

IV, intravenous.

and route of administration must be individualized. If parenteral agents are used initially, oral medications should be administered shortly thereafter to facilitate rapid weaning from parenteral therapy.

○ **Sodium nitroprusside**, a direct-acting arterial and venous vasodilator, is the drug of choice for most hypertensive emergencies (see Table 3-3). It reduces BP rapidly and is easily titratable, and its action is short lived when discontinued. Patients should be monitored very closely to avoid an exaggerated hypotensive response. Therapy for more than 48 to 72 hours with a high cumulative dose or renal insufficiency may cause accumulation of thiocyanate, a toxic metabolite. Thiocyanate toxicity may cause paresthesias, tinnitus, blurred vision, delirium, or seizures. Serum thiocyanate levels should be kept at <10 mg/dL. Patients on high doses (>2 to 3 mg/kg/min) or those with renal dysfunction should have serum levels of thiocyanate drawn after 48 to 72 hours of therapy. In patients with normal renal function or those receiving lower doses, levels can be drawn after 5 to 7 days. Hepatic dysfunction may result in accumulation of cyanide, which can cause metabolic acidosis, dyspnea, vomiting, dizziness, ataxia, and syncope. Hemodialysis should be considered for thiocyanate poisoning. Nitrites and thiosulfate can be administered intravenously for cyanide poisoning.

○ **Nitroglycerin** given as a continuous intravenous (IV) infusion (see Table 3-3) may be appropriate in situations in which sodium nitroprusside is relatively contraindicated, such as in patients with severe coronary insufficiency or advanced renal or hepatic disease. It is the preferred agent for patients with moderate hypertension in the setting of acute coronary ischemia or after coronary artery bypass surgery because of its more favorable effects on pulmonary gas exchange and collateral coronary blood flow. In patients with severely elevated BP, sodium nitroprusside remains the agent of choice. Nitroglycerin reduces preload more than afterload and should be used with caution or avoided in patients who have inferior MI with right ventricular infarction and are dependent on preload to maintain cardiac output.

○ **Labetalol** can be administered parenterally (see Table 3-3) in hypertensive crisis, even in patients in the early phase of an acute MI, and is the drug of choice in hypertensive emergencies that occur during pregnancy. When given intravenously, the β-adrenergic antagonist effect is greater than the α-adrenergic antagonist effect. Nevertheless, symptomatic postural hypotension may occur with IV use; thus, patients should be treated in a supine position. Labetalol may be particularly beneficial during adrenergic excess (e.g., clonidine withdrawal, pheochromocytoma, post–coronary bypass grafting). As the half-life of labetalol is 5 to 8 hours, intermittent IV bolus dosing may be preferable to IV infusion. IV infusion can be discontinued before oral labetalol is begun. When the supine DBP begins to rise, oral dosing can be initiated at 200 mg PO, followed in 6 to 12 hours by 200 to 400 mg PO, depending on the BP response.

○ **Esmolol** is a parenteral, short-acting, cardioselective β-adrenergic antagonist (see Table 3-3) that can be used in the treatment of hypertensive emergencies in patients in whom β-blocker intolerance is a concern. Esmolol is also useful for the treatment of aortic dissection. β-Adrenergic antagonists may be ineffective when used as monotherapy in the treatment of severe hypertension and are frequently combined with other agents (e.g., with sodium nitroprusside in the treatment of aortic dissection).

○ **Nicardipine** is an effective IV calcium antagonist preparation (see Table 3-3) approved for use in postoperative hypertension. Side effects include headache, flushing, reflex tachycardia, and venous irritation. Nicardipine should be administered via a central venous line. If it is given peripherally, the IV site should be changed q12h. Fifty percent of the peak effect is seen within the first 30 minutes, but the full peak effect is not achieved until after 48 hours of administration.

○ **Enalaprilat** is the active de-esterified form of enalapril (see Table 3-3) that results from hepatic conversion after an oral dose. Enalaprilat (as well as other ACE inhibitors) has been used effectively in cases of severe and malignant hypertension. However, variable and unpredictable results have also been reported. ACE inhibition can cause rapid BP reduction in hypertensive patients with high renin states such as renovascular hypertension, concomitant use of vasodilators, and scleroderma renal crisis; thus, Enalaprilat should be used cautiously to avoid precipitating hypotension. Therapy can be changed to an oral preparation when IV therapy is no longer necessary.

○ **Diazoxide and hydralazine** are only rarely used in hypertensive crises and offer little or no advantage to the agents discussed previously. It should be noted, however, that hydralazine is a useful agent in pregnancy-related hypertensive emergencies because of its established safety profile.

○ **Fenoldopam** is a selective agonist to peripheral dopamine-1 receptors, and it produces vasodilation, increases renal perfusion, and enhances natriuresis. Fenoldopam has a short duration of action; the elimination half-life is <10 minutes. The drug has important application as parental therapy for high-risk hypertensive surgical patients and the perioperative management of patients undergoing organ transplantation.

• **Oral loading of antihypertensive agents** has been used successfully in patients with hypertensive crisis when urgent but not immediate reduction of BP is indicated.

○ **Oral clonidine loading** is achieved by using an initial dose of 0.2 mg PO followed by 0.1 mg PO q1h to a total dose of 0.7 mg or a reduction in diastolic pressure of 20 mm Hg or more. BP should be checked at 15-minute intervals over the first hour, 30-minute intervals over the second hour, and then hourly. After 6 hours, a diuretic can be added, and an 8-hour clonidine dosing interval can be begun. Sedative side effects are significant.

○ Sublingual nifedipine has an onset of action within 30 minutes but can produce wide fluctuations and excessive reductions in BP. Because of the potential for adverse cardiovascular events (stroke/MI), sublingual nifedipine should be avoided in the acute management of elevated BP. Side effects include facial flushing and postural hypotension.

Lifestyle/Risk Modification

Lifestyle modifications should be encouraged in all hypertensive patients regardless of whether they require medication. These changes may have beneficial effects on other cardiovascular risk factors. Some of these lifestyle modifications include cessation of smoking, reduction in body weight if the patient is overweight, judicious consumption of alcohol, adequate nutritional intake of minerals and vitamins, reduction in sodium intake, and increased physical activity.

General considerations and goals. The goal of treatment for hypertension is to prevent long-term sequelae (i.e., target organ damage). Barring an overt need for immediate pharmacologic therapy, most patients should be given the opportunity to achieve a reduction in BP over an interval of 3 to 6 months by applying nonpharmacologic modifications and pharmacologic therapies if needed. The primary goal is to reduce BP to <140/90 mm Hg while concurrently controlling other modifiable cardiovascular risk factors. As isolated systolic hypertension is also associated with increased cerebrovascular and cardiac events, the therapeutic goal in this subset of patients should be to lower BP to <140 mm Hg systolic. Treatment should be more aggressive in patients with chronic kidney disease or diabetes, with a goal BP of <130/80 mm Hg. Discretion is warranted in prescribing medication to lower BP that may affect cardiovascular risk adversely in other ways (e.g., glucose control, lipid metabolism, uric acid levels). In the absence of hypertensive crisis, BP should be reduced gradually to avoid end-organ (e.g., cerebral) ischemia.

SPECIAL CONSIDERATIONS

- **Protocol**
  - **Hypertensive crisis.** In hypertensive emergency, control of acute or ongoing end-organ damage is more important than the absolute level of BP. BP control with a rapidly acting parenteral agent should be accomplished as soon as possible (within 1 hour) to reduce the chance of permanent organ dysfunction and death. A reasonable goal is a 20% to 25% reduction of mean arterial pressure or a reduction of the diastolic pressure to 100 to 110 mm Hg over a period of minutes to hours. A precipitous fall in BP may occur in patients who are elderly, volume depleted, or receiving other antihypertensive agents, and caution should be used to avoid cerebral hypoperfusion. BP control in hypertensive urgencies can be accomplished more slowly. The initial goal of therapy in urgency should be to achieve a DBP of 100 to 110 mm Hg. Excessive or rapid decreases in BP should be avoided to minimize the risk of cerebral hypoperfusion or coronary insufficiency. Normal BP can be attained gradually over several days as tolerated by the individual patient.
- **Aortic dissection**
  - Acute, proximal aortic dissection (type A) is a surgical emergency, whereas uncomplicated, distal dissection (type B) can be treated successfully with medical therapy alone. All patients, including those treated surgically, require acute and chronic antihypertensive therapy to provide initial stabilization and to prevent complications (e.g., aortic rupture, continued dissection). Medical therapy of chronic stable aortic dissection should seek to maintain SBP at or below 130 to 140 mm Hg if tolerated. Antihypertensive agents with negative inotropic properties, including calcium channel antagonists, β-adrenergic antagonists, methyldopa, clonidine, and reserpine, are preferred for management in the post-acute phase.
    - **Sodium nitroprusside** is considered the initial drug of choice because of the predictability of response and absence of tachyphylaxis. The dose should be titrated to achieve an SBP of 100 to 120 mm Hg or the lowest possible BP that permits adequate organ perfusion. Nitroprusside alone causes an increase in left ventricular contractility and subsequent arterial shearing forces, which contribute to ongoing intimal dissection. Thus, when using sodium nitroprusside, adequate simultaneous **β-adrenergic antagonist therapy** is essential, regardless of whether systolic hypertension is present. Traditionally, propranolol has been recommended. **Esmolol**, a cardioselective IV β-adrenergic antagonist with a very short duration of action, may be preferable, especially in patients with relative contraindications to β-antagonists. If esmolol is tolerated, a longer acting β-adrenergic antagonist should be used.

- **IV labetalol** has been used successfully as a single agent in the treatment of acute aortic dissection. Labetalol produces a dose-related decrease in BP and lowers contractility. It has the advantage of allowing for oral administration after the acute stage of dissection has been managed successfully.
- **Trimethaphan camsylate**, a ganglionic blocking agent, can be used as a single IV agent if sodium nitroprusside or β-adrenergic antagonists cannot be tolerated. Unlike sodium nitroprusside, trimethaphan reduces left ventricular contractility. Because trimethaphan is associated with rapid tachyphylaxis and sympathalgia (e.g., orthostatic hypotension, blurred vision, and urinary retention), other drugs are preferable.
- **Individual patient considerations.** Cultural and other individual differences among patients must be considered in planning a therapeutic regimen. Although classification of adult BP is somewhat arbitrary, it may nevertheless be useful in making clinical decisions (Table 3-4).
  - **The elderly hypertensive patient** (older than age 60 years) is generally characterized by increased vascular resistance, decreased plasma renin activity, and greater LVH than in younger patients. Often, elderly hypertensive patients have coexisting medical problems that must be considered when initiating antihypertensive therapy. Drug doses should be increased slowly to avoid adverse effects and hypotension. Diuretics as initial therapy have been shown to decrease the incidence of stroke,

Table 3-4	Classification of Blood Pressure for Adults Aged 18 Years and Older[a]	
Category	**Systolic Pressure (mm Hg)**	**Diastolic Pressure (mm Hg)**
Normal[b]	<120 and	<80
Prehypertension	120–139 or	80–89
Hypertension[c]		
Stage 1	140–159 or	90–99
Stage 2	>160 or	>100

Isolated systolic hypertension is defined as a systolic blood pressure (BP) of 140 mm Hg or more and a diastolic BP of <90 mm Hg and staged appropriately (e.g., 170/85 mm Hg is defined as stage 2 isolated systolic hypertension). In addition to classifying stages of hypertension on the basis of average BP levels, the clinician should specify the presence or absence of target organ disease and additional risk factors. This specificity is important for risk classification and management.

[a]Not taking antihypertensive drugs and not acutely ill. When systolic and diastolic pressures fall into different categories, the higher category should be selected to classify the individual's BP status.

[b]Optimal BP with respect to cardiovascular risk is <120 mm Hg systolic and <80 mm Hg diastolic. However, unusually low readings should be evaluated for clinical significance.

[c]Based on the average of two or more readings taken at each of two or more visits after an initial screening.

From National High Blood Pressure Education Program. The Seventh Report of the Joint National Committee on Prevention, Detection, Evaluation, and Treatment of High Blood Pressure. Bethesda (MD): National Heart, Lung, and Blood Institute (US), 2004.

fatal MI, and overall mortality in this age group (*JAMA 1991;265:3255*). Calcium channel antagonists decrease vascular resistance, have no adverse effects on lipid levels, and are also good choices for elderly patients. ACE inhibitors and ARBs may be effective agents in this population.

○ **African American hypertensive patients** generally have a lower plasma renin level, higher plasma volume, and higher vascular resistance than do Caucasian patients. Thus, African American patients respond well to diuretics, alone or in combination with calcium channel antagonists. ACE inhibitors, ARBs, and β-adrenergic antagonists are also effective agents in this population, particularly when combined with a diuretic.

○ **The obese hypertensive patient** is characterized by more modest elevations in vascular resistance, higher cardiac output, expanded intravascular volume, and lower plasma renin activity at any given level of arterial pressure. Weight reduction is the primary goal of therapy and is effective in reducing BP and causing regression of LVH.

○ **The diabetic patient** with nephropathy may have significant proteinuria and renal insufficiency, which can complicate management (see Chapter 13, Renal Diseases). Control of BP is the most important intervention shown to slow loss of renal function. ACE inhibitors should be used as first-line therapy, as they have been shown to decrease proteinuria and to slow progressive loss of renal function independent of their antihypertensive effects. ACE inhibitors may also be beneficial in reducing the rates of death, MI, and stroke in diabetics who have cardiovascular risk factors but lack left ventricular dysfunction. Hyperkalemia is a common side effect in diabetic patients treated with ACE inhibitors, especially in those with moderate to severe impairment of their GFR. ARBs are also effective antihypertensive agents and have been shown to slow the rate of progression to ESRD, thus supporting a renal protective effect (*N Engl J Med 2001;345(12): 861*).

○ **The hypertensive patient with chronic renal insufficiency** has hypertension that usually is partially volume dependent. Retention of sodium and water exacerbates the existing hypertensive state, and diuretics are important in the management of this problem. With a serum creatinine >2.5 mg/dL, loop diuretics are the most effective class.

○ **The hypertensive patient with LVH** is at increased risk for sudden death, MI, and all-cause mortality. Although there is no direct evidence, regression of LVH could be expected to reduce the risk for subsequent complications. ACE inhibitors appear to have the greatest effect on regression.

○ **The hypertensive patient with CAD** is at increased risk for UA and MI. β-Adrenergic antagonists can be used as first-line agents in these patients as they can decrease cardiac mortality and subsequent reinfarction in the setting of acute MI and can decrease progression to MI in those who present with UA. β-Adrenergic antagonists also have a role in secondary prevention of cardiac events and in increasing long-term survival after MI. Care should be exercised in those with cardiac conduction system disease. Calcium channel antagonists should be used with caution in the setting of acute MI, as studies have shown conflicting results from their use. ACE inhibitors are also useful in patients with CAD and decrease mortality in individuals who present with acute MI, especially those with left ventricular dysfunction, and more recently have been shown to decrease mortality in patients without left ventricular dysfunction.

○ **The hypertensive patient with HF** is at risk for progressive left ventricular dilatation and sudden death. In this population, ACE inhibitors decrease mortality (*N Engl J Med 1992;327:685*), and in the setting of acute MI, they decrease the risk of recurrent MI, hospitalization for HF, and mortality (*N Engl J Med 1992;327:669*). ARBs have similar beneficial effects, and they appear to be an effective alternative in patients who are unable to tolerate an ACE inhibitor (*N Engl J Med 2001;345:1667*). Nitrates and hydralazine also decrease mortality in patients with HF irrespective of hypertension, but hydralazine can cause reflex tachycardia and worsening ischemia in patients with unstable coronary syndromes and should be used with caution. Calcium channel antagonists should generally be avoided in patients in whom negative inotropic effects would affect their status adversely.

• **Pregnancy and hypertension**
  ○ Hypertension in the setting of pregnancy is a special situation because of the potential for maternal and fetal morbidity and mortality associated with elevated BP and the clinical syndromes of preeclampsia and eclampsia. The possibility of teratogenic or other adverse effects of antihypertensive medications on fetal development also should be considered.
  ○ **Classification of hypertension** during pregnancy has been proposed by the American College of Obstetrics and Gynecology (*N Engl J Med 1996;335: 257*).
    ▪ **Preeclampsia or eclampsia.** Preeclampsia is a condition defined by pregnancy, hypertension, proteinuria, generalized edema, and occasionally, coagulation and liver function abnormalities after 20 weeks' gestation. Eclampsia encompasses these parameters in addition to generalized seizures.
    ▪ **Chronic hypertension.** This disorder is defined by a BP >140/90 mm Hg before the 20th week of pregnancy.
    ▪ **Transient hypertension.** This condition results in increases in BP without associated proteinuria or CNS manifestations. BP returns to normal within 10 days of delivery.
  ○ **Therapy.** Treatment of hypertension in pregnancy should begin if the DBP is >100 mm Hg.
    ▪ Nonpharmacologic therapy, such as weight reduction and vigorous exercise, is not recommended during pregnancy.
    ▪ Alcohol and tobacco use should be strongly discouraged.
    ▪ Pharmacologic intervention with methyldopa is recommended as first-line therapy because of its proven safety. Hydralazine and labetalol are also safe and can be used as alternative agents; both can be used parenterally.
    ▪ Other antihypertensives have theoretical disadvantages, but none except the ACE inhibitors have been proven to increase fetal morbidity or mortality.
    ▪ If a patient is suspected of having preeclampsia or eclampsia, urgent referral to an obstetrician who specializes in high-risk pregnancy is recommended.
    ▪ Monoamine oxidase inhibitors (MAOIs). MAOIs used in association with certain drugs or foods can produce a catecholamine excess state and accelerated hypertension. Interactions are common with tricyclic antidepressants, meperidine, methyldopa, levodopa, sympathomimetic agents, and antihistamines. Tyramine-containing foods that can lead to this syndrome include certain cheeses, red wine, beer, chocolate, chicken liver, processed meat, herring, broad beans, canned figs, and yeast. Nitroprusside, labetalol, and phentolamine have been used effectively in the treatment of accelerated hypertension associated with monoamine oxidase inhibitor use (see Table 3-3).

COMPLICATIONS

Withdrawal syndrome associated with discontinuation of antihypertensive therapy. In substituting therapy in patients with moderate-to-severe hypertension, it is reasonable to increase doses of the new medication in small increments while tapering the previous medication to avoid excessive BP fluctuations. On occasion, an AWS develops, usually within the first 24 to 72 hours. Occasionally, BP rises to levels that are much higher than those of baseline values. The most severe complications of AWS include encephalopathy, stroke, MI, and sudden death. The AWS is associated most commonly with centrally acting adrenergic agents (particularly clonidine) and β-adrenergic antagonists but has been reported with other agents as well including diuretics. Rarely should BP medications be withdrawn; rather, in discontinuing therapy, these drugs should be tapered over several days to weeks unless other medications are used to substitute in the interim. Discontinuation of antihypertensive medications should be done with caution in patients with preexisting cerebrovascular or cardiac disease. Management of AWS by reinstitution of the previously administered drug is generally effective. Sodium nitroprusside (see Table 3-2) is the treatment of choice when parenteral administration of an antihypertensive agent is required or when the identity of the previously administered agent is unknown. In the AWS caused by clonidine, β-adrenergic antagonists should not be used because unopposed α-adrenergic activity will be augmented and may exacerbate hypertension. However, labetalol (see Table 3-2) may be useful in this situation.

PATIENT EDUCATION

Patient education is an essential component of the treatment plan and promotes patient compliance. Physicians should emphasize the following:
• Lifelong treatment is usually required.
• Symptoms are an unreliable gauge of severity of hypertension.
• Prognosis improves with proper management.
• Lifestyle modifications are essential.

MONITORING/FOLLOW-UP

• BP measurements should be performed on multiple occasions under nonstressful circumstances (e.g., rest, sitting, empty bladder, comfortable temperature) to obtain an accurate assessment of BP in a given patient.
• Hypertension should not be diagnosed on the basis of one measurement alone, unless it is >210/120 mm Hg or accompanied by target organ damage. Two or more abnormal readings should be obtained, preferably over a period of several weeks, before therapy is considered.
• Care should also be used to exclude pseudohypertension, which usually occurs in elderly individuals with stiff, noncompressible vessels. A palpable artery that persists after cuff inflation (Osler sign) should alert the physician to this possibility.
• Home and ambulatory BP monitoring can be used to assess a patient's true average BP, which correlates better with target organ damage. Circumstances in which ambulatory BP monitoring might be of value include:
  ○ Suspected "white-coat hypertension" (increases in BP associated with the stress of physician office visits) should be evaluated carefully.
  ○ Evaluation of possible "drug resistance" where suspected.

Dyslipidemia

GENERAL PRINCIPLES

- Lipids are sparingly soluble molecules that include cholesterol, fatty acids, and their derivatives.
- Plasma lipids are transported by lipoprotein particles composed of proteins called **apolipoproteins**, and **phospholipids, free cholesterol, cholesterol esters**, and **triglycerides**.
- Human plasma lipoproteins are separated into **five major classes** based on density:
  - Chylomicrons (least dense)
  - Very low–density lipoproteins (VLDLs)
  - Intermediate-density lipoproteins (IDLs)
  - LDLs
  - HDLs
  - A sixth class, lipoprotein(a) [Lp(a)], resembles LDL in lipid composition and has a density that overlaps LDL and HDL
- Physical properties of plasma lipoproteins are summarized in Table 3-5.
- **Atherosclerosis and lipoproteins.** Increased levels of LDL cholesterol, remnant lipoproteins, and Lp(a) as well as decreased levels of HDL cholesterol have all been associated with an increased risk of premature vascular disease (*J Am Coll Cardiol 1992;19:792; JAMA 1999;282:2043; Circulation 2011;123:2292; J Clin Endocrinol Metab 2012;97:2969*).
- **Clinical dyslipoproteinemias**
  - Most dyslipidemias are multifactorial in etiology and reflect the effects of genetic influences coupled with diet, activity, smoking, alcohol use, and comorbid conditions such as obesity and DM.
  - Differential diagnoses of the major lipid abnormalities are summarized in Table 3-6.

Table 3-5	Physical Properties of Plasma Lipoproteins		
Lipoprotein	Lipid Composition	Origin	Apolipoproteins
Chylomicrons	TG, 85%; chol, 3%	Intestine	B-48; A-I, A-IV, C-I, C-II, C-III; E
VLDL	TG, 55%; chol, 20%	Liver	B-100; C-I, C-II, C-III; E
IDL	TG, 25%; chol, 35%	Metabolic product of VLDL	B-100; C-I, C-II, C-III; E
LDL	TG, 5%; chol, 60%	Metabolic product of IDL	B-100
HDL	TG, 5%; chol, 20%	Liver, intestine	A-I, A-II; C-I, C-II, C-III; E
Lp(a)	TG, 5%; chol, 60%	Liver	B-100; Apo(a)

Chol, cholesterol; HDL, high-density lipoprotein; IDL, intermediate-density lipoprotein; LDL, low-density lipoprotein; Lp(a), lipoprotein(a); TG, triglyceride; VLDL, very low–density lipoprotein.

Table 3-6	Differential Diagnosis of Major Lipid Abnormalities	
Lipid Abnormality	**Primary Disorders**	**Secondary Disorders**
Hypercholesterolemia	Polygenic, familial hypercholesterolemia, familial defective apo B-100	Hypothyroidism, nephrotic syndrome, anorexia nervosa
Hypertriglyceridemia	Lipoprotein lipase deficiency, apo C-II deficiency, familial hypertriglyceridemia, dysbetalipoproteinemia	Diabetes mellitus, obesity, metabolic syndrome, alcohol use, oral estrogen, renal failure, hypothyroidism, retinoic acid, lipodystrophies
Combined hyperlipidemia	Familial combined hyperlipidemia, dysbetalipoproteinemia	Diabetes mellitus, obesity, metabolic syndrome, hypothyroidism, nephrotic syndrome, lipodystrophies
Low HDL	Familial alpha lipoproteinemia, Tangier disease (ABCA1 deficiency), apoA1 mutations, lecithin:cholesterol acyltransferase deficiency	Diabetes mellitus, metabolic syndrome, hypertriglyceridemia, smoking, anabolic steroids

HDL, high-density lipoprotein.

○ The major genetic dyslipoproteinemias are reviewed in Table 3-7 (*Circulation 1974;49:476; J Clin Lipidol 2011;5:S9; Circulation 2011;123:2292; J Clin Endocrinol Metab 2012;97:2969*).
○ Familial hypercholesterolemia and familial combined hyperlipidemia are disorders that contribute significantly to premature cardiovascular disease.
  ▪ Familial hypercholesterolemia is an underdiagnosed, autosomal codominant condition with a prevalence of at least 1 in 500 people and that causes elevated LDL cholesterol levels from birth. It is associated with significantly increased risk of early cardiovascular disease when untreated (*J Clin Lipidol 2011;5:133*).
  ▪ Familial combined hyperlipidemia has a prevalence of 1% to 2% and typically presents in adulthood, although obesity and high dietary fat and sugar intakes have led to increased presentation in childhood and adolescence (*J Clin Endocrinol Metab 2012;97:2969*).
• **Standards of care for hyperlipidemia**
○ LDL cholesterol–lowering therapy, particularly with hydroxymethylglutaryl-coenzyme A (HMG-CoA) reductase inhibitors, lowers the risk of CHD-related death, morbidity, and revascularization procedures in hypercholesterolemic patients with (secondary prevention) (*Lancet 1994;344:1383; N Engl J Med 1996;335:1001; N Engl J Med 1998;339:1349; Lancet 2002;360:7; N Engl J Med*

Table 3-7   Review of Major Genetic Dyslipoproteinemias

Type of Genetic Dyslipidemia	Typical Lipid Profile	Type of Inheritance pattern	Phenotypic Features	Other Information
Familial hypercholesterolemia (FH)	• Increased total (>300 mg/dL) and LDL (>250 mg/dL) cholesterol • Homozygous form (rare) can have total cholesterol >600 mg/dL and LDL >550 mg/dL	Autosomal dominant	• Premature CAD • Tendon xanthomas • Premature arcus corneae (full arcus before age 40 yr)	Due to mutations of the LDL receptor that lead to defective uptake and degradation of LDL
Familial combined hyperlipidemia (FCH)	• High levels of VLDL, LDL, or both • LDL apo B-100 level >130 mg/dL	Autosomal dominant	• Premature CAD • Patients do not develop tendon xanthomas	Genetic and metabolic defects are not established.
Familial defective apolipoprotein B-100	• Similar to familial hypercholesterolemia		• Similar to familial hypercholesterolemia	Most all cases are due to a glutamine for arginine mutation at amino acid 3500 of apo B-100. *(continued)*

Table 3-7 Review of Major Genetic Dyslipoproteinemias (Continued)

Type of Genetic Dyslipidemia	Typical Lipid Profile	Type of Inheritance pattern	Phenotypic Features	Other Information
Dysbetalipoproteinemia	• Symmetric elevations of cholesterol and triglycerides (300–500 mg/dL) • Elevated VLDL to triglyceride ratio (>0.3)	Autosomal recessive	• Premature CAD • Tuberous or tubereoruptive xanthomas • Planar xanthomas of the palmar creases are essentially pathognomonic.	Mutation of ApoE gene Many homozygotes are normolipidemic, and emergence of hyperlipidemia often requires a secondary metabolic factor such as diabetes mellitus, hypothyroidism, or obesity.
Chylomicronemia syndrome	• Most patients have triglycerides >150 mg/dL • Clinical manifestations occur when triglycerides exceed 1,500 mg/dL	• Onset before puberty indicates deficiency of lipoprotein lipase or apo C-II, both autosomal recessive. • Familial hypertriglyceridemia is an autosomal dominant disorder caused by overproduction of VLDL triglycerides and manifests in adults.	• Eruptive xanthomas • Lipemia retinalis • Pancreatitis • Hepatosplenomegaly	Familial hypertriglyceridemia and FCH patients may develop chylomicronemia syndrome in the presence of secondary factors such as obesity, alcohol use, or diabetes.

CAD, coronary artery disease; LDL, low-density lipoprotein; VLDL, very low–density lipoprotein.

2004;350:1495; N Engl J Med 2005;352:1425) or without (primary prevention) known CHD (*Lancet 2002;360:7; N Engl J Med 1995;333:1301; JAMA 1998;279:1615; Lancet 2003;361:1149; Lancet 2004;364:685; N Engl J Med 2008;359:2195*).

○ Identification and management of high LDL cholesterol is the primary goal of the National Cholesterol Education Program's (NCEP's) third expert report on cholesterol management in adults, or Adult Treatment Program III (ATP III) (*JAMA 2001;285:2486; Circulation 2002;106:3143*).

○ The ATP III executive summary and full report can be viewed online at *www.nhlbi.nih.gov/guidelines/cholesterol/*.

DIAGNOSIS

Screening

- Screening for hypercholesterolemia should begin **in all adults aged 20 years or older**.
- Screening is best performed with a lipid profile (total cholesterol, LDL cholesterol, HDL cholesterol, and triglycerides) obtained after a 12-hour fast.
- If a fasting lipid panel cannot be obtained, total and HDL cholesterol should be measured.
- Measurement of fasting lipids is indicated if the total cholesterol is ≥200 mg/dL or HDL cholesterol is ≤40 mg/dL.
- If lipids are unremarkable and the patient has no major risk factors for CHD (Table 3-8), then screening can be performed every 5 years (*JAMA 2001;285: 2486*).
- Patients hospitalized for an acute coronary syndrome (ACS) or coronary revascularization should have a lipid panel obtained within 24 hours of admission if lipid levels are unknown.

Table 3-8	Major Risk Factors that Modify Low-Density Lipoprotein Goals

Cigarette smoking
Hypertension (blood pressure ≥140/90 mm Hg or on antihypertensive medication)
Low HDL cholesterol (<40 mg/dL)[a]
Family history of premature CHD (CHD in male first-degree relative <age 55 yr; CHD in female first-degree relative <age 65 yr)
Age (men ≥45 yr; women ≥55 yr)

[a]HDL cholesterol ≥60 mg/dL counts as a "negative" risk factor; its presence removes one risk factor from the total count.
CHD, coronary heart disease; HDL, high-density lipoprotein.
Modified from Expert Panel on Detection, Evaluation, and Treatment of High Blood Cholesterol in Adults. Executive summary of the third report of the National Cholesterol Education Program (NCEP) Expert Panel on Detection, Evaluation, and Treatment of High Blood Cholesterol in Adults (Adult Treatment Panel III). JAMA 2001;285:2486–2497.

- Individuals with hyperlipidemia should be evaluated for potential **secondary causes**, including hypothyroidism, DM, obstructive liver disease, chronic renal disease, or nephrotic syndrome, or medications such as estrogens, progestins, anabolic steroids, corticosteroids, retinoids, cyclosporine, and antiretroviral medications.

TREATMENT

- **Therapeutic lifestyle change**
  - ATP III thresholds for initiating cholesterol-lowering therapy with **therapeutic lifestyle change** (TLC, diet, and exercise) and **hypolipidemic drugs** are summarized in Table 3-9 (*Circulation 2004;110:227*).
    - All patients requiring cholesterol treatment should implement a diet restricted in total and saturated fat intake in accordance with ATP III recommendations (Table 3-10) (*JAMA 2001;285:2486*).
    - Moderate exercise and weight reduction is also recommended.
    - A registered dietitian may be helpful to plan and start a saturated fat–restricted and weight loss–promoting diet.
- **Treatment targets**
  - **High risk and very high risk**
    - The ATP III LDL cholesterol treatment target for all high-risk patients is <100 mg/dL (*JAMA 2001;285:2486*).
    - For CHD patients in the **very high–risk** category, an LDL cholesterol <70 mg/dL is a therapeutic option (*Circulation 2004;110:227*).
    - An LDL cholesterol of ≥100 mg/dL is identified as the threshold for simultaneous treatment with TLC and lipid-lowering agents (*Circulation 2004;110: 227*).

Table 3-9	ATP III Low-Density Lipoprotein Cholesterol Goals and Thresholds for Therapeutic Lifestyle Changes and Drug Therapy		
Category	**LDL-C Goal**	**Start TLC**	**Start Drug Therapy**
Very high risk	<70 mg/dL	Any LDL-C	LDL-C ≥70 mg/dL
High risk	<100 mg/dL	≥100 mg/dL	≥100 mg/dL (consider if baseline LDL-C <100 mg/dL)
Moderately high risk	<130 mg/dL (<100 mg/dL optional)	≥130 mg/dL	≥130 mg/dL (optional if baseline LDL-C 100–129 mg/dL)
Moderate risk	<130 mg/dL	≥130 mg/dL	≥160 mg/dL
Lower risk	<160 mg/dL	≥160 mg/dL	≥190 mg/dL (optional if baseline LDL-C 160–189 mg/dL)

ATP III, Adult Treatment Panel III; LDL-C, low-density lipoprotein cholesterol; TLCs, therapeutic lifestyle changes.
Modified from Grundy SM, Cleeman C, Merz NB, et al. Implications of recent clinical trials for the National Cholesterol Education Program Adult Treatment Panel III Guidelines. *Circulation* 2004;110:227–239.

Table 3-10	Nutrient Composition of the Therapeutic Lifestyle Change Diet

Nutrient	Recommended Intake
Saturated fat[a]	<7% of total calories
Polyunsaturated fat	Up to 10% of total calories
Monounsaturated fat	Up to 20% of total calories
Total fat	25%–35% of total calories
Carbohydrate[b]	50%–60% of total calories
Fiber	20–30 g/d
Protein	Approximately 15% of total calories
Cholesterol	<200 mg/d
Total calories (energy)[c]	Balance energy intake and expenditure to maintain desirable body weight/prevent weight gain

[a]Trans fatty acids are another low-density lipoprotein (LDL), raising fat that should be kept at a low intake.
[b]Carbohydrate should be derived predominantly from foods rich in complex carbohydrates, including grains (especially whole grains), fruits, and vegetables.
[c]Daily energy expenditure should include at least moderate physical activity (contributing approximately 200 kcal/d).
From Expert Panel on Detection, Evaluation, and Treatment of High Blood Cholesterol in Adults. Executive summary of the third report of the National Cholesterol Education Program (NCEP) Expert Panel on Detection, Evaluation, and Treatment of High Blood Cholesterol in Adults (Adult Treatment Panel III). *JAMA.* 2001;285:2486–2497, with permission.

- Based on outcomes in the Heart Protection Study (HPS), lipid-lowering drug therapy is also an option for patients with CHD and baseline LDL cholesterol <100 mg/dL (*Lancet 2002;360:7*).
- Based on the Cholesterol Treatment Trialists meta-analyses, greater LDL cholesterol reduction with a statin is associated with decreased reduction of cardiovascular risk (*Lancet 2012;380:581*; *Lancet 2010;376:1670*).

○ **Moderately high risk**
  - Patients with two or more non-LDL cholesterol risk factors and a Framingham score predicting a 10-year CHD risk of 10% to 20% are considered at **moderately high risk** of CHD.
  - Pharmacotherapy should be initiated if LDL cholesterol is ≥130 mg/dL.
  - ATP III identifies an LDL cholesterol target <100 mg/dL as optional for this group, with drug therapy to be considered for patients with baseline LDL cholesterol 100 to 129 mg/dL.
  - Patients with two or more risk factors and a 10-year risk <10% are candidates for drug therapy when LDL cholesterol remains ≥160 mg/dL despite TLC (*Circulation 2004;110:227*).

○ **Low risk**
  - For **low-risk patients** (zero to one risk factors), cholesterol-lowering therapy should be considered if the LDL cholesterol is ≥190 mg/dL, especially for patients who have undergone a 3-month trial of TLC.
  - Patients with very high LDL concentrations (≥190 mg/dL) often have a hereditary dyslipidemia and require treatment with multiple lipid-lowering agents.

Table 3-11	Adult Treatment Program III Diagnostic Criteria for the Metabolic Syndrome
Risk Factor	**ATP III[a] Definition**
Carbohydrate metabolism	Fasting glucose >110 mg/dL (modified to >100 mg/dL)[c]
Abdominal obesity[b]	Men, waist >40 in.
	Women, waist >35 in.
Dyslipidemia	Triglycerides ≥150 mg/dL
	Men, HDL cholesterol <40 mg/dL
	Women, HDL cholesterol <50 mg/dL
Hypertension	BP ≥130/85 mm Hg

[a]To qualify for the diagnosis of metabolic syndrome by ATP III criteria, a patient must meet at least three of the five criteria (hyperglycemia, abdominal obesity, high triglycerides, low HDL cholesterol, high blood pressure).
[b]Waist circumferences in Asian and South Asian patients may require different cut points.
Modified from Expert Panel on Detection, Evaluation, and Treatment of High Blood Cholesterol in Adults Executive Summary of the Third Report of the National Cholesterol Education Program (NCEP) Expert Panel on Detection, Evaluation, and Treatment of High Blood Cholesterol in Adults (Adult Treatment Panel III). *JAMA.* 2001;285:2486–2497.
[c]*Circulation* 2009;120:1640–1645.
ATP III, Adult Treatment Panel III; BP, blood pressure; HDL, high-density lipoprotein.

These patients should be referred to a lipid specialist, and family members should be screened with a fasting lipid battery.

- When LDL cholesterol is 160 to 189 mg/dL, drug therapy should be considered if the patient has a significant risk factor for cardiovascular disease, such as heavy tobacco use, poorly controlled hypertension, strong family history of early CHD, or low HDL cholesterol (*Circulation 2004;110:227*).

- **Assessing response to therapy**
  - **Response to therapy should be assessed after 6 weeks** and the dose of medication titrated if the LDL cholesterol treatment target is not achieved.
  - The initial dose of a cholesterol-lowering drug should be sufficient to achieve a 30% to 40% reduction in LDL cholesterol.
  - Patients with familial hypercholesterolemia should have LDL cholesterol lowered by at least 50% from baseline (*J Clin Lipidol 2011;5:S18–S29*).
  - If target LDL cholesterol has not been reached after 12 weeks, current therapy should be intensified by further dose titration, adding another lipid-lowering agent, or referral to a lipid specialist.
  - Patients at goal should be monitored every 4 to 6 months.

- **Metabolic syndrome**
  - The constellation of abdominal obesity, hypertension, glucose intolerance, and an atherogenic lipid profile (hypertriglyceridemia; low HDL cholesterol; and small, dense LDL cholesterol) characterizes a condition called the **metabolic syndrome**. ATP III diagnostic criteria for the metabolic syndrome are summarized in Table 3-11 (*JAMA 2001;285:2486; Circulation 2009;120:1640*).
  - At least 22% of Americans qualify for a diagnosis of the metabolic syndrome by ATP III criteria. Prevalence is increased in older individuals, women, Hispanic Americans, and African Americans (*JAMA 2002;287:356*).

○ Multiple studies have demonstrated an association between cardiovascular events and death and all-cause mortality with the metabolic syndrome (*Am J Med 2006;119:812*).

○ ATP III recognizes the metabolic syndrome as a **secondary treatment** target after LDL cholesterol is controlled (*JAMA 2001;285:2486*).

○ The report recommends treating the underlying causes of metabolic syndrome (overweight/obesity, physical inactivity) by implementing weight loss and aerobic exercise and managing cardiovascular risks, such as hypertension, that may persist despite lifestyle changes (*JAMA 2001;285:2486*).

• **Hypertriglyceridemia**

○ Hypertriglyceridemia may be an **independent cardiovascular risk factor** (*Circulation 2007;115:450*; *Ann Intern Med 2007;147:377*; *Circulation 2011; 123:2292*).

○ Hypertriglyceridemia is often observed in the metabolic syndrome, and there are many potential etiologies for hypertriglyceridemia including obesity, DM, renal insufficiency, genetic dyslipidemias, and therapy with oral estrogen, glucocorticoids, retinoic acid, or β-blockers (*Circulation 2011;123:2292*).

○ The ATP III classification of serum triglyceride levels is as follows (*JAMA 2001;285:2486*):

  ▪ Normal: <150 mg/dL
  ▪ Borderline high: 150 to 199 mg/dL
  ▪ High: 200 to 499 mg/dL
  ▪ Very high: ≥500 mg/dL

○ Severe (triglycerides 1,000 to 1,999 mg/dL) and very severe (triglycerides ≥2,000 mg/dL) hypertriglyceridemia greatly increase the risk for pancreatitis (*J Clin Endo Metab 2012;96:2969*).

○ Treatment of hypertriglyceridemia depends on the degree of severity.

  ▪ For patients with very high triglycerides, triglyceride reduction through a very low-fat diet (≤15% of calories), exercise, weight loss, and drugs (fibrates, niacin, omega-3 fatty acids) is the primary goal of therapy to prevent acute pancreatitis.
  ▪ When patients have a lesser degree of hypertriglyceridemia, control of LDL cholesterol is the primary aim of initial therapy. TLC is emphasized as the initial intervention to lower triglycerides (*JAMA 2001;285:2486*).

• **Non-HDL cholesterol**

○ Non-HDL cholesterol is a secondary treatment target.

○ A patient's non-HDL cholesterol is calculated by subtracting HDL cholesterol from total cholesterol.

○ Target non-HDL cholesterol is 30 mg/dL higher than the LDL cholesterol target.

○ LDL and non-HDL cholesterol treatment targets for various degrees of cardiovascular risk are summarized in Table 3-12 (*JAMA 2001;285:2486*; *Circulation 2004;110:227*).

• **Low HDL cholesterol**

○ Low HDL cholesterol is an **independent CHD risk factor** that is identified as a non-LDL cholesterol risk and included as a component of the Framingham scoring algorithm (*JAMA 1986;256:2835*).

○ Etiologies for low HDL cholesterol include physical inactivity, obesity, insulin resistance, DM, hypertriglyceridemia, cigarette smoking, and certain medications (β-blockers, anabolic steroids, progestins).

○ Because therapeutic interventions for low HDL cholesterol are of limited efficacy, ATP III identifies **LDL cholesterol as the primary target of therapy for patients with low HDL cholesterol.**

Table 3-12	Comparison of Low-Density Lipoprotein Cholesterol and Non–High-Density Lipoprotein Cholesterol Goals by Coronary Heart Disease Risk Category	
Category	LDL-C Target (mg/dL)	Non–HDL-C Target (mg/dL)
Very high risk	<70	<100
High risk	<100	<130
Moderately high risk	<130	<160
Moderate risk	<130	<160
Low risk	<160	<190

HDL-C, high-density lipoprotein cholesterol; LDL-C, low-density lipoprotein cholesterol.
Modified from Grundy SM, Cleeman C, Merz NB, et al. Implications of recent clinical trials for the National Cholesterol Education Program Adult Treatment Panel III Guidelines. *Circulation* 2004;110:227–239.

- Low HDL cholesterol often occurs in the setting of hypertriglyceridemia and metabolic syndrome. Management of these conditions may result in improvement of HDL cholesterol.
- Aerobic exercise, weight loss, smoking cessation, menopausal estrogen replacement, and treatment with niacin or fibrates may elevate low HDL cholesterol (*JAMA 2001;285:2486*).
- There are no clinical trial data showing a benefit of pharmacologic methods of elevating HDL cholesterol.
- **Lipid-lowering therapy and age**
  - The risk of a fatal or nonfatal cardiovascular event increases with age, and most cardiovascular events occur in patients aged 65 years and older.
  - Secondary prevention trials with the HMG-CoA reductase inhibitors have demonstrated significant clinical benefit for patients aged 65 to 75 years.
  - The HPS failed to show an age threshold for primary or secondary prevention with statin therapy. Patients aged 75 to 80 years at study entry experienced a nearly 30% reduction in major vascular events (*Lancet 2002;360:7*).
  - The Prospective Study of Pravastatin in the Elderly (PROSPER) trial found a significant reduction in major coronary events among patients aged 70 to 82 years with vascular disease or CHD risks treated with pravastatin (*Lancet 2002;360:1623*).
  - **ATP III does not place age restrictions** on treatment of hypercholesterolemia in elderly adults.
  - ATP III recommends TLC for young adults (men aged 20 to 35 years; women aged 20 to 45 years) with an LDL level ≥130 mg/dL. Drug therapy should be considered in the following high-risk groups:
    - Men who both smoke and have elevated LDL levels (160 to 189 mg/dL)
    - All young adults with an LDL ≥190 mg/dL
    - Those with an inherited dyslipidemia (*JAMA 2001;285:2486*).
- **Treatment of elevated LDL cholesterol**
  - **HMG-CoA reductase inhibitors (statins)**
    - Statins (Table 3-13) are the treatment of choice for elevated LDL cholesterol (*JAMA 2001;285:2486*; *Circulation 2002;106:1024*; *Lancet 2012;380:581*;

| Table 3-13 | Low-Density Lipoprotein Cholesterol Lowering Effect of Currently Available Statins |

Name	Atorvas-tatin	Fluvas-tatin	Lovas-tatin	Pravas-tatin	Rosuvas-tatin	Simvas-tatin	Pitavas-tatin
Dose range (mg PO/d)	10–80	20–80	10–80	10–80	5–40	10–80*	1–4
LDL effect (%)	↓ 38–54	↓ 17–36	↓ 21–40	↓ 19–34	↓ 41–65	↓ 28–46	↓ 32–43

LDL, low-density lipoprotein; ↑, increased; ↓, decreased.
*Simvastatin 80 mg should not be used.

Lancet 2010;376:1670; J Clin Lipidol 2011;5:S18; J Clin Lipidol 2011;5:S38; Atheroscler Suppl 2011;12:221).

- The lipid-lowering effect of statins appears within the first week of use and becomes stable after approximately 4 weeks of use.
- Common side effects (5% to 10% of patients) include gastrointestinal (GI) upset (e.g., abdominal pain, diarrhea, bloating, constipation) and muscle pain or weakness, which can occur without creatinine kinase elevations. Other potential side effects include malaise, fatigue, headache, and rash (*N Engl J Med 1999;341:498; Endocrinol Metab Clin North Am 2009;38:79*).
- Muscle problems are the most common cause of discontinuation of statin therapy. Muscle problems are often dose dependent as well as being affected by factors such as age, renal function, body size, and use of multiple medications. Changing or decreasing the statin dosage or using less than daily statin may allow for the use of a statin in patients who otherwise would be intolerant of this therapy (*Endocrinol Metab Clin North Am 2009;38:121*).
- Elevations of liver transaminases two to three times the upper limit of normal are dose dependent and reversible with discontinuation of the drug.
  In 2012, the U.S. Food and Drug Administration (FDA) stated that liver enzyme tests should be performed before starting statin therapy and as clinically indicated thereafter. The FDA concluded that serious liver injury with statins is rare and unpredictable in individual patients, and that routine periodic monitoring of liver enzymes does not appear to be effective in detecting or preventing serious liver injury (*http://www.fda.gov/Drugs/DrugSafety/ucm293101.htm*)
- Because some of the statins undergo metabolism by the cytochrome P450 enzyme system, taking them in combination with other drugs metabolized by this enzyme system increases the risk of **rhabdomyolysis** (*N Engl J Med 1999;341:498; Circulation 2002;106:1024*).
  - Among these drugs are fibrates (greater risk with gemfibrozil), itraconazole, ketoconazole, erythromycin, clarithromycin, cyclosporin, nefazodone, and protease inhibitors (*Circulation 2002;106:1024*).
  - Statins may also interact with large quantities of grapefruit juice to increase the risk of myopathy.
  - Simvastatin can increase levels of warfarin and digoxin. There are also significant interactions with amiodarone and other medications requiring the use of lower dosages of simvastatin. Maximum dosage of simvastatin is 40 mg,

and 80 mg should not be used unless the patient has taken this dose for more than 1 year (*http://www.fda.gov/Drugs/DrugSafety/ucm293101.htm*).
- Rosuvastatin may also increase warfarin levels.
- Statins should not be used during pregnancy or lactation.
○ **Bile acid sequestrant resins**
  - Currently available bile acid sequestrant resins include the following:
    □ **Cholestyramine:** 4 to 24 g PO per day in divided doses before meals
    □ **Colestipol:** tablets, 2 to 16 g PO per day; granules, 5 to 30 g PO per day in divided doses before meals
    □ **Colesevelam:** 625-mg tablets; three tablets PO bid or six tablets PO daily with food (maximum, seven tablets PO per day); suspension, one packet per day.
  - Bile acid sequestrants typically lower LDL levels by 15% to 30% and thereby lower the incidence of CHD (*N Engl J Med 1999;341:498*; *JAMA 1984; 251:351*). These agents should not be used as monotherapy in patients with triglyceride levels >250 mg/dL because they can raise triglyceride levels. They may be combined with nicotinic acid or statins (*Endocrinol Metab Clin North Am 2009;38:79*).
  - Common side effects of resins include constipation, abdominal pain, bloating, nausea, and flatulence.
  - Bile acid sequestrants may decrease oral absorption of many other drugs, including warfarin, digoxin, thyroid hormone, thiazide diuretics, amiodarone, glipizide, and statins.
    □ Colesevelam interacts with fewer drugs than the older resins.
    □ Other medications should be given 1 hour before or 4 hours after resins.
○ **Nicotinic acid (Niacin)**
  - Niacin can lower LDL cholesterol levels by ≥15%, lower triglyceride levels 20% to 50%, and raise HDL cholesterol levels by up to 35% (*Arch Intern Med 1994;154:1586*).
  - Crystalline niacin is given 1 to 3 g PO per day in two to three divided doses with meals. Extended-release niacin is dosed at night. The starting dose is 500 mg PO, and the dose may be titrated monthly in 500-mg increments to a maximum of 2,000 mg PO (administer dose with milk or crackers).
  - Common side effects of niacin include flushing, pruritus, headache, nausea, and bloating. Other potential side effects include elevation of liver transaminases, hyperuricemia, and hyperglycemia.
    □ Flushing may be decreased with use of aspirin 30 minutes before the first few doses.
    □ Hepatotoxicity associated with niacin is partially dose dependent and appears to be more prevalent with some over-the-counter time-release preparations.
  - Avoid use of niacin in patients with gout, liver disease, active peptic ulcer disease, and uncontrolled DM.
    □ Niacin can be used with care in patients with well-controlled DM (HgA$_{1c}$ ≤7%).
    □ Serum transaminases, glucose, and uric acid levels should be monitored every 6 to 8 weeks during dose titration, then every 4 months.
○ **Ezetimibe**
  - Ezetimibe is currently the only available cholesterol absorption inhibitor.
  - It appears to act at the brush border of the small intestine and inhibits cholesterol absorption.

- The recommended dosing is 10 mg PO once daily. No dosage adjustment is required for renal insufficiency, mild hepatic impairment, or in elderly patients.
- Ezetimibe may provide an additional 25% mean reduction in LDL cholesterol when combined with a statin and provides an approximately 18% decrease in LDL cholesterol when used as monotherapy (*Am J Cardiol 2002;90:1092*; *Mayo Clin Proc 2004;79:620*; *Endocrinol Metab Clin North Am 2009;38:79*).
- It is not recommended for use in patients with moderate-to-severe hepatic impairment.
- Side effects are infrequent and include GI symptoms and myalgias.
  - In clinical trials, there was no excess of rhabdomyolysis or myopathy when compared with statin or placebo alone.
  - There is a low incidence of diarrhea and abdominal pain compared to placebo. Liver function monitoring is not required with monotherapy because there appears to be no significant impact on liver enzymes when this drug is used alone.
  - Liver enzymes should be monitored when used in conjunction with a statin, as there appears to be a slight increased incidence of enzyme elevations with combination therapy.
- Long-term clinical outcome trials of ezetimibe are ongoing. One clinical outcome trial showed decreased reduction of cardiovascular events with the combination of simvastatin and ezetimibe compared to placebo in patients with chronic renal failure (*Lancet 2011;377:2181*). The effect on cardiovascular events of ezetimibe when added to a statin compared with statin alone has not been demonstrated.
- **Treatment of hypertriglyceridemia**
  - **Nonpharmacologic treatment**
    - Nonpharmacologic treatments are important in the therapy of hypertriglyceridemia.
    - Nonpharmacologic approaches include the following:
      - Changing oral estrogen replacement to transdermal estrogen
      - Decreasing alcohol intake
      - Encouraging weight loss and exercise
      - Controlling hyperglycemia in patients with DM
      - Avoiding simple sugars and very high-carbohydrate diets
    - Patients with severe hypertriglyceridemia (triglycerides over 1,000 mg/dL) require reduction of fat and simple carbohydrate intakes in addition to medication in order to decrease the risk of pancreatitis.
  - **Pharmacologic treatment**
    - Pharmacologic treatment of moderate-to-severe hypertriglyceridemia consists of fibric acid derivative, niacin, or omega-3 fatty acids. Patients who have triglyceride-induced pancreatitis should be treated with a fibric acid derivative (*J Clin Endo Metab 2012;96:2969*).
    - Statins may be effective for patients with mild-to-moderate hypertriglyceridemia and concomitant LDL cholesterol elevation (*N Engl J Med 2007;357:1009*).
    - **Fibric acid derivatives**
      - Currently available fibric acid derivatives include **gemfibrozil**: 600 mg PO bid before meals; **fenofibrate**: typically 48 to 145 mg PO per day.
      - Fibrates generally lower triglyceride levels 30% to 50% and increase HDL levels 10% to 35%. They can lower LDL cholesterol levels by 5% to 25%

in patients with normal triglyceride levels but may actually increase LDL cholesterol levels in patients with elevated triglyceride levels.

▫ Common side effects include dyspepsia, abdominal pain, cholelithiasis, rash, and pruritus. Fibrates may potentiate the effects of warfarin (*N Engl J Med 1999;341:498*).

▫ Gemfibrozil given in conjunction with statins may increase the risk of rhabdomyolysis (*Am J Cardiol 2005;95:120*).

- **Omega-3 fatty acids**
  ▫ Omega-3 fatty acids from fish oil can lower triglycerides in high doses (*J Clin Endo Metab 2012;96:2969*).
  ▫ The active ingredients are eicosapentaenoic acid (EPA) and docosahexaenoic acid (DHA).
  ▫ To lower triglyceride levels, 1 to 6 g of EPA plus DHA is needed daily.
  ▫ Main side effects are burping, bloating, and diarrhea.
  ▫ A prescription form of omega-3 acid fatty acids is available and is indicated for triglycerides over 500 mg/dL; four tablets contain about 3.6 g of omega-3 acid ethyl esters and can lower triglycerides by 30%.
  ▫ In practice, omega-3 fatty acids are being used as an adjunct to statin or other drugs in patients with moderately elevated triglyceride levels.
  ▫ The combination of omega-3 fatty acids plus statin has the advantage of avoiding the risk of myopathy seen in the statin–fibrate combination (*Am J Cardiol 2008;102:429*; *Am J Cardiol 2008;102:1040*).

- **Treatment of low HDL cholesterol**
  ○ Low HDL cholesterol often occurs in the setting of hypertriglyceridemia and metabolic syndrome. Management of accompanying high LDL cholesterol, hypertriglyceridemia, and the metabolic syndrome may result in improvement of HDL cholesterol.
  ○ Nonpharmacologic therapies are the mainstay of treatment including:
    - Smoking cessation
    - Exercise
    - Weight loss
  ○ In addition, medications known to lower HDL cholesterol levels should be avoided such as β-blockers (except carvedilol), progestins, and androgenic compounds.
  ○ There are no cardiovascular clinical outcomes trials that have shown a clear benefit of raising HDL cholesterol.

Lifestyle/Risk Modification

Risk Assessment

- ATP III recognizes **five categories of CHD risk**: very high, high, moderately high, moderate, and lower risk. These CHD risk categories are defined in Table 3-12.
- DM, noncoronary atherosclerosis (symptomatic cerebrovascular disease, peripheral artery disease, abdominal aortic aneurysm), or multiple risk factors conferring a 10-year CHD risk of more than 20% are considered **CHD risk equivalents in ATP III** (*Circulation 2004;110:227*).
- Risk assessment for patients without known CHD or CHD risk equivalents begins with consideration of five risk factors (see Table 3-8) (*JAMA 2001;285:2486*).
- A Framingham score should be determined for any individual with two or more non-LDL cholesterol risk factors (*JAMA 2001;285:2486*; *Circulation 2004;*

110:227). An online calculator using continuous variables is available at *www.nhlbi.nih.gov*.

- Patients with multiple non-LDL cholesterol CHD risk factors are then divided into those with a **10-year CHD risk >20%, 10% to 20%, or <10%.**
- Presently, emerging risk factors (e.g., obesity, sedentary lifestyle, prothrombotic and proinflammatory factors, and impaired fasting glucose) do not impact risk assessment, although they may influence clinical judgment when determining therapeutic options.

4

Ischemic Heart Disease

Mohammad Kizilbash, Jeffrey R. Parker,
Muhammad A. Sarwar, and Jason D. Meyers

Coronary Heart Disease and Stable Angina

GENERAL PRINCIPLES

Definition

- Coronary artery disease (CAD) refers to the luminal narrowing of a coronary artery, usually due to atherosclerosis. CAD is the leading contributor to coronary heart disease (CHD). CHD includes angina pectoris, myocardial infarction (MI), and silent myocardial ischemia.
- Cardiovascular disease (CVD) is commonly defined to include CHD, heart failure, arrhythmia, hypertension, cerebrovascular accident (CVA), diseases of the aorta, peripheral vascular disease (PVD), valvular heart disease, and congenital heart disease.

Epidemiology

- In the United States, CHD is the cause of 1 of every 6 deaths.
- The lifetime risk of CHD, after 40 years of age, is 49% for men and 32% for women.
- The average number of years of life lost because of a MI is 16.6.
- Of those who die suddenly of CHD, 64% of women and 50% of men had no previous symptoms (*Circulation 2012;125:e2*).

Etiology

- CAD most commonly results from luminal accumulation of atheromatous plaque.
- Other causes of obstructive CAD include congenital coronary anomalies, myocardial bridging, vasculitis, and prior radiation therapy.
- Apart from obstructive CAD, other causes of angina include cocaine use, aortic stenosis, hypertrophic cardiomyopathy, left ventricular hypertrophy (LVH), malignant hypertension, dilated cardiomyopathy, spontaneous coronary dissection (most often noted in pregnant women), variant angina, and syndrome X.

Pathophysiology

- Common CAD manifestations include stable angina, acute coronary syndromes (ACS), sudden cardiac death, and heart failure.
- Notably, angiographically insignificant (<50% luminal stenosis) lesions account for the majority of acute MIs, which has led to the concept of the vulnerable plaque (*JACC 1988;12:56*; *Circulation 2003;108:1664*).
  - Rupturing/erosion of a vulnerable plaque leads to acute obstruction of coronary blood flow.
  - ACS represents a clinical continuum from unstable angina (UA), non–ST-segment MI (NSTEMI) when ischemia is severe enough to cause release of cardiac biomarkers, and ST-segment elevation MI (STEMI).

- Stable angina results from luminal obstruction of angiographically visible epicardial coronary arteries, which results in a mismatch between myocardial oxygen supply and demand causing inadequate distal microvascular perfusion. In contrast, syndrome X is disease of the microvascular circulation, not visible at angiography.
  - The coronary lesions responsible for stable angina differ from the vulnerable plaque associated with acute MI. The stable angina lesion is fixed and is less prone to fissuring, hence producing symptoms that are more predictable (*Circulation 2012;125:1147*).
  - Epicardial coronary lesions causing less than 50% luminal obstruction do not significantly impair coronary flow (with the exception of left main disease) and generally should not cause angina under normal circumstances but may under extremes of duress (e.g., septic shock).
  - Exertional angina generally develops when a stenosis reaches >70%, and a stenosis of >90% is expected to be associated with rest angina.

Risk Factors

- Of CHD events, >90% can be attributed to elevations in at least one major risk factor (*JAMA 2003;290:891*).
- Assessment of traditional CVD risk factors:
  - Age.
  - Blood pressure (BP).
  - Blood sugar (NOTE: Diabetes is considered a CHD risk equivalent).
  - Lipid profile (low-density lipoprotein [LDL], high-density lipoprotein [HDL], triglycerides). Direct LDL for nonfasting samples or very high triglycerides.
  - Tobacco use (NOTE: Smoking cessation restores the risk of CHD to that of a nonsmoker within approximately 15 years) (*Arch Intern Med 1994;154(2):169*).
  - Family history of premature CAD: Defined as first-degree male relative with CHD before age 55 years or female relative before age 65 years.
  - Measures for obesity, particularly central obesity. Body mass index goal is between 18.5 to 24.9 kg/m^2. Waist circumference goal is <40 inches for men and <35 inches for women.
  - Assessment for physical inactivity and poor diet.
  - Assessment of CHD risk equivalents (PVD, CVA, aortic aneurysm, diabetes).
  - Assess for chronic kidney disease or history of systemic autoimmune collagen-vascular diseases.
  - In women, assess for history of preeclampsia or gestational diabetes.
- A Global Risk Score (GRS) should be calculated to determine the absolute risk for CHD **or** CVD in the next 10 years based on the presence of individual risk factors in all individuals without known CHD or CHD risk equivalent.
  - Most validated is the Framingham Risk Score (see section on hyperlipidemia) for major CHD events (MI or coronary death) (*http://hp2010.nhlbihin.net/ATPiii/calculator.asp?usertype=prof*).
  - **Note the availability of the *updated* Framingham CVD Risk Profile for major CVD events.** Given women have a higher stroke burden, estimation of CVD risk is superior to CHD risk only (*JACC 2011;57:1404*). (*http://www.framinghamheartstudy.org/risk/gencardio.html#*)
  - Other GRS methods include Systemic Coronary Risk Evaluation (SCORE) for CVD death and the Reynolds Risk Score for major CVD events.

- ○ Based on the GRS patients can be categorized as low, intermediate, or high risk for CHD or CVD over the next 10 years.
  - ■ Low (<10% CHD risk) risk patients are not appropriate further testing or pharmaceuticals. Lifestyle interventions are stressed.
  - ■ Intermediate (10% to 20% CHD risk) risk patients could be appropriate for further testing to better delineate risk. Testing may aid in determining whether a patient may benefit from statin or aspirin (ASA) therapy, or serve as a catalyst for the patient to make necessary lifestyle changes. Further testing could include:
    - □ Coronary Artery Calcium scoring by computed tomography (CT), a score >400 would reclassify to high risk.
    - □ Ankle-Brachial Index (ABI) ratios (blood pressure ratio of legs over the arms) <0.9 or >1.3 suggests presence of PVD and would reclassify to high risk.
    - □ Carotid intima media thickness (assessed by ultrasound) levels >75 percentile would reclassify to high risk.
    - □ High Sensitive C-reactive protein (hs-CRP) could be considered in men older than 50 years and women older than 60 years with LDL-cholesterol (LDL-C) <130 mg/dL with hs-CRP levels >2 mg/dL used as criteria to begin statin therapy.
  - ■ High (>20% CHD risk **or** >10% risk for CVD events) risk patients are not appropriate for further risk assessment and need intensive risk factor modification.
- • Lifetime risk: It is important to note that individuals at low/moderate 10-year risk may still be at high risk over a longer period of time (e.g., 1 in 25 person risk over 10 years, but a 1 in 2 person risk over the long term) due to the cumulative time effect of even a single elevated risk factor or multiple nonoptimal risk factors (*JACC 2011;57:1404*).
  - ○ Ten-year GRS underestimates risk in younger adults.
  - ○ Maintaining ideal cardiovascular risk factors early in adult life, prior to any need for pharmaceutical or other intervention is the key in primary prevention of CVD (Table 4-1).

Table 4-1	Ideal Cardiovascular Health Includes All of the Following
Risk Factor	**Criteria**
Total cholesterol	<200 mg/dL without treatment
Blood pressure	<120/80 mm Hg without treatment
Fasting blood glucose	<100 mg/dL
Body mass index	<25 kg/m^2
Tobacco use	Never used
Physical activity	>150 min/wk of moderate intensity or >75 min of high intensity
Diet	Maintaining a healthy diet (e.g., DASH diet)

DASH, Dietary Approaches to Stop Hypertension.
Adapted from Mosca L, Benjamin EJ, Berra K, et al. Effectiveness-Based Guidelines for the Prevention of Cardiovascular Disease in Women—2011 Update: A Guideline From the American Heart Association. *J Am Coll Cardiol* 2011;57:1404.

Prevention

- ASA (75 to 162 mg/d) should be considered in men with >10% risk CVD event risk over 10 years. ASA (75 to 162 mg/d) should be considered in women at high risk (>20% CVD event risk). Risk of ASA-related bleeding should not outweigh its potential benefit.
- Cholesterol and blood pressure should be managed (see Chapter 3, Preventive Cardiology).
- Physical activity of >150 min/wk of moderate intensity or >75 min/wk of vigorous activity should be encouraged.
- A healthy DASH-like diet can be beneficial. See *www.nhlbi.nih.gov/health/public/heart/hbp/dash/new_dash.pdf*
- Tobacco products should be avoided.
  - Assess willingness to quit.
  - Develop a quitting plan.
  - Consider available pharmacotherapy.
    - Nicotine patch, nicotine gum, nicotine spray, or nicotine inhalers.
    - Bupropion alone or in combination with nicotine replacement therapy.
    - 150 mg PO daily for 3 days, followed by 150 mg PO twice daily for 8 to 12 weeks. The patient is instructed to avoid smoking on days 5 to 7. It is contraindicated in patients at risk for seizures.
    - Varenicline is used for 12 to 24 weeks. Patients need to be monitored for risk of depression and suicide ideation. Also, its use is associated with a slight increase risk of CVD events.
- Hormone replacement therapy, antioxidants, and folic acid are not indicated for primary or secondary CAD prevention (*JACC 2011;57:1404*).

Clinical Presentation

History

- Angina: **Typical angina has three features**: (1) substernal chest discomfort with a characteristic quality and duration that is (2) provoked by stress or exertion and (3) relieved by rest or nitroglycerin (NTG).
  - **Atypical angina** has two of these three characteristics.
  - **Noncardiac chest pain** meets one or none of these characteristics.
- Chronic stable angina is reproducibly precipitated in a predictable manner by exertion or emotional stress and relieved within 5 to 10 minutes by sublingual nitroglycerin or rest.
- The severity of angina may be quantified using the Canadian Cardiovascular Society (CCS) classification system (Table 4-2).
- Associated symptoms may include dyspnea, diaphoresis, nausea, vomiting, and dizziness.
- Female patients and those with diabetes or chronic kidney disease may have minimal or atypical symptoms that serve as anginal equivalents. Such symptoms include dyspnea (most common), epigastric pain, and nausea.
- It is important to determine the pretest probability of CAD in patients with angina. Pretest probability will guide testing as well as test interpretation in patients with suspected angina (Table 4-3). For example, a young patient with complaints of typical angina is unlikely to have significant CAD on testing, while atypical cardiac pain in an older adult may warrant noninvasive testing. An older man or woman with typical angina, however, especially in association with cardiac risk factors, may be better served with an angiogram due to the risk of a false negative study with a noninvasive stress test.

Table 4-2	Canadian Cardiovascular Society Classification System

Class	Definition
CCS 1	Angina with strenuous or prolonged activity
CCS 2	Angina with moderate activity (walking greater than two level blocks or one flight of stairs)
CCS 3	Angina with mild activity (walking less than two level blocks or one flight of stairs)
CCS 4	Angina that occurs with any activity or at rest

Anginal symptoms may include typical chest discomfort or anginal equivalents.
CCS, Canadian Cardiovascular Society.
From Sangareddi V, Anand C, Gnanavelu G, et al. Canadian Cardiovascular Society classification of effort angina: an angiographic correlation. *Coronary Artery Dis* 2004;15:111–114.

Physical Examination
- Clinical exam should include measurement of blood pressure, heart rate, and arterial pulses.
- Exam findings of a mitral regurgitation (MR) murmur, which is new or worsening, is a high risk exam finding, other murmurs may clue the presence of aortic stenosis or hypertrophic cardiomyopathy with the latter murmur being the only one to worsening with Valsalva.
- Stigmata of hyperlipidemia such as corneal arcus and xanthelasmas should be noted.
- Signs of heart failure including an S_3 gallop, inspiratory crackles on lung exam, elevated jugular venous pulsation, and peripheral edema are also high risk exam findings.

Differential Diagnosis
- A wide range of disorders may manifest with chest discomfort and may include both cardiovascular and noncardiovascular etiologies (Table 4-4).

Table 4-3	Pretest Probability of Coronary Artery Disease by Age, Gender, and Symptoms

Age (yr)	Asymptomatic		Nonanginal Chest Pain		Atypical/ Probable Angina Pectoris		Typical/ Definite Angina Pectoris	
Gender	Women	Men	Women	Men	Women	Men	Women	Men
30–39	<5	<5	2	4	12	34	26	76
40–49	<5	<10	3	13	22	51	55	87
50–59	<5	<10	7	20	31	65	73	93
60–69	<5	<5	14	27	51	72	86	94
	Very Low <5%		Low <10%		Intermediate 10%–80%		High >80%	

Data from Gibbons RJ, Balady GJ, Bricker JT, et al. ACC/AHA 2002 guideline update for exercise testing: Summary article. A report of the ACC/AHA Task Force on Practice Guidelines (Committee to Update the 1997 Exercise Testing Guidelines). *Circulation* 2002;106:1883.

Table 4-4	Differential Diagnosis of Chest Pain
Diagnosis	**Comments**
Cardiovascular	
Aortic stenosis	Anginal episodes can occur with severe aortic stenosis.
HCM	Subendocardial ischemia may occur with exercise and/or exertion.
Prinzmetal angina	Coronary vasospasm that may be elicited by exertion or emotional stress.
Syndrome X	Ischemic chest pain in the presence of normal coronary arteries that is thought to be related to microvascular disease.
Pericarditis	Pleuritic chest pain associated with pericardial inflammation from infectious or autoimmune disease.
Aortic dissection	May mimic anginal pain and/or involve the coronary arteries.
Cocaine use	Results in coronary vasospasm and/or thrombus formation.
Other	
Anemia	Marked anemia can result in a myocardial O_2 supply–demand mismatch.
Thyrotoxicosis	Increase in myocardial demand may result in an O_2 supply–demand mismatch.
Esophageal disease	GERD and esophageal spasm can mimic angina (responsive to NTG).
Biliary colic	Gallstones can usually be visualized on abdominal sonography.
Respiratory diseases	Pneumonia with pleuritic pain. Pulmonary embolism. Pulmonary hypertension.
Musculoskeletal	Costochondritis, cervical radiculopathy.

GERD, gastroesophageal reflux disease; HCM, hypertrophic cardiomyopathy; NTG, nitroglycerin.

- A careful history focused on cardiac risk factors, physical exam, and initial laboratory evaluation usually narrows the differential diagnosis.

Diagnostic Testing
- **Stress testing and indications**
  - Patients without known CAD:
    - Not indicated in asymptomatic patients as a screening test.
    - Patients with anginal symptoms.
    - Asymptomatic intermediate-risk patients who plan on beginning a vigorous exercise program or those with high-risk occupations (e.g., airline pilot).
    - Asymptomatic high-risk patients with risk factors such as diabetes or PVD.
  - Patients with known CAD:
    - Post-MI risk stratification (see section on STEMI).
    - Preoperative risk assessment.

Table 4-5	Exercise Stress Testing: Duke Treadmill Score

Duke Treadmill Score (DTS) = Minutes exercised − [5 × maximum ST-segment deviation] − [4 × angina score]. Angina score: 0 = none, 1 = not test limiting, 2 = test limiting

DTS Score

5	Annual mortality 0.25%	Low-risk study
−10 to 4	Annual mortality 1.25%	Intermediate-risk study
<−10	Annual mortality >5%	High-risk study

In general, β-blockers, other nodal blocking agents, and nitrates should be discontinued prior to stress testing.
Data from *N Engl J Med* 1991;325:849.

- Recurrent anginal symptoms despite medical therapy or revascularization.
- Routine screening in asymptomatic patients after revascularization is controversial.
- **Exercise stress testing**
  - The test of choice for evaluating most patients of intermediate risk for CAD (Table 4-3).
  - Bruce Protocol: Consists of 3-min stages of increasing treadmill speed and incline. BP, heart rate, and electrocardiogram (ECG) are monitored throughout the study and the recovery period.
  - Specificity and sensitivity of 70% to 80% if the patient has a normal resting ECG and reaches the target heart rate (85% of maximal predicted heart rate for age).
  - The study is considered positive if:
    - New ST-segment depressions of >1 mm in multiple leads
    - Hypotensive response to exercise
    - Sustained ventricular arrhythmias are precipitated by exercise
  - The Duke Treadmill Score provides prognostic information for patients presenting with chronic angina (Table 4-5).
- **Stress testing with imaging**
  - Recommended for patients with the following baseline ECG abnormalities:
    - Preexcitation (Wolf–Parkinson–White syndrome)
    - LVH
    - Left bundle branch block (LBBB) or paced rhythm
    - Intraventricular conduction delay (IVCD)
    - Digoxin effects
    - Resting ST-segment or T-wave changes
  - **Myocardial perfusion imaging.** Commonly utilizes tracers Thallium-201 or technetium-99m in conjunction with exercise or pharmacologic stress. Perfusion imaging allows the diagnosis and localization of areas of ischemia and allows determination of ejection fraction (EF). Myocardial viability can also be assessed via this technique. Nuclear perfusion stress imaging has a sensitivity of 85% to 90% and specificity of 70%.
  - **Echocardiographic imaging.** Exercise or dobutamine stress testing can be performed with echocardiography to aid in the diagnosis of CAD. As with nuclear imaging, echocardiography adds to the sensitivity and specificity of the test by

revealing areas with wall motion abnormalities. The technical quality of this study can be limited by imaging quality (i.e., obesity). Stress echocardiography has a sensitivity of 75% and specificity of 85% to 90%.

- ○ **Magnetic resonance perfusion imaging** with adenosine utilizing contrast enhancement is another tool to evaluate myocardial ischemia and viability.
- **Pharmacologic stress testing**
  - ○ In patients who are unable to exercise, pharmacologic stress testing may be preferable.
  - ○ Dipyridamole, adenosine, and regadenoson are vasodilators that are commonly used in conjunction with myocardial perfusion scintigraphy. These agents are the agents of choice in patients with LBBB or paced rhythm on ECG due to the increased incidence of false-positive stress tests with either exercise or dobutamine infusion.
  - ○ Dobutamine is a positive inotrope commonly used with echocardiographic stress tests.
- **Contraindications to stress testing**
  - ○ Acute MI within 2 days
  - ○ UA not previously stabilized by medical therapy
  - ○ Cardiac arrhythmias causing symptoms or hemodynamic compromise
  - ○ Symptomatic severe aortic stenosis
  - ○ Symptomatic heart failure
  - ○ Acute pulmonary embolus, myocarditis, pericarditis, or aortic dissection

Diagnostic Procedures
- **Coronary Angiography**
  - ○ The gold standard for evaluating epicardial coronary anatomy since it quantifies the presence and severity of atherosclerotic lesions.
  - ○ Coronary angiography is invasive and is associated with a small risk of death, MI, CVA, bleeding, arrhythmia, and vascular complications. Therefore, it is reserved for patients whose risk benefit ratio favors an invasive approach such as:
    - ▪ STEMI patients
    - ▪ Most UA/NSTEMI patients
    - ▪ Symptomatic patients with high-risk stress tests who are expected to benefit from revascularization
    - ▪ Class III and IV angina despite medical therapy
    - ▪ Survivors of sudden cardiac death or those with serious ventricular arrhythmias
    - ▪ Signs or symptoms of heart failure or decreased LV EF
    - ▪ Angina, that from the patients perspective, is inadequately controlled with medical therapy alone for their particular lifestyle
    - ▪ Previous coronary artery bypass grafting (CABG) or percutaneous coronary intervention (PCI)
    - ▪ Suspected/known left main (≥50% stenosis) or severe three-vessel CAD
    - ▪ To diagnosis CAD in patients with angina who have not undergone stress testing due to a very high pretest probability of having CAD (see Table 4-3).
  - ○ Can be both diagnostic and therapeutic if PCI is needed.
  - ○ Can be used to evaluate patients who are suspected of having a nonatherosclerotic cause of ischemia (e.g., coronary anomaly, coronary dissection, radiation vasculopathy).
  - ○ Intravascular ultrasound (IVUS) can be employed to further assess plaque burden, providing definitive assessment of the coronary vasculature at time of catheterization.

○ Functional significance of a stenotic lesion can further be assessed by fractional flow reserve (FFR) at the time of the catheterization. This can be useful in evaluation of coronary lesions of questionable clinical severity or discovered incidentally with an FFR ≤0.8 considered flow limiting.

○ LV catheterization also allows measurement of LV filling pressures (diastolic function), aortic and mitral valve gradients, assessment of regional wall motion and LV function, and assessment for certain aortopathies.

- **Contrast-induced nephropathy (CIN)** occurs in up to 5% of patients and is more common in patients with baseline renal insufficiency and diabetics. In most patients, creatinine returns to baseline within 7 days. The following are considerations in the prevention of CIN:

○ The volume of contrast media used should be minimized, and consideration for staged interventions in those with a creatinine clearance <60 mL/min.

○ Adequate hydration should be given prior to angiography.

○ Nonionic low osmolal contrast agents should be used. N-acetyl-L-cysteine and intravenous (IV) bicarbonate are not useful in the prevention of CIN, regardless of baseline risk.

- **Cardiac computed tomography**

○ A noninvasive technique used to establish a diagnosis of CAD. Like cardiac catheterization, it exposes the patient to both radiation and contrast material. Its current role in the management of CAD is under investigation.

○ It has a high negative predictive value and hence better suited for symptomatic patients with low to intermediate pretest probability for CAD to rule out disease. Such as patient with repeated emergency room admissions for chest pain or patients with equivocal stress test results.

○ May aid in identification of congenital anomalies of the coronary arteries.

○ Due to diminished study quality, it is not useful in patients with extensive coronary calcification, coronary stents, or small caliber vessels.

TREATMENT

- The major goal of treatment is to prevent MI, cardiac death, and to reduce symptoms.
- A combination of lifestyle modification, medical therapy, and coronary revascularization can be employed. A recommended strategy for the evaluation and management of the patient with stable angina can be found in Figure 4-1.
- **Medical treatment** is aimed at improving myocardial oxygen supply, reducing myocardial oxygen demand, controlling exacerbating factors (anemia, valvular disease), and limiting the development of further atherosclerotic disease. Medical treatment often is sufficient to control anginal symptoms in chronic stable angina and, as compared to coronary revascularization, produces similar long-term results.

Medications

- ASA (75 to 162 mg/d) reduces cardiovascular events including repeat revascularization, MI, and cardiac death by approximately 33% (*BMJ 1994;308:81*; *Lancet 1992;114:1421*).

○ 81 mg ASA appears to be sufficient for most patients (primary or secondary prevention for both CHD and CVA).

○ ASA desensitization may be performed in patients with ASA allergy.

○ Clopidogrel (75 mg/d) can be used in those allergic/intolerant of ASA.

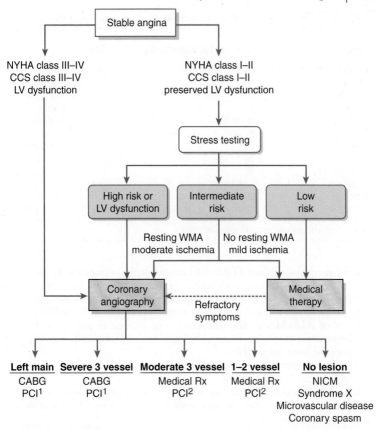

Figure 4-1. Approach to the evaluation and management of the patient of stable angina. Patients with clinical heart failure, severe limiting angina, and those with LV dysfunction should undergo coronary angiography to define underlying coronary artery disease. Patients without these features may undergo further risk stratification with stress testing. Following stress testing, patients may undergo either coronary angiography or empiric medical therapy depending on their risk profile. Patients initially treated with medical therapy who have refractory symptoms should undergo angiography. [1]CABG generally preferred due to known survival advantage over medical therapy alone; however, if the coronary lesions are not complex, PCI may offer similar results to CABG but with a higher need for future revascularizations. [2]PCI should be reserved for patients who have high-grade lesions, severe ischemia, and are refractory to medical therapy. CABG, coronary artery bypass grafting; CCS, Canadian Cardiovascular Society Classification (angina); LV, left ventricle; NICM, nonischemic cardiomyopathy; NYHA, New York Heart Association; PCI, percutaneous coronary intervention; WMA, wall motion abnormality.

Table 4-6	β-Blockers Commonly Used for Ischemic Heart Disease	
Drug	**β-Receptor Selectivity**	**Dose**
Propranolol	β_1 and β_2	20–80 mg bid
Metoprolol	β_1	50–200 mg bid
Atenolol	β_1	50–200 mg daily
Nebivolol	β_1	5–40 mg daily
Nadolol	β_1 and β_2	40–80 mg daily
Timolol	β_1 and β_2	10–30 mg tid
Acebutolol*	β_1	200–600 mg bid
Bisoprolol	β_1	10–20 mg daily
Esmolol (IV)	β_1	50–300 mcg/kg/min
Labetalol	Combined α, β_1, β_2	200–600 mg bid
Pindolol*	β_1 and β_2	2.5–7.5 mg tid
Carvedilol	Combined α, β_1, β_2	3.125–25 mg bid

*β-blockers with intrinsic sympathomimetic activity

- ○ β-Adrenergic antagonists (Table 4-6) control anginal symptoms by decreasing heart rate and myocardial work leading to reduced myocardial oxygen demand.
  - ■ β-Blockers with intrinsic sympathomimetic activity should be avoided.
  - ■ Dosage can be adjusted to result in a resting heart rate of 50 to 60 bpm.
  - ■ Use of β-blockers is used with caution or avoided in patients with active bronchospasm, atrioventricular (AV) block, resting bradycardia, or poorly compensated heart failure (HF).
  - ■ β-Blockers may worsen coronary vasospasm and should be avoided in vasospastic or Prinzmetal variant angina.
- ○ Calcium channel blockers can be used either in conjunction with or in lieu of β-blockers in the presence of contraindications or adverse effects as a second-line agent (Table 4-7).
  - ■ Calcium antagonists are often used in conjunction with β-blockers if the latter are not fully effective at relieving anginal symptoms. Both long-acting dihydropyridines and nondihydropyridine agents can be used.
  - ■ Calcium channel blockers are effective agents for the treatment of coronary vasospasm.
  - ■ Nondihydropyridine agents (verapamil/diltiazem) are avoided in patients with systolic dysfunction due to their negative inotropic effects.
  - ■ The use of short-acting dihydropyridines (nifedipine) should be avoided due to the potential to increase the risk of adverse cardiac events.
- ○ Nitrates, either long-acting formulations for chronic use or sublingual/topical preparations for acute anginal symptoms. More often used as adjunctive antianginal agents (Table 4-8).
  - ■ Sublingual preparations should be used at the first indication of angina or prophylactically before engaging in activities that are known to precipitate angina. Patients should seek prompt medical attention if angina occurs at rest or fails to respond to the third sublingual dose.
  - ■ Nitrate tolerance resulting in reduced therapeutic response may occur with all nitrate preparations. The institution of a nitrate-free period of 10 to 12 hours (usually at night) can enhance treatment efficacy.

Table 4-7	Calcium Channel Blockers Commonly Used for Ischemic Heart Disease		
Drug	**Duration of Action**		**Usual Dosage**
Dihydropyridines			
Nifedipine			
Slow release	Long		30–180 mg/d
Amlodipine	Long		5–10 mg/d
Felodipine (SR)	Long		5–10 mg/d
Isradipine (SR)	Medium		2.5–10 mg/d
Nicardipine	Short		20–40 mg tid
Nondihydropyridines			
Diltiazem			
Immediate release	Short		30–80 mg qid
Slow release	Long		120–360 mg/d
Verapamil			
Immediate release	Short		80–160 mg tid
Slow release	Long		120–480 mg/d

- For patients with CAD, nitrates have not shown a mortality benefit.
- Nitrates are contraindicated (even in patients with ACS) for use in patients who are on phoshodiesterase-5 inhibitors due to risk of severe hypotension. A washout period of 24 hours for sildenafil and vardenafil and 48 hours for tadalafil is required prior to nitrate use.
  - ACE inhibitors (ACEIs) may have additive benefit in the treatment of stable angina.
  - ACEI therapy or angiotensin receptor blockers (ARBs) in those intolerant to ACEI, should be used in all in patients with an LV EF <40%, and in those with hypertension, diabetes, or chronic kidney disease.
  - It is reasonable to use ACEI in all stable angina patients.
  - ACEI use can be associated with life-threatening angioedema and cough and may worsen kidney function (particularly in the setting of dehydration, strict

Table 4-8	Nitrate Preparations Commonly Used for Ischemic Heart Disease		
Preparation	**Dosage**	**Onset (min)**	**Duration**
Sublingual nitroglycerin	0.3–0.6 mg prn	2–5	10–30 min
Aerosol nitroglycerin	0.4 mg prn	2–5	10–30 min
Oral isosorbide dinitrate	5–40 mg tid	30–60	4–6 hr
Oral isosorbide mononitrate	10–20 mg bid	30–60	6–8 hr
Oral isosorbide mononitrate SR	30–120 mg daily	30–60	12–18 hr
2% Nitroglycerin ointment	0.5–2.0 in. tid	20–60	3–8 hr
Transdermal nitroglycerin patches	5–15 mg daily	>60	12 hr
Intravenous nitroglycerin	10–200 mcg/min	<2	During infusion

sodium retention, concomitant use of nonsteroidal anti-inflammatory drug [NSAID] and in 5% to 10% of patients with bilateral renal artery stenosis).
- ACEI associated cough and angioedema are rare with use of ARBs.
○ Ranolazine is an antianginal agent that does not depend on reductions in heart rate or BP. Generally not used as a first- or second-line agent.
○ Cholesterol-lowering agents including statins, fibrates, bile acid sequestrants, and niacin (see Chapter 3, Preventive Cardiology). Note, in secondary prevention of CHD apart from statins, no other cholesterol agents have proven consistent mortality benefit.

Surgical Management

- **Coronary revascularization**
  ○ In general, medical therapy with at least two, and preferably three classes of antianginal agents should be attempted before medical therapy is considered a failure and coronary revascularization pursued.
  ○ In patients with stable angina and no high-risk features (e.g., high-risk stress test or low LV function), medical therapy results in similar cardiovascular outcomes when compared to PCI, except that PCI offers greater short- and long-term relief of angina symptoms. Patients should be aware, as part of the informed consent, that their risk for MI or death is not altered (*N Engl J Med 2007;256:1503; Lancet 1997;350:461*). However, patients with certain coronary lesions have a survival advantage with revascularization as compared to medical therapy alone (see the following text).
  ○ The choice between PCI and CABG surgery is dependent on the coronary anatomy, medical comorbidities, and patient preference.
    ■ In general, patients with complex and diffuse disease do better with CABG; while PCI in select patients with the proper coronary anatomy can provide comparable results as CABG. Due to the more extensive nature of CABG, patient comorbidities often necessitate PCI for revascularization.
    ■ The decision between medical therapy, PCI and CABG should consider whether both symptom and mortality benefit is sought or symptom relief alone is sufficient. PCI and CABG are both effective at symptom relief of angina.
    ■ We recommend that the decision between CABG or PCI, when both are feasible, take into consideration risk of surgery using the Society of Thoracic Surgeons (STS) risk score as well as the Syntax score to determine how suitable the coronary antimony is for PCI. (*http://riskcalc.sts.org/STSWebRiskCalc273/, http://www.syntaxscore.com/*)
  ○ Revascularization is shown to **improve survival** in the following circumstances as compared to medical therapy in:
    ■ CABG for >50% left main disease. PCI is a reasonable alternative for patients with left main disease if the patient is a poor surgical candidate and has a favorable morphology for PCI. PCI, in the right clinical context, can offer rates of MI, CVA, or death similar to CABG (*N Engl J Med 2009;360:961*).
    ■ CABG for three-vessel disease or disease in the proximal left anterior descending (LAD) and one other artery in patients with an LV EF of >35% when either reversible ischemia or viable myocardium is noted on noninvasive stress testing.
    ■ Survival advantage for CABG in patients with an LV EF <35% (with or without viability) might be superior to medical therapy (*N Engl J Med 2011;364:1607*). PCI has not been evaluated as compared to CABG with decreased LV EF and the choice between CABG and PCI should be based on anatomy, presence of diabetes or chronic kidney disease, and other surgical comorbidities.

- CABG for two-vessel disease in the setting of severe ischemia observed on stress imaging (e.g., >20% of myocardium ischemic or significant viable myocardium present on cardiac imaging).
- Patients with isolated proximal LAD disease *may* have a survival advantage with PCI or CABG (*JACC 2008;1:483*; *Ann Thorac Surg 2006;82:1420*).
- CABG, as compared to PCI or medical therapy, in patients with multivessel disease and diabetes, if a left internal mammary artery (LIMA) to the LAD can be placed (*N Engl J Med 1996;335:217*). PCI *may* offer similar survival outcomes in diabetics with multivessel disease and a low syntax score (<22) but with a higher need for repeat revascularization (*JACC 2010;55:1067*).
- PCI or CABG in patients who have survived sudden cardiac death due to ischemic ventricular tachycardia.
- PCI or CABG in patients with ACS.

○ Due to the morbidity of a repeat CABG, PCI is often used to improve symptoms in patients with recurrent angina after CABG.
○ CABG carries a 1% to 3% mortality rate, 5% to 10% incidence of periopera-tive MI, and a small risk of perioperative stroke. The use of internal mammary artery grafts is associated with 90% graft patency at 10 years, compared with 40% to 50% for saphenous vein grafts. The long-term patency of a radial artery graft is 80% at 5 years. After 10 years of follow-up, 50% of patients develop recurrent angina or other adverse cardiac events related to late vein graft failure or progression of native CAD (*N Engl J Med 1996;334:216*).
○ The risks of elective PCI include <1% mortality, a 2% to 5% rate of nonfatal MI, and <1% need for emergent CABG for an unsuccessful procedure. Patients undergoing PCI have shorter hospitalizations. PCI does have a higher rate of target lesion restenosis requiring repeated procedures and, as compared to CABG, a higher rate of CVD events attributed to the latter. Use of drug eluting stents has shown decreased rates of restenosis, but need for repeat procedure is still higher than observed post-CABG (*N Engl J Med 2009;360:961*; *N Engl J Med 2005;352:2174*). **NOTE:** In some patients with stable angina and multivessel disease who have a low syntax score (score based on lesion complexity, length, and location) of less than 22, PCI might be equal to CABG in terms of survival and is associated with less procedure related risk of stroke.
○ Post-PCI, patients need to take ASA and a P2Y12 antagonist for 12 months; however, patients who receive a bare metal stent may stop the P2Y12 antagonist after a minimum of 1 month of therapy. This may be necessary and a planned option in patients who may need surgery within the year or is at high risk of bleeding. **NOTE:** Patients who are expected to be nonadherent or unable to tolerate dual antiplatelet therapy with ASA and a P2Y12 antagonist for the minimum time period for the type of stent they receive should not be offered PCI with coronary stenting.

PATIENT EDUCATION

- Compliance with medications, diet, and exercise should be stressed to patients. All patients should be encouraged to participate in cardiac rehab as well as meet with a registered dietician.
- Patients with known CAD should present for evaluation if any change in chest pain pattern, frequency, or intensity develops.
- Patients should also be reevaluated if they report the presence of any HF symptoms.

MONITORING/FOLLOW-UP

- Close patient follow-up is a critical component of the treatment of CAD as lifestyle modification and secondary risk factor reduction require serial reassessment and interventions.
- Relatively minor changes in anginal symptoms can be safely treated with titration and/or addition of antianginal medications.
- Significant changes in anginal complaints (frequency, severity, or time to onset with activity) should be evaluated by either stress testing (usually in conjunction with an imaging modality) or cardiac catheterization as warranted.
- Cardiac rehabilitation or an exercise program should be offered or instituted.
- All primary prevention efforts (discussed earlier) are also valid in secondary prevention

Acute Coronary Syndromes, Unstable Angina, and Non–ST-Segment Elevation Myocardial Infarction

GENERAL PRINCIPLES

- NSTEMI and UA are closely related conditions whose pathogenesis and clinical presentations are similar but differ in severity.
- If coronary flow is not severe enough or the occlusion does not persist long enough to cause myocardial necrosis (as indicated by positive cardiac biomarkers), the syndrome is labeled UA.
- NSTEMI is defined by an elevation of cardiac enzymes (creatine kinase MB [CK-MB] or troponin) and the absence of ST-segment elevation. Of NSTEMI patients, 25% develop Q wave MIs.
- The management of ACS should focus on risk stratification based on history, angina characteristics, physical examination, ECG, and cardiac enzymes.

Epidemiology

- The annual incidence of MI is 785,000 new events, and 470,000 recurrent attacks (*Circulation 2011;123:e18*).
- Among patients with ACS, approximately 60% have UA and 40% have MI (one-third of MIs present with an acute STEMI).
- At 1 year, patients with UA/NSTEMI are at considerable risk for death (~6%), recurrent MI (~11%), and need for revascularization (~50% to 60%). It is important to note that although the short-term mortality of STEMI is greater than that of NSTEMI, the long-term mortality is similar (*JACC 2007;50:e1*; *JAMA 1996;275:1104*).
- The incidence of CHD in women lags behind men by 10 years and by 20 years for more serious clinical events such as MI and sudden death.

Pathophysiology

- Myocardial ischemia results from decreased myocardial oxygen supply and/or increased demand. In the majority of cases, NSTEMI is due to a sudden decrease in blood supply via partial occlusion of the affected vessel. In some cases, marked increased myocardial oxygen demand may lead to NSTEMI (demand ischemia), as seen in severe anemia or a hypertensive crisis.

- UA/NSTEMI most often represents severe coronary artery narrowing or acute atherosclerotic plaque rupture/erosion and superimposed thrombus formation. Alternatively, it may also be due to progressive mechanical obstruction from advancing atherosclerotic disease, in-stent restenosis (ISR), or bypass graft disease.
- Plaque rupture may be triggered by local and/or systemic inflammation as well as shear stress. Rupture leads to exposure of lipid-rich subendothelial components to circulating platelets and inflammatory cells, serving as a potent substrate for thrombus formation.
- Less common causes include dynamic obstruction of the coronary artery due to vasospasm (Prinzmetal angina, cocaine), coronary artery dissection (consider in peripartum women), coronary vasculitis, and embolus.

Clinical Presentation

History

- ACS symptoms include all the qualities of typical angina except the episodes are more severe and of longer duration and may occur at rest.
- The three principal presentations for UA are **rest angina** (angina occurring at rest and prolonged, usually >20 minutes), **new-onset angina**, and **progressive angina** (previously diagnosed angina that has become more frequent, lasts longer, or occurs with less exertion). New-onset and progressive angina should occur with at least mild to moderate activity, CCS class III severity.
  - Female sex, diabetes, HF, end-stage kidney disease, and older age are traits that have been associated a higher chance of atypical ACS symptoms.
  - Dyspnea is the most common presentation in silent MIs.
  - Jaw, neck, arm, back, or epigastric pain can be angina equivalents.

Physical Examination

Physical examination should be directed at identifying hemodynamic instability, pulmonary congestion, and other causes of acute chest discomfort.

- Objective evidence of HF, including peripheral hypoperfusion, heart murmur (particularly MR murmur), elevated jugular venous pulsation, pulmonary edema, hypotension, and peripheral edema, worsen the prognosis and affect management.
- Examination may also give clues to other causes of ischemia such as thyrotoxicosis or aortic dissection (see Table 4-4).

Diagnostic Testing

Electrocardiography

- A baseline ECG should be obtained in all patients with suspected ACS, prior to or immediately on arrival to the emergency department. A normal tracing does not exclude the presence of disease.
- The presence of Q waves, ST-segment changes, or T-wave inversions are suggestive of CAD.
- Isolated Q waves in lead III only are a normal finding.
- Serial ECGs should be obtained to assess for dynamic ischemic changes.
- Comparison to prior ECGs is important when evaluating an ECG for dynamic changes.
- Approximately 50% of patients with UA/NSTEMI have significant ECG abnormalities, including transient ST-segment elevations, ST depressions, and T-wave inversions (*JACC 2007;50:e1*).
  - ST-segment depression in two contiguous leads is a sensitive indicator of myocardial ischemia, especially if dynamic and associated with symptoms.

- Threshold value for abnormal J-point depression should be −0.05 mm in leads V_2 and V_3 and −1 mm in all other leads.
- ST-segment depression in multiple leads with ST-segment elevation in aVR and/or V_1 suggests ischemia due to multivessel or left main disease.
  - Deeply inverted T waves (>5 mm) with QT prolongation in leads V2 to V4 (Wellens' waves) are strongly suggestive of a particularly worrisome critical lesion in the LAD artery distribution or recent intracranial hemorrhage.
  - Nonspecific ST-segment changes or T-wave inversions (those that do not meet voltage criteria) are nondiagnostic and unhelpful in management of acute ischemia but are associated with a higher risk for future cardiac events.

Laboratories
- A complete blood count, basic metabolic panel, fasting glucose, and lipid profile should be obtained in all patients with suspected CAD. Other conditions may be found to be contributing to ischemia (e.g., anemia), mimicking ischemic (e.g., hyperkalemia-related ECG changes), or may alter management (e.g., severe thrombocytopenia).
- Cardiac biomarkers are essential in the diagnosis of UA/NSTEMI and should be obtained in all patients who present with chest discomfort suggestive of ACS. In patients with negative cardiac markers within 6 hours of the onset of pain, a second sample should be drawn 8 to 12 hours after symptom onset. The most commonly measured markers are troponins, CK-MB, and myoglobin (Table 4-9).

Table 4-9	Cardiac Biomarkers		
	Detectable	**Peak**	**Return to Baseline**
Troponin I, T	3–6 hr	24–36 hr	5–14 d
CK-MB	2–6 hr	12–18 hr	24–48 hr
Myoglobin	1–2 hr	6–8 hr	12–24 hr

CK-MB, creatine kinase MB.

- Cardiac-specific troponin is the preferred marker and should be measured in all patients.
  - Troponin T and I assays are highly specific and sensitive markers of myocardial necrosis. Serum troponin levels are usually undetectable in normal individuals, and any elevation is considered abnormal.
  - MI size and prognosis are directly proportional to the increase in troponin (*N Engl J Med 1996;335:1333*; *Circulation 1998;98:1853*).
- CK-MB is also an acceptable marker of myocardial necrosis, but lacks specificity, as it is present in both skeletal and cardiac muscle cells.
  - Specificity can be improved by using the CK-MB/total CK fraction. A CK-MB fraction greater than 2.5% is suggestive of myocardial injury.
  - CK-MB is a useful assay for detecting postinfarct ischemia, as a fall and subsequent rise in enzyme levels suggests reinfarction, especially if accompanied by recurrent ischemic symptoms or ECG changes.
  - Similarly, CK-MB levels are often followed after percutaneous revascularization. Small rises in CK-MB often represent distal microembolization, while large rises suggest more significant complications, such as acute stent thrombosis.
    - For patients with a normal baseline troponin, a threefold increase post-PCI is suggestive of post-PCI MI; if the baseline level was elevated but stable/decreasing, an increase of 20% is used. However, CK-MB is preferred over troponin in diagnosing post-PCI infarction (*JACC 2011;57:653*).
- Myoglobin is released more rapidly following myocardial damage than either CK-MB, troponin T, or troponin I, but lacks specificity. Measurement can be useful in patients presenting in the first few hours of symptom onset.

TREATMENT

- The approach to clinical testing, pharmacologic treatment, and timing of possible invasive therapy is guided by the probability of progression to acute MI, risk of reinfarction, and risk of subsequent mortality.
- Risk of death or MI progression is elevated with the following ***high-risk ACS characteristics***:
  - Recurrent/accelerating angina despite adequate medical therapy
  - Signs or symptoms of new heart failure, pulmonary edema, or shock
  - New or worsening MR
  - New LBBB
  - Ventricular tachycardia noted on monitoring
- These findings (on presentation **or anytime during the index hospitalization**) should prompt the performance of an urgent heart catheterization with intention to offer revascularization.
- Several clinical tools can estimate a patient's risk of MI and cardiac mortality, such as the Thrombolysis in Myocardial Infarction (TIMI) and Global Registry of Acute Coronary Events (GRACE) risk scores. The TIMI risk score can be used to determine the patient's 14-day risk of death or nonfatal MI (*JAMA 2000;284:835*). Patients can be classified as low, intermediate, or high risk on the basis of their clinical profile (Figure 4-2).
  - Low-risk patients (TIMI 0 or 1) may be observed with cardiac monitoring in a chest pain or observation unit.
  - Intermediate- and high-risk patients should be admitted to the hospital for observation and management.

TIMI risk score (1 point for each)

1. Age >65 years
2. Known CAD (stenosis >50%)
3. 2+ episodes of chest pain in 24 hours
4. ST-segment or T-wave changes
5. Elevated cardiac biomarkers
6. ASA in the last 7 days
7. 3+ CAD risk factors

Conservative strategy	Early invasive strategy

β-Blocker, nitrates, oxygen ⟶
UFH, LMWH ⟶
ASA ⟶
Dual antiplatelet therapy ⟶
Triple antiplatelet therapy ⟶

TIMI risk score

Figure 4-2. Fourteen-day rates of death, MI, or urgent revascularization from the TIMI 11B and ESSENCE trials based on increasing TIMI risk score. Coronary artery disease (CAD) risk factors include family history of CAD, diabetes, hypertension, hyperlipidemia, and tobacco use. ASA, aspirin; MI, myocardial infarction; TIMI, Thrombolysis in Myocardial Infarction; UFH, unfractionated heparin. (Adapted from *JAMA 2000;284:835–842*.)

- In the stabilized patient, two treatment strategies are accepted: the **initial conservative approach** versus **the initial invasive approach**. The planned approach should always be individualized to each particular patient (Figure 4-3).
  - In the **initial conservative strategy**, maximal medical therapy is utilized, and if effective, a noninvasive stress test is obtained prior to discharge.

- May be considered in low-TIMI/GRACE risk patients and select intermediate-risk patients with expected outcomes similar to the direct invasive strategy.
- If the patient does not develop high-risk ACS features, has normal subsequent cardiac enzymes, and no dynamic ECG changes, a noninvasive stress test should be obtained for further risk stratification.
  - Patients should be angina free for at least 12 hours prior to stress testing.
  - If a patient with positive cardiac enzymes is selected for noninvasive testing, a submaximal or pharmacologic stress test 72 hours after the peak value may be performed.
- Coronary angiography is reserved for patients who develop high-risk ACS features, have a high-risk stress test, develop angina at low levels of stress, or are noted to have a LV EF <40%.
  - In the **initial invasive strategy**, the patient is planned for a coronary angiography with intent to revascularize (within 12 to 48 hours) without first obtaining a stress test or ascertaining if medical therapy failed to control symptoms (*Lancet 1999;354:708; N Engl J Med 2001;344:1879; JAMA 2003;290:1593; Lancet 2002; 360:743; N Engl J Med 2009;360:2165; JAMA 2005;293:2908*).
    - Features, other than earlier mentioned high-risk ACS characteristics, which make an invasive strategy preferable, include:
      - Elevated cardiac enzymes.
      - New ST-segment depression.
      - History of CABG or recent PCI (6 months).
      - LV EF <40%.
      - Presence of diabetes mellitus.
      - Presence of mild-to-moderate renal insufficiency.
        Patients with a creatinine clearance less than 30 or those receiving dialysis may not benefit from an invasive approach (*Circulation 2009;120:851*).
      - High TIMI or GRACE risk score.
        An early invasive strategy (angiography within 12 to 24 hours) in stabilized patients with a GRACE score >140 should be considered (*N Engl J Med 2009; 360:2165*).
      - An early invasive strategy is also warranted in low- or intermediate-risk patients with repeated ACS presentations despite appropriate therapy.

Medications

Patients presenting with UA/NSTEMI should receive medications that reduce myocardial ischemia through reduction in myocardial oxygen demand, improvement in coronary perfusion, and prevention of further thrombus formation.

- This approach should include antiplatelet, anticoagulant, and antianginal medications.
- Supplemental oxygen should be provided if the patient is hypoxemic (<90%) or having difficulty breathing. Routine use of oxygen is not needed and possibly harmful (*HEART 2009;95:198*).
- **Antiplatelet therapy**
  - **Aspirin** blocks platelet aggregation within minutes (Table 4-10).
    - A chewable 162- to 325-mg dose ASA should be administered immediately at symptom onset or at first medical contact, unless a contraindication exists. Followed by 81 mg ASA daily indefinitely.
    - If an ASA allergy is present (e.g., bronchospasm in asthma patients with nasal polyps), clopidogrel (with bolus doing) may be substituted. An allergy consultation should be obtained for possible desensitization, preferably prior to the need of a cardiac stent.

□ Guidelines suggest a maintenance ASA dose of 162 to 325 mg for 1 month for ACS patients who receive a bare metal stent and up to 6 months for drug eluting stents, followed by 75 to 162 mg daily indefinitely.

- However 81 mg ASA daily for all patients post-PCI is also reasonable. Doses of ASA higher than 100 mg in patients taking a second antiplatelet agent increase risk of bleeding without added benefit (*N Engl J Med 2010;363:930*).

○ Oral antiplatelet agents, **clopidogrel**, **ticlopidine**, **prasugrel**, are thienopyridine P2Y12 receptor antagonists and **ticagrelor** is the only reversible ***non*-thienopyridine** P2Y12 receptor antagonist. They inhibit platelet activation and aggregation by blocking the ADP receptor site on platelets.

▪ **Clopidogrel** is a prodrug whose metabolite blocks the P2Y12 receptor; therefore, maximal platelet activity is not seen for several hours.

□ As compared to other agents in its class it has less risk of bleeding. Patients who also need to be on warfarin and ASA, clopidogrel may be safer than ticagrelor and prasugrel. International normalized ratio (INR) goal should be between 2.0 and 2.5.

□ It is part of the early conservative and early invasive pathways (given on initial presentation or during PCI).

□ Efficacy has also been proven in treatment of STEMI patients (*Lancet 2005;366:1607*; *N Engl J Med 2005;352:1179*; *JAMA 2005;294:1224*).

□ TTP is a rare side effect, and platelets should be monitored.

□ It has largely supplanted ticlopidine (less risk of TTP or neutropenia). NOTE: Although dual antiplatelet therapy is necessary for ACS and mandatory in patients who receive PCI, the combination of ASA and clopidogrel is contraindicated in patients with a prior TIA/CVA per stroke guidelines (*Lancet 2004;364:331*).

▪ **Prasugrel** is also a prodrug; its conversion to its active metabolite occurs faster and to a greater extent than clopidogrel.

□ Results in faster, greater, and more uniform platelet inhibition compared to clopidogrel at the expense of higher risk of bleeding.

← _____

Figure 4-3. Diagnostic and therapeutic approach to patients presenting with ACS focusing on antiplatelet and antithrombotic therapy. *Bivalirudin is an appropriate alternative to UFH and LMWH, or at time of PCI patients on UFH may be switched to bivalirudin. †Choose either clopidogrel, ticagrelor, or prasugrel as the second antiplatelet agent. GPIIb/IIIa inhibitors can be used as an alternative if need for CABG seems highly possible. ††GPIIb/IIIa inhibitors can be administered at time of PCI in addition to ASA and a P2Y12 inhibitor in high-risk patients or as add-on therapy in patients who have recurrent or worsening symptoms. #Indicators of recurrent ischemia include worsening chest pain, increasing cardiac enzymes, heart failure signs/symptoms, arrhythmia (VT/VF), and dynamic ECG changes. ¹GPIIb/IIIa inhibitors should be used selectively or bivalirudin may be used whether UFH was given prior or not. ²UFH for 48 hours or LMWH or fondaparinux until discharge pr up to 8 days and clopidogrel or ticagrelor for 1 year. P2Y12 inhibitor includes antiplatelet agents clopidogrel, ticagrelor, or prasugrel. ASA, aspirin; CABG, coronary artery bypass grafting; CAD, coronary artery disease; ECG, electrocardiogram; EF, ejection fraction; GPIIb/IIIa, glycoprotein IIb/IIIa inhibitor; LMWH, low–molecular-weight heparin; NSTEMI, non–ST-segment elevation myocardial infarction; PCI, percutaneous coronary intervention; Rx, treatment; STEMI, ST-segment elevation myocardial infarction; UA, unstable angina; UFH, unfractionated heparin; VT/VF, ventricular tachycardia/ventricular fibrillation; WMA, wall motion abnormality. (Adapted from the ACC/AHA 2007 Guidelines for the Management of Patients With Unstable Angina/Non-ST-Elevation Myocardial Infarction.)

Table 4-10	Antiplatelet Agents in Unstable Angina/NSTEMI	

Medication	Dosage	Comments
Aspirin (ASA)	162–325 mg initial, then 75–100 mg	In patients taking ticagrelor, the maintenance dose of ASA *should not* exceed 100 mg.
Clopidogrel	300–600 mg loading dose, 75 mg daily	In combination with ASA, clopidogrel (300–600 mg loading dose, then 75 mg/d) decreased the composite end point of cardiovascular death, MI, or stroke by 18%–30% in patients with UA/NSTEMI (*N Engl J Med 2001;345:494; Lancet 2001;358: 527; JAMA 2002;288:2411*).
Ticagrelor	180 mg loading dose, then 90 mg bid	Ticagrelor reduced incidence of vascular death, MI, or CVA (9.8% vs. 11.0%) but with higher major bleeding not related to CABG (4.5% vs. 3.8%) as compared to clopidogrel (*N Engl J Med 2009;361:1045*).
Prasugrel	60 mg loading dose, 10 mg daily	Prasugrel has increased antiplatelet potency compared to clopidogrel. Prasugrel reduced the incidence of cardiovascular death, MI, and stroke (9.9% vs. 12.1%) at the expense of increased major (2.4% vs. 1.1%) and fatal bleeding (0.4% vs. 0.1%), compared to clopidogrel (*N Engl J Med 2007;357:2001*).
Eptifibatide	180 mcg/kg IV bolus, 2 mcg/kg/min[a]	Eptifibatide reduces the risk of death or MI in patients with ACS undergoing either invasive or noninvasive therapy in combination with ASA and heparin (*N Engl J Med 1998;339:436; Circulation 2000;101:751*). Compared to abciximab and tirofiban, eptifibatide has the most consistent effects on platelet inhibition with shortest on-time and drug half-life (*Circulation 2002;106:1470–1476*).
Tirofiban	0.4 mcg/kg IV bolus, 0.1 mcg/kg/min[a]	Tirofiban reduces the risk of death or MI in patients with ACS undergoing either invasive or noninvasive therapy in combination with ASA and heparin (*Circulation 1997;96:1445; N Engl J Med 1998;338:1498; N Engl J Med 1998;338:1488*).

(continued)

Table 4-10	Antiplatelet Agents in Unstable Angina/NSTEMI (*Continued*)	

Medication	Dosage	Comments
Abciximab	0.25 mg/kg IV bolus, 10 mcg/min[b]	Abciximab reduces the risk of death or MI in patients with ACS undergoing coronary intervention (*N Engl J Med 1994;330:956; Lancet 1997;349: 1429; N Engl J Med 1997;336: 1689*). It should not be used in patients in whom percutaneous intervention is not planned (*Lancet 2001;357:1915*). Platelet inhibition may be reversed by platelet transfusion.

[a]Infusion doses should be decreased by 50% in patients with a GFR less than 30 mL/min and avoided in patients on HD.
[b]Abciximab may be used in patients with ESRD, as it is not cleared by the kidney.
ACS, acute coronary syndrome; CABG, coronary artery bypass grafting; CVA, cerebrovascular accident; ESRD, end-stage renal disease; GFR, glomerular filtration rate; HD, hemodialysis; MI, myocardial infarction; NSTEMI, non–ST-segment elevation myocardial infarction; UA, unstable angina.

- It decreases risk of CVD death, MI, CVA, and acute stent thrombosis as compared to clopidogrel in ACS patients, including STEMI patients.
- It should be used with caution or avoided in patients older than 75 years and who weigh less than 60 kg. It is ***contraindicated*** in those with prior stroke or TIA.
- Used only in the invasive approach of ACS, and preferably only after coronary anatomy is known and PCI is planned.
- **Ticagrelor** is not a prodrug, and thus metabolic conversion is not needed.
  - Reduces the risk of death, MI, CVA, and stent thrombosis as compared to clopidogrel in ACS patients, including STEMI patients (*N Engl J Med 2009; 361:1045*).
  - Ticagrelor as compared to clopidogrel is associated with higher risk of major bleeding (non-CABG related).
  - After the loading dose of ASA, the maintenance dose of ASA **must be below 100 mg** (*Circulation 2011;124:544*).
  - Can be used as part of the protocol in both the early conservative and early invasive pathways (on initial presentation or during PCI) (*BMJ 2011; 342:d3527*).
- Use of **proton pump inhibitors (PPIs)** with P2Y12 receptor antagonists.
  - PPIs should be used in patients who will require both ASA therapy and a P2Y12 antagonist with prior history of gastrointestinal bleeding and may be considered in those at increased risk of bleeding (such as older individuals, patients with known ulcers or *Helicobacter pylori* infection, and in patients also on warfarin, steroids, or NSAIDs (*Circulation 2010;122:2619*).
  - Pharmacologic studies have raised concerns about the potential of PPIs to blunt the efficiency of clopidogrel. However, in a prospective, randomized trial, no apparent cardiovascular interaction was noted between PPIs and clopidogrel (*N Engl J Med 2010;363:1909*).

- ○ **Glycoprotein IIb/IIIa (GPIIb/IIIa) antagonists** (abciximab, eptifibatide, or tirofiban) block the interaction between platelets and fibrinogen, thus targeting the final common pathway for platelet aggregation (*JAMA 2006;295:1531; Circulation 2001;104:2767; N Engl J Med 2009;360:2176*).
  - Much of the data for use of GPIIb/IIIa agents comes from an era before availability of P2Y12 receptor blockers and bivalirudin. Overall current data is most supportive for use in patients who are troponin positive.
  - GPIIb/IIIa agents (based on recent trials) is most beneficial with selective use in certain patients:
    - Patients who need add on therapy for *worsening* ischemia any time prior to angiography or as part of conservative therapy even if the patient is already being treated with clopidogrel and/or bivalirudin.
    - Troponin-positive patients, administered during PCI (even if clopidogrel given upstream). Routine use GPIIb/IIIa inhibitors in patients along the initial invasive pathway treated upstream with clopidogrel (at least 6 hours prior to PCI) and bivalirudin is not necessary even if troponin positive.
    - Discretional use during PCI due to the presence of complex coronary lesions or coronary thrombus.
  - Routine use of GPIIb/IIIa antagonist on initial presentation, before angiography, in patients undergoing the invasive approach *should be avoided* due to increased risk of major bleeding with
    - Routine use in patients already being treated with dual antiplatelet agents *unless* there is significant ST depression, positive troponin, TIMI score >3, or diabetes.
    - Routine use with bivalirudin and clopidogrel.
    - Patients at increased risk of bleeding.
  - Abciximab is reserved only for use only during PCI, started no sooner than 4 hours prior to the planned procedure.
  - Thrombocytopenia, which can be severe, is an uncommon complication of these agents and should prompt discontinuation.
- ○ **Antiplatelet agents and timing of CABG**
  - Due to increased risk of bleeding, it is currently recommended that clopidogrel be withheld for at least 5 days prior to CABG, and 7 days prior for prasugrel. Ticagrelor should be withheld 3 to 5 days prior to CABG; however, since CABG-related bleeding may not be increased, timing/need of discontinuation is unclear.
  - GPIIb/IIIa agents have a short plasma half-life, and thus CABG is only delayed 4 hours. These agents can be an alternative to clopidogrel, ticagrelor, and prasugrel for upstream use (prior to angiography) in appropriate patients with UA/NSTEMI that may ultimately require surgical revascularization.
- ○ **Individual variability in response to clopidogrel**
  - A polymorphism in the CYP2C19 gene has been associated with decreased platelet inhibition and increased risk of major adverse cardiovascular outcomes in patients receiving clopidogrel (*N Engl J Med 2009;360:354; N Engl J Med 2009;360:363*).
  - Reduced CYP2C19 activity leads to impaired conversion of clopidogrel to its active metabolite. Patients with an enhanced CYP2C17 allele, on the other hand, create excess active metabolite.
  - Clopidogrel resistance can be screened for using point-of-care platelet inhibition assays or genotyping.

- Proposed strategies to combat clopidogrel resistance include higher clopidogrel dosing, use of GPIIb/IIIa antagonist, or use of prasugrel/ticagrelor. Prasugrel and ticagrelor platelet activity may not similarly affected by these alleles.
- **Anticoagulant therapy**
  - Available therapeutic agents include the indirect thrombin inhibitors (**unfractionated heparin (UFH)** and **low–molecular-weight heparin [LMWH] enoxaparin**), the direct thrombin inhibitor (**bivalirudin**), and the selective factor Xa inhibitor (**fondaparinux**) (Table 4-11).
  - Anticoagulation accompanied by dual antiplatelet therapy is required for all UA/NSTEMI patients, whether along the early invasive or conservative pathway.
  - UFH is given through a continuous IV infusion and partial thromboplastin times (PTTs) must be monitored to determine degree of anticoagulation. Of the other agents, UFH carries the highest risk of immune-mediated heparin-induced thrombocytopenia (HIT). Due to risk of HIT, extended use of UFH (>48 hours) should be avoided.
  - LMWH offers an ease of administration (weight based, twice daily subcutaneous dose), and since PTT levels are generally not affected they are not followed. The risk of HIT is lower but not absent.
    - As compared to UFH it has a more predictable anticoagulant effect.
    - It has a similar efficacy as UFH but is associated with a higher risk of bleeding in patients also treated with dual antiplatelet agents (*JAMA 2004;292:45*).
    - For patients in the conservative pathway, enoxaparin is preferred to UFH.
  - Fondaparinux is administered subcutaneously once daily and generally does not affect PTT levels, so PTT monitoring is not required.
    - It is not associated with HIT.
    - As compared to enoxaparin, it was studied to be associated with less combined death, MI, or refractory ischemia with less risk of major bleeding (*N Engl J Med 2006;354:1464*).
    - It can be used as part of the conservative or invasive strategies. For patients in the conservative pathway, fondaparinux is preferred to UFH.
    - It is associated with catheter-related thrombosis, so patients undergoing PCI must be coadministered UFH.
  - **Bivalirudin** is also given as a continuous IV infusion and does prolong PTT levels.
    - It does not cause HIT and is used in the treatment of patients who develop HIT or patients with ACS who have history of HIT.
    - Bivalirudin can be given in conjunction with ASA and clopidogrel in patients presenting with UA/NSTEMI who will undergo an early invasive strategy. It has not been studied for use in the conservative pathway.
    - Bivalirudin with dual antiplatelet therapy is as effective as the combination of UFH/LMWH + GPIIb/IIIa inhibitor but is associated with less bleeding risk (*N Engl J Med 2006;355:2203*).
    - **Thrombolytic therapy** is not indicated in UA/NSTEMI.
- **Anti-ischemic therapy** (please also refer to Treatment section of stable angina)
  - **Nitroglycerin**
    - Treatment can be initiated at the time of presentation with sublingual nitroglycerin. Note, 40% of patients with chest pain *not* due to CAD will get relief with nitroglycerin (Table 4-12) (*Ann Intern Med 2003;139:979*).
    - Ongoing ischemic symptoms in patients or those who require additional agents to control significant hypertension can be treated with IV nitroglycerin until pain relief, hypertension control, or both are achieved.

Table 4-11	Anticoagulant Medications	
Medication	Dosage	Comments
Heparin (UFH)	60 U/kg IV bolus (maximum dose: 4,000 units), 12–14 U/kg/hr	Heparin therapy, when used in conjunction with ASA, has been shown to reduce the early rate of death or MI by up to 60% (*JAMA 1996;276:811*). The aPTT should be adjusted to maintain a value of 1.5–2.0 times control.
Enoxaparin (LMWH)	1 mg/kg SC bid[a]	LMWH is at least as efficacious as UFH and may further reduce the rate of death, MI, or recurrent angina (*N Engl J Med 1997;337:447*). LMWH may increase the rate of bleeding (*JAMA 2004;292:45*) and cannot be reversed in the setting of refractory bleeding. LMWH does not require monitoring for clinical effect. If cardiac catheterization is planned, then the dose should be withheld on the morning of procedure.
Fondaparinux	2.5 mg SC daily	Fondaparinux has efficacy similar to that of LMWH with possibly reduced bleeding rates (*N Engl J Med 2006;354:1464*).
Bivalirudin[b]	0.75 mg/kg IV bolus, 1.75 mg/kg/hr	When used in conjunction with ASA and clopidogrel, bivalirudin is at least as effective as the combination of ASA, UFH, clopidogrel, and GPIIb/IIIa antagonists with decreased bleeding rates (*N Engl J Med 2006;355:2203*). Monitoring is required with a goal aPTT of 1.5–2.5 times control.

[a]LMWH should be given at reduced dose (50%) in patients with a serum creatinine >2 mg/dL or GFR <30 mL/min.
[b]Bivalirudin requires dosage adjustment in patients with a GFR less than 30 mL/min or those on hemodialysis.
aPTT, activated partial thromboplastin time; ASA, aspirin; GFR, glomerular filtration rate; GP, glycoprotein; LMWH, low–molecular-weight heparin; MI, myocardial infarction; UFH, unfractionated heparin.

Table 4-12	Antianginal Medications	

Medication	Dosage	Comments
Nitroglycerin (NTG)	SL: 0.4 mg every 5 min Topical: 0.5–2.0 in. IV: 10–200 mcg/min	Significant antianginal effects are not seen above 200 mcg/min, but doses of up to 400 mcg/min can be used for BP control. NTG is contraindicated in patients who have used PDE5 inhibitors (e.g., within 24 hr of sildenafil or 48 hr of tadalafil) given the risk of severe hypotension. Appropriate timing for vardenafil dosing with nitrates is unknown and should be avoided. Nitrates are relatively contraindicated in patients who are preload dependent, including those with severe aortic stenosis and hypertrophic obstructive cardiomyopathy.
Morphine	2–4 mg IV	IV narcotics are effective agents for relief of anginal symptoms and should be used if NTG does not provide complete relief or cannot be titrated further due to hypotension or headache.
β-Blockers	25 mg PO qid Bisoprolol: 10–20 mg PO daily Carvedilol: 3.125–25 mg PO bid Atenolol: 50–200 mg PO daily Propranolol: 20–80 mg PO bid Esmolol: 50–300 mcg/kg/min Nebivolol: 5–40 mg PO daily	β-Adrenergic blockade reduces the risk of recurrent ischemia, MI, and mortality in patients with UA/NSTEMI (*J Interv Cardiol 2003;16:299*). The efficacy of β-blockade is limited by the development of cardiogenic shock. Those at risk include patients greater than 70 yr of age, SBP <120 mm Hg, and heart rate >110 bpm or <60 bpm. In such cases, oral agents at reduced doses may be cautiously used (*Lancet 2005;366:1622*).
Calcium channel blockers	Nifedipine 30–180 mg daily Amlodipine 5–10 mg daily Diltiazem 30–80 mg qid Verapamil 80–160 mg tid	Short-acting nifedipine preparations should be avoided in the absence of adequate concurrent β-blocker therapy because of increased risk of MI and death. Verapamil and diltiazem should be avoided in patients with evidence of severe LV dysfunction, pulmonary congestion, or AV block.

AV, atrioventricular; BP, blood pressure; LV, left ventricular; MI, myocardial infarction; NSTEMI, non–ST-segment elevation myocardial infarction; SBP, systolic blood pressure; UA, unstable angina.

- Rule out right-sided infarct prior to administration of nitrates as this can precipitate profound hypotension.
  ○ **β-Adrenergic blockers (BBL)** (please also refer to the Treatment section for stable angina)
    - Should be started early in the absence of contraindications.
    - Treatment with an IV preparation should be reserved for treatment of arrhythmia, ongoing chest pain, or advanced hypertension rather than routine use.
    - The goals of therapy are to reduce the heart rate to 60 bpm and maintain an systolic blood pressure (SBP) greater than 90 to 100 mm Hg.
    - Contraindications to β-blocker therapy include advanced AV block, active bronchospasm, decompensated HF, cardiogenic shock, hypotension, and bradycardia.
  ○ **Calcium channel blockers** (please also refer to Treatment section for stable angina) can be used as third-line agents in patients continuing to have chest pain in the setting of adequate β-blocker and nitrate therapy.
    - Nifedipine, amlodipine, diltiazem, and verapamil appear to have similar coronary dilatory properties. Neither of these agents has demonstrated an effect on mortality or recurrent MI.
    - Diltiazem and verapamil may worsen cardiac output.
- **Other medications**
  ○ **ACEIs** (please also refer to Treatment section for stable angina) are effective antihypertensive agents and have been shown to reduce mortality in patients with CAD and LV systolic dysfunction. ACEIs should be used in patients with LV dysfunction (EF <40%), hypertension, or diabetes presenting with ACS. **ARBs** are appropriate in patients who cannot tolerate ACEIs (*N Engl J Med 2003; 349:1893*).
  ○ **Aldosterone antagonists** should be added if no contraindication (potassium >5 mEq/L or CrCl <30 mL/min) after initiation of ACEIs to patients with diabetes or an LV EF <40%.
  ○ **HMG-CoA reductase inhibitors (statins)** are potent lipid-lowering agents that reduce the incidence of ischemia, MI, and death in patients with CAD. High-dose statins should be routinely administered within 24 hours of presentation in patients presenting with ACS. A lipid profile should be obtained in all patients.
    - Statin therapy reduces adverse outcomes through lipid lowering and potentially through pleiotropic effects (anti-inflammatory/atherosclerotic plaque–stabilizing effects).
    - Aggressive statin therapy reduces the risk of recurrent ischemia, MI, and death in patients presenting with ACS (*JAMA 2001;285:1711*).
    - A reduction in adverse CVD outcomes following early initiation of high-dose station with achievement of an LDL less than 70 mg/dL can be seen in as early 30 days following initial presentation with ACS (*N Engl J Med 2004;350:1495*). Aggressive LDL lowering also reduces the incidence of periprocedural MI following PCI (*JACC 2007;49:1272*).
  ○ **NSAIDs** are associated with an increased risk of death, MI, myocardial rupture, hypertension, and HF in large meta-analyses (*Circulation 2006;113:2906*). Adverse outcomes have been observed for both nonselective and COX-2 selective agents.
    - NSAIDs should be discontinued in patients presenting with UA/NSTEMI.
    - Acetaminophen is an acceptable alternative for the treatment of osteoarthritis and other musculoskeletal pain.

- **Other nonpharmacological therapies**
  - **Blood transfusion** improves oxygen-carrying capacity and myocardial oxygen supply. The potential benefit of routine blood transfusions in patients presenting with an NSTEMI is based on limited clinic data (*N Engl J Med 2001;345:1230*).
    - The recommended target hemoglobin and hematocrit is 10 mg/dL and 30%, respectively.
    - Patients presenting with UA/NSTEMI who are actively bleeding and/or significantly anemic should be transfused routinely.

Other Nonmedical Therapies

- **Revascularization**
  - The indications for PCI and CABG in patients with UA/NSTEMI are similar to those for individuals with chronic stable angina (please see section on revascularization in chronic stable angina).
    - Patients who are optimally managed with CABG include those with
      - Significant left main CAD
      - Three-vessel disease with LV dysfunction
      - Two-vessel disease with a significant proximal LAD artery stenosis and complicated disease
      - Diabetes and multivessel disease
    - Patients with multivessel coronary disease requiring revascularization can be treated with CABG or PCI. Patients who are treated with CABG tend to have less need for subsequent revascularization but have an increased risk of stroke. Survival advantage of CABG compared to PCI also depends on syntax score. While the preferred treatment of unprotected left main disease remains CABG, a role for PCI is also present (*Circulation 2008;118:1146; N Engl J Med 2009; 360:961*).
    - The decision between PCI and CABG should be based on the extent and complexity of coronary disease, medical comorbidities, and patient preference.
  - If there is uncertainty regarding the hemodynamic significance of a coronary lesion, FFR can be performed to quantify the functional severity of blood flow limitation. This modality has been shown to reduce death, recurrent MI, or revascularization compared to conventional PCI at 1 year in patients with multivessel CAD (*N Engl J Med 2009;360:213*).
  - Drug eluting stents (DES) significantly reduce the rate of ISR and some adverse cardiac outcomes compared to bare metal stents (BMS) (*N Engl J Med 2003; 349:1315; Circulation 2003;108:788*). However, DES imparts an additional risk of late stent thrombosis, most notably following the premature discontinuation of clopidogrel therapy in the 1 year following stent placement (*JAMA 2007; 297:159*).

Monitoring/Follow-up

The highest rate of progression to MI or development of recurrent MI is in the first 2 months after presentation with the index episode. Beyond that time, most patients have a clinical course similar to those with chronic stable angina.

- Patients should be discharged on earlier recommended antiplatelet therapies and β blockers, and statin therapy.
- Most patients should be discharged on ACEIs.
- Evaluate need of aldosterone antagonists.
- Screen for life stressors and depression. Refer for depression treatment as needed.
- Smoking cessation should be stressed and risk factor modification.
- Referral to cardiac rehabilitation should also be pursued.

ST-Segment Elevation Myocardial Infarction

GENERAL PRINCIPLES

- STEMI is a medical emergency caused by acute total occlusion of an epicardial coronary artery, most often due to atherosclerotic plaque rupture/erosion and subsequent thrombus formation.
- Compared to UA/NSTEMI, STEMI is associated with a higher in-hospital and 30 day morbidity and mortality. Left untreated, the mortality rate of STEMI can exceed 30%, and the presence of mechanical complications (papillary muscle rupture, ventricular septal defect [VSD], and free wall rupture) increases the mortality rate to 90%. Over the past several decades, there has been a dramatic improvement in short-term mortality to the current rate of 6% to 10%.
- Ventricular fibrillation accounts for approximately 50% of mortality and often occurs within the first hour from symptom onset.
- Keys to treatment of STEMI include rapid recognition and diagnosis, coordinated mobilization of health care resources, and prompt reperfusion therapy.
- Mortality is directly related to total ischemia time.

Prevention

Secondary prevention. The strategies outlined for primary prevention and the management of stable angina have also been shown to decrease the rates of repeat infarction, progression to HF, and incidence of cardiovascular deaths in patients with known CAD (see earlier sections).

DIAGNOSIS

Clinical Presentation

- Multiple risk assessment tools have been developed to stratify patients presenting with acute STEMI into low-, intermediate-, and high-risk groups based on history, physical exam, and hemodynamic monitoring (Figure 4-4).
- The Killip classification system utilizes history and physical exam findings (S_3 gallop, pulmonary congestion, and cardiogenic shock) to predict 30-day mortality in the absence of reperfusion therapy (*Am J Cardiol 1967;20:457*). In contrast, the TIMI risk score for STEMI incorporates a combination of history and physical to predict 30-day mortality in patients who receive thrombolytic therapy (*Circulation 2000;102:2031*). The Forrester classification system uses invasive hemodynamic data including cardiac index and pulmonary capillary wedge pressure (*N Engl J Med 1976;295:1356*).

History

- Chest pain from STEMI resembles angina, but lasts longer, is more intense, and is not relieved by rest or sublingual nitroglycerin. Chest discomfort may be accompanied by dyspnea, diaphoresis, palpitations, nausea, vomiting, fatigue, and/or syncope.
- It is imperative to determine the time of symptom onset, as this is critical in determining the appropriate means of reperfusion (Table 4-13).
- STEMI may have atypical presentations particularly in women, elderly, and postoperative patients, as well as those with diabetes and chronic or end-stage kidney

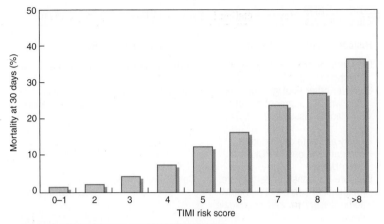

TIMI risk score	Points
1. Age 65–74 years	2
2. Age >75 years	3
3. Diabetes, HTN, or angina	1
4. Systolic BP <100 mm Hg	3
5. Heart rate >100	2
6. Killip class II–IV	2
7. Anterior STEMI or LBBB	1
8. Time to reperfusion >4 hr	1
9. Weight <67 kg	1

Killip class	Definition	Mortality (%)
I	No signs of congestive heart failure	6
II	Presence of an S_3 and/or lung rales	17
III	Pulmonary edema	30–40
IV	Cardiogenic shock	60–80

Figure 4-4. Risk indices for ST-segment elevation myocardial infarction (MI). Killip classification in acute MI. **Top.** TIMI risk score for STEMI (*Circulation 2000;102:2031*). **Bottom.** Killip classification system (*Am J Cardiol 1967;20:457*). The TIMI risk score incorporates prognosis following coronary reperfusion with thrombolytic therapy. The Killip classification system was devised before reperfusion therapy was routinely used. BP, blood pressure; HTN, hypertension; LBBB, left bundle branch block.

disease. Such patients may experience atypical or no chest pain and may instead present with confusion, dyspnea, unexplained hypotension, or HF.
• If the patient has a history of previous cardiac catheterization or revascularization, it is important to obtain these records, as these can provide valuable information with respect to PCI planning, particularly in the setting of previous CABG. However, this should not delay definitive therapy.

Table 4-13	Key Information in the Patient Presenting with STEMI	
History and Physical Exam	**Laboratory Values**	**Records**
Inquire about the exact time of chest pain onset	Complete blood cell count	Prior ECGs
Consider other etiologies of chest pain with ST-segment elevation (i.e., aortic dissection, cocaine use)	Basic chemistry panel	Last cardiac catheterization
Identify absolute and relative contraindications to PCI and thrombolysis	PTT, PT, and INR	CABG operative report
Evaluate for signs of heart failure, mechanical complications of MI, aortic dissection, and neurologic disease	Cardiac enzymes	Prior echocardiogram

CABG, coronary artery bypass grafting; ECG, electrocardiogram; INR, international normalized ratio; MI, myocardial infarction; PCI, percutaneous coronary intervention; PT, prothrombin time; PTT, partial thromboplastin time; STEMI, ST-segment elevation myocardial infarction.

- Assess for absolute and relative contraindications to thrombolytic therapy (see the following text) and potential issues complicating primary PCI (IV contrast allergy, PVD/peripheral revascularization, renal dysfunction, central nervous system [CNS] disease, pregnancy, bleeding diathesis, or severe comorbidity).
- Inquire about recent cocaine use. In this setting, aggressive medical therapy with nitroglycerin, coronary vasodilators, and benzodiazepines should be administered before reperfusion therapy is considered.

Physical Examination
Physical examination should be directed at identifying hemodynamic instability, pulmonary congestion, mechanical complications of MI, and other causes of acute chest discomfort.
- The identification of a new systolic murmur may suggest the presence of ischemic MR or a VSD.
- A limited neurologic exam to detect baseline cognitive and motor deficits and a vascular examination (lower extremity pulses and bruits) will aid in determining candidacy and planning for reperfusion treatment.
- Cardiogenic shock due to right ventricular myocardial infarction (RVMI) may be clinically suspected by the presence of hypotension, elevated jugular venous pressure, and absence of pulmonary congestion. While RVMI may be seen in isolation, it more commonly complicates inferior/posterior MI.
- Bilateral arm BPs should be obtained to assess for the presence of aortic dissection.

Diagnostic Criteria
STEMI diagnosis and initiation of treatment is made in a patient who reports prolonged chest discomfort or anginal equivalent with qualifying ECG findings. Attempting to wait for results of cardiac biomarkers will add unnecessary delay. ECG finding include ST-segment elevation in two consecutive ECG leads, new LBBB, or evidence of posterior MI (see ECG section).

Diagnostic Testing

Laboratories

Blood samples should be sent for cardiac enzymes (Troponin, CK-MB), complete blood cell count, coagulation studies (PTT, prothrombin time [PT], INR), creatinine, electrolytes including magnesium, and type and screen. A fasting lipid profile should be obtained in all patients with STEMI for secondary prevention (note, however, that lipid levels may be falsely lowered during the acute phase of MI).

- Initial cardiac enzymes (including troponin assays) may be normal, depending upon the time in relation to symptom onset. Myoglobin is the first enzyme to rise.
- CK-MB can be used to confirm that myocardial injury occurred within the previous 48 hours, as troponin levels may remain elevated for several days after MI.
- The risk of subsequent cardiac death is directly proportional to the increase in cardiac-specific troponins, even when CK-MB levels are not elevated. Measuring enzymes until the peak level has been attained can be used to determine infarct size.
- Routine use of cardiac noninvasive imaging is not recommended for the initial diagnosis of STEMI. When the diagnosis is in question, a transthoracic echocardiogram (TTE) can be performed to document regional wall motion abnormalities. If not adequately evaluated by TTE, a transesophageal echocardiogram (TEE) can be obtained to assess for acute complications of MI and presence of aortic dissection.
- A portable chest radiograph is useful to assess for pulmonary edema and evaluate for other causes of chest pain including aortic dissection. Importantly, a normal mediastinal width does not exclude aortic dissection, especially if clinically suspected.

Electrocardiography

The ECG is paramount to the diagnosis of STEMI and should be obtained within 10 minutes of presentation. If the diagnosis of STEMI is in doubt, serial ECGs may help elucidate the diagnosis. Classic findings include (Table 4-14):

- Peaked upright T waves is the first ECG manifestation of myocardial injury.
- ST elevations correlate with the territory of injured myocardium (Figure 4-5).
- **Diagnostic ECG criteria for STEMI** (*JACC 2009;53:1003*)
  - When ST elevations reach threshold values in two or more anatomically contiguous leads, a diagnosis of STEMI can be made.
  - In men >40 years of age, threshold value for abnormal ST-segment elevation at the J point is ≥2 mm in leads V2 and V3 and >1 mm in all other leads. In

Table 4-14	Electrocardiogram-Based Anatomic Distribution	
ST Elevation	**Myocardial Territory**	**Coronary Artery**
V_1–V_6 or LBBB	Anterior and septal walls	Proximal LAD or left main
V_1–V_2	Septum	Proximal LAD or septal branch
V_2–V_4	Anterior wall	LAD
V_5–V_6	Lateral wall	LCX
II, III, aVF	Inferior wall	RCA or LCX
I, aVL	High lateral wall	Diagonal or proximal LCX

LAD, left anterior descending artery; LBBB, left bundle branch block; LCX, left circumflex artery; RCA, right coronary artery.

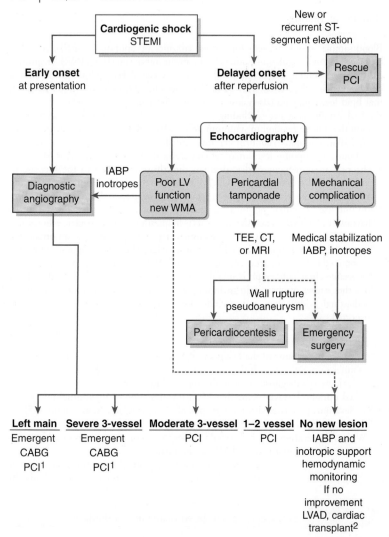

Figure 4-5. Recommended diagnostic and therapeutic strategy for patients presenting with STEMI and cardiogenic shock. [1]PCI may be preferable if CABG cannot be readily performed or if surgery imposes unacceptable risk. [2]Advanced heart therapy modalities including percutaneous LV assist devices (TandemHeart, Impella), external ventricular assist devices, and extracorporeal membrane oxygenation (ECMO) may be required prior to placement of a permanent LVAD or cardiac transplant. CABG, coronary artery bypass graft; CT, computed tomography; IABP, intra-aortic balloon pump; LVAD, left ventricular assist device; PCI, percutaneous coronary intervention; STEMI, ST-segment elevation myocardial infarction; TEE, transesophageal echocardiography; WMA, wall motion abnormality.

men <40 years of age, threshold value for abnormal ST-segment elevation at the J point in leads V2 and V3 is >2.5 mm.

o In women, the threshold value of abnormal is ST-segment elevation at the J point is >1.5 mm in leads V2 and V3 and >1 mm in all other leads.

o In right-sided leads (V3R and V4R), the threshold for abnormal ST elevation at the J point is 0.5 mm, except in males <30 years in whom it is 1 mm. Right-sided leads should be obtained in all patients with evidence of inferior wall ischemia to rule out right ventricular (RV) ischemia. RV infarction can occur with proximal right coronary artery (RCA) lesions.

o In posterior leads (V7, V8, and V9), the threshold for abnormal ST elevation at the J point is 0.5 mm.

▪ All patients with ST-segment depression in leads V1 to V3, inferior wall ST elevation, or tall R waves in V1 to V3 should have posterior leads placed in order to diagnosis a posterior wall MI. Posterior STEMIs are usually due to occlusion of the circumflex artery and are often misdiagnosed as UA/NSTEMI. R waves in V1 or V2 represent Q waves of the posterior territory.

▪ Ischemia of the circumflex artery may also be electrocardiographically silent.

o The presence of reciprocal ST-segment depression opposite of the infarct territory increases the specificity for acute MI.

o New LBBB. Suggests a large anterior wall MI with a worse prognosis.

o ECG criteria for STEMI in patients with preexisting LBBB or RV-pacing can be found in Table 4-15. Above criteria do not apply.

o **ECG changes that mimic MI.** ST-segment elevation and Q waves may result from numerous etiologies other than acute MI, including prior MI with aneurysm formation, aortic dissection, LV hypertrophy, pericarditis, myocarditis, pulmonary embolism, or may be a normal finding (Table 4-16). It is critical to obtain prior ECGs to clarify the diagnosis.

o **Q waves.** Development of new pathologic Q waves is considered diagnostic for transmural MI but may occur in patients with prolonged ischemia or poor collateral supply. The presence of Q waves only is not an indication for acute reperfusion; however, it is very helpful to have an old ECG to compare to on order to determine chronicity. Diagnostic criteria include:

▪ In leads V2 and V3, a pathologic Q wave is ≥0.02 s, or a QS complex in V2 or V3. An isolated Q wave in lead V1 or lead III is normal.

Table 4-15	Criteria for ST-segment Elevation for Prior LBBB or RV-paced Rhythm

ECG change

ST-segment elevation greater than 1 mm in the presence of a positive QRS complex (concordant with the QRS)

ST-segment elevation greater than 5 mm in the presence of a negative QRS complex (disconcordant with the QRS)

ST-segment depression greater than 1 mm in V_1-V_3

ECG, electrocardiogram; LBBB, left bundle branch block; RV, right ventricular.
Sgarbossa's (GUSTO) criteria: *Am J Cardiol 1996;77:423; N Engl J Med 1996;334:481; PACE 2001;24:1289.*

Table 4-16	Differential Diagnosis of ST-Segment Elevation

Cardiac Etiologies	Other Etiologies
Prior MI with aneurysm formation	Pulmonary embolism
Aortic dissection with coronary involvement	Hyperkalemia
Pericarditis	
Myocarditis	
LV hypertrophy or aortic stenosis (with strain)[a]	
Hypertrophic cardiomyopathy	
Coronary vasospasm (cocaine, Prinzmetal angina)	
Early repolarization (normal variant)	
Brugada syndrome	

[a]Strain may occur in numerous settings including systemic hypertension, hypotension, tachycardia, exercise, and sepsis.
LV, left ventricular; MI, myocardial infarction.

- In leads other than V1 through V3, presence of a Q wave ≥0.03 s and ≥0.1 mV deep or a QS complex in any two contiguous leads suggest prior MI.
- R wave ≥0.04 s in V1 and V2 and R/S ratio ≥1 with a positive T wave suggest prior posterior MI (in the absence of RVH or right bundle branch block [RBBB])
- **ECG changes that mimic MI.** ST-segment elevation and Q waves may result from numerous etiologies other than acute MI including prior MI with aneurysm formation, aortic dissection, LV hypertrophy, pericarditis, myocarditis, pulmonary embolism, or may be a normal finding (see Table 4-15). It is critical to obtain prior ECGs to clarify the diagnosis.

TREATMENT

- **Before presentation to the hospital.** The general public should be informed of the signs and symptoms consistent with an acute MI that should lead them to seek urgent medical care. Availability of "911" access and emergency medical services facilitates delivery of patients to emergency medical care.
- **Acute management.** Prompt treatment should be initiated as soon as the diagnosis is suspected, as mortality and risk of subsequent HF is directly related to ischemia time (Figure 4-6).
- All medical centers should have in place and utilize an American Heart Association/American College of Cardiology (AHA/ACC) guideline–based STEMI protocol. Centers that are not primary PCI capable should have protocols in place to meet accepted time to therapy guidelines, with either rapid transfer to a PCI-capable facility or administer thrombolytics with subsequent transfer to a PCI center.
- **In the emergency department**, an acute MI protocol should be activated that includes a targeted clinical examination and a 12-lead ECG completed within 10 minutes of arrival.
- **Immediate management.** The goal of immediate management in patients with STEMI is to identify candidates for reperfusion therapy and to immediately initiate that process. Other priorities include relief of ischemic pain, as well as recognition and treatment of hypotension, pulmonary edema, and arrhythmia.

Figure 4-6. The benefit of coronary reperfusion is inversely related to ischemia time. **Top.** Graphic representation of mortality benefit of coronary reperfusion as a function of ischemia time. (Adapted from *JAMA 2005;293:979.*) **Bottom.** Recommended timeline of events following chest pain onset according to AHA/ACC guidelines (*Circulation 2008;117:296*). ACC/AHA, American Heart Association/American College of Cardiology; ECG, electrocardiogram; EMS, emergency medical service; ER, emergency room; PCI, percutaneous coronary intervention; STEMI, ST-segment elevation myocardial infarction.

- **General measures**
  - Supplemental oxygen should be administered if saturations are <90%. If necessary, institution of mechanical ventilation decreases the work of breathing and reduces myocardial oxygen demand.
  - Two peripheral IV catheters should be inserted upon arrival.
  - Serial ECGs should be obtained for patients who do not have ST-segment elevation on the initial ECG but experience ongoing chest discomfort as they may have an evolving STEMI. Telemetry monitoring for arrhythmias.

Medications

Upstream medical therapy should include administration of ASA and anticoagulants as well as agents that reduce myocardial ischemia (Table 4-17).

- Chewable 162 to 325 mg **ASA** should be given immediately to <u>all</u> patients with suspected acute MI; 325 mg is preferred for those who are ASA naïve. After PCI, the subsequent dose of ASA is 81 mg a day is acceptable and is to be given indefinitely (*Eur Heart J 2009;30:900*).
- A loading dose of a **P2Y12 inhibitor** should be given to all STEMI patients, as part of dual antiplatelet therapy, as soon as possible after presentation. Cost and bleeding risk can be taken into consideration when choosing which agent. *Please also refer to the antiplatelet section on UA/NSTEMI for background information on agents listed in the following text.*
  - If the patient is to receive fibrinolytic therapy, along with ASA and an anticoagulant, patients should receive
    - Clopidogrel 300 mg loading dose if given during the first 24 hours of therapy; if started 24 hours after administration of fibrinolytics, a 600 mg loading dose is preferred. Maintenance is 75 mg a day.
    - Patients older than 75 years should not be given the loading dose.
  - If the patient is going for PCI, **one** of the following should be added to ASA and anticoagulant:
    - **Clopidogrel** 600 mg loading, then 75 mg daily for 12 months. Can be given prior to diagnostic angiography.
    - **Prasugrel** 60 mg loading, then 10 mg daily for minimum of 12 months (contraindicated in patients with prior CVA and avoided in those >75 years and weight <60 kg). Prasugrel generally should be given after diagnostic angiography (or within an hour of PCI) when it is certain the patient will not need CABG surgery given a higher incidence of bleeding related to surgery as compared to clopidogrel (*Lancet 2009;373:723*).
    - **Ticagrelor** 180 mg loading dose, then 90 mg bid (NOTE: maintenance ASA is 81 or 100 mg daily <u>only</u>) for a minimum of 12 months. Can be given on admission. It is not associated with higher risk of CABG-related bleeding; although, nonprocedural related major bleeding was higher when compared to clopidogrel.
- **GPIIb/IIIa inhibitors** most of the trials with these agents were conducted prior to the routine use of P2Y12 blockers. They do not have a role in the initial presentation of STEMI patients or as part of adjunctive therapy with thrombolytics.
  - GPIIb/IIIa antagonists are most useful when given at the time of PCI in patients treated with UFH and in patients not considered at higher risk of bleeding.
  - GPIIb/IIIa antagonists should be used *selectively* during PCI, in patients adequately treated with clopidogrel and UHF or clopidogrel and bivalirudin (e.g., presence of large thrombus, large anterior MI, or poor coronary flow post-PCI).
  - It may be reasonable to use GPIIb/IIIa inhibitors as an alternative to a P2Y12 antagonist in patients who present with acute complications of MI requiring surgery (ischemic MR, ruptured papillary muscle, or VSD).
  - Double bolus eptifibatide and high bolus dose tirofiban may have similar efficacy to abciximab (*Am J Cardiol 2004;94:35*; *JAMA 2008;299:1788*; *JACC 2008; 51:529*).
- **Anticoagulant therapy** should be initiated on presentation in all patients with STEMI regardless of the choice of PCI or thrombolytic therapy. *Please also refer to the medication section on UA/NSTEMI for background information on agents listed in the following text.*

Table 4-17	Upstream Medical Therapy	

Medication	Dosage	Comments
Aspirin (ASA)	162–325 mg	Nonenteric coated formulations (chewed or crushed) given orally or rectally facilitate rapid drug absorption and platelet inhibition.
Clopidogrel	600 mg loading dose, 75–150 mg daily	600 mg loading dose followed by 7 d of 150 mg maintenance dose for 7 d may reduce the incidence of stent thrombosis and MI compared to the standard 300 mg loading dose and 75 mg maintenance dose. Caution should be used in the elderly as clinical trials validating clopidogrel use in STEMI either did not include elderly patients or did not use a loading dose.
Prasugrel	60 mg loading dose, 10 mg daily	Compared to clopidogrel, prasugrel is a quicker acting and more potent antiplatelet agent with improved efficacy but did significantly increase CABG bleeding rates. Prasugrel should not be used in patients greater than 75 yr old, less than 60 kg, or with a history of stroke/TIA.
Ticagrelor	180 mg loading, then 90 mg bid	ASA dose should not exceed 100 mg. Ticagrelor has shown mortality benefit over clopidogrel at the expense of higher bleeding rates.
Unfractionated heparin (UFH)	60 U/kg IV bolus, 12 U/kg/hr	UFH should be given to all patients undergoing PCI and those receiving thrombolytics with the exception of streptokinase. The maximum IV bolus is 4,000 units.
Enoxaparin (LMWH)	30 mg IV bolus, 1 mg/kg SC bid	Patients greater than 75 yr of age should not be given a loading dose and receive 0.75 mg SC bid. An additional loading dose of 0.3 mg/kg should be given if the last dose of LMWH was more than 8 hr prior to PCI. The use of LMWH is only validated in thrombolysis and rescue PCI.

(continued)

Table 4-17	Upstream Medical Therapy (*Continued*)	
Medication	Dosage	Comments
Bivalirudin	0.75 mg/kg IV bolus, 1.75 mg/kg/hr	Bivalirudin has been validated in patients undergoing PCI and has not been studied in conjunction with thrombolysis. Patients who received a heparin bolus prior to bivalirudin had a lower incidence of stent thrombosis than those who only received bivalirudin.
Fondaparinux	2.5 mg IV bolus, 2.5 mg SC daily	Shown to be superior to UFH when used during thrombolysis with decreased bleeding rates. Fondaparinux increases the risk of catheter thrombosis when used during PCI (*JAMA 2006;295:1519*).
Nitroglycerin	0.4 mg SL or aerosol infusion: 10–200 mcg/min	Sublingual or aerosol nitroglycerin can be given every 5 min for a total of three doses in the absence of hypotension. IV nitroglycerin can be used for uncontrolled chest discomfort.
Metoprolol	25 mg PO qid, uptitrate as needed	β-Blockers should also be avoided in patients with evidence of heart failure, hemodynamic instability, marked first-degree AV block, advanced heart block, and bronchospasm.

AV, atrioventricular; CABG, coronary artery bypass grafting; LMWH, low–molecular-weight heparin; MI, myocardial infarction; PCI, percutaneous coronary intervention; STEMI, ST-segment elevation myocardial infarction; TIA, transient ischemic attack.

○ **Patients who will receive fibrinolytic therapy should be started on either:**
  ■ UFH for 48 hours. Given it is preferable to continue anticoagulation for the duration of the hospitalization (not greater than 8 days), use of UFH is less desirable due to its risk of inducing HIT. Studies suggest an advantage of enoxaparin or fondaparinux over UFH (*Lancet 2001;358:605; Circulation 2002;105:1642; N Engl J Med 2006;354:1477; JAMA 2006;295:1519*).
    □ If angiography with intent to perform PCI is anticipated to occur early postfibrinolysis, then UFH may be preferable.
    □ Dosing for UFH: bolus dose of 60 U/kg (max 4,000 U) then 12 U/kg/hr (maximum 1,000 U/hr) to keep PTT at 50 to 70 seconds.
  ■ Enoxaparin, if the serum creatinine is less than 2.5 mg/dL in men or 2.0 mg/dL in women, an initial 30 mg IV bolus is given followed 15 minutes later with 1 mg/kg subcutaneous given bid. Give for the entirety of the index hospitalization but not to exceed 8 days.

   ▫ Patients 75 years or older, no bolus is given and subcutaneous dose is 0.75 mg/kg bid.
   ▫ If CrCL <30 mL/min, the subcutaneous dose is 1 mg/kg daily.
 ▪ Fondaparinux, if the serum creatinine is less than 3 mg/dL, the initial IV dose is 2.5 mg, followed by subcutaneous 2.5 mg daily. Give for the entirety of the index hospitalization but not to exceed 8 days.
• **Anticoagulant choice for patients who will receive primary PCI:**
   ○ UFH is often preferred during PCI by many operators due to the availability as real-time therapeutic monitoring with activating clotting times (ACTs) in the catheterization laboratory (Figure 4-7). Additional bolus doses of UFH are given at PCI, with the dose and ACT goal dependent on whether a GPIIb/IIIa antagonist has been given.
   ○ Enoxaparin use in STEMI patients as an anticoagulant for PCI is unclear.
      ▪ Additional IV dose may be needed at PCI depending on timing of the last dose and total number of doses given.
      ▪ Patients on therapeutic enoxaparin should not be given UFH.
   ○ **Bivalirudin** can be given to patients already treated with ASA and clopidogrel on presentation (see Figure 4-7).

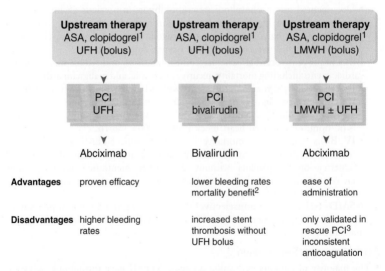

Figure 4-7. Recommended strategies for upstream therapy prior to PCI. [1]Prasugrel or ticagrelor may be used in place of clopidogrel in patients undergoing PCI. GPIIb/IIIa inhibitors may be used instead of clopidogrel, prasugrel, or ticagrelor in patients who present with mechanical complications of MI and require urgent cardiac surgery. [2]In comparison to UFH + GPIIb/IIIa inhibitor, bivalirudin improves mortality and decreases bleeding in patients presenting with STEMI. A heparin bolus and/or 600 mg clopidogrel loading dose should be given prior to bivalirudin to decrease the rate of stent thrombosis (*N Engl J Med 2008;358:2218*). [3]LMWH has only been studied in rescue PCI and has not been validated for primary PCI (*N Engl J Med 2006;354:1477*). ASA, aspirin; GP, glycoprotein; LMWH, low–molecular-weight heparin; PCI, percutaneous coronary intervention; STEMI, ST-segment elevation myocardial infarction; UFH, unfractionated heparin.

- Bivalirudin is an acceptable alternative to the use of combined heparin and GPIIb/IIIa inhibitor during PCI with lower bleeding rates but high rate of stent thrombosis (*N Engl J Med 2008;358:2218*; *JAMA 2003;19:853*).
- It is the agent of choice in patients with known HIT.
- It can be given with or without prior treatment with UFH. If patient is being treated with UFH, discontinue UFH for 30 minutes prior to starting bivalirudin.
- It is the preferred agent in patients at higher risk of bleeding.
- Risk of stent thrombosis *may* be lower if patients are pretreated with a 600 mg loading dose of clopidogrel or UFH.
- Dose is 0.75 mg/kg bolus, then 1.75 mg/kg/hr infusion.
  - **Fondaparinux** is not indicated for use in STEMI patients as a sole anticoagulant and has to be given along with UFH due to risk of catheter-related thrombosis.
- **Anti-ischemic therapy.** (Also refer to the Medications section for UA/NSTEMI for background information on agents listed here.)
  - **Nitroglycerin** should be administered to patients with ischemic chest pain, aid in control of hypertension, or as part of the management of HF. Nitroglycerin should either be avoided or used with caution in patients with
    - Hypotension (SBP <90 mm Hg)
    - Right ventricular infarct
    - HR >100 bpm or <50 bpm
    - Documented use of phosphodiesterase inhibitors in previous 48 hours
  - **Morphine** (2 to 4 mg IV) can be used for refractory chest pain that is not responsive to nitroglycerin. Adequate analgesia decreases levels of circulating catecholamines and reduces myocardial oxygen consumption.
  - **BBLs** improve myocardial ischemia, limit infarct size, and reduce major adverse cardiac events including mortality, recurrent ischemia, and malignant arrhythmias.
    - BBLs should be started in all patients with STEMI within the first 24 hours who do not have signs of new HF, evidence of cardiogenic shock (Killip II or greater), age older than 70 years, SBP <120 mm Hg, pulse >110, pulse <60 bpm, or advanced heart block (*Lancet 2005;366:1622*).
    - IV BBLs can increase mortality in patients with STEMI and should be reserved for management of arrhythmias or acute treatment of accelerated hypertension in patients without the earlier mentioned features. Sinus tachycardia in the setting of an STEMI may be a compensatory response to maintain cardiac output.
  - **NSAIDs (selective and nonselective)** should not be given during hospitalization due to an associated increase risk of MI, HF, hypertension, myocardial rupture, and death.

Acute Coronary Reperfusion

- The majority of patients who suffer an acute STEMI have thrombotic occlusion of a coronary artery. Early restoration of coronary perfusion limits infarct size, preserves LV function, and reduces mortality.
- All other therapies are secondary and should not delay the timely goal of achieving coronary reperfusion.
- Unless spontaneous resolution of ischemia occurs (as determined by resolution of chest discomfort and normalization of ST elevation), the choice of reperfusion strategy includes thrombolysis, primary PCI, or emergent CABG (Figure 4-8).
  - Normalization of the ECG and symptoms should not preclude the patient being referred for urgent diagnostic angiography. Morphine may mask ongoing ischemic symptoms.

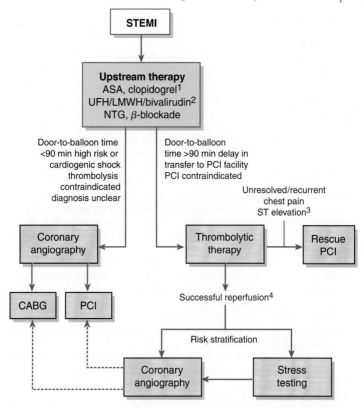

Figure 4-8. Strategies for coronary reperfusion and risk assessment. [1]If fibrinolytics are to be given, use clopidogrel only. If primary PCI is planned give either ticagrelor, prasugrel, or clopidogrel. [2]UFH may be used with either PCI or thrombolytic therapy, while bivalirudin has only been studied with PCI and LMWH has only been validated for fibrinolytic therapy and rescue PCI. Patients who are to get fibrinolysis LMWH and fondaparinux are preferred to UFH. [3]Patients who do not experience chest pain relief, have recurrent chest pain, unstable arrhythmias, development of heart failure, or ST-segment do not normalize 60 to 90 minutes following fibrinolysis should undergo rescue PCI. [4]Signs of successful reperfusion include chest pain relief, 50% reduction in ST-segment elevation, and idioventricular rhythm. P2Y12 inhibitors include antiplatelet agents: clopidogrel, prasugrel, and ticagrelor. ASA, aspirin; CABG, coronary artery bypass graft; LMWH, low–molecular-weight heparin; NTG, nitroglycerin; PCI, percutaneous coronary intervention; STEMI, ST-segment elevation myocardial infarction; UFH, unfractionated heparin.

○ **NOTE:** Ongoing symptoms are not criteria for treatment of STEMI in the first 12 hours of symptom onset. Patients who arrive within 12 hours of their symptoms, despite symptom resolution, but with continued ECG changes of STEMI are still candidates for immediate reperfusion (either primary PCI or fibrinolytics). Although we recommend angiography with intent for PCI/CABG in such a circumstance.

- The choice of reperfusion therapy should almost be considered of secondary importance to the overall goal of achieving reperfusion in a timely manner.
  - **Primary PCI**
    - Primary PCI is the preferred reperfusion strategy when available within 90 minutes of first medical contact. Compared to fibrinolytic therapy, PCI offers superior vessel patency and perfusion (TIMI 3 flow) with less reinfarction, less risk of intracranial hemorrhage, and improved survival regardless of lesion location or patient age (*N Engl J Med 1997;336:1621*; *Lancet 2003;361:13*).
    - STEMI patients with symptom onset less than 12 hours prior have a better prognosis and outcome after PCI. However, PCI should still be offered to patients with STEMI who have ongoing symptoms, which began 12 to 24 hours prior because they will still likely benefit from revascularization. PCI may also be considered, although evidence of benefit is limited, in patients who are now asymptomatic but had symptoms in previous 12- to 24-hour period. Asymptomatic patients who are hemodynamically and electrically stable without evidence of ischemia, whose symptoms began more than 24 hours prior, should not be offered PCI of a totally occluded infarct artery (*Circulation 2011;22:2320*).
    - **PCI** is preferred over fibrinolysis in the following situations:
      - Patients who present with severe heart failure or cardiogenic shock should receive primary PCI (even if transfer to a PCI center may cause delays beyond current time goals for reperfusion).
        - Killip class III/IV or TIMI risk score ≥5, represent a high-risk groups where PCI is preferred despite a potential time delay (*Eur Heart J 2010;31:676*; *Circulation 2005;112:2017*).
        - Patients in cardiogenic shock who do not quickly stabilize should be offered a hemodynamic support device.
      - Have a contraindication to fibrinolytic therapy.
      - Have had recent PCI or prior CABG.
      - PCI is generally preferred to fibrinolysis in patients with symptom onset greater than 12 hours prior (*N Engl J Med 1997;336:1621*; *Lancet 2003;361:13*).
    - Optimally, operators should perform greater than 75 PCIs per year at experienced centers with a volume that exceeds 200 PCIs per year (36 of the PCIs should have been in STEMI patients).
    - If the patient has multivessel coronary disease, only the infarct-related artery (IRA) should be revascularized, unless revascularization of a non-IRA is expected to benefit a patient in shock. Otherwise, it is more appropriate to delay complete revascularization, generally after the IRA is revascularized and the patient is stabilized for 24 hours. Complete revascularization is often performed in a staged manner to minimize contrast-mediated renal toxicity.
    - Coronary stenting is superior to balloon angioplasty alone and reduces the rates of target vessel revascularization (*N Engl J Med 1999;341:1949*; *N Engl J Med 2002;346:957*). DES further reduce the need for target vessel revascularization without increasing the incidence of stent thrombosis (*Circulation 2009;120:964*; *JACC 2008;51:618*; *JAMA 2008;299:1788*).
    - Facilitated PCI, a strategy of reduced dose of a GPIIb/IIIa inhibitors and/or fibrinolytic agent just prior to PCI, should not be routinely employed as it does not improve efficacy and significantly increases bleeding rates (*Lancet 2006;367:569*; *N Engl J Med 2008;358:2205*; *Lancet 2006;367:579*).

○ **Fibrinolytic therapy**
  ▪ Fibrinolytic therapy has the main advantages of widespread availability and ease of delivery. The primary disadvantage of fibrinolytic therapy is the risk of intracranial hemorrhage, uncertainty of whether normal coronary flow has been restored, and risk of reocclusion of the IRA. It is used when PCI is not available in a timely fashion.
  ▪ Fibrinolytic therapy is indicated for use if given within 12 hours of the symptom onset with qualifying ECG changes of ST elevation, new LBBB, or true posterior MI. When given, it should be administered within 30 minutes of initial patient contact.
    □ Fibrinolytic therapy is most successful when given in the first 3 hours of symptom onset after which the benefit tapers.
    □ Patients presenting to a hospital without PCI capability should be transferred for primary PCI, rather than being given fibrinolytics if time from first medical contact to PCI will not be greater than 120 minutes (however, system goals should continue to strive for <90 minutes). This seems particularly relevant to patients arriving 3 to 12 hours from symptom onset (*J Am Coll Cardiol 2011;57:272*; *Circulation 2007;116:721*; *Circulation 2008;117:1145*). In patients transferred for PCI, primary PCI significantly lowered the incidence of death, MI, or stroke compared to on-site thrombolysis (*N Engl J Med 2003;249:733*; *JACC 2002;39:1713*; *Eur Heart J 2000;21:823*).
  ▪ Available thrombolytic agents include the fibrin-selective agents such as **alteplase** (recombinant tissue plasminogen activator, rt-PA), **reteplase** (r-PA), and **tenecteplase** (TNK-tPA). **Streptokinase** is the only nonselective agent in use. Further details and dosing information can be found in Table 4-18.
    □ TNK-tPA is the current agent of choice due to similar efficacy, lower risk of bleeding and convenient single bolus administration as compared to rt-PA. Streptokinase is the cheapest and still widely used worldwide.
    □ Fibrin-selective agents should be used in combination with anticoagulant therapy, ASA, and clopidogrel (see earlier). GPIIb/IIIa inhibitors should not be used in conjunction. Prasugrel and ticagrelor have not been studied for use with fibrinolytics.
  ▪ Fibrinolytic therapy is contraindicated in patients:
    □ ST-segment depression (unless posterior MI suspected).
    □ In patients who are asymptomatic with initial symptoms occurring more than 24 hours ago (*this in contrast to patients who are asymptomatic with symptom onset less than 12 hours prior; see earlier*).
    □ Other contraindications to fibrinolysis are listed in Table 4-19.
    □ Presence of five or more risk factors for intracranial hemorrhage.
  ▪ The most common complication of fibrinolytic therapy is bleeding. Intracranial hemorrhage occurs in >4% of patients with five or more of the following risk factors for intracranial hemorrhage (*Stroke 2000;31:1802*).
    □ Age ≥75 years
    □ Weight ≤65 kg in women and ≤80 kg in men
    □ Female gender
    □ Black race
    □ Prior history of stroke
    □ SBP ≥160 mm Hg
    □ INR >4 or PT >24
    □ Use of alteplase

Table 4-18	Fibrinolytic Agents	
Medication	**Dosage**	**Comments**
Streptokinase (SK)	1.5 million U IV over 60 min	Produces a generalized fibrinolytic state (not clot specific). SK reduces mortality following STEMI: 18% relative risk reduction and 2% absolute risk reduction (*Lancet 1987;2:871*). Allergic reactions including skin rashes, fever, and anaphylaxis may be seen in 1%–2% of patients. Isolated hypotension occurs in 10% of patients and usually responds to volume expansion. Because of the development of antibodies, patients who were previously treated with SK should be given an alternate thrombolytic agent.
Recombinant tissue plasminogen activator (rt-PA)	15 mg IV bolus 0.75 mg/kg over 30 min (maximum 50 mg) 0.50 mg/kg over 60 min (maximum 35 mg)	Fibrin selective agent with improved clot specificity compared to SK. Does not cause allergic reactions or hypotension. Mortality benefit compared to SK at the expense of an increased risk of intracranial hemorrhage (*N Engl J Med 1993;329:673*).
Reteplase (r-PA)	Two 10-U IV boluses administered 30 min apart	Fibrin selective agent with a longer half-life but reduced clot specificity compared to rt-PA. Mortality benefit equivalent to that of rt-PA (*N Engl J Med 1997;337:1118*).
Tenecteplase (TNK-tPA)	0.50 mg/kg IV bolus (total dose 30–50 mg)	Genetically engineered variant of rt-PA with slower plasma clearance, improved fibrin specificity, and higher resistance to PAI-1. Mortality benefit equivalent to that of rt-PA with reduced bleeding rates (*Lancet 1999;354:716*). Monitoring is required with a goal aPTT of 1.5–2.5 times control.

aPTT, activated partial thromboplastin time; PAI-1, plasminogen activator inhibitor-1; STEMI, ST-segment elevation myocardial infarction.

Table 4-19	Contraindications to Thrombolytic Therapy

Absolute Contraindications	Relative Contraindications
History of intracranial hemorrhage or hemorrhagic stroke	Prior ischemic stroke more than 3 mo ago
Ischemic stroke within 3 mo	Allergy or previous use of streptokinase (greater than 5 d ago)[a]
Known structural cerebrovascular lesion (AVMs, aneurysms, tumor)	Recent internal bleeding (2–4 wk)
Closed head injury within 3 mo	Prolonged/traumatic CPR more than 10 min
Aortic dissection	Major surgery within 3 wk
Severe uncontrolled hypertension (SBP >180 mm Hg, DBP >110 mm Hg)	Active peptic ulcer disease
Active bleeding or bleeding diathesis	Noncompressible vascular punctures
Acute pericarditis	History of intraocular bleeding
	Pregnancy
	Uncontrolled hypertension
	Use of oral anticoagulants

[a]Thrombolytics other than streptokinase may be used.
AVM, arteriovenous malformation; CPR, cardiopulmonary resuscitation; DBP, diastolic blood pressure; SBP, systolic blood pressure.

- Any patient who experiences a sudden change in neurologic status should undergo urgent head CT and all anticoagulant and thrombolytic therapies discontinued. Fresh frozen plasma should be given to patients with intracerebral hemorrhage. Cryoprecipitate may also be used to replenish fibrinogen and factor VIII levels. Platelet transfusions and Protamine can be useful in patients with markedly prolonged bleeding times. Neurologic and neurosurgical consultation should be obtained immediately. Major bleeding complications that require blood transfusion occur in approximately 10% of patients.

- **Postfibrinolysis Care**
  □ Postfibrinolysis, patients should be transferred to a PCI-capable facility with the intention to perform PCI 3 to 24 hours after initiating fibrinolytic therapy even if fibrinolysis was successful and patient is hemodynamically stable.
  □ Routine coronary angiography within 24 hours of thrombolysis has reduced adverse cardiac events compared to rescue PCI (*Lancet 2004;264:1045*). Immediate transfer for angiography (3 to 24 hours postfibrinolysis) at a PCI-capable facility is also proven to be beneficial (*Lancet 2008;371:559*). This strategy, known as the pharmacoinvasive strategy, should be differentiated from facilitated PCI where thrombolytic agents are administered immediately before primary PCI.
  □ Facilitated PCI, however, was associated with higher mortality, stroke, and free wall rupture.

- **Rescue PCI post failed fibrinolysis**
  □ Thrombolytic therapy does not achieve coronary artery patency in 30% of patients. In contrast, primary PCI results in restoration of normal coronary flow (TIMI 3) in greater than 95% of cases.
  □ Patients with failed fibrinolytic therapy should be referred for rescue PCI.

□ Rescue PCI reduces the incidence of death, reinfarction, and HF by nearly 50% (*Circulation 1994;90:2280; N Engl J Med 2005;353:2758*).
□ Evidence of failed fibrinolysis includes:
  - Persistence or reoccurrence of ischemic symptoms
  - ST segments resolve less than 50%, 90 minutes postfibrinolysis
  - Electrical or hemodynamic instability
  - Development of HF symptoms
- **Emergency CABG** is a high-risk procedure that should be considered only if the patient has severe left main disease or refractory ischemia in the setting of failed PCI or coronary anatomy that is not amenable to PCI. Emergency surgery should also be considered for patients with acute mechanical complications of MI including papillary muscle rupture, severe ischemic MR, VSD, ventricular aneurysm formation in the setting of intractable ventricular arrhythmias, or ventricular free wall rupture.

Peri-Infarct Management

- **The coronary care unit (CCU)** was the first major advance in the modern era of treatment of acute MI. The majority of patients benefit from the specialized training of the nursing and support staff in the CCU. Most patients with acute MI should be observed for 24 to 48 hours in the CCU.
- Bed rest is appropriate intermediate care for the first 24 hours after presentation with an acute MI. After 24 hours, clinically stable patients can progressively advance their activity as tolerated.
- Patients should have continuous telemetry monitoring to detect for recurrent ischemia and arrhythmias. Daily evaluation should include assessment for recurrent chest discomfort, new HF symptoms, and routine ECGs. Physical exam should focusing on new murmurs and any evidence of HF.
- A baseline echocardiogram should be obtained to document EF, wall motion abnormalities, valvular lesions, and presence of ventricular thrombus.
- **Hemodynamic monitoring** may be useful to optimize medical therapy in unstable patients (see the following text).
- **Cardiac pacing** may be required in the setting of an acute MI. Rhythm disturbance may be transient in nature in which case temporary pacing is sufficient until a stable rhythm returns (see the following text). As compared to inferior wall MIs where AV block is transient and stable, AV block with anterior wall MIs can be unstable with wide QRS escape rhythms with an 80% mortality and usually requiring temporary and then permanent pacemakers.

Post-STEMI Medical Therapy

- See also Medications section for UA/NSTEMI.
- **ASA** should continued indefinitely. Dose of 81 mg/d has been shown to be effective post-PCI; however, the range of 75 to 162 mg/d has also been endorsed.
- **Clopidogrel** (75 mg/d), **prasugrel** (10 mg/d), or **ticagrelor** (90 mg bid) should be given for a minimum of 12 months regardless of whether a BMS or DES was employed (*this is in contrast to non-ACS patients who receive a BMS and the minimum duration of therapy is 1 month*).
- **BBLs** confer a mortality benefit following acute MI. Treatment should begin as soon as possible (preferably within the first 24 hours) and continued indefinitely unless contraindicated.
- **ACEIs** provide a reduction in short-term mortality, incidence of HF, and recurrent MI when initiated within the first 24 hours of an acute MI (*Lancet 1994;343:1115; Lancet 1995;345:669*).

- ○ Patients with EF <40%, large anterior MI, and prior MI derive the most benefit from ACEI therapy.
- ○ Contraindications include hypotension, history of angioedema with use, pregnancy, acute renal failure, and hyperkalemia. Care must be taken to avoid hypotension and use in bilateral renal artery stenosis.
- ○ Angiotensin II receptor blockers can be used in patients who are intolerant of ACEIs.
- **HMG-CoA reductase inhibitors** should be started in all patients in the absence of contraindications. Several trials have shown the benefit of early and aggressive use of high-dose statins following AMI. The goal is at least 50% reduction in LDL or LDL <70 mg/dL.
- **Aldosterone receptor antagonists (Aldactone and eplerenone)** have shown benefit in post-MI patients with LV EF <40% and in diabetics (*N Engl J Med 1999;341:709*; *N Engl J Med 2003;348:1309*). Caution should be used in patients with hyperkalemia and renal insufficiency.
- All patients should be referred for cardiac rehabilitation.

SPECIAL CONSIDERATIONS

Risk Assessment

- Asymptomatic patients who present greater than 24 hours after symptom onset, patients who receive medical therapy alone, and patients who receive an incomplete revascularization should undergo further risk assessment. Patients may be evaluated using either a noninvasive stress testing or invasive (coronary angiography) strategy.
- **Stress testing** can be used to determine prognosis, residual ischemia, and functional capacity. Patients who are successfully revascularized do not need stress testing prior to discharge unless needed for referral to cardiac rehabilitation.
  - ○ A submaximal exercise stress test can be performed as early as 2 to 3 days following MI in stable patients who have had no further ischemic signs/symptoms or signs of HF.
  - ○ Alternatively, stress testing can be performed after hospital discharge (2 to 6 weeks) for low-risk patients and for patients starting cardiac rehabilitation.
  - ○ Coronary angiography should be performed in patients with limiting angina, significant ischemic burden, and those with poor functional capacity.
- Patients treated medically or with fibrinolytics who experience complications of MI, including recurrent angina/ischemia, HF, significant ventricular arrhythmia, or a mechanical complication of the MI, should proceed directly to coronary angiography to define their anatomy and offer an appropriate revascularization strategy.
- **Special clinical situations**
  - ○ **RV myocardial infarction** is seen in approximately 50% of patients with an acute inferior MI. Roughly half of these patients have hemodynamic compromise as a result of right ventricular involvement.
    - ▪ Clinical signs may include hypotension, cardiogenic shock, elevated jugular venous pulsation, Kussmaul sign (an increase in jugular venous pressures with inspiration), and right-sided third or fourth heart sounds. The lung fields are often clear (unless HF or MR develop, as well).
    - ▪ LV filling pressures are typically normal or decreased, the right atrial pressures are elevated (>10 mm Hg), and the cardiac index is depressed. In some patients, elevated right atrial pressures may not be evident until IV fluids are administered.

- Initial therapy is IV fluids. If hypotension persists, inotropic support with dobutamine and/or an intra-aortic balloon pump (IABP) may be necessary. Invasive hemodynamic monitoring is critical in the persistently hypotensive patient as it guides volume status and the need for inotropic and mechanical support.
- In patients with heart block and AV dyssynchrony, sequential AV pacing has a marked beneficial effect.
○ **ISR and stent thrombosis** are disease entities unique to patients who have previously undergone coronary angioplasty with stent placement. Risk factors for ISR and stent thrombosis can be found in Table 4-20.
- ISR is a result of intimal hyperplasia and occurs within 6 to 9 months following balloon angioplasty and stent deployment. Progressive exertional angina is the typical presenting symptom. Prior to BMS, the incidence of target lesion restenosis 1 year following balloon angioplasty was 35% to 40%. BMS placement reduced the rate of angiographic restenosis to 20% to 30%, and DES further reduced the 1-year restenosis rate to 3% to 5%.
  □ DES placement is the treatment of choice for ISR (*N Engl J Med 2002; 346:1773*; *N Engl J Med 2003;349:1315*; *JAMA 2005;294:1215*).
  □ Other proposed treatments for ISR including rotational atherectomy and brachytherapy produce inferior results compared to DES placement, and in the case of brachytherapy, increase the risk of stent thrombosis (*JAMA 2006;295:1264*; *JAMA 2006;295:1253*).
- Stent thrombosis occurs with BMS or DES and is due to poor endothelial repair or patient nonadherence to P2Y12 inhibitors. Stent thrombosis commonly presents either as an ACS or as sudden cardiac death and is associated with a high mortality rate. The etiology of stent thrombosis is based on the time from prior coronary intervention (*JAMA 2005;293:2126*; *JACC 2009; 53:1399*).

Table 4-20	Risk Factors for In-Stent Restenosis and Stent Thrombosis
ISR	**Stent Thrombosis**
Diabetes	Clopidogrel discontinuation
Chronic kidney disease	Clopidogrel resistance
Prior restenosis	Diabetes
Prior stent placed in the setting of ACS	Chronic kidney disease
Small luminal diameter (<2.5 mm)	Malignancy
Long lesion length	Prior brachytherapy
Proximal LAD lesion	Small luminal diameter
Saphenous vein graft lesion	(<3 mm)
Residual stenosis following prior intervention	Long lesion length
	Bifurcation lesion
	Margin dissection
	Incomplete wall apposition
	Overlapping stents

ACS, acute coronary syndrome; ISR, in-stent restenosis; LAD, left anterior descending artery.

□ Acute stent thrombosis occurs within 24 hours and is due to mechanical procedural complications as well as inadequate anticoagulation and antiplatelet therapies.

□ Subacute stent thrombosis (24 hours to 30 days) is a consequence of inadequate platelet inhibition and mechanical stent complications. Cessation of P2Y12 inhibitor (clopidogrel, prasugrel, ticagrelor) therapy during this time yields a 30- to 100-fold risk of stent thrombosis.

□ Late (30 days to 1 year) stent thrombosis occurs principally with DES and is associated with P2Y12 inhibitor cessation (fourfold to sixfold increased risk if discontinued early) and/or resistance.

- In general, PCI with thrombus aspiration and repeat stent deployment is recommended. Screening for clopidogrel resistance and initiation of more potent antiplatelet regimens such as prasugrel, ticagrelor, or clopidogrel 150 mg in combination with cilostazol can be considered (*JACC 2005;46:1833; Circulation 2009;119:3207*).

○ **Ischemic MR** is a poor prognostic indicator following MI that can present with HF or acute pulmonary edema without LV dysfunction. It is associated with posterior infarcts and resultant posterior papillary muscle involvement/rupture. The anterior papillary muscle has a dual blood supply, so is less vulnerable to rupture. The presence of MR following MI significantly increases mortality (*Ann Intern Med 1992;117:10; Am J Med 2006;119:103*).

▪ The mechanism of acute MR includes papillary muscle dysfunction or leaflet tethering due to posterior wall akinesis.

▪ Progressive MR following MI may develop as a result of LV chamber dilation, apical remodeling, or posterior wall dyskinesis. These changes lead to leaflet tethering or mitral annular dilation.

▪ Echocardiography is the diagnostic modality of choice. *Acute* ischemic MR, as compared to slowly developing MR, is not always readily identified on physical exam, and may produce little or no murmur in cases of acute MR. Similarly, TTEs may also miss acute severe MR and a high clinical suspicion should prompt obtaining a TEE to access the severity and mechanism of MR. Patients with acute severe MR will present in acute pulmonary edema without an obvious cause. MR should be considered in such patients and TEE obtained if an apparent cause of pulmonary congestion is not present or if LV function appears hyperdynamic.

▪ Initial treatment of MR involves aggressive afterload reduction and revascularization. *Stable* patients should receive a trial of medical therapy and undergo surgery only if they fail to improve. Early surgical intervention is warranted for patients with severe ischemic MR due to papillary muscle rupture.

○ **STEMI** in the setting of recent **cocaine use** presents a unique and challenging management situation (*Circulation 2008;117:1897–1907*). ST elevation can result from myocardial ischemia due to coronary vasospasm, in situ thrombus formation, and/or increased myocardial oxygen demand. The common pathophysiology is excessive stimulation of α- and β-adrenergic receptors. Chest pain due to cocaine use usually occurs within 3 hours but may be seen several days following use.

▪ Oxygen, ASA, and heparin (UFH or LMWH) should be administered to all patients with cocaine-associated STEMI.

▪ Nitrates should be used preferentially to treat vasospasm. Additionally, benzodiazepines may confer additional relief by decreasing sympathetic tone.

- **BBLs** are contraindicated; both selective and nonselective BBLs should be avoided.
- Phentolamine (α-adrenergic antagonist) and calcium channel blockers may reverse coronary vasospasm and are recommended as second-line agents.
- The use of reperfusion therapy is controversial and should be reserved for those patients whose symptoms persist despite initial medical therapy.
  - Primary PCI is the preferred approach for the patient with persistent symptoms and ECG changes despite aggressive medical therapy. It is important to note that coronary angiography and intervention carry a significant risk of worsening vasospasm.
  - Fibrinolytic therapy should be reserved for patients who are clearly having an STEMI who cannot undergo PCI.

COMPLICATIONS

Myocardial damage predisposes the patient to several potential adverse consequences and complications that should be considered if the patient experiences new clinical signs and/or symptoms. These include recurrent chest pain, cardiac arrhythmias, cardiogenic shock, and mechanical complications of MI.

- **Recurrent chest pain** may be due to ischemia in the territory of the original infarction, pericarditis, myocardial rupture, or pulmonary embolism.
  - Recurrent angina is experienced by 20% to 30% of patients after MI who receive fibrinolytic therapy and up to 10% of patients in the early time period following percutaneous revascularization. These symptoms may represent recurrence of ischemia or infarct extension.
    - Assessment of the patient may include evaluation for new murmurs or friction rubs, ECG to assess for new ischemic changes, cardiac enzymes (troponin and CK-MB), echocardiography, and repeat coronary angiography if indicated.
    - Patients with recurrent chest pain should continue to receive ASA, P2Y12 inhibition, heparin, nitroglycerin, and BBL therapy.
    - If recurrent angina is refractory to medical treatment, repeat coronary angiography and intervention should be considered along with possible placement of an IABP.
  - **Acute pericarditis** occurs 24 to 96 hours after MI in approximately 10% to 15% of patients. The associated chest pain is often pleuritic and may be relieved in the upright position. A friction rub may be noted on clinical examination, and the ECG may show diffuse ST-segment elevation and PR-segment depression. Lead AVR may have PR elevation. Treatment is directed at pain management.
    - High-dose ASA (up to 650 mg qid maximum) is generally considered a first-line agent. NSAIDs such as ibuprofen may be used if ASA is not effective but should be avoided early post–acute MI.
    - Colchicine along with ASA may also be beneficial for recurrent symptoms and may also be superior to each agent alone.
    - Glucocorticoids (prednisone, 1 mg/kg daily) may be useful if symptoms are severe and refractory to initial therapy. Steroids should be used sparingly as they may lead to an increased risk of recurrence of pericarditis. Use should also be deferred until at least 4 weeks after acute MI due to their adverse impact on infarct healing and risk of ventricular aneurysm (*Am Heart J 1981;101:750*).
    - Heparin should be avoided in the setting of pericarditis with or without effusion as it may lead to pericardial hemorrhage.

○ **Dressler syndrome** is thought to be an autoimmune process characterized by malaise, fever, pericardial pain, leukocytosis, elevated sedimentation rate, and often a pericardial effusion. In contrast to acute pericarditis, Dressler syndrome occurs 1 to 8 weeks after MI. Treatment is identical to acute pericarditis.

• **Arrhythmias.** Cardiac rhythm abnormalities are common following MI and may include conduction block, atrial arrhythmias, and ventricular arrhythmias. Arrhythmias that result in hemodynamic compromise require prompt, aggressive intervention. If the arrhythmia precipitates refractory angina or HF, urgent therapy is warranted. For all rhythm disturbances, exacerbating conditions should be addressed, including electrolyte imbalances, hypoxia, acidosis, and adverse drug effects. (Details on specific arrhythmias can be found in Table 4-21.)

○ **Transcutaneous and transvenous pacing.** Conduction system disease that progresses to complete heart block or results in symptomatic bradycardia can be effectively treated with cardiac pacing. A transcutaneous pacing device can be used under emergent circumstances; however, a temporary transvenous system should be used for longer duration therapy.

  ▪ Absolute indications for temporary transvenous pacing include asystole, symptomatic bradycardia, recurrent sinus pauses, complete heart block, and incessant VT.

  ▪ Temporary transvenous pacing may also be warranted for new trifascicular block, new Mobitz II block, and for patients with LBBB who require a pulmonary artery catheter, given the risk of developing complete heart block.

○ **Implantable cardioverter-defibrillators (ICDs)** should not routinely be implanted in patients with reduced LV function following MI or those with ventricular tachycardia/fibrillation (VT/VF) in the setting of ischemia or immediately following reperfusion.

  ▪ Routine insertion of ICDs into patients with reduced LV function immediately following MI does not improve outcomes (*N Engl J Med 2004;351:2481*).

  ▪ In contrast, patients who continue to have depressed LV function (EF <35% and New York Heart Association [NYHA] 2 or 3 or EF <30% regardless of NYHA class) greater than 40 days following MI benefit from ICD therapy (*N Engl J Med 2005;352:225; N Engl J Med 2002;346:877*).

  ▪ ICD therapy is also indicated for patients with recurrent episodes of sustained VT or VF despite coronary reperfusion.

• **Cardiogenic shock** is an infrequent, but serious, complication of MI and is defined as hypotension in the setting of inadequate ventricular function to meet the metabolic needs of the peripheral tissue. Risk factors include prior MI, older age, diabetes, and anterior infarction. Organ hypoperfusion may manifest as progressive renal failure, dyspnea, diaphoresis, or mental status changes. Hemodynamic monitoring reveals elevated filling pressures (wedge pressure >20 mm Hg), depressed cardiac index (<2.5 L/kg/min), and hypotension (see Figure 4-5).

○ Patients with cardiogenic shock in the setting of MI have a mortality in excess of 50%. Such patients may require invasive hemodynamic monitoring and advanced therapeutic modalities including inotropic and mechanical support (see Figure 4-5).

○ **Dobutamine** is the inotrope of choice for patients with relatively preserved SBP (>90 mm Hg) as it both increases myocardial contractility and decreases ventricular afterload.

Table 4-21	Arrhythmias Complicating Myocardial Infarction	
Arrhythmia	**Treatment**	**Comments**
Intraventricular conduction delays	None	The left anterior fascicle is most commonly affected because of isolated coronary blood supply. Bifascicular and trifascicular block may progress to complete heart block and other rhythm disturbances.
Sinus bradycardia	None Atropine 0.5 mg Temporary pacing[a]	Sinus bradycardia is common in patients with RCA infarcts. In the absence of hypotension or significant ventricular ectopy, observation is indicated.
AV block	Temporary pacing[a]	First-degree AV block usually does not require specific treatment. Mobitz I second-degree block occurs more often with inferior MI. The block is usually within the His bundle and does not require treatment unless symptomatic bradycardia is present. Mobitz II second-degree AV block originates below the His bundle and is more commonly associated with anterior MI. Because of the significant risk of progression to complete heart block, patients should be observed in the CCU and treated with temporary pacing if symptomatic. Third-degree AV block complicates large anterior and RV infarcts. In patients with anterior MI, third-degree heart block often occurs 12–24 hr after initial presentation and may appear suddenly. Temporary pacing is recommended because of the risk of progression to ventricular asystole.
Sinus tachycardia	None[b]	Sinus tachycardia is common in patients with acute MI and is often due to enhanced sympathetic activity resulting from pain, anxiety, hypovolemia, anxiety, heart failure, or fever.

(continued)

Table 4-21	Upstream Medical Therapy (*Continued*)	
Arrhythmia	**Treatment**	**Comments**
		Persistent sinus tachycardia suggests poor underlying ventricular function and is associated with excess mortality.
Atrial fibrillation and flutter	β-Blockers Anticoagulation Cardioversion	Atrial fibrillation and flutter are observed in up to 20% of patients with acute MI. Because atrial fibrillation and atrial flutter are usually transient in the acute MI period, long-term anticoagulation is often not necessary after documentation of stable sinus rhythm.
Accelerated junctional rhythm	None	Accelerated junctional rhythm occurs in conjunction with inferior MI. The rhythm is usually benign and warrants treatment only if hypotension is present. Digitalis intoxication should be considered in patients with accelerated junctional rhythm.
Ventricular premature depolarizations (VPDs)	β-Blockers if symptomatic[c]	VPDs are common in the course of an acute MI. Prophylactic treatment with lidocaine or other antiarrhythmics has been associated with increased overall mortality and is not recommended (*N Engl J Med 1989;321:406*).
Accelerated idioventricular rhythm (AIVR)	None	Commonly seen within 48 hr of successful reperfusion and is not associated with an increased incidence of adverse outcomes. If hemodynamically unstable, sinus activity may be restored with atropine or temporary atrial pacing.
Ventricular tachycardia (VT)	Cardioversion for sustained VT Lidocaine or amiodarone for 24–48 hr[d]	Nonsustained ventricular tachycardia (NSVT, <30 sec) is common in the first 24 hr after MI and is only associated with increased mortality when occurring late in the post-MI course. Sustained VT (>30 sec) during the first 48 hr after acute MI is associated with increased in-hospital mortality.

(*continued*)

Table 4-21	Upstream Medical Therapy (*Continued*)	
Arrhythmia	**Treatment**	**Comments**
Ventricular fibrillation (VF)	Unsynchronized cardioversion Lidocaine or amiodarone for 24–48 hr[d]	VF occurs in up to 5% of patients in the early post-MI period and is life threatening.

[a]Atropine and temporary pacing should only be used for symptomatic or hemodynamically unstable patients.
[b]The use of β-blockers in the setting of sinus tachycardia and poor left ventricular (LV) function may result in decompensated heart failure.
[c]β-Blockers should be used with caution in the setting of bradycardia and frequent VPDs as they may increase the risk of polymorphic VT.
[d]Lidocaine should be used as a 1 mg/kg bolus followed by a 1–2 mg/kg/hr infusion. Amiodarone should be given as a 150–300 mg bolus followed by an infusion of 1 mg/kg/hr for 6 hours and then 0.5 mg/kg/hr for 18 hours.
AV, atrioventricular; CCU, coronary care unit; MI, myocardial infarction; RCA, right coronary artery; RV, right ventricular.

- **Dopamine** is the preferred therapeutic agent in patients with an SBP less than 80 mm Hg. Addition of norepinephrine or phenylephrine may be required in markedly hypotensive patients (SBP <70 mm Hg).
- **Milrinone** should be added in patients who are either not responding to dobutamine or who are experiencing excessive tachycardia in response to dobutamine. It should not be routinely used in patients with renal insufficiency.
- Patients in whom contraindications do not exist should be considered for insertion of an IABP, as inotropes increase myocardial oxygen consumption and may worsen ischemia or fail to augment cardiac output (Table 4-22).

Table 4-22	Intra-Aortic Balloon Counterpulsation	
Indications	**Contraindications**	**Monitoring**
Cardiogenic shock, pump failure	Aortic insufficiency	Daily chest X-ray, platelet count, and creatinine
Papillary muscle rupture	Severe peripheral vascular disease	
Severe ischemic mitral regurgitation	Systemic infection, sepsis	Regular evaluation of lower extremity pulses
VSD		
Facilitation of unprotected left main and LAD angioplasty or CABG		Heparin infusion (PTT)
Complex PCI with severe underlying CAD		

CABG, coronary artery bypass grafting; LAD, left anterior descending artery; PCI, percutaneous coronary intervention; PTT, partial thromboplastin time; VSD, ventricular septal defect.

- In some patients, other circulatory support devices can be considered. Most are surgically placed (see Chapter 5, Heart Failure and Cardiomyopathy), except for the percutaneous transvalvular LVAD, which can be placed in the cardiac catheterization laboratory, and offers up to 3.5 L per minute of cardiac output support.
  - All patients with cardiogenic shock should undergo echocardiography to evaluate for mechanical complications of MI (see the following text).
  - Select patients with refractory HF who fail to respond to inotropes and require prolonged mechanical support may be considered for either cardiac transplant or surgical placement of an LV assist device (LVAD) or extracorporeal membrane oxygenation.
- Patients with documented LV thrombus, LV aneurysm, or chronic atrial fibrillation should receive continued anticoagulant therapy. Heparin (UFH or LMWH) can be used until a therapeutic INR is achieved. Patients on ASA and a P2Y12 inhibitor should keep their INR between 2.0 and 2.5.
  - Patients with documented LV thrombus as assessed by echocardiography at the time of discharge should receive warfarin for 3 to 6 months unless other indications warrant its continued use.
  - Patients in sinus rhythm and an EF <35% and no evidence of thrombus use of warfarin decreases risk of ischemic stroke; however, that benefit was offset by increased risk of bleeding. The decision to add warfarin to ASA needs to be individualized (*N Engl J Med 2012;366*).
- **Mechanical complications**
  - **Aneurysm.** After MI, the affected area of the myocardium may undergo infarct expansion and thinning, forming an aneurysm. The wall motion may become dyskinetic, making the endocardial surface susceptible for mural thrombus formation.
    - LV aneurysm is suggested by persistent ST elevation on the ECG and may be diagnosed by imaging studies including ventriculography, echocardiography, and MRI.
    - Anticoagulation is warranted to lower the risk of embolic events, especially if a mural thrombus is present.
    - Surgical intervention may be appropriate if the aneurysm results in HF or ventricular arrhythmias that are not satisfactorily managed with medical therapy.
  - **Ventricular pseudoaneurysm.** Incomplete rupture of the myocardial free wall can result in formation of a ventricular pseudoaneurysm. In this case, blood escapes through the myocardial wall and is contained within the visceral pericardium. In the post-CABG patient, hemorrhage from frank ventricular rupture may be contained within the fibrotic pericardial space producing a pseudoaneurysm.
    - Echocardiography (TTE with contrast or TEE) is the preferred diagnostic test to assess for a pseudoaneurysm, often allowing differentiation from a true aneurysm.
    - Prompt surgical intervention for pseudoaneurysms is advised because of the high incidence of myocardial rupture.
  - **Free wall rupture** represents a catastrophic complication of acute MI, accounting for 10% of early deaths. Rupture typically occurs within the first week after MI and presents with sudden hemodynamic collapse. This complication can occur after anterior or inferior MI and is more commonly seen in hypertensive women

with their first large transmural MI, in patients receiving late therapy with fibrinolytics, and patients given NSAIDs or glucocorticoids.

- Echocardiography may identify patients with particularly thinned ventricular walls at risk for rupture.
- Emergent surgical correction is necessary.
- Despite optimal intervention, mortality of free wall rupture remains greater than 90%.

○ **Papillary muscle rupture** (*please also refer to MR section earlier*) is a rare complication after MI and is associated with abrupt clinical deterioration. The posterior medial papillary muscle is most commonly affected due to its isolated vascular supply, but anterolateral papillary muscle rupture has been reported. Of note, papillary muscle rupture may be seen in the setting of a relatively small acute MI or even NSTEMI.

- The diagnostic test of choice is echocardiography with Doppler imaging and/or TEE as physical exam reveals a murmur in only ~50% of cases.
- Initial medical therapy should include aggressive afterload reduction. Patients with refractory HF and those with hemodynamic instability may require inotropic support with dobutamine and/or intra-aortic balloon counterpulsation. Surgical repair is indicated in the majority of patients.

○ **Ventricular septal rupture** is most commonly associated with anterior MI occurring 3 to 5 days post-MI. The perforation may follow a direct course between the ventricles or a serpiginous route through the septal wall.

- Diagnosis can be made by echocardiography with Doppler imaging and often requires TEE.
- Diagnosis should be suspected in the postinfarct patient who develops HF symptoms and a new holosystolic murmur.
- Stabilization with afterload reduction, inotropic support, and/or IABP may be necessary for hemodynamically unstable patients until definitive therapy with surgical repair can be performed.
- In hemodynamically stable patients, surgery is best deferred for at least a week to improve patient outcome. Left untreated, mortality approaches 90%.
- Percutaneous device closure in the cardiac catheterization laboratory can be performed in select patients with an unacceptable surgical risk.

MONITORING/FOLLOW-UP

Routine office visits 1 month after discharge and every 3 to 12 months thereafter are suggested for the patient presenting with an acute MI.

- Patients should be instructed to seek more frequent or urgent follow-up evaluation if they experience any noticeable change in their clinical status.
- Specific plans for long-term follow-up care should be individualized based on clinical status, anatomy, prior interventions, and change in symptoms.

5

Heart Failure and Cardiomyopathy

Shane J. LaRue, Susan M. Joseph, and
Gregory A. Ewald

HEART FAILURE

GENERAL PRINCIPLES

Definition

Heart failure (HF) is a **clinical syndrome** in which either structural or functional abnormalities in the heart impair its ability to meet the metabolic demands of the body. HF is a progressive disorder and is associated with extremely high morbidity and mortality.

Classification

- HF may be due to abnormalities in myocardial contraction (systolic dysfunction), relaxation and filling (diastolic dysfunction), or both.
- Almost half of patients admitted to the hospital with HF have preserved ejection fraction (EF).
- HF may be classified either by American College of Cardiology/American Heart Association (ACC/AHA) HF stage or by New York Heart Association (NYHA) Functional Class (Tables 5-1 and 5-2).

Epidemiology

- In the United States, there are nearly 6 million people living with HF.
- Over 550,000 new cases of HF are diagnosed each year.
- HF accounts for over 1 million hospitalizations per year.
- Estimated 1- and 5-year mortality is 30% and 50%, respectively (*Circulation 2010;123(4):410–528*).

Etiology

- Coronary artery disease (CAD) is the most frequent cause of HF in the United States, accounting for over 50% of cases (*Arch Intern Med 2001;161:996*). Diabetes and hypertension are other major contributors.
- Other causes include valvular heart disease, toxin induced (alcohol, cocaine, chemotherapy), myocarditis (infectious or autoimmune), familial cardiomyopathy, infiltrative disease (amyloidosis, sarcoidosis, hemochromatosis), peripartum cardiomyopathy (PPCM), hypertrophic cardiomyopathy (HCM), constrictive pericardial disease, high-output states (i.e., arteriovenous malformation or fistula), generalized myopathy (Duchenne or Becker muscular dystrophy), tachycardia-induced cardiomyopathy, and idiopathic cardiomyopathy.

Table 5-1	American College of Cardiology/American Heart Association Guidelines of Evaluation and Management of Chronic Heart Failure in Adults	

Stage	Description	Treatment
A	No structural heart disease and no symptoms but risk factors: CAD, HTN, DM, cardio toxins, familial cardiomyopathy	Lifestyle modification—diet, exercise, smoking cessation; treat hyperlipidemia and use ACEI for HTN
B	Abnormal LV systolic function, MI, valvular heart disease but no HF symptoms	Lifestyle modifications, ACEI, β-adrenergic blockers
C	Structural heart disease and HF symptoms	Lifestyle modifications, ACEI, β-adrenergic blockers, diuretics, digoxin
D	Refractory HF symptoms to maximal medical management	Therapy listed under A, B, C, and mechanical assist device, heart transplantation, continuous IV inotropic infusion, hospice care in selected patients

ACEI, angiotensin-converting enzyme inhibitor; CAD, coronary artery disease; DM, diabetes mellitus; HF, heart failure; HTN, hypertension; IV, intravenous; LV, left ventricular; MI, myocardial infarction.

From Hunt SA, Abraham WT, Chin MH, et al. ACC/AHA guidelines for the evaluation and management of chronic heart failure in the adult: executive summary. *J Am Coll Cardiol* 2005;46:1116–1143.

• HF exacerbations are often precipitated by dietary and medication noncompliance; however, myocardial ischemia, hypertension (HTN), arrhythmias (particularly atrial fibrillation), infection, volume overload, alcohol/toxins, thyroid disease, drugs (nonsteroidal anti-inflammatory drugs [NSAIDs], calcium channel blockers [CCBs], doxorubicin), and pulmonary embolism are also potential triggers.

Table 5-2	New York Heart Association Functional Classification

NYHA Class	Symptoms
I (mild)	No symptoms or limitation while performing ordinary physical activity (walking, climbing stairs, etc.).
II (mild)	Mild symptoms (mild shortness of breath, palpitations, fatigue, and/or angina) and slight limitation during ordinary physical activity.
III (moderate)	Marked limitation in activity due to symptoms, even during less than ordinary activity (walking short distances [20–100 m]). Comfortable only at rest.
IV (severe)	Severe limitations with symptoms even while at rest. Mostly bedbound patients.

Pathophysiology

- HF begins with an initial insult leading to myocardial injury.
- Regardless of etiology, the myocardial injury leads to a pathologic remodeling, which manifests as an increase in left ventricular (LV) size (dilation) and/or mass (hypertrophy).
- Compensatory adaptations initially maintain cardiac output; specifically, there is activation of the renin-angiotensin-aldosterone system (RAAS) and vasopressin (antidiuretic hormone), which lead to increased sodium retention and peripheral vasoconstriction. The sympathetic nervous system is also activated, with increased levels of circulating catecholamines, resulting in increased myocardial contractility. Ultimately, these neurohormonal pathways result in direct cellular toxicity, fibrosis, arrhythmias, and pump failure.
- Reduction in cardiac output results in organ hypoperfusion and pulmonary and systemic venous congestion.

DIAGNOSIS

Clinical Presentation

History
- Affected patients most commonly present with symptoms of HF including:
  - Dyspnea (on exertion and/or at rest)
  - Fatigue
  - Exercise intolerance
  - Orthopnea, paroxysmal nocturnal dyspnea (PND)
  - Systemic or pulmonary venous congestion (lower extremity swelling or cough/wheezing)
  - Presyncope, palpitations, and angina may also be present
- Other presentations include incidental detection of asymptomatic cardiomegaly or symptoms related to coexisting arrhythmia, conduction disturbance, thromboembolic complications, or sudden death.
- Clinical manifestations of HF vary depending on the rapidity of cardiac decompensation, underlying etiology, age, and comorbidities of the patient.
- Extreme decompensation may present as cardiogenic shock, characterized by hypoperfusion of vital organs, leading to renal failure (decreased urine output), mental status changes (confusion and lethargy), or "shock liver" (elevated liver function tests [LFTs]).

Physical Examination
- Systemic and pulmonary venous congestion result in lower extremity edema, pulmonary rales, jugular venous distension (JVD), pleural and pericardial effusions, hepatic congestion, and ascites.
- In the setting of systolic dysfunction, a third (S3) or fourth (S4) heart sound as well as the holosystolic murmurs of tricuspid or mitral regurgitation (MR) may be present; carotid upstrokes may also be diminished.

Diagnostic Testing

Laboratories
- Initial laboratory studies should include complete blood count (CBC); comprehensive metabolic panel (CMP) including electrolytes, blood urea nitrogen (BUN),

creatinine, calcium, magnesium, fasting glucose, and LFTs; fasting lipid profile; urinalysis; and thyroid function tests.

- B-type natriuretic peptide (BNP) is released by myocytes in response to stretch, volume overload, and increased filling pressures. Elevated BNP is present in patients with asymptomatic LV dysfunction as well as symptomatic HF.
  - BNP levels have been shown to correlate with HF severity and to predict survival (*N Engl J Med 2002;347:161*). A serum BNP >400 is consistent with HF; however, specificity is reduced in patients with renal dysfunction. A serum BNP level <100 has a good negative predictive value to exclude HF in patients presenting with dyspnea (*Curr Opin Cardiol 2006;21:208*).
- Additional laboratory testing in a patient with new-onset HF without CAD should include diagnostic tests for HIV, hepatitis, and hemochromatosis. When clinically suspected, serum tests for rheumatologic diseases (antinuclear antibody [ANA], antineutrophil cytoplasmic antibody [ANCA], etc.), amyloidosis (serum protein electrophoresis [SPEP], urine protein electrophoresis [UPEP]), or pheochromocytoma (catecholamines) should be considered (*Circulation 2009;119:1977*).

Electrocardiography

An electrocardiogram (ECG) should be performed to look for evidence of ischemia (ST-T wave abnormalities), previous myocardial infarction (MI) (Q waves), conduction delays, and arrhythmias (supraventricular and ventricular).

Imaging

- Chest radiography should be performed to evaluate the presence of pulmonary edema or cardiomegaly and rule out other etiologies of dyspnea (e.g., pneumonia, pneumothorax). It should be noted that the majority of patients admitted to the hospital with acute decompensated HF will not have overt pulmonary edema.
- An echocardiogram should be performed to assess ventricular and valvular structure and function and to exclude cardiac tamponade.
- LV function may also be evaluated using radionuclide ventriculography (i.e., multigated acquisition [MUGA] scan) or cardiac catheterization with ventriculography.
- Cardiac magnetic resonance imaging (MRI) may also be useful in assessing ventricular function and evaluating the presence of valvular heart disease, infiltrative cardiomyopathies (amyloid and sarcoid), myocarditis, and previous MI.

Diagnostic Procedures

- Coronary angiography should be performed in patients with angina or evidence of ischemia by ECG or stress testing, unless the patient is not a candidate for revascularization (*Circulation 2009;119:1977*).
- Right heart catheterization with placement of a pulmonary artery (PA) catheter may help guide therapy in patients with hypotension and evidence of shock.
- Cardiopulmonary exercise testing with measurement of peak oxygen consumption (VO$_2$) is useful in assessing functional capacity and in identifying candidates for heart transplantation (*J Heart Lung Transplant 2003;22:70*; *Circulation 2009;83:778*).
- Endomyocardial biopsy may be useful in making the diagnosis of infiltrative cardiomyopathy if suspected; however, in most cases of nonischemic cardiomyopathy (NICM), only nonspecific findings of hypertrophy or fibrosis are seen and biopsy results rarely alter management (*Eur Heart J 2007;28:3076*; *Circulation 2009; 119:1977*).

TREATMENT

Medications

- In general, pharmacologic therapy in chronic HF is aimed at blocking the neurohormonal pathways that contribute to negative remodeling and the progression of HF, while reducing symptoms, hospitalizations, and mortality.
- The cornerstone of medical therapy for HF includes vasodilators, β-adrenergic blockade, and diuretic therapy for volume overload.
- **β-Adrenergic receptor antagonists (β-blockers)** (Table 5-3). β-Blockers are a critical component of HF therapy and work by blocking the toxic effects of chronic adrenergic stimulation on the heart.
  - Many large randomized trials have documented the beneficial effects of β-blockers on functional status, disease progression, and survival in patients with NYHA class II–IV symptoms.
  - Improvement in EF, exercise tolerance, and functional class are common after the institution of a β-blocker.
  - Typically, 2 to 3 months of therapy is required to observe significant effects on LV function, but reduction of cardiac arrhythmia and incidence of sudden cardiac death (SCD) may occur much earlier (*JAMA 2003;289:712*).
  - β-Blockers should be instituted at a low dose and titrated with careful attention to blood pressure (BP) and heart rate. Some patients experience volume retention and worsening HF symptoms that typically respond to transient increases in diuretic therapy.
  - Individual β-blockers have unique properties, and the beneficial effect of β-blockers may not be a class effect. Therefore, one of three β-blockers with proven benefit on mortality in large clinical trials should be used (*Circulation 2005;112:e154*; *Circulation 2009;119:1977*):
    - **Carvedilol** (*N Engl J Med 2001;344:1651*; *Lancet 2003;362:7*)
    - **Metoprolol succinate** (*JAMA 2000;283:1295*)
    - **Bisoprolol** (*Lancet 1999;353:9*)
- **Vasodilator therapy** is another mainstay of treatment in patients with HF. The RAAS and sympathetic nervous system, as well as increased secretion of arginine vasopressin, increases arterial vasoconstriction (afterload) and venous vasoconstriction (preload) in patients with HF. Agents with predominantly venodilatory properties decrease preload and ventricular filling pressures. In the absence of LV outflow tract obstruction, arterial vasodilators reduce afterload by decreasing systemic vascular resistance (SVR), resulting in increased cardiac output, decreased ventricular filling pressure, and decreased myocardial wall stress. The efficacy and toxicity of vasodilator therapy depend on intravascular volume status and preload. Vasodilators should be used with caution in patients with a fixed cardiac output (e.g., aortic stenosis [AS] or HCM) or with predominantly diastolic dysfunction.
  - **Oral vasodilators** should be the initial therapy in patients with symptomatic chronic HF and in patients in whom parenteral vasodilators are being discontinued. When treatment with oral vasodilators is being initiated in hypotensive patients, it is prudent to use agents with a shorter half-life.
- **Angiotensin-converting enzyme (ACE) inhibitors** (Table 5-3) attenuate vasoconstriction, vital organ hypoperfusion, hyponatremia, hypokalemia, and fluid retention attributable to compensatory activation of the renin–angiotensin system. They are the first choice for antagonism of the RAAS.

Table 5-3	Drugs Commonly Used for Treatment of Heart Failure	
Drug	Initial Dose	Target
Angiotensin-Converting Enzyme Inhibitors		
Captopril	6.25–12.5 mg q6–8h	50 mg tid
Enalapril	2.5 mg bid	10 mg bid
Fosinopril	5–10 mg daily; can use bid	20 mg daily
Lisinopril	2.5–5.0 mg daily; can use bid	10–20 mg bid
Quinapril	2.5–5.0 mg bid	10 mg bid
Ramipril	1.25–2.5 mg bid	5 mg bid
Trandolapril	0.5–1.0 mg daily	4 mg daily
Angiotensin Receptor Blockers		
Valsartan[a]	40 mg bid	160 mg bid
Losartan	25 mg daily; can use bid	25–100 mg daily
Irbesartan	75–150 mg daily	75–300 mg daily
Candesartan[a]	2–16 mg daily	2–32 mg daily
Olmesartan	20 mg daily	20–40 mg daily
Thiazide Diuretics		
HCTZ	25–50 mg daily	25–50 mg daily
Metolazone	2.5–5.0 mg daily or bid	10–20 mg total daily
Loop Diuretics		
Bumetanide	0.5–1.0 mg daily or bid	10 mg total daily (maximum)
Furosemide	20–40 mg daily or bid	400 mg total daily (maximum)
Torsemide	10–20 mg daily or bid	200 mg total daily (maximum)
Aldosterone Antagonists		
Eplerenone	25 mg daily	50 mg daily
Spironolactone	12.5–25.0 mg daily	25 mg daily
β-Blockers		
Bisoprolol	1.25 mg daily	10 mg daily
Carvedilol	3.125 mg q12h	25–50 mg q12h
Metoprolol succinate	12.5–25.0 mg daily	200 mg daily
Digoxin	0.125–0.25 mg daily	0.125–0.25 mg daily

[a]Valsartan and candesartan are the only U.S. Food and Drug Administration–approved angiotensin II receptor blockers in the treatment of heart failure.
HCTZ, hydrochlorothiazide.

- Multiple large clinical trials have clearly demonstrated that ACE inhibitors improve symptoms and survival in patients with LV systolic dysfunction (*Circulation 2005;112:e154; Circulation 2009;119:1977*).
- ACE inhibitors may also prevent the development of HF in patients with asymptomatic LV dysfunction and in those at high risk of developing structural heart

disease or HF symptoms (i.e., patients with CAD, diabetes mellitus [DM], HTN). Currently, no consensus has been reached regarding the optimal dosing of ACE inhibitors in HF, although higher doses have been shown to reduce morbidity without improving overall survival (*Circulation 1999;100:2312*).

○ Absence of an initial beneficial response to treatment with an ACE inhibitor does not preclude long-term benefit.

○ Most ACE inhibitors are excreted by the kidneys, necessitating careful dose titration in patients with renal insufficiency. Acute renal insufficiency may occur in patients with bilateral renal artery stenosis. Additional adverse effects include cough, rash, angioedema, dysgeusia, increases in serum creatinine, proteinuria, hyperkalemia, and leukopenia.

○ Oral potassium supplements, potassium salt substitutes, and potassium-sparing diuretics should be used with caution during treatment with an ACE inhibitor.

○ Agranulocytosis and angioedema are more common with captopril than with other ACE inhibitors, particularly in patients with associated collagen vascular disease or serum creatinine >1.5 mg/dL.

○ **ACE inhibitors are contraindicated in pregnancy.**

• **Angiotensin II receptor blockers (ARBs)** (Table 5-3) inhibit the renin–angiotensin system via specific blockade of the angiotensin II receptor.

○ ARBs reduce morbidity and mortality associated with HF in patients who are not receiving an ACE inhibitor (*Lancet 2000;355:1582*; *N Engl J Med 2001;345:1667*; *Lancet 2003;362:777*) and therefore should be instituted when ACE inhibitors are not tolerated (*Circulation 2009;119:1977*).

○ In contrast to ACE inhibitors, they do not increase bradykinin levels and therefore are not associated with cough.

○ Caution should be exercised when ARBs are used in patients with renal insufficiency and bilateral renal artery stenosis because hyperkalemia and acute renal failure can develop.

○ Renal function and potassium levels should be periodically monitored.

○ **ARBs are contraindicated in pregnancy.**

• **Hydralazine** acts directly on arterial smooth muscle to produce vasodilation and to reduce afterload. In combination with nitrates, hydralazine improves survival in patients with HF (*N Engl J Med 1986;314:1547*).

○ A *combination of hydralazine and isosorbide dinitrate* (starting dose: 37.5/20.0 mg three times daily), when added to standard therapy with β-blockers and ACE inhibitors, has been shown to reduce mortality in African American patients (*N Engl J Med 2004;351:2049*).

○ Reflex tachycardia and increased myocardial oxygen consumption may occur, requiring cautious use in patients with ischemic heart disease.

• **Nitrates** are predominantly venodilators and help relieve symptoms of venous and pulmonary congestion. They reduce myocardial ischemia by decreasing ventricular filling pressures and by directly dilating coronary arteries. Nitrate therapy may precipitate hypotension in patients with reduced preload.

• **Parenteral vasodilators** should be reserved for patients with severe HF or those who are unable to take oral medications. Intravenous (IV) vasodilator therapy may be guided by central hemodynamic monitoring (PA catheterization) to assess efficacy and avoid hemodynamic instability. Parenteral agents should be started at low doses, titrated to the desired hemodynamic effect, and discontinued slowly to avoid rebound vasoconstriction.

- **Nitroglycerin** is a potent vasodilator with effects on venous and, to a lesser extent, arterial vascular beds. It relieves pulmonary and systemic venous congestion and is an effective coronary vasodilator. Nitroglycerin is the preferred vasodilator for treatment of HF in the setting of acute MI or unstable angina.
- **Sodium nitroprusside** is a direct arterial vasodilator with less potent venodilatory properties. Its predominant effect is to reduce afterload, and it is particularly effective in patients with HF who are hypertensive or who have severe aortic or mitral valvular regurgitation. Nitroprusside should be used cautiously in patients with myocardial ischemia because of a potential reduction in regional myocardial blood flow (**coronary steal**).
  - The initial dose of **0.25 mcg/kg/min** can be titrated (**maximum dose of 10 mcg/kg/min**) to the desired hemodynamic effect or until hypotension develops.
  - The half-life of nitroprusside is 1 to 3 minutes, and its metabolism results in the release of cyanide, which is metabolized by the liver to thiocyanate and is then excreted via the kidney.
  - Toxic levels of thiocyanate (>10 mg/dL) may develop in patients with renal insufficiency. Thiocyanate toxicity may manifest as nausea, paresthesias, mental status changes, abdominal pain, and seizures.
  - **Methemoglobinemia** is a rare complication of treatment with nitroprusside.
- **Recombinant BNP (nesiritide)** is an arterial and venous vasodilator.
  - IV infusion of nesiritide reduces right atrial and LV end-diastolic pressures (LVEDPs) and SVR and results in an increase in cardiac output.
  - It is administered as a 2-mcg/kg IV bolus, followed by a continuous IV infusion starting at 0.01 mcg/kg/min. Nesiritide is approved for use in acute HF exacerbations and relieves HF symptoms early after its administration (*JAMA 2002; 287:1531*). It does not have an effect on survival or rehospitalization in patients with HF (*N Engl J Med 2011;365:32*).
  - It should not be used to improve renal function or to enhance diuresis.
  - *Hypotension* is the most common side effect of nesiritide, and its use should be avoided in patients with systemic hypotension (systolic BP <90 mm Hg) or evidence of cardiogenic shock. Episodes of hypotension should be managed with discontinuation of nesiritide and cautious volume expansion or pressor support if necessary.
- **Enalaprilat** is an active metabolite of the ACE inhibitor enalapril that is available for IV administration. Its onset of action is more rapid, and its pharmacologic half-life is shorter than that of enalapril. The initial dosage is 1.25 mg IV q6h, which can be titrated to a maximum dosage of 5 mg IV q6h. Patients who take diuretics or those with impaired renal function (serum creatinine >3 mg/dL, creatinine clearance <30 mL/min) should initially receive 0.625 mg IV q6h. Because its actions may be variable and unpredictable, its use is not common in HF patients.
- **α-Adrenergic receptor antagonists** have not been shown to improve survival in HF, and hypertensive patients treated with doxazosin as first-line therapy had an increased risk of developing HF (*JAMA 2000;283:1967*).
- **Aldosterone antagonists**
  - **Spironolactone** is an aldosterone receptor antagonist that has been shown to improve survival and decrease hospitalizations in NYHA class III–IV patients with low EF (*N Engl J Med 1999;341:709*) and is therefore indicated in such

patients if the creatinine is <2.5 mg/dL and potassium is <5.0 mEq/L (Table 5-3) (*Circulation 2009;119:1977*).

- ○ **Eplerenone** is a selective aldosterone receptor antagonist without the hormonal side effects of spironolactone. It has proven beneficial in patients with HF following MI (*N Engl J Med 2003;348:1309*) and in less symptomatic patients with reduced EF (*N Engl J Med 2011;364:11*).
- ○ The potential for development of life-threatening hyperkalemia exists with the use of these agents. Gynecomastia may develop in 10% to 20% of men treated with spironolactone. Serum potassium must be monitored closely after initiation; concomitant use of ACE inhibitors and NSAIDs and the presence of renal insufficiency increase the risk of hyperkalemia.
- **Digitalis glycosides** increase myocardial contractility and may attenuate the neuro-hormonal activation associated with HF. Digoxin decreases the number of HF hospitalizations without improving overall mortality (*N Engl J Med 1997;336:525*).
  - ○ Discontinuation of digoxin in patients who are stable on a regimen of digoxin, diuretics, and an ACE inhibitor may result in clinical deterioration (*N Engl J Med 1993;329:1*).
  - ○ The usual daily dose is 0.125 to 0.25 mg and should be decreased in patients with renal insufficiency. Clinical benefits may not be related to the serum levels, and although serum digoxin levels of 0.8 to 2.0 ng/mL are considered "therapeutic," toxicity can occur in this range.
  - ○ It has **narrow therapeutic index**, and serum levels should be followed closely, particularly in patients with unstable renal function.
  - ○ Observations suggest that women and patients with higher serum digoxin levels (1.2 to 2.0 ng/mL) have an increased mortality risk (*N Engl J Med 2002;347:1403; JAMA 2003;289:871*).
  - ○ Drug interactions with digoxin are common. Oral antibiotics such as erythromycin and tetracycline may increase digoxin levels by 10% to 40%. Quinidine, verapamil, flecainide, and amiodarone also increase digoxin levels significantly.
  - ○ Digoxin toxicity may be caused or exacerbated by drug interactions, electrolyte abnormalities (particularly hypokalemia), hypoxemia, hypothyroidism, renal insufficiency, and volume depletion.
- **Diuretic therapy** (Table 5-3), in conjunction with restriction of dietary sodium and fluids, often leads to clinical improvement in patients with symptomatic HF. Frequent assessment of the patient's weight along with careful observation of fluid intake and output is essential during initiation and maintenance of therapy. Frequent complications of therapy include hypokalemia, hyponatremia, hypomagnesemia, volume contraction alkalosis, intravascular volume depletion, and hypotension. Serum electrolytes, BUN, and creatinine levels should be followed after institution of diuretic therapy. Hypokalemia may be life threatening in patients who are receiving digoxin or in those who have severe LV dysfunction that predisposes them to ventricular arrhythmias. Potassium supplementation or a potassium-sparing diuretic should be considered in addition to careful monitoring of serum potassium levels.
  - ○ **Thiazide diuretics (hydrochlorothiazide, chlorthalidone)** can be used as initial agents in patients with normal renal function in whom only a mild diuresis is desired. **Metolazone**, unlike other thiazides, exerts its action at the proximal as well as the distal tubule and may be useful in combination with a loop diuretic in patients with a low glomerular filtration rate.

- ○ **Loop diuretics (furosemide, torsemide, bumetanide, ethacrynic acid)** should be used in patients who require significant diuresis and in those with markedly decreased renal function.
  - ■ Furosemide reduces preload acutely by causing direct venodilation when administered intravenously, making it useful for managing severe HF or acute pulmonary edema.
  - ■ Use of loop diuretics may be complicated by hyperuricemia, hypocalcemia, ototoxicity, rash, and vasculitis. Furosemide and bumetanide are sulfa derivatives and may rarely cause drug reactions in sulfa-sensitive patients. Ethacrynic acid can generally be used safely in such patients.
- ○ **Potassium-sparing diuretics** do not exert a potent diuretic effect when used alone.
- • **Inotropic agents**
  - ○ **Sympathomimetic agents** are potent drugs that are primarily used to treat severe HF. Beneficial and adverse effects are mediated by stimulation of myocardial β-adrenergic receptors. The most important adverse effects are related to the arrhythmogenic nature of these agents and the potential for exacerbation of myocardial ischemia. Treatment should be guided by careful hemodynamic and ECG monitoring. Patients with refractory chronic HF may benefit symptomatically from continuous ambulatory administration of IV inotropes as palliative therapy or as a bridge to mechanical ventricular support or cardiac transplantation. However, this strategy may increase the risk of life-threatening arrhythmias or indwelling catheter-related infections (*Circulation 2005;112:e154*; *Circulation 2009;119:1977*).
    - ■ **Dopamine** (Table 5-4) should be used primarily for stabilization of the hypotensive patient.
    - ■ **Dobutamine** (Table 5-4) is a synthetic analog of dopamine. Dobutamine tolerance has been described, and several studies have demonstrated increased mortality in patients treated with continuous dobutamine. Dobutamine has no significant role in the treatment of HF resulting from diastolic dysfunction or a high-output state.

Table 5-4	Inotropic Agents		
Drug	**Dose**	**Mechanism**	**Effects/Side Effects**
Dopamine	1–3 mcg/kg/min	Dopaminergic receptors	Splanchnic vasodilation
	2–8 mcg/kg/min	β_1-receptor agonist	+Inotropic
	7–10 mcg/kg/min	α-receptor agonist	↑ SVR
Dobutamine	2.5–15.0 mcg/kg/min	β_1- >β_2- >α- Receptor agonist	+Inotropic, ↓ SVR, tachycardia
Milrinone[a]	50-mcg/kg bolus IV over 10 min, 0.375–0.75 mcg/kg/min	↑ cAMP	↓ SVR, +inotropic; atrial and ventricular tachyarrhythmias

[a]Needs dose adjustment for creatinine clearance.
cAMP, cyclic adenosine monophosphate; IV, intravenous; SVR, systemic vascular resistance; ↑, increased; ↓, decreased.

- **Phosphodiesterase inhibitors** increase myocardial contractility and produce vasodilation by increasing intracellular cyclic adenosine monophosphate (cAMP). **Milrinone** is currently available for clinical use and is indicated for treatment of refractory HF. Hypotension may develop in patients who receive vasodilator therapy or have intravascular volume contraction, or both. Milrinone may improve hemodynamics in patients who are treated concurrently with dobutamine or dopamine. Data suggest that in-hospital short-term milrinone administration in addition to standard medical therapy does not reduce the length of hospitalization or the 60-day mortality or rehospitalization rate when compared with placebo (*JAMA 2002;287:1541*).

Other Nonpharmacologic Therapies

- **Coronary revascularization** reduces ischemia and may improve systolic function in some patients with CAD.
- **Cardiac resynchronization therapy** or **biventricular pacing** (see Chapter 7, Cardiac Arrhythmias) appears to be beneficial in some patients with an EF of ≤35%, NYHA class III–IV HF, and conduction abnormalities (left bundle branch block and atrioventricular delay). It has been demonstrated to improve quality of life and reduce the risk of death in carefully selected patients (*N Engl J Med 2005;352:1539*).
- **Implantable cardiac defibrillator (ICD)** placement is recommended for selected HF patients with an EF ≤35% for primary prevention of SCD. Sudden death occurs six to nine times more often in patients with HF compared to the general population and is the leading cause of death in ambulatory HF patients.
  - Multiple large randomized trials have demonstrated a survival benefit of 1.0% to 1.5% per year in patients with both ischemic and NICM (*N Engl J Med 2005;352:1539; Circulation 2009;119:1977*).
  - Patients should receive at least 3 months of optimal medical therapy prior to reassessment of EF and implantation of an ICD.
  - Following an acute MI or revascularization, EF should be assessed following 40 days of optimal therapy prior to ICD implantation.
  - ICD therapy should be deferred in patients with advanced age, life-shortening co-morbidities, and end-stage HF patients who are not candidates for transplantation.
- An **intra-aortic balloon pump (IABP)** can be considered for patients who have failed other therapies, have transient myocardial dysfunction, or are awaiting a definitive procedure such as left ventricular assist device (LVAD) or transplantation. Severe aortoiliac atherosclerosis and moderate-to-severe aortic valve insufficiency are contraindications to IABP placement.
- **Percutaneous LVADs** are now available to provide short-term support for patients in cardiogenic shock and have been shown to have superior hemodynamic effects compared to the IABP. However, use of percutaneous LVADs did not improve 30-day survival in critically ill patients (*Eur Heart J 2009;30:2012*).

Surgical Management

- **Ventricular assist devices (VADs)** are surgically implanted devices that shuttle blood from the left ventricle to the aorta to augment cardiac output. They may be indicated for patients with severe HF after cardiac surgery, individuals with intractable cardiogenic shock after acute MI, as a "bridge to transplantation" for patients awaiting heart transplantation, and as permanent or "destination" therapy

for select patients with refractory end-stage HF and an estimated 1-year mortality over 50% with medical therapy (*Circulation 2009;119:1977*).
- ○ Currently available devices vary with regard to degree of mechanical hemolysis, intensity of anticoagulation required, and difficulty of implantation. The decision to institute VAD circulatory support must be made in consultation with an HF cardiologist and a cardiac surgeon who have experience with this technology.
- **Cardiac transplantation** is an option for selected patients with severe end-stage HF that has become refractory to aggressive medical therapy and for whom no other conventional treatment options are available.
- ○ Approximately 2,200 heart transplants are performed each year in the United States.
- ○ Candidates considered for transplantation should generally be younger than age 65 years (although selected older patients may also benefit), have advanced HF (NYHA class III–IV), have a strong psychosocial support system, have exhausted all other therapeutic options, and be free of irreversible extracardiac organ dysfunction that would limit functional recovery or predispose them to posttransplant complications (*J Am Coll Cardiol 1993;22:1*).
- ○ Survival rates post-heart transplant are approximately 90%, 70%, and 50% at 1, 5, and 10 years, respectively, since the induction of calcineurin inhibitor-based immunosuppression. Annual statistics can be found on the United Network for Organ Sharing Web site (*www.unos.org*).
- ○ In general, functional capacity and quality of life improve significantly after transplantation.
- ○ **Posttransplant complications** include acute and chronic rejection, typical and atypical infections, and adverse effects of immunosuppressive agents. Cardiac allograft vasculopathy (CAD/chronic rejection) and malignancy are the leading causes of death after the first posttransplant year.

Lifestyle/Risk Modification
- Dietary counseling for sodium and fluid restriction should be provided.
- Smoking cessation should be strongly encouraged.
- Abstinence from alcohol is recommended in symptomatic HF patients with low EF.
- Exercise training is recommended in stable HF patients as an adjunct to pharmacologic treatment. Exercise training in patients with HF has been shown to improve exercise capacity (peak VO_2 max as well as 6-minute walk time), improve quality of life, and decrease neurohormonal activation (*JAMA 2009;301:1439; JAMA 2009;301:1451*). Treatment programs should be individualized and include a warm-up period, 20 to 30 minutes of exercise at the desired intensity, and a cool-down period 3 to 5 days a week (*Circulation 2003;107:1210*).
- Weight loss should be recommended when appropriate.

SPECIAL CONSIDERATIONS

- **Fluid and free water restriction** (<1.5 L/d) is especially important in the setting of hyponatremia (serum sodium <130 mEq/L) and volume overload.
- **Minimization of medications** with deleterious effects in HF should be attempted.
- ○ **Negative inotropes** (e.g., verapamil, diltiazem) should be avoided in patients with impaired ventricular contractility, as should over-the-counter β stimulants (e.g., compounds containing ephedra, pseudoephedrine hydrochloride).

- o **NSAIDs**, which antagonize the effect of ACE inhibitors and diuretic therapy, should be avoided if possible.
- **Administration of supplemental oxygen** may relieve dyspnea, improve oxygen delivery, reduce the work of breathing, and limit pulmonary vasoconstriction in patients with hypoxemia but is not routinely recommended in patients without hypoxemia.
- **Sleep apnea** has a prevalence as high as 37% in the HF population. Treatment with nocturnal positive airway pressure improves symptoms and EF (*Am J Respir Crit Care Med 2001;164:2147*; *N Engl J Med 2003;348:1233*).
- **Dialysis** or **ultrafiltration** may be beneficial in patients with severe HF and renal dysfunction who cannot respond adequately to fluid and sodium restriction and diuretics (*J Am Coll Cardiol 2007;49:675*). Other mechanical methods of fluid removal such as therapeutic thoracentesis and paracentesis may provide temporary symptomatic relief of dyspnea. Care must be taken to avoid rapid fluid removal and hypotension.
- **End-of-life considerations** may be necessary in patients with advanced HF who are refractory to therapy. Discussions regarding the disease course, treatment options, survival, functional status, and advance directives should be addressed early in the treatment of the patient with HF. For those with end-stage disease (stage D, NYHA class IV) with multiple hospitalizations and severe decline in their functional status and quality of life, hospice and palliative care should be considered.

Acute Heart Failure and Cardiogenic Pulmonary Edema

GENERAL PRINCIPLES

Cardiogenic pulmonary edema (CPE) occurs when the pulmonary capillary pressure exceeds the forces that maintain fluid within the vascular space (serum oncotic pressure and interstitial hydrostatic pressure).

- Increased pulmonary capillary pressure may be caused by LV failure of any cause, obstruction to transmitral flow (e.g., mitral stenosis [MS], atrial myxoma), or rarely, pulmonary veno-occlusive disease.
- Alveolar flooding and impairment of gas exchange follow accumulation of fluid in the pulmonary interstitium.

DIAGNOSIS

Clinical Presentation

- Clinical manifestations of CPE may occur rapidly and include dyspnea, anxiety, cough, and restlessness.
- The patient may expectorate pink frothy fluid.
- Physical signs of decreased peripheral perfusion, pulmonary congestion, hypoxemia, use of accessory respiratory muscles, and wheezing are often present.

Diagnostic Testing

- Radiographic abnormalities include cardiomegaly, interstitial and perihilar vascular engorgement, Kerley B lines, and pleural effusions.

- The radiographic abnormalities may follow the development of symptoms by several hours, and their resolution may be out of phase with clinical improvement.

TREATMENT

- **Supplemental oxygen** should be administered initially to raise the arterial oxygen tension to **>60 mm Hg**.
  - ○ **Mechanical ventilation** is indicated if oxygenation is inadequate by noninvasive means or if hypercapnia coexists.
  - ○ Placing the patient in a sitting position improves pulmonary function.
  - ○ Bed rest, pain control, and relief of anxiety can decrease cardiac workload.
- **Precipitating factors** should be identified and corrected, as resolution of pulmonary edema can often be accomplished with correction of the underlying process. The most common precipitants are as follows:
  - ○ Severe HTN
  - ○ MI or myocardial ischemia (particularly if associated with MR)
  - ○ Acute valvular regurgitation
  - ○ New-onset tachyarrhythmias or bradyarrhythmias
  - ○ Volume overload in the setting of severe LV dysfunction

Medications

- **Morphine sulfate** reduces anxiety and dilates pulmonary and systemic veins. Two to 5 mg can be given intravenously over several minutes and can be repeated every 10 to 25 minutes until an effect is seen.
- **Furosemide** is a venodilator that decreases pulmonary congestion within minutes of IV administration well before its diuretic action begins. An initial dose of 20 to 80 mg IV should be given over several minutes and can be increased based on response to a maximum of 200 mg in subsequent doses.
- **Nitroglycerin** is a venodilator that can potentiate the effect of furosemide. IV administration is preferable to oral and transdermal forms as it can be rapidly titrated.
- **Nitroprusside** is an effective adjunct in the treatment of acute CPE and is useful when CPE is brought on by acute valvular regurgitation or HTN (see Chapter 6, Pericardial and Valvular Heart Disease). Pulmonary and systemic arterial catheterization should be considered to guide titration of nitroprusside therapy.
- **Inotropic agents**, such as dobutamine or milrinone, may be helpful after initial treatment of CPE in patients with concomitant hypotension or shock.
- **Recombinant BNP (nesiritide)** is administered as an IV bolus followed by an IV infusion.
  - ○ Nesiritide reduces intracardiac filling pressures by producing vasodilation and indirectly increases the cardiac output.
  - ○ In conjunction with furosemide, nesiritide produces natriuresis and diuresis.

SPECIAL CONSIDERATIONS

- **Right heart catheterization** (e.g., Swan-Ganz catheter) may be helpful in cases in which a prompt response to therapy does not occur by allowing differentiation between cardiogenic and noncardiogenic causes of pulmonary edema via measure-

ment of central hemodynamics and cardiac output. It may then be used to guide subsequent therapy.
- **Acute hemodialysis and ultrafiltration** may be effective, especially in the patient with significant renal dysfunction and diuretic resistance (*J Am Coll Cardiol 2007;49:675*; *Congest Heart Fail 2008;14:19*).

CARDIOMYOPATHY

Dilated Cardiomyopathy

GENERAL PRINCIPLES

Definition
Dilated cardiomyopathy (DCM) is a disease of heart muscle characterized by dilation of the cardiac chambers and reduction in ventricular contractile function.

Epidemiology
DCM is the most common form of cardiomyopathy and is responsible for approximately 10,000 deaths and 46,000 hospitalizations each year. The lifetime incidence of DCM is about 30 cases per 100,000 persons.

Pathophysiology
- DCM may be secondary to progression of any process that affects the myocardium, and dilation is directly related to neurohormonal activation. The majority of cases are idiopathic (*Am J Cardiol 1992;69:1458*).
- Dilation of the cardiac chambers and varying degrees of hypertrophy are anatomic hallmarks. Tricuspid and MR are common due to the effect of chamber dilation on the valvular apparatus.
- **Atrial and ventricular arrhythmias** are present in as many as one-half of these patients and are likely responsible for the high incidence of sudden death in this population.

DIAGNOSIS

Clinical Presentation
- Symptomatic HF (dyspnea, volume overload) is often present.
- A portion of patients with clinical disease may be asymptomatic.
- The ECG is usually abnormal, but changes are typically nonspecific.

Diagnostic Testing
Imaging
- Diagnosis of DCM can be confirmed with echocardiography or radionuclide ventriculography.
- Two-dimensional and Doppler echocardiography are helpful in differentiating this condition from hypertrophic or restrictive cardiomyopathy (RCM), pericardial disease, and valvular disorders.

Diagnostic Procedures

Endomyocardial biopsy provides little information that affects treatment of patients with dilated cardiomyopathies and is not routinely recommended (*Eur Heart J 2007;28:3076; Circulation 2009;119:1977*).

TREATMENT

Medications

- The medical management of symptomatic patients is identical to that for HF from other causes.
- Therapeutic strategies include control of total body sodium and volume in addition to appropriate preload and afterload reduction using vasodilator therapy.
- β-Adrenergic antagonists and ACE inhibitors should be used unless contraindicated.
- Immunizations against influenza and pneumococcal pneumonia are recommended.
- Chronic oral anticoagulation has not been shown to decrease the risk of ischemic stroke, intracerebral hemorrhage, or mortality in patients with LV dysfunction (*N Engl J Med 2012;366:1859*). Anticoagulation should be individualized and considered in patients with a history of thromboembolic events, atrial fibrillation, or evidence of an LV thrombus. The level of anticoagulation recommended varies but is generally targeted to an international normalized ratio (INR) of 2.0 to 3.0.
- Immunosuppressive therapy with agents such as prednisone, azathioprine, and cyclosporine for biopsy-proven myocarditis has been advocated by some, but efficacy has not been established, with the possible exception of the very rare patient with giant cell myocarditis (*N Engl J Med 1995;333:269; Circulation 2009;119:1977*).

Other Nonpharmacologic Therapies

- DCM (of nonischemic origin) is associated with an increased incidence of **SCD** and **ventricular arrhythmia**. In comparison to NYHA class IV HF patients who are more likely to die of progressive pump failure, SCD is relatively more common in patients with mild-to-moderate symptoms.
- Suppression of asymptomatic ventricular premature beats or nonsustained ventricular tachycardia (NSVT) using antiarrhythmic drugs in patients with HF does not improve survival and may increase mortality as a result of the proarrhythmic effects of the drugs (*N Engl J Med 1989;321:406; N Engl J Med 1995;333:77; N Engl J Med 2005;352:225*).
- Primary prevention of SCD is recommended by implantation of an ICD in patients with DCM who have an EF of ≤35% and NYHA class II–III symptoms despite maximal medical therapy for 3 months.
- Cardiac resynchronization therapy is beneficial in selected patients (NYHA class II–IV; EF ≤30% to 35%; intraventricular conduction delay QRS ≥120 ms) with symptomatic HF (*N Engl J Med 2004;350:2140; N Engl J Med 2005; 352:1539*).

Surgical Management

- Cardiac transplantation should be considered for selected patients with HF due to DCM that is refractory to medical therapy.
- IABP or LVAD placement may be necessary for stabilization of patients in whom cardiac transplantation is an option.

- Mitral valve annuloplasty or replacement can be used for symptomatic relief in patients with severe MR.

Heart Failure with Preserved Ejection Fraction

GENERAL PRINCIPLES

Definition
- Heart failure with preserved ejection fraction (HFpEF), also called diastolic heart failure, refers to the clinical syndrome of HF in the presence of preserved systolic function (LV EF >40).
- Diastolic dysfunction refers to abnormality in the mechanical function of the heart during diastole or the relaxation phase of the cardiac cycle. Usually, this involves elevated filling pressures and impairment of ventricular filling.

Epidemiology
- Almost half of patients admitted to the hospital with HF have a normal or near-normal EF.
- HFpEF is most prevalent in elderly women, most of whom have HTN and/or DM. Many of these women also have CAD and/or atrial fibrillation.

Etiology
- The vast majority of patients with HFpEF have hypertension and LV hypertrophy.
- Myocardial disorders associated with HFpEF include RCM, obstructive and nonobstructive HCM, infiltrative cardiomyopathies, and constrictive pericarditis.

Pathophysiology
- Reduced ventricular compliance plays a major role in the pathophysiology of HFpEF.
- Abnormal sodium handling by the kidneys and arterial stiffness also contribute.

DIAGNOSIS

- Differentiating between diastolic and systolic HF cannot be reliably accomplished without two-dimensional echocardiography.
- Diagnosis is based on echocardiographic criteria and Doppler findings of normal LV systolic function with impaired diastolic relaxation and elevated filling pressures.

TREATMENT

In contrast to systolic heart failure, treatment remains largely empiric and is directed toward improving the symptoms with diuretic therapy and correcting the precipitating factors (e.g., hypertension, ischemia, tachycardia).

Hypertrophic Cardiomyopathy

GENERAL PRINCIPLES

Definition
HCM is a myocardial disorder characterized by ventricular hypertrophy, diminished LV cavity dimensions, normal or enhanced contractile function, and impaired ventricular relaxation in the absence of an identifiable cause.

Epidemiology

- HCM is the most common inherited heart defect, occurring in 1 out of 500 individuals.
- Approximately 500,000 people have HCM in the United States, yet most are unaware. An estimated 36% of young athletes who die suddenly have probable or definite HCM, making it the leading cause of SCD in young people in the United States, including trained athletes (*Circulation 2009;119:1977*).
- The idiopathic form of HCM has an early onset (as early as the first decade of life) without associated HTN.
- An acquired form also occurs in elderly patients with chronic HTN.

Pathophysiology

- The pathophysiologic change in HCM is myocardial hypertrophy that is typically predominant in the ventricular septum (asymmetric septal hypertrophy) but may involve all ventricular segments.
- Many cases of HCM have a genetic component, with mutations in the myosin heavy-chain gene that follow an autosomal dominant transmission with variable phenotypic expression and penetrance.
- HCM can be classified according to the presence or absence of LV outflow tract obstruction.
- LV outflow obstruction may occur at rest but is enhanced by factors that increase LV contractility or decrease ventricular volume.
- Delayed ventricular diastolic relaxation and decreased compliance are common and may lead to pulmonary congestion.
- Myocardial ischemia is frequently secondary to a myocardial oxygen supply–demand mismatch.
- Systolic anterior motion (SAM) of the anterior leaflet of the mitral valve is often associated with MR and may contribute to LV outflow tract obstruction.

DIAGNOSIS

Clinical Presentation

- Presentation varies but may include dyspnea, angina, arrhythmias, syncope, cardiac failure, or sudden death.
- Sudden death is most common in children and young adults between the ages of 10 and 35 years and often occurs during periods of strenuous exertion.

History
Family history of HCM or sudden death is suggestive of the familial subtype.

Physical Examination
- Physical findings include bisferious (double peak per cardiac cycle) carotid pulse (in the presence of obstruction).
- Forceful double or triple apical impulse and a coarse **systolic outflow murmur** localized along the left sternal border that is **accentuated by maneuvers that decrease preload** (e.g., standing, Valsalva maneuver) may also be found.

Diagnostic Testing

Electrocardiography
The ECG of HCM is usually abnormal and invariably so in symptomatic patients with LV outflow tract obstruction. The most common abnormalities are ST-segment

and T-wave abnormalities, followed by evidence of LV hypertrophy (*Am J Cardiol 2002;90:1020*).

Imaging
- Two-dimensional echocardiography and Doppler flow studies can establish the presence of a significant LV outflow gradient at rest or with provocation.
- Additional risk stratification should be pursued with 24- to 48-hour Holter monitoring and exercise testing.

TREATMENT

- Management is directed toward relief of symptoms and prevention of endocarditis, arrhythmias, and sudden death.
- Treatment in asymptomatic individuals is controversial, and no conclusive evidence has been found that medical therapy is beneficial.
- All individuals with HCM should avoid strenuous physical activity, including most competitive sports.

Medications
- β-Blockers may reduce symptoms of HCM by reducing myocardial contractility and heart rate. However, symptoms may recur during long-term therapy.
- Calcium channel antagonists, particularly verapamil and diltiazem, may improve the symptoms of HCM, primarily by augmentation of diastolic ventricular filling. Therapy should be initiated at low doses, with careful titration in patients with outflow obstruction. The dose should be increased gradually over several days to weeks if symptoms persist. Dihydropyridines should be avoided in patients with LV outflow tract obstruction as a result of their vasodilatory properties.
- Diuretics may improve pulmonary congestive symptoms in patients with elevated pulmonary venous pressures. These agents should be used cautiously in patients with severe LV outflow obstruction because excessive preload reduction worsens the obstruction.
- Nitrates and vasodilators should be avoided because of the risk of increasing the LV outflow gradient.
- **Treatment of arrhythmias.** Atrial and ventricular arrhythmias occur commonly in patients with HCM. Supraventricular tachyarrhythmias are tolerated poorly and should be treated aggressively. Cardioversion is indicated if hemodynamic compromise develops.
  - **Digoxin is relatively contraindicated** because of its positive inotropic properties and potential for exacerbating ventricular outflow obstruction.
  - Atrial fibrillation should be converted to sinus rhythm when possible, and anticoagulation is recommended if paroxysmal or chronic atrial fibrillation develops.
  - **Diltiazem, verapamil, or β-blockers** can be used to control the ventricular response before cardioversion. Procainamide, disopyramide, or amiodarone (see Chapter 7, Cardiac Arrhythmias) may be effective in the chronic suppression of atrial fibrillation.
  - Patients with NSVT detected on ambulatory monitoring are at increased risk for sudden death. However, the benefit of suppressing these arrhythmias with medical therapy has not been established, and there is a risk of proarrhythmic effects from antiarrhythmic drugs.

- ○ ICD placement should be considered in high-risk patients:
  - Those with genetic mutations associated with SCD (*JAMA 2007;298:405*);
  - Prior SCD or sustained ventricular tachyarrhythmia;
  - History of syncope or near-syncope, recurrent or exertional, in young patients;
  - Multiple NSVTs on Holter recordings;
  - Hypotensive response to exercise;
  - LV hypertrophy with a wall thickness >30 mm in young patients; and
  - History of sudden, premature death in close relatives.
  - ○ There is very limited benefit for invasive electrophysiologic testing for the risk stratification of patients with HCM.
- Symptomatic ventricular arrhythmias should be treated as outlined in Chapter 7, Cardiac Arrhythmias.
- Dual-chamber pacing (see Chapter 7, Cardiac Arrhythmias) improves symptoms in some patients with HCM. Alteration of the ventricular activation sequence via right ventricular (RV) pacing may minimize LV outflow tract obstruction secondary to asymmetric septal hypertrophy.
- Only 10% of the patients with HCM meet the criteria for pacemaker implantation, and the effect on decreasing the left ventricular outflow tract (LVOT) gradient is only 25%. A subset of patients with HCM may derive symptomatic benefit from dual chamber pacing without an affect on survival (*Heart 2010;96(5):352*).

Surgical Management

- Surgical therapy is useful in the treatment of symptoms but has not been shown to alter the natural history of HCM.
- The most frequently used operative procedure involves septal myotomy–myectomy with or without mitral valve replacement (MVR).
- Alcohol septal ablation, a catheter-based alternative to surgical myotomy–myectomy, seems to be equally effective at reducing obstruction and providing symptomatic relief when compared to the gold standard surgical procedure (*J Am Coll Cardiol 2007;50:831*).
- Cardiac transplantation should be reserved for patients with end-stage HCM with symptomatic HF.

PATIENT EDUCATION

Genetic counseling and family screening are recommended for first-degree relatives of patients at high risk for SCD because the disease is transmitted as an autosomal dominant trait.

Restrictive Cardiomyopathy

GENERAL PRINCIPLES

Definition

- RCM is characterized by a rigid heart with poor ventricular filling.
- Both infiltrative (amyloidosis or sarcoidosis) and noninfiltrative (diabetic or idiopathic) forms exist.
- Pericardial disease (constrictive pericarditis) can present in a similar fashion but carries a different prognosis and treatment options and thus must be excluded.

Pathophysiology

- In amyloidosis, amyloid deposits in the interstitium replace the normal myocardial contractile units and cause restriction.
- Approximately 5% of sarcoidosis cases have cardiac involvement in which scar formation leads to restriction.
- Other etiologies include hemochromatosis, Gaucher's and Hurler's cardiomyopathies (rare, inherited glycogen storage diseases), hypereosinophilic syndrome, and carcinoid heart disease.

DIAGNOSIS

Diagnostic Testing

Electrocardiography
The classic ECG finding in amyloidosis is low voltage (despite echocardiographically evident ventricular thickening) with poor R-wave progression. In sarcoidosis, conduction disease is often present.

Imaging
- In RCM, echocardiography with Doppler analysis may demonstrate thickened myocardium with normal or abnormal systolic function, abnormal diastolic filling patterns, and elevated intracardiac pressure.
- Cardiac MRI, position emission tomography (PET), and computed tomography (CT) are emerging as useful diagnostic tools for patients with cardiac sarcoid as granulomas, inflammation, and edema may be seen, which appear to improve with therapy (*Am Heart J 2009;157:746*).

Diagnostic Procedures
- On cardiac catheterization, elevated RV and LV filling pressures are seen with a classic dip-and-plateau pattern in the RV and LV pressure tracing.
- RV endomyocardial biopsy may be diagnostic and should be considered in patients in whom a diagnosis is not established.

TREATMENT

- Specific therapy aimed at amelioration of the underlying cause should be initiated.
- Cardiac hemochromatosis may respond to reduction of total body iron stores via phlebotomy or chelation therapy with deferoxamine.
- Cardiac sarcoidosis may respond to glucocorticoid therapy, but prolongation of survival with this approach has not been established.
- In those with syncope and/or ventricular arrhythmias, placement of an ICD is indicated. Patients with high-grade conduction disease warrant pacemaker placement.
- No therapy is known to be effective at reversing the progression of cardiac amyloidosis.
- Digoxin should be avoided in patients with cardiac amyloidosis because digoxin is bound extracellularly by amyloid fibrils and may cause hypersensitivity and toxicity (*Circulation 1981;63:1285*).

Peripartum Cardiomyopathy

GENERAL PRINCIPLES

Definition
- PPCM is defined as LV systolic dysfunction diagnosed in the last month of pregnancy up to 5 months postpartum.
- The incidence of PPCM is 1 in 3,000 to 4,000 pregnancies in the United States.

Etiology
- The etiology of PPCM remains unclear. There is evidence to support **viral triggers**, including coxsackievirus, parvovirus B19, adenovirus, and herpesvirus, which may replicate unchecked in the reduced immunologic state brought on by pregnancy.
- **Fetal microchimerism**, wherein fetal cells escape into the maternal circulation and induce an autoimmune myocarditis, has also been suggested as a cause (*Lancet 2006;368:687*).
- Recently, a cleavage product of **prolactin** has also been implicated in the development of PPCM (*Cell 2007;128:589*).

Risk Factors
Risk factors that predispose a woman to PPCM include advanced maternal age, multiparity, multiple pregnancy, preeclampsia, and gestational hypertension. There is a higher risk in African American women, but this may be confounded by the higher prevalence of hypertension in this population.

DIAGNOSIS

Clinical Presentation
- Clinically, women with PPCM present with the signs and symptoms of HF.
- As dyspnea on exertion and lower extremity edema are common in late pregnancy, PPCM may be difficult to recognize. Cough, orthopnea, and PND are warning signs that PPCM may be present, as is the presence of a displaced apical impulse and a new MR murmur on exam.
- Most commonly, patients present with NYHA class III and IV HF, although more mild cases and sudden cardiac arrest also occur.

Diagnostic Testing
Electrocardiography
On ECG, LVH is often present, as are ST-T wave abnormalities.

Imaging
Diagnosis requires an echocardiogram with a depressed EF and/or LV dilatation.

TREATMENT

Medications
- The mainstay of treatment is afterload and preload reduction.
- **ACE inhibitors** are used in the postpartum patient, while hydralazine is used in the patient who is still pregnant.

- **β-Blockers** are used to reduce tachycardia, arrhythmia, and risk of SCD and are relatively safe, although β_1-selective blockers (metoprolol and atenolol) are preferred because they avoid peripheral vasodilation and uterine relaxation.
- **Digoxin** is also safe during pregnancy and should be used to augment contractility and rate control, although levels need to be closely monitored.
- **Diuretics** are used for preload reduction and symptom relief and are also safe.
- In those with thromboembolism, **heparin** is required, followed by **Coumadin** after delivery.

OUTCOME/PROGNOSIS

- The prognosis in PPCM is better than that seen in other forms of NICM.
- The extent of ventricular recovery at 6 months postdelivery can predict overall recovery, although continued improvement has been seen 2 to 3 years after diagnosis.
- Subsequent pregnancies in patients with PPCM may be associated with significant deterioration in LV function and can even result in death. Family planning counseling is essential after the diagnosis of PPCM is made, and women who do not recover their LV function should be encouraged to consider foregoing future pregnancy.

6 Pericardial and Valvular Heart Disease

Jay Shah and Brian R. Lindman

PERICARDIAL DISEASE

Constrictive Pericarditis

GENERAL PRINCIPLES

- Constrictive pericarditis, as a cause of right-sided heart failure (HF), often goes undiagnosed.
- Constrictive pericarditis is often difficult to distinguish from restrictive cardiomyopathies (RCMs).
- Multiple imaging modalities and invasive hemodynamics are often needed to confirm the diagnosis.

Etiology

- **Common**
  - Idiopathic
  - Viral pericarditis (chronic or recurrent)
  - Postcardiotomy
  - Chest irradiation
- **Less common**
  - Autoimmune connective tissue disorders
  - End-stage renal disease, uremia
  - Malignancy (e.g., breast, lung, lymphoma)
  - Tuberculosis (most common cause in developing countries)

Pathophysiology

The pericardium is a fibrous sac surrounding the heart consisting of two layers: a thin visceral layer attached to the pericardium and a thicker parietal layer. The pericardial space is normally filled with 15 to 50 mL of fluid, and the two layers slide smoothly against each other, allowing for normal expansion and contraction of the heart. In the setting of chronic inflammation, the pericardial layers become thickened, scarred, and calcified; the pericardial space is obliterated and the pericardium becomes noncompliant, which impairs ventricular filling and leads to an equalization of pressures in all four chambers and subsequent HF symptoms.

DIAGNOSIS

Clinical Presentation

History

The clinical presentation of constrictive pericarditis is insidious, with gradual development of fatigue, exercise intolerance, and venous congestion. If it goes undiagnosed for a long period, it is not unusual for patients to have undergone an extensive gastrointestinal (GI)/liver evaluation, including a liver biopsy (showing "nutmeg liver" [also known as cardiac cirrhosis or congestive hepatopathy]) before the diagnosis is made.

Physical Examination
- Features of right-sided HF
  - Lower extremity edema
  - Hepatomegaly
  - Ascites
  - Elevated jugular venous pressure (JVP)
- Features more specific for constriction
  - Increased JVP with prominent y descent
  - Kussmaul's sign: lack of expected decrease or obvious increase of JVP upon inspiration
  - Pericardial knock: early, loud, high-pitched S_3

Differential Diagnosis
- **Pericardial constriction**
  - Ventricular interdependence **present**
  - Abnormal pericardial features (thickened, adherent, and/or calcified)
  - Preserved (or increased) tissue Doppler velocities on echo
  - Pulmonary hypertension (PH) mild or absent
  - Septal bounce seen on noninvasive imaging
  - Equalization of pressures in all cardiac chambers (left ventricular end-diastolic pressure [LVEDP] − right ventricular end-diastolic pressure [RVEDP] <5 mm Hg)
  - RVEDP/right ventricular systolic pressure (RVSP) >1/3
  - B-type natriuretic peptide (BNP) low or mildly elevated (usually <200, unless postcardiotomy or radiation with concomitant left ventricular [LV] dysfunction)
- **Restrictive cardiomyopathy**
  - Ventricular interdependence **absent**
  - Abnormal myocardial features (infiltration, thickened, fibrotic, conduction system disease)
  - Decreased tissue Doppler velocities on echo
  - PH present
  - Normal septal motion
  - LVEDP − RVEDP >5 mm Hg
  - RVEDP/RVSP <1/3
  - BNP elevated (>200)

Diagnostic Testing
- **Echocardiogram**
  - First-line diagnostic test
  - Helpful for distinguishing constriction from restriction (see earlier)
  - Ventricular systolic function is often normal and can lead to the false assessment that the heart function is "normal" and not a cause of the patient's symptoms
  - May require a fluid bolus to elicit some of the hemodynamic findings of constriction
  - Features suggestive of constriction include:
    - Thickened, echogenic pericardium

- Tethering of the pericardium to the myocardium
- Dilated, incompressible inferior vena cava (IVC)
- Septal bounce
- Inspiratory variation in mitral flow velocity curves
- Expiratory reversal of hepatic vein flow
- Preserved (or increased) tissue Doppler velocities of the mitral annulus.
- **Cardiac catheterization**
  - Often required to make the diagnosis of constriction
  - Method of choice for an accurate hemodynamic assessment
    - Simultaneous measurement of RVEDP and LVEDP
    - Right atrial (RA) pressure will be very high
    - Pulmonary artery pressures will be near normal
    - Cardiac output (CO)/cardiac index (CI) may be clinically helpful
- **Cardiac computed tomography (CT) and magnetic resonance imaging (MRI)**
  - Provide excellent anatomy of the pericardium (thickness and calcification)
  - An MRI and gated CT can show evidence of ventricular interdependence (septal bounce); this may be particularly important if echo images are poor
  - Can provide other anatomic information that may be helpful in making the diagnosis of constriction (i.e., engorgement of IVC and hepatic veins) and its etiology (i.e., lymph nodes, tumors)

TREATMENT

- Limited role for medical therapy: diuretics and low-salt diet to alleviate edema
- Patients with constriction often have a resting sinus tachycardia
  - Cardiac output (CO = heart rate [HR] × stroke volume [SV]) is dependent on HR, because diastolic filling and augmentation of SV is significantly impaired
  - Avoid β-blockers and calcium channel blockers (CCBs) to slow the HR.

Surgical Management

- **Surgical pericardiectomy is the only definitive treatment** and should be pursued once the diagnosis is made
- Operative mortality is 5%–15%; more advanced congestive heart failure (CHF) symptoms confer higher operative risk
- A significant majority experience a symptomatic benefit from surgery

Cardiac Tamponade

GENERAL PRINCIPLES

Cardiac tamponade is a **clinical diagnosis** and is considered a medical emergency.

Etiology

- More likely to cause tamponade:
  - Procedural complications during percutaneous coronary intervention, pacemaker/defibrillator lead insertion, and electrophysiology (EP) ablations.
  - Idiopathic pericarditis
  - Infection (bacterial, including mycobacteria; fungal; and viral, including HIV)
  - Neoplasms (sometimes initially diagnosed during a workup for a pericardial effusion)

- Postcardiotomy
- Autoimmune connective tissue disorders
- Uremia
- Trauma
- Radiation
- Myocardial infarction (MI) (subacute)
- Drugs (hydralazine, procainamide, isoniazid, phenytoin, minoxidil)
- Hypothyroidism

Pathophysiology

Fluid accumulation in the pericardial space increases the pericardial pressure. The pressure depends on the amount of fluid, the rate of accumulation, and the compliance of the pericardium. Rapid accumulation of a small volume (50 to 60 mL) of fluid (e.g., trauma or perforation during percutaneous coronary intervention [PCI]) can raise the pericardial pressure substantially. If the accumulation of fluid is more insidious, the pericardium can stretch to accommodate a large amount of fluid and remain at a lower pressure. Tamponade develops when the pressure in the pericardial space is sufficiently high to interfere with adequate cardiac filling, resulting in a decrease in CO.

DIAGNOSIS

Clinical Presentation

History
- The diagnosis of cardiac tamponade should be suspected in patients with elevated JVP, hypotension, and distant heart sounds (**Beck's triad**).
- Symptoms can include dyspnea, fatigue, anxiety, presyncope, chest discomfort, abdominal fullness, lethargy, and a vague sense of being "uncomfortable"; patients often feel more comfortable sitting forward.

Physical Examination
- Pulsus paradoxus >10 mm Hg
- Jugular venous distention
- Diminished heart sounds
- Tachycardia, hypotension, and signs of shock

Diagnostic Testing
- **Electrocardiogram (ECG)**
  - Low voltage (more likely with larger effusions)
  - Tachycardia
  - Electrical alternans (due to the swinging of the heart within the pericardium; specific but not sensitive)
- **Transthoracic echocardiogram (TTE)**
  - First-line diagnostic test to diagnose an effusion and evaluate its hemodynamic significance
  - The size of the effusion can be misleading; its hemodynamic impact depends on the rate of fluid accumulation
  - Important to assess the location of the effusion and determine whether it is loculated or free flowing; this has implications for the approach taken to drain the fluid
  - Features suggestive of a hemodynamically significant effusion:
    - Dilated, incompressible IVC
    - Significant respiratory variation of tricuspid and mitral inflow velocities

- Early diastolic collapse of the right ventricle (RV) and systolic collapse of the right atrium
- Usually the effusion is circumferential
- **Transesophageal echocardiogram (TEE)**
  Helpful when TTE images are poor or when there is a suspicion for a loculated effusion (particularly those that might develop posteriorly, adjacent to the atria, after cardiac surgery).
- **CT and MRI**
  - Can be helpful in assessing the anatomic location of the effusion (particularly if loculated)
  - May be helpful in determining the etiology of the effusion and the content of the pericardial fluid
  - Should be avoided in an unstable patient
- **Right heart catheterization (RHC)**
  - Usually not necessary to establish the diagnosis
  - Hemodynamic assessment showing equalization of atrial and ventricular diastolic pressures

TREATMENT

- Limited role for medical therapy
- Maintain adequate filling pressures with intravenous (IV) fluids
- Avoid diuretics, nitrates, and any other preload-reducing medications
- Avoid efforts to slow sinus tachycardia; it compensates for a reduced SV to try to maintain adequate CO
- If intubation is to be performed for respiratory distress before the fluid is drained, make sure volume status is replete and a pericardiocentesis needle is immediately available before any sedatives are given (a patient in particularly "severe tamponade" can arrest with the preload reduction from sedation)

Other Nonoperative Therapies

Percutaneous pericardiocentesis with echocardiographic guidance can be a relatively safe and effective way to drain the pericardial fluid if there is an adequate amount of fluid; the approach should be guided by where the predominant collection of fluid is located and is usually easiest when the effusion is anterior.

Surgical Management

- Open pericardiocentesis with the creation of a window is a minimally invasive procedure and is preferred for recurring effusions, loculated effusions, or those not safely accessible percutaneously
- Allows pericardial biopsies to be taken, which may be helpful in making a diagnosis

VALVULAR HEART DISEASE

Mitral Stenosis

GENERAL PRINCIPLES

- Mitral stenosis (MS) is characterized by incomplete opening of the mitral valve during diastole, which limits antegrade flow and yields a sustained diastolic pressure gradient between the left atrium (LA) and the LV.

- Due to the widespread use of antibiotics, the incidence of rheumatic heart disease (and MS) has decreased in the developed world.

Etiology

- **Rheumatic**
  - ○ Predominant cause of MS
  - ○ Two-thirds are females
  - ○ May be associated with mitral regurgitation (MR)
  - ○ Stenotic orifice often shaped like a "fish mouth"
  - ○ Rheumatic fever can cause fibrosis, thickening, and calcification leading to fusion of the commissures, leaflets, chordae, and/or papillary muscles
- **Other causes**
  - ○ Systemic lupus erythematosus (SLE)
  - ○ Rheumatoid arthritis
  - ○ Congenital
  - ○ Substantial mitral annular calcification
  - ○ Mitral valve prosthesis dysfunction or "patient-prosthesis" mismatch
  - ○ Oversewn or small mitral annuloplasty ring
  - ○ "Functional MS" may occur with obstruction of left atrial outflow due to
    - Tumor, particularly myxoma
    - LA thrombus
    - Endocarditis with a large vegetation
    - Congenital membrane of the LA (i.e., cor triatriatum)

Pathophysiology

Physiologic states that either increase the transvalvular flow (enhance CO) or decrease diastolic filling time (via tachycardia) can increase symptoms at any given valve area. Pregnancy, exercise, hyperthyroidism, atrial fibrillation (AF) with rapid ventricular response, and fever are examples in which either or both of these conditions occur. Symptoms are often first noticed at these times (Figure 6-1).

DIAGNOSIS

Clinical Presentation

History

After a prolonged asymptomatic period, depending on when they present, patients may report any of the following: dyspnea, decreased functional capacity, orthopnea and/or paroxysmal nocturnal dyspnea (PND), fatigue, palpitations (often due to AF), systemic embolism, hemoptysis, chest pain, and/or signs and symptoms of infective endocarditis.

Physical Examination

Findings on physical exam will depend on the severity of valve obstruction and the associated adaptations that have had time to develop in response to it; they may include

- Accentuation of S_1 may occur when the leaflets are flexible.
- Opening snap (OS) caused by sudden tensing of the valve leaflets; the A_2-OS interval varies inversely with the severity of stenosis (shorter interval = more severe stenosis).
- Mid-diastolic rumble: low-pitched murmur heard best at the apex with the bell of the stethoscope; the severity of stenosis is related to the duration of the murmur, not intensity (more severe = longer duration).

Figure 6-1. Pathophysiology of mitral stenosis. CO, cardiac output; HR, heart rate; HTN, hypertension; LA, left atrium; LAE, left atrial enlargement; LAP, left atrial pressure; LV, left ventricle; PVR, pulmonary vascular resistance; RV, right ventricle; RVH, right ventricular hypertrophy.

- Loud P_2, tricuspid regurgitation (TR) murmur, pulmonary artery (PA) tap, and/or RV heave can indicate PH.
- Higher JVP, hepatic congestion, and peripheral edema can indicate varying degrees of right heart failure.

Diagnostic Testing

- **ECG**
  - P mitrale (P-wave duration in lead II ≥0.12 seconds indicating left atrial enlargement [LAE])
  - AF
  - RVH
- **CXR**
  - LAE
  - Enlarged RA/RV and/or enlarged pulmonary arteries
  - Calcification of the mitral valve (MV) and/or annulus
- **TTE**
  - Assess etiology of MS
  - Assess leaflets and subvalvular apparatus to determine candidacy for percutaneous mitral balloon valvotomy (PMBV)
  - Determine mitral valve area and mean transmitral gradient
  - Estimate PA systolic pressure and evaluate RV size and function
- **Exercise testing by TTE or RHC**
  - Helpful in clarifying functional capacity of those with an unclear history
  - Assess transmitral gradient and PA pressure with exercise when there is a discrepancy between resting Doppler findings, clinical findings, signs, and symptoms
- **TEE**
  - Assess presence or absence of clot and severity of MR in patients being considered for PMBV
  - Evaluate MV morphology and hemodynamics in patients with MS for whom TTE was suboptimal
- **Cardiac catheterization**
  - Indicated to determine severity of MS when clinical and echo assessment are discordant
  - Reasonable in patients with MS to assess the cause of severe PH when out of proportion to the severity of MS as determined by noninvasive testing; can also assess the reversibility of PH
- **Severe MS**
  - Mean gradient (mm Hg) >10
  - Pulmonary artery systolic pressure (PASP) (mm Hg) >50
  - Valve area (cm^2) <1.0

TREATMENT

Medical Management

- Reduce CHF symptoms with intermittent diuretics and low-salt diet
- Reducing the risk for endocarditis with antibiotic prophylaxis for rheumatic MS is no longer recommended by the American College of Cardiology/American Heart Association (ACC/AHA)
- Managing AF and risk of thromboembolism
- For patients who develop symptoms only with exercise, negative chronotropic agents such as β-blockers or nondihydropyridine CCBs may be of benefit
- Prompt recognition and treatment of rheumatic fever

- **Atrial fibrillation**
  - Therapy is mostly aimed at rate control and prevention of thromboembolism.
  - About 30%–40% of patients with MS develop AF or atrial flutter.
  - AF may worsen symptoms (particularly when there is a rapid ventricular response) due to a shortened diastolic filling period and loss of the atrial contribution to diastolic filling.
  - Rate control using β-blockers or nondihydropyridine CCBs tend to be more effective than digoxin for tachycardia associated with exertion.
  - **ACC/AHA Guidelines—Class I indications for anticoagulation** for prevention of systemic embolization in patients with mitral stenosis:
    - MS and AF (paroxysmal, persistent, or permanent)
    - MS and a prior embolic event, even in sinus rhythm
    - MS with left atrial thrombus
  - Target INR range is unclear; traditionally, an international normalized ratio (INR) of 2.5 to 3.5 was recommended, although recently there has been more evidence that an INR of 2.0 to 3.0 provides similar rates of prevention of thromboembolism.
  - Efforts to maintain sinus rhythm (through direct current cardioversion [DCCV], ablation, or with drugs) are focused on those patients with symptoms from their AF but can be particularly challenging in patients with MS.

Other Nonoperative Therapies
Percutaneous Mitral Balloon Valvotomy
- **ACC/AHA Guidelines—Class I indications for PMBV**
  - Symptomatic (New York Heart Association [NYHA] Class II, III, or IV) with moderate or severe MS and valve morphology favorable for PMBV in the absence of LA thrombus or moderate-to-severe MR
  - Asymptomatic with moderate or severe MS and valve morphology favorable for PMBV in those who have PH (PASP >50 mm Hg at rest or >60 mm Hg with exercise) in the absence of LA thrombus or moderate-to-severe MR
- Balloon inflation separates the commissures and fractures some of the nodular calcium in the leaflets, yielding an increased valve area.
- Hemodynamic results often observed: transmitral gradient ↓50% to 60%, CO ↑10% to 20%, and valve area increases from 1.0 to 2.0 cm^2.
- Contraindications: LA thrombus, moderate-to-severe MR, and an echo score of >8 (this score reflects the thickening, mobility, and calcification of the leaflets and subvalvular apparatus; a relative contraindication).
- **Complications:** death (~1%), stroke, cardiac perforation, severe MR requiring surgical correction, and residual atrial septal defect (ASD) requiring closure.
- When done in patients with favorable MV morphology, event-free survival (freedom from death, repeat valvotomy, or MV replacement) is 80% to 90% at 3 to 7 years (*Circulation 1992;85:448*).
- It compares favorably with surgical mitral commissurotomy (open or closed) and is the valvotomy procedure of choice in experienced centers in patients without contraindications.

Surgical Management
- **ACC/AHA Guidelines—Class I indications for surgery for mitral stenosis**
  - MV surgery (repair if possible) is indicated in symptomatic patients (NYHA Class III or IV) with moderate or severe MS in a patient with acceptable operative risk when:

- PMBV is unavailable,
- PMBV is contraindicated because of LA thrombus despite anticoagulation or because concomitant moderate-to-severe MR is present, or
- Valve morphology is not favorable for PMBV.
  - Symptomatic patients with moderate or severe MS who also have moderate-to-severe MR should receive valve replacement unless valve repair is possible at the time of surgery.
- Surgical treatment is usually reserved for those who are not candidates for PMBV because of the presence of one or more contraindications to PMBV or because the percutaneous option is unavailable.
- Surgical valvotomy can be done either closed (bypass unnecessary) or open (done under direct visualization on bypass).

OUTCOME/PROGNOSIS

MS usually progresses slowly with a long latent period (several decades) between rheumatic fever and the development of stenosis severe enough to cause symptoms. Ten-year survival of untreated patients with MS depends on the severity of symptoms at presentation: asymptomatic or minimally symptomatic patients have an 80% 10-year survival, whereas those with significant limiting symptoms have a 0% to 15% 10-year survival. Once severe PH develops, mean survival is 3 years. The mortality of untreated patients is due mostly to progressive pulmonary and systemic congestion, systemic embolism, pulmonary embolism, and infection (in order of frequency).

Aortic Stenosis

GENERAL PRINCIPLES

- **Aortic stenosis** (AS) is the most common cause for obstruction of flow from the LV into the aorta; it is present in 2% of those >65 years of age and 4% of those >85 years of age.
- Other causes of obstruction occur above the valve (supravalvular) and below the valve (subvalvular), both fixed (i.e., subaortic membrane) and dynamic (i.e., hypertrophic cardiomyopathy [HCM] with obstruction).
- **Aortic sclerosis** is thickening of the aortic valve leaflets that cause turbulent flow through the valve and a murmur but no significant gradient; over time it can develop into AS.

Epidemiology

- **Calcific/degenerative**
  - Most common cause in United States
  - Trileaflet calcific AS usually presents in the seventh to ninth decades (mean age, mid-70s)
  - Risk factors similar to coronary artery disease (CAD)
  - Active biologic process with fibrosis and bone formation in the valve
  - Calcification leading to stenosis affects both trileaflet and bicuspid valves
- **Bicuspid**
  - Occurs in 1% to 2% of population (congenital lesion)

○ Usually presents in the sixth to eighth decades (mean age, mid–late 60s)
○ ~50% of patients needing aortic valve replacement (AVR) for AS have a bicuspid valve
○ More prone to endocarditis than trileaflet valves
○ Associated with aortopathies (i.e., dissection, aneurysm) in a significant proportion of patients

• **Rheumatic**
  ○ More common cause worldwide, much less common in the United States
  ○ Usually presents in the third to fifth decades
  ○ Almost always accompanied by mitral valve disease

Pathophysiology

The pathophysiology for calcific AS involves both the valve and the ventricular adaptation to the stenosis. Within the valve, there is growing evidence for an active biologic process that begins much like the formation of an atherosclerotic plaque and eventually leads to calcified bone formation (Figure 6-2).

DIAGNOSIS

Clinical Presentation

History

• The classic triad of symptoms includes **angina, syncope, and HF**.
• Frequently, patients will gradually limit themselves in ways that mask the presence of symptoms but indicate a progressive and premature decline in functional capacity. In the setting of severe AS, these patients should be viewed as symptomatic.

Physical Examination

• Harsh systolic crescendo–decrescendo murmur heard best at the right upper sternal border and radiating to both carotids; time to peak intensity correlates with severity (later peak = more severe)
• Diminished or absent A_2 (soft S_2) suggests severe AS
• An ejection click suggests bicuspid AS
• S_4 reflects atrial contraction on a poorly compliant ventricle
• Pulsus parvus et tardus: late-peaking and diminished carotid upstroke in severe AS
• Gallavardin phenomenon is an AS murmur heard best at the apex (could be confused with MR). It does not radiate to the left axilla and is accentuated by a slowing of the heart rate whereas the MR murmur does not change.
• Between extremes, it is often difficult to assess AS severity on exam

Diagnostic Testing

• **ECG:** LAE and left ventricular hypertrophy (LVH)
• **CXR:** LVH, cardiomegaly, and calcification of the aorta, aortic valve, and/or coronaries
• **TTE**
  ○ Leaflet number, morphology, and calcification
  ○ Calculate valve area using continuity equation and measure transvalvular mean and peak gradients
  ○ **Severe AS**
    ▪ Peak jet velocity (m/s) >4.0
    ▪ Mean gradient (mm Hg) >40
    ▪ Valve area (cm^2) <1.0

Figure 6-2. Pathophysiology of aortic stenosis. CO, cardiac output; EF, ejection fraction; LVEDP, left ventricular end-diastolic pressure; LVH, left ventricular hypertrophy.

- **Further evaluation in selected patients**
  - **TEE**
    - Clarify whether there is a bicuspid valve if unclear on TTE
    - Occasionally needed to evaluate for other or additional causes of left ventricular outflow tract (LVOT) obstruction
  - **Exercise testing:** Performed in the patient presumed to be asymptomatic or in whom symptoms are unclear; evaluate for exercise capacity, abnormal blood pressure response (<20 mm Hg increase with exercise), or exercise-induced symptoms
  - **Dobutamine stress echo:**
    - Useful to assess the patient with a reduced SV (which may occur with a reduced or preserved ejection fraction [EF]) with a small calculated valve area (suggesting severe AS) but a low (<30 to 40 mm Hg) mean transvalvular gradient (suggesting less severe AS)
    - Can help distinguish truly severe AS from pseudo-severe AS
    - Assess for the presence of contractile reserve
  - **Cardiac catheterization**
    - In patients undergoing AVR who are at risk for CAD
    - Evaluate for CAD in patients with moderate AS and symptoms of angina

- Hemodynamic assessment of severity of AS in patients in whom noninvasive tests are inconclusive or when there is discrepancy between noninvasive tests and clinical findings regarding AS severity (utilizes the Gorlin formula)
  - **Computerized Tomographic Angiography (CTA):** May be an alternative to catheterization to evaluate coronary anatomy prior to valve surgery, particularly in those considered lower risk for CAD
  - **BNP or N-terminus ProBNP (NT-proBNP)**
    - Predicts symptom-free survival in asymptomatic patients and preoperative level predicts postoperative survival, functional class, and LV function (*Circulation 2004;109:2302*).
    - BNP is higher in patients with truly severe AS versus pseudo-severe AS and predicts survival among patients with low-flow, low-gradient AS (*Circulation 2007;115:2848*).

TREATMENT

- Severe symptomatic AS is a surgical disease; **currently, there are no medical treatments proven to decrease mortality or to delay surgery**.
- **Hypertension (HTN):** Do not undertreat HTN in patients with AS because inadequately treated HTN imposes an additional load on the LV. Treat with appropriate antihypertensive agents.
- **Angiotensin-converting enzyme (ACE) inhibitor:** Some data suggest that ACE inhibition may advantageously interfere with the valvular biology that leads to valve calcification.
- **Statins:** Most prospective, randomized clinical trials have not demonstrated that statins slow the progression of valvular stenosis; they are not recommended for the sole purpose of delaying the progression of AS.
- **Diuretics:** Can help reduce pulmonary congestion and may relieve symptoms in patients with AS. However, symptoms generally imply that AVR is indicated. Avoid overdiuresis and loss of preload which may precipitate hypotension.
- **Severe AS with decompensated HF**
  - Patients with severe AS and LV dysfunction may experience decompensated HF; depending on the clinical scenario, several options may help bridge the patient to definitive surgical management (e.g., AVR):
    - Intra-aortic balloon pump (IABP) (contraindicated in patients with moderate-to-severe AR)
    - Sodium nitroprusside
    - Balloon aortic valvuloplasty
  - Each of the above measures provides some degree of afterload reduction, either at the level of the valve (valvuloplasty) or systemic vascular resistance (SVR) (IABP, Nipride), which can facilitate forward flow; as the HF becomes more compensated and transient end-organ damage is reversed (i.e., renal failure, respiratory failure), operative mortality likely decreases.

Other Nonoperative Therapies
Percutaneous
- Balloon aortic valvuloplasty has a limited role in the treatment of patients with severe AS; the improvement in valve area is modest and the clinical improvement that it provides usually lasts weeks to months.

- **Transcatheter aortic valve replacement (TAVR)**
  - Recently introduced as an option for patients at high risk for AVR or those considered inoperable
  - Requires a team of cardiologists and cardiac surgeons, using fluoroscopic and echocardiographic guidance to place a stented bioprosthetic valve within the stenotic valve. This can be performed either via a transfemoral or transapical (using a left thoracotomy) approach.
  - These less invasive catheter-based techniques for valve replacement are rapidly evolving and are being investigated in ongoing clinical trials and clinical registries

Surgical Management

- Symptomatic severe AS is a deadly disease; AVR is the only currently effective treatment
- Certain associated high-risk features or the need for another cardiac surgical intervention may lead to the recommendation for an AVR even when the patient is asymptomatic or has less than severe AS
- Operative mortality varies significantly depending on age, comorbidities, surgical experience, and concurrent surgical procedures to be performed
- **ACC/AHA Guidelines—Class I indications for AVR**
  - Symptomatic patients with severe AS
  - Patients with severe AS undergoing coronary artery bypass graft (CABG)
  - Patients with severe AS undergoing surgery on the aorta or other heart valves
  - Patients with severe AS and LV systolic dysfunction (EF <50%)

OUTCOME/PROGNOSIS

AS is a progressive disease typically characterized by an asymptomatic phase until the valve area reaches a minimum threshold, generally <1 cm^2. In the absence of symptoms, patients with AS have a good prognosis with a risk of sudden death estimated to be <1% per year. Predictors of decreased event-free survival (free of AVR or death) include higher peak aortic jet velocity, extent of valve calcification, and coexistent CAD. Once patients experience symptoms, their average survival is 2 to 3 years with a high risk of sudden death.

Mitral Regurgitation

GENERAL PRINCIPLES

- Prevention of MR is dependent on the integrated and proper function of the mitral valve (annulus and leaflets), subvalvular apparatus (chordae tendineae and papillary muscles), LA and the ventricle; abnormal function or size of any one of these components can lead to MR.
- **Organic MR** refers to MR caused primarily by lesions to the valve leaflets and/ or chordae tendineae (i.e., myxomatous degeneration, endocarditis, rheumatic).
- **Functional MR** refers to MR caused primarily by ventricular dysfunction usually with accompanying annular dilatation (i.e., dilated cardiomyopathy [DCM] and ischemic MR).
- It is critical to define the mechanism of MR and the time course (acute vs. chronic) as these significantly impact clinical management.

Etiology

- **Degenerative** (overlap with mitral valve prolapse syndrome)
  - Usually occurs as a primary condition (Barlow's disease or fibroelastic deficiency) but has also been associated with heritable diseases affecting the connective tissue including Marfan's syndrome, Ehlers–Danlos syndrome, osteogenesis imperfecta, etc.
  - May be familial or nonfamilial
  - Occurs in 1.0% to 2.5% of the population (based on stricter echo criteria)
  - Female to male 2:1
  - Either one or both leaflets may prolapse
  - Most common reason for MV surgery
  - Myxomatous proliferation and cartilage formation can occur in the leaflets, chordae tendineae, and/or annulus
- **DCM**
  - Mechanism of MR is due to both
    - Annular dilatation from ventricular enlargement and
    - Papillary muscle displacement due to ventricular enlargement and remodeling prevents adequate leaflet coaptation
  - May occur in the setting of nonischemic DCM or ischemic DCM (there is often an overlap of mechanism for MR in the setting of previous infarction)
- **Ischemic**
  - **Ischemic MR is mostly a misnomer**, as this is primarily postinfarction MR, not MR caused by active ischemia (although MR can be due to ischemia alone or postinfarct MR can be exacerbated by ischemia)
  - Mechanism of MR usually involves one or both of the following:
    - Annular dilatation from ventricular enlargement
    - Local LV remodeling with papillary muscle displacement (both the dilatation of the ventricle and the akinesis/dyskinesis of the wall to which the papillary muscle is attached can prevent adequate leaflet coaptation)
  - Rarely, MR may develop acutely from papillary muscle rupture (more commonly of the posteromedial papillary muscle)
- **Rheumatic**
  - May be pure MR or combined MR/MS
  - Caused by thickening and/or calcification of the leaflets and chords
- **Infective endocarditis:** Usually caused by destruction of the leaflet tissue (i.e., perforation)
- **Other causes**
  - Congenital (cleft, parachute, or fenestrated mitral valves)
  - Infiltrative diseases (i.e., amyloid)
  - SLE (Libman–Sacks lesion)
  - HCM with obstruction
  - Mitral annular calcification
  - Paravalvular prosthetic leak
  - Drug toxicity (e.g., Fen-phen)
- **Acute causes**
  - Ruptured papillary muscle
  - Ruptured chordae tendineae
  - Infective endocarditis

Figure 6-3. Acute mitral regurgitation. CO, cardiac output; EF, ejection fraction; HR, heart rate; LA, left atrium; LAP, left atrial pressure; LV, left ventricle; LVEDP, left ventricular end-diastolic pressure; SV, stroke volume.

Pathophysiology
- Acute MR (Figure 6-3)
- Chronic MR (Figure 6-4)

DIAGNOSIS

Clinical Presentation

History
- Acute MR
  - Most prominent symptom is relatively rapid onset of significant shortness of breath, which may lead quickly to respiratory failure
  - Symptoms of reduced forward flow may also be present depending on the patient's ability to compensate for the regurgitant volume
- Chronic MR
  - The etiology of MR and the time at which the patient presents will influence the symptoms reported.
  - In degenerative MR that has gradually progressed, the patient may be asymptomatic even when the MR is severe. As compensatory mechanisms fail, patients may note
    - Dyspnea on exertion (may be due to PH and/or pulmonary edema)
    - Palpitations (from an atrial arrhythmia)
    - Fatigue
    - Volume overload

Figure 6-4. Chronic mitral regurgitation. CO, cardiac output; EF, ejection fraction; LA, left atrium; LAP, left atrial pressure; LV, left ventricle; LVEDP, left ventricular end-diastolic pressure; MR, mitral regurgitation; PH, pulmonary hypertension; SV, stroke volume.

- Patients with ischemic MR and MR due to a DCM may report similar symptoms; in general, these patients will tend to be more symptomatic because almost all of them have associated LV dysfunction

Physical Examination
- Acute MR
  - Tachypnea with respiratory distress
  - Tachycardia
  - Systolic murmur, usually at the apex (may not be holosystolic and may be absent)
  - Relative hypotension (even shock)

- Chronic MR
  - Apical holosystolic murmur that radiates to the axilla
  - The murmur may radiate to the anterior chest wall if the posterior leaflet is prolapsed or toward the back if the anterior leaflet is prolapsed
  - In mitral valve prolapse, there is a midsystolic click heard before the murmur
  - S_2 may be widely split due to an early A_2
  - Other signs of CHF (lower extremity [LE] edema, ↑ central venous pressure, crackles, etc.)

Diagnostic Testing

- **ECG**
  - LAE, LVH/Left ventricular enlargement (LVE)
  - AF
  - Pathologic Q waves from previous MI in ischemic MR
- **CXR**
  - Enlarged LA
  - Pulmonary edema
  - Enlarged pulmonary arteries
  - Cardiomegaly
- **TTE**
  - Assess etiology of MR
  - LA size and LV dimensions (should be dilated in chronic severe MR of any etiology)
  - EF (LV dysfunction is present if EF ≤60%)
  - Qualitative and quantitative measures of MR severity
- **TEE**
  - Provides better visualization of the valve to help define anatomy, presence of endocarditis, and feasibility of repair
  - May help determine severity of MR when TTE is nondiagnostic, particularly in the setting of an eccentric jet
- **3D echocardiogram**
  May provide additional and more accurate anatomic insights that can guide repair, especially for periprosthetic valve MR
- **Exercise testing with echocardiogram**
  - Helpful in clarifying functional capacity of those with an unclear history
  - Assess severity of MR with exercise in patients with exertional symptoms that seem discordant with the assessment of MR severity at rest
  - Assess pulmonary artery pressure with exercise
- **Cardiac catheterization**
  - RHC:
    - PH in patients with chronic severe MR
    - LA filling pressure in patients with unclear symptoms
    - Giant "V" waves on pulmonary capillary wedge pressure (PCWP) tracing may suggest severe MR
  - Left heart catheterization (LHC):
    - May influence therapeutic strategy in ischemic MR
    - Evaluation of CAD in patients with risk factors undergoing MV surgery
  - Left ventriculogram can evaluate LV function and severity of MR

- **MRI**
  - Assess EF in patients with severe MR but with an inadequate assessment of EF by echo
  - Assess quantitative measures of MR severity when echo is nondiagnostic
  - Viability assessment may play a role in considering therapeutic strategy in ischemic MR
- **Nuclear**
  - Assess EF in patients with severe MR but with an inadequate assessment of EF by echo
  - Viability assessment may play a role in considering therapeutic strategy in ischemic MR
- **CTA**
  - CTA may be an alternative to LHC to evaluate coronary anatomy prior to valve surgery

TREATMENT

Acute MR

- While awaiting surgery, aggressive afterload reduction with IV nitroprusside or an IABP can diminish the amount of MR and stabilize the patient by promoting forward flow and reducing pulmonary edema.
- These patients are usually tachycardic, but attempts to slow their HR should be avoided as they are often HR dependent for an adequate forward CO.

Chronic MR

The role for medical therapy may differ depending on the etiology of the MR.

- **Degenerative MR:**
  - In the asymptomatic patient with normal LV function and chronic severe MR due to leaflet prolapse, there is generally no accepted medical therapy.
  - In the absence of systemic HTN, there is no established indication for vasodilating drugs.
  - Whether ACE inhibitors or β-blockers delay ventricular remodeling and the need for surgery is being investigated in prospective studies.
- **Functional MR:**
  - Treat as other patients with LV dysfunction
  - ACE inhibitors and β-blockers are indicated and have been shown to reduce mortality and the severity of MR
  - Some patients may also qualify for cardiac resynchronization therapy, which has also been shown to reduce the severity of MR

Other Nonoperative Therapies

Percutaneous

- Various approaches target each of the interrelated components that can contribute to MR: annular dilatation, lack of leaflet coaptation, and ventricular remodeling causing papillary muscle displacement
- Currently, the most developed device may be the placement of a mitral clip, which pinches the leaflets together in an attempt to enhance coaptation (a percutaneous treatment analogous to the surgical Alfieri stitch), creating a figure eight orifice
  - This procedure is performed via femoral venous access, and a transseptal puncture is employed to position the delivery system in the LA.

○ Using fluoroscopy and TEE guidance, the clip is advanced and attempts are made to grasp the leaflet tips of the anterior and posterior MV leaflets and clip them together.

○ This is a rapidly developing field with new devices and several trials in progress.

Surgical Management

• **ACC/AHA Guidelines—Class I indications for surgery in mitral regurgitation**
  ○ Symptomatic acute severe MR
  ○ Chronic severe MR and NYHA functional Class II, III, or IV symptoms in the absence of severe LV dysfunction (EF <30%) and/or end-systolic dimension (ESD) >55 mm
  ○ Asymptomatic with chronic severe MR and mild–moderate LV dysfunction (EF 30% to 60%) and/or ESD ≥40 mm
  ○ MV repair is recommended over MV replacement in the majority of patients with severe chronic MR who require surgery, and patients should be referred to surgical centers experienced in MV repair

• Surgery for MR is most commonly performed in patients with degenerative mitral valve disease

• Advances in surgical technique and lower operative mortality are causing some centers to operate earlier on patients with severe MR, even when they are asymptomatic

• Preoperative factors that increase operative and/or postoperative mortality include: worse NYHA functional Class, LV dysfunction (EF <60%), age, associated CAD, and AF

• Surgery for patients with ischemic MR and MR due to a DCM is more controversial and potentially more complex; the MR is largely due to a ventricular problem, so an isolated annuloplasty likely will not solve the problem; this is an active area of research and debate

• Patients with AF should be considered for a concomitant surgical MAZE procedure

Aortic Regurgitation

GENERAL PRINCIPLES

• Aortic regurgitation (AR) may result from pathology of the aortic valve, the aortic root, or both; it is important that both the valve and the root are evaluated to determine the appropriate management and treatment.

• AR usually progresses insidiously with a long asymptomatic period; when it occurs acutely, patients are often very sick and must be managed aggressively.

Etiology

• **More common**
  ○ Bicuspid aortic valve
  ○ Rheumatic disease
  ○ Calcific degeneration
  ○ Infective endocarditis
  ○ Idiopathic dilatation of the aorta
  ○ Myxomatous degeneration
  ○ Systemic HTN

Figure 6-5. Acute aortic regurgitation. CO, cardiac output; HR, heart rate; LAP, left atrial pressure; LV, left ventricle; LVEDP, left ventricular end-diastolic pressure; SV, stroke volume.

- ○ Dissection of the ascending aorta
- ○ Marfan's syndrome
- **Less common**
  - ○ Traumatic injury to the aortic valve
  - ○ Collagen vascular diseases (ankylosing spondylitis, rheumatoid arthritis, reactive arthritis, giant cell aortitis, and Whipple's disease)
  - ○ Syphilitic aortitis
  - ○ Discrete subaortic stenosis
  - ○ Ventricular septal defect (VSD) with prolapse of an aortic cusp
- **Acute**
  - ○ Infective endocarditis
  - ○ Dissection of the ascending aorta
  - ○ Trauma

Pathophysiology
- Acute AR (Figure 6-5)
- Chronic AR (Figure 6-6)

DIAGNOSIS

Clinical Presentation

History
- **Acute:** Patients with acute AR may present with **symptoms of cardiogenic shock and severe dyspnea**. Other presenting symptoms may be related to the cause of acute AR.

Figure 6-6. Chronic aortic regurgitation. CO, cardiac output; CHF, congestive heart failure; EF, ejection fraction; LV, left ventricle; LVED, left ventricular end-diastolic; LVEDP, left ventricular end-diastolic pressure; LVH, left ventricular hypertrophy; SV, stroke volume.

- **Chronic:** Symptoms depend on the presence of LV dysfunction and whether the patient is in the **compensated versus decompensated stage**. Compensated patients are typically asymptomatic, whereas those in the decompensated stage may note decreased exercise tolerance, dyspnea, fatigue, and/or angina.

Physical Examination
- Acute
  - **Tachycardia**
  - Wide pulse pressure may be present, but is often not present because forward SV (and therefore systolic blood pressure) is reduced
  - Brief soft diastolic murmur heard best at 3rd left intercostal space (often not heard)
  - Systolic flow murmur (due to volume overload and hyperdynamic LV)
  - Look for evidence of aortic dissection, infective endocarditis, and Marfanoid characteristics

- Chronic
  - LV heave, and point of maximal impulse (PMI) is laterally displaced
  - Diastolic decrescendo murmur heard best at left sternal border (LSB) leaning forward at end-expiration (severity of AR correlates with duration, not intensity, of the murmur)
  - Systolic flow murmur (due mostly to volume overload; concomitant AS may also be present)
  - Austin Flint murmur
  - Widened pulse pressure (often >100 mm Hg) with a low diastolic pressure; there are numerous eponyms for the characteristic signs related to a wide pulse pressure

Diagnostic Testing

The diagnostic evaluation depends somewhat on the acuity of the presentation but will likely include
- **ECG**
  - Tachycardia
  - LVH and LAE (more common in chronic AR)
  - New conduction block may suggest an aortic root abscess
- **CXR**
  Look for pulmonary edema, widened mediastinum, and cardiomegaly
- **TTE**
  - LV systolic function
  - LV dimensions at end systole and end diastole
  - Leaflet number and morphology
  - Assessment of the severity of AR
  - Look for evidence of endocarditis or aortic dissection
  - Dimension of aortic root
- **TEE**
  - Clarify whether there is a bicuspid valve if unclear on TTE
  - Better sensitivity and specificity for aortic dissection than TTE
  - Clarify whether there is endocarditis ± root abscess if unclear on TTE
  - Better visualization of aortic valve in patients with a prosthetic aortic valve
- **Cardiac catheterization**
  - In patients undergoing AVR who are at risk for CAD
  - Assessment of LV pressure, LV function, and severity of AR (via aortic root angiography) is indicated in symptomatic patients in whom the severity of AR is unclear on noninvasive imaging or discordant with clinical findings
- MRI/CT
  - Depending on the institution, either of these may be the imaging modality of choice for evaluating aortic dimensions and/or for evaluation of aortic dissection.
  - If echo assessment of the severity of AR is inadequate, MRI is useful for assessing the severity of AR.
  - CTA may be an alternative to catheterization to evaluate coronary anatomy prior to valve surgery.

TREATMENT

- **The role of medical therapy in patients with AR is limited**; there are currently no randomized, placebo-controlled data showing that vasodilator therapy delays the development of symptoms or LV dysfunction warranting surgery.

- **Vasodilator therapy (i.e., nifedipine, ACE inhibitor, hydralazine)** is indicated to reduce systolic blood pressure in hypertensive patients with AR.
- Other than for treating HTN, vasodilator therapy has a potential role in three situations:
  ○ As chronic therapy in patients with severe AS who have symptoms or LV dysfunction but are not surgical candidates
  ○ As a short-term therapy to improve hemodynamics in patients with severe HF and severe LV dysfunction prior to surgery
  ○ May be considered for long-term therapy in asymptomatic patients with severe AS who have some LV dilatation but normal LV systolic function
- Retrospective data suggest that β-blocker use may be associated with a survival benefit in patients with severe AR, but prospective studies are needed.
- When endocarditis is suspected or confirmed, appropriate antibiotic coverage is critical.

Surgical Management

- **ACC/AHA Guidelines—Class I indications for AVR for AR**
  ○ **Symptomatic with severe AR irrespective of LV systolic function.**
  ○ Asymptomatic with chronic severe AR and LV systolic dysfunction (EF ≤50%).
  ○ Chronic severe AR while undergoing CABG, surgery on the aorta, or other valve surgery.
- Acute, severe AR is almost universally symptomatic and is treated surgically.
- If the aortic root is dilated, it may be repaired or replaced at the time of AVR. For patients with a bicuspid valve, Marfan's syndrome (or related genetically triggered aortopathy), surgery on the aorta should occur at the time of AVR if the aortic root or ascending aorta is >4.5 cm.
- Although worse NYHA functional Class, LV dysfunction, and the chronicity of these abnormalities are predictors of higher operative and postoperative mortality, AVR is usually a better alternative than medical therapy in improving overall mortality and morbidity.

OUTCOME/PROGNOSIS

- Asymptomatic patients with normal LV systolic function (*J AM Coll Cardiol 2006;48(3):e1–e148*)
  ○ Progression to symptoms and/or LV dysfunction <6% per year
  ○ Progression to asymptomatic LV dysfunction <3.5% per year
  ○ Sudden death <0.2% per year
- Asymptomatic patients with LV dysfunction
  ○ Progression to cardiac symptoms >25% per year
- Symptomatic patients
  ○ Mortality rate >10% per year

Prosthetic Heart Valves

GENERAL PRINCIPLES

The choice of valve prosthesis depends on many factors including the patient, surgeon, cardiologist, and clinical scenario. With improvements in bioprosthetic valves, the recommendation for a mechanical valve in patients <65 years of age is no longer as firm and bioprosthetic valve use has increased in younger patients.

- **Mechanical**
  - Ball-and-cage (Starr–Edwards): rarely, if ever, used today
  - Bileaflet (i.e., St. Jude, Carbomedics): most commonly used
  - Single-tilting disk (i.e., Björk–Shiley, Medtronic Hall, Omnicarbon)
  - **Advantages:** structurally stable, long-lasting, relatively hemodynamically efficient (particularly bileaflet)
  - **Disadvantages:** need for anticoagulation, risk of bleeding, risk of thrombosis/embolism despite anticoagulation, severe hemodynamic compromise if disk thrombosis or immobility occurs (single-tilting disk), risk of endocarditis
- **Bioprosthetic**
  - Porcine aortic valve tissue (i.e., Hancock, Carpentier–Edwards)
  - Bovine pericardial tissue (i.e., Carpentier–Edwards Perimount)
  - Stented or stentless
  - **Advantages:** no need for anticoagulation, low thromboembolism risk, low risk of catastrophic valve failure
  - **Disadvantages:** structural valve deterioration, imperfect hemodynamic efficiency, risk of endocarditis, still a small risk (0.7% per year) of thromboembolism without anticoagulation
- **Homograft (cadaveric)**
  - Rarely used for AV surgery; the only remaining use for aortic valve/root homograft may be in the setting AV endocarditis, particularly complex aortic root endocarditis
  - Most commonly used to replace the pulmonic valve

Table 6-1	Antithrombotic Therapy for Patients with Prosthetic Heart Valves			
Valve and Duration	Aspirin (75–100 mg)	Warfarin (INR 2–3)	Warfarin (INR 2.5–3.5)	No Warfarin
Mechanical				
AVR—low risk				
<3 months	Class I	Class I	Class IIa	
>3 months	Class I	Class I		
AVR—high risk	Class I		Class I	
MVR	Class I		Class I	
Biologic				
AVR—low risk				
<3 months	Class I	Class IIa		Class IIb
>3 months	Class I			Class IIa
AVR—high risk	Class I	Class I		
MVR—low risk				
<3 months	Class I	Class IIa		
>3 months	Class I			Class IIa
MVR—high risk	Class I	Class I		

AVR, aortic valve replacement; INR, international normalized ratio; MVR, mitral valve replacement.

TREATMENT

Risk factors include AF, previous thromboembolism, LV dysfunction, and hypercoagulable condition. Low risk means no risk factors. INR should be maintained between 2.5 and 3.5 for aortic disk valves and Starr–Edwards valves regardless of risk factors (Table 6-1) (*J AM Coll Cardiol 2006;48(3):e1*).

7

Cardiac Arrhythmias

Shivak Sharma, Daniel H. Cooper, and
Mitchell N. Faddis

TACHYARRHYTHMIAS

Approach to Tachyarrhythmias

GENERAL PRINCIPLES

- Tachyarrhythmias are commonly encountered in the inpatient setting.
- Approaching these rhythms in a prompt and stepwise manner will facilitate early recognition of the underlying arrhythmia and timely initiation of appropriate therapy.
- Clinical decision making is guided by patient symptoms and signs of hemodynamic stability.

Definition

Cardiac rhythms whose ventricular rate exceeds **100 beats per minute** (bpm).

Classification

Tachyarrhythmias are broadly classified based on the width of the QRS complex on the electrocardiogram (ECG):
- Narrow-Complex tachyarrhythmia (QRS <120 ms): Arrhythmia (supraventricular tachycardia) originates within or above the atrioventricular (AV) node and rapidly activates ventricles via the normal His–Purkinje system.
- Wide-Complex tachyarrhythmia (QRS ≥120 ms): Arrhythmia originates outside the normal conduction system (ventricular tachycardia [VT]) or travels via an abnormal His–Purkinje system (supraventricular tachycardia with aberrancy) activating the ventricles in an abnormally slow manner.

Etiology

Mechanism divided into disorders of **impulse conduction** and **impulse formatioten**:
- **Disorders of impulse conduction:** Reentry accounts for the majority of tachyrrhythmias. It refers to conduction of the electrical activation wavefront retrograde into a myocardial region that was initially refractory to antegrade conduction of the wavefront. Differential refractory periods of myocardial tissue are a necessary component to allow reentry to occur. As a result of reentry, propagation of the activation wavefront around a myocardial circuit sustains the arrhythmia (e.g., VT).
- **Disorders of impulse formation:** Enhanced automaticity (e.g., accelerated junctional and accelerated idioventricular rhythm) **and triggered activity** (e.g., long QT syndrome and digitalis toxicity) are other less common mechanisms of tachyarrhythmias.

DIAGNOSIS

Clinical Presentation

- Tachyarrhythmias can be the cause of initial presentation at an outpatient or acute care setting.
- They can be associated with systemic illnesses in patients who are being evaluated in the emergency department or are being treated in an inpatient setting.

History

- Symptoms are an important facet of what guides clinical decision making.
- **Dyspnea, angina, lightheadedness or syncope, and decreased level of consciousness** are alarming symptoms likely to guide the physician to a more immediate therapeutic option.
- Baseline symptoms that reflect **poor left ventricular (LV) function**, such as dyspnea on exertion (DOE), orthopnea, paroxysmal nocturnal dyspnea (PND), and lower extremity swelling, are critical to elucidate.
- **Palpitations:** Commonly associated with tachyarrhythmias but important to inquire about the nature of their onset and termination.
  - ○ Sudden onset and termination is highly suggestive of a tachyarrhythmia.
  - ○ Symptom abatement with breath holding or Valsalva maneuver is suggestive of a supraventricular tachyarrhythmia. AV node is critical in the maintenance of this arrhythmia.
- History of **organic heart disease** (i.e., ischemic, nonischemic, valvular cardiomyopathy) or **endocrinopathy** (i.e., thyroid disease, pheochromocytoma) should be sought.
- History of **familial or congenital causes of arrhythmias** such as hypertrophic cardiomyopathy (HCM), congenital long QT syndrome, or other congenital heart disease should be addressed as well.
  - ○ **Hypertrophic obstructive cardiomyopathy** (HOCM) is associated with atrial arrhythmias (atrial fibrillation [AF] in 20% to 25%), as well as malignant ventricular arrhythmias.
  - ○ **Mitral valve prolapse** (MVP) is associated with supraventricular and ventricular arrhythmias.
- **Medications:** Critical to obtain a complete list, including over-the-counter and herbal medications.

Physical Examination

- Signs of clinical stability or instability, including vital signs, mental status, peripheral perfusion, etc., are critical in guiding initial decision making.
- If clinically stable, then physical exam should be focused on determining underlying cardiovascular abnormalities that may make certain rhythms more or less likely.
- Findings of **congestive heart failure (CHF)**, including elevated jugular venous pressure (JVP), pulmonary rales, peripheral edema, and S_3 gallop, make the diagnosis of malignant ventricular arrhythmias more likely.
- If arrhythmia is sustained, here are some special considerations during physical exam:
  - ○ **Palpate the pulse** and assess for rate and regularity.
    - ▪ If rate is about 150 bpm, suspect atrial flutter (AFl) with 2:1 block.
    - ▪ If rate is >150 bpm, suspect atrioventricular nodal reentrant tachycardia (AVNRT) or atrioventricular reentrant tachycardia (AVRT).
    - ▪ Ventricular arrhythmia rates are more variable.

- If pulse is irregular with no pattern, suspect AF.
- Irregular pulse with a discernible pattern (group beating) suggests the presence of second-degree heart block.
  - **"Cannon" A waves:** Revealed on inspection of JVP and reflect atrial contraction against a closed tricuspid valve.
    - If irregular, then suggestive of underlying AV dissociation and clue for VT.
    - If regular in 1:1 ratio with peripheral pulse, then suggestive of AVNRT, AVRT, or a junctional tachycardia, all leading to retrograde atrial activation occurring simultaneously with ventricular contraction.

Diagnostic Testing

Laboratories

Serum electrolytes, complete blood count (CBC), thyroid function tests, serum concentration of digoxin (when applicable), and a urine toxicology screen should be considered for all patients.

Electrocardiography

- **A 12-lead ECG** is critical for the initial evaluation; may need to be repeated several times depending on changes in patient's clinical course.
- If the patient is clinically stable, obtain a 12-lead ECG and a **continuous rhythm strip** with leads that best demonstrate atrial activation (e.g., V_1, II, III, aVF).
- Examine the ECG for evidence of conduction abnormalities, such as preexcitation or bundle branch block, or signs of structural heart disease such as prior myocardial infarction (MI).
- Comparison of the ECG obtained during arrhythmia with that at baseline can highlight subtle features of the QRS deflection that indicate the superposition of atrial and ventricular depolarization.
- Rhythm strip is very useful to document the response to interventions (e.g., vagal maneuvers, antiarrhythmic drug therapy, electrical cardioversion).

Imaging

Chest radiographs and **transthoracic echocardiograms** can help provide evidence of structural heart disease that may make ventricular arrhythmias more likely.

Diagnostic Procedures

- **Continuous ambulatory ECG monitoring**
  - One or more days; useful for documenting symptomatic transient arrhythmias that occur with sufficient frequency.
  - Recording mode useful for assessment of patient's heart rate response to daily activities or antiarrhythmic drug treatment.
  - Correlation between patient-reported symptoms in a time-marked diary and heart rhythm recordings is the key to determining if symptoms are attributable to an arrhythmia.
- **In-hospital telemetry monitoring**
  Mainstay of surveillance monitoring during the course of hospitalization for cardiac arrhythmia patients who are seriously ill or are having life-threatening arrhythmias.
- **Event recorders**
  - Weeks to months; useful for documenting symptomatic transient arrhythmias that occur infrequently.
  - A "loop recorder" is worn by the patient and continuously records the ECG. When activated by the patient or with an autodetection feature, the ECG recording is saved with several minutes of preceding rhythm data.

- An "event monitor" is connected only when the patient experiences symptoms.
- An **implantable loop recorder or insertable loop recorder (ILR)** is a subcutaneous monitoring device, to provide automated or patient-activated recording of significant arrhythmic events that occur very infrequently over several months or for patients who are unable to activate external recorders.
- **Exercise ECG**
  Useful for studying exercise-induced arrhythmias or to assess the sinus node response to exercise.
- **Electrophysiology study (EPS)**
  - Invasive, catheter-based procedure that is used to study a patient's susceptibility to arrhythmias or to investigate the mechanism of a known arrhythmia.
  - EPS is also combined with catheter ablation for curative treatment of many arrhythmia mechanisms.
  - The efficacy of EPS to induce and study arrhythmias is highest for reentrant mechanisms.

TREATMENT

Please refer to the treatment of individual tachyarrhythmias for hemodynamically stable patients and advanced cardiac life support (ACLS) algorithm for tachycardias in Appendix C.

Supraventricular Tachyarrhythmias

GENERAL PRINCIPLES

- **Supraventricular tachyarrhythmias (SVTs)** are often recurrent, occasionally persistent, and a frequent cause of visits to emergency departments and primary care physician offices.
- The evaluation of patients with SVT should always begin with prompt assessment of hemodynamic stability and clinical "substrate." Young and healthy adults usually tolerate tachyarrhythmias better than patients with a significant cardiopulmonary comorbidity.
- The diagnostic and therapeutic discussion that follows is aimed at the hemodynamically stable patient. If a patient is deemed clinically unstable based on clinical signs, symptoms, or hemodynamics, one should immediately proceed to cardioversion per ACLS guidelines.

Definition

- Tachyarrhythmias that require atrial or AV nodal tissue, or both, for their initiation and maintenance are termed SVT.
- The QRS complex in most SVTs is narrow (QRS <120 ms). However, they can certainly present as wide-complex tachycardia (WCT) (QRS ≥120 ms) in SVT with aberrancy or preexcited tachycardia.

Classification

- SVT can be classified in several ways—ECG appearance, underlying mechanism, AV node dependence, etc.

• A diagnostic approach to tachyarrhythmias as summarized in Figure 7-1 is a clinically useful classification to approach these patients.

Epidemiology

Published incidence data can vary widely between studies and is difficult to quantify because of a high rate of asymptomatic episodes in patients.

DIAGNOSIS

What are the odds?—When approaching any diagnostic dilemma, it is always helpful to have a rough idea of how commonly or rarely a particular diagnosis presents in your patient population.

• **AF** is the most common narrow-complex tachycardia seen in the inpatient setting. **AFl** can often accompany AF and is diagnosed one-tenth as often as AF but is twice as prevalent as the paroxysmal SVTs. The other atrial tachyarrhythmias are far less common.

• In one case series, **AVNRT** was reported as the most common diagnosis of the paroxysmal SVTs (60%) followed by AVRT (30%) (*Crit Care Med 2000; 28(10 suppl):N129*).

• However, if the patient is younger than age 40, then AVRT, often in the context of Wolff–Parkinson–White (WPW) syndrome, is more likely.

• Please refer to Figure 7-1 for the diagnostic approach to tachyarrhythmias.

Clinical Presentation

The clinical presentation for SVT is similar to tachyarrhythmias in general and has been previously outlined in this section.

Differential Diagnosis

• **AF**

The most common sustained tachyarrhythmia and is discussed as a separate topic in this section.

• **AFl**

○ The second most common atrial arrhythmia, with estimated 200,000 new cases in the United States annually, is associated with increasing age, underlying heart disease, and male gender (*J Am Coll Cardiol 2000;36:2242*).

○ AFl usually presents as a **regular rhythm** but can be **irregularly irregular** when associated with variable AV block (2:1 to 4:1 to 3:1, etc.).

○ **Mechanism:** Reentrant circuit around functional or structural conduction barriers within the atria. Atrial rate is 250 to 350 bpm with conduction to ventricle that is usually not 1:1; most often 2:1. (**SVT with regular ventricular rate of 150 bpm should raise suspicion for AFl.**)

○ Like AF, AFl is commonly associated with the post–cardiac surgery period, pulmonary disease, thyrotoxicosis, and atrial enlargement.

○ **ECG:** In typical AFl, "saw tooth" pattern best visualized in leads II, III, and aVF with negative deflections in V_1.

• **Multifocal atrial tachycardia (MAT)**

○ **Irregularly irregular** SVT seen generally in elderly hospitalized patients with multiple comorbidities.

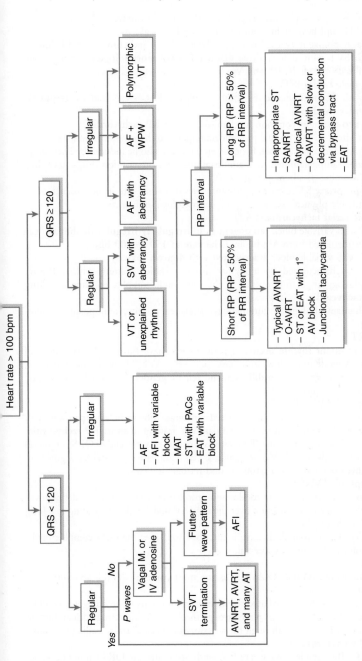

Figure 7-1. Diagnostic approach to tachyarrhythmias. AF, atrial fibrillation; AFI, atrial flutter; AV, atrioventricular; AVRT, atrioventricular reentrant tachycardia; AVNRT, atrioventricular nodal reentrant tachycardia; EAT, ectopic atrial tachycardia; MAT, multifocal atrial tachycardia; O-AVRT, orthodromic AVRT; PAC, premature atrial complex; SANRT, Sinoatrial nodal reentrant tachycardia; ST, sinus tachycardia; SVT, supraventricular tachyarrhythmia; VT, ventricular tachycardia; WPW, Wolff–Parkinson–White.

- ○ MAT is most often associated with chronic obstructive pulmonary disease (COPD) and heart failure but also associated with glucose intolerance, hypokalemia, hypomagnesemia, drugs (e.g., theophylline), and chronic renal failure.
- ○ **ECG:** SVT with at least **three distinct P-wave morphologies**, generally best visualized in leads II, III, and V_1.
- **Sinus tachycardia (ST)**
  - ○ ST with frequent premature atrial complexes (PACs) can lead to **irregularly irregular rhythm**.
  - ○ It is also the most common mechanism of **long RP tachycardia**.
  - ○ Most often, ST is a normal physiologic response to hyperadrenergic states (fever, pain, hypovolemia, anemia, hypoxia, etc.) but can also be induced by illicit drugs (cocaine, amphetamines, methamphetamine) and prescription drugs (theophylline, atropine, β-adrenergic agonists).
  - ○ **Inappropriate ST** refers to persistently elevated sinus rate in the absence of an identifiable physical, pathologic, or pharmacologic influence.
- **Ectopic atrial tachycardia (EAT)**
  - ○ EAT with variable block can present as an **irregularly irregular** rhythm and can be distinguished from AFl by an **atrial rate of 150 to 200 bpm**.
  - ○ EAT with variable block is associated with **digoxin toxicity**.
  - ○ EAT is characterized by a regular atrial activation pattern with a P-wave morphology originating outside of the sinus node complex resulting in a **long RP tachycardia**.
  - ○ **Mechanism:** Enhanced automaticity, triggered activity, and possibly micro-reentry.
- **AVNRT**
  - ○ This reentrant rhythm occurs in patients who have functional dissociation of their AV node into "slow" and "fast" pathways. AVNRT can occur at any age, with a predilection for **middle age** and **female gender**. Structural heart disease is not a prerequisite.
  - ○ **"Typical" AVNRT**
    - ▪ More common; conduction proceeds antegrade down the slow pathway with retrograde conduction up the fast pathway, leading to **short RP tachycardia**.
    - ▪ **ECG:** P waves hidden in QRS complexes or buried at the end of QRS complexes creating a pseudo-r″ (V_1) or pseudo-s′ (II). Compare QRS and ST segment in tachycardia and sinus rhythm to find retrograde P waves.
  - ○ **"Atypical" AVNRT**
    - ▪ Less common; antegrade conduction proceeds over the fast AV nodal pathway with retrograde conduction over the slow AV nodal pathway, leading to a **long RP tachycardia**.
    - ▪ **ECG:** The retrograde P wave is inscribed well after the QRS complex in the second half of the RR interval.
- **AVRT**
  - ○ **Orthodromic AVRT (O-AVRT)** is the most common AVRT accounting for about 95% of all AVRT.
    - ▪ Accessory pathway-mediated reentrant rhythm occurs when antegrade conduction to the ventricle takes place through the AV node and retrograde conduction to the atrium occurs through the accessory or "bypass" tract, leading to a **short RP tachycardia**.
    - ▪ **ECG:** Retrograde P waves are frequently seen after the QRS complex and are usually distinguishable from the QRS (i.e., separated by >70 ms).

- O-AVRT is the most common mechanism of SVT in patients with preexcitation syndromes, like WPW syndrome (defined by short PR and a delta wave on upstroke of QRS) present on sinus rhythm ECG.
- O-AVRT can occur without preexcitation in which conduction through the bypass tract occurs only during tachycardia in a retrograde fashion ("concealed pathway").
- Less commonly, retrograde conduction over the accessory pathway to the atrium proceeds slowly enough for atrial activation to occur in the second half of the RR interval, leading to a **long RP tachycardia**. The associated incessant tachycardia can cause tachycardia-induced cardiomyopathy.
  - ○ **Antidromic AVRT:** This reentrant form of SVT occurs when conduction to the ventricle is down an accessory bypass tract with retrograde conduction through the AV node or a second bypass tract.
    - **ECG:** The QRS seems consistent with VT; however, the presence of preexcitation on the baseline QRS should be diagnostic for WPW syndrome.
    Antidromic AVRT is seen in <5% of patients with WPW syndrome.
- **Junctional tachycardia**
  - ○ Arises from enhanced automaticity within the AV junction as the electrical impulses conduct to the ventricle and atrium simultaneously, similar to typical AVNRT, so that the retrograde P waves are frequently buried in the QRS complex.
  - ○ Common in young children particularly after cardiac surgery.
- **Sinoatrial nodal reentrant tachycardia (SANRT)**
  - ○ Reentrant circuit is localized at least partially within the sinoatrial (SA) node.
  - ○ Abrupt onset and termination, triggered by a PAC.
  - ○ **ECG:** P-wave morphology and axis are identical to the native sinus P wave during normal sinus rhythm.

TREATMENT

- Please refer to Table 7-1 for general therapeutic approach to common SVTs.
- Acute treatment of symptomatic SVT should follow the **ACLS protocol** as outlined in Appendix C.
- Chronic treatment should be aimed at either prevention of recurrence or prevention of the complications associated with the specific SVT.
- Many SVTs can be terminated by **AV nodal blocking agents or techniques** (Table 7-2), whereas AF, AFl, and some atrial tachycardias will persist with a slowing of the ventricular rate due to partial AV nodal blockade.
- **Correction of electrolyte abnormalities** like hypokalemia and hypomagnesemia may have therapeutic and preventive value in the treatment of some SVTs.
- **Radiofrequency ablation (RFA):** Definitive cure with high success rates from 85% to 95% for many SVTs, including AVNRT, accessory bypass tract–mediated tachycardias, focal atrial tachycardia, and AFl.
- Complication rates are dependent on the particular procedure and are usually <1% and include bleeding, groin hematomas, cardiac perforation or tamponade, stroke, pulmonary embolism, and complete heart block requiring permanent pacemaker (PPM).
- There is growing evidence but lack of large randomized trials with long-term follow-up, which suggests that catheter ablation as compared to antiarrhythmic therapy improves quality of life and is more cost-effective in the long term (*Am J Cardiol 1998;82:589*).

Table 7-1	Treatment of Common Supraventricular Tachyarrhythmias

Treatment Strategies

Atrial flutter (AFl)	Anticoagulation similar to AF; risk of thromboembolic complications is similar.
	Rate control with same agents as AF.
	If highly symptomatic or rate control difficult, electrical or chemical cardioversion is appropriate.
	If pacemaker present, overdrive atrial pacing can achieve cardioversion.
	Catheter ablation of typical right AFl with long-term success above 90% and rare complications.
Multifocal atrial tachycardia (MAT)	Therapy targeted at treatment of underlying pathophysiologic process.
	Maintain potassium and magnesium electrolyte balance.
	Antiarrhythmic, if symptomatic rapid ventricular response. Individualize β-adrenergic blockers vs. calcium channel blocker therapy.
	DC cardioversion is not effective.
Sinus tachycardia (ST)	Therapy targeted at treatment of underlying pathophysiologic process.
Ectopic atrial tachycardia (EAT)	**Acute therapy:** Identify and treat precipitating factors like digoxin toxicity; if hemodynamically stable, then β-blockers and calcium channel blockers. In rare cases, amiodarone, flecainide, or sotalol.
	Chronic therapy: Rate control with β-adrenergic blockers and calcium channel blockers. If unsuccessful, options include catheter ablation (86% success rate), flecainide, propafenone, sotalol, or amiodarone.
AV nodal re-entrant tachycardia (AVNRT)	Catheter ablation highly successful (96%) but has to be individualized to each patient.
	If medical therapy more desirable—β-adrenergic blockers, calcium channel blockers, and digoxin; then consider propafenone, flecainide, etc.
Orthodromic AV reentrant tachycardia (O-AVRT)	**Acute therapy:** Vagal maneuvers, adenosine, calcium channel blockers. If ineffective, then procainamide or β-blockers.
	Chronic suppressive therapy: Catheter ablation highly successful (95%) but has to be individualized to each patient. If medical therapy more desirable for prevention, flecainide and procainamide are indicated.
Antidromic AV reentrant tachycardia (A-AVRT)	**Acute therapy:** Avoid adenosine or other AV node–specific blocking agents. Consider ibutilide, procainamide, or flecainide.
	Chronic suppressive therapy: Accessory pathway catheter ablation is preferred and successful (95%). If medical therapy desired, consider flecainide and propafenone.

AF, atrial fibrillation; DC, direct current.
From Blomström-Lundqvist C, Scheinman MM, Aliot EM, et al. ACC/AHA/ESC guidelines for the management of patients with supraventricular arrhythmias—executive summary: a report of the American college of cardiology/American heart association task force on practice guidelines and the European society of cardiology committee for practice guidelines. *J Am Coll Cardiol.* 2003;42:1493.

Table 7-2 Common Vagal Maneuvers and Adenosine

	Patient Preparation[a]	Mechanism	Dose/Duration/Details	Toxicity	Contraindication	Potentiators/Antagonists	Common Side Effects
Valsalva	Describe the procedure.	Vagal stimulation during relaxation phase.	Exhale forcefully against a closed airway for several seconds followed by relaxation.	Well tolerated.	Patient unable to follow commands.	—	—
Carotid sinus massage	Check for carotid bruits and history of CVA; then place in recumbent position with neck extended.	Vagal stimulation.	First, apply enough pressure to simply feel carotid pulse with index and middle fingers. If no effect, then use rotating motion for 3–5 s	Well tolerated. Risk of embolizing carotid plaque. **Never massage both carotids.**	Recent TIA or stroke, or ipsilateral significant carotid artery stenosis or carotid artery bruit.	—	—
Adenosine	Explain the potential side effects to the patient.	AV nodal blocking agent. Short-acting (serum half-life 4–8 min).	Initial: 6 mg IV rapid bolus via antecubital vein, followed by 10–30 mL saline flush. If desired, effect not achieved, can repeat 12 mg followed by 12 mg after 1–2 min intervals. Central venous line: 3 mg IV initial dose.	Precipitate prolonged asystole in patients with sick sinus syndrome or second- or third-degree AV block.	Significant bronchospasm.	Potentiators: Dipyridamole and carbamazepine. **Effect pronounced in heart transplant recipients.** Antagonists: Caffeine and theophylline.	Facial flushing, palpitations, chest pain, hypotension, exacerbation of bronchospasm.

Atrioventricular nodal reentrant tachycardia, atrioventricular reentrant tachycardia, and many atrial tachycardias will terminate with vagal maneuvers or adenosine and in atrial flutter, the appearance of flutter waveform will help diagnosis.

Water immersion, eyeball pressure, coughing, gagging, deep breathing, etc., are other alternative vagal maneuvers.

[a]Patients should be under continuous electrocardiogram monitoring for each of these procedures. To enhance diagnostic value of rhythm strip, use leads V_1, II (atrial activity).

AV, atrioventricular; CVA, cerebrovascular accident; IV, intravenous; TIA, transient ischemic attack.

Atrial Fibrillation

GENERAL PRINCIPLES

The medical management of **AF** requires careful consideration of three issues: **rate control, prevention of thromboembolic events, and rhythm control**.

Definition

AF is an atrial tachyarrhythmia characterized by the predominantly uncoordinated activation of the atria with the consequent deterioration of atrial mechanical function. AF has a pattern on 12-lead ECG indicated by the absence of consistent P waves. Instead, there are rapid, low-amplitude oscillations or fibrillatory waves that vary in size, shape, and timing across the baseline of the ECG recording. The ventricular response to AF is characteristically irregular and often rapid in the presence of intact AV conduction. AF is the most common cardiac arrhythmia.

Classification

AF has been classified into four forms based upon the clinical presentation: first occurrence, paroxysmal, persistent, and permanent forms.
- **First occurrence** may be symptomatic or asymptomatic. The spontaneous conversion rate is high, measured >60% in hospitalized patients.
- **Paroxysmal** AF describes a recurrent form of AF in which individual episodes are <7 days and usually <48 hours in duration.
- **Persistent** AF describes a recurrent form of AF in which individual episodes are >7 days in duration or require electrical cardioversion to terminate.
- **Permanent** AF describes the form of long-lasting AF, which has failed attempts at cardioversion, electrical or pharmacologic, or has been accepted due to contraindications for cardioversion or a lack of symptoms.

Epidemiology

- AF is the most common sustained tachyarrhythmia for which patients seek treatment and the most likely etiology for an irregularly irregular rhythm discovered on an inpatient ECG. AF is typically a disease of the elderly, affecting >10% of those >75 years old.
- Independent risk factors for AF in addition to advanced age include male sex, diabetes mellitus, cardiovascular disease such as CHF, valvular heart disease, hypertension (HTN), and previous MI (*JAMA 1994;271:840*). Below age 65, obesity and obstructive sleep apnea are important risk factors for new-onset AF (*J Am Coll Cardiol 2007;49(5):565*). Although clinical hyperthyroidism is associated with new-onset AF, the prevalence is low in a population of patients with AF (*J Epidemiol 2008;18(5):209*).
- Following cardiothoracic surgery, AF occurs in 20% to 50% of patients (*J Am Coll Cardiol 2006;48(4):8540*).

Pathophysiology

The precise mechanisms giving rise to AF are incompletely understood. The initiation of AF is commonly due to rapid, repetitive firing of an ectopic focus within the pulmonary veins with fibrillatory conduction to the bodies of the atria. The mainte-nance of persistent AF likely requires multiple reentrant circuits varying in location and timing to explain the self-perpetuating characteristic of AF. Structural and electrical remodeling of the left atrium associated with cardiovascular disease promotes ectopic activity and heterogeneous conduction patterns that provide the substrate for AF. AF, when present, also promotes structural and electrical remodeling in the atria that stabilizes the rhythm. Inflammation and fibrosis may play a major role in initiation and maintenance of AF. Inflammatory markers, such as interleukin-6 and C-reactive protein, are raised in AF and correlate with the duration of AF, success of cardioversion, and thrombogenesis.

Prevention

- Currently, there is a lack of prospective clinical trials that examine the value of primary prevention of non–postoperative AF through treatment of associated conditions or risk factor modification. Some analyses suggest that the statins may reduce recurrent AF by 61%, independent of their lipid-lowering effect (*J Am Coll Cardiol 2008;51:828*). Angiotensin-converting enzyme inhibitor (**ACE-I**) and angiotensin receptor blockers (**ARBs**) have been shown to prevent atrial remodeling in animals via suppression of the renin–angiotensin system. A meta-analysis of patients with CHF and HTN treated with either ACE-I or ARBs demonstrated a reduction in new-onset AF by 20% to 30% (*J Am Coll Cardiol 2005;45:1832*).
- A number of pharmacologic and nonpharmacologic strategies have been evaluated to prevent postoperative AF. Perioperative continuation of **β-adrenergic antago-nists** has been shown to reduce postoperative AF rates. **Amiodarone, sotalol, magnesium, or omega-3 fatty acids** used in the perioperative period have demon-strated a reduction in postoperative AF (*Ann Pharmacother 2007;41:587*).

DIAGNOSIS

AF is diagnosed by 12-lead ECG with a stereotypical pattern of an irregularly fluctuating baseline with an irregular, and often rapid, ventricular rate (>100 bpm). AF should be distinguished from other tachycardia mechanisms with an irregular ventricular response such as MAT and AFl with variable conduction.

Clinical Presentation

Symptoms associated with AF can range from severe (acute pulmonary edema, palpitations, angina, syncope) to nonspecific (fatigue) to none at all. Symptoms are usually secondary to the rapid ventricular response to AF rather than the loss of atrial systole. However, patients with significant ventricular systolic or diastolic dysfunction can have symptoms directly attributable to the loss of atrial systole. Prolonged episodes of tachycardia due to AF may lead to a **tachycardia-induced cardiomyopathy**.

TREATMENT

The medical management of AF is directed at three therapeutic goals: **rate control, prevention of thromboembolic events, and rhythm control** through maintenance of sinus rhythm. Recent studies have shown that there is no mortality advantage to a management strategy aimed at maintaining sinus rhythm (*N Engl J Med 2002;347:1825*). Therefore, the approach to the treatment of AF in the minimally symptomatic patient is devoted to prevention of thromboembolus and pharmacologic control of the ventricular response to AF. Pharmacologic maintenance of sinus rhythm is reserved for patients who remain symptomatic despite efforts to optimize the ventricular response to AF.

Medications

Medical management of AF should start with a consideration of appropriate anti-thrombotic therapy. Warfarin has been shown to be consistently superior to aspirin (ASA) or ASA in combination with clopidogrel for prevention of thromboembolus. Both dabigatran and rivaroxaban have been directly compared to warfarin in random-ized prospective trials that documented a lower rate of systemic or cerebrovascular emboli with a similar rate of bleeding complications as warfarin. Rate control of the ventricular response to AF is achieved with medications that limit conduction through the AV node such as **verapamil, diltiazem, β-adrenergic antagonists, and digoxin**. Rhythm control through maintenance of sinus rhythm can be attempted with selected antiarrhythmic drugs. Pharmacologic control with antiarrhythmic drugs is most effective at preventing recurrence of AF and less effective at chemical cardioversion of AF (Table 7-3).

First Line
- **Prevention of thromboembolic complications** is a central tenet of AF manage-ment and should begin with individual risk assessment of each patient. Chronic anticoagulation with warfarin, dabigatran, or rivaroxaban are the most effective therapies for attenuating the risk of stroke associated with AF; however, the use of any one of these agents requires a careful risk–benefit analysis to identify the patients who are at sufficient risk for embolic cerebrovascular accident (CVA) to outweigh the increased risk of hemorrhagic complications.
  - The **CHADS$_2$ score** is a validated, risk stratification tool that can categorize nonvalvular AF patients as low, intermediate, or high risk for stroke based on the presence of these risk factors: **C**HF, **H**TN, **A**ge >75 years, **D**iabetes mellitus, or prior **S**troke/transient ischemic attacks (TIAs) (Table 7-4).
  - In one study, high-risk patients have a 6% to 7% per year stroke risk that can be reduced to 3.6% per year if placed on ASA 325 mg/d or reduced further to 2.3% per year if placed on therapeutic doses of warfarin (*Circulation 1991;84:527*). A general consensus exists that patients younger than 65 years without structural heart disease or HTN (i.e., "lone AF") are at low risk (approximately 1% per year) and can be managed with daily ASA alone. The current American Heart Association (AHA)/American College of Cardiology (ACC)/European Society of Cardiology (ESC) recommendations for chronic antithrombotic therapy in AF are summarized in Table 7-5.
  - The role of antithrombotic therapy leading up to and after restoration of sinus rhythm is discussed in the following text in the context of cardioversion.
- **Rate control** of AF can be achieved with agents that prolong conduction through the AV node. These include the nondihydropyridine calcium channel blockers (diltiazem, verapamil), β-adrenergic blockers, and digoxin. Refer to Table 7-3 for loading and dosing recommendations.
  - **Digoxin** is useful in controlling the resting ventricular rate in AF in the setting of LV dysfunction and CHF and may be useful as adjunctive therapy in combina-tion with calcium channel antagonists or β-adrenergic antagonists for optimum rate control of chronic AF. It is less useful for rate control during exertion.

Table 7-3 Pharmacologic Agents Used for Heart Rate Control in Atrial Fibrillation

Drug	Loading Dose	Onset of Action	Maintenance Dose	Major Side Effects	Recommendation
Without evidence of accessory pathway					
Esmolol[a]	IV: 0.5 mg/kg over 1 min	5 min[b]	0.06–0.2 mg/kg/min	↓BP, ↓HR, HB, HF, bronchospasm	I
Metoprolol[a]	IV: 2.5–5.0 mg bolus over 2 min (up to three doses)	5 min	NA	↓BP, ↓HR, HB, HF, bronchospasm	I
	PO: Same as maintenance	4–6 h	25–100 mg bid		
Propranolol[a]	IV: 0.15 mg/kg	5 min	NA	↓BP, ↓HR, HB, HF, bronchospasm	I
	PO: Same as maintenance	60–90 min	80–240 mg/d in divided doses		
Diltiazem	IV: 0.25 mg/kg over 2 min	2–7 min	5–15 mg/hr	↓BP, HB, HF	I
	PO: Same as maintenance	2–4 hr	120–360 mg/d in divided doses; slow release available		
Verapamil	IV: 0.075–0.15 mg/kg over 2 min	3–5 min	NA	↓BP, HB, HF	I
	PO: Same as maintenance	1–2 hr	120–360 mg/d in divided doses; slow release available		
With evidence of accessory pathway[c]					
Amiodarone	IV: 150 mg over 10 min	Days	1 mg/min × 6 h, then 0.5 mg/min	See below	IIa

(continued)

Table 7-3	Pharmacologic Agents Used for Heart Rate Control in Atrial Fibrillation (Continued)				
Drug	**Loading Dose**	**Onset of Action**	**Maintenance Dose**	**Major Side Effects**	**Recommendation**
In patients with heart failure and without accessory pathway					
Digoxin	IV: 0.25 mg q2h, up to 1.5 mg PO: 0.5 mg/d	60 min or more 2 days	0.125–0.375 mg/d IV or orally	Digoxin toxicity, HB, ↓HR	I
Amiodarone[d]	IV: 150 mg over 10 min PO: 800 mg/d for 1 wk, 600 mg/d for 1 wk, 400 mg/d for 1 wk,	Days 1–3 wk	1 mg/min × 6 h, then 0.5 mg/min 100–400 mg PO daily	↓BP, HB, ↓HR, warfarin interaction; see text for description of dermatologic, thyroid, pulmonary, corneal, and liver side effects	Acute setting: IIa(IV); nonacute/chronic: IIb(PO)

[a]Only representative members of the type of β-blockers are included in the table, but other similar agents could be used for this indication in appropriate doses.

[b]Onset is variable and some effects occur earlier.

[c]Conversion to sinus rhythm and catheter ablation of the accessory pathway are generally recommended; pharmacologic therapy for rate control may be appropriate therapy in certain patients. See text for discussion of atrial fibrillation in setting of preexcitation/WPW syndrome.

[d]Amiodarone can be useful to control the heart rate in patients with atrial fibrillation when other measures are unsuccessful or contraindicated.

↓BP, hypotension; ↓HR, bradycardia; HB, heart block; HF, heart failure; IV, intravenous; NA, not applicable.

Adapted from Fuster V, Ryden LE, Cannom DS, et al. ACC/AHA/ESC 2006 guidelines for the management of patients with atrial fibrillation: a report of the American College of Cardiology/American Heart Association Task Force on Practice Guidelines and the European Society of Cardiology Committee for Practice Guidelines (Writing Committee to Revise the 2001 Guidelines for the Management of Patients With Atrial Fibrillation). Circulation. 2006;114:e257–e354.

Table 7-4	Stroke Risk in Patients with Nonvalvular Atrial Fibrillation Not Treated with Anticoagulation According to the CHADS$_2$ Index

CHADS$_2$ risk criteria	Score
Prior stroke or TIA	2
Age >75 yr	1
Hypertension	1
Diabetes mellitus	1
Heart failure	1

Patients (N = 1,733)	Adjusted stroke Rate (%/yr)[a] (95% CI)	CHADS$_2$ score	Risk category	Recommended Antithrombotic Therapy
120	1.9 (1.2–3.0)	0	Low	→ Aspirin 81–325 mg PO daily
463	2.8 (2.0–3.8)	1	Moderate	→ Aspirin or Warfarin
523	4.0 (3.1–5.1)	2	Moderate	→ Previous CVA/TIA/embolism?
337	5.9 (4.6–7.3)	3	High	- Yes = Warfarin
220	8.5 (6.3–11.1)	4	High	- No = Aspirin or Warfarin
65	12.5 (8.2–17.5)	5	High	→ Warfarin (INR 2.0–3.0)
5	18.2 (10.5–27.4)	6	High	

Aspirin, 81–325 mg PO daily. Warfarin, international normalized ratio (INR), 2.0–3.0.
[a]The adjusted stroke rate was derived from multivariate analysis assuming no aspirin usage.
AF, atrial fibrillation; CHADS$_2$, **c**ardiac failure, **h**ypertension, **a**ge, **d**iabetes, and **s**troke (doubled); CI, confidence interval; CVA, cerebrovascular accident; TIA, transient ischemic attack.
Adapted from Fuster V, Ryden LE, Cannom DS, et al. ACC/AHA/ESC 2006 guidelines for the management of patients with atrial fibrillation: a report of the American College of Cardiology/ American Heart Association Task Force on Practice Guidelines and the European Society of Cardiology Committee for Practice Guidelines (Writing Committee to Revise the 2001 Guidelines for the Management of Patients With Atrial Fibrillation). *Circulation.* 2006;114:e257–e354. Data from Gage BF, Waterman AD, Shannon W, et al. Validation of clinical classification schemes for predicting stroke: results from the National Registry of Atrial Fibrillation. *JAMA.* 2001;285:2864–2870.

- **Digitalis toxicity** is usually diagnosed clinically with presenting symptoms including **nausea, abdominal pain, vision changes, confusion, and delirium**. It is often seen in patients with renal dysfunction or in those patients on agents known to increase digoxin levels (verapamil, diltiazem, erythromycin, cyclosporine, etc.). **Paroxysmal atrial tachycardia with varying degrees of AV block and bidirectional VT** are the most commonly seen arrhythmias in association with digitalis toxicity. Treatment is supportive, by withholding the drug, insertion of temporary pacemakers for AV block, and **intravenous (IV) phenytoin for bidirectional VT**.
- **Nonpharmacologic rate control** of AF can be accomplished by AV nodal ablation in association with PPM implantation. This strategy should be reserved for patients who have failed pharmacologic rate control, and rhythm control is either ineffective or contraindicated.

Table 7-5	Appropriate Anticoagulation in Various Atrial Fibrillation Populations	
Patient Features	**Antithrombotic Therapy**	**Class of Recommendation**
Age <60 yr, no heart disease (lone AF)	Aspirin (81–325 mg/d) or no therapy	I
Age <60 yr, heart disease but no RF[a]	Aspirin (81–325 mg/d)	I
Age 60–74 yr, no RF[a]	Aspirin (81–325 mg/d)	I
Age 65–74 yr with diabetes mellitus or CAD	Oral anticoagulation (INR 2.0–3.0)	I
Age 75 yr or older, women	Oral anticoagulation (INR 2.0–3.0)	I
Age 75 yr or older, men, no other RF	Oral anticoagulation (INR 2.0–3.0) or aspirin (81–325 mg/d)	I
Age 65 yr or older, heart failure	Oral anticoagulation (INR 2.0–3.0)	I
LV ejection fraction <35% or fractional shortening <25%, and hypertension	Oral anticoagulation (INR 2.0–3.0)	I
Rheumatic heart disease (mitral stenosis)	Oral anticoagulation (INR 2.0–3.0)	I
Prosthetic heart valves; prior thromboembolism	Oral anticoagulation (INR 2.0–3.0 or higher)	I
Persistent atrial thrombus on TEE	Oral anticoagulation (INR 2.0–3.0 or higher)	IIa

[a]Risk factors for thromboembolism include heart failure (HF), LV ejection fraction <35%, and history of hypertension.

AF, atrial fibrillation; CAD, coronary artery disease; INR, international normalized ratio; LV, left ventricular; RF, risk factor; TEE, transesophageal echocardiography.

Adapted from Fuster V, Ryden LE, Cannom DS, et al. ACC/AHA/ESC 2006 guidelines for the management of patients with atrial fibrillation: a report of the American College of Cardiology/American Heart Association Task Force on Practice Guidelines and the European Society of Cardiology Committee for Practice Guidelines (Writing Committee to Revise the 2001 Guidelines for the Management of Patients With Atrial Fibrillation). *Circulation.* 2006;114:e257–e354.

Second Line

Rhythm control of AF is accomplished pharmacologically with antiarrhythmic drugs that modify impulse formation or propagation to prevent initiation of AF. Antiarrhythmic drugs are less effective at restoration of sinus rhythm through **pharmacologic cardioversion. The risk of thromboembolus associated with a pharmacologic cardioversion should be considered before beginning antiarrhythmic drug therapy.** Guidelines for anticoagulation are discussed in the following text:

- **Pharmacologic cardioversion** should be done in the hospital setting with continuous ECG monitoring because of a small risk of life-threatening tachyarrhythmias or bradyarrhythmias. **Ibutilide** is the only drug that is approved by the U.S. Food and Drug Administration for pharmacologic cardioversion. Clinical trials have shown a 45% conversion rate for AF and a 60% conversion rate for AFl. Ibutilide is associated with a 4% to 8% risk for Torsades de pointes (TdP), especially in the first 2 to 4 hours after administration of the drug. Because of this risk, patients must be monitored on telemetry with an external defibrillator immediately available during ibutilide infusion and for at least 4 hours after the infusion. The risk for TdP is higher in patients with cardiomyopathy and CHF. Ibutilide is given via an IV, at a dosage of 1 mg (0.01 mg/kg if patient is <60 kg), **infused slowly over 10 minutes**. Faster administration can promote TdP. The efficacy of antiarrhythmics to achieve pharmacologic conversion drops sharply when AF is >7 days in duration. For shorter duration AF episodes, dofetilide, sotalol, flecainide, and propafenone have some efficacy, while amiodarone has limited efficacy to achieve pharmacologic cardioversion.

- **Maintenance of sinus rhythm** with antiarrhythmic agents is associated with a small risk for life-threatening proarrhythmia. As a result, antiarrhythmic therapy should be reserved for patients who have highly symptomatic AF in spite of adequate rate control. Antiarrhythmic agents are grouped by the predominant mechanism of action according to the Vaughan Williams classification. **Class I agents** inhibit the fast sodium channel, **class II agents** are β-adrenergic antagonists, **class III agents** primarily block potassium channels, and **class IV agents** are calcium channel antagonists. Commonly used antiarrhythmic agents, their major route of elimination, and dosing regimen are listed in Table 7-6. The most effective agents for maintenance of sinus rhythm are flecainide, propafenone, sotalol, dofetilide, and amiodarone.

  ○ **Flecainide** and **propafenone** are **class Ic** antiarrhythmic drugs that are useful for maintenance of sinus rhythm in patients with **structurally normal hearts**. In patients with structural heart disease, class Ic agents are associated with an increased mortality rate (*N Engl J Med 1989;321:406*), and both agents are potent negative inotropes that can provoke or exacerbate heart failure. Both agents prolong the QRS duration as an early manifestation of toxicity. The toxic drug levels correlate with heart rate due to preferential blockade of active sodium channels. This property is described as **use dependence**. Exercise ECG can be used to give additional information about dose safety at higher heart rates. Flecainide should be used with caution without concomitant dosing with an AV nodal blocker because a paradoxical increase in the ventricular rate may occur due to drug-induced conversion of AF to AFl. Propafenone is less prone to this phenomenon due to intrinsic β-adrenergic antagonism.

  ○ **Sotalol** is a **class III** antiarrhythmic agent that is useful for the maintenance of sinus rhythm. Sotalol is a mixture of stereoisomers (DL-); D-sotalol is a potassium channel blocker, while L-sotalol is a β-antagonist. Side effects reflect both mechanisms of action. In addition to QT interval prolongation leading to TdP, DL-sotalol may result in sinus bradycardia or AV conduction abnormalities. Sotalol should not be used in patients with decompensated CHF (due to the negative inotropic effect) or with a prolonged QT interval.

  ○ **Dofetilide** is a **class III** antiarrhythmic agent that is useful for the maintenance of sinus rhythm. Dofetilide blocks the rapid component of the delayed rectifier potassium current, I_{Kr}. As a result, dofetilide increases the QT interval at clinically effective doses. QT prolongation is intensified by bradycardia, a characteristic known as "**reverse use dependence.**" The main risk of dofetilide is TdP. Dofetilide is contraindicated in patients with a baseline corrected QT interval (QT_c) >440

Table 7-6 Commonly Used Antiarrhythmic Drugs

Class	Drug	Route of Administration (Elimination)[a]	Initial/Loading Dose	Maintenance Dose	Major Adverse Effects[a]/Comments
Ia	Procainamide	IV (R, H) PO (R, H)	15–18 mg/kg at 20 mg/min 50 mg/kg/24 h, Max: 5 g/24 h	1–4 mg/min IR: 250–500 mg q3–6h; SR: 500 mg q6; Procanbid: 1,000–2,500 mg q12h	GI, CNS, +ANA/SLE-like syndrome, fever, hematologic, anticholinergic. Follow QT_c, serum procainamide (4–8 mg/L) and NAPA levels (<20 mg/mL)
	Quinidine	PO (H)	Sulfate, 200–400 mg q6h; gluconate, 324–972 mg q8–12h	NA	↑QT, TdP, ↓BP, thrombocytopenia, cinchonism, GI upset. Anticholinergic, HF.
	Disopyramide	PO (H, R)	300–400 mg	IR: 100–200 mg q6h; SR: 200–400 mg q12h	
Ib	Lidocaine	IV (H)	1 mg/kg over 2 min (may repeat × 2 up to 3 mg/kg total)	1–4 mg/min	↓HR, CNS, GI. Adjust dose in patients w/hepatic failure, AMI, HF, or shock.
	Mexiletine	PO (H)	400 mg one time dose	200–300 mg q8h	GI, CNS.
Ic	Flecainide	PO (H, R)	50 mg q12h	Increase by 50–100 mg/d every 4 days to max 400 mg/d	HF, GI, CNS, blurred vision.
	Propafenone	PO (H)	IR: 150 mg q8h ER: 225 mg q12h	IR: Increase at 3–4 day intervals up to 300 mg q8h; ER: may increase in 5 day intervals, up to 425 mg q12h	GI, dizziness.

III				
Sotalol	PO (R)	80 mg q12h	May increase every 3 days up to 240–320 mg/d in two to three divided doses	↓HR, ↓BP, CHF, CNS. Limit QT$_c$ prolongation to <550 ms.
Dofetilide	PO (R, H)	CrCl (mL/min): Dose (mcg bid): >60: 500 40–60: 250 20–39: 125 <20: Contraindicated	Dose adjusted based on QT$_c$ 2–3 hr after inpatient doses 1 through 5 Chronic therapy requires calculation of QT$_c$ and CrCl every 3 months with adjustment as necessary	↑QT, VT/TdP, HA, dizziness. See text for further details on initiating and monitoring treatment.
Ibutilide	IV (H)	1 mg (0.01 mg/kg if patient <60 kg) over 10 min; can repeat if no response 10 min after initial infusion	NA	↑QT, TdP, AV block, GI, HA.
Amiodarone	IV (H) PO (H)	IV: 150 mg over 10 min PO: 800 mg/d for 1 wk, then 600 mg/d for 1 wk, then 400 mg/d for 1 wk	1 mg/min × 6 h, then 0.5 mg/min 100–400 mg PO daily	↓BP, HB, ↓HR, warfarin interaction; see text for description of dermatologic, thyroid, pulmonary, corneal, and liver effects.

[a]Either common or life-threatening adverse effects of these medications are listed. This is not a comprehensive list of all possible adverse effects. AMI, acute myocardial infarction; ANA, antinuclear antibodies; ↓BP, hypotension; CNS, central nervous system; CHF, congestive heart failure; CrCl, creatinine clearance; ER, extended release; GI, gastrointestinal; H, hepatic; HA, headache; HB, heart block; HF, heart failure; ↓HR, bradycardia; IR, immediate release; IV, intravenous; NA, not applicable; NAPA, N-Acetylprocainamide; R, renal; SLE, systemic lupus erythematosus; SR, sustained release; TdP, Torsades de pointes; VT, ventricular tachycardia.

ms, or 500 ms in patients with bundle branch block. Initial dosing of dofetilide is based on the creatinine clearance. A 12-lead ECG should be obtained before the first dose of dofetilide and 1 to 2 hours after each dose. If the QT_c interval after the first dose prolongs by 15% of the baseline or exceeds 500 milliseconds, a 50% dosage reduction is indicated. If the QT_c exceeds 500 milliseconds after the second dose, dofetilide must be discontinued. Several medications block the renal secretion of dofetilide (verapamil, cimetidine, prochlorperazine, trimethoprim, megestrol, ketoconazole) and are contraindicated with dofetilide. The advantages of dofetilide are that it is not associated with increased CHF or mortality in patients with LV dysfunction (*N Engl J Med 1999;341:857*), and dofetilide does not cause sinus node dysfunction or conduction abnormalities.

○ **Dronedarone** is the newest antiarrhythmic agent approved for treatment of AF. Like amiodarone, from which it was derived, dronedarone shares properties with Vaughan Williams classes I to IV antiarrhythmic drugs. Dronedarone has been shown to be more effective than placebo at maintaining sinus rhythm after cardioversion but less effective than amiodarone at maintenance of sinus rhythm. The incidence of proarrhythmia is low with dronedarone as is the incidence of organ toxicity. A trend toward increased mortality has been shown in patients with advanced heart failure symptoms, and it is contraindicated in this patient group. Dronedarone is metabolized in the liver and should not be used in patients with significant hepatic dysfunction. Dronedarone can be used in patients with significant renal dysfunction because clearance is predominantly in the feces.

○ **Amiodarone** has the properties of class I to IV drugs and is arguably the most effective antiarrhythmic agent for maintenance of sinus rhythm. **Because of the extensive toxicity profile of amiodarone, it should not be considered as a first-line agent for rhythm control of AF in patients in whom an alternative antiarrhythmic can be safely used.** IV amiodarone has a low efficacy for acute conversion of AF, although conversion after several days of IV amiodarone has been observed. Given its common use and relative high incidence of side effects, a more detailed discussion of these effects is required.

▪ Adverse effects of oral amiodarone are partially dose dependent and may occur in up to 75% of patients treated at high doses for 5 years. At lower dosages (200 to 300 mg/d), adverse effects that require discontinuation occur in approximately 5% to 10% of patients per year.

▪ **Pulmonary toxicity** occurs in 1% to 15% of treated patients but appears less likely in those who receive <300 mg/d (*Circulation 1990;82:580*). Patients characteristically have a dry cough and dyspnea associated with pulmonary infiltrates and rales. The process appears to be reversible if detected early, but undetected cases may result in a mortality of up to 10% of those affected. A chest radiograph and pulmonary function tests should be obtained at baseline and every 12 months or when patients complain of shortness of breath. The presence of interstitial infiltrates on the chest radiograph and a decreased diffusing capacity raise concern of amiodarone pulmonary toxicity.

▪ **Photosensitivity** is a common adverse reaction, and in some patients, a violaceous skin discoloration develops in sun-exposed areas. The blue-gray discoloration may not resolve completely with discontinuation of therapy.

▪ **Thyroid dysfunction** is a common adverse effect. Hypothyroidism and hyperthyroidism have been reported, with an incidence of 2% to 5% per year. Thyroid-stimulating hormone should be obtained at baseline and monitored every 6 months. If hypothyroidism develops, concurrent treatment with levothyroxine may allow continued amiodarone use.

- **Corneal microdeposits**, detectable on slit-lamp examination, develop in virtually all patients. These deposits rarely interfere with vision and are not an indication for discontinuation of the drug. Optic neuritis, leading to blindness, is rare but has been reported in association with amiodarone.
- The most common **ECG changes** are lengthened PR intervals and bradycardia; however, high-grade AV block may occur in patients who have preexisting conduction abnormalities. Amiodarone may prolong QT intervals, although usually not extensively, and **TdP is rare**. Other agents that prolong the QT interval, however, should be avoided in patients who are taking amiodarone.
- **Liver dysfunction** usually manifests in an asymptomatic and transient rise in hepatic transaminases. If the increase exceeds three times normal or doubles in a patient with an elevated baseline level, amiodarone should be discontinued or the dose should be reduced. Aspartate transaminase (AST) and alanine transaminase (ALT) should be monitored every 6 months in patients who are receiving amiodarone.
- **Drug interactions.** Amiodarone may raise the blood levels of warfarin and digoxin; therefore, these drugs should be reduced routinely by one-half when amiodarone is started, and levels should be followed closely.

Other Nonpharmacologic Therapies

Nonpharmacologic methods of rhythm control include catheter or surgical ablation techniques that block the initiation and maintenance of AF.

- **DC Cardioversion (DCCV)** is the safest and most effective method of acutely restoring sinus rhythm. Prior to cardioversion, consideration of thromboembolic risk and anticoagulation is critical, when possible, to minimize thromboembolic events triggered by the cardioversion process. AF with a rapid ventricular response in the setting of ongoing myocardial ischemia, MI, hypotension, or respiratory distress should receive prompt cardioversion regardless of the anticoagulation status.
  - If the duration of AF is documented to be **<48 hours**, cardioversion may proceed without anticoagulation. If AF has persisted for **>48 hours** (or for an unknown duration), patients should be anticoagulated with warfarin, with an international normalized ratio (INR) of 2.0 to 3.0, for at least 3 weeks before cardioversion, and anticoagulation should be continued in the same therapeutic range following successful cardioversion.
  - An alternative to anticoagulation for 3 weeks before cardioversion is to perform a **transesophageal echocardiogram** to rule out left atrial appendage thrombus before cardioversion. This method is safe and has the advantage of shorter time to cardioversion than warfarin and therefore is indicated in patients who are not able to wait weeks before cardioversion. Therapeutic anticoagulation with warfarin is indicated after the cardioversion for a minimum of 4 weeks (*Am J Cardiol 1998;82:1545*), although the AFFIRM trial (*N Engl J Med 2002;347:1825*) suggests that in patients with high risk for stroke, warfarin should be continued indefinitely.
  - When practical, sedation should be accomplished with midazolam (1 to 2 mg IV q2min to a maximum of 5 mg), methohexital (25 to 75 mg IV), etomidate (0.2 to 0.6 mg/kg IV), or propofol (initial dose, 5 mg/kg/hr IV).
  - Proper synchronization to the QRS is critical to avoid induction of VT by a cardioversion shock delivered during a vulnerable period. Synchronization of the

external cardioverter-defibrillator should be confirmed by noting the presence of a synchronization marker superimposed on the QRS complex.

○ For cardioversion of atrial arrhythmias, the anterior patch electrode should be positioned just right of the sternum at the level of the third or fourth intercostal space, with the second electrode positioned just below the left scapula posteriorly. **Care should be taken to position patch electrodes at least 6 cm from PPM or defibrillator generators.** If electrode paddles are used, firm pressure and conductive gel should be applied to minimize contact impedance. Direct contact with the patient or the bed should be avoided. Atropine (1 mg IV) should be readily available to treat prolonged pauses. Reports of serious arrhythmias, such as VT, VF, or asystole, are rare and are more likely in the setting of improperly synchronized cardioversions, digitalis toxicity, or concomitant antiarrhythmic drug therapy.

- **Curative catheter ablation of AF** has been shown to be highly effective in young patients with structurally normal hearts and a paroxysmal pattern of their AF. Cure rates in this patient category are in the range of 80% to 90%. Cure rates are diminished in patients with structural heart disease, advanced age, and persistent AF. A significant fraction of patients require more than one ablation procedure to achieve cure. The goal of the catheter ablation procedure in paroxysmal AF patients is to achieve electrical isolation of the pulmonary veins. In patients with persistent AF, this goal is frequently combined with substrate modification strategies whereby regions of the atria are targeted for ablation to block reentry or extrapulmonary vein triggers. Because of potential complications and modest success, patients should undergo at least one trial of an antiarrhythmic drug for maintenance of sinus rhythm. If this trial is ineffective or poorly tolerated, curative catheter ablation can be contemplated.

Surgical Management

Surgical techniques for cure of AF have been evaluated since the 1980s. Of these techniques, the Cox Maze procedure has the highest demonstrated efficacy and the most substantial published follow-up data documenting sustained efficacy. Including patients with persistent AF and structural heart disease, cure rates approach 90%. Because of its highly invasive nature, surgical treatment is usually reserved for patients who have failed a catheter ablation strategy or who have planned concomitant cardiac surgery.

Ventricular Tachyarrhythmias

GENERAL PRINCIPLES

- Ventricular tachyarrhythmias should be initially approached with the assumption that they will have a malignant course until proven otherwise.
- Characterization of the arrhythmia involves consideration of hemodynamic stability, duration, morphology, and the presence or lack of underlying structural heart disease.
- Ultimately, this characterization will aid in determining the patient's risk for **sudden cardiac arrest** and need for device or ablation-based therapy.

Definition

- **Nonsustained VT** is defined as three or more consecutive ventricular complexes (>100 bpm) that terminates spontaneously within 30 seconds without significant hemodynamic consequences or need for intervention.
- **Sustained monomorphic VT** is defined as a tachycardia composed of ventricular complexes of a single QRS morphology that lasts longer than 30 seconds or requires cardioversion due to hemodynamic compromise.
- **Polymorphic VT** is characterized by an ever-changing QRS morphology. **TdP** is a variant of polymorphic VT that is typically preceded by a prolonged QT interval in sinus rhythm. Polymorphic VT is usually associated with hemodynamic collapse or instability.
- **VF** is associated with disorganized mechanical contraction, hemodynamic collapse, and sudden death. The ECG reveals irregular and rapid oscillations (250 to 400 bpm) of highly variable amplitude without uniquely identifiable QRS complexes or T waves.
- Ventricular arrhythmias are the major cause of **sudden cardiac death (SCD)**. **SCD** is defined as the death that occurs within 1 hour of the onset of symptoms. In the United States, 350,000 cases of SCD occur annually. Among patients with aborted SCD, ischemic heart disease is the most common associated cardiac structural abnormality. Most cardiac arrest survivors do not evolve evidence of an acute MI; however, >75% have evidence of previous infarcts. A nonischemic cardiomyopathy is also associated with an elevated risk for SCD.

Etiology

- **VT associated with structural heart disease**
  - Most ventricular arrhythmias are associated with structural heart disease, typically related to active ischemia or history of infarct.
    - Scar and the peri-infarct area provide the substrate for reentry that produces sustained monomorphic VT.
    - Polymorphic VT and VF are commonly associated with ischemia and are the presumed cause of most out-of-hospital SCDs.
  - Nonischemic cardiomyopathy typically involves progressive dilation and fibrosis of the ventricular myocardium, providing an arrhythmogenic substrate.
  - Infiltrative cardiomyopathies (sarcoid, hemochromatosis, amyloid) represent a smaller patient population that is at significant risk for ventricular arrhythmias whose management is less clearly defined.
  - Adults with prior repair of congenital heart disease are commonly afflicted with both VT and SVT.
  - Arrhythmogenic right ventricular dysplasia or cardiomyopathy is marked by fibrofatty replacement of the right ventricular (RV) (and sometimes LV) myocardium that gives rise to left bundle branch block (LBBB) morphology VT and is associated with sudden death, particularly in young athletes.
  - Bundle branch reentry VT (BBRVT) is a form of VT that utilizes the His-Purkinje system in a reentrant circuit and is typically associated with cardiomyopathy and an abnormal conduction system.
- **VT in the absence of structural heart disease**
  - Inherited ion channelopathies, such as those seen in Brugada and long QT syndromes, can lead to polymorphic VT and sudden death in patients without evidence of structural heart disease on imaging.

- Catecholaminergic polymorphic VT (CPVT) involves familial, exercise-induced VT that is related to irregular calcium processing.
- **Idiopathic VT** is a diagnosis of exclusion that requires the documented absence of structural heart disease, genetic disorders, and reversible etiologies (i.e., ischemia, electrolyte/metabolic abnormalities).
  - Most idiopathic VTs originate from the right ventricular outflow tract (RVOT) and are amenable to ablation. Less commonly, left ventricular outflow tract VT (LVOT-VT) or fascicular VT (utilizing anterior and posterior divisions of the left bundle branch) may be discovered on EPS.

DIAGNOSIS

Clinical Presentation

- The evaluation of wide-complex tachyarrhythmias (WCT) should always begin with prompt assessment of vital signs and clinical symptoms. If the arrhythmia is poorly tolerated, postpone further detailed evaluation and proceed to acute management per ACLS guidelines. If stable, there are several important questions to address that can guide one toward the most likely diagnosis. A common mistake is the assumption that hemodynamic stability supports the diagnosis of SVT over VT.
- VT represents the vast majority of WCT seen in the inpatient setting with reported prevalence upward of 80%. With that in mind, one can then proceed to elicit several historical points of emphasis and scrutinize electrocardiographic properties of the arrhythmia to further delineate the mechanism of the underlying rhythm disturbance. Begin with the following questions:
  - Does the patient have a history of structural heart disease?
    - Patients with structural heart disease are much more likely to have VT rather than SVT as the etiology of a WCT. In one report, 98% of patients with WCT who had prior MI proved to have VT (*Am J Med 1988;84:53*).
  - Does the patient have a pacemaker, implantable cardiac defibrillator (ICD), or wide QRS at baseline (i.e., right bundle branch block [RBBB], LBBB, intraventricular conduction delay [IVCD])?
    - The presence of either a pacemaker or an ICD should raise suspicion for a device-mediated WCT.
    - **Device-mediated WCT** can be due to ventricular pacing at a rapid rate either due to device tracking of an atrial tachyarrhythmia or an "endless loop tachycardia" created by tracking of the retrograde atrial impulses created by the preceding ventricular paced beat. In either case, the tachycardia rate is a clue to the mechanism as this is typically equal to the programmed upper rate limit (URL) of the device. A commonly programmed URL is 120 paces per minute (ppm). A tachycardia rate above the URL effectively excludes a device-mediated WCT.
    - History of device implantation can be confirmed by inspection of the chest wall (usually left chest for right-handed patients), chest X-ray (CXR), or by the presence of pacing spikes seen on ECG. Typically, the wide QRS induced by right ventricular pacing leads has an LBBB pattern and is preceded by a short pacing spike. Most modern devices utilize bipolar pacing, which is often difficult to recognize on the 12-lead ECG due to the small size of the electrical artifact. Therefore, one should not exclude the presence of a device-mediated

tachycardia mechanism by the absence of visible pacing spikes during the tachycardia.

- Patients with known RBBB, LBBB, or IVCD at baseline who present with WCT will have a QRS morphology identical to baseline in the presence of SVT. In addition, some patients with a narrow QRS at baseline will manifest a WCT due to SVT when a rate-related bundle branch block is present. This phenomenon is referred to as SVT with aberrancy and can be distinguished from VT reliably with the criteria described in the following text.

  ○ What medications is the patient taking?

  - The medication list should be scanned for any medication with proarrhythmic side effects, especially those that can prolong the baseline QT interval and increase the risk for polymorphic VT or TdP. These medicines include many of the class I and III antiarrhythmics, certain antibiotics, antipsychotics, and many more. The University of Arizona–sponsored Web site, *http://www.qtd rugs.org*, provides a comprehensive list of QT-prolonging agents.
  - Medications that can lead to electrolyte abnormalities, such as loop and potassium-sparing diuretics, ACEIs, ARBs, etc., should be ascertained. Also, digoxin toxicity is always an important consideration in the setting of any arrhythmia.

Differential Diagnosis

- Diagnosis of VT requires knowledge of the general approach to WCTs.
- WCT may be due to either SVT with aberrant conduction (presence of bundle branch block) or VT. The differentiation between these mechanisms is of the utmost importance. **The pharmacologic agents utilized in the management of SVT (i.e., adenosine, β-blockers, calcium channel blockers) can cause severe hemodynamic instability if used erroneously in the setting of VT.** Therefore, all WCTs are considered to be ventricular in origin until clearly proven otherwise.

  ○ Other, less common mechanisms of WCT include **antidromic AVRT, hyperkalemia-induced arrhythmia, or pacemaker-induced tachycardia**.

- **Telemetry artifact** due to poor lead contact or repetitive patient motion (tremor, shivering, brushing teeth, chest physical therapy, etc.) can mimic VT or VF.

Diagnostic Testing

Laboratories

Laboratory studies should include basic metabolic panel, magnesium, CBC, and serial troponins.

Electrocardiography

- **Differentiation of SVT with aberrancy from VT** on the basis of analysis of the surface ECG is critical in the determination of appropriate acute and chronic therapy. Features that are diagnostic of VT are **AV dissociation**, **capture or fusion beats**, an absence of RS morphology in the precordial leads (V_1–V_6), and **LBBB morphology with right axis deviation**. In the absence of these features, examination of an RS complex in a precordial lead for an RS interval >100 ms is consistent with VT. In addition, characteristic QRS morphologies that are suggestive of VT may be sought, as shown in Figure 7-2A and B.
- **ECG pearls**
  ○ **Classic Brugada pattern:**
    - Baseline: Pseudo-RBBB with ST-segment elevation and T-wave inversion in V_1, V_2.
    - May be unmasked by stress, illness, fever, illicit drug use, etc.

A

Figure 7-2. A and B. Brugada criteria for distinguishing ventricular tachycardia from supraventricular tachycardia with aberrancy in wide-complex tachycardias. LBBB, left bundle branch block; RBBB, right bundle branch block; SVT, supraventricular tachyarrhythmia; VT, ventricular tachycardia. (From Cuculich PS. Advanced electrocardiogram interpretation [ECG 201]. In: Cuculich PS, Kates AM, eds. *The Washington manual cardiology subspecialty consult.* 2nd ed. Philadelphia, PA: Lippincott Williams & Wilkins; 2009.)

	LBBB		RBBB	
	VT	**SVT**	**VT**	**SVT**
Lead V₁	In V₁, V₂ any of: (a) r ≥ 0.04 sec (b) Notched S downstroke (c) Delayed S nadir >0.06 sec	In V₁, V₂ absence of: (a) r ≥ 0.04 sec (b) Notched S downstroke (c) Delayed S nadir >0.06 sec	Taller left peak Biphasic RS or QR	Triphasic rsR′ or rR′
Lead V₆	Monophasic QS 		Biphasic rS 	Triphasic qRs

B

Figure 7-2. *(Continued).*

- ○ **Arrhythmogenic RV dysplasia:**
  - ▪ Baseline: Epsilon wave (late potential just after QRS), ± wide QRS, ± T-Wave inversion (TWI) (V₁, V₂).
  - ▪ VT: Reflects RV origin, likely LBBB configuration. May present with polymorphic VT.
- ○ **Bundle branch reentrant VT:**
  - ▪ Baseline: IVCD
  - ▪ VT: LBBB morphology typically ("down" the right bundle; "up" the left bundle)
- ○ **Fascicular VT:**
  - ▪ VT: Superior axis, RBBB morphology
- ○ **Long QT syndrome:**
  - ▪ Baseline: QT >50% of the RR interval if HR 60 to 100. QTc ≥440 ms.
  - ▪ VT: TdP degenerating into VF.
- ○ **Outflow tract VT:**
  - ▪ VT: Inferior axis, LBBB morphology. R/S transition in the precordial leads can aid in localization. Early transition (V₁ or V₂) suggests an LVOT origin; later transition (V₄) suggests RVOT origin.

Imaging
- The presence or absence of structural heart disease should be initially evaluated by transthoracic echocardiography.
- Further imaging (cardiac MRI, noninvasive stress test, coronary angiogram, etc.) should be obtained based on suspected etiology.

TREATMENT

- **Differentiation of SVT with aberrancy from VT** on the basis of analysis of the surface ECG is critical in the determination of appropriate acute and chronic therapy.
  - For acute therapy of SVT, IV medications such as adenosine, calcium channel blockers, or β-blockers are used. However, calcium channel blockers and β-blockers can produce hemodynamic instability in patients with VT.
  - Chronically, many SVTs are amenable to RFA, whereas most VTs are malignant and require an antiarrhythmic agent and/or ICD implantation.
- Immediate unsynchronized DC cardioversion is the primary therapy for pulseless VT and VF.

Other Nonpharmacologic Therapies

- **ICDs** provide automatic recognition and treatment of ventricular arrhythmias. ICD implantation improves survival in patients resuscitated from ventricular arrhythmias (secondary prevention of SCD) and in individuals without prior symptoms who are at high risk for SCD (primary prevention of SCD).
  - **Secondary prevention of SCD** with ICD implantation is indicated for most patients who survive SCD outside of the peri-MI setting. The superiority of ICD therapy to chronic antiarrhythmic drug therapy has been demonstrated (*AVID trial. N Engl J Med 1997;337:1576*).
  - **Primary prevention of SCD** with ICD implantation is indicated for patients who are at high risk of SCD. The efficacy of ICD implantation for primary prevention of SCD in the setting of cardiomyopathy has been established in multiple prospective clinical trials (see Multicenter Automatic Defibrillator Implantation Trial [**MADIT**], *N Engl J Med 1996;335:1933*; Multicenter Un-Sustained Tachycardia Trial [**MUSTT**], *N Engl J Med 1999;341:1882*; **MADIT II** Trial, *N Engl J Med 2002;346:877*; and **SCD-HeFT**, *N Engl J Med 2005;352(3):225*). Most patients with an LV ejection fraction (LVEF) of <35% for more than 3 months on optimal medical therapy meet current indications for prophylactic ICD implantation.
  - **Other indications for ICD:**
    - Phenotypes associated with **HCM, arrhythmogenic right ventricular cardiomyopathy, congenital long QT syndrome, or Brugada syndrome have a high risk of SCD**. ICD implantation is indicated if patients with one of these syndromes have had a resuscitated cardiac arrest or documented ventricular arrhythmias. Prophylactic ICD implantation for asymptomatic patients is generally considered appropriate particularly in patients who have had syncope or with a family history of sudden death.
    - Patients who are awaiting cardiac transplantation are at high risk for SCD, especially if they are receiving an intravenous inotrope. Prophylactic ICD implantation is reasonable to protect against SCD prior to transplantation.

- ○ ICDs are **contraindicated** in patients who have incessant VT, recent MI <40 days in the case of primary prevention, significant psychiatric illnesses, or life expectancy of less than 12 to 24 months.
- **Radiofrequency catheter ablation of VT** is most successfully performed in patients with hemodynamically stable forms of idiopathic VT that is not associated with structural heart disease. Long-term cure rates in these patients are similar to those achieved for catheter ablation of SVT. In the presence of structural heart disease, and particularly with hemodynamically unstable VT, catheter ablation is generally reserved for drug-refractory VT due to a lower efficacy and a higher morbidity associated with the ablation procedure.
  - ○ **Idiopathic VT is usually associated with a structurally normal heart, but an associated tachycardia-mediated cardiomyopathy has been described.**
    - ▪ **Right ventricular outflow tract VT (RVOT-VT)** often presents as repetitive, nonsustained bursts of VT that can be exercise induced. RVOT-VT is usually responsive to β-adrenergic blockers, diltiazem or verapamil, and adenosine.
    - ▪ **LVOT-VT** is frequently responsive to verapamil.
    - ▪ Both forms of idiopathic VT are thought to be benign in the absence of structural heart disease. Therefore, ICD implantation is not appropriate. All forms of idiopathic VT are amenable to treatment with RFA or drug therapy.
  - ○ **BBRVT** is a form of VT that involves the His–Purkinje system in a reentrant circuit. BBRVT can be treated successfully by catheter ablation of the right bundle branch. Because BBRVT usually occurs in patients with cardiomyopathy and an abnormal conduction system, an ICD is generally implanted in conjunction with ablation.
  - ○ **VT associated with ischemic heart disease** can also be treated by catheter ablation; however, success rates are lower compared to idiopathic VT. The reasons for the lower success rate include the hemodynamic instability of VT and the multiple different VT circuits that are often present. Catheter ablation of ischemic VT in patients with antiarrhythmic drug-refractory VT and an implanted ICD has been successful in reducing frequent ICD shocks (*Circulation 1997;96:1525*).
  - ○ **Ablation of VT in nonischemic cardiomyopathy** is also reasonable, particularly in drug-refractory patients, but VT circuits may be intramyocardial or epicardial. As a result, success rates are typically lower than those associated with ischemic VT and referral to a center that routinely performs both endocardial and epicardial ablations should be considered.

Medications

- VF that is resistant to external defibrillation requires the addition of IV antiarrhythmic agents.
  - ○ IV lidocaine is frequently used; however, IV amiodarone appears to be more effective in increasing survival of VF when used in conjunction with defibrillation (*N Engl J Med 2002;346:884*).
  - ○ After successful cardioversion, continuous IV infusion of effective antiarrhythmic therapy should be maintained until any reversible causes have been corrected.
- Chronic antiarrhythmic drug therapy is indicated for the treatment of recurrent symptomatic ventricular arrhythmias. In the setting of hemodynamically unstable ventricular arrhythmias treated with an ICD, antiarrhythmic drug therapy is often necessary to suppress frequent device discharges.

First Line

- **Amiodarone** is safe and well tolerated for the acute management of ventricular arrhythmias. Amiodarone has complex pharmacokinetics and is associated with significant toxicities arising from chronic therapy (*Am Heart J 1993;125:109*).
  - After oral loading, amiodarone prevents the recurrence of sustained VT or VF in up to 60% of patients. A therapeutic latency of more than 5 days exists before beneficial antiarrhythmic effects are observed with oral dosing, and full suppression of arrhythmias may not occur for 4 to 6 weeks after therapy is initiated. Unfortunately, recurrence of ventricular arrhythmias during long-term follow-up is common.
  - Amiodarone has become the most studied antiarrhythmic agent in the treatment of SCD and the main drug against which ICDs are compared, in secondary and in primary prevention trials.
  - The balance of multiple prospective clinical trials does not support the prophylactic use of amiodarone for prevention of SCD in cardiomyopathy patients.
- **Class II** agents, the β-adrenergic antagonists, are the only class of antiarrhythmic agents to have consistently shown improved survival in post-MI patients.
  - β-Adrenergic blockers reduce postinfarction total mortality by 25% to 40% and SCD by 32% to 50% (*Lancet 1981;2:823*; *Lancet 1999; 353:9*; *Lancet 1999; 353:2001*; *N Engl J Med 2001;344:1651*; *Lancet 2001; 357:1385*).
  - After acute therapy of VT/VF and stabilization, β-adrenergic blockers should be initiated and titrated as blood pressure and heart rate allow.
  - Idiopathic VT often responds to AV nodal blocking agents.
- **ACE inhibitors** have also been shown to reduce sudden death and overall mortality in patients with coronary artery disease (CAD) or CHF.

Second Line

- **Sotalol** is a **class III** agent indicated for the chronic treatment of VT/VF. Sotalol prevents the recurrence of sustained VT and VF in 70% of patients (*N Engl J Med 1993;329:452*) but must be used with caution in individuals with CHF.
- **Class I** agents in general have not been shown to reduce mortality in patients with VT/VF. In fact, the class Ic agents, **flecainide** and **propafenone**, are associated with increased mortality in patients with ventricular arrhythmias (*N Engl J Med 1991;324:781*).
  - **Lidocaine** is a **class Ib** agent available only in IV form with efficacy in the management of sustained and recurrent VT/VF. The prophylactic use of lidocaine for suppression of PVCs and NSVT in the otherwise uncomplicated post-MI setting is not indicated and may lead to an increase in mortality from bradyarrhythmias (*Arch Intern Med 1989;149:2694*). Toxicities of lidocaine include CNS effects (convulsions, confusion, stupor, and, rarely, respiratory arrest), all of which resolve with discontinuation of therapy. Negative inotropic effects are seen only at high drug levels.
  - **Mexiletine** is similar to lidocaine but is available in oral form. **Mexiletine is most often used in combination with either amiodarone or sotalol for chronic treatment of refractory ventricular arrhythmias.** Mexiletine may have a limited role in the treatment of some patients with congenital long QT syndromes. CNS toxicity includes tremor, dizziness, and blurred vision. Higher levels may result in dysarthria, diplopia, nystagmus, and an impaired level of consciousness. Nausea and vomiting are common.

○ **Phenytoin** is used primarily in the treatment of **digitalis-induced ventricular arrhythmias**. It may have a limited role in the treatment of ventricular arrhythmias associated with congenital long QT syndromes. The IV loading dose is 250 mg given over 10 minutes (maximum rate of 50 mg/min). Subsequent doses of 100 mg can be given q5min as necessary and as blood pressure (BP) tolerates, to a total of 1,000 mg. Frequent monitoring of the ECG, BP, and neurologic status is required. Continuous infusion is not recommended (see Chapter 26, Neurologic Disorders).

SPECIAL CONSIDERATIONS

- **Class IV** agents have no role in the chronic management of VT. IV calcium channel blockers should never be used in the acute management of VT, as they may cause hemodynamic collapse. Oral calcium channel blockers are not effective in the management of VT. Short-acting nifedipine is associated with a trend toward increasing mortality when used in the post-MI patient (*Arch Intern Med 1993;153:345*).
- Primary VF that occurs within the first 72 hours of an acute MI is not associated with an elevated risk of recurrence and does not require chronic antiarrhythmic therapy.
- In the case of **TdP associated with long QT syndrome**, acute therapy is immediate DC cardioversion.
  ○ Bolus administration of magnesium sulfate in 1- to 2-g increments up to 4 to 6 g IV is highly effective.
  ○ In cases of acquired long QT syndrome, identification and treatment of the underlying condition should be undertaken, if possible.
  ○ Elimination of long–short triggering sequences and shortening of the QT interval can be achieved by increasing the heart rate to the range of 90 to 120 bpm by either IV isoproterenol infusion (initial rate at 1 to 2 mcg/min) or temporary transvenous pacing.

BRADYARRHYTHMIAS

GENERAL PRINCIPLES

- Bradyarrhythmias are commonly encountered rhythms in the inpatient setting that result in a ventricular rate of <60 bpm.
- Bradyarrhythmias can be attributed to dysfunction somewhere within the native conduction system; therefore, review of the normal propagation of the wave of depolarization, the respective vascular supply to each section, and the intrinsic and extrinsic influences on the conduction system is useful.
- **Anatomy of the conduction system**
  ○ The **sinus node** is a collection of specialized pacemaker cells located in the high right atrium. Under normal conditions, it initiates a wave of depolarization that spreads inferiorly and leftward via atrial myocardium and intranodal tracts, producing atrial systole.
    ▪ The typical resting rate of the sinus node is between 50 and 90 bpm, is inversely related to age, and is determined by the relative balance of sympathetic and parasympathetic inputs.

- Arterial blood is supplied to the sinus node via the sinus node artery, which has variable anatomic origins: right coronary artery (RCA), 65%; circumflex, 25%; or dual (RCA and circumflex), 10%.
o The wave of depolarization then reaches another grouping of specialized cells, the **AV node**, located in the right atrial side of the interatrial septum. Normally, the AV node should serve as the lone electrical connection between the atria and ventricles.
  - Conduction through the AV node is decremental, producing a delay typically in the range of 55 to 110 ms and accounts for the majority of the PR interval measured on ECG.
  - The AV node consists of slow-response fibers that, like the sinus node, possess inherent pace making properties that produce rates of 40 to 50 bpm. Because of its slower rate of depolarization, this only becomes clinically relevant in the setting of sinus node dysfunction or complete AV nodal block.
  - Ventricular response to atrial depolarization is modulated by the effects of the autonomic nervous system on the AV node.
  - Blood supply to the AV node is primarily via the AV nodal artery that typically originates from the proximal portion of the posterior descending artery (PDA, 80%), but can also come off the circumflex (10%) or both (10%). In addition, it receives collateral flow from the left anterior descending (LAD) artery. This makes the AV node relatively protected against vascular compromise.
o From the AV node, the wave of depolarization travels down the **His bundle**, located in the membranous septum, and into the **right and left bundle branches** before reaching the **Purkinje fibers** that depolarize the rest of the ventricular myocardium.
  - The His and right bundle receive blood via the AV nodal artery and from septal perforators off the LAD.
  - The left bundle divides further into an anterior fascicle that is supplied by septal perforators and a posterior fascicle, which runs posterior and inferior to the anterior fascicle, which is supplied by branches off the PDA and septal perforators off the LAD.

Etiology

Common causes of bradycardia are listed in Table 7-7.

DIAGNOSIS

Clinical Presentation

When evaluating a suspected bradyarrhythmia, one should efficiently utilize the history, physical exam, and available data to address the following "five S" approach to an **SSSSS**low heart rate:
- **S**TABLE: Is the patient hemodynamically unstable?
- **S**YMPTOMS: Does the patient have symptoms and do the symptoms correlate with the bradycardia?
- **S**HORT TERM: Are the circumstances surrounding the arrhythmia reversible or transient?
- **S**OURCE: Where in the conduction system is the dysfunction? Has the bradyarrhythmia been captured on electrocardiographic monitoring?
- **S**CHEDULE A PACEMAKER: Does the patient require a PPM?

Table 7-7	Causes of Bradycardia

Intrinsic

Congenital disease (may present later in life)
Idiopathic degeneration (aging)
Infarction or ischemia
Cardiomyopathy
Infiltrative disease: sarcoidosis, amyloidosis, hemochromatosis
Collagen vascular diseases: systemic lupus erythematosus,
   rheumatoid arthritis, scleroderma
Surgical trauma: valve surgery, transplantation
Infectious disease: endocarditis, Lyme disease, Chagas disease

Extrinsic

Autonomically mediated
Neurocardiogenic syncope
Carotid sinus hypersensitivity
Increased vagal tone: coughing, vomiting, micturition, defecation,
   intubation
Drugs: β-blockers, calcium channel blockers, digoxin,
   antiarrhythmic agents
Hypothyroidism
Hypothermia
Neurologic disorders: increased intracranial pressure
Electrolyte imbalances: hyperkalemia, hypermagnesemia
Hypercarbia/obstructive sleep apnea
Sepsis

From Cooper DH. Bradyarrhythmias and permanent pacemakers. In: Cuculich PS, Kates AM, eds. *The Washington manual cardiology subspecialty consult.* 2nd ed. Philadelphia, PA: Lippincott Williams & Wilkins; 2009.

Physical Examination
- If the bradycardia is ongoing, the initial history and physical examination should be truncated, focusing on assessing the hemodynamic stability of the arrhythmia.
  - If the patient is demonstrating signs of poor perfusion (hypotension, confusion, decreased consciousness, cyanosis, etc.) then immediate management per ACLS protocol should be initiated.
  - If stable, a more thorough evaluation can be performed.
  - The clinical manifestations of bradyarrhythmias are variable, ranging from asymptomatic to nonspecific (lightheadedness, fatigue, weakness, exercise intolerance) to overt (syncope). Tolerance for bradyarrhythmias is largely dictated by the patient's ability to augment cardiac output in response to the decreased heart rate.
- Emphasis should be placed on delineating **whether the presenting symptoms have a direct temporal relationship to underlying bradycardia**. Other historical points of emphasis include the following:
  - Ischemic heart disease, particularly involving the right-sided circulation, can precipitate a number of bradyarrhythmias. Therefore, symptoms of acute coronary syndrome should always be sought.

○ **Precipitating circumstances** (micturition, coughing, defecation, noxious smells) surrounding episodes may help identify a neurocardiogenic etiology.

○ **Tachyarrhythmias**, particularly in patients with underlying sinus node dysfunction, can be followed by long pauses due to sinus node suppression during tachycardia. Therefore, symptoms of palpitations may reveal the presence of an underlying tachy-brady syndrome. Given that the agents used to treat tachyarrhythmias are designed to promote decreased heart rates, this syndrome leads to management dilemmas.

○ History of structural heart disease, hypothyroidism, obstructive sleep apnea, collagen vascular disease, infections (bacteremia, endocarditis, Lyme, Chagas), infiltrative diseases (amyloid, hemochromatosis, and sarcoid), neuromuscular diseases, and prior cardiac surgery (valve replacement, congenital repair) should be sought.

○ **Medications** should be reviewed with particular emphasis on those that affect the sinus and AV nodes (i.e., calcium channel blockers, β-adrenergic blockers, digoxin).

• After hemodynamic stability is confirmed, a more thorough examination with particular emphasis on the cardiovascular exam and any findings consistent with the aforementioned comorbidities is appropriate (Figure 7-3).

Diagnostic Testing

Laboratories

Laboratory studies should include serum electrolytes and thyroid function tests in most patients. Digoxin levels and serial troponins should be drawn when clinically appropriate.

Electrocardiography

• The **12-lead ECG** is the cornerstone for diagnosis in any workup where arrhythmia is suspected.

○ Rhythm strips from leads that provide the best view of atrial activity (II, III, AVF, or V_1) should be examined.

○ Emphasis should be placed on identifying evidence of **sinus node dysfunction** (P-wave intervals) or **AV conduction abnormalities** (PR interval).

○ Evidence of both old and acute manifestations of ischemic heart disease should be sought as well.

• The analysis of ECGs in the setting of bradycardia should also focus on localizing the likely site of dysfunction along the conduction system. Along with correlating symptoms to the arrhythmia, localization of the block will help determine if pacemaker implantation is necessary.

• **Sinus node dysfunction**, or sick sinus syndrome, represents the most common reason for pacemaker implantation in the United States. Manifestations of sick sinus syndrome include (Figure 7-4):

○ **Sinus bradycardia** is defined as a regular rhythm with QRS complexes preceded by "sinus" P waves (upright in II, III, AVF) at a rate <60 bpm. Young patients and athletes often have resting sinus bradycardia that is well tolerated. Nocturnal heart rates are lower in all patients but the elderly tend to have higher resting heart rates and sinus bradycardia is a far less common normal variant.

○ **Sinus arrest** and **sinus pauses** refer to failure of the sinus node to depolarize, which manifest as periods of atrial asystole (no P waves). This may be accompanied by ventricular asystole or escape beats from junctional tissue or ventricular myocardium. Pauses of 2 to 3 seconds can be found in healthy, asymptomatic people,

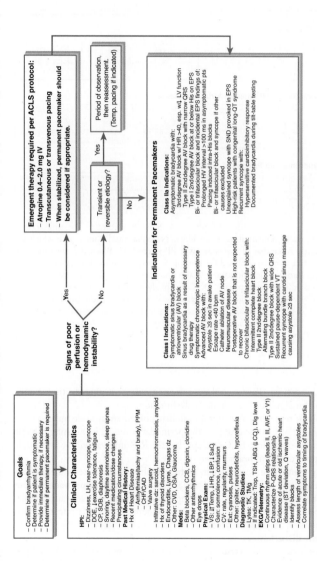

Figure 7-3. Approach to bradyarrhythmias. ABG, arterial blood gas; ACLS, advanced cardiac life support; ↓BP, hypotension; CAD, coronary artery disease; CCB, calcium channel blocker; CHF, congestive heart failure; CP, chest pain; CVD, cerebrovascular disease; DOE, dyspnea on exertion; EPS, electrophysiologic study; HPI, history of present illness; ↓HR, bradycardia; ↑K, hyperkalemia; LH, lightheadedness; ↑Mg, hypermagnesemia; OSA, obstructive sleep apnea; PPM, permanent pacemaker; ↓SaO$_2$, hypoxia; SND, sinus node dysfunction; SOB, shortness of breath; TSH, thyroid-stimulating hormone; VT, ventricular tachycardia. (From Cooper DH. Bradyarrhythmias and permanent pacemakers. In: Cuculich PS, Kates AM, eds. *The Washington manual cardiology subspecialty consult.* 2nd ed. Philadelphia, PA: Lippincott Williams & Wilkins; 2009.)

Sinus Bradycardia

Sinoatrial Node Exit Block

Sinus Rhythm with Blocked Premature Atrial Complexes

Tachy-Brady Syndrome with Prolonged Sinus Pause

Figure 7-4. Examples of sinus node dysfunction. **A.** Sinus bradycardia. The sinus rate is approximately 45 bpm. **B.** Sinoatrial node exit block. Note that the PP interval in which the pause occurs is exactly twice that of the nonpaused PP interval. **C.** Blocked premature atrial complexes. This rhythm is often confused for sinus node dysfunction or atrioventricular (AV) block. Note the premature, nonconducted P waves inscribed in the T wave that resets the sinus node leading to the observed pauses. **D.** Tachy-brady syndrome. Note the termination of the irregular tachyarrhythmia followed by a prolonged 4.5-second pause prior to the first sinus beat. (From Cooper DH. Bradyarrhythmias and permanent pacemakers. In: Cuculich PS, Kates AM, eds. *The Washington manual cardiology subspecialty consult.* 2nd ed. Philadelphia, PA: Lippincott Williams & Wilkins; 2009.)

especially during sleep. Pauses >3 seconds, particularly during daytime hours, raise concern for significant sinus node dysfunction.

- ○ **Sinus exit block** represents the appropriate firing of the sinus node but the wave of depolarization fails to traverse past the perinodal tissue. It is indistinguishable from sinus arrest on surface ECGs except that the R-R interval will be a multiple of the R-R preceding the bradycardia.
- ○ **Tachy-brady syndrome** occurs when tachyarrhythmias alternate with bradyarrhythmias, especially AF. The rapid atrial rate suppresses sinus node output leading to sinus node dysfunction following termination of the tachyarrhythmia.
- ○ **Chronotropic incompetence** is the inability to increase the heart rate appropriately in response to metabolic need.
- **AV conduction disturbances**
  - ○ AV conduction can be **diverted** (fascicular or bundle branch blocks), **delayed** (first-degree AV block), **occasionally interrupted** (second-degree AV block), **frequently, but not always, interrupted** (advanced or high-degree AV block), or **completely absent** (third-degree AV block). Assignment of the bradyarrhythmia under investigation to one of these categories allows one to better determine prognosis and, therefore, guide therapy.

- **First-degree AV block** describes a conduction delay, usually localized to the AV node, that results in a PR interval >200 ms on the surface ECG. "Block" is a misnomer because, by definition, there are no dropped beats (i.e., there is a P wave for every QRS complex).
- **Second-degree AV block** is present when there are periodic interruptions (i.e., "dropped beats") in AV conduction. Distinction between Mobitz I and II is important because they possess differing natural histories of progression to complete heart block.
  - **Mobitz type I block (Wenckebach)** is represented by a progressive delay in AV conduction with successive atrial impulses until an impulse fails to conduct, followed by reiterations of the sequence. On surface ECG, classic Wenckebach block manifests as:
    - Progressive prolongation of the PR interval of each successive beat, before the dropped beat.
    - Shortening of each subsequent RR interval before the dropped beat. Therefore, the RR interval of the dropped beat will equal less than 2× the shortest RR on the tracing.
    - A regularly, irregular grouping of QRS complexes (group beating).
    - Type I block is usually within the AV node and portends a more benign natural history with progression to complete heart block unlikely.
  - **Mobitz type II block** carries a less favorable prognosis and is characterized by abrupt AV conduction block without evidence of progressive conduction delay.
    - On ECG, the PR intervals remained unchanged preceding the nonconducted P wave.
    - The presence of type II block, particularly if a bundle branch block is present, often antedates progression to complete heart block.
  - The presence of **AV 2:1 block** makes the differentiation between Mobitz type I or II mechanisms difficult. Diagnostic clues to the site of block include the following:
    - Concomitant first-degree AV block, periodic AV Wenckebach, or improved conduction (1:1) with enhanced sinus rates or sympathetic input suggests a more proximal interruption of conduction (i.e., Mobitz type 1 mechanism).
    - Concomitant bundle branch block, fascicular block, or worsened conduction (3:1, 4:1, etc.) with enhanced sympathetic input localizes the site of block more distally (Mobitz type II mechanism).
- **Third-degree (complete) AV block** is present when all atrial impulses fail to conduct to the ventricles. There is complete dissociation between the atria and ventricles ("A > V" rates). This should be distinguished from dissociation with competition at the AV node ("V > A" rates).
- **Advanced or high-degree AV block** is present when more than one consecutive atrial depolarization fails to conduct to the ventricles (i.e., 3:1 block or greater). On ECG, consecutive P waves will be seen without associated QRS complexes. However, there will be demonstrable P:QRS conduction somewhere on the record to avoid a "third degree" designation (Figure 7-5).

Imaging
- The presence or absence of structural heart disease should be initially evaluated by transthoracic echocardiography.
- Further imaging should be obtained based on suspected etiology.

First-Degree AV Block

A

Second-Degree AV Block-Mobitz type I (Wenckebach Block)

B

Second-Degree AV Block-Mobitz type II

C

Second-Degree AV Block

D

Third-Degree (Complete) AV Block

E

Figure 7-5. Examples of atrioventricular block (AVB). **A.** First-degree AVB. There are no dropped beats and the PR interval is >200 ms. **B.** 3:2 Second-degree AVB-Mobitz I. Note the "group beating" and the prolonging PR interval prior to the dropped beat. The third P wave in the sequence is subtly inscribed in the T wave of the preceding beat. **C.** Second-degree AVB-Mobitz II. Note the abrupt AV conduction block without evidence of progressive conduction delay. **D.** 2:1 AVB. This pattern makes it difficult to distinguish between Mobitz I versus II type mechanisms of block. Note the narrow QRS complex which supports a more proximal origin of block (type I mechanism). A wider QRS (concomitant bundle branch or fascicular block) would suggest a type II mechanism. **E.** Complete heart block. Note the independent regularity of both the atrial and ventricular rhythms (junctional escape) with no clear association with each other throughout the rhythm strip. (From Cooper DH. Bradyarrhythmias and permanent pacemakers. In: Cuculich PS, Kates AM, eds. *The Washington manual cardiology subspecialty consult.* 2nd ed. Philadelphia, PA: Lippincott Williams & Wilkins; 2009.)

TREATMENT

Pharmacologic therapy

- Bradyarrhythmias that lead to significant symptoms and hemodynamic instability are considered cardiovascular emergencies and should be managed as outlined in ACLS guidelines (see Appendix C).
- **Atropine**, an anticholinergic agent given in doses of 0.5 to 2.0 mg IV, is the cornerstone pharmacologic agent for emergent bradycardia treatment.
  - Dysfunction localized more proximally in the conduction system (i.e., symptomatic sinus bradycardia, first-degree AV block, Mobitz I second-degree AV block) tends to be atropine responsive.
  - Distal disease is not responsive and can be worsened by atropine.

- Reversible causes of bradyarrhythmias should be identified as previously described and any agents (digoxin, calcium channel blockers, β-adrenergic blockers) that caused or exacerbated the underlying dysrhythmia should be withheld.

Other Nonpharmacologic Therapies

- For bradyarrhythmias that have irreversible etiologies or that are secondary to medically necessary pharmacologic therapy, pacemaker therapy should be considered.
  - Temporary pacing is indicated for symptomatic second-degree or third-degree heart block caused by transient drug intoxication or electrolyte imbalance and complete heart block or Mobitz II second-degree AV block in the setting of an acute MI.
  - Sinus bradycardia, AF with a slow ventricular response, or Mobitz I second-degree AV block should be treated with temporary pacing only if significant symptoms or hemodynamic instability is present.
  - Temporary pacing is achieved preferably via insertion of a transvenous pacemaker. Transthoracic external pacing can be utilized, although the lack of reliability of capture and patient discomfort clearly makes this a second-line modality.
- Once hemodynamic stability has been established, attention turns to the indications for PPM placement.
  - In symptomatic patients, the key determinants include **potential reversibility of causative factors** and **temporal correlation of symptoms to the arrhythmia**.
  - In asymptomatic patients, the key determinant is based on whether the **discovered conduction abnormality has a natural history of progression to higher degrees of heart block** that portends a poor prognosis.
- **Permanent pacing**
  - Permanent pacing involves the placement of anchored, intracardiac pacing leads for the purpose of maintaining a heart rate sufficient to avoid the aforementioned symptoms and hemodynamic consequences of certain bradyarrhythmias. In addition, advances in pacemaker technology allow contemporary pacers, through maintenance of AV synchrony and rate-adaptive programming, to more closely mimic normal physiologic heart rate behavior.
    - Class I (general agreement/evidence for benefit) and IIa (weight of conflicting opinion/evidence in favor of benefit) indications for permanent pacing are listed in Figure 7-3.
    - Pacemakers are designed to provide an electrical stimulus to the heart whenever the rate drops below a preprogrammed **lower rate limit**. Therefore, the ECG appearance of a PPM varies depending on the pacer dependence of the individual heart rate.
    - The pacing spike produced by contemporary pacemakers are low-amplitude, sharp, and immediately preceding the generated P wave or QRS complex indicating capture of the chamber.
      - Atrial leads are typically placed in the right atrial appendage and therefore generate P waves of normal (sinus) morphology.
      - However, the QRS complexes generated by a typical right ventricular pacing lead are wide and typically assume an "LBBB-like" morphology.
      - Figure 7-6 illustrates some common ECG appearances of normally and abnormally functioning pacemakers.
  - The pacemaker generator is commonly placed subcutaneously in the pectoral region on the side of the nondominant arm. The electronic lead(s) is placed in the cardiac chamber(s) via central veins. Complications of placement include

Figure 7-6. Pacemaker rhythms. **A.** Normal dual-chamber (DDD) pacing. First two complexes are atrioventricular (AV) sequential pacing, followed by sinus with atrial sensing and ventricular pacing. **B.** Normal single-chamber (VVI) pacing. The underlying rhythm is atrial fibrillation (no distinct P waves), with ventricular pacing at 60 bpm. **C.** Pacemaker malfunction. The underlying rhythm is sinus (P) at 80 bpm with 2:1 heart block and first-degree AV block (long PR). Ventricular pacing spikes are seen (V) after each P wave, demonstrating appropriate sensing and tracking of the P waves; however, there is failure to capture. **D.** Pacemaker-mediated tachycardia. A, paced atrial events; V, paced ventricular events; P, sensed atrial events; R, sensed ventricular events. (**A–C.** From Cooper DH, Faddis MN. Cardiac arrhythmias. In: Cooper DH, et al., eds. *The Washington manual of medical therapeutics*. 32nd ed. Philadelphia, PA: Lippincott Williams & Wilkins; 2007; **D.** From Cooper DH. Bradyarrhythmias and permanent pacemakers. In: Cuculich PS, Kates AM, eds. *The Washington manual cardiology subspecialty consult*. 2nd ed. Philadelphia, PA: Lippincott Williams & Wilkins; 2009.)

pneumothorax, device infection, bleeding, and rarely, cardiac perforation with tamponade.

- Before implantation, the patient must be free of any active infections and anticoagulation issues must be carefully considered. Hematomas in the pacemaker pocket develop most commonly in patients who are receiving IV heparin or subcutaneous low–molecular-weight heparin. In severe cases, surgical evacuation is required.

- Following implantation, a **posteroanterior (PA) and lateral CXR** are obtained to confirm appropriate lead placement. The pacemaker is interrogated at appropriate intervals: typically, before discharge, 2 to 6 weeks following discharge, and every 6 to 12 months thereafter.
- **Pacing modes** are classified by a sequence of three to five letters. Most pacemakers are referred to by the three-letter code alone.
  - **Position I denotes the chamber that is paced:** A for atria, V for ventricle, or D for dual (A + V).
  - **Position II refers to the chamber that is sensed:** A for atria, V for ventricle, D for dual (A + V), or O for none.
  - **Position III denotes the type of response the pacemaker will have to a sensed signal:** I for inhibition, T for triggering, D for dual (I + T), or O for none.
  - **Position IV is utilized to signify the presence of rate-adaptive pacing (R)** in response to increased metabolic need. Almost all contemporary pacers implanted have rate-modulating capabilities.
  - **Position V identifies the presence or absence of multisite pacing:** O for none, A for multiple sites within the atria, V for multiple ventricular sites, or D for both (A + V). Biventricular pacing for resynchronization therapy in heart failure is the most common application of this position.
- The most common pacing systems utilized today include VVIR, DDDR, or AAIR.
  - AAI systems should be utilized only for sinus node dysfunction in the absence of any AV conduction abnormalities.
  - The presence of AV nodal or His–Purkinje disease makes a dual chamber device (i.e., DDD) more appropriate.
  - Patients in chronic AF warrant a single ventricular lead with VVI programming.
  - The 2008 ACC/AHA/HRS guidelines for device-based therapy provide an algorithm to help guide pacing system decisions.
- Modern-day pacemakers also have the capability of **mode switching.** This is useful in patients with DDD pacers who have paroxysmal tachyarrhythmias. When these patients develop an atrial arrhythmia faster than a programmed mode switch rate, the device will switch to a mode (i.e., VVI) that does not track atrial signals. It will return to DDD when the tachyarrhythmia resolves.
- **Pacemaker malfunction** is a potentially life-threatening situation, particularly for patients who are pacemaker dependent. The workup of suspected malfunction should begin with a 12-lead ECG.
  - If no pacing activity is seen, one can place a magnet over the pacemaker to assess for output failure and ability to capture. **Application of the magnet switches the pacemaker to an asynchronous pacing mode.** For example, VVI mode becomes VOO (ventricular asynchronous pacing), and DDD mode becomes DOO (asynchronous AV pacing).
  - If malfunction is obvious or if the ECG is unrevealing and malfunction is still suspected, then a formal interrogation of the device should be done. **Patients are given a card to carry upon implantation that will identify the make and model of the device to facilitate this evaluation.**
  - **Chest radiograph (two views)** should also be obtained to assess for evidence of overt lead abnormalities (dislodgement, fracture, migration, etc.).
- General categories of pacemaker malfunction include failure to pace (output failure), failure to capture, failure to sense (undersensing), and pacemaker-mediated dysrhythmias.

- **Failure to pace** refers to situations where a pacemaker does not deliver a stimulus when it should.
  - **Oversensing** of environmental noise, myopotentials, or electrical artifact from a failing lead can cause long pauses in a pacemaker-dependent patient.
  - Also, atrial leads can misinterpret or oversense ventricular depolarizations as atrial activity leading to inhibition of atrial outputs that is referred to as "cross-talk."
  - Lead fracture or dislodgment, battery failure, and generator failure are less common causes of output failure.
- **Failure to capture** refers to those situations where the pacing stimulus is delivered but fails to generate evidence of myocardial depolarization (i.e., P or QRS complex).
  - Elevation in the threshold voltage required to initiate a wave of depolarization due to changes in the tissue surrounding the electrode is often at fault. This phenomenon is referred to as "exit block."
- **Undersensing** occurs when the preprogrammed amplitude and/or frequency thresholds for sensing are too high to identify native cardiac activity.
  - This may lead to pacing spikes being identified on top of native P, QRS, or T complexes.
- **Pacemaker-mediated tachycardias** are WCTs caused by ventricular pacing at a rapid rate either due to device tracking of an atrial tachyarrhythmia or an "endless loop tachycardia" created by tracking of retrograde atrial impulses created by the previous ventricular paced beat.
  - The rate of the arrhythmia provides a clue to diagnosis because it is typically at or below the programmed URL. A rate exceeding the URL excludes the diagnosis.
  - Similarly, pacemakers with rate-modulation programming can misinterpret febrile illness, external vibrations, hyperventilation, and other external stimuli and cause a **sensor-mediated, paced tachycardia**.

SPECIAL CONSIDERATIONS

- Often, episodes of bradycardia are transient and episodic; therefore, a baseline ECG may not be sufficient to capture the bradycardia. Some form of continuous monitoring is often required.
  - In the inpatient setting, **continuous central telemetry monitoring** can be utilized.
  - If further workup is done as an outpatient, **24- to 72-hour Holter monitoring** can be used if the episodes occur somewhat frequently. If infrequent, **an event recorder** or **ILR** should be considered.
  - Again, it is vital to correlate symptoms with the rhythm disturbances discovered via continuous monitoring—a task easily accomplished during inpatient care but more difficult as an outpatient. Therefore, the importance of accurate symptom diaries in the ambulatory setting should be emphasized to patients.
- To evaluate the sinus node's response to exertion (chronotropic competence), walking the patient in the hallway or up a flight of stairs under appropriate supervision is easy and inexpensive. A formal **exercise ECG** can be ordered if necessary.
- An **EPS** can also be used to assess sinus node function and AV conduction, but it is rarely necessary if the rhythm is already discovered via noninvasive modalities.

- The role of **tilt-table testing** will be discussed in the following text in the setting of a syncope evaluation.

SYNCOPE

GENERAL PRINCIPLES

Syncope is a common clinical problem, and a primary goal of evaluation is to determine whether the patient is at increased risk of death.

Definition
Sudden, self-limited loss of consciousness and postural tone caused by transient global cerebral hypoperfusion and followed by spontaneous, complete, and prompt recovery.

Classification
Syncope can be classified into four major categories based on etiology:
- **Neurocardiogenic** (most common): vasovagal, carotid sinus hypersensitivity, and situational.
- **Orthostatic hypotension:** hypovolemia, medication induced (iatrogenic), and autonomic dysfunction.
- **Cardiovascular:**
  ○ **Arrhythmia:** sinus node dysfunction, AV nodal block, pacemaker malfunction, VT, SVT, WPW syndrome, and long QT syndrome.
  ○ **Mechanical:** HCM, valvular stenosis, aortic dissection, myxomas, pulmonary embolism, pulmonary HTN, acute MI, subclavian steal, etc.
- **Miscellaneous** (not true syncope): seizures, stroke/TIA, hypoglycemia, hypoxia, psychogenic, etc.
  ○ Atherosclerotic cerebral artery disease is a rare cause of true syncope; exception is severe obstructive four-vessel cerebrovascular disease (expect focal neurologic findings prior to syncope).

Epidemiology
- Common in the general population—**6% of medical admissions and 3% of emergency room visits**.
- Incidence is similar among men and women; one of the largest epidemiologic studies revealed an 11% incidence during an average follow-up for 17 years, with a sharp rise after age 70 years (*N Engl J Med 2002;347:878*).

Pathophysiology
- The two components of **neurocardiogenic syncope** are described as **cardioinhibitory**, in which bradycardia or asystole results from increased vagal outflow to the heart, and **vasodepression**, where the peripheral vasodilation results from sympathetic withdrawal to peripheral arteries. Most patients have a combination of both components as the mechanism of their syncope.
- Specific stimuli may evoke a neurocardiogenic mechanism, leading to **situational syncope** (e.g., micturition, defecation, coughing, swallowing).

Risk Factors
Cardiovascular disease, history of **stroke or TIA**, and **HTN**. Also, low body mass index, increased alcohol intake, and diabetes are associated with syncope (*Am J Cardiol 2000;85:1189*; *N Engl J Med 2002;347:878*).

DIAGNOSIS

- A syncopal event may herald an otherwise unsuspected, potentially lethal cardiac condition, and therefore, a careful evaluation of the patient with syncope is warranted.
- A meticulous history and physical exam is the key to an accurate diagnosis of the etiology of syncope. In 40% of episodes, the mechanism of syncope remains unexplained (*Ann Intern Med 1997;126:989*).

Clinical Presentation

History

Special attention should be focused on the **events or symptoms** that **precede and follow** the syncopal event, **eyewitness** accounts during the event, the **time course** of loss and resumption of consciousness (abrupt vs. gradual), and the patient's **medical history**.

- A characteristic prodrome of nausea, diaphoresis, visual changes, or flushing suggests neurocardiogenic syncope, as does the identification of a particular emotional or situational trigger and postepisode fatigue.
- Alternatively, an unusual sensory prodrome, incontinence, or a decreased level of consciousness that gradually clears suggests a seizure as a likely diagnosis.
- With transient ventricular arrhythmias, an abrupt loss of consciousness may occur, with a rapid recovery.
- Syncope with exertion is a matter of concern for structural heart disease, pulmonary HTN, and CAD.

Physical Examination

The **cardiovascular** and **neurologic** exams should be the primary focus of initial evaluation.

- Orthostatic vital signs are critical in assessing for orthostatic hypotension. All patients should have BP checked in both arms.
- Cardiac exam findings may help detect valvular heart disease, LV dysfunction, pulmonary HTN, etc.
- Neurologic findings are often absent but if present may point to a possible neurologic etiology of the syncopal event.
- Carotid sinus massage for 5 to 10 seconds with reproduction of symptoms and consequent ventricular pause >3 seconds is considered positive for carotid sinus hypersensitivity. It is critical to take proper precautions of telemetry monitoring, availability of bradycardia treatments, and avoiding the procedure in patients with known or suspected carotid disease.

Diagnostic Testing

- The presence of known **structural heart disease**, **abnormal ECG**, **age older than 65 years**, **focal neurologic findings**, and **severe orthostatic hypotension** suggest a potentially more ominous etiology. Therefore, these patients should be admitted for their workup to avoid delay and adverse outcomes.
- After the history and physical exam, the ECG is the most important diagnostic tool in the evaluation of the patient. It will be abnormal in 50% of cases but alone will yield a diagnosis in only 5% of these patients.
- If the patient has no history of heart disease or baseline ECG abnormalities, **tilt-table testing** can be used to evaluate a patient's hemodynamic response during

transition from supine to upright state for diagnosis of neurally mediated processes. In an unselected population, the predictive value of this test is low.
- Please refer to Figure 7-7 with regards to the diagnostic approach to syncope.

TREATMENT

In general, therapy is tailored to the underlying etiology of syncope with goals of preventing recurrence and reducing risk of injury or death.
- **Neurocardiogenic syncope:**
  - **Counsel** patients to take precautionary steps to avoid injury by being aware of prodromal symptoms and maintaining a **horizontal position** at those times.
  - Avoid known precipitants and maintain adequate **hydration**.
  - Employ **isometric muscle contraction** during prodrome to abort episode.
  - Evidence suggests that β-adrenergic blockers are probably unhelpful (*Circulation 2006;113:1164*); **Selective serotonin reuptake inhibitor (SSRI) antidepressants** and **fludrocortisone** have a debatable effect; and **midodrine** (start at 5 mg PO tid and can be increased to 15 mg tid) is probably helpful in the treatment of neurocardiogenic syncope (*Am J Cardiol 2001;88:80*; *Heart Rhythm 2008;5:1609*).
  - In general, **PPMs** have no proven benefit (*JAMA 2003;289:2224*); however, permanent dual-chamber pacemakers with a hysteresis function (high-rate pacing in response to a detected sudden drop in heart rate) have been shown to be useful in highly selected patients with recurrent neurocardiogenic syncope with a prominent cardioinhibitory component (*J Am Coll Cardiol 1990;16:165*).
  - **Cardiac pacing** for **carotid sinus hypersensitivity** is appropriate in syncopal patients.
  - In general, neurocardiogenic syncope is not associated with increased risk of mortality.
- **Orthostatic hypotension:**
  - **Adequate hydration** and elimination of offending drugs.
  - Salt supplementation, compressive stockings, and counseling on standing slowly.
  - Midodrine and fludrocortisone can help by increasing systolic BP and expanding plasma volume, respectively.
- **Cardiovascular (arrhythmia or mechanical):**
  - Treatment of **underlying disorder** (valve replacement, antiarrhythmic agent, coronary revascularization, etc.)
  - **Cardiac pacing** for sinus node dysfunction or high-degree AV block.
  - Discontinuation of QT-prolonging drugs.
  - Catheter **ablation** procedures in select patients with syncope associated with SVT.
- **ICD** for documented VT without correctable cause and for syncope with ejection fraction (EF) <35% even in absence of documented arrhythmia.

CARDIAC RESYNCHRONIZATION THERAPY

GENERAL PRINCIPLES

- CHF is complicated by a significant interventricular conduction delay in about 30% of heart failure patients. In this patient group, dyssynchronous ventricular contraction of the septum and lateral wall complicate systolic dysfunction. The consequences of ventricular dyssynchrony include a loss of mechanical energy for

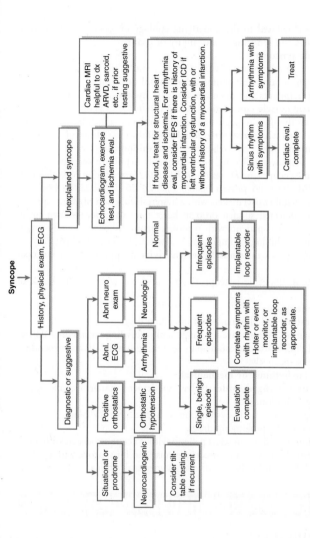

Figure 7-7. Algorithm for the evaluation of syncope. ARVD, arrhythmogenic right ventricular dysplasia; ECG, echocardiogram; ICD, implantable cardioverter-defibrillator; MRI, magnetic resonance imaging. (Data from Holley C. Evaluation of syncope. In: Cooper DH, et al., eds. *The Washington manual of medical therapeutics.* 32nd ed. Philadelphia, PA: Lippincott Williams & Wilkins; 2007; and Strickberger SA, Benson DW, Biaggioni I, et al.; American Heart Association Councils on Clinical Cardiology, Cardiovascular Nursing, Cardiovascular Disease in the Young, and Stroke; Quality of Care and Outcomes Research Interdisciplinary Working Group; American College of Cardiology Foundation; Heart Rhythm Society; American Autonomic Society. AHA/ACCF Scientific Statement on the evaluation of syncope: from the American Heart Association Councils on Clinical Cardiology, Cardiovascular Nursing, Cardiovascular Disease in the Young, and Stroke, and the Quality of Care and Outcomes Research Interdisciplinary Working Group; and the American College of Cardiology Foundation: in collaboration with the Heart Rhythm Society: endorsed by the American Autonomic Society. *Circulation. 2006;113(2):316–327.*)

blood ejection due to wasted motion of a partially relaxed opposing wall, an expansion of the isovolumetric phases of the cardiac cycle at the expense of systolic ejection and diastolic filling periods, and excessively high wall strains that can contribute to myopathic changes. The result is a worse prognosis than heart failure uncomplicated by conduction system disease.

- Biventricular pacing was first proposed as a way to restore, to some degree, electrical synchronization of the septum and lateral wall of the left ventricle in the setting of interventricular conduction delay leading to improvement in LV systolic function and heart failure symptoms. Randomized clinical trials have consistently verified these clinical benefits as well as providing evidence for a modification of the natural history of severe heart failure in patients treated with a "state-of-the-art" heart failure medical regimen manifested by a reduction in mortality and incidence of heart failure decompensation (*N Engl J Med 2004;350:2140*; *N Engl J Med 2005;352:1539*).

- As a result, cardiac resynchronization therapy (CRT) has become a standard of care for the treatment of patients with LV conduction delay and concomitant systolic heart failure that has become unresponsive to medical therapy.

Definition

- CRT is indicated for treatment of the patients with an LVEF of <35% and QRS duration of >0.12 seconds in the presence of medically refractory advanced heart failure symptoms quantified by New York Heart Association (NYHA) Class III or IV. CRT can also be considered in patients with LVEF <35% who are relatively asymptomatic. In this patient group, the benefits seem to be restricted to patients with a QRS duration of >150 ms (*N Engl J Med 2009;361:1329*). Patients who have an indication for ventricular pacing and an LVEF of <35% with NYHA Class I or II heart failure symptoms can also be considered as candidates for implantation of a CRT device.

- CRT can be delivered by a dedicated pacemaker system, or through a combination pacemaker/ICD system. Because most patients who are candidates for CRT also qualify for ICD implantation as primary prevention of SCD, the combination CRT pacemaker/ICD units are usually implanted.

8

Critical Care

Anthony Boyer, Scott T. Micek, and
Marin H. Kollef

Respiratory Failure

GENERAL PRINCIPLES

- **Hypercapnic respiratory failure** occurs with acute carbon dioxide retention (arterial carbon dioxide tension [$PaCO_2$] >45 mm Hg), producing a respiratory acidosis (pH <7.35).
- **Hypoxemic respiratory failure** occurs when normal gas exchange is seriously impaired, resulting in hypoxemia (arterial oxygen tension [PaO_2] <60 mm Hg or arterial oxygen saturation [SaO_2] <90%). Usually, this type of respiratory failure is associated with tachypnea and hypocapnia; however, its progression can lead to hypercapnia as well. Hypoxemic respiratory failure can result from various insults (Table 8-1).
  - The **acute respiratory distress syndrome (ARDS)** is a form of hypoxemic respiratory failure caused by acute lung injury. The common end result is disruption of the alveolocapillary membrane, leading to increased vascular permeability and accumulation of inflammatory cells and protein-rich edema fluid within the alveolar space.
  - The **American-European Consensus Conference** has defined ARDS as follows: (a) acute bilateral pulmonary infiltrates, (b) ratio of PaO_2 to inspired oxygen concentration (FIO_2) <200, and (c) no evidence for heart failure or volume overload as the principal cause of the pulmonary infiltrates (*N Eng J Med 2000;342:1334*).

Pathophysiology

- **Hypercapnic respiratory failure** occurs in conjunction with an elevated $PaCO_2$:

$$PaCO_2 = \frac{\dot{V}CO_2}{\dot{V}_A} = \frac{\dot{V}CO_2}{\dot{V}_E - \dot{V}_D}$$

where $\dot{V}CO_2$ = CO_2 production, $\dot{V}_A$ = alveolar ventilation, $\dot{V}_E$ = expired total ventilation, and $\dot{V}_D$ = dead space ventilation. Therefore, any of the three following processes can result in hypercapnia.
  - **Increased carbon dioxide production** can be precipitated by fever, sepsis, seizures, and excessive carbohydrate loads in patients with underlying lung disease.
  - **Increased dead space** occurs when areas of the lung are ventilated but not perfused or when decreases in regional perfusion exceed decreases in ventilation. Examples include intrinsic lung diseases (e.g., chronic obstructive pulmonary disease [COPD], asthma, cystic fibrosis, pulmonary fibrosis) and chest wall disorders associated with parenchymal abnormalities (e.g., scoliosis). Usually, these disorders are associated with a widened $P(A-a)O_2$ gradient.

Table 8-1	Causes of Shunts and Hypoxemic Respiratory Failure
Clinical Presentation	**Causes**
Cardiogenic pulmonary edema (low permeability, high hydrostatic pressure)	Acute myocardial infarction Left ventricular failure Mitral regurgitation Mitral stenosis Diastolic dysfunction
Noncardiogenic pulmonary edema (high permeability, low hydrostatic pressure)	Aspiration Sepsis Multiple trauma Pancreatitis Near drowning Pneumonia Reperfusion injury Inhalational injury Drug reaction (aspirin, narcotics, interleukin-2)
Mixed pulmonary edema (high permeability, high hydrostatic pressure)	Myocardial ischemia or volume overload associated with sepsis, aspiration, etc. High-altitude exposure
Pulmonary edema of unclear etiology	Upper airway obstruction Neurogenic cause Lung reexpansion

- **Decreased minute ventilation** (i.e., expired total ventilation) can result from central nervous system (CNS) disorders (e.g., spinal cord lesions), peripheral nerve diseases (e.g., Guillain-Barré syndrome, botulism, myasthenia gravis, amyotrophic lateral sclerosis), muscle disorders (e.g., polymyositis, muscular dystrophy), chest wall abnormalities (e.g., thoracoplasty, scoliosis), drug overdoses, metabolic abnormalities (e.g., myxedema, hypokalemia), and upper airway obstruction. These disorders are usually associated with a normal $P(A–a)O_2$ gradient unless accompanying lung disease is also present.
- **Hypoxemic respiratory failure** usually is the result of the lung's reduced ability to deliver oxygen across the alveolocapillary membrane. The severity of gas exchange impairment is determined by calculating the $P(A–a)O_2$ gradient using the alveolar gas equation:

$$PAO_2 = FIO_2 (P_{ATM} - P_{H_2O}) - \frac{PACO_2}{R}$$

where FIO_2 = the fraction of inspired oxygen, P_{ATM} = atmospheric pressure, P_{H_2O} = water vapor pressure, and R = the respiratory quotient. The following six processes can result in hypoxemia:
- **Shunt:** This term refers to the fraction of mixed venous blood that passes into the systemic arterial circulation after bypassing functioning lung units. Congenital shunts are due to developmental anomalies of the heart and great vessels. Acquired shunts usually result from diseases that affect lung units, although acquired cardiac

and peripheral vascular shunts also can occur (Table 8-1). Shunts are associated with a widened $P(A–a)O_2$ gradient, and the resultant hypoxemia is resistant to correction with supplemental oxygen alone when the shunt fraction of the cardiac output (CO) is >30%.

○ **Ventilation–perfusion mismatch:** Diseases associated with airflow obstruction (e.g., COPD, asthma), interstitial inflammation (e.g., pneumonia, sarcoidosis), or vascular obstruction (e.g., pulmonary embolism) often produce lung regions with abnormal ventilation-to-perfusion relationships. In ventilation–perfusion mismatch, unlike shunt physiology, increases in FIO_2 result in increases in PaO_2.

○ **Low inspired oxygen:** The partial pressure of inspired oxygen is reduced at high altitude secondary to decreased barometric pressure. Inhaled toxic gas decreases FIO_2.

○ **Hypoventilation:** A decrease in minute ventilation results in an increase in $PACO_2$ displacing oxygen. Usually, oxygen therapy improves hypoxemia but could worsen hypoventilation, especially in the setting of chronic airflow obstruction. In pure hypoventilation, the $P(A–a)O_2$ gradient is normal. Primary treatment is directed at correcting the cause of hypoventilation.

○ **Diffusion impairment:** Hypoxemia due to diffusion impairments usually responds to supplemental oxygen therapy, as is seen in patients with interstitial lung diseases.

○ **Low mixed venous oxygenation:** Normally, the lungs fully oxygenate pulmonary arterial blood, and mixed venous oxygen tension (PvO_2) does not affect PaO_2 significantly. However, a decreased PvO_2 can lower the PaO_2 significantly when either intrapulmonary shunting or ventilation–perfusion mismatch is present. Factors that can contribute to low mixed venous oxygenation include anemia, hypoxemia, inadequate CO, and increased oxygen consumption. Improving oxygen delivery to tissues by increasing hemoglobin or CO usually decreases oxygen extraction and improves mixed venous oxygen saturation (SvO_2).

• **Mixed respiratory failure** is seen most commonly after surgery, particularly in patients with underlying lung disease who are undergoing upper abdominal procedures. Abnormalities in oxygenation usually occur on the basis of atelectasis, which often is multifactorial in origin-decreased lung volumes and cough due to the effects of anesthesia, abnormal diaphragmatic function resulting from the surgery or associated pain, and interstitial edema causing small airways to close. Hypoventilation can also result from abnormal diaphragmatic function, particularly when complete paralysis occurs, as with phrenic nerve injury.

• **Blood gas analysis** (see Acid–Base Disturbances in Chapter 12, Fluid and Electrolyte Management).

Noninvasive Oxygen Therapy

GENERAL PRINCIPLES

• **Nasal prongs** allow patients to eat, drink, and speak during oxygen administration. Their disadvantage is that the exact FIO_2 delivered is not known, as it is influenced by the patient's peak inspiratory flow demand. As an approximation, 1 L/min of nasal prong oxygen flow is roughly equivalent to FIO_2 of 24%, with each additional liter of flow increasing the FIO_2 by approximately 4%. Flow rates should be limited to <5 L/min.

- **Venturi masks** allow the precise administration of oxygen. Usual FIO_2 values delivered are 24%, 28%, 31%, 35%, 40%, and 50%. Often, Venturi masks are useful in patients with COPD and hypercapnia because one can titrate the PaO_2 to minimize carbon dioxide retention.
- **Nonrebreathing masks** achieve higher oxygen concentrations (approximately 80% to 90%) than do partial rebreathing systems. A one-way valve prevents exhaled gases from entering the reservoir bag in a nonrebreathing system, thereby maximizing the FIO_2.
- A **continuous positive airway pressure (CPAP) mask** can be used if the PaO_2 is <60 to 65 mm Hg with a nonrebreathing mask, and the patient is conscious and cooperative, able to protect the lower airway, and hemodynamically stable (*N Engl J Med 1998;339:429*). CPAP is delivered by a tight-fitting mask equipped with pressure-limiting valves. Many patients cannot tolerate a CPAP mask because of persistent hypoxemia, hemodynamic instability, or feelings of claustrophobia or aerophagia. In these patients, endotracheal intubation should be performed. Initially, 3 to 5 cm H_2O of CPAP should be applied and, if the PaO_2 is still 60 mm Hg (SaO_2 <90%), the level of CPAP should be increased in steps of 3 to 5 cm H_2O up to a level of 10 to 15 cm H_2O.
- **Bilevel positive airway pressure (BiPAP)** is a method of noninvasive ventilation whereby both inspiratory and expiratory pressures can be applied. The inspiratory support decreases the patient's work of breathing. The expiratory support (CPAP) improves gas exchange by preventing alveolar collapse. Noninvasive ventilation using face or nasal masks has been successfully performed in patients with neuromuscular disease, COPD, congestive heart failure (CHF), and postoperative respiratory insufficiency as a means of decreasing the need for endotracheal intubation and mechanical ventilation (*Crit Care Clin 2007;23:201*). In using BiPAP, an inspiratory pressure of 5 to 10 cm H_2O and an expiratory pressure of 3 to 5 cm H_2O are reasonable starting points. The inspiratory pressure can be increased in increments of 3 to 5 cm H_2O in order to achieve adequate ventilation.

Airway Management and Tracheal Intubation

GENERAL PRINCIPLES

- **Airway management**
  - **Head and jaw positioning:** The oropharynx should be inspected, and all foreign bodies should be removed. For patients with inadequate respirations, the jaw thrust or head tilt–chin lift maneuvers should be performed (see Acute Upper Airway Obstruction in Chapter 27, Medical Emergencies).
  - **Oral and nasopharyngeal airways:** When head and jaw positioning fail to establish a patent airway or when more permanent airway maintenance is desired, an oral or nasopharyngeal airway can be used. Initially, oral airways are positioned with the concave curve of the airway facing up into the roof of the mouth. The oral airway then is turned 180 degrees so that the concave curve of the airway follows the natural curve of the tongue. A tongue depressor can also be used to displace the tongue inferiorly and laterally to allow direct positioning of the oral airway. Careful monitoring of airway patency is required, as malpositioning of oral airways can push the tongue posteriorly and can result in obstruction of the oropharynx. Nasopharyngeal airways are made of soft plastic and are passed easily

down one of the nasal passages to the posterior pharynx after topical nasal lubrication and anesthesia with viscous lidocaine jelly.

○ **Mask-to-face ventilation:** Ineffective respiratory efforts can be augmented with simple mask-to-face ventilation. Proper fitting and positioning of the mask ensure a tight seal around the mouth and nose. Additionally, proper head positioning and the use of airway adjuncts (e.g., oral or nasopharyngeal airways) optimize ventilation with a mask-to-face system.

○ **Laryngeal mask airway (LMA):** The LMA is an endotracheal tube with a small mask on one end that can be passed orally over the larynx to provide ventilatory assistance and prevent aspiration. Placement of the LMA is more easily performed than endotracheal intubation. However, it should be considered a temporary airway for patients who require prolonged ventilatory support.

• **Endotracheal intubation** (*Int Anesthesiol Clin 2000;38:1*)

○ **Indications** include
  ▪ Initiation of mechanical ventilation
  ▪ Airway protection
  ▪ Inadequate oxygenation using less invasive methods
  ▪ Prevention of aspiration
  ▪ Suctioning of pulmonary secretions
  ▪ Hyperventilation for the treatment of increased intracranial pressure

○ **Techniques** include
  ▪ Direct laryngoscopic orotracheal intubation
  ▪ Video laryngoscopic orotracheal intubation
  ▪ Blind nasotracheal intubation
  ▪ Flexible fiberoptically guided orotracheal or nasotracheal intubation depending on the skill of the operator and the urgency.
  ▪ The direct laryngoscopic technique allows for the most rapid intubation of the trachea with the largest endotracheal tube. Nasotracheal intubation often requires smaller endotracheal tubes that are more susceptible to kinking and is associated with a higher incidence of otitis media and sinusitis. Before endotracheal intubation is attempted, a systematic evaluation of the patient's head and neck positioning must be performed. The oral, pharyngeal, and tracheal axes should be aligned before any intubation attempts. This "sniffing" position is achieved by flexing the patient's neck and extending the head. A small pillow or several towels placed under the occiput can assist in maintaining this position. A step-by-step approach to performing successful orotracheal intubation is essential (Table 8-2). After successful intubation of the trachea, the tracheal tube cuff pressures should be monitored at regular intervals and should be maintained below capillary filling pressure (i.e., <25 mm Hg) to prevent ischemic mucosal injury.

○ **Verification of correct endotracheal tube positioning:** Proper tube positioning must be ensured by
  ▪ Direct view of the endotracheal tube entering the trachea through the vocal cords
  ▪ Fiberoptic inspection of the airways through the endotracheal tube
  ▪ Use of an end-tidal carbon dioxide monitor. Clinical evaluation of the patient (i.e., listening for bilateral breath sounds over the chest and the absence of ventilation over the stomach) and radiographic evaluation (e.g., standard portable chest radiograph) can be unreliable for establishing correct endotracheal tube positioning.

Table 8-2	Procedure for Direct Orotracheal Intubation

1. Administer oxygen by face mask.
2. Ensure that basic equipment is present and easily accessible (oxygen source, bag-valve device, suctioning device, endotracheal [ET] tube, blunt stylet, laryngoscope, 20-mL syringe).
3. Place patient on nonmobile rigid surface.
4. If patient is in hospital bed, remove backboard and adjust bed height.
5. Depress patient's tongue with tongue depressor and administer topical anesthesia to patient's pharynx.
6. Position patient's head in sniffing position.
7. Administer intravenous (IV) sedation and neuromuscular blocker if necessary.[a]
8. Have assistant apply Sellick maneuver (compressing cricothyroid cartilage posteriorly against vertebral bodies) to prevent regurgitation and aspiration of stomach contents from esophagus.
9. Grasp laryngoscope handle in left hand while opening patient's mouth with gloved right hand.
10. Insert laryngoscope blade on right side of patient's mouth and advance to base of tongue, displacing tongue to the left.
11. Lift laryngoscope away from patient's at a 45-degree angle using arm and shoulder strength. Do not use patient's teeth as a fulcrum.
12. Suction oropharynx and hypopharynx if necessary.
13. Grasp ET tube with inserted stylet in right hand and insert it into right corner of patient's mouth, avoiding obscuration of epiglottis and vocal cords.
14. Advance ET tube through vocal cords until cuff is no longer visible and remove stylet.
15. Inflate cuff with enough air to prevent significant air leakage.
16. Verify correct ET tube positioning by auscultation of both lungs and the abdomen.
17. Obtain a chest radiograph or use end-tidal CO_2 monitor to verify correct position of the ET tube.

---

[a]Neuromuscular blockade can result in complete airway collapse and airway obstruction. Personnel who are skillful in establishment of an emergency surgical airway should be available if paralysis is used.

○ **Complications:** Improper endotracheal tube positioning is the most important immediate complication to be recognized and corrected. Ideally, the tip of the endotracheal tube should be 3 to 5 cm above the carina, depending on head and neck positioning. Esophageal or right main-stem intubation should be suspected if hypoxemia, hypoventilation, or cardiac decompensation occurs. Abdominal distention, lack of breath sounds over the thorax, and regurgitation of stomach contents through the endotracheal tube indicate an esophageal intubation. Other complications associated with endotracheal intubation include dislodgment of teeth, trauma to the upper airway, and increased intracranial pressure.

- **Surgical airways**
  - **Tracheostomy**
    - **Indications** include
      - The need for prolonged respiratory support
      - Potentially life-threatening upper airway obstruction (due to epiglottitis, facial burns, or worsening laryngeal edema)
      - Obstructive sleep apnea that is unresponsive to less invasive therapies
      - Congenital abnormalities (e.g., Pierre Robin syndrome)
    - Tracheostomy sites usually require at least 72 hours to mature. Tube dislodgment before site maturation followed by blind attempts at tube reinsertion can lead to tube malpositioning within a false channel in the pretracheal space. This misplacement can result in complete loss of the airway. If a tracheostomy tube cannot be reinserted easily, standard direct orotracheal intubation should be performed (Table 8-2), with the exception being after head and neck surgeries that have obliterated the connection between the oral cavity and the trachea (e.g., total laryngectomy). Optimal timing of surgical tracheostomy is controversial. While a previous randomized controlled trial suggested benefits of early tracheostomy regarding mortality, rate of ventilator-associated pneumonia, and intensive care unit (ICU) length of stay (*Crit Care Med 2004;32:1689*), these findings were not confirmed in a recent meta-analysis (*Chest 2011;140:1456*). Therefore, tracheostomy should be considered after 7 to 14 days of mechanical ventilation if prolonged ventilation is anticipated.
  - **Cricothyrotomy:** This procedure is indicated for the establishment of an emergency airway when direct tracheal intubation cannot be performed owing to upper airway obstruction. A pillow or towel roll should be placed under the patient's shoulders to extend the neck. The thyroid cartilage superiorly and the cricoid cartilage inferiorly should be located where they border the cricothyroid membrane. The thumb and second finger of the surgeon's nondominant hand should grasp and stabilize the lateral aspects of the cricothyroid membrane. With a scalpel, a transverse skin incision is made over the entire distance of the membrane. The incision then is deepened to the cricothyroid membrane, avoiding injury to surrounding structures. Standard tracheostomy tubes or endotracheal tubes can be inserted into the stoma to ventilate the patient. Alternatively, prepackaged kits using the Seldinger technique with progressive dilation of the stoma can be used.
  - **Cricothyroid needle cannulation:** In emergency settings when standard endotracheal intubation cannot be performed and placement of a surgical airway is not immediately possible, needle cannulation of the cricothyroid membrane can be performed as an intermediate procedure until a more definitive airway can be established. The ends of the cricothyroid membrane are grasped with the nondominant hand, and a 22-gauge needle is inserted into the airway, aspirating air to confirm positioning. Lidocaine is then injected into the trachea to blunt the patient's cough reflex before the needle is withdrawn. By the same technique, a 14-gauge (or larger) needle-through-cannula device can be passed through the cricothyroid membrane at a 45-degree angle to the skin. When air is aspirated freely, the outer cannula is passed into the airway caudally, and the needle is removed. A 3-mL syringe barrel can then be attached to the catheter, and a 7-mm inner-diameter endotracheal tube adapter is attached to the syringe to allow bag-valve ventilation. Alternatively, the cannula can be attached directly to high-flow oxygen (i.e., 10 to 15 L/min).

Mechanical Ventilation

GENERAL PRINCIPLES

- **Initiation of mechanical ventilation:** Certain variables should be considered when initiating mechanical ventilation.
  - ○ **Ventilator type:** Often, ventilator selection is dictated by what is available at a particular hospital. A volume-cycled ventilator is used in most clinical circumstances.
  - ○ **Mode of ventilation:**
    - ▪ **Assist-control ventilation (ACV)** should be the initial mode of ventilation used in most patients with respiratory failure. It produces a ventilator-delivered breath for every patient-initiated inspiratory effort. Controlled ventilator-initiated breaths are delivered automatically when the patient's spontaneous rate falls below the selected backup rate. Respiratory alkalosis is a potential concern when using ACV for patients with tachypnea.
    - ▪ **Intermittent mandatory ventilation (IMV)** allows patients to breathe at a spontaneous rate and tidal volume without triggering the ventilator, while the ventilator adds additional mechanical breaths at a preset rate and tidal volume.
    - ▪ **Synchronized intermittent mandatory ventilation (SIMV)** allows the ventilator to become sensitized to the patient's respiratory efforts at intervals determined by the frequency setting. This capability allows coordination of the delivery of the ventilator-driven breath with the respiratory cycle of the patient to prevent inadvertent stacking of a mechanical breath on top of a spontaneous inspiration. Potential advantages include less respiratory alkalosis, fewer adverse cardiovascular effects due to lower intrathoracic pressures, less requirement for sedation and paralysis, maintenance of respiratory muscle function, and facilitation of long-term weaning. However, considerable patient-initiated respiratory muscle work may contribute to respiratory muscle fatigue and failure to wean from mechanical ventilation in some patients. This nonphysiologic work of spontaneous breathing can be alleviated by the addition of low levels of pressure support ventilation (PSV).
    - ▪ **PSV** augments each patient-triggered respiratory effort by an operator-specified amount of pressure that is usually between 5 and 50 cm H_2O. PSV is used primarily to augment spontaneous respiratory efforts during IMV modes of ventilation or during weaning trials. PSV can also be used as a primary form of ventilation in patients who can trigger the ventilator spontaneously. Increased airway resistance, decreased lung compliance, and decreased patient effort result in diminished tidal volumes and, frequently, in decreased minute ventilation. PSV is not recommended as a primary ventilatory mode in patients in whom any of the aforementioned parameters are expected to fluctuate widely.
    - ▪ **Inverse ratio ventilation (IRV)** uses an inspiratory-to-expiratory ratio that is greater than the standard 1:2 to 1:3 ratio (i.e., ≥1:1) to recruit alveoli and improve gas exchange primarily for patients with ARDS (*Crit Care Clin 1998;14:707*). The goals of IRV are to decrease peak airway pressures, to maintain adequate alveolar ventilation, and to improve oxygenation. The use of IRV can be considered in patients with a low PaO_2:FIO_2 ratio (i.e., <300),

peak airway pressures >40 to 45 cm H_2O, or the need for positive end-expiratory pressure (PEEP) of >15 cm H_2O. However, lung strain may be greater in acute lung injury when IRV is employed (*Am J Respir Crit Care Med 2004;169:239*).

- **Lung-protective, pressure-targeted ventilation** is a method whereby controlled hypoventilation is allowed to occur with elevation of the $PaCO_2$ (i.e., permissive hypercapnia) to minimize the detrimental effects of excessive airway pressures. This form of ventilation has been used traditionally in patients with respiratory failure due to ARDS as the application of tidal volumes ≤6 mL/kg is associated with improved outcomes (*Crit Care Med 2005;33:S223*). However, the use of smaller tidal volumes should be considered in all mechanically ventilated patients to prevent iatrogenic lung injury. Additional methods for improving oxygenation while minimizing lung injury during mechanical ventilation in ARDS include prone positioning (*N Engl J Med 2001;345:568*) and the administration of nitric oxide (NO) or inhaled epoprostenol, although these interventions have not been associated with a survival advantage. When administered early in the course of ARDS (i.e., <14 days), corticosteroids can improve oxygenation and cardiopulmonary physiology (*Chest 2007;131:954*), but a mortality benefit has not been demonstrated (*N Engl J Med 2006;354:1671*). Neuromuscular blockade can improve ventilator synchrony and may increase survival at the potential cost of critical illness myoneuropathy (*N Engl J Med 2010;363:1107*). Extracorporeal membrane oxygenation can be considered for refractory hypoxemic respiratory failure, but further evidence is required to elucidate the safety and efficacy of this intervention (*Lancet 2009;374:1351*).
- **Independent lung ventilation** uses two independent ventilators and a double-lumen endotracheal tube. Usually, this modality is reserved for severe unilateral lung disease, such as unilateral pneumonia, respiratory failure associated with hemoptysis, or a bronchopleural fistula.
- **High-frequency ventilation** uses rates that are substantially faster (60 to 300 breaths/min) than those for conventional ventilation with small tidal volumes (2 to 4 mL/kg). The use of high-frequency ventilation is controversial except during upper airway surgery.
- **Airway pressure release ventilation (APRV)** uses CPAP with an intermittent pressure release phase. APRV applies CPAP to maintain adequate lung volume and promote alveolar recruitment. A time-cycled release phase to a lower set pressure allows ventilation to occur. APRV allows spontaneous breathing to be integrated independent of the ventilator cycle, making mechanical ventilation more comfortable for some patients (*Crit Care Med 2005;33:S228*).
- **Mechanical ventilation with inhaled NO** has been demonstrated to improve gas exchange in adults and children with respiratory failure, including patients with ARDS, pulmonary arterial hypertension, cor pulmonale secondary to congenital heart disease, and after cardiac surgery or heart or lung transplantation. Inhaled NO acts as a selective pulmonary artery (PA) vasodilator, decreasing PA pressures (without decreasing systemic blood pressure [BP] or CO) and improving oxygenation by reducing intrapulmonary shunt (*JAMA 2004;291:1603*). Generally, 5 to 20 ppm NO is administered, and the level of methemoglobin is monitored periodically.
- **Heliox**, a mixture of helium and oxygen, may result in improved lung mechanics compared to the use of oxygen alone, particularly in the setting of asthma

exacerbation and upper airway obstruction (*Am J Respir Crit Care Med 2002;165:1317*).

○ **Ventilator management**

▪ **FIO_2:** Hypoxemia is more dangerous than brief exposure to high inspired levels of oxygen. The initial FIO_2 should be 100%. Adjustments in the FIO_2 can be made to achieve a PaO_2 of >60 mm Hg or a SaO_2 of >90%.

▪ **Minute ventilation** is determined by the respiratory rate and the tidal volume. In general, a respiratory rate of 10 to 15 breaths/min is an appropriate rate with which to begin. Close monitoring of minute ventilation is especially important in ventilating patients with COPD and carbon dioxide retention. In these individuals, the minute ventilation should be adjusted to achieve the patient's baseline $PaCO_2$ and not necessarily a normal $PaCO_2$. Inadvertent hyperventilation with resultant metabolic alkalosis in these patients may be associated with serious serum electrolyte shifts and arrhythmias. Initial tidal volumes usually can be set at 6 to 8 mL/kg in order to minimize airway pressures and resultant barotrauma.

▪ **PEEP** is defined as the maintenance of positive airway pressure at the end of expiration. It can be applied to the spontaneously breathing patient in the form of CPAP or to the patient who is receiving mechanical ventilation. The appropriate application of PEEP usually increases lung compliance and oxygenation while decreasing the shunt fraction and the work of breathing. PEEP increases peak and mean airway pressures, which can increase the likelihood of barotrauma and cardiovascular compromise. PEEP is used primarily in patients with hypoxemic respiratory failure (e.g., ARDS, cardiogenic pulmonary edema). Low levels of PEEP (3 to 5 cm H_2O) may also be useful in patients with COPD to prevent dynamic airway collapse during expiration. The main goal of PEEP is to achieve a PaO_2 of >55 to 60 mm Hg with an FIO_2 of ≤60% while avoiding significant cardiovascular sequelae. Usually, PEEP is applied in 3 to 5 cm H_2O increments during monitoring of oxygenation, organ perfusion, and hemodynamic parameters. The plateau pressure should be kept <30 cm H_2O to avoid barotrauma. Patients who receive significant levels of PEEP (i.e., >10 cm H_2O) should not have their PEEP removed abruptly, which can result in collapse of distal lung units, the worsening of shunt, and potentially life-threatening hypoxemia. When lung-protective ventilation strategies are employed in severe ARDS, higher levels of PEEP (i.e., >12 cm H_2O) may improve survival and time to liberation from mechanical ventilation (*JAMA 2010;303:865*). PEEP should be weaned in 3 to 5 cm H_2O increments while oxygenation is monitored closely.

▪ **Inspiratory flow rate:** Flow rates set inappropriately low can be associated with prolonged inspiratory times that can lead to the development of auto-PEEP. The resultant lung hyperinflation can affect patient hemodynamics adversely by impairing venous return to the heart. Patients with severe airflow obstruction are at the greatest risk for development of lung hyperinflation when improper flow rates are used. Increasing the inspiratory flow rate usually allows for longer expiratory times that help to reverse this process.

▪ **Trigger sensitivity:** Most mechanical ventilators use pressure triggering either to initiate a machine-assisted breath or to permit spontaneous breathing during IMV or PSV. The patient must generate a decrease in the airway circuit pressure equal to the selected pressure sensitivity. Most patients do not tolerate a trigger sensitivity less than −2 cm because of autocycling of the ventilator. Alternatively, excessive trigger sensitivity can increase the patient's work of breathing, contributing to failure to wean from mechanical ventilation. In general, the smallest trigger sensitivity should be selected, allowing the patient to initiate mechanical or spontaneous breaths without causing the ventilator to autocycle.

- **Flow triggering:** To decrease the patient's work of breathing, flow by can be used as an adjunct to conventional modes of mechanical ventilation. Flow by refers to triggering of the ventilator by changes in airflow as opposed to changes in airway pressures. A continuous base flow of gas is provided through the ventilator circuit at a preselected flow rate (5 to 20 L/min). A flow sensitivity (i.e., patient rate of inhaled flow that triggers the ventilator to switch from base flow to either a machine delivered or a spontaneous breath) is selected (usually 2 L/min). Flow-triggered systems are more responsive than are pressure-triggered systems and result in a decreased work of breathing.

- **Management of problems and complications**
  - **Airway malpositioning and occlusion** (see Airway Management and Tracheal Intubation section).
  - **Worsening respiratory distress or arterial oxygen desaturation** may develop suddenly as a result of changes in the patient's cardiopulmonary status or secondary to a mechanical malfunction. The first priority is to ensure patency and correct positioning of the patient's airway so that adequate oxygenation and ventilation can be administered during the ensuing evaluation.
    - **Note ventilator alarms, airway pressures, and tidal volume.** Low-pressure alarms with decreased exhaled tidal volumes may suggest a leak in the ventilator circuit.
    - **Disconnect the patient from the ventilator and manually ventilate with an anesthesia bag using 100% oxygen.** For patients receiving PEEP, manual ventilation with a PEEP valve should be used to prevent atelectasis and hypoxemia.
    - **If manual ventilation is difficult,** check airway patency by passing a suction catheter through the endotracheal tube or tracheostomy. Listen for prolonged expiration continuing up to the point of the next manual breath. This suggests the presence of gas trapping and auto-PEEP.
    - **Check vital signs and perform a rapid physical examination with attention to the patient's cardiopulmonary status.** Be attentive to asymmetry in breath sounds or tracheal deviation suggesting tension pneumothorax. Note other parameters including cardiac rhythm and hemodynamics.
    - **Treat appropriately on the basis of the foregoing evaluation.** Treatment should be specific to the identified problems. If the presence of gas trapping and auto-PEEP is suspected, a reduction in the minute ventilation is appropriate. In some circumstances, periods of hypoventilation (4 to 6 breaths/min) or even apnea for 30 to 60 seconds may be necessary to reverse the sequelae of auto-PEEP.
    - **Return the patient to the ventilator only after checking its function.** Increase the level of support provided by the ventilator after an episode of respiratory distress or arterial oxygen desaturation. Usually, this adjustment means increasing the FIO_2 and the delivered minute ventilation unless significant auto-PEEP is present.
  - **An acute increase in the peak airway pressure** usually implies either a decrease in lung compliance or an increase in airway resistance. At a minimum,

considerations that should be entertained include pneumothorax, hemothorax, or hydropneumothorax; occlusion of the patient's airway; bronchospasm; increased accumulation of condensate in the ventilator circuit tubing; mainstem intubation; worsening pulmonary edema; or the development of gas trapping with auto-PEEP. Measurement of the peak-to-plateau pressure gradient ($P_{PEAK} - P_{PLATEAU}$) can differentiate between a decrease in lung compliance (stable gradient) and an increase in airway resistance (increased gradient). Some of these possibilities will be addressed in more detail in the following text.

o **Loss of tidal volume**, as evidenced by a difference between the tidal volume setting and the delivered tidal volume, implies a leak in either the ventilator or the inspiratory limb of the circuit tubing. A difference between the delivered tidal volume and the expired tidal volume implies the presence of a leak at the patient's airway due either to cuff malfunction or to malpositioning of the airway (e.g., positioning of the cuff at or above the level of the glottis) or a leak within the patient (e.g., presence of a bronchopleural fistula in a patient with a chest tube).

o **Asynchronous breathing ("fighting" or "bucking" the ventilator)** occurs when a patient's breathing coordinates poorly with the ventilator. This difficulty may indicate unmet respiratory demands. A careful evaluation is mandated, with attention focused at the identification of leaks in the ventilator system or airway, inadequate FIO_2, or inadequate ventilatory support. The problem can be alleviated by adjustments in the mode of mechanical ventilation, rate, tidal volume, inspiratory flow rate, and level of PEEP. The identification of gas trapping with auto-PEEP may require changing multiple settings to allow adequate time for exhalation (e.g., decreasing rate and tidal volume, increasing inspiratory flow rate, switching from assist-control to SIMV in selected cases). Additionally, measures aimed at reducing the work of breathing with mechanical ventilation may resolve the problem (e.g., low levels of PSV to patients taking spontaneous breaths). If these adjustments are unsuccessful, sedation should be attempted. Muscle paralysis should be reserved for patients in whom effective gas exchange and ventilation cannot be achieved with other measures.

o **Organ hypoperfusion or hypotension** can occur. Positive-pressure ventilation can result in decreased CO and BP by decreasing venous return to the right ventricle, increasing pulmonary vascular resistance, and impairing diastolic filling of the left ventricle because of increased right-sided heart pressures. Increasing the preload to the left ventricle with fluid administration should increase stroke volume and CO in most cases. Occasionally, the administration of dobutamine (after appropriate preload replacement) or vasopressors becomes necessary. Under these circumstances, consideration should be given to reducing airway pressures (peak airway pressures <40 cm H_2O) at the expense of relative hypoventilation (i.e., pressure-targeted ventilation).

o **Auto-PEEP** is the development of end-expiratory pressure caused by airflow limitation in patients with airway disease (emphysema, asthma), excessive minute ventilation, or an inadequate expiratory time. Graphic tracings on modern ventilators can suggest the presence of gas trapping by demonstrating persistent airflow at end expiration. The level of auto-PEEP can be estimated in the spontaneously breathing patient by occluding the expiratory port of the ventilator briefly just before inspiration and measuring the end-expiratory pressure reading on the ventilator's manometer. The presence of auto-PEEP can increase the work of breathing, contribute to barotrauma, and result in organ hypoperfusion by impairing CO. Appropriate adjustments to the ventilator can reduce or eliminate the presence of auto-PEEP.

- **Barotrauma or volutrauma** in the form of subcutaneous emphysema, pneumo peritoneum, pneumomediastinum, pneumopericardium, air embolism, and pneumothorax is associated with high peak airway pressures, PEEP, and auto-PEEP. Subcutaneous emphysema, pneumomediastinum, and pneumoperitoneum seldom threaten the patient's well-being. However, the occurrence of these disorders usually indicates a need to reduce peak airway pressures and the total level of PEEP. The occurrence of a pneumothorax is a potentially life-threatening complication and should be considered whenever airway pressure rises acutely, breath sounds are diminished unilaterally, or BP falls abruptly (for treatment, see Pneumothorax in Chapter 27, Medical Emergencies).
- **Positive fluid balance and hyponatremia** in mechanically ventilated patients often develop from several factors, including applied PEEP, humidification of inspired gases, administration of hypotonic fluids and diuretics, and increased levels of circulating antidiuretic hormone.
- **Cardiac arrhythmias**, particularly multifocal atrial tachycardia and atrial fibrillation, are common in respiratory failure and should be treated as outlined in Chapter 7, Cardiac Arrhythmias.
- **Aspiration** commonly occurs despite the use of a cuffed endotracheal tube, especially in patients who are receiving enteral nutrition. Elevating the head of the bed and avoiding excessive gastric distention help to minimize the occurrence of aspiration. Additionally, pooling of secretions around the cuff of the endotracheal tube requires suctioning of these secretions before deflation or manipulation of the cuff.
- **Ventilator-associated pneumonia (VAP)** is a frequent complication connected with increased patient morbidity and mortality. Prevention of VAP is aimed at avoiding colonization of pathogenic bacteria in the patient and their subsequent aspiration into the lower airway (*Semin Respir Crit Care Med 2006;27:5*).
- **Upper gastrointestinal (GI) hemorrhage** may develop secondary to gastritis or ulceration. The prevention of stress bleeding requires ensuring hemodynamic stability and, in high-risk patients (e.g., those receiving prolonged mechanical ventilation [>48 to 72 hours] or with a coagulopathy), the administration of proton pump inhibitors, H_2-receptor antagonists, antacids, or sucralfate.
- **Acid–base complications** are common in the critically ill patient
  - **Nonanion gap metabolic acidosis** may render weaning difficult, as minute ventilation must increase to normalize pH.
  - **Metabolic alkalosis** may compromise weaning by blunting ventilatory drive to maintain a normal pH. In patients with chronic ventilatory insufficiency (e.g., emphysema, cystic fibrosis), correction of metabolic alkalosis usually is inappropriate and can cause an unsustainable minute ventilation requirement. Under these circumstances, a patient should be allowed to adjust minute ventilation gradually to a more appropriate level. This change may be facilitated by switching from ACV to SIMV or PSV.
  - **Respiratory alkalosis** may develop rapidly during mechanical ventilation. When severe, it can lead to arrhythmias, CNS disturbances (including seizures), and a decrease in CO. Changing the ventilator settings to reduce the minute ventilation or changing the mode of ventilation (ACV to SIMV) usually corrects the alkalosis. However, some patients (such as those with ARDS, interstitial lung disease, pulmonary embolism, asthma) are driven to high respiratory rates

by local pulmonary stimuli. In such patients, sedation with or without paralysis may be indicated briefly during the acute phase of the respiratory compromise.

○ **Oxygen toxicity** commonly is accepted to occur when an FIO_2 of >0.6 is administered, particularly for more than 48 hours. However, the highest FIO_2 necessary should be used initially to maintain the SaO_2 at >0.9. The application of PEEP or other maneuvers that increase mean airway pressure (e.g., IRV) can be used to reduce FIO_2 requirements. However, an FIO_2 of 0.6 to 0.8 should be accepted before a plateau pressure above 30 cm H_2O is accepted. This caution-ary note is due to the greater risk of morbidity associated with plateau pressures above this level (*N Engl J Med 1998;338:347*).

• **Weaning from mechanical ventilation:** Weaning is the gradual withdrawal of mechanical ventilatory support (*Thorax 2005;60:175*). Successful weaning depends on the condition of the patient and on the status of the cardiovascular and respiratory systems. In patients who have had brief periods of mechanical ventilation, the manner in which ventilatory support is discontinued often is not crucial. In patients with marginal respiratory function, chronic underlying lung disease, or incompletely resolved respiratory impairment, the approach to weaning may be critical to obtain-ing a favorable outcome. In general, the level of supported ventilation (minute ventilation) is decreased gradually, and the patient assumes more of the work of ventilation with each of the techniques described. However, it is important not to fatigue the patient excessively, which can prolong the duration of mechanical ventilation.

○ **IMV** allows a progressive change from mechanical ventilation to spontaneous breathing by decreasing the ventilator rate gradually. However, the weaning process may be prolonged if ventilator changes are not made often enough. Prolonged periods at low rates (<6 breaths/min) may promote a state of respiratory muscle fatigue because of the imposed work of breathing through a high-resistance ventilator circuit. The addition of PSV may alleviate this fatigue but can prolong the weaning process if not titrated appropriately. Very often, tachypnea that occurs during weaning of the IMV rate represents a problem related to the imposed work from the ventilator circuit and the endotracheal tube rather than a diagnosis of persistent respiratory failure. In circumstances in which this problem is suspected, a trial of extubation may be appropriate.

○ **T-tube technique** intersperses periods of unassisted spontaneous breathing through a T tube (or other continuous-flow circuit) with periods of ventilator support. A once-daily spontaneous breathing trial using this technique resulted in faster extubation when compared to IMV and PSV (*N Engl J Med 1995;332:345*). Intermittent trials of spontaneous breathing (5 to 15 minutes two to four times per day followed by a progressive increase in duration) can also be used. Small amounts of CPAP (3 to 5 cm H_2O) during these periods may prevent distal airway closure and atelectasis, although the effects on weaning success appear to be negligible (*Chest 1991;100:1655*). Similar to IMV weaning, small amounts of pressure support (4 to 8 cm H_2O) can be used to decrease inspiratory resistance imposed by the ventilator circuit and the endotracheal tube. Extubation may be appropriate when the patient can comfortably tolerate more than 30 to 90 minutes of T-tube ventilation. More prolonged periods of T-tube breathing may produce fatigue, especially when small endotracheal tubes (<8 mm internal diameter) are used.

○ **PSV** is preferred by some practitioners when respiratory muscle weakness appears to be compromising weaning success (*Am J Respir Crit Care Med 1994;150:896*).

PSV can reduce the patient's work of breathing through the endotracheal tube and the ventilator circuit. The optimal level of PSV is selected by increasing the PSV level from a baseline of 15 to 20 cm H_2O in increments of 3 to 5 cm H_2O. A decrease in respiratory rate with achieved tidal volumes of 10 to 12 mL/kg signals that the optimal PSV level has been reached. When the patient is ready to begin weaning, the level of PSV is reduced gradually by 3- to 5-cm H_2O increments. Once a PSV level of 5 to 8 cm H_2O is reached, the patient can be extubated without further decreases in PSV.

○ **Protocol-guided weaning of mechanical ventilation** has been safely and successfully used by nonphysicians (*J Trauma 2004;56:943*). The use of protocols or guidelines can reduce the duration of mechanical ventilation by expediting the weaning process.

• **Failure to wean:** Patients who do not wean from mechanical ventilation after 48 to 72 hours of the resolution of their underlying disease process need further investigation. Key factors should be considered when weaning failure occurs. The acronym **"WEANS NOW"** (Table 8-3) has been developed to aid in addressing

Table 8-3	Factors to be Considered in the Weaning Process

Weaning parameters
See Table 8-4.
Endotracheal tube
Use largest tube possible.
Consider use of supplemental pressure-support ventilation.
Suction secretions.
Arterial blood gases
Avoid or treat metabolic alkalosis.
Maintain PaO_2 at 60–65 mm Hg to avoid blunting of respiratory drive.
For patients with carbon dioxide retention, keep $PaCO_2$ at or above the baseline level.
Nutrition
Ensure adequate nutritional support.
Avoid electrolyte deficiencies.
Avoid excessive calories.
Secretions
Clear regularly.
Avoid excessive dehydration.
Neuromuscular factors
Avoid neuromuscular-depressing drugs.
Avoid unnecessary corticosteroids.
Obstruction of airways
Use bronchodilators when appropriate.
Exclude foreign bodies within the airway.
Wakefulness
Avoid oversedation.
Wean in morning or when patient is most awake.

$PaCO_2$, arterial carbon dioxide tension; PaO_2, arterial oxygen tension.

Table 8-4	Guidelines for Assessing Withdrawal of Mechanical Ventilation

Patient's mental status: awake, alert, cooperative
PaO_2 >60 mm Hg with an FIO_2 <50%
PEEP ≤5 cm H_2O
$PaCO_2$ and pH acceptable
Spontaneous tidal volume >5 mL/kg
Vital capacity >10 mL/kg
MV <10 L/min
Maximum voluntary ventilation double of MV
Maximum negative inspiratory pressure >25 cm H_2O
Respiratory rate <30 breaths/min
Static compliance >30 mL/cm H_2O
Rapid shallow breathing index (ratio of respiratory rate to tidal volume) <100 breaths/min/L
Stable vital signs after a 1- to 2-hr spontaneous breathing trial

FIO_2, inspired oxygen concentration; MV, minute ventilation; $PaCO_2$, arterial carbon dioxide tension; PaO_2, arterial oxygen tension; PEEP, positive end-expiratory pressure.

each of these factors. Commonly used parameters can be assessed in predicting weaning success (Table 8-4).

- **Extubation**
  - Usually, extubation should be performed early in the day, when full ancillary staff are available. The patient should be clearly educated about the procedure, the need to cough, and the possible need for reintubation. Elevation of the head and trunk to more than 30 to 45 degrees improves diaphragmatic function. Equipment for reintubation should be available, and a high-humidity, oxygen-enriched gas source with a higher-than-current FIO_2 setting should be available at the bedside. The patient's airway and the oropharynx above the cuff should be suctioned. The cuff of the endotracheal tube should be deflated partially, and airflow around the outside of the tube—a cuff-leak indicating the absence of airway obstruction—should be detected. After the cuff is deflated completely, the patient should be extubated, and high-humidity oxygen should be administered by a face mask. Coughing and deep breathing should be encouraged while the examiner monitors the patient's vital signs and upper airway for stridor. Postextubation stridor may result from glottic and subglottic edema, and the lack of a cuff-leak prior to extubation increases the risk for this complication. Intravenous corticosteroids can reduce the rate of postextubation stridor in high-risk patients (*Crit Care Med 2006;34:1345*). If stridor occurs and clinical status permits, treatment with nebulized 2.5% racemic epinephrine (0.5 mL in 3 mL normal saline) should be administered. If upper airway obstruction persists or worsens, reintubation should be performed.
  - Extubation should not be reattempted for 24 to 72 hours after reintubation for upper airway obstruction. Otolaryngology consultation may be beneficial to exclude other causes of upper airway obstruction and to perform tracheostomy if upper airway obstruction persists.

○ Patients with chronic lung disease may benefit from noninvasive positive-pressure ventilation after extubation especially if hypercapnia develops during an otherwise successful spontaneous breathing trial (*Lancet 2009;374:1082*).

• **Medications:** Drugs are commonly used in the ICU to facilitate tracheal intubation and mechanical ventilation (Table 8-5). Daily sedation holidays to avoid oversedation and delirium should occur and be paired with spontaneous breathing trials when appropriate (*Lancet 2008;371:1226*). Nondepolarizing muscle relaxants have been implicated in muscle dysfunction and prolonged weakness after their use in ICU patients (*Curr Opin Crit Care 2004;10:47*). Some reports suggest a drug interaction between muscle relaxants and glucocorticoids, potentiating this effect. To minimize the chances of this complication, the use of muscle relaxants should be limited to as brief a period as possible. Peripheral nerve stimulators should be used to titrate the dose of the muscle relaxant to the lowest effective dose. Glucocorticoids should be avoided in patients who are receiving muscle relaxants unless their use is clearly indicated (e.g., for status asthmaticus, anaphylactic shock).

Shock

GENERAL PRINCIPLES

Circulatory shock is a process in which blood flow and oxygen delivery to tissues are disturbed. This event leads to tissue hypoxia, with resultant compromise of cellular metabolic activity and organ function. Oliguria, diminished mental status, and decreased peripheral pulses represent the major clinical manifestations of circulatory shock. Survival from shock is related to the adequacy of the initial resuscitation and the degree of subsequent organ system dysfunction. The main goal of therapy is rapid cardiovascular resuscitation with the reestablishment of tissue perfusion using fluid therapy and vasoactive drugs. The definitive treatment of shock requires reversal of the underlying etiologic process.

• **Resuscitative principles**
  ○ **Fluid resuscitation** is usually the first treatment used. All patients in shock should receive an initial IV fluid challenge. Determination of fluid responsiveness should be based on changes in clinical parameters, including arterial BP, urine output, cardiac filling pressures, and CO. The amount of fluid required to maintain tissue perfusion is variable, and exuberant resuscitation without clinical response can lead to pulmonary edema and increased intracranial pressure. Recent evidence in African children challenges traditional fluid resuscitation guidelines (*N Engl J Med 2011;364:2483*). Crystalloid fluid solutions (0.9% sodium chloride or Ringer's lactate) are usually administered, owing to their lower cost and comparable efficacy compared to colloid solutions (5% and 25% albumin, 6% hetastarch, dextran 40, and dextran 70). Blood products should be administered to patients with significant anemia or active hemorrhage. Young, adequately resuscitated patients usually tolerate hematocrits of 20% to 25%. In older patients, individuals with atherosclerosis, and patients who exhibit ongoing anaerobic metabolism, hematocrits of 30% or greater may be required to optimize oxygen delivery to tissues.
  ○ **Vasopressors and inotropes** play a crucial role in the management of shock states. Their use usually requires monitoring with intra-arterial and/or PA catheters (PACs).

Table 8-5	Intensive Care Unit Drugs to Facilitate Endotracheal Intubation and Mechanical Ventilation			
Drug	Bolus Dosages (IV)	Continuous-infusion Dosages[a]	Onset	Duration after Single Dose
Succinylcholine[b]	0.3–1 mg/kg	—	45–60 s	2–10 min
Pancuronium	0.05–0.1 mg/kg	1–2 mcg/kg/min	2–4 min	60–90 min
Vecuronium	0.08–0.1 mg/kg	0.3–1 mcg/kg/min	2–4 min	30–45 min
Atracurium	0.2–0.6 mg/kg	5–15 mcg/kg/min	2–4 min	20–35 min
Lorazepam[a]	0.03–0.1 mg/kg	0.01–0.1 mg/kg/hr, titrate to effect	5–20 min	2–6 hr[c]
Midazolam[a]	0.02–0.08 mg/kg	0.04–0.2 mg/kg/hr, titrate to effect	1–5 min	30–60 min[c]
Morphine	0.01–0.15 mg/kg	0.1–0.5 mg/kg/hr, titrate to effect	2–10 min	2–4 hr[c]
Fentanyl	0.35–1.5 mcg/kg	1–10 mcg/kg/hr, titrate to effect	30–60 s	30–60 min[c]
Thiopental	50–100 mg; repeat up to 20 mg/kg	—	20 s	10–20 min
Methohexital	1–1.5 mg/kg	—	15–45 s	5–20 min
Etomidate[b]	0.3–0.4 mg/kg	—	10–20 s	4–10 min
Propofol	0.25–0.5 mg/kg	25–80 mcg/kg/min	15–60 s	3–10 min[c]
Dexmedetomidine	1 mcg/kg	0.2–0.7 mcg/kg/hr	10 min	30 min

[a]A continuous infusion should be started or titrated upward only after the desired level of sedation is achieved with bolus administration.

[b]Use only in the process of rapid sequence intubation.

[c]Duration is prolonged with continuous intravenous administration. Frequent titration to the minimum effective dose is required to prevent accumulation of drug.

- **Dopamine** is capable of stimulating cardiac β_1-receptors, peripheral α-receptors, and dopaminergic receptors in renal, splanchnic, and other vascular beds. The effects of dopamine are dose dependent. At dosages of <5 mcg/kg/min, dopamine primarily acts as a vasodilator, increasing renal and splanchnic blood flow. At dosages of 5 to 10 mcg/kg/min, dopamine increases cardiac contractility and CO via the activation of cardiac β_1-receptors. At higher dosages (>10 mcg/kg/min), dopamine increases the BP by activation of peripheral α-receptors.
- **Dobutamine** is an inotropic agent that is generally considered a selective β_1-agonist. It exerts powerful inotropic effects, reduces afterload by indirect (reflex) peripheral vasodilation, and is a relatively weak chronotropic agent, accounting for its favorable hemodynamic response (increased stroke volume with modest increases in heart rate unless used in high dose or in the setting of hypovolemia).
- **Epinephrine** has α_1- and nonselective β-adrenergic activity. It is the agent of choice for anaphylactic shock. Like dopamine, its effects are dose dependent.
- **Norepinephrine** also has α_1- and β_1-adrenergic activity but primarily is a potent vasoconstricting agent. It is the preferred agent in septic shock.
- **Vasopressin** is a vasoconstrictor mediated by three different G-peptide receptors called V_{1a}, V_{1b}, and V_2. The usual dose of vasopressin for hypotension is 0.01 to 0.04 U/min (*Crit Care Med 2008;36:296*).
- **Milrinone** is a noncatecholamine inhibitor of phosphodiesterase III that acts as an inotrope and a direct peripheral vasodilator to increase CO.

Classification

- **Hypovolemic shock** results from a decrease in effective intravascular volume that decreases venous return to the right ventricle (Table 8-6). Significant hypovolemic shock (i.e., >40% loss of intravascular volume) that lasts for more than several hours is often associated with a fatal outcome despite resuscitative efforts. Therapy

Table 8-6	Hemodynamic Patterns Associated with Specific Shock States							
Type of Shock	**CI**	**SVR**	**PVR**	**SvO₂**	**RAP**	**RVP**	**PAP**	**PAOP**
Cardiogenic (e.g., MI, cardiac tamponade[a])	↓	↑	N	↓	↑	↑	↑	↑
Hypovolemic (e.g., hemorrhage)	↓	↑	N	↓	↓	↓	↓	↓
Distributive (e.g., septic)	N–↑	↓	N	N–↑	N–↓	N–↓	N–↓	N–↓
Obstructive (e.g., massive pulmonary embolism)	↓	↑–N	↑	N–↓	↑	↑	↑	N–↓

[a]Equalization of RAP, PAOP, diastolic PAP, and diastolic RVP establishes a diagnosis of cardiac tamponade.
CI, cardiac index; MI, myocardial infarction; N, normal; PAOP, pulmonary artery occlusion pressure; PAP, pulmonary artery pressure; PVR, pulmonary vascular resistance; RAP, right atrial pressure; RVP, right ventricular pressure; SvO₂, mixed venous oxygen saturation; SVR, systemic vascular resistance.

of hypovolemic shock usually is aimed at reestablishing the adequacy of the intravascular volume. At the same time, ongoing sources of volume loss, such as bleeding, may require surgical intervention. Crystalloid solutions are used initially for the resuscitation of patients in hypovolemic shock. Fluid resuscitation must be prompt and should be given through large-bore catheters placed in large peripheral veins. Rapid infusers can be used to increase the rate of fluid resuscitation. In the absence of overt signs of CHF, the patient should receive a 500- to 1,000-mL initial bolus of normal saline or Ringer's lactate, with further infusions adjusted to achieve adequate BP and tissue perfusion. When shock is due to hemorrhage, packed red blood cells (RBCs) should be given as soon as feasible. When hemorrhage is massive, type-specific unmatched blood can be given safely. Rarely, type O-negative blood is needed.

- **Cardiogenic shock** is seen most commonly after acute myocardial infarction (see Chapter 4, Ischemic Heart Disease) and usually is the result of pump failure. Other causes of cardiogenic shock include septal wall rupture, acute mitral regurgitation, myocarditis, dilated cardiomyopathy, arrhythmias, pericardial tamponade, and right ventricular failure due to pulmonary embolism. Cardiogenic shock secondary to acute myocardial infarction usually is associated with hypotension (mean arterial BP [MAP] <60 mm Hg), decreased cardiac index (<2.0 L/min/m^2), elevated intracardiac pressures (pulmonary artery occlusive pressure [PAOP] >18 mm Hg), increased peripheral vascular resistance, and organ hypoperfusion (e.g., decreased urine output, altered mentation).

  ○ **Certain general measures should be undertaken.** A PaO$_2$ of >60 mm Hg should be achieved, and the hematocrit should be maintained at ≥30%. Endotracheal intubation and mechanical ventilation should be considered to reduce the work of breathing and to increase juxtacardiac pressure (P$_{JC}$), which may improve cardiac function. Noninvasive mechanical ventilation with BiPAP can be used to accomplish similar end points in patients who are able to sustain spontaneous breathing. Careful attention to fluid management is necessary to ensure that an adequate preload is present to optimize ventricular function (especially in the presence of right ventricular infarction) and to avoid excessive volume administration with resultant pulmonary edema.

  ○ **Pharmacologic treatment** usually involves two classes of drugs: inotropes and vasopressors. Vasodilators generally are not used in patients with cardiogenic shock due to severe hypotension. The use of vasodilators can be considered after the patient's hemodynamics have stabilized as a means of improving left ventricular function. **Dopamine** has historically been administered first in patients with cardiogenic shock because it has inotropic and vasopressor properties. However, more side effects (e.g., arrhythmia) along with an increased mortality rate in a subgroup of patients with cardiogenic shock were noted when dopamine was compared to levophed (*N Engl J Med 2010;362:779*). A PAC can guide additional interventions, including inotropic support (dobutamine, milrinone), afterload reduction (nitroprusside), and fluid administration or diuresis for changes in intravascular volume.

  ○ **Mechanical circulatory assist devices** are required in patients who do not respond to medical therapy or who have specific conditions identified as the cause of shock (e.g., acute mitral valve insufficiency, ventricular septal defect). Intra-aortic balloon counterpulsation usually is performed with the device inserted percutaneously. The balloon filling is controlled electronically so that it is synchronized with the patient's electrocardiogram (ECG). The balloon inflates during diastole, improving coronary artery perfusion, and deflates during systole, reducing afterload and improving CO. In addition to intra-aortic balloon pumps, ventricular assist devices can be placed percutaneously to augment cardiac ouput. Both of these options should be considered only as an interim step to more definitive therapy.

○ **Definitive treatment** must be considered for any patient with cardiogenic shock. This treatment can take the form of relatively noninvasive procedures (e.g., angioplasty and/or percutaneous coronary intervention) or more invasive surgical procedures (e.g., coronary artery bypass surgery, valve replacement, heart transplantation).

• **Obstructive shock** usually is caused by massive pulmonary embolism. Occasionally, air embolism, amniotic fluid embolism, or tumor embolism also may cause obstructive shock. When shock complicates pulmonary embolism, therapy is directed toward preserving peripheral organ perfusion and removing the vascular obstruction. Fluid administration and the use of vasoconstrictors (e.g., norepinephrine, dopamine) may preserve BP while more definitive measures, such as thrombolytic therapy or surgical embolectomy, are considered.

• **Distributive shock** occurs primarily as septic shock or anaphylactic shock. These two forms are associated with significant decreases in vascular tone.

○ **Septic shock** is caused by the systemic release of mediators that is usually triggered by circulating bacteria or their products, although the systemic inflammatory response syndrome can be seen without evidence of infection (e.g., pancreatitis, crush injuries, and certain drug ingestions such as salicylates) (*N Engl J Med 2001;344:759*). Septic shock is characterized primarily by hypotension due to decreased vascular tone. CO is increased, owing to increased heart rate and end-diastolic volumes despite overall myocardial depression. The main goals of treatment of septic shock include initial fluid resuscitation, adequate treatment of underlying infection, and interruption of the mediator-associated systemic inflammatory response (Figure 8-1).

▪ **Fluid administration and vasoactive agents:** Initial goals of therapy include achieving a MAP >65 mm Hg, a central venous pressure (CVP) >8 mm Hg, and a central venous blood oxygen saturation ($ScvO_2$) >70% in order to promote adequate oxygen delivery and maintain tissue perfusion (*N Engl J Med 2001;345:1368*). Aggressive fluid resuscitation should be utilized early in the course of sepsis, but fluid responsiveness should be monitored closely to avoid overhydration. In fact, patients with acute lung injury (without evidence of organ hypoperfusion) may benefit from a more conservative fluid management strategy (*Chest 2005;128:3098*; *N Engl J Med 2006;354:2564*). Although a targeted CVP remains a component of early goal-directed therapy, pulse pressure variation, estimated stroke volume by esophageal Doppler, and direct measurement of CO via a PAC are probably more accurate predictors of volume responsiveness (*Chest 2008;134:172*). Vasopressors and inotropes may be required to achieve treatment goals. Catecholamines remain the first-line vasoconstrictor agents for hypotension refractory to fluid resuscitation, as no mortality benefit has been demonstrated for low-dose vasopressin (*N Engl J Med 2008;358:877*).

▪ **Relative adrenal insufficiency** can be associated with septic shock. Low-dose corticosteroids can shorten the time to shock reversal and the duration of vasopressor support, but their effect on survival remains controversial. Among patients with septic shock who were classified as nonresponders to a corticotropin test, a

Figure 8-1. Sepsis protocol.

7-day course of hydrocortisone and fludrocortisone was associated with a significant 28-day survival advantage (*JAMA 2002;288:862*). However, the mortality benefit noted earlier was not duplicated in a second multicenter trial (*N Engl J Med 2008;358:111*). Therefore, while a definitive recommendation cannot be made, corticosteroids should at least be considered in fluid-resuscitated, vasopressor-dependent patients.

- **Anaphylactic shock** is discussed further in the section Anaphylaxis in Chapter 11, Allergy and Immunology.

Hemodynamic Monitoring

GENERAL PRINCIPLES

- **Pulmonary artery catheterization**
  - **Indications**
    - The PAC allows measurement of intravascular and intracardiac pressures, CO, and PvO_2 and SvO_2.
    - A PAC can be placed to differentiate between cardiogenic and noncardiogenic forms of pulmonary edema, to identify the etiology of shock, to evaluate acute renal failure or unexplained acidosis, to evaluate cardiac disorders, or to monitor high-risk surgical patients in the perioperative setting.
  - **Method**
    - The PAC is advanced through a central vein after the distal balloon is inflated. Bedside waveform analysis is used to determine successful passage of the catheter through the right atrium, right ventricle, and PA into a PAOP position. Fluoroscopy should be used when difficulty is encountered in positioning the PAC.
    - If at any time after passage into the PA, the tracing is found to move off the scale of the graph, overwedging of the catheter has occurred. An overwedged catheter should be withdrawn immediately 2 to 3 cm after balloon deflation, and catheter positioning should then be rechecked with reinflation of the balloon. Overwedging of a PAC increases the likelihood of serious complications (e.g., PA rupture, pulmonary infarct).
    - Respiratory variation on the waveform, atrial pressure characteristics (including a and v waves), mean value of the PAOP tracing obtained at end expiration at less than the mean value of the PA pressure measurement, and the aspiration of highly oxygenated blood with the catheter in the PAOP position all indicate an accurate reading.
- **Transmural pressure:** When PEEP is present (applied or auto-PEEP), the positive intra-alveolar pressure at end expiration is transmitted through the lung to the pleural space. In these circumstances, the measured PAOP reflects the sum of the hydrostatic pressure within the vessel and the P_{JC}. When significant levels of total PEEP are present (>10 cm H_2O), it is more appropriate to use the transmural pressure as a measure of left ventricular filling (transmural pressure = PAOP – P_{JC}). For patients with normal lung compliance, one-half of the total PEEP can be used as an estimate of P_{JC}. When lung compliance is depressed significantly (e.g., in ARDS), one-third of the total PEEP can be used as an estimate for P_{JC}.
- **Cardiac output:** PACs are equipped with a thermistor to measure CO. At least two measurements that differ by $<10\%$ to 15% should be obtained. Injections should be synchronized with the respiratory cycle to minimize variability between results. Often, thermodilution measurements of CO are inaccurate at an extremely low CO (e.g., <1.5 L/min) or an extremely high CO (e.g., >7.0 L/min), in the presence of significant valvular disease (e.g., severe tricuspid insufficiency), or when large intracardiac shunts are present. Calculation of the CO using the **Fick formula** may be more accurate in these circumstances.
- **Interpretation of hemodynamic readings:** PAOP can be used as an index of left ventricular filling (preload) and as an index of the patient's propensity for development of pulmonary edema.

○ **Optimizing cardiac function:** Improving cardiac function by optimizing preload is more efficient in terms of myocardial oxygen consumption than similar improvements in cardiac function by use of inotropes when preload is inadequate. As a general rule, preload should be optimized before inotropic agents (which can increase myocardial oxygen consumption) or vasodilators (which can cause hypotension when preload is inadequate) are used. Fluid boluses should be administered in patients who are suspected of having inadequate cardiac filling pressures (i.e., inadequate preload) and should be followed by repeat measurements of PAOP, CO, heart rate, and stroke volume. In low CO states, if the PAOP increases by <5 mm Hg without significant changes in heart rate, CO, and stroke volume, additional fluid boluses may have to be given. An increase in the PAOP by >5 mm Hg usually signals that adequate ventricular filling is being achieved. Once the patient's preload has been optimized, cardiac performance can be reassessed and, if necessary, further therapy with inotropes or with vasodilators can be initiated to achieve further improvements in cardiac performance and tissue perfusion.

○ **Reducing unnecessary lung water:** PAOP is a reflection of the lung's tendency to develop pulmonary edema. Decreased left ventricular compliance results in a "critical pressure" being reached sooner for similar volume changes as compared to a normally compliant left ventricle. This difference is due to the increased stiffness of the noncompliant ventricle that causes higher pressures to be achieved for similar changes in volume. To optimize cardiac performance and to minimize the tendency for pulmonary edema formation, PAOP should be kept at the lowest point at which cardiac performance is acceptable.

○ **Differentiating hydrostatic from nonhydrostatic pulmonary edema:** The management of pulmonary edema depends in large part on whether the excessive accumulation of lung water is due to increased hydrostatic pressures (e.g., left ventricular failure, mitral stenosis, acute volume overload), increased permeability of the alveolocapillary barrier (e.g., ARDS due to sepsis, aspiration, or trauma), or a combination of these factors. Clinical and radiographic criteria alone often are insufficient to determine the underlying mechanisms of pulmonary edema. In general, a PAOP of <18 mm Hg suggests that the primary mechanism of pulmonary edema is nonhydrostatic. Values >18 mm Hg support a hydrostatic cause for the increased lung water.

○ **Adequacy of organ perfusion:** Oxygen delivery to tissues depends on an intact respiratory system to provide oxygen for hemoglobin saturation, the concentration of hemoglobin, CO, tissue microcirculation, and the unloading of oxygen from hemoglobin for diffusion into the tissue beds. Oxygen delivery can be measured as the product of CO and arterial oxygen content (CaO_2). CaO_2 is the sum of hemoglobin-bound and dissolved oxygen. Inadequate organ perfusion generally is associated with elevated blood lactate levels and decreased SvO_2 (usually <0.6). Factors that contribute to a low SvO_2 include anemia, hypoxemia, inadequate CO, and increased oxygen consumption. Factors that may elevate measured SvO_2 despite tissue hypoxia include peripheral arteriovenous shunting, the blood flow maldistribution of sepsis or cirrhosis, and cellular poisoning, such as that associated with cyanide toxicity. In general, optimization of gas exchange and CO along with adequate hemoglobin (usually ≥10 g/dL) results in improved oxygen delivery to tissues.

• **Noninvasive hemodynamic monitoring:** The PAC remains the reference for hemodynamic monitoring, although the utility of this method is often limited by invasiveness and risks associated with catheter placement. Several noninvasive approaches have emerged as alternatives for CO monitoring, one of which is the esophageal Doppler that has become increasingly utilized in the ICU setting (*Crit Care Med 2002;6:216*). This method is based upon measurement of aortic blood flow velocity over time via a flexible esophageal probe containing a Doppler transducer (marketed as CardioQ, Deltex Medical Ltd., Chichester, UK). The measured aortic velocity–time integral and estimated aortic cross-sectional area are used to calculate stroke volume, CO, and systemic vascular resistance (SVR). Accuracy and reproducibility of the method is dependent upon proper probe positioning during data acquisition. Esophageal Doppler–derived measurements have been shown to correlate well with thermodilution values, although the method appears to systematically underestimate CO when compared to PAC-based measurements (*Am J Respir Crit Care Med 1998;158:77*).

9

Obstructive Lung Disease

Jeffrey J. Atkinson, Robert M. Senior, Ajay Sheshadri, and Mario Castro

Chronic Obstructive Pulmonary Disease

GENERAL PRINCIPLES

Definition

Chronic obstructive pulmonary disease (COPD) is a mostly preventable and treatable disorder characterized by expiratory airflow limitation that is not fully reversible. The airflow limitation is often progressive and associated with an abnormal inflammatory response of the lungs to noxious particles or gases, principally cigarette smoke (*GOLD Global Strategy for the Diagnosis, Management, and Prevention of Chronic Obstructive Pulmonary Disease [Updated 2011]. Available at www.goldcopd.com*). **The airflow obstruction in COPD is caused by emphysema and airway disease.**

- Emphysema is defined pathologically as permanent enlargement of air spaces distal to the terminal bronchiole accompanied by destruction of the alveolar walls and absence of associated fibrosis.
- The airway disease in COPD occurs principally in small airways (i.e., those with an internal diameter of less than 2 mm. Chronic bronchitis is a common feature of COPD. Chronic bronchitis is defined clinically as productive cough on most days for at least 3 consecutive months per year for at least 2 consecutive years, in the absence of other lung disease that could account for this symptom. Individuals with chronic bronchitis but without airflow obstruction do not have COPD.

Epidemiology

- Although the prevalence of COPD is difficult to determine, it is estimated to affect 10 to 24 million Americans.
- COPD and other chronic lower respiratory diseases represent the third leading cause of death in the United States (*Nat Vital Stat Reports 2011;59(4)*).
- In the United States, the age-adjusted mortality rate remains higher among Caucasians compared with African Americans, Hispanics, or Pacific Islanders, but rate differences between men and women have closed.

Etiology

- Most cases of COPD are attributable to **cigarette smoking**. Although only a minority of cigarette smokers develops clinically significant COPD, a much higher proportion develops abnormal lung function (*Lancet 2011;378:991*).
- **Environmental (e.g., wood-burning stoves) and occupational dusts, fumes, gases, and chemicals** are other etiologic agents of COPD. Household indoor air pollution is a major cause of fatal COPD in underdeveloped countries (*Science 2011;334:180*).

- **α_1-Antitrypsin deficiency** is found in 1% to 2% of COPD patients. Clinical characteristics of affected patients may include a minimal smoking history, early-onset COPD (e.g., younger than 45 years of age), a family history of lung disease, or lower lobe–predominant emphysema. Despite its relative rarity, some authorities recommend diagnostic testing for this condition in all patients with COPD (*Am J Respir Crit Care Med 2003;168:818*).

Pathophysiology

- Processes in the lungs and airways important in the pathogenesis of COPD include inflammation, immune reactions, imbalance of proteinases and antiproteinases, turnover of extracellular matrix, oxidative stress, and apoptosis.
- Pathologic features include destruction of alveolar tissue and small airways, airway wall inflammation, edema and fibrosis, and intraluminal mucus.
- Pulmonary function changes include decreased maximal expiratory airflow, hyperinflation, air trapping, and alveolar gas exchange abnormalities.
- An increased incidence of osteoporosis, skeletal muscle dysfunction, and coronary artery disease occur in COPD, perhaps indicating a systemic component of inflammation (*Chest 2005;128:2640*).

Prevention

- **Abstinence from smoking is the most effective measure for preventing COPD.**
- In patients with COPD, smoking cessation may result in a reduction in the rate of lung function decline (*Am J Respir Crit Care Med 2002;166:675*) and improves survival (*Ann Intern Med 2005;142:233*).
- Tobacco dependence warrants repeated treatment until patients stop smoking (*N Engl J Med 2011;365:1222*). Most smokers fail initial attempts at smoking cessation, and relapse reflects the nature of the dependence and not the failure of the patient or the physician.
- A multimodality approach is recommended to optimize smoking quit rates.
  - Counseling on the preventable health risks of smoking, providing advice to stop smoking, and encouraging patients to make further attempts to stop smoking even after previous failures
  - Providing smoking cessation materials to patients
  - Prescribing pharmacotherapy (Table 9-1)
- Formal smoking cessation programs, often administered in a group setting, can be effective (*Cochrane Database Syst Rev 2002;(3):CD001007*).
- The U.S. Department of Health and Human Services has developed a telephone-based support system (1-800-QUIT NOW) with an Internet analog (1800quitnow.cancer.gov).

DIAGNOSIS

Clinical Presentation

History

- Common symptoms of COPD are dyspnea on exertion, cough, sputum production, and wheezing.
- Typically, dyspnea on exertion progresses gradually over years.
- Significant nocturnal symptoms should lead to a search for comorbidities, such as gastroesophageal reflux, congestive heart failure, or sleep-disordered breathing.
- Clinicians should obtain a lifelong smoking history and quantify exposure to environmental and occupational risk factors.

Table 9-1	Pharmacotherapy for Smoking Cessation

Nicotine Replacement Therapy[a]

Product	Dosing	Side Effects/Precautions
Transdermal patch	7, 14, or 21 mg/24 hr Usual regimen = 21 mg/d × 6 wk, 14 mg/d × 2 wk, 7 mg/d × 2 wk[b]	(Apply to all nicotine products) Headache, insomnia, nightmares, nausea, dizziness, blurred vision
Chewing gum, lozenges	2–4 mg q1–8h Gradually taper use	
Inhaler	10 mg/cartridge (4 mg delivered dose) 6–16 cartridges/d	
Nasal spray	0.5 mg/spray 1–2 sprays in each nostril q1h	

Nonnicotine Pharmacotherapy

Bupropion ER (*Zyban*)	150 mg/d × 3 d, then bid × 7–12 wks Start 1 wk before quit date	Dizziness, headache, insomnia, nausea, xerostomia, hypertension, seizure Avoid monoamine oxidase inhibitors
Varenicline (*Chantix*)	0.5 mg/d × 3 d, bid × 4 d, then 1 mg bid × 12–24 wk Start 1 wk before quit date	Nausea, vomiting, headache, insomnia, abnormal dreams Worsening of underlying psychiatric illness

[a]Combination therapy is often employed. A long-acting product (e.g., patch) is used for basal nicotine replacement, with a short-acting product (e.g., inhaler) used for breakthrough cravings.
[b]If patient smokes less than a half pack per day, start at 14-mg dose.
See also *N Engl J Med* 365;1222;2011 for strategies and approach.

- Weight loss often occurs in patients with end-stage COPD, but other etiologies, such as malignancy and depression, should be sought.
- Although dyspnea contributes predominantly to the morbidity of COPD, death in patients with COPD commonly results from cardiovascular disease, lung cancer, or nonlung cancers (*Chest 2005;128:2640*).

Physical Examination
- Until significant reduction of lung function occurs (e.g., forced expiratory volume in 1 second [FEV_1] <50% predicted), physical signs of COPD are usually not present.
- Patients with severe COPD may exhibit prolonged (>6 seconds) breath sounds on a maximal forced exhalation, decreased breath sounds, use of accessory muscles of respiration, and hyperresonance to chest percussion. Expiratory wheezing may or may not be present.
- Signs of pulmonary hypertension (PH) and right heart failure may be present.

- **Clubbing is not a feature of COPD**, so its presence should prompt an evaluation for other conditions, especially lung cancer.

Differential Diagnosis

Airway tumors, asthma, bronchiectasis, chronic pulmonary thromboembolic disease, congestive heart failure, cystic fibrosis, constrictive bronchiolitis, diffuse panbronchiolitis, eosinophilic granuloma, ischemic heart disease, lymphangioleiomyomatosis, mycobacterial infection (tuberculous and nontuberculous), tracheobronchomalacia, and tracheal stenosis all must be considered as part of the differential in the workup of COPD.

Diagnostic Testing

- Consider the diagnosis of COPD in any patient with chronic cough, dyspnea, or sputum production as well as any patient with a history of exposure to COPD risk factors, especially cigarette smoking (*GOLD Global Strategy for the Diagnosis, Management, and Prevention of Chronic Obstructive Pulmonary Disease [Updated 2011]. Available at www.goldcopd.com*).
- **Pulmonary function testing**
  - A definite diagnosis of COPD requires the presence of expiratory airflow limitation on spirometry, measured as the forced expiratory volume in the first second/forced vital capacity (FEV_1/FVC) ratio. Although 0.7 is taken as the lower limit of normal for all adults, with advancing age, the ratio may decrease below 0.7 in individuals who are asymptomatic and have never smoked. Therefore, a reduced ratio should not be interpreted automatically as diagnostic of COPD. The FEV_1 is usually reduced.
  - The FEV_1 relative to the predicted normal defines the severity of expiratory airflow obstruction (Table 9-2) and is a predictor of mortality.
  - The FEV_1 is often used to assess the clinical course and response to therapy.
  - Spirometry may assist in the evaluation of worsened symptoms of unclear etiology.
  - The total lung capacity, functional residual capacity, and residual volume often increase to supernormal values in patients with COPD, indicating lung hyperinflation and air trapping.
  - The diffusing capacity for carbon monoxide (DLCO) may be reduced.

Laboratories

- A baseline arterial blood gas (ABG) is recommended for patients with severe COPD to assess for the presence and severity of hypoxemia and hypercapnia. Annual monitoring may be considered.
- An elevated venous bicarbonate may signify chronic hypercapnia.
- Polycythemia may reflect a physiologic response to chronic hypoxemia and inadequate supplemental oxygen use.

Imaging

- Chest radiographs are not sensitive for determining the presence of COPD, but they are useful for evaluating alternative diagnoses.
- Chest computed tomography (CT) without contrast can detect emphysema and other conditions associated with tobacco smoking and COPD, especially lung cancer (see Complications section). However, routine diagnostic chest CT adds little to management and is not required to exclude many alternative diagnoses, unless historical or examination findings suggest occult thromboembolic or interstitial lung disease.

Table 9-2	GOLD Classification of Chronic Obstructive Pulmonary Disease Severity[a]
Stage I: Mild	FEV_1/FVC <0.70 FEV_1 ≥80% predicted
Stage II: Moderate	FEV_1/FVC <0.70 FEV_1 50%–79% predicted
Stage III: Severe	FEV_1/FVC <0.70 FEV_1 30%–49% predicted
Stage IV: Very severe	FEV_1/FVC <0.70 FEV_1 <30% predicted or FEV_1 <50% predicted plus chronic respiratory failure[b]

[a]Based on postbronchodilator FEV_1.
[b]Chronic respiratory failure defined as arterial partial pressure of oxygen <60 mm Hg (8.0 kPa) with or without arterial partial pressure of CO_2 >50 mm Hg (6.7 kPa) while breathing air at sea level.
FEV_1, forced expiratory volume in 1 second; FVC, forced vital capacity.
Data from Global Initiative for Chronic Obstructive Lung Disease (GOLD) Global Strategy for the Diagnosis, Management, and Prevention of Chronic Obstructive Pulmonary Disease (Updated 2011). Available at www.goldcopd.com.

- With increasing severity of COPD, patients often develop radiographic signs of thoracic hyperinflation, including flattening of the diaphragm, increased retrosternal/retrocardiac air spaces, and lung hyperlucency with diminished vascular markings. Bullae may be visible. In severe disease, chest CT is utilized to determine candidacy for lung volume reduction surgery (LVRS) (see Treatment: Surgical Therapy section).

TREATMENT

- Long-term management of patients with COPD aims to improve quality of life, decrease the frequency and the severity of acute exacerbations, slow the progression of disease, and prolong survival.
- Of all chronic medical therapies, **only smoking cessation and the correction of hypoxemia with supplemental oxygen have been shown to improve survival** (*Ann Intern Med 2005;142:233*; *Cochrane Database Syst Rev 2005;(4):CD001744*). Among surgical interventions, LVRS improves survival in select patients (*Am J Respir Crit Care Med 2011;184:763*).
- COPD should be treated in a stepwise approach (Table 9-3).

Medications

A pharmacologic treatment plan (Table 9-4) is based on a patient's disease severity, response to specific medications, frequency of exacerbations, drug availability, affordability, and patient compliance.

- **Inhaled bronchodilators**
  - Inhaled bronchodilators are the foundation of COPD pharmacotherapy. They work mainly by relaxing airway smooth muscle tone. This results in a reduction in expiratory airflow obstruction.

Table 9-3	Stepwise Approach to Chronic Obstructive Pulmonary Disease Therapy
GOLD Stage	**Intervention**
Mild	Smoking cessation Vaccinations (influenza, pneumococcus) Short-acting β-agonist prn
Moderate	All of the above plus: Long-acting bronchodilator (one or more) Pulmonary rehabilitation Consider macrolide if frequent exacerbations
Severe	All of the above plus: Combination inhaled corticosteroid if repeated exacerbations Oxygen if needed Consider PDE4 inhibitor if chronic bronchitis and frequent exacerbations not controlled with inhaled therapies
Very severe	All of the above plus: Consider surgical treatments

PDE4, phosphodiesterase 4.
Data from Global Initiative for Chronic Obstructive Lung Disease (GOLD) Global Strategy for the Diagnosis, Management, and Prevention of Chronic Obstructive Pulmonary Disease (Updated 2011). Available at www.goldcopd.com.

○ Proper use of a metered-dose inhaler (MDI) results in equally effective drug delivery as use of a nebulizer in most patients (*Health Technol Assess 2001;5*). Health care providers should routinely assess patient MDI technique and provide training.

○ Long-acting inhaled anticholinergic agents result in significant improvements in lung function, quality of life, and COPD exacerbations, although the rate of decline of FEV_1 is unaffected (*N Engl J Med 2008;359:1543*).

○ Long-acting β-adrenergic agonists (LABAs) offer improvements that are at least similar to long-acting anticholinergic agents and inhaled corticosteroids (ICSs) (*Cochrane Database Syst Rev 2011;12*).

• **Inhaled corticosteroids**
  ○ The rationale for using ICSs stems from the central role of inflammation in the pathogenesis of COPD.
  ○ ICSs may increase the FEV_1, reduce the frequency of COPD exacerbations, and improve quality of life. They do not slow the rate of decline of lung function over time (*N Engl J Med 1999;340:1948*; *BMJ 2000;320:1297*; *Eur Respir J 2003;21:68*).

• **Combination therapy:** Compared to single-agent therapy, a combination of medications may yield superior efficacy while reducing the potential for toxicity. Some examples follow:
  ○ The combination of an ICS and a LABA is effective in reducing the rate of COPD exacerbations, but this benefit must be balanced against an increased risk of pneumonia (*N Engl J Med 2007;356:775*).

Table 9-4	Inhalational Pharmacotherapy for Stable Chronic Obstructive Pulmonary Disease[a]

Short-acting β-Agonists

Name	Dose	Side Effects[b]
Albuterol	MDI: 2 puffs q4–6h Nebulizer: 2.5 mg q6–8h MDI: 2 puffs q4–6h	Palpitations, tremor, anxiety, nausea/vomiting, throat irritation, dyspepsia, tachycardia, arrhythmia, hypertension
Levalbuterol (Xopenex)	Nebulizer: 0.63–1.25 mg q6–8h	Cardiovascular effects may be less common with levalbuterol

Long-acting β-Agonists

Salmeterol (Serevent)	DPI: 1 puff (50 mcg) bid MDI: 1 capsule (75 mcg) od	Headache, upper respiratory tract infection, cough, palpitations, fatigue, diarrhea
Formoterol (Foradil)	DPI: 1 puff (12 mcg) bid	
Arformoterol (Brovana)	Nebulizer: 15 mcg bid	
Indacaterol[c] (Arcapta)	MDI: 1 capsule (75 mcg) qd	

Anticholinergics[d]

Ipratropium (Atrovent)	MDI: 2 puffs q4–6h	Xerostomia, cough, nausea/vomiting, diarrhea, urinary retention
Tiotropium (Spiriva)	Nebulizer: 0.5 mg q6–8h DPI: 1 puff (18 mcg) qd	

Combination Medications

Albuterol/ Ipratropium (Combivent, DuoNeb)	MDI: 2 puffs qid Nebulizer: one 3-mL vial qid (each vial contains 2.5 mg Albuterol and 0.5 mg Ipratropium)	As above
Fluticasone/ Salmeterol (Advair)	DPI: 1 puff bid Recommended dose is 250 mcg Fluticasone/50 mcg Salmeterol Reduced exacerbations at 500 mcg Fluticasone/ 50 mcg Salmeterol	As above, plus lower respiratory tract infection (pneumonia) and oral candidiasis

(continued)

Table 9-4	Inhalational Pharmacotherapy for Stable Chronic Obstructive Pulmonary Disease[a] (Continued)

Name	Dose	Side Effects[b]
	Combination Medications (Continued)	
Budesonide/ Formoterol (Symbicort)	DPI: 2 puffs bid 160 mcg Budesonide/ 4 mcg Formoterol	

[a]Commonly used medications are listed. This table is not exhaustive.
[b]Only the most common side effects are listed.
[c]Indacaterol dosage approved in United States is lower than other countries including Canada.
[d]Short-acting anticholinergic therapy (e.g., ipratropium) is usually discontinued with initiation of long-acting anticholinergic therapy (e.g., tiotropium), since minimal additional benefit is expected, side effects may increase, and use of two inhaled anticholinergic agents has had limited evaluation.
DPI, dry powder inhaler; MDI, metered-dose inhaler.

○ Combination therapy with a LABA and a long-acting anticholinergic agent sustains improved lung function compared to either agent alone (*Eur Respir J 2005;26:214*).
○ Combining a short-acting β-agonist (SABA) with a short-acting anticholinergic agent results in a greater increase in FEV_1 than using either medication alone (*Chest 1994;105:1411*).
○ Questions remain regarding the value of the incremental gains of adding long-acting anticholinergic therapy to LABA/ICS combinations, suggesting a stepwise approach with individualized therapy based on symptoms and exacerbation frequency (*Cochrane Database Syst Rev 2011;9*).
• **Macrolide antibiotics** (e.g., azithromycin 250 mg q day)
○ May function as an anti-infective or direct anti-inflammatory in COPD
○ In patients with previous exacerbations, the frequency of subsequent exacerbations decreased by 19%. Improvement in clinical symptoms was modest but significant (*N Engl J Med 2011;365:689*).
○ The benefit may be greater in older individuals (>65 years) and milder disease (GOLD stage II) but may be absent in current smokers.
○ Hearing loss in the absence of tinnitus was reported, suggesting routine monitoring with audiometry should be considered with chronic therapy.
• **Phosphodiesterase 4 (PDE4) inhibitors** (e.g., roflumilast 500 mcg q day)
○ U.S. Food and Drug Administration (FDA) approved for a relatively narrow indication of severe chronic obstructive lung disease ($FEV_1 < 50\%$) and chronic bronchitis with frequent exacerbations, demonstrating a 17% reduction in exacerbations (*Lancet 2009;374:685*).
○ Appears to be safe when used as an additional therapy to chronic bronchodilators
○ Did not result in improvements in clinical symptoms possibly due to a higher frequency of side effects, particularly gastrointestinal, that limit the dose tolerated
○ Limited long-term data and the possibility of weight loss and increased psychiatric symptoms suggest close monitoring is indicated.

- **Theophylline**
  - Theophylline is a xanthine derivative with bronchodilator properties. Patients not responding adequately to inhaled bronchodilator therapy may benefit from the addition of theophylline, but potential toxicities and lack of data regarding efficacy in patients already on long-acting inhaled combination therapies limit its use.
  - Sustained-release theophylline is dosed once or twice a day. Serum levels should be maintained between 8 and 12 mcg/mL to avoid toxicity.
  - Side effects include anxiety, tremor, headache, insomnia, nausea, vomiting, dyspepsia, tachycardia, tachyarrhythmia, and seizure.
  - In the event of suspected toxicity, theophylline should be stopped and a serum level measured.
  - Patients with severe COPD may experience clinical deterioration with discontinuation of theophylline.
  - Theophylline clearance is increased in current smokers and reduced in the elderly and patients with liver disease or congestive heart failure.
- **Systemic corticosteroids** are not recommended for the long-term management of COPD due to an unfavorable side effect profile and limited efficacy. However, they are sometimes used in patients with severe disease who are not responding to other therapies. If used, chronic oral steroid therapy should be administered at the minimum effective dose and discontinued as soon as is feasible. Routine bone mineral density assessment to prevent complications of osteoporosis should be incorporated.
- **Intravenous (IV) α-1 antitrypsin (A1AT)** augmentation therapy may benefit select patients with severe A1AT deficiency and COPD (*Am J Respir Crit Care Med 2012;185:246*). Weekly infusion of 60 mg/kg is the standard treatment.
- For the treatment of stable COPD, antibiotics, mucolytics, antioxidants, immunoregulators, antitussives, vasodilators, respiratory stimulants, narcotics, and leukotriene inhibitors have not shown significant benefit.

Other Nonpharmacologic Therapies

- **Supplemental oxygen** decreases mortality and improves physical and mental functioning in hypoxemic patients with COPD.
  - A room-air resting ABG is the gold standard test for determining the need for supplemental oxygen. Pulse oximetry may be useful for routine checks after a baseline oxyhemoglobin saturation is assessed and compared for accuracy with the measured arterial oxyhemoglobin saturation (SaO_2).
  - Oxygen therapy is indicated for patients with an arterial partial pressure of oxygen (PaO_2) ≤ 55 mm Hg or an SaO_2 $\leq 88\%$, or if a patient has a PaO_2 < 60 mm Hg or an SaO_2 $< 90\%$ and evidence of PH, polycythemia (hematocrit $> 55\%$), or heart failure.
  - Supplemental oxygen requirements are typically greatest during exertion and least at rest while awake. Patients who require supplemental oxygen during exertion often need it during sleep as well. Although the exact amount of supplemental oxygen required during sleep can be measured with pulse oximetry, it is reasonable to initially estimate the amount needed by setting the oxygen flow rate at 1 L/min greater than that required during rest while awake.
  - The oxygen prescription should include the delivery system (compressed gas, liquid, or concentrator) and the required oxygen flow rates (liters per minute) for rest, sleep, and exercise.

- ○ Patients receiving long-term oxygen therapy should undergo reevaluation to assess oxygen requirements at least once a year.
- **Pulmonary rehabilitation** is a multidisciplinary intervention that improves symptoms and quality of life and reduces the frequency of exacerbations in patients with COPD (*Am J Respir Crit Care Med 2006;173:1390*). Components of a rehabilitation program include exercise training, nutritional counseling, and psychosocial support. Pulmonary rehabilitation should be considered for all patients with moderate-to-very severe COPD (*N Engl J Med 2009;360:1329*).
- **Vaccinations**
  - ○ Annual influenza vaccination reduces the incidence of influenza-related acute respiratory illnesses in COPD patients (*Chest 2004;125:2011*).
  - ○ Although pneumococcal vaccination has not been shown to significantly reduce morbidity and mortality in COPD patients, it is reasonable to give this vaccination every 5 years (*Cochrane Database Syst Rev 2006;(4):CD001390*).

Surgical Therapy

- **Lung transplantation** for severe COPD can improve quality of life and functional capacity. The data are conflicting regarding survival, and a consistent survival benefit has not been demonstrated.
  - ○ Selection criteria for transplantation for COPD patients include a BODE score (Table 9-8) (see Outcome/Prognosis section) of 7 to 10 or at least one of the following: history of hospitalization for a COPD exacerbation associated with acute hypercapnia ($PaCO_2$ >50); PH; right heart failure, or both, despite supplemental oxygen therapy; FEV_1 <20%; and either a DLCO <20% or homogeneous distribution of emphysema (*J Heart Lung Transplant 2006;25:745*).
- **LVRS** may provide quality of life and survival benefits in a specific subset of patients with upper lobe-predominant emphysema and significantly reduced exercise capacity (*Am J Respir Crit Care Med 2011;184(7):763*).

SPECIAL CONSIDERATIONS

Acute Exacerbation of COPD

- Increased dyspnea, often accompanied by increased cough, sputum production, sputum purulence, wheezing, chest tightness, or other symptoms (and signs) of acutely worsened respiratory status, in the absence of an alternative explanation, define a COPD exacerbation.
- Respiratory infections (viral and bacterial) and air pollution cause most exacerbations (*Thorax 2006;61:250*).
- The differential diagnosis includes pneumothorax, pneumonia, pleural effusion, congestive heart failure, cardiac ischemia, and pulmonary embolism.
- In addition to the history and physical examination, assessment of a patient with a suspected COPD exacerbation should include oxyhemoglobin saturation, ABG, electrocardiogram, and chest radiograph.
- Criteria for hospital admission include a significant increase in symptom severity, severe underlying COPD, significant comorbidities, failure to respond to initial medical management, diagnostic uncertainty, and insufficient home support (*GOLD Global Strategy for the Diagnosis, Management, and Prevention of Chronic Obstructive Pulmonary Disease [Update 2011]. Available at www.goldcopd.com*).

- Criteria for admission to an intensive care unit include the need for invasive mechanical ventilation, hemodynamic instability, severe dyspnea that does not adequately respond to therapy, mental status changes, and persistent or worsening hypoxemia, hypercapnia, or respiratory acidosis despite supplemental oxygen and noninvasive ventilation (*GOLD Global Strategy for the Diagnosis, Management, and Prevention of Chronic Obstructive Pulmonary Disease [Updated 2011]. Available at www.goldcopd.com*).
- **Pharmacotherapy** (Table 9-5)
  - ○ **SABAs are the first-line therapy for COPD exacerbations**. Short-acting anticholinergic agents can be added in the event of inadequate response to SABAs.

Table 9-5	Pharmacotherapy for Acute Exacerbations of Chronic Obstructive Pulmonary Disease
Medication Name	**Dose**
Albuterol	MDI: 2–4 puffs q1–4h Nebulizer: 2.5 mg q1–4h
Ipratropium	MDI: 2 puffs q4h Nebulizer: 0.5 mg q4h
Prednisone	30–40 mg/d × 7–10 d[a]

Antibiotics

Patient Characteristics	Pathogens to Consider	Antibiotic[b] (One of the Following)
No risk factors for poor outcome or drug-resistant pathogen[c]	*Haemophilus influenzae* *Streptococcus pneumoniae* *Moraxella catarrhalis*	Macrolide, second- or third-generation cephalosporin, Doxycycline, trimethoprim/sulfamethoxazole
Risk factors present	As above, plus gram-negative rods, including *Pseudomonas*	Antipseudomonal fluoroquinolone or β-lactam

[a]Indicated for all inpatients and most outpatients. Dosing recommendation from Global Initiative for Chronic Obstructive Lung Disease. *Global Strategy for the Diagnosis, Management, and Prevention of Chronic Obstructive Pulmonary Disease.* http://www.goldcopd.com. Updated 2011.
[b]Treat for 3 to 7 days. If recent antibiotic exposure, select an agent from an alternative class. Take local resistance patterns into account.
[c]Risk factors: age >65 years, comorbid conditions (especially cardiac disease), forced expiratory volume in 1 second (FEV_1) <50%, >3 exacerbations/yr, antibiotic therapy within the past 3 months (*Thorax 2006;61:337*).
MDI, metered-dose inhaler.

○ Many patients experiencing an acute exacerbation of COPD have difficulty performing optimal MDI technique. Therefore, numerous clinicians opt to deliver bronchodilators via nebulization.

○ Due to the risk of serious side effects, clinicians typically avoid using methylxanthines (e.g., theophylline) for acute exacerbations. However, if a patient uses methylxanthines chronically, discontinuation during an exacerbation is discouraged due to the risk of decompensation.

○ **Systemic corticosteroids** produce improvement in hospital length of stay, lung function, and the incidence of relapse. They are recommended for all inpatients and most outpatients experiencing an exacerbation of COPD (*N Engl J Med 2003;348:2618*; *N Engl J Med 1999;340:1941*; *Lancet 1999;354:456*).

○ **Antibiotic therapy** is routinely administered but most often benefits patients with sputum purulence as well as patients with a need for mechanical ventilation (*Ann Intern Med 1987;106:196*; *Chest 2000;117:1638*; *Lancet 2001;358:2020*).

• **Supplemental oxygen** should be administered with a target oxygen saturation of 88% to 92%.

• **Noninvasive ventilation** (Table 9-6) reduces intubation rate, improves respiratory acidosis, decreases respiratory rate, and decreases hospital length of stay (*BMJ 2003;326:185*).

• **Endotracheal intubation** and invasive mechanical ventilation are required in some patients (Table 9-7).

• Discharge criteria for patients with acute exacerbations of COPD include the need for inhaled bronchodilators less frequently than every 4 hours; clinical and ABG stability for at least 12 to 24 hours; the ability to eat, sleep, and ambulate fairly comfortably; adequate patient understanding of home therapy; and adequate home arrangements.

Table 9-6	Indications and Contraindications for Noninvasive Ventilation in Acute Exacerbations of Chronic Obstructive Pulmonary Disease

Indications	Contraindications
Moderate-to-severe dyspnea with evidence of increased work of breathing	Respiratory arrest
	Hemodynamic instability
	Altered mental status, inability to cooperate
Acute respiratory acidosis with pH ≤7.35 and/or $PaCO_2$ >45 mm Hg (6.0 kPa)	High risk of aspiration
	Viscous or copious secretions
	Recent facial or gastroesophageal surgery
Respiratory rate >25	Craniofacial trauma
	Fixed nasopharyngeal abnormalities
	Burns
	Extreme obesity

Data from Global Initiative for Chronic Obstructive Lung Disease (GOLD) Global Strategy for the Diagnosis, Management, and Prevention of Chronic Obstructive Pulmonary Disease (Updated 2011). Available at www.goldcopd.com.

Table 9-7	Indications for Invasive Mechanical Ventilation in Acute Exacerbations of Chronic Obstructive Pulmonary Disease

Failure to improve with or not a candidate for noninvasive ventilation (see Table 9-6)

Severe dyspnea with evidence of increased work of breathing

Acute respiratory acidosis with pH <7.25 and/or $PaCO_2$ >60 mm Hg (8.0 kPa)

PaO_2 <40 mm Hg (5.3 kPa)

Respiratory rate >35

Coexisting conditions such as cardiovascular disease, metabolic abnormalities, sepsis, pneumonia, pulmonary embolism, pneumothorax, large pleural effusion

Data from Global Initiative for Chronic Obstructive Lung Disease (GOLD) Global Strategy for the Diagnosis, Management, and Prevention of Chronic Obstructive Pulmonary Disease (Updated 2011). Available at www.goldcopd.com.

- Prior to discharge from the hospital, chronic therapy issues should be readdressed, including supplemental oxygen requirements, vaccinations, smoking cessation, assessment of inhaler technique, and pulmonary rehabilitation.

COMPLICATIONS

- Patients with severe COPD and chronic hypoxemia may develop PH and right-sided heart failure.
- COPD patients are at increased risk for lung cancer, ischemic heart disease, pneumothorax, arrhythmias, osteoporosis, and psychiatric disorders such as anxiety and depression.
  - Annual low-dose CT screening of heavy smokers (age >55 years, >30-pack year history) provides a 20% reduction in mortality from lung cancer. This must be balanced with the risk of invasive procedures from false-positive tests that were seen in approximately 40% of screened individuals (*N Engl J Med 2011;365:395*). In the largest screening trial, the majority of false-positive results could be resolved with repeat imaging.
  - Many patients with mild and moderate (GOLD stage I and II) COPD will die of cardiovascular disease. Therefore, cardioselective β-blockers should be utilized when indicated.
  - Osteoporosis and vitamin D deficiency are common in COPD and should be monitored and treated.
- Sleep disturbances are estimated to affect 50% of patients with COPD (*http://aarc.org/resources/confronting_copd/exesum.pdf*). Newer non-benzodiazepines medications such as zolpidem appear to be safe in patients with less severe COPD (*Proc Am Thorac Soc 2008;5:536*).

OUTCOME/PROGNOSIS

The BODE index (Table 9-8) is a composite of body mass index, airflow obstruction, dyspnea, and exercise tolerance that has been validated as a more accurate predictor of COPD mortality than FEV_1 alone (*N Engl J Med 2004;350:1005*).

Table 9-8	BODE Index			

Points on BODE Index[a]

Variable	0	1	2	3
FEV$_1$ (% of predicted)	≥65	50–64	36–49	≤35
Distance walked in 6 min (meters)	≥350	250–349	150–249	≤149
MMRC dyspnea scale	0–1	2	3	4
Body mass index	>21	≤21		

[a]The total possible cumulative values range from 0 to 10.
FEV$_1$, forced expiratory volume in 1 second; MMRC, Modified Medical Research Council.
From *N Engl J Med* 2004 Mar 4;350(10):1005–1012.

Asthma

GENERAL PRINCIPLES

Definition

- Asthma is an airway disease characterized by chronic inflammation, hyperresponsiveness with exposure to a wide variety of stimuli, and variable airflow obstruction. As a consequence, patients have paroxysms of cough, dyspnea, chest tightness, and wheezing.
- **Asthma is a chronic disease with episodic acute exacerbations that are interspersed with symptom-free periods.** Exacerbations are characterized by a progressive increase in asthma symptoms that can last minutes to hours. They are associated with viral infections, allergens, and occupational exposures and occur when airway reactivity is increased and lung function becomes unstable.

Classification

- Asthma severity should be classified based on both level of impairment (symptoms, lung function, and rescue medication use) and risk (exacerbations, lung function decline, medication side effects).
- At the initial evaluation, this assessment will determine the level of severity in patients not on controller medications (Table 9-9). The level of severity is based upon the most severe category in which any feature appears. On subsequent visits, or if the patient is on a controller medication, this assessment is based on the lowest step of therapy to maintain clinical control (Table 9-10). Control of asthma is based upon the most severe impairment or risk category.
- During an exacerbation, the acute severity of the attack should be classified based upon symptoms, signs, and objective measures of lung function (Table 9-11).
- Patients who have had two or more exacerbations requiring systemic corticosteroids in the past year may be considered in the same category as those who have persistent asthma, regardless of level of impairment.

Epidemiology

In the United States,

- Asthma is the leading chronic illness among children (20% to 30%) (*NCHS Data Brief 2012;1*).

Table 9-9	Classification of Severity on Initial Assessment			
	Intermittent	Mild Persistent	Moderate Persistent	Severe Persistent
Daytime symptoms	≤2 days/wk	≥2 days/wk but not daily	Daily	Throughout the day
Nighttime symptoms	≤2×/mo	3–4×/mo	≥1×/wk but not nightly	Nightly
Activity limitations	None	Minor	Some	Extreme
Reliever medicine use	≤2 days/wk	≥2 days/wk but not daily	Daily	Several times per day
FEV$_1$ or PEF	≥80%	≥80%	60×80%	<60%
Exacerbations	0–1×/yr	≥2×/yr	≥2×/yr	≥2×/yr
Management	Step 1	Step 2	Step 3 and consider short-course OCS	Step 4 or 5 and consider short-course OCS

FEV$_1$, forced expiratory volume in 1 second; OCS, oral corticosteroids PEF, peak expiratory flow.
Data from Global Initiative for Asthma. GINA report, global strategy for asthma management and prevention. http://www.ginasthma.org. 2011; National Asthma Education and Prevention Program. Expert Panel Report 3. http://www.nhlbi.nih.gov/guidelines/asthma/asthgdln.pdf. 2007.

Table 9-10	Assessment of Asthma Control		
	Well Controlled	Not Well Controlled	Very Poorly Controlled
Daytime symptoms	≤2 days/wk	>2 days/wk	Throughout the day
Nighttime symptoms	None	1–3×/wk	≥4×/wk
Activity limitations	None	Some	Extreme
Reliever medicine use	≤2×/wk	>2×/wk	Frequent
FEV$_1$ or PEF	≥80%	60%–80%	≤60%
Validated questionnaire	ACT ≥20 ACQ <0.75	ACT 16–19 ACQ >1.5	ACT ≤15
Exacerbations	0–1/yr	≥2×/yr	≥2×/yr
Management	Maintain at lowest step possible	Step up one step	Step up one to two steps and consider short-course OCS
Follow-up	1–6 mo	2–6 wk	2 wk

ACT, Asthma Control Test; ACQ, Asthma Control Questionnaire; FEV$_1$, forced expiratory volume in 1 second; OCS, oral corticosteroids PEF, peak expiratory flow.
Data from Global Initiative for Asthma. GINA report, global strategy for asthma management and prevention. http://www.ginasthma.org. 2011; National Asthma Education and Prevention Program. Expert Panel Report 3. http://www.nhlbi.nih.gov/guidelines/asthma/asthgdln.pdf

Table 9-11	Classification of Asthma Exacerbation Severity		
	Moderate	Severe	Impending Respiratory Arrest
FEV₁ or PEF predicted or personal best	40%–69%	<40%	<25% or unable to measure
Symptoms	DOE or SOB with talking	SOB at rest	Severe SOB
Exam	Expiratory wheeze	Inspiratory and expiratory wheeze	Wheeze may become absent
	Some accessory muscle use	Increased accessory muscle use Chest retraction	Accessory muscle use with paradoxical thoracoabdominal movement
		Agitation or confusion	Depressed mental status
Vitals	RR <28/min HR <110 O₂sat >91% RA No pulsus paradoxus	RR >28/min HR >110 O₂sat <91% RA Pulsus paradoxus >25 mm Hg	Same as severe but could develop respiratory depression and/or bradycardia
PaCO₂	Normal to hypocapnia	>42 mm Hg	Hypercapnia is a late sign

DOE, dyspnea on exertions; FEV₁, forced expiratory volume in 1 second; HR, heart rate; O₂sat, oxygen saturation; PEF, peak expiratory flow; RA, room air; RR, respiratory rate; SOB, shortness of breath.
Data from Global Initiative for Asthma. GINA report, global strategy for asthma management and prevention. http://www.ginasthma.org. 2011; National Asthma Education and Prevention Program. Expert Panel Report 3. http://www.nhlbi.nih.gov/guidelines/asthma/asthgdln.pdf. 2007.

- The prevalence of asthma and asthma-related mortality had been increasing from 1980 to the mid-1990s, but since the 2000s, a stabilization in prevalence and decrease in mortality has occurred. Currently, an estimated 300 million individuals are affected worldwide. An estimated 250,000 individuals worldwide die every year due to asthma (*GINA Report, Global Strategy for Asthma Management and Prevention, 2011, www.ginasthma.org*; National Asthma Education and Prevention Program Expert Panel Report 3, 2007, *http://www.nhlbi.nih.gov/guidelines/asthma/asthgdln.pdf*).
- African Americans are more likely than Caucasians to be hospitalized and have a higher rate of mortality due to asthma.

Etiology

Possible factors for asthma development can be broadly divided into host, genetic, and environmental factors.
- There have been multiple genes and chromosomal regions associated with the development of asthma. Racial and ethnic differences have also been reported

in asthma and are likely the result of a complex interaction between genetic, socioeconomic, and environmental factors.

- There are multiple environmental factors that contribute to the development and persistence of asthma. Severe viral infections early in life, particularly respiratory syncytial virus (RSV) and rhinovirus, are associated with the development of asthma in childhood and play a role in its pathogenesis.
- Childhood exposure and sensitization to a variety of allergens and irritants (e.g., cigarette smoke, mold, pet dander) may play a role in the development of asthma, but the exact nature of this relationship is not yet fully elucidated. The prevalence of asthma in children raised in a rural setting is reduced, although the reason for this is not fully known.

Pathophysiology

Asthma is characterized by airway obstruction, hyperinflation, and airflow limitation resulting from multiple processes:

- Acute and chronic airway inflammation characterized by infiltration of the airway wall, mucosa, and lumen by activated eosinophils, mast cells, macrophages, and T lymphocytes.
- Bronchial smooth muscle contraction resulting from mediators released by a variety of cell types including inflammatory, local neural, and epithelial cells.
- Epithelial damage manifested by denudation and desquamation of the epithelium leading to mucous plugs that obstruct the airway.
- Airway remodeling characterized by the following findings:
  ○ Subepithelial fibrosis, specifically thickening of the lamina reticularis from collagen deposition
  ○ Smooth muscle hypertrophy and hyperplasia
  ○ Goblet cell and submucosal gland hypertrophy and hyperplasia resulting in mucus hypersecretion
  ○ Airway angiogenesis
  ○ Airway wall thickening due to edema and cellular infiltration

Risk Factors

A number of factors increase airway hyperresponsiveness and can cause an acute and chronic increase in the severity of the disease:

- Allergens such as dust mites, cockroaches, pollens, molds, and pet dander in susceptible patients
- Viral upper respiratory tract infections
- Many occupational allergens and irritants such as perfumes, cleaners, or detergents, even in small doses
- Changes in weather (i.e., from warm to cold), strong emotional stimuli, and exercise
- Irritants, such as tobacco and wood smoke, can trigger acute bronchospasm and should be avoided by all patients.
- Medications such as β-blockers (including ophthalmic preparations), aspirin, and nonsteroidal anti-inflammatory drugs (NSAIDs) can cause the sudden onset of severe airway obstruction.

Prevention

- Strict compliance and appropriate follow-up can help prevent worsening of asthma control.

- Identification and avoidance of risk factors (allergens, irritants) that exacerbate symptoms play a key role in prevention.
- All patients with asthma should receive a yearly influenza vaccination.

Associated Conditions

- **Rhinosinusitis**, with or without nasal polyps, is frequently present and should be treated with intranasal corticosteroids, saline rinses, and/or antihistamines.
- **Vocal cord dysfunction (VCD)** can coexist or masquerade severe, uncontrolled asthma. Treatment consists of speech and, if needed, behavioral therapy.
- Symptomatic **gastroesophageal reflux disease (GERD)** can cause cough and wheezing in some patients and may benefit from treatment with H2 blockers or proton pump inhibitors. Empiric treatment of GERD in asymptomatic patients with uncontrolled asthma is not an effective strategy.
- **Obesity** is increasingly being recognized as a comorbid condition as well as possibly playing a role in worsening asthma control. This may be related to altered lung mechanics, altered respiratory patterns, or an increase in systemic inflammation. Obese patients should be strongly encouraged to focus on weight loss through diet and exercise.
- Smoking prevalence in patients with asthma is the same as the general population. Although no convincing evidence links tobacco use with developing asthma, it may make patients less responsive to ICSs and more difficult to control. Tobacco cessation should be encouraged in all patients.
- **Obstructive sleep apnea (OSA)** may make asthma more difficult to control and should be addressed with an overnight polysomnogram if suspected.

DIAGNOSIS

Clinical Presentation

History

- Recurring episodes of cough, dyspnea, chest tightness, and wheezing are suggestive of asthma. Symptoms occur most often at night or early morning, in the presence of potential triggers, and/or in a seasonal pattern.
- A personal or family history of atopy can increase the likelihood of asthma.
- Patients presenting for the first time over 50 years old or with >20-pack years of smoking are features that make asthma less likely as the sole cause of respiratory symptoms.

Physical Examination

- Auscultation of wheezing and a prolonged expiratory phase can be present on exam, but a normal chest exam does not exclude asthma.
- Signs of atopy, such as eczema, rhinitis, or nasal polyps, often coexist with asthma.
- During a suspected asthma exacerbation, a rapid assessment should be performed to identify those patients who require immediate intervention (Table 9-11).
  - Respiratory distress and/or peak expiratory flow (PEF) <25% of predicted.
  - The presence or intensity of wheezing is an unreliable indicator of the severity of an attack.
  - Subcutaneous emphysema should alert the examiner to the presence of a pneumothorax or pneumomediastinum.

Table 9-12	Conditions that Can Present as Refractory Asthma

Upper airway obstruction
Tumor
Epiglottitis
Vocal cord dysfunction
Obstructive sleep apnea
Lower airway disease
Allergic bronchopulmonary aspergillosis
Chronic obstructive pulmonary disease
Cystic fibrosis
Bronchiectasis
Bronchiolitis obliterans
Tracheomalacia
Endobronchial lesion
Foreign body
Herpetic tracheobronchitis

Congestive heart failure
Gastroesophageal reflux
Sinusitis
Hypersensitivity pneumonitis
Churg–Strauss syndrome
Eosinophilic pneumonia
Adverse drug reaction
Aspirin
β-Adrenergic antagonist
Angiotensin-converting enzyme
 inhibitors
Inhaled pentamidine
Hyperventilation with panic attacks
Dysfunctional breathlessness

Diagnostic Criteria

- In general, the diagnosis is supported by the presence of symptoms consistent with asthma combined with demonstration of variable expiratory airflow obstruction.
- Adequate response to asthma treatment is a valid method to assist with making the diagnosis.

Differential Diagnosis

Other conditions may present with wheezing and must be considered, especially in patients who are not responsive to therapy (Table 9-12).

Diagnostic Testing

Laboratories

- Routine laboratory tests are not indicated for the diagnosis of asthma and should not delay the initiation of treatment.
- During an exacerbation, monitor oxygen saturation. ABG measurement should be considered in patients in severe distress or with an FEV_1 of <40% of predicted values after initial treatment.
  - A PaO_2 <60 mm Hg is a sign of severe bronchoconstriction or of a complicating condition, such as pulmonary edema or pneumonia.
  - Initially, the $PaCO_2$ is low due to an increase in respiratory rate. With a prolonged attack, the $PaCO_2$ may rise as a result of severe airway obstruction, increased dead space ventilation, and respiratory muscle fatigue. **A normal or increased $PaCO_2$ is a sign of impending respiratory failure and necessitates hospitalization.**

Imaging

- Obtaining a chest radiograph is not routinely required and is performed only if a complicating pulmonary process, such as pneumonia or pneumothorax, is suspected or to rule out other causes of respiratory symptoms in patients being evaluated for asthma.
- Computerized tomography of the chest can be considered in patients with severe asthma refractory to treatment to evaluate for alternative diagnosis.

Diagnostic Procedures

- **Pulmonary function tests (PFTs)** are essential to the diagnosis of asthma. In patients with asthma, PFTs demonstrate an obstructive pattern—the hallmark of which is a decrease in expiratory flow rates.
  - A reduction in FEV_1 and a proportionally smaller reduction in the FVC occur. This produces a decreased FEV_1/FVC ratio (generally <0.7). With mild obstructive disease that involves only the small airways, the FEV_1/FVC ratio may be normal, with the only abnormality being a decrease in airflow at midlung volumes (forced expiratory flow 25% to 75%).
  - The clinical diagnosis of asthma is supported by an obstructive pattern that improves after bronchodilator therapy. **Improvement is defined as an increase in FEV_1 of >12% and 200 mL after two to four puffs of a short-acting bronchodilator.** Most patients will not demonstrate reversibility at each assessment.
  - In patients with chronic, severe asthma, the airflow obstruction may no longer be completely reversible. In these patients, the most effective way to establish the maximal degree of airway reversibility is to repeat PFTs after a course of oral corticosteroids (usually 40 mg/d for 10 to 14 days). The lack of demonstrable airway obstruction or reactivity does not rule out a diagnosis of asthma.
  - In cases in which spirometry is normal, the diagnosis can be made by showing heightened airway responsiveness to a **methacholine challenge**. A methacholine challenge is considered positive when a provocative concentration of 8 mg/mL or less causes a drop in FEV_1 of 20% (PC_{20}).
- An objective measurement of airflow obstruction is essential to the evaluation of an exacerbation. The severity of the exacerbation should be classified as
  - Mild (PEF or FEV_1 >70% of predicted or personal best)
  - Moderate (PEF or FEV_1 40% to 69%)
  - Severe (PEF or FEV_1 <40%)
  - Life-threatening/impending respiratory arrest (PEF or FEV_1 <25%)

TREATMENT

- Medical management involves chronic management and a plan for acute exacerbations, otherwise known as the **asthma action plan**. Most often, it includes the daily use of an anti-inflammatory, disease-modifying medication (long-term control medications) and as needed use of a short-acting bronchodilator (quick-relief medications).
- The goals of daily management are to **avoid impairment** (lack of symptoms while maintaining normal activity and pulmonary function) and to **minimize risk** (preventing exacerbations, loss of lung function, medication side effects). Successful management requires patient education, objective measurement of airflow obstruction, and a medication plan for daily use and for exacerbations.
- When initiating therapy for a patient not already on controller medicine, one should assess patient's severity and assign the patient to the highest level in which any one feature has occurred over the previous 2 to 4 weeks (Table 9-9).
- Assessment of control on subsequent visits is used to modify therapy when following patients already on controller medication (Table 9-10).
- The goal of the stepwise approach is to gain control of symptoms as quickly as possible. At the same time, level of control varies over time and, consequently,

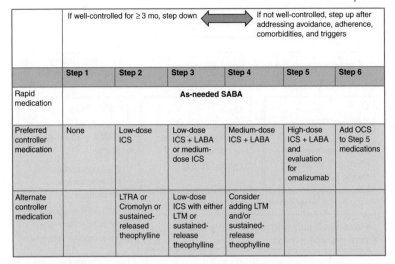

	Step 1	Step 2	Step 3	Step 4	Step 5	Step 6
					If well-controlled for ≥ 3 mo, step down ⟷ If not well-controlled, step up after addressing avoidance, adherence, comorbidities, and triggers	
Rapid medication	As-needed SABA					
Preferred controller medication	None	Low-dose ICS	Low-dose ICS + LABA or medium-dose ICS	Medium-dose ICS + LABA	High-dose ICS + LABA and evaluation for omalizumab	Add OCS to Step 5 medications
Alternate controller medication		LTRA or Cromolyn or sustained-released theophylline	Low-dose ICS with either LTM or sustained-release theophylline	Consider adding LTM and/or sustained-release theophylline		

Figure 9-1. Management algorithm based on level of control. ICS, inhaled corticosteroid; LABA, long-acting β_2-agonist; LTM, leukotriene modifier; LTRA, leukotriene receptor antagonist; OCS, oral corticosteroid; SABA, short-acting β_2-agonist. (From Global Initiative for Asthma. GINA Report, global strategy for asthma management and Prevention. http://www.ginasthma.org. 2011; National Asthma Education and Prevention Program. Expert panel report 3. http://www.nhlbi.nih.gov/guidelines/asthma/asthgdln.pdf. 2007.)

medication requirements as well, so therapy should be reviewed every 3 months to check whether stepwise reduction is possible (Figure 9-1).
- **Management of an exacerbation** requiring hospital-based care should follow a treatment algorithm to triage patients based on response to treatment (Figure 9-2).
  - The response to initial treatment (three treatments with a short-acting bronchodilator every 20 minutes for 60 to 90 minutes) can be a better predictor of the need for hospitalization than the severity of an exacerbation.
  - Patients at high risk of asthma-related death (see Outcome/Prognosis section) should be advised to seek medical attention early in the course of an exacerbation.
  - A low threshold for admission is appropriate for patients with recent hospitalization, a failure of aggressive outpatient management (with oral corticosteroids), or a previous life-threatening attack.

Medications
First Line
- **Short-acting bronchodilators**
  - Quick-relief medications used on an as-needed basis for long-term management of all severities of asthma as well as for rapid treatment of exacerbations given via either MDI or nebulization
  - For long-term management, a **SABA** used on an as-needed basis (e.g., albuterol, two to three puffs q6h) is appropriate.
  - During an exacerbation, reversal of airflow obstruction is achieved most effectively by frequent administration of an inhaled SABA.

Figure 9-2. Treatment algorithm for asthma exacerbation. CS, corticosteroid; d/c, discharge; FEV_1, forced expiratory volume in 1 second; f/u, follow-up; ICS, inhaled corticosteroid; PEF, peak expiratory flow; SABA, short-acting β_2-agonist. (From Global Initiative for Asthma. GINA Report, global strategy for asthma management and prevention. http://www.ginasthma.org. 2011; National Asthma Education and Prevention Program. Expert panel report 3. http://www.nhlbi.nih.gov/guidelines/asthma/asthgdln.pdf. 2007.)

- For a **mild-to-moderate exacerbation**, initial treatment starts with two to six puffs of albuterol via MDI or 2.5 mg via nebulizer and is repeated q20min until improvement is obtained or toxicity is noted.

- For a **severe exacerbation**, albuterol 2.5 to 5.0 mg q20min with ipratropium bromide 0.5 mg q20min should be administered via nebulizer. Alternatively, albuterol 10.0 to 15.0 mg, administered continuously over an hour, may be more effective in severely obstructed adults. If used, telemetry monitoring is necessary.

- Levalbuterol four to eight puffs or nebulized 1.25 to 2.5 mg q20min can be substituted for albuterol but has not been associated with fewer side effects in adults.

- The subsequent dosing schedule is adjusted according to the patient's symptoms and clinical presentation. Often, patients require a SABA q2-4h during an acute attack. The use of an MDI with a spacer device under supervision of trained personnel is as effective as aerosolized solution by nebulizer. Cooperation may not be possible in the patient with severe airflow obstruction.

- Subcutaneous administration of a β_2-adrenergic agonist is unnecessary if inhaled medications can be administered quickly with an adequate response. In rare settings, aqueous epinephrine (0.3 to 0.5 mL of a 1:1,000 solution SC q20min) or terbutaline (0.25 mg SC q20min) for up to three doses can be used. However, there has been no evidence to suggest their superiority over aerosolized therapy. Their use is contraindicated if the patient has had a myocardial infarction within the last 6 months or is having active angina. If used, electrocardiograph monitoring is necessary.

  ○ All SABAs now use hydrofluoroalkane (HFA) as a propellant. They should be primed with four puffs when first used and again if not used over 2 weeks.

- **ICSs**
  ○ ICSs are safe and effective for the treatment of persistent asthma. They are generally administered via a dry powder inhaler (DPI), MDI with a spacing device, or nebulized.
  ○ Dosing depends on assessment of severity and control (Table 9-13).
  ○ Once-daily dosing of ICS may be as effective as twice-daily dosing in the management of mild persistent asthma and may improve adherence.
  ○ Systemic corticosteroid absorption can occur in patients who use high doses of ICS. Consequently, prolonged therapy with high-dose ICS should be reserved for patients with severe disease or for those who otherwise require oral corticosteroids.
  ○ Attempts should be made to decrease the dose of ICS every 2 to 3 months to the lowest possible dose to maintain control.

- **LABAs**
  ○ Recommended for moderate and severe persistent asthma in patients not adequately controlled with ICS
  ○ Salmeterol or the more fast-acting formoterol added to ICS have consistently been shown to improve lung function, both day and nighttime symptoms; reduce exacerbations; and minimize the required dose of ICS.
  ○ LABA should only be used in combination with ICS in patients with asthma (salmeterol/fluticasone, budesonide/formoterol).
  ○ The benefits of adding LABAs are more substantial than those achieved by leukotriene modifiers (LTMs), theophylline, or increased doses of ICS.

Table 9-13	Comparative Daily Adult Dosages for Inhaled Corticosteroids		
Drug	**Low Dose**	**Medium Dose**	**High Dose**
Triamcinolone HFA (75 mcg/puff)	300–750 mcg	>750–1,500 mcg	>1,500 mcg
Beclomethasone HFA (40 or 80 mcg/puff)	80–240 mcg	>240–480 mcg	>480 mcg
Budesonide DPI (90, 180, or 200 mcg/dose)	180–600 mcg	>600–1,200 mcg	>1,200 mcg
Budesonide nebulized respules (250, 500, or 1,000 mcg/respules)	250–500 mcg	>500–1000 mcg	>1,000 mcg
Ciclesonide HFA (80 or 160 mcg/puff)	160–320 mcg	>320–640 mcg	>640 mcg
Flunisolide HFA (80 mcg/puff)	320 mcg	>320–640 mcg	>640 mcg
Fluticasone HFA (44, 110, or 220 mcg/puff)	88–264 mcg	>264–440 mcg	>440 mcg
Fluticasone DPI (50, 100, or 250 mcg/dose)	100–300 mcg	>300–500 mcg	>500 mcg
Mometasone furoate DPI (110 or 220 mcg/puff)	220 mcg	440 mcg	>440 mcg
Combination agents			
Budesonide/formoterol (MDI: 80/4.5 or 160/4.5 mcg/puff)	2 puffs bid: 80/4.5 mcg/puff	2 puffs bid: 80/4.5 to 160/4.5 mcg/puff	2 puffs bid: 160/4.5 mcg/puff
Fluticasone/salmeterol (MDI: 45/21, 115/21, or 230/21 mcg/puff) (DPI: 100/50, 250/50, or 500/50 mcg/dose)	1 inhalation bid: 100/50 mcg	1 inhalation bid: 250/50 mcg	1 inhalation bid: 500/50 mcg
Mometasone/formoterol (MDI: 100/5 or 200/5 mcg/puff)	2 inhalations bid: 100/5 mcg/puff	2 inhalations bid: 100/5 mcg/puff to 200/5 mcg/puff	2 inhalations bid: 200/5 mcg/puff

bid, twice daily; DPI, dry powder inhaler; MDI, metered-dose inhaler.
Data from Global Initiative for Asthma. GINA Report, global strategy for asthma management and prevention. http://www.ginasthma.org. 2011; National Asthma Education and Prevention Program. Expert panel report 3. http://www.nhlbi.nih.gov/guidelines/asthma/asthgdln.pdf. 2007.

- **Systemic corticosteroids**
  - May be necessary to gain control of disease quickly via either oral or IV route.
  - If chronic symptoms are severe and accompanied by nighttime awakening, or PEF is <70% of predicted values, a short course of oral corticosteroid (prednisone 40 to 60 mg/d for 5 to 7 days) might be necessary.
  - Long-term therapy is occasionally necessary and should be started at prednisone 2 mg/kg/d, not to exceed 60 mg/d, and repeated attempts should be made to reduce the dose while they are receiving high-dose ICS.

- ○ **During an exacerbation, systemic corticosteroids speed the resolution of exacerbations of asthma and should be administered to all patients.**
  - ▪ The ideal dose of corticosteroid needed to speed recovery and limit symptoms is not well defined. Oral corticosteroid administration seems to be as effective as IV if given in equivalent doses (prednisone, 40 to 80 mg PO daily).
  - ▪ IV methylprednisolone, 125 mg, given on initial presentation decreases the rate of return to the ED of those patients who are discharged.
  - ▪ For maximal therapeutic response, tapering of high-dose corticosteroids should not take place until objective evidence of clinical improvement is observed (usually 36 to 48 hours or when PEF >70%). Initially, patients are given a daily dose of oral prednisone, which is then reduced slowly.
  - ▪ A 7- to 14-day tapering dose of prednisone is usually successful in combination with an ICS instituted at the beginning of the tapering schedule. In patients with severe disease or with a history of respiratory failure, a slower reduction in dose is appropriate.
  - ▪ Patients discharged from the ED should receive oral corticosteroids. A dose of prednisone, 40 mg/d for 5 to 7 days, can be substituted for a tapering schedule in selected patients. Either regimen should be accompanied by the initiation of an ICS or an increase in the previous dose of ICS.

Second Line
- • **LTMs**
  - ○ **Montelukast** (10 mg PO daily) and **zafirlukast** (20 mg PO bid) are oral leukotriene-receptor antagonists (LTRAs), and **zileuton** (extended-release 1,200 mg bid) is an oral 5-lipoxygenase inhibitor. The LTRAs are recommended as an alternative first-line medication for mild persistent asthma and as an add-on to ICS for more severe forms of asthma.
  - ○ As add-on therapy to ICS, these agents have been shown to improve lung function, lead to improved quality of life, and lead to fewer exacerbations. However, in comparison to ICS + LABA, they are not as effective in improving asthma outcomes.
  - ○ **An LTM should be strongly considered for patients with aspirin-induced asthma or for individuals who cannot master the use of an inhaler.**
- • **Cromolyn sodium**
  - ○ Anti-inflammatory inhaled medication is an alternative to ICS in children with mild persistent asthma or **first-line for exercised-induced asthma**. The usual dosage is 8 to 12 puffs q day in three to four divided doses. Maximum improvement may be delayed for 4 to 6 weeks after initiation of therapy.
  - ○ Little additional benefit accrues from using cromolyn with an ICS.
- • **Anti-IgE therapy**
  - ○ **Omalizumab** is a monoclonal antibody against IgE that is approved for the management of patients with moderate-to-severe persistent allergic asthma with a demonstrable sensitivity to a perennial aeroallergen and incomplete control with ICS.
  - ○ Omalizumab can decrease airway inflammation through its effects on IgE. Treatment with omalizumab decreases eosinophil counts in sputum and biopsy specimens and attenuates lymphocyte proliferation and cytokine production.
  - ○ Omalizumab is administered subcutaneously q2–4wk and dosed based upon the patient's baseline IgE level (if between 30 and 700 IU/mL) and weight.
  - ○ Addition of omalizumab in adults and children 12 years of age or older has been shown to reduce exacerbation rates and need for corticosteroids in patients on a

controller medication regimen. Rescue medication use is often reduced and asthma-related quality of life is improved. Health care utilization (emergency department [ED] visits, hospital admissions) is decreased with omalizumab use in severe asthmatics.

○ Allergic rhinitis symptoms often improve with omalizumab therapy. In one controlled trial, omalizumab use reduced nasal symptom severity scores and rescue antihistamine use in a dose-dependent manner (*JAMA 2001;286(23):2956*).

• **Methylxanthines:** Sustained-release theophylline at low doses (300 mg/d) may be useful as adjuvant therapy to an anti-inflammatory agent in persistent asthma, especially for controlling nighttime symptoms.

• **IV magnesium sulfate:** During a severe exacerbation refractory to standard treatment over 1 hour, one dose of 2 g IV over 20 minutes in the ED should be considered. It has been shown to acutely improve lung function especially in those with severe, life-threatening exacerbations (*Ann Emerg Med 2000;36:181*).

• **Inhaled heliox:** During a severe exacerbation refractory to standard treatment over 1 hour, heliox-driven albuterol nebulization in a mixture with oxygen (70:30) should be considered. It has been shown to acutely improve lung function, especially in those with severe, life-threatening exacerbations (*Acad Emerg Med 2005;12(9): 820*).

• **Antibiotics:** Antibiotic therapy has not been shown to have any benefit when used to treat exacerbations. Antibiotics can only be recommended as needed for treatment of comorbid conditions, such as pneumonia or bacterial sinusitis.

• **Bronchial thermoplasty:** Bronchial thermoplasty is a novel therapy for severe asthma in which a specialized radiofrequency catheter is introduced through a bronchoscope to deliver thermal energy to smaller airways in order to reduce smooth muscle mass surrounding the airways. Although asthma symptoms worsen immediately after the procedure, long-term asthma-related quality of life and health care utilization improves with bronchial thermoplasty (*Am J Respir Crit Care Med 2010; 181(2):116*). Bronchial thermoplasty should be performed by experienced bronchoscopists in conjunction with an asthma specialist.

Other Nonpharmacologic Therapies

• **Supplemental oxygen** should be administered to the patient who is awaiting an assessment of arterial oxygen tension and should be continued to maintain an O_2sat >92% (95% in patients with coexisting cardiac disease or pregnancy).

• **Mechanical ventilation** may be required for respiratory failure.

○ General principles include use of a **large endotracheal tube (≥7.5 mm), low tidal volumes, prolonged expiratory time with high inspiratory flows, low respiratory rate and low positive end-expiratory pressure (PEEP)**, and in some patients, **permissive hypercapnia**, with the goal to avoid dynamic hyperinflation. Patients with asthma who are intubated often have elevated plateau pressures and intrinsic PEEP.

○ Heavy sedation may be needed and should be maximized before the use of paralytics, given their adverse side effects.

○ Evidence is lacking to suggest modes of noninvasive ventilation are beneficial.

• Subcutaneous injection **allergen immunotherapy** can be considered in allergic patients with mild-to-moderate disease with persistent symptoms despite adherence to allergen avoidance and medication.

Lifestyle/Risk Modification

Diet

There is no general diet that is known to improve asthma control. However, a small percentage of patients may have reproducible deterioration after exposure to dietary sulfites used to prevent discoloration in foods such as beer, wine, processed potatoes, and dried fruit and should therefore be avoided in these patients.

Activity

Patients should be encouraged to lead an active lifestyle. If their asthma is well controlled, they should expect to be as physically active as they desire. If exercise is a trigger, patients should be advised to continue physical activity after prophylactic use of an LTM or an inhaled β_2-adrenergic agonist (two to four puffs, 15 to 20 minutes before exposure).

SPECIAL CONSIDERATIONS

- During pregnancy, patients should have more frequent follow-up as the severity often changes and requires medication adjustment. **There is more potential risk to the fetus with poorly controlled asthma compared to asthma medication exposure, most of which are generally considered safe.** A recent birth cohort study of ICSs in pregnant women with asthma confirmed their safety (*Am J Resp Crit Care Med 2012;185(5):557*).
- Occupational asthma requires a detailed history of occupational exposure to a sensitizing agent, lack of asthma symptoms prior to exposure, and a documented relationship with symptoms and the workplace. Beyond standard asthma medical treatment, exposure avoidance is crucial.
- Patients with aspirin sensitivity and nasal polyps typically have the onset of asthma in the third or fourth decade of life. A precipitous onset of symptoms should raise the possibility of reaction to acute ingestion of aspirin or an NSAID.

COMPLICATIONS

Medication side effects
- **SABA:** Sympathomimetic symptoms (tremor, anxiety, tachycardia), decrease in serum potassium and magnesium, mild lactic acidosis, prolonged QT_c
- **ICS**
  - Increased risk for systemic effects at high doses (equivalent >1,000 mcg/d of beclomethasone) including skin bruising, cataracts, elevated intraocular pressure, and accelerated loss of bone mass
  - Pharyngeal and laryngeal effects are common such as sore throat, hoarse voice, and oral candidiasis. **Patients should be instructed to rinse their mouth after each administration to reduce the possibility of thrush.** A change in the delivery method and/or use of a valved holding chamber/spacer may alleviate the other side effects.
- **LABA**
  - Fewer sympathomimetic-type side effects
  - Associated with an increased risk of severe asthma exacerbations and asthma-related death when used without ICS based on the Salmeterol Multicenter Asthma Research Trial (SMART), which showed a very low but significant increase in

asthma-related deaths in patients receiving salmeterol (0.01% to 0.04%) (*Chest 2006;129(1):15*)
  ○ Should only be used in combination with ICS.
- **LTM**
  ○ Cases of newly diagnosed Churg–Strauss vasculitis after exposure to LTRA have been described, but it is unclear if it is related to unmasking of a preexisting case with concurrent corticosteroid tapering or if there is a causal relationship.
  ○ Zileuton can cause a reversible hepatitis, so it is recommended that hepatic function be monitored at initiation once a month during the first 3 months, every 3 months for the first year, and then periodically.
- **Omalizumab (anti-IgE) therapy:** Anaphylaxis occurs in 1 to 2 per 1,000, usually within 2 hours of the first doses. For this reason, patients should be medically observed 2 hours after the initial doses and then 30 minutes for subsequent dosing. Patients should possess self-administered epinephrine to be used as needed for anaphylaxis.
- **Methylxanthines**
  ○ Theophylline has a narrow therapeutic range with significant toxicities, such as arrhythmias and seizures, as well as many potential drug interactions, especially with antibiotics.
  ○ Serum concentrations of theophylline should be monitored on a regular basis, aiming for a level of 5 to 10 mcg/mL; however, at the lower doses used for asthma, toxicity is much less likely.

REFERRAL

Referral to a specialist should be considered in the following situations:
- Patients who require step 4 (Figure 9-1) or higher treatment, or if they have had a life-threatening asthma exacerbation
- Patients being considered for anti-IgE therapy, bronchial thermoplasty, or other alternative treatments
- Patients with atypical signs or symptoms that make the diagnosis uncertain
- Patients with comorbidities such as chronic sinusitis, nasal polyposis, allergic bronchopulmonary aspergillosis (ABPA), VCD, severe GERD, severe rhinitis, or significant psychiatric or psychosocial difficulties interfering with treatment
- Patients requiring additional diagnostic testing, such as rhinoscopy or bronchoscopy, bronchoprovocation testing, or allergy skin testing
- Patients with a need to be evaluated for allergen immunotherapy

PATIENT EDUCATION

- Patient education should focus on the chronic and inflammatory nature of asthma, with identification of factors that contribute to increased inflammation.
  ○ The consequences of ongoing exposure to chronic irritants or allergens and the rationale for therapy should be explained. Patients should be instructed to avoid factors that aggravate their disease, on how to manage their daily medications, and on how to recognize and deal with acute exacerbations (known as an asthma action plan).
  ○ The use of a **written daily management plan** as part of the education strategy is recommended for all patients with persistent asthma.

- It is important for patients to recognize signs of poorly controlled disease.
  - These signs include an increased or daily need for bronchodilators, limitation of activity, waking at night because of asthma symptoms, and variability in the PEF.
  - Specific instructions about handling these symptoms, including criteria for seeking emergency care, should be provided.

MONITORING/FOLLOW-UP

- PEF monitoring provides an objective measurement of airflow obstruction and can be considered in patients with moderate-to-severe persistent asthma. However, symptom-based asthma action plans are equivalent to PEF-based plans in terms of overall self-management and control (*Respirology 2001 Dec;6(4):297*).
  - The personal best PEF (the highest PEF obtained when the disease is under control) is identified, and the PEF is checked when symptoms escalate or in the setting of an asthma trigger. This should be incorporated into an asthma action plan, setting 80% to 100% of personal best PEF as the "green" zone, 50% to 80% as the "yellow" zone, and <50% as the "red" zone.
- Patients should learn to anticipate situations that cause increased symptoms. For most individuals, monitoring symptoms instead of PEF is sufficient (symptom-based asthma action plan).
- Questionnaires can also provide objective monitoring of asthma control. The Asthma Control Test (ACT) or Asthma Control Questionnaire (ACQ) are useful instruments to rapidly assess patient-reported asthma control.

OUTCOME/PROGNOSIS

- Most patients with asthma can be effectively treated and achieve good control of their disease when following the stepwise treatment approach. Goals should include to be free from troublesome symptoms, minimal use of reliever medication, near-normal lung function, absence of serious attacks, and ability to lead a physically active life.
- Previous exacerbations that have required the use of oral corticosteroids or led to respiratory failure as well as the use of more than two canisters per month of inhaled short-acting bronchodilator and seizures with asthma attacks, have been associated with severe and potentially fatal asthma.

10 Pulmonary Diseases

Murali Chakinala, Colleen McEvoy, Tonya D. Russell, Rachel Bardowell, Alexander Chen, and Daniel B. Rosenbluth

Pulmonary Hypertension

GENERAL PRINCIPLES

Definition

Pulmonary hypertension (PH) is the sustained elevation of the mean pulmonary artery pressure (mPAP) (≥ 25 mm Hg at rest).

Classification

- PH is subcategorized into five major groups (Table 10-1):
  - Group I—**Pulmonary arterial hypertension (PAH)**
  - Group II—**PH due to left heart disease**
  - Group III—**PH due to lung diseases and/or hypoxemia**
  - Group IV—**Chronic thromboembolic pulmonary hypertension (CTEPH)**
  - Group V—**PH with unclear multifactorial mechanisms**
- **PAH** represents a specific group of disorders with similar pathologies and clinical presentation, with a propensity for right heart failure in the absence of elevated left-sided pressures.

Epidemiology

- PH is most often due to left heart disease (Group II) or parenchymal lung disease (Group III).
- **Idiopathic pulmonary arterial hypertension (IPAH)** (Group I) is a rare disorder with an estimated prevalence of 6 to 9 cases per million compared to an overall PAH prevalence of 15 to 26 cases per million (*Am J Respir Crit Care Med 2006;173:1023*; *Eur Respir J 2007;30:104*). The average age of PAH patients in modern registries is ~50 years (*Am J Respir Crit Care Med 2006;173:1023*; *Eur Respir J 2007;30:1103*). IPAH patients tend to be even younger, with mean age ~35 years (*Ann Intern Med 1987;107:216*).
- Despite increased awareness, PAH continues to be diagnosed late in its course, with a reported delay of 27 months from symptom onset and majority in advanced World Health Organization (WHO) functional Class III or IV (*Am J Respir Crit Care Med 2006;173:1023*).
- IPAH and PAH associated with systemic sclerosis are the most common sub-types of PAH (*Eur Respir J 2007;30:1103*).
- Incidence of **CTEPH** (Group IV) may be as high as 4% among survivors of acute pulmonary embolism (*N Engl J Med 2004;350:2257*).

Pathophysiology

- Complex origins of PAH include infectious/environmental insults or comorbid conditions that "trigger" the condition in individuals susceptible due to a genetic predisposition.

Table 10-1	Clinical Classification of Pulmonary Hypertension: Dana Point (2008) Classification System of Pulmonary Hypertension

I. Pulmonary arterial hypertension (PAH)
Idiopathic PAH
Heritable:
  BMPR-II
  ALK1 or endoglin
  Unknown
Associated with:
  Connective tissue diseases
  HIV infection
  Portal hypertension
  Congenital heart diseases
  Schistosomiasis
  Chronic hemolytic anemia
  Persistent PH of the newborn
Pulmonary veno-occlusive disease and/or pulmonary capillary
  hemangiomatosis

II. Pulmonary hypertension due to left heart disease
Systolic dysfunction
Diastolic dysfunction
Valvular disease

III. Pulmonary hypertension due to lung diseases and/or hypoxemia
Chronic obstructive lung disease
Interstitial lung disease
Other pulmonary diseases with mixed obstructive and restrictive pattern
Sleep-disordered breathing
Alveolar hypoventilation disorders
Chronic exposure to high altitude
Developmental abnormalities

IV. Chronic thromboembolic pulmonary hypertension (CTEPH)

V. Pulmonary hypertension with unclear multifactorial mechanisms
Hematologic disorders:
  Myeloproliferative disorders
  Postsplenectomy
Systemic diseases:
  Sarcoidosis
  Pulmonary Langerhans cell histiocytosis
  Lymphangioleiomyomatosis
  Neurofibromatosis
  Vasculitis
Metabolic disorders:
  Glycogen storage disease
  Gaucher disease
  Thyroid disorders
Miscellaneous:
  Tumoral obstruction
  Fibrosing mediastinitis
  Chronic renal failure on hemodialysis

BMPR-II, bone morphogenetic protein receptor II.
From Simonneau G, Robbins IM, Beghetti M, et al. Updated clinical classification of pulmonary hypertension. *J Am Coll Cardiol* 2009;54(1 Suppl):S43–S54.

- ○ Known **genetic mutations** include bone morphogenetic protein receptor II (BMPR-II), activin-like kinase receptor I, endoglin, and caveolin.
- ○ 70% of familial PAH and 10% to 40% of sporadic or anorexigen-associated cases are found to have mutations in BMPR-II (*Circulation 2010;122:156*).
- PAH involves a complex interplay of factors resulting in progressive vascular remodeling with endothelial cell and smooth-muscle proliferation, vasoconstriction, as well as thrombosis of arterioles. As a result of vessel wall changes and luminal narrowing, flow of blood is restricted yet high pressure is generated and quantifiable as an elevated pulmonary vascular resistance (PVR) (*Circulation 2009;119:2252*).
  - ○ Elevated PVR results in increased afterload to the right ventricle (RV), which over time impacts RV contractility.
  - ○ Initially, cardiac output diminishes during strenuous exercise. As PH severity worsens, maximal cardiac output is achieved at progressively lower workloads; ultimately, resting cardiac output is reduced.
  - ○ Unlike the left ventricle (LV), the RV has limited ability to hypertrophy and tolerates high afterload poorly, causing "vascular–ventricular uncoupling" and eventual RV failure, the most common cause of death.
  - ○ In very advanced stages, pulmonary artery pressures decline as the failing RV cannot generate enough blood flow to maintain high pressures.
- Mechanisms of PH in Groups II–V vary and include high postcapillary pressures, hypoxemia-mediated vasoconstriction and remodeling, parenchymal destruction, thromboembolic narrowing or occlusion of large arteries, and compression of proximal vasculature.

Prevention

Yearly screening transthoracic echocardiogram (TTE) is indicated for high-risk groups including individuals with known BMPR-II mutation, scleroderma spectrum of disease, portal hypertension (HTN) undergoing liver transplantation evaluation, and congenital systemic-to-pulmonary shunts.

DIAGNOSIS

Clinical Presentation

- **Symptoms** include **dyspnea** (most common), exercise intolerance, fatigue, palpitations, exertional dizziness, **syncope**, chest pain, lower extremity swelling, increased abdominal girth (ascites), and hoarseness (impingement of recurrent laryngeal nerve by enlarging pulmonary artery).
- Explore for underlying risk factors (i.e., anorectic drugs, methamphetamines) or associated conditions (e.g., connective tissue diseases, left ventricular heart failure [congestive heart failure (CHF)], obstructive sleep apnea syndrome [OSAS], and venous thromboembolism [VTE]).
- Auscultatory signs of PH include **prominent second heart sound** (loud S_2) with loud P_2 component, right ventricular S_3, tricuspid regurgitation, and pulmonary insufficiency murmurs.
- **Signs of right heart failure**
  - ○ Elevated jugular venous pressure
  - ○ Hepatomegaly
  - ○ Pulsatile liver
  - ○ Pedal edema
  - ○ Ascites

- Physical examination should focus on identifying underlying conditions linked to PH: skin changes of scleroderma, stigmata of liver disease, clubbing (congenital heart disease), and abnormal breath sounds (parenchymal lung disease).

Diagnostic Testing

- **The purpose of diagnostic testing is to confirm clinical suspicion of PH, determine etiology of PH, and gauge severity of condition, which assists with treatment planning.**
- **Acute illnesses** (e.g., pulmonary edema, pulmonary embolism, pneumonia, adult respiratory distress syndrome) can cause **mild PH** (pulmonary artery systolic pressure [PASP] <50) or aggravate preexisting PH.
- Evaluation of **chronic PH** becomes necessary if pulmonary artery pressures remain elevated after resolution of the acute process.
- If chronic PH is considered based on clinical suspicion or during the evaluation of a vulnerable population (see Prevention section), **TTE should be the initial test**.

Transthoracic Echocardiogram with Doppler and Agitated Saline Injection

- **Estimate PASP** by Doppler interrogation of tricuspid valve regurgitant jet. The absence of tricuspid regurgitation does not exclude elevated pulmonary artery pressure. Sensitivity for PH is 80% to 100% and correlation coefficient with invasive measurement is 0.6 to 0.9 (*Chest 2004;126:14S*). **Invasive measurement is recommended if suspicion remains despite a normal estimation by echocardiogram.**
- **Assess RV characteristics**, looking for pressure overload and dysfunction (e.g., RV hypertrophy and/or dilation, RV hypokinesis, displaced intraventricular septum, paradoxical septal motion, left ventricular compression, and pericardial effusion from impaired pericardial drainage). Absence of any RV abnormalities makes moderate or severe PH very unlikely.
- **Identify causes of PH** (e.g., left ventricular systolic or **diastolic dysfunction**, left-sided valvular disease, left atrial structural anomalies, and congenital systemic to pulmonary shunts). Left atrial enlargement, elevated LV filling pressures, and Grade II–III diastolic dysfunction are important clues for LV diastolic heart disease that frequently leads to PH, especially in the elderly (*J Am Coll Cardiol 2009;53:1119*).
- Transesophageal echocardiogram (TEE) is indicated to exclude intracardiac shunts suspected by TTE, although majority of such shunts are a patent foramen ovale.
- Additional studies, as outlined in the following text and in Figure 10-1, should be completed if PH is unexplained by TTE, or if PAH is still a consideration after echocardiography (*Chest 2004;126:14S*).

Laboratories

- Evaluate for causative conditions and gauge degree of cardiac impairment.
  - Complete blood counts (CBCs)
  - Blood urea nitrogen, serum creatinine
  - Hepatic function tests
  - B-type natriuretic peptide (BNP)
  - Human immunodeficiency virus (HIV) serology
  - Thyroid-stimulating hormone (TSH)
  - Antinuclear antibody (ANA)
  - Antitopoisomerase antibodies and anticentromere antibodies

Figure 10-1. Algorithm for diagnostic workup of pulmonary hypertension. CTEPH, chronic thromboembolic pulmonary hypertension; ECG, electrocardiogram; HRCT, high-resolution computed tomography; HTN, hypertension; LFT, liver function test; PCH, pulmonary capillary hemangiomatosis; PFT, pulmonary function test; PH, pulmonary hypertension; PVOD, pulmonary veno-occlusive disease; RA, rheumatoid arthritis; SLE, systemic lupus erythematosis.

- Additional laboratory studies, based on initial findings, include complete thyroid function studies, hepatitis B and C serologies, hemoglobin electrophoresis, extractable nuclear antigen (ENA), antiphospholipid antibody, and lupus anticoagulant.

Electrocardiography

Signs of **right heart enlargement** include right ventricular hypertrophy, right atrial enlargement, right bundle branch block, and right ventricular strain pattern (S wave in lead I with Q wave and inverted T wave in lead III), but these findings have low sensitivity in milder PH.

Pulmonary Function Testing

- **Spirometry and lung volumes** to assess for obstructive (e.g., **chronic obstructive lung disease**) or restrictive (e.g., interstitial lung disease [ILD]) ventilatory abnormalities.
- **Diffusing capacity for carbon monoxide (DLCO)** is usually reduced with parenchymal lung diseases, but isolated mild–moderate reduction is often encountered in PAH.
- **Arterial blood gas (ABG):** Elevated $PaCO_2$ is an important clue for a hypoventilation syndrome.
- **Six-minute walk (6MW) or simple exercise test**
  - Unexplained exercise-induced desaturation could indicate PH.
  - Distance walked correlates with WHO functional classification and provides intermediate prognosis (*Am J Respir Crit Care Med 2000;161:487*).
- **Nocturnal oximetry:** Nocturnal desaturations could indicate OSAS. PH patients with symptoms of sleep-disordered breathing should undergo **polysomnography**. Nocturnal desaturations are common in PAH and should be treated with nocturnal supplemental oxygen (*Chest 2007;131:109*).

Imaging

- General findings include enlarged central pulmonary arteries as well as RV enlargement with opacification of retrosternal space, seen best on lateral view.
- Clues to specific PH diagnosis include:
  - Decreased peripheral vascular markings or pruning (PAH)
  - Very large pulmonary vasculature throughout lung fields (congenital-to-systemic shunt)
  - Regional oligemia of pulmonary vasculature (chronic thromboembolic disease)
  - Interstitial infiltrates (ILD)
  - Hyperinflated lungs (chronic obstructive lung disease).
- **Ventilation–Perfusion (V/Q) lung scan**
  - Critical for excluding chronic thromboembolic disease but could also be abnormal in pulmonary veno-occlusive disease and fibrosing mediastinitis.
  - **Heterogeneous perfusion patterns** are associated with PAH.
  - Presence of one or more segmental mismatches raises concern for chronic thromboembolic disease and should be investigated with computed tomography and pulmonary angiography (*N Engl J Med 2001;345:145*).
- **Pulmonary angiography** can be done safely in the setting of severe PH and should be performed
  - Confirm chronic thromboembolic disease
  - Determine surgical accessibility of thrombotic material
  - Inferior vena cava filter can be deployed at the same time
- **Chest computed tomography (CT) scan**
  - Evaluates lung parenchyma and mediastinum
  - High-resolution images to assess for interstitial or bronchiolar disease
- **Cardiac magnetic resonance imaging (MRI)**
  - Investigate cardiac anomalies leading to the development of PAH, especially if TEE is contraindicated
  - Provides anatomic and functional information on the RV, including contractility measures

Diagnostic Procedures

- **Lung biopsy**
  - Lung biopsy is rarely performed but useful if lung disease requires histologic confirmation (e.g., pulmonary vasculitis or veno-occlusive disease).
  - The risk of surgery is usually prohibitive in the setting of severe PH or RV dysfunction.
- **Right heart catheterization: Essential investigation if PAH is suspected and treatment is being considered.**
  - **Confirm noninvasive estimate of PASP**, as TTE can under- and overestimate PASP (*Am J Respir Crit Care Med 2009;179:615*).
  - **Measure cardiac output and mean right atrial pressure (RAP) to gauge severity of condition and predict future course.** Increased RAP is an indicator of RV dysfunction and has greatest odds ratio for predicting mortality (*Ann Intern Med 1987;107:216*).
  - **Investigate etiologies of PH**, including left heart disease (by measuring pulmonary artery occlusion pressure [PAOP]) or missed systemic-to-pulmonary shunts (by noting "step-ups" in oxygen saturations).
  - Exercise hemodynamics can elicit PH occurring during exercise or also confirm suspicion of diastolic heart failure, but exercise protocols and methods of measurement are not standardized.
- **Acute vasodilator testing** is recommended if PAH is suspected.
  - Performed with a **short-acting vasodilator**, such as intravenous adenosine, intravenous epoprostenol, or inhaled nitric oxide. **Long-acting calcium channel blockers (CCBs) should not be used for initial vasodilator testing** due to risk of sustained systemic hypotension (*Chest 2004;26:35S*).
  - **Not recommended for patients in extreme right heart failure** (mean RAP >20).
  - Definition of a **responder** is **decline in mPAP ≥10 mm Hg *and* concluding mPAP ≤40 mm Hg** (*Chest 2004;126:35S*).
  - Responders should undergo a CCB trial with pulmonary artery catheter in place. If vasoresponsiveness is recapitulated, chronic CCB therapy can be prescribed (see Treatment section).
- **Left heart catheterization** should be done to directly measure **left ventricular end-diastolic pressure** (LVEDP) if PAOP cannot reliably exclude left heart disease, especially in patients older than 65 years.

TREATMENT

- **Management of PH depends on the specific category of PH**.
  - Patients with PH due to left heart disease should receive appropriate therapy for the underlying causative condition with the goal of minimizing postcapillary pressures.
  - Patients with underlying lung diseases should be treated as appropriate for specific condition. Examples include: bronchodilators (e.g., obstructive lung disease), immunomodulators (e.g., ILDs), noninvasive ventilation (e.g., OSAS), and supplemental oxygen.
  - CTEPH may be treated by **pulmonary thromboendarterectomy** at specialized centers and requires careful screening to determine resectability and expected hemodynamic response (*N Engl J Med 2001;345:1465*).
- Regardless of PH diagnosis, normoxemia should be maintained to avoid hypoxic vasoconstriction and further aggravation of pulmonary artery pressures. **Supplemental oxygen** to maintain adequate arterial saturations (>89%) 24 hours a day

is recommended. However, normoxemia may not be possible in the presence of a significant right-to-left shunt (e.g., intracardiac right-to-left shunt).

- **In-line filters** should be used to prevent paradoxical air emboli from intravenous catheters in PH patients with large right-to-left shunts.
- **Pneumovax and influenza vaccination** should be given to avoid respiratory tract infections.
- Patients with severe PH and RV dysfunction should **minimize behaviors** that can acutely decrease RV preload and/or increase RV afterload, which could cause circulatory collapse:
  - **Deep Valsalva** maneuvers can raise intrathoracic pressure and induce syncope through diminished central venous return (e.g., vigorous exercise, severe coughing paroxysm, straining during defecation or micturition).
  - **High altitudes** (>5,000 ft) due to low inspired concentration of oxygen.
  - **Cigarette smoking**, because of nicotine's vasoactive effects.
  - **Pregnancy**, due to hemodynamic alterations that further strain the heart.
  - Systemic **sympathomimetic** agents, such as decongestants and cocaine.

Medications

- **PAH patients are candidates for vasomodulator/vasodilator** therapy (Figure 10-2 and Table 10-2).
  - There are three categories of PAH-specific therapies with unique mechanisms of actions:
    - **Endothelin receptor antagonists** block the binding of endothelin-1 to its receptors on pulmonary artery smooth muscle cells, which would typically cause vasoconstriction and cellular hypertrophy/growth.
    - **Phosphodiesterase-5 inhibitors** block the enzyme that shuts down nitric oxide–mediated vasodilation and platelet inhibition.
    - **Prostanoids** induce vasodilation, inhibit cellular growth, and inhibit platelet aggregation.
  - Initial choice of PAH-specific therapy should be individualized to the severity of one's condition (see Figure 10-2).
  - **Predictors of poor prognosis** include: (*Chest 2011;141:354*)
    - PAH subtype: scleroderma, porto-pulmonary hypertension, familial PAH
    - Men older than 60 years
    - Renal insufficiency
    - BNP >180
    - PVR >32 Wood units
    - RAP >20
    - DLCO ≤32%
    - Pericardial effusion
    - Systolic blood pressure <110
    - Resting heart rate >92
    - New York Heart Association (NYHA) functional Class IV
    - 6MW distance <165 meters
  - Due to the complexity of some therapies, an individual's comorbid conditions, cognitive abilities, and psychosocial makeup must also be heavily factored.
  - Because current therapies for PAH are palliative and not curative, patients require close follow-up as deterioration often occurs, requiring alternative/additional medical and possibly surgical intervention (see Figure 10-2). While there is no consensus follow-up strategy, periodic functional (e.g., 6MW and WHO

Figure 10-2. Algorithm for treatment management of pulmonary hypertension. CCB, calcium channel blocker; ERA, endothelin receptor antagonist; IV, intravenous; PDE-5 I, phosphodiesterase-5 inhibitor; SC, subcutaneous.

Functional Classification) and cardiac (e.g., TTE, MRI, or right heart catheterization) assessments provide the most sound strategy.
- Patients with suboptimal treatment responses to single drugs should be considered for combination therapy regimens with medications from more than one therapeutic class.
- **Diuretic therapy** (loop diuretic ± aldosterone antagonist ± thiazides)
  - Alleviates **right heart failure** and improves symptoms.

Table 10-2 Vasomodulator/Vasodilatory Therapy for Pulmonary Arterial Hypertension

Drug	Therapeutic Class	Indication	Route of Delivery	Dosing Range	Adverse Effects	Cautions
Nifedipine, amlodipine, diltiazem	Calcium channel blockers	Vasoresponders	PO	Varies by patient tolerance	Peripheral edema, hypotension, fatigue	**Use in patients who are vasoresponsive during acute vasodilator challenges**; avoid with low cardiac output or decompensated right heart failure.
Sildenafil/tadalafil	Phosphodiesterase-5 inhibitor	Functional class II–IV	PO	20 mg tid/40 mg/d	Headache, hypotension, dyspepsia, myalgias, visual disturbances	Avoid using with **nitrates** or **protease inhibitors.**
Bosentan	Endothelin receptor antagonist	Functional class II–IV	PO	125 mg bid	Hepatotoxicity, teratogen, peripheral edema	**Monthly liver function monitoring;** avoid using with glyburide and glipizide.
Ambrisentan	Endothelin receptor antagonist	Functional class II–III	PO	5–10 mg/d	Hepatotoxicity, teratogen, peripheral edema, nasal congestion	**Monthly liver function monitoring;** avoid using with glyburide and glipizide.

(continued)

Table 10-2 Vasomodulator/Vasodilatory Therapy for Pulmonary Arterial Hypertension *(Continued)*

Drug	Therapeutic Class	Indication	Route of Delivery	Dosing Range	Adverse Effects	Cautions
Sitaxsentan	Endothelin receptor antagonist	Functional class II–III	PO	100 mg/d	Hepatotoxicity, teratogen, peripheral edema	**Strong interaction with warfarin; monthly liver function monitoring;** not available in United States.
Iloprost	Prostanoid	Functional class III–IV	IH	2.5–5.0 mcg 6–8/d	Cough, flushing, headache, trismus	**Suboptimal compliance due to dosing frequency;** overnight drug holiday.
Treprostinil	Prostanoid	Functional class II–IV	SQ or IV	Varies by patient tolerance	Headache, jaw pain, diarrhea, extremity pain	**Continuous parenteral agent;** catheter-related complications (IV); **site pain/reaction (SQ).**
Epoprostenol	Prostanoid	Functional class III–IV	IV	Varies by patient tolerance	Headache, jaw pain, diarrhea, extremity pain	**Continuous parenteral agent; very short half-life;** catheter-related complications (IV); **high-output state at higher doses.**

IH, inhaled; IV, intravenous; PO, oral; SQ, subcutaneous.

○ Over diuresis or too rapid of a diuresis can be poorly tolerated due to **preload dependency** of the RV and limited ability of the cardiac output to compensate for systemic hypotension.

• **Anticoagulation** (warfarin)
  ○ Chronic anticoagulation improves survival, based on limited data in IPAH patients (*N Engl J Med 1992;327:76; Circulation 1984;70:580*).
  ○ Warfarin is dosed to **target international normalized ratio (INR) of 1.5 to 2.5** (*Chest 2004;126:35S*).
  ○ Anticoagulant therapy is not urgent and can be stopped for invasive procedures or active bleeding.

• **Inotropic agents** (dobutamine, milrinone, digoxin)
  ○ Modestly improves right heart function, cardiac output, and symptoms.
  ○ Dobutamine and milrinone are best suited for **short-term use** in extremely decompensated states.
  ○ Digoxin's effects on right ventricular contractility are limited, and its use is quite variable (*Chest 1998;114:787*).

Surgical Management

• **Lung transplantation or heart–lung transplantation**
  ○ Reserved for suitable patients with PAH who **remain in advanced functional Class III–IV despite maximal medical therapy**.
  ○ The **Lung Allocation Score** (LAS), derived from multiple clinical variables, takes into consideration PH diagnosis and provides a mechanism for prioritizing PAH patients beyond their imputed LAS. This improves the likelihood for IPAH to received transplants; however, mortality on the waiting list is high compared to other diagnoses.
  ○ Since the RV recovers after isolated lung transplantation, heart–lung transplantation is usually reserved for complex congenital heart defects that cannot be repaired.
  ○ Median survival after lung transplantation is ~5 years and **survival for IPAH patients at 5 years is ~50%** (*J Heart Lung Transplant 2005;24:956*).

• **Atrial septostomy**
  ○ Palliative procedure performed in cases of right heart failure (i.e., syncope, hepatic congestion, prerenal azotemia) refractory to medical therapy.
  ○ Percutaneous creation of a right-to-left shunt across the interatrial septum in patients whose RAPs are greater than left atrial pressures.
  ○ Despite arterial oxyhemoglobin desaturation and hypoxemia, oxygen delivery increases from improved left ventricular filling and cardiac output.

• **Septal defect closure**
  ○ In select cases of intracardiac defects that still have significant left-to-right shunting, closure can be undertaken by **percutaneous or surgical** means.
  ○ Criteria for closure include net left-to-right shunt with flow ratio (pulmonary flow/systemic flow) ≥ 1.5, resistance ratio (pulmonary vascular resistance/systemic vascular resistance) ≤ 0.6, and pressure ratio (pulmonary artery pressure/systemic pressure) ≤ 0.6 (*Circulation 2008;118:2395*).

Prognosis

One, 3-, and 5-year survival rates in PAH are 85%, 70%, and 55%, respectively, with median survival of 3.6 years (*Circulation 2010;122:156; Eur Respir J 2007;30:1103*).

Obstructive Sleep Apnea–Hypopnea Syndrome

GENERAL PRINCIPLES

Definition

Obstructive sleep apnea–hypopnea syndrome (OSAHS) is a disorder in which patients experience apneas or hypopneas due to upper airway narrowing. It is associated with excessive daytime somnolence (*Sleep 1999;22:667*).

Classification

- **Apneas** represent complete cessation of airflow.
  - ○ Obstructive events are associated with continued respiratory effort.
  - ○ Central events are associated with no respiratory effort.
- **Hypopneas** represent diminished airflow associated with at least a 4% oxygen desaturation.
- **Respiratory effort related arousals (RERAs)** represent changes in airflow that lead to an arousal but do not meet criteria for an apnea or hypopnea.
- **Apnea-hypopnea index (AHI)** is the number of apneas and hypopneas per hour of sleep.
- **Respiratory disturbance index (RDI)** is the number of apneas, hypopneas, and RERAs per hour of sleep.

Epidemiology

- Lack of recognition and diagnosis of OSAHS is a significant problem.
- The prevalence of OSAHS in the general population is estimated to be about 4%, with men being twice as likely as women to be affected (*Eur Respir J 2009;33:907*; *JAMA 2004;291:2013*).

Etiology

- **Obstructive sleep apnea (OSA)**
  Narrowing of the upper airway due to excessive soft tissue or structural abnormalities
- **Central sleep apnea (CSA)**
  Disturbance of central control of respiration during sleep

Pathophysiology

OSA occurs due to narrowing of the upper airway, which results in diminished airflow or cessation of airflow leading to arousals that fragment sleep.

Risk Factors

Risk factors for OSAHS include obesity, nasal obstruction, adenoidal or tonsillar hypertrophy, and mandibular size and positioning (*Otolaryngol Clin North Am 1990;23:727*). Potential risk factors also include family history and smoking (*JAMA 2004;291:2013*).

Prevention

- Weight loss
- Avoiding sedatives such as hypnotic medications or alcohol

Associated Conditions

- **Cardiovascular disease**, including systemic hypertension, heart failure, arrhythmia, myocardial infarction, and stroke (*Circulation 2008;118:1080*). OSA has been

Table 10-3	Symptoms Associated with Obstructive Sleep Apnea–Hypopnea Syndrome
Excessive daytime sleepiness	Enuresis
Snoring	Awakening without feeling refreshed
Nocturnal arousals	Morning headaches
Nocturnal apneas	Impaired memory and concentration
Nocturnal gasping, grunting, and choking	Irritability and depression
Nocturia	Impotence

established as an independent risk factor for hypertension (*Eur Resp J 2007;29: 156*).

- **Increased risk of death**, mainly due to cardiovascular events (*Sleep 2008;31:1071; Sleep 2008;31:1079; N Engl J Med 2005;353:2034*).
- Increased prevalence of **diabetes** has been noted in patients with OSAHS, independent of the effect of obesity (*Am J Respir Crit Care Med 2005;172:1590; J Clin Endocrinol Metab 2000;85:1151*).
- Higher risk of motor vehicle accidents (*Sleep 1997;20:608*).

DIAGNOSIS

Clinical Presentation

History
- **Habitual loud snoring** is the most common symptom of OSAHS, although not all people who snore have this syndrome. Patients with OSA may experience snore arousals along with a sensation of gasping or choking.
- Excessive daytime sleepiness (**hypersomnolence**) is a classic symptom of OSAHS (Table 10-3). Patients may describe falling asleep while driving or having difficulty concentrating at work.
- Patients may also complain of personality changes, intellectual deterioration, morning headaches, nocturnal angina, loss of libido, and chronic fatigue.
- Subjective sleepiness can be assessed by a validated scale, such as the **Epworth Sleepiness Scale** (Table 10-4) (*Sleep 1991;14:540*).

Physical Examination
- All patients should have a thorough nose and throat examination to detect sources of upper airway obstruction that are surgically correctable (e.g., septal deviation, enlarged tonsils), especially if continuous positive airway pressure (CPAP) (see Nonoperative Therapies section) is poorly tolerated.
- Increased severity of OSA has been associated with a higher **Mallampati class** (Table 10-5) (*Eur Respir J 2003;21:248*).

Diagnostic Criteria
Polysomnogram demonstrating obstructive events with an RDI >15 or RDI >5 associated with daytime sleepiness, sleep that is not refreshing, awakening gasping, or witnessed apneas is diagnostic.

Table 10-4	Epworth Sleepiness Scale

How likely are you to doze off or fall asleep in the following situations, in contrast to just feeling tired? This refers to your usual way of life in recent times. Even if you have not done some of these things recently, try to work out how they would have affected you. Use the following scale to choose the most appropriate number for each situation:

0 = would never doze   2 = moderate chance of dozing
1 = slight chance of dozing   3 = high chance of dozing

Situation:
Sitting and reading
Watching TV
Sitting, inactive, in a public place
Sittfing as a passenger in a car for an hour
Lying down in the afternoon
Sitting and talking to someone
Sitting quietly after a lunch without alcohol
Sitting in a car, while stopped for a few minutes in traffic

Note: The scores for each situation are summed to obtain the Epworth score. An Epworth score >10 suggests that significant daytime sleepiness is present.
Adapted from Johns MW. A New Method For Measuring Daytime Sleepiness: The Epworth Sleepiness Scale. *Sleep* 1991;14:540–545.

Differential Diagnosis
- In addition to OSAHS and sleep-related hypoventilation, the differential diagnosis for daytime sleepiness includes sleep deprivation, periodic limb movement disorder, narcolepsy, and medication side effects.
- Patients should also be evaluated for other medical conditions that may cause nighttime awakenings and dyspnea and thus mimic OSAHS, such as chronic lung disease, CHF, and gastroesophageal reflux disease.

Diagnostic Testing
- The gold standard for the diagnosis of OSAHS is **overnight polysomnography** (PSG, or "sleep study") with direct observation by a qualified technician (*Am Rev Respir Dis 1989;139:559*). Sleep studies are typically performed in the outpatient setting.

Table 10-5	Mallampati Airway Classification

Class	Visible Structures with Mouth Maximally Open and Tongue Protruded
I	Hard palate, soft palate, uvula, tonsillar pillars
II	Hard palate, soft palate, uvula
III	Hard palate, soft palate, base of uvula
IV	Hard palate

From Mallampati SR, Gatt SP, Gugino LD, et al. A clinical sign to predict difficult tracheal intubation: a prospective study. *Can Anaesth Soc J* 1985;32(4):429–434. With kind permission from Springer Science Business & Media B.V.

- Typical indications for a sleep study include snoring with excessive daytime sleepiness, titration of optimal positive airway pressure therapy, and assessment of objective response to therapeutic interventions.
- PSG involves determination of sleep stages using electroencephalography, electromyography, and electro-oculography and assessment of respiratory airflow and effort, oxyhemoglobin saturation, cardiac electrical activity (e.g., electrocardiogram [ECG]), and body position.
- Data are analyzed for sleep staging, the frequency of respiratory events, limb movements, and abnormal behaviors. Respiratory events are categorized as obstructive or central.
- Most sleep studies are performed as "split studies," where the first few hours of the study are diagnostic and the latter part of the study is used for CPAP titration if the AHI is consistent with moderate-to-severe OSA.
- Some patients only have significant events when lying in certain positions (usually supine) or during rapid eye movement (REM) sleep. These patients may require a complete overnight study for diagnosis and a second study for initiation of therapy.
- Recognizing the cost, required manpower, and limited availability of PSG, the American Academy of Sleep Medicine supports the use of unattended portable monitoring as an alternative to PSG for patients with a high pretest probability of moderate-to-severe OSA without significant comorbid medical conditions or other suspected sleep disorders. The portable device must record airflow, respiratory effort, and blood oxygenation, and results should be reviewed by a sleep specialist (*J Clin Sleep Med 2007;3:737*).

TREATMENT

The therapeutic approach to OSAHS depends on the severity of the disease, comorbid medical conditions, and patient preference and expected compliance. Treatment must be highly individualized, with special attention paid to correcting potentially reversible exacerbating factors.

Medications
- No pharmacologic agent has sufficient efficacy to warrant replacement of positive airway pressure as the primary therapeutic modality for OSAHS.
- **Modafinil** may improve daytime sleepiness in patients with persistent symptoms despite adequate CPAP use (*Sleep 2006;29:31*).

Nonpharmacologic Therapies
- **Positive airway pressure**
  - **CPAP** delivers air via a facemask at a constant pressure level throughout the respiratory cycle with the goal of pneumatically splinting open the upper airway, thus preventing collapse and airflow obstruction.
  - The PSG determines the positive airway pressure (expressed in cm H_2O) required to optimize airflow. The pressure setting is gradually increased until obstructive events, snoring, and oxygen desaturations are minimized.
  - The benefits of positive airway pressure include consolidated sleep and decreased daytime sleepiness. Hypertension, nocturia, peripheral edema, polycythemia, and PH may also improve. Additionally, CPAP is a highly cost-effective intervention (*Can J Physiol Pharmacol 2007;85:179*) that appears to reduce the risk of cardiovascular events (*Am J Respir Crit Care Med 2007;176:1274*), and may also improve the metabolic syndrome associated with OSA (*N Engl J Med 2011; 365:2277*).

○ **Nasal CPAP (nCPAP) is the current treatment of choice for most patients with OSAHS.**
   ▪ The compliance rate with nCPAP is approximately 50%.
   ▪ Compliance can be improved with education, instruction, follow-up, adjustment of the mask for fit and comfort, humidification of the air to decrease dryness, and treatment of nasal or sinus symptoms.
   ▪ Use of a full facemask (oronasal) has not been shown to improve compliance compared to the use of nCPAP. However, full facemasks are frequently used in patients who "mouth breathe" or patients who require higher CPAP pressures, as they will often experience air leak through the mouth when using nCPAP.
○ Autotitrating or "smart" CPAP machines use flow and pressure transducers to sense airflow patterns and then automatically adjust the pressure setting in response. Small studies have shown that autotitrating CPAP may be as effective as traditional CPAP and appears to be preferred by patients (*Respiration 2007; 74:279*; *Chest 2006;129:638*).
○ **Bilevel positive airway pressure (BiPAP)** can be used to treat patients with OSAHS. BiPAP is more expensive than CPAP and does not improve patient compliance. Patients with intolerance of very high levels of CPAP, a poor response to CPAP, or concomitant alveolar hypoventilation may respond well to noninvasive mechanical ventilation with BiPAP or volume ventilation.
○ All noninvasive positive pressure ventilation devices may induce dryness of the airway, nasal congestion, rhinorrhea, epistaxis, skin reactions to the mask, nasal bridge abrasions, and aerophagia. Some of these nasal symptoms may be treated with nasal saline and decongestants, which may help to improve compliance.
○ Some patients, such as those with concomitant COPD, require supplemental oxygen to maintain adequate nocturnal oxygen saturations ($SaO_2 \geq 90\%$).
• **Oral appliances**
○ Used for mild OSAHS, with aim to increase airway size to improve airflow. These devices, such as the mandibular repositioning device, can be fixed or adjustable, and most require customized fitting. Many devices have not been well studied.
○ Contraindications include temporomandibular joint disease, bruxism, full dentures, and inability to protrude the mandible.
• **Nasal expiratory resistance device**
○ Nasal plugs increase resistance with expiration, creating a back pressure to stent open the upper airway.
○ Most effective for milder OSA. Should not be used in patients with significant comorbid conditions such as lung disease.

Surgical Management
• **Tracheostomy**
○ Tracheostomy is very effective in treating OSAHS but is rarely used since the advent of positive airway pressure therapy.
○ Tracheostomy should be reserved for patients with life-threatening disease (cor pulmonale, arrhythmias, or severe hypoxemia) or significant alveolar hypoventilation that cannot be controlled with other measures.
• **Uvulopalatopharyngoplasty**
○ Uvulopalatopharyngoplasty (UPPP) is the most common surgical treatment of mild-to-moderate OSAHS in patients who do not respond to medical therapy.
○ UPPP enlarges the airway by removing tissue from the tonsils, tonsillar pillars, uvula, and posterior palate. UPPP may be complicated by change in voice,

nasopharyngeal stenosis, foreign body sensation, velopharyngeal insufficiency with associated nasal regurgitation during swallowing, and CPAP tolerance problems.
  ○ The success rate of UPPP for treatment of OSAHS is only approximately 50%, when defined as a 50% reduction of the AHI, and improvements related to UPPP may diminish over time (*Sleep 1996;19:156*). Thus, UPPP is considered a second-line treatment for patients with mild-to-moderate OSAHS who cannot successfully use CPAP and who have retropalatal obstruction.
- **Staged Procedures**
  In experienced centers, other staged procedures for OSA can be performed, including mandibular osteotomy with genioglossus advancement, hyoid myotomy with suspension, and maxillomandibular advancement (MMA) (*Sleep Breath 2000;4:137*). Significant reductions in AHI have been reported with MMA, but more research is needed (*Sleep 2010;33:1396*).

Lifestyle/Risk Modification
- Weight reduction for the obese is recommended (*Chest 1987;92:631*).
- Weight loss, both surgical and through reduced caloric intake, has been shown to reduce the severity of OSA by reduction in AHI (*Am J Respir Crit Care Med 2009;179:320*; *Am J Med 2009;122:535*).
- OSAHS patients should avoid use of alcohol, tobacco, and sedatives.
- Clinicians should counsel patients with OSAHS regarding the increased risk of driving and operating dangerous equipment.

SPECIAL CONSIDERATIONS

- Patients with a body mass index (BMI) >40 are at increased risk for concomitant sleep-related hypoventilation due to morbid obesity.

COMPLICATIONS

- When OSAHS is associated with disorders such as obesity and chronic lung disease, patients may develop hypoxemia, hypercapnia, polycythemia, PH, and cor pulmonale (*Mayo Clin Proc 1990;65:1087*).
- Patients with OSAHS are at greater risk for perioperative complications due to intubation difficulty and/or impaired arousal secondary to the effects of anesthetics, narcotics, and sedatives (*Otolaryngol Clin North Am 2007;40:877*).
- The risk of death, hypertension, and poor neuropsychological functioning rises with increasing severity of OSA.

REFERRAL

- Patients with risk factors and symptoms or sequelae of OSAHS should be referred to a sleep specialist and sleep laboratory for further evaluation.

Interstitial Lung Disease

GENERAL PRINCIPLES

This section focuses on subacute and chronic ILDs, with emphasis on **idiopathic pulmonary fibrosis (IPF)** and **sarcoidosis**.

Definition

ILDs are a heterogeneous group of disorders, pathologically characterized by infiltration of the lung interstitium with cells, fluid, and/or connective tissue.

Classification

- ILD of known etiology:
  - ○ Medication (e.g., bleomycin, amiodarone, nitrofurantoin, methotrexate)
  - ○ Connective tissue disease (e.g., rheumatoid arthritis, scleroderma, polymyositis/dermatomyositis)
  - ○ Pneumoconiosis (e.g., coal worker's pneumoconiosis, silicosis, asbestosis)
  - ○ Radiation
  - ○ Toxic inhalation (e.g., cocaine, talc)
  - ○ Lymphangitic carcinomatosis
- Idiopathic interstitial pneumonias:
  - ○ IPF, usual interstitial pneumonia (UIP)
  - ○ Nonspecific interstitial pneumonia (NSIP)
  - ○ Desquamative interstitial pneumonia (DIP)
  - ○ Respiratory bronchiolitis interstitial lung disease (RB-ILD)
  - ○ Cryptogenic organizing pneumonia (COP)
  - ○ Lymphocytic interstitial pneumonia (LIP)
  - ○ Acute interstitial pneumonia (AIP)
- Granulomatous ILD (e.g., sarcoidosis, hypersensitivity pneumonitis)
- Other (e.g., lymphangioleiomyomatosis [LAM], pulmonary Langerhans cell histiocytosis [LCH], eosinophilic pneumonia)

Epidemiology

- IPF
  - ○ Incidence is 4.6 to 16.3/100,000
  - ○ Incidence is higher in males than females, with the exception of a family history of ILD, where the incidence is equivalent between both.
  - ○ Patients often present in sixth or seventh decade (*Am J Respir Crit Care Med 2011;183:788*).
- Sarcoidosis
  - ○ Incidence rate in the United States is 35.5/100,000 for African Americans and 10.9/100,000 for Caucasians (*Am J Respir Crit Care Med 1999;160:736*).
  - ○ Incidence is higher in females than males.

Etiology

- The cause of IPF is unknown.
  - ○ There is a familial form of pulmonary fibrosis.
  - ○ Mutations in telomerase RNA component (TERC), telomerase reverse transcriptase (TERT), pulmonary surfactant protein C (SFTPC), and surfactant protein A2 have been identified (*Am J Med Sci 2011;341:439*).
- The exact cause of sarcoidosis has not been identified, although there may be environmental and genetic factors. Abnormalities of HLA genes may be involved in some phenotypes (*Am J Respir Crit Care Med 2011;183:573*).

Pathophysiology

- The major pathophysiologic consequence of ILD is impaired gas exchange, caused by alteration of the alveolar–capillary interface.

- Interstitial infiltration leads to a restrictive ventilatory defect characterized by decreased lung compliance.
- Some ILDs (e.g., sarcoidosis, hypersensitivity pneumonitis) can have significant bronchiolar involvement with resulting expiratory airflow obstruction and preserved lung volumes.
- Pulmonary vascular abnormalities due to long-standing ILD may lead to the development of PH.

Risk Factors

- Smoking is strongly associated with DIP, RB-ILD, LCH. It is also a risk factor for IPF.
- Family history can increase the risk for a given ILD, especially IPF.
- Work- or environment-related exposures (e.g., birds, molds, silica, coal dust, asbestos, metal dust, wood dust).
- Underlying connective tissue disease can predispose to some ILDs (e.g., NSIP, organizing pneumonia, UIP, LIP).

DIAGNOSIS

Clinical Presentation

History

- Patients typically present with gradually progressive dyspnea on exertion. A subset of ILDs have an acute presentation (e.g., AIP, acute eosinophilic pneumonia), and urgent evaluation is warranted in these cases.
- Persistent dry cough is a common complaint with ILD, especially IPF.
- The history should focus on possible causes of lung injury, such as medications, occupational exposures, and environmental exposures. Comorbid conditions (e.g., connective tissue disease) may be relevant.
- Smoking history is important given the connection between smoking and certain ILDs.

Physical Examination

The physical examination findings depend on the type of ILD but may include inspiratory crackles, clubbing, and signs of PH with right ventricular failure.

Diagnostic Criteria

- IPF
- Either a definite radiographic pattern for UIP on high resolution chest CT (see Imaging section) or UIP pattern on surgical lung biopsy without another known cause (*Am J Respir Crit Care Med 2011;183:788*).
- Sarcoidosis
  - The diagnosis of sarcoidosis is made in a patient with consistent clinical and radiographic findings (Table 10-6) and histologic evidence of noncaseating granulomas, in the absence of an alternate etiology of granulomatous disease (e.g., mycobacterial or fungal infection, berylliosis, granulomatous vasculitis, cancer with a local sarcoid reaction).
  - Biopsy is not required in all patients, such as with Löfgren syndrome (see Table 10-6 and Special Considerations section) (*Am J Respir Crit Care Med 2011;183: 573*).

Differential Diagnosis

The differential diagnosis typically includes other entities within the ILD category.

Table 10-6	Imaging Findings in Selected Interstitial Lung Diseases (ILDs)		
ILD	**Distribution**[a]	**CXR Findings**[b]	**HRCT Findings**[b]
IPF/UIP	Lower, subpleural	• Reticular infiltrates • Honeycombing • Decreased lung volume	• Reticular infiltrates • Honeycombing • Traction bronchiectasis • Minimal ground-glass opacities (may increase during acute exacerbation)
NSIP	Lower	• Reticular infiltrates • Ill-defined opacities • Consolidation	• Reticular infiltrates • Ground-glass opacities • Patchy consolidation • Minimal honeycombing
COP	Usually lower; peripheral, peribronchial	• Patchy consolidation • Nodular opacities	• Patchy consolidation • Patchy ground-glass opacities • Nodules (small or large)
Sarcoidosis	Upper, middle	• Stage 0: Normal • Stage 1: Hilar or mediastinal lymphadenopathy • Stage 2: Hilar or mediastinal lymphadenopathy with pulmonary infiltrates • Stage 3: Pulmonary infiltrates • Stage 4: End-stage fibrosis	• Perilymphatic nodules • Patchy ground-glass opacities • Reticular infiltrates • Traction bronchiectasis • Progressive massive fibrosis • Hilar or mediastinal lymphadenopathy

[a]Refers to the predominant distribution of radiographic abnormalities, e.g., upper lung zone, lower lung zone, diffuse.
[b]All findings listed may not be present in a given patient.
COP, cryptogenic organizing pneumonia; CXR, chest X-ray; HRCT, high-resolution computed tomography; IPF, idiopathic pulmonary fibrosis; NSIP, nonspecific interstitial pneumonia; UIP, usual interstitial pneumonia.
From Webb RW, Higgins CB. *Thoracic Imaging: Pulmonary and Cardiovascular Radiology*. Philadelphia, PA: Lippincott Williams & Wilkins, 2005.

Diagnostic Testing

Laboratories

Blood testing is rarely diagnostic. The laboratory workup should be directed by the history and physical exam, and may provide supportive evidence for certain ILDs. Some examples follow:

- Peripheral eosinophilia may be present in entities such as eosinophilic pneumonia and drug-induced ILD.
- Autoimmune serologies can assist in the diagnosis of connective tissue disease–related ILD.
- Positive serum precipitating antibody testing indicates host sensitization to certain antigens and may support the diagnosis of hypersensitivity pneumonitis.

Electrocardiography

- No particular findings are associated with most ILDs. Evidence of right heart strain in end-stage ILD associated with cor pulmonale may be present.
- Sarcoidosis can have cardiac involvement, so a baseline ECG should be obtained.
  - Conduction abnormalities or bundle branch blocks may be present.
  - Evidence of right heart strain if PH is present.

Imaging

- ILDs typically result in abnormal imaging (chest radiograph or high-resolution CT [HRCT]), although some patients initially have normal studies (see Table 10-6).
- **HRCT** is the test of choice in patients with suspected ILD.
- Comparison should be made with prior studies, when available, to assess the radiographic progression of disease.
- Imaging studies are not always diagnostic. Rather, they usually show nonspecific radiographic patterns, which help narrow the differential diagnosis. Additionally, they may reveal complications of ILD (e.g., infection, malignancy) and provide guidance for biopsy.
- IPF. The American Thoracic Society has published guidelines of the features required to make definite diagnosis of UIP, the radiographic and histopathologic pattern associated with IPF, on HRCT (*Am J Respir Crit Care Med 2011;183: 788*).

Diagnostic Procedures

- **Bronchoalveolar lavage (BAL)** is most often used to evaluate for infection and malignancy, and otherwise has a very limited diagnostic role.
- **Lung biopsy**
  - Transbronchial lung biopsy has the highest yield in bronchocentric ILDs in which small biopsy samples may suffice for diagnosis, such as sarcoidosis and hypersensitivity pneumonitis (Table 10-7) (*Thorax 2008;63(suppl 5):v1*).
  - Surgical lung biopsy can be performed by video-assisted thoracoscopic surgery (VATS) or open thoracotomy. HRCT is used to target areas of active disease and avoid lung regions with end-stage fibrosis.
  - Most patients tolerate lung biopsy well, although certain subgroups of patients are more predisposed to complications. For example, a requirement for mechanical ventilation and an immunocompromised state have been associated with higher mortality following surgical lung biopsy (*Chest 2005;127:1600*).
- All stable patients with suspected ILD should undergo **pulmonary function testing**.
  - Spirometry, lung volumes, and diffusing capacity (DL_{CO})

Table 10-7	Indications for Lung Biopsy in Interstitial Lung Disease

- Atypical clinical features (e.g., age <50 years, fever, weight loss, hemoptysis, signs of vasculitis)
- Progressive disease course
- Normal, atypical, or rapidly changing CXR or HRCT
- Unexplained extrapulmonary manifestations
- Pulmonary vascular disease of unclear etiology
- Assessment of disease activity
- Concern for cancer or infection
- To identify a more treatable process than originally suspected
- To obtain definitive diagnostic and prognostic information before beginning therapy with the potential for significant side effects

CXR, chest X-ray; HRCT, high-resolution computed tomography.
Data from Raghu G. Interstitial lung disease: a diagnostic approach. Are CT scan and lung biopsy indicated in every patient? *Am J Respir Crit Care Med* 1995;151:909–914.

- ○ Resting ABG
- ○ Exercise assessment of arterial oxygenation
- Most patients with ILD have abnormal pulmonary function tests.
  - ○ Restrictive ventilatory defect is characterized by a decrease in total lung capacity with preservation of a normal forced expiratory volume in 1 second (FEV_1)/forced vital capacity (FVC) ratio.
  - ○ As previously mentioned, certain ILDs may manifest an obstructive pattern on pulmonary function testing, defined by an FEV_1/FVC ratio <0.70 (see Pathophysiology section).
- Gas exchange abnormalities are common with ILD, and may be detected by a decrease in DL_{CO}, a widening of the alveolar–arterial oxygen gradient at rest, or a significant decrease in the PaO_2 or SaO_2 with exercise. Hypercapnia may occur in severe ILD.

TREATMENT

The decision to treat ILD is collaboratively made by the patient and his/her physician based on symptoms, lung function, extrapulmonary manifestations, comorbid conditions, potential treatment side effects, and the potential benefit of the proposed treatment plan.

Medications

- Treatment of ILD varies depending on the underlying etiology but usually involves immunosuppression and/or avoidance of offending agents (Table 10-8).
  - ○ Patients receiving immunosuppressive therapy often require regular laboratory monitoring to assess for the development of common adverse drug effects.
  - ○ *Pneumocystis jirovecii* pneumonia prophylaxis should be considered in patients receiving immunosuppressive therapy (*Mayo Clin Proc 1996;71:5*).
- **IPF**
  - ○ **No approved therapies at this time.**
  - ○ Consideration for participation in a clinical trial.

Table 10-8	Medical Treatment of Selected Interstitial Lung Diseases
ILD	**Potential Therapeutic Interventions[a]**
Medication-induced ILD	• Discontinue culprit medication • Corticosteroids
Connective tissue disease–associated ILD, UIP, NSIP, COP	• Corticosteroids • Cytotoxic therapy (e.g., cyclophosphamide, azathioprine)
IPF	• Currently no approved therapies • Consideration for participation in a clinical trial
DIP, RB-ILD	• Smoking cessation • Corticosteroids (likely of limited benefit)
Sarcoidosis	• Corticosteroids • Cytotoxic therapy (e.g., methotrexate, azathioprine) • Hydroxychloroquine • Infliximab
Hypersensitivity pneumonitis	• Avoid offending antigens • Corticosteroids • Cytotoxic therapy

[a]Lung transplantation is a consideration for select patients with end-stage interstitial lung disease.
COP, cryptogenic organizing pneumonia; DIP, desquamative interstitial pneumonia; ILD, interstitial lung disease; IPF, idiopathic pulmonary fibrosis; NSAIDs, nonsteroidal anti-inflammatory drugs; NSIP, nonspecific interstitial pneumonia; RB-ILD: respiratory bronchiolitis-interstitial lung disease.

• **Sarcoidosis**
  For Stage 1 and 2 disease, therapy may not be needed as there can be spontaneous remission.

Nonpharmacologic Therapies
• Bone density assessment is recommended for patients receiving chronic systemic corticosteroid therapy and periodic reassessment (e.g., every 1 to 2 years) should be performed.
• Isoniazid prophylaxis should be considered prior to the initiation of immunosuppressive therapy in patients with a positive PPD.
• All patients with ILD should be offered pulmonary rehabilitation, as well as influenza and pneumococcal vaccinations.
• Patients with ILD should undergo evaluation of need for supplemental oxygen.

Surgical Management
Select patients with end-stage ILD may benefit from lung transplantation (Table 10-9).

Lifestyle/Risk Modification
Depends on underlying ILD, but avoidance of potential causative agents (hypersensitivity pneumonitis) and cigarette smoke (IPF, DIP, RB-ILD) is important.

Table 10-9	Criteria for Listing for Lung Transplantation in Idiopathic Pulmonary Fibrosis and Sarcoidosis

IPF

Histologic or radiographic evidence of UIP and any of the following:
- DL_{CO} <39% predicted
- ≥10% decrement in FVC during 6 months of follow-up
- SpO_2 <88% during a 6-minute walk test
- Honeycombing on HRCT (fibrosis score >2)

Sarcoidosis

NYHA functional Class III or IV and any of the following:
- Hypoxemia at rest
- Pulmonary hypertension
- Right atrial pressure >15 mm Hg

DL_{CO}, diffusing capacity of the lung for carbon monoxide; FVC, forced vital capacity; HRCT, high-resolution computed tomography; IPF, idiopathic pulmonary fibrosis; NYHA, New York Heart Association; SpO_2, oxyhemoglobin saturation by pulse oximetry; UIP, usual interstitial pneumonia.
Modified from Orens JB, Estenne M, Arcasoy S, et al. International Guidelines for the Selection of Lung Transplant Candidates: 2006 Update— A Consensus Report From the Pulmonary Scientific Council of the International Society for Heart and Lung Transplantation. *J Heart Lung Transplant* 2006;25:745–755.

SPECIAL CONSIDERATIONS

- **IPF**
  - Acute exacerbations of IPF (Table 10-10) carry a high mortality rate. Systemic corticosteroids are often used to treat acute exacerbations, although their benefit has not been systematically proven (*Chest 2007;132:1652*).

Table 10-10	Diagnostic Criteria for Acute Exacerbation of Idiopathic Pulmonary Fibrosis

- Previous or concurrent diagnosis of IPF
- Unexplained development or worsening of dyspnea within 30 days
- HRCT showing new bilateral ground-glass abnormality and/or consolidation superimposed on a background reticular or honeycomb pattern consistent with UIP
- No evidence of pulmonary infection
- Exclusion of alternative causes, including left heart failure, pulmonary embolism, and other identifiable causes of acute lung injury

HRCT, high-resolution computed tomography; IPF, idiopathic pulmonary fibrosis; UIP, usual interstitial pneumonia.
Data from Raghu G, Collard HR, Egan JJ, et al. An Official ATS/ERS/JRS/ALAT Statement: Idiopathic Pulmonary Fibrosis: Evidence-based Guidelines for Diagnosis and Management. *Am J Respir Crit Care Med* 2011;183:788–824.

- ○ Patients with IPF are at increased risk for lung cancer (*Curr Opin Pulm Med 2005;11:431*).
- **Sarcoidosis**
  Extrapulmonary manifestations:
  - ○ Constitutional symptoms (e.g., fever, fatigue, malaise, weight loss).
  - ○ Typical extrapulmonary manifestations include skin and eye lesions, peripheral lymphadenopathy, and hepatosplenomegaly.
  - ○ Cutaneous manifestations of sarcoidosis include **erythema nodosum** (raised, red, tender bumps or nodules on the anterior legs) and **lupus pernio** (indurated plaques with associated discoloration of the nose, cheeks, lips, and ears).
  - ○ **Uveitis** is the most common eye lesion in sarcoidosis (*Am J Respir Crit Care Med 1999;160:736*). Patients with sarcoidosis should see an ophthalmologist for a thorough exam due to the potential for eye involvement.
  - ○ **Löfgren syndrome** is defined as an acute presentation of sarcoidosis characterized by arthritis, erythema nodosum, and bilateral hilar lymphadenopathy (*Am J Respir Crit Care Med 2011;183:573*).
  - ○ Myocardial involvement may result in cardiomyopathy, arrhythmia, and sudden death (*Am Heart J 2009;157:9*).
  - ○ Endocrinologic involvement can manifest as hypercalcemia and hypercalciuria secondary to dysregulated production of calcitriol (*Am J Respir Crit Care Med 1999;160:736*).

COMPLICATIONS

- In general, some ILDs can progress to end-stage lung disease with associated PH and right heart failure.
- Sarcoidosis in particular can have direct cutaneous, ophthalmologic, cardiac, endocrinologic, and neurologic manifestations (see Special Considerations section).
  - ○ Chronic uveitis can lead to glaucoma and blindness.
  - ○ Renal failure can develop due to hypercalcemia.
  - ○ Arrhythmias and cardiomyopathy can occur with cardiac involvement.

REFERRAL

- If severe pulmonary impairment, consider referral for lung transplant evaluation.
- If concern for underlying connective tissue disease, consider referral to rheumatology.
- Patients with sarcoidosis should be referred to ophthalmology for regular eye exam.
- Consider referring sarcoidosis patients with evidence of other organ involvement to specialists in those areas for evaluation and monitoring.
- Consideration should be given to referring patients with IPF to centers participating in clinical trials given the lack of effective therapy at this time.

MONITORING/FOLLOW-UP

Monitoring of patients with ILD involves periodic assessment of clinical, radiographic, and physiologic parameters, as well as surveillance for medication toxicity in patients receiving pharmacotherapy.

OUTCOMES/PROGNOSIS

- Varies depending upon the specific ILD and severity of underlying lung disease.
- **IPF**
  - Mean survival from the time of diagnosis is approximately 3 to 5 years.
  - There can be variability in patient progression. Some patients progress very rapidly, while others can remain stable for longer periods of time. However, most patients have a slow, steady progression of symptoms and decline in lung function, which can be precipitously worsened by an acute exacerbation (see Special Considerations section).
- **Sarcoidosis**
  - Highly variable course across patient populations. Many patients either have spontaneous remission or good response to steroids.
    - Patients with radiographic stage 1 or 2 disease (see Table 10-6) have a spontaneous remission rate of 40% to 90% with stage 1 disease being more likely to spontaneously remit.
    - Stage 3 and 4 disease are unlikely to spontaneously remit.
    - Symptoms of erythema nodosum and Löfgren syndrome portend good prognosis.
    - Extrapulmonary manifestations such as lupus pernio, cardiac involvement, neurosarcoidosis, or nephrocalcinosis portend worse prognosis.
    - African American patients tend to have more extrapulmonary manifestations and a more progressive course.
  - Relapses can occur in 16% to 74% of patients (*Am J Respir Crit Care Med 1999;160:736*).

Solitary Pulmonary Nodule

GENERAL PRINCIPLES

- The goal of a careful evaluation of the solitary pulmonary nodule (SPN) is to determine if the lesion is more likely **malignant or benign**.
- **A lesion greater than 3 cm has a high likelihood of malignancy and should be treated as such, whereas lesions less than 3 cm need more careful assessment.**
- Benign nodules with low-risk characteristics should be closely followed so that invasive procedures with associated risks can be avoided.
- Identifying early lung cancer is of the utmost importance as there is a >60% survival rate of patients who have a malignant SPN removed (*Chest 1997;111:1710*).

Definition

- **A solitary pulmonary nodule is defined as an asymptomatic rounded lesion less than 3 cm in diameter.** It is completely surrounded by lung parenchyma, unaccompanied by atelectasis, intrathoracic adenopathy, or pleural effusion.
- Pulmonary nodules less than 8 to 10 mm (subcentimeter nodules) remain within this definition; however, there is evidence to suggest that these nodules undergo a less rigorous evaluation due to lower overall malignancy risk (*Chest 2007;132(3 suppl):945*).

Epidemiology

- Approximately 150,000 SPNs are identified each year in the United States.
- It has been estimated that such a nodule is noted on 0.09% to 0.20% of all chest radiographs.

Etiology

- Although underlying etiologies for pulmonary nodules are varied, the most important designation clinically is deciphering between a malignant and a nonmalignant process.
- **Malignancy accounts for approximately 40% of SPNs.**
- **Granulomas** (both infectious and noninfectious) account for 50% of undiagnosed SPNs.
- The remaining 10% are composed of **benign neoplasms**, such as **hamartomas** (5%) and a multitude of other causes.

Risk Factors

- **Smoking** is the most important associated risk factor for almost all malignant SPNs.
- For infectious etiologies, an immunocompromised state promotes an increased risk.

Lung Cancer Screening

Screening high-risk patients using low-dose chest CT resulted in a 20% relative reduction in mortality from lung cancer compared to screening with chest X-ray (*N Engl J Med 2011;365:395*).

DIAGNOSIS

- Diagnosis of the SPN is made radiographically, usually via chest X-ray or CT scan.
- Most frequently, the nodule is noted incidentally on a study performed for other reasons (e.g., chronic cough, chest pain).

Clinical Presentation

- As stated previously, the majority of SPNs are diagnosed incidentally by radiographic tests done for other reasons so there may not be overt symptoms.
- There are instances when a nodule may precipitate cough, chest pain, hemoptysis, or sputum production depending on the etiology and location of the SPN.

History

- Ask typical screening questions for malignancy including **weight loss and night sweats**.
- **Hemoptysis** may indicate malignancy but may also prompt investigations for antineutrophil cytoplasmic antibody (ANCA)-associated vasculitis, tuberculosis (TB), and hereditary hemorrhagic telangiectasia (HHT).
- Ask about arthritis and arthralgias for possible undiagnosed rheumatoid arthritis or sarcoidosis.
- Take an exposure history including recent travel history related to endemic mycoses (histoplasmosis, coccidioidomycosis, etc.) as well as possible TB exposures.
- A history of previous malignancies increases the risk of metastatic disease of the lung.
- Patients who are immunosuppressed from HIV, organ transplant, or chronic steroids have increased risk of infectious causes.
- Smoking is linked to 85% of lung cancers. A patient's risk of lung cancer decreases significantly 5 years after smoking cessation, but it never truly returns to normal.
- An occupational history is important including possible asbestosis exposure (associated with not only mesothelioma, but also non–small cell lung cancer), silica, beryllium, radon, ionizing radiation, among others.

Physical Examination
- Although there are no specific physical exam findings related to SPNs, evidence for underlying etiologies may be discovered with a thorough exam.
- Note signs of weight loss or cachexia, suggestive of malignancy.
- Do a thorough lymph node exam. **A cervical lymph node might provide an easy diagnostic target to determine the etiology of an SPN.**
- Perform a breast exam in women and testicular exam in young men.
- A careful skin examination may reveal telangiectasias, erythema nodosum, rheumatoid nodules, or other findings that might suggest a cause.

Diagnostic Criteria
- As mentioned previously, an SPN is identified as a rounded lesion less than 3 cm in circumference. It is completely surrounded by lung parenchyma, unaccompanied by atelectasis, intrathoracic adenopathy, or pleural effusion.
- The first step in managing an SPN is to stratify the patient in terms of malignancy risk: low-, intermediate-, or high-risk categories (Table 10-11).
- Risk stratification can be accomplished either qualitatively via clinical judgment or quantitatively using validated risk assessment tools (*Arch Intern Med 1997;157:849*).
- Once the risk of malignancy has been established, further management can proceed, as outlined in Figure 10-3.

Differential Diagnosis
Pulmonary nodules are divided primarily into malignant or benign etiologies, with benign processes further divided into infectious or noninfectious causes (Table 10-12).

Diagnostic Testing
Laboratories
- Routine laboratory testing is seldom helpful unless the history and physical exam strongly suggest an etiology.
- If connective tissue diseases or vasculitides are suggested, perform appropriate testing.
- Hyponatremia may suggest syndrome of inappropriate antidiuretic hormone (SIADH) associated with primary lung cancer, as well as other pulmonary processes.

Table 10-11	Risk Stratification of a Solitary Pulmonary Nodule		
Variable	**Low Risk**	**Intermediate Risk**	**High Risk**
Lesion diameter (cm)	<1.5	1.5–2.2	>2.2
Patient age (years)	<45	45–60	>60
Smoking status	Never smoked or quit >7 yr ago	Current smoker of <20 cigarettes/d or quit <7 yr ago	Current smoker of >20 cigarettes/d
Lesion margin characteristics	Smooth and rounded	Scalloped	Spiculated or corona radiata
Densitometry in Hounsfield Units (HU)	<15 HU	>15 HU	>15 HU

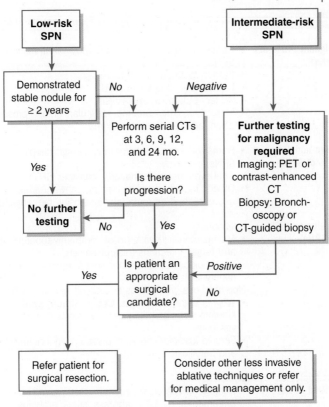

Figure 10-3. Diagnostic and therapeutic management of low- and intermediate-risk pulmonary nodules. CT, computed tomography; PET, positron emission tomography; SPN, solitary pulmonary nodule.

- Hypercalcemia might suggest lung cancer as well as sarcoidosis.
- Anemia may indicate chronic pulmonary hemorrhage (e.g., HHT) or a chronic inflammatory disease.
- Microbiologic studies, particularly sputum culture, may aid in the diagnosis of an infectious SPN.
- Sputum cytology has limited use, as yield is low for peripherally located, small lesions.

Imaging

The mainstay of diagnostic evaluation of the SPN is via radiographic studies, primarily **chest X-ray, chest CT, and positron emission tomography (PET) scan**.

- **Chest X-ray**
  - A previous chest radiograph is an important tool in the initial evaluation of an SPN.
  - If an SPN has been present and unchanged on chest radiograph for more than 2 years, then further evaluation may not be warranted. Ground glass lesions may

Table 10-12	Differential Diagnosis of the Solitary Pulmonary Nodule
Malignant (40% of SPNs)	• Primary pulmonary carcinoma (80% of all malignant SPNs) • Primary pulmonary lymphoma • Primary pulmonary carcinoid • Solitary pulmonary metastasis • Melanoma, osteosarcoma, testicular, breast, prostate, colon, and renal cell carcinoma
Benign neoplasms (5% of SPNs)	• Hamartoma (accounts for most benign neoplastic SPNs) • Arteriovenous malformations (consider HHT) • Others, including neural tumors (schwannoma, neurofibroma), fibroma, and sclerosing hemangioma
Granulomas (50% of SPNs)	Infectious • Mycobacterial disease (most commonly tuberculosis) and fungal infections (histoplasmosis, coccidioidomycosis, blastomycosis, cryptococcosis, aspergillosis) Noninfectious granulomas associated with vasculitis • Wegner's granulomatosis, Churg–Strauss syndrome • Noninfectious granulomas not associated with vasculitis • Sarcoid granulomatosis, hypersensitivity pneumonitis, and berylliosis
Other etiologies (5% of SPNs)	Infectious • Bacterial (nocardiosis, actinomycosis, round pneumonia), measles, abscess, septic embolus Noninfectious • Lipoid pneumonia, amyloid, subpleural lymph node, rheumatoid nodule, pulmonary scar or infarct, congenital malformations (bronchogenic cyst, sequestration), skin nodule, rib fracture, pleural thickening from mass or fluid

HHT, hereditary hemorrhagic telangiectasia; SPN, solitary pulmonary nodule.

be followed for longer periods of time as the volume-doubling time may be extended in certain types of non–small cell lung cancer.

○ If an SPN appears on a new radiograph in less than 30 days, it is likely not malignant and most likely infectious or inflammatory.

○ There are radiographic findings that make it more likely that a lesion is **benign: calcifications, a laminated appearance**; or, more likely **malignant: spiculated, irregular border** (see Table 10-11).

○ The chest X-ray is easy to obtain and delivers a low dose of radiation; however, it has limitations in the initial characterization and careful comparisons over time required for SPN evaluation.

- **Chest CT**
  - Chest CT is now considered the most important radiologic exam for SPN evaluation. With few exceptions, an SPN requires assessment by CT.
  - Accurate volumetric measurement of lesion size allows precise comparison to determine stability or growth.
  - Imaging allows a careful examination of mediastinal lymph nodes.
  - Thin cuts through the lesion are more sensitive than chest X-ray for characterizing calcifications and lamination as well as the margins of the lesion.
- **PET scan**
  - 18-Flourodeoxyglucose positron emission tomography (FDG-PET) can help distinguish malignant and benign lesions because cancers are metabolically active and take up FDG avidly.
  - Sensitivity of 80% to 100% and specificity of 79% to 100% of detecting malignancy.
  - **False negatives** can occur in bronchoalveolar carcinoma, carcinoid, and mucinous neoplasms while **false positives** are common in nonmalignant "inflammatory" conditions (infectious and autoimmune processes).
  - Higher incidence of both false-positive and false-negative results occurs in nodules <10 mm, thus discouraging the use of PET scan in this situation (*Lung Cancer 2004;45:19*).
  - PET scan is most commonly utilized in the evaluation of low-to-moderate risk indeterminate nodules for further risk stratification (see Figure 10-3).
- **Contrast-enhanced CT**
  - Technique utilizing contrast enhancement and measurement of Hounsfield units to risk stratify an SPN for malignancy.
  - A multicenter analysis demonstrates high sensitivity but relatively low specificity for identifying malignant nodules (*Radiology 2000;214:73*).
  - This method may be an important tool for risk assessment of an indeterminate SPN in centers that have experience with the technique.

Diagnostic Procedures
- **If a nodule is considered high risk, and the patient is an appropriate surgical candidate, then the best approach is to forego biopsy and pursue resection.**
- Any change of an SPN on serial imaging warrants resection or invasive biopsy.
- If a lesion has low-risk characteristics, there is no indication to pursue biopsy and subjecting a patient to unneeded risk.
- **Biopsy** is most often pursued when there is discordance between clinical risk stratification and imaging tests. For example, when pretest suspicion for malignancy is significant but PET imaging is negative, biopsy may be indicated.
- Also, for patients where surgery represents significant risk secondary to comorbidities, using a less invasive biopsy strategy to determine the presence of malignancy is appropriate.
- There are primarily two options for biopsy of an SPN: transthoracic needle aspiration (TTNA) and fiber optic flexible bronchoscopy.
  - **Transthoracic needle aspiration**
    - This technique is usually performed under the guidance of fluoroscopy, ultrasound, or CT (more common).
    - This approach is most commonly employed for nodules with a peripheral location and without anatomic impediment to a biopsy needle.

- Specificity for identifying malignancy is high with TTNA; however, there is a significant rate of nondiagnostic biopsies, and sensitivity depends on many factors, including nodule size.
- A nondiagnostic biopsy does not rule out malignancy.
- The main complication of TTNA is pneumothorax with 25% incidence of minor pneumothorax and 5% major requiring chest tube drainage.
  ○ **Bronchoscopy**
    - Conventional flexible bronchoscopy has traditionally been used to access central airway lesions, mediastinal lymph nodes, and large parenchymal masses, leaving only a limited role in the evaluation of an SPN.
    - However, with the recent use of **endobronchial ultrasound (EBUS)**, evaluating an SPN with bronchoscopy has developed into an important modality, providing diagnostic yields over 80% regardless of lesion size (*Am J Respir Crit Care Med 2007;176:36*).
- Other interventional techniques, including electromagnetic navigation and CT virtual bronchoscopy, also show promise in improving the use of bronchoscopy in the management of SPN.

TREATMENT

- Management of low- and intermediate-risk SPNs is outlined in Figure 10-3.
- Overall treatment strategy is to identify lesions with significant malignancy risk and pursue surgical resection when possible.
- If a nodule has low-risk characteristics and has demonstrated stability over a period of 2 years, then no further treatment is warranted. Further follow-up of ground glass lesions may be necessary, as the volume-doubling times of these lesions may be prolonged.
- If a specific etiology for the SPN is diagnosed (e.g., a connective tissue disease or infection), then treatment is targeted toward the underlying process.

Other Nonpharmacologic Therapies

- Although **surgical resection is preferable in patients with either a high-risk lesion or biopsy proven malignancy**, if surgical resection is not an option, there are other less effective therapies.
- **Stereotactic radiation** is currently the most widely utilized therapy in this clinical situation. This mode of external beam therapy aims to decrease collateral radiation-induced damage to adjacent lung tissue.
- There are more experimental approaches, including brachytherapy and radiofrequency ablation, that are currently under development.

Surgical Management

- Surgical resection of an indeterminate SPN is indicated in the following situations:
  ○ The clinical probability of malignancy is moderate to high (>60%).
  ○ The nodule is hypermetabolic by PET imaging.
  ○ The nodule has been proven malignant by biopsy.
- A combination of surgical techniques, including VATS, mediastinoscopy, and thoracotomy, can lead to diagnosis (via intraoperative frozen section), staging, and potential cure during a single induction of anesthesia.

MONITORING/FOLLOW-UP

- For a low- or intermediate-risk pulmonary nodule for which resection is either not warranted (see Figure 10-3), desired, or possible, routine follow-up with chest CT is standard practice.
- The typical practice for following an SPN is with serial chest CT performed at intervals of **3, 6, 12, 18, and 24 months** from initial detection, assessing for any evidence of growth.

Pleural Effusion

GENERAL PRINCIPLES

Definition
The accumulation of fluid in the pleural space.

Classification
Diagnosis and management is based on classifying a pleural effusion as either a **transudate or exudate**.

Etiology
- **Most common causes** (*Pleural Disease. 4th ed. Philadelphia: Lippincott, Williams and Wilkins, 2001*):
  - Left heart failure (36%)
  - Pneumonia (22%)
  - Malignancy (14%): lung, breast, lymphoma
  - Pulmonary embolism (11%)
  - Viral disease (7%)
- **Less common but important causes:** rheumatologic/collagen vascular disease, hepatic cirrhosis, hepatic hydrothorax, pancreatitis, esophageal rupture, lymphatic obstruction, "trapped" lung

Pathophysiology
- **Normal pleural physiology:**
  - Each pleural space produces and reabsorbs up to 15 mL of fluid per day and **contains about 10 mL of fluid at any one time** not apparent on imaging.
  - **Normal pleural fluid chemistries:** lactate dehydrogenase (LDH) <0.6 of serum, protein <0.5 of serum, glucose 0.6 to 0.8 of serum, pH 7.60.
- **Transudative effusion: alteration of hydrostatic and/or oncotic factors** that increase the formation and/or decrease reabsorption of pleural fluid.
  - CHF: increased venous pressures and lung edema
  - Hepatic cirrhosis and nephrotic syndrome: hypoalbuminemia
  - Malignancy: infiltration/obstruction of pleural capillaries and/or lymphatics (up to 10% of malignant effusions are transudative)
- **Exudative effusion:** either direct or cytokine-induced disruption of normal pleural membranes and/or vasculature leading to **increased capillary permeability**.
  - Infection/pneumonia
  - Malignancy

- ○ Inflammatory disease (i.e., systemic lupus erythematosis [SLE] or rheumatoid arthritis [RA])
- ○ Trauma/surgery
- ○ Pulmonary embolus
- **Fluid markers of pleural infection, inflammation, and/or obstruction** often coexist.
  - ○ **Low glucose and pH levels**
    - ▪ Byproducts of microorganism and/or inflammatory cell metabolism
    - ▪ Decreased acid removal due to pleural disruption from inflammation or malignancy
  - ○ **High LDH level**
    Cell turnover and lysis

DIAGNOSIS

The clinical setting, combined with pleural fluid analysis, is crucial to establishing a proper diagnosis.

Clinical Presentation

Symptoms and signs may be directly related to the pleural effusion itself, and/or to any underlying disease process.

History

- **Dyspnea** due to abnormal pulmonary mechanics: most common symptom, usually develops with greater than 500 to 1,000 mL of pleural fluid but may not correlate
- **Often asymptomatic**
- Pleurisy or referred chest/back/shoulder pain from pleural inflammation
- Should include survey of potential underlying causes

Physical Examination

- Vital signs: Assess for fever, hemodynamic instability, hypoxemia.
- Chest exam: **Dullness to percussion, decreased breath sounds, and tactile fremitus.** These signs are more sensitive with larger effusions, but the chest exam is often unreliable and should not be used solely to diagnose and approximate size (*Clev Clin J Med 2008;75:297*).
- A thorough system-based exam should evaluate for CHF, malignancy, pneumonia, hepatic cirrhosis, venous thrombosis, and other potential causes of pleural effusion.

Diagnostic Criteria

- **Analysis of pleural fluid obtained by thoracentesis** is the mainstay of diagnosing an etiology.
- **Transudate: Presence of ALL of Light's criteria** (*Ann Intern Med 1972;77:507*).
  - ○ Fluid: serum protein ratio <0.5
  - ○ Fluid: serum LDH ratio <0.6
  - ○ Pleural fluid LDH <0.67 of upper limit of normal for serum LDH
- **Exudate: Presence of ANY of Light's criteria** (*Ann Intern Med 1972;77:507*).
  - ○ Fluid: serum protein ratio >0.5
  - ○ Fluid: serum LDH ratio >0.6
  - ○ Pleural fluid LDH >0.67 of upper limit of normal for serum LDH
- **Pseudo exudate:** An effusion that meets one or more of Light's criteria but is actually a transudate.

- ○ **Usually due to diuretic-treated CHF**, cirrhosis, or nephrotic kidney disease.
- ○ **Serum to pleural fluid albumin gradient** >1.2.
- • **Simple parapneumonic effusion:** A sterile, small (encompassing less than one-half the hemithorax), free-flowing pleural effusion in the setting of pneumonia, with pH >7.20 and glucose >60 mg/dL.
- • **Complicated parapneumonic effusion: ANY one of the following** (*Chest 2000;118:1158*):
  - ○ Large (encompassing more than one-half of the hemithorax), free flowing
  - ○ Effusion of any size with loculations
  - ○ Thickened parietal pleura on chest CT
  - ○ Positive-gram stain or culture
  - ○ pH <7.20 or glucose <60 mg/dL
- • **Empyema: Gross pus in the pleural space or positive gram stain.** Positive culture is NOT required for diagnosis (high false-negative rate).

Differential Diagnosis
See Table 10-13.

Diagnostic Testing
- • Pleural effusion is detected by chest imaging and characterized through sampling by thoracentesis.
- • **All parapneumonic effusions, and new, undiagnosed effusions should be sampled.**

Laboratories
- • **Pleural fluid** (see Table 10-13):
  - ○ Note color and consistency
  - ○ Chemistries: Protein, albumin, LDH, glucose, pH
  - ○ Cell count with differential
  - ○ Hematocrit if suspicion for hemothorax (>0.5 of serum is diagnostic)
  - ○ Microbiologic stains and culture per suspicion
  - ○ Cytology (yield approximately 60%)
  - ○ Consider triglyceride, amylase, adenosine deaminase (ADA) as indicated
- • Serum: CBC, CMP, LDH, urinalysis, coagulation studies, BNP
- • Additional labs guided by suggestion of underlying illness

Electrocardiography
Assess for structural heart disease. Otherwise usually nonspecific and noncontributory.

Imaging
- • Standard upright **PA/lateral chest X-ray (CXR)**:
  - ○ Diagnostic for a suspected pleural effusion and approximates size (*Radiology: Diagnosis, Imaging, Intervention. Philadelphia: Lippincott, 2000:1*).
    - ▪ 75 mL obscures the posterior costophrenic sulcus
    - ▪ 175 mL obscures the lateral costophrenic sulcus
    - ▪ 500 mL obscures the entire diaphragmatic contour
    - ▪ 1,000 mL reaches the level of the anterior 4th rib
  - ○ Helps suggest associated conditions (CHF, pneumonia).
- • **Lateral decubitus radiograph**
  - ○ **Demonstrates fluidity.**
  - ○ Usually amenable for thoracentesis if fluid layers to >1 cm.

Table 10-13	Clues to Diagnosing the Cause of a Pleural Effusion Based on Fluid Analysis

Gross appearance

- **Clear/serous/light yellow:** Transudate of any etiology (cardiac, liver, kidney disease) Urinothorax (consider if smells like ammonia)
- **Bloody/serosanguineous:** Hemothorax (surgery/trauma); PE; malignancy
- **Purulent/turbid/brown:** Infectious/empyema; esophageal rupture

Nucleated cells

- **Total >50,000, neutrophilia:** Infectious/empyema
- **Total <5,000:** Transudate of any etiology; chronic malignant; tuberculous
- **Lymphocytosis (>85%):** Tuberculous; lymphoma; chronic rheumatoid; sarcoid; pseudo-exudates
- **Eosinophilia (>10%):** Pneumothorax; hemothorax; fungal; parasitic; meds; malignancy; benign asbestos effusion
- **Mesothelial cells (>5%):** Normal; transudate

Chemical analysis

- **Elevated protein: >3 g/dL:** Most exudates; pseudo-exudates (serum-fluid albumin gradient >1.2 g/dL)
- **>4 g/dL:** Tuberculous
- **>7–8 g/dL:** Blood cell dyscrasias
- **Elevated LDH: >1,000 IU/L:** Empyema; rheumatoid; paragonimiasis; high burden malignant
- **Fluid:serum ratio >1:** Pneumocystis or urinothorax
- **Glucose <60 mg/dL:** Infectious/empyema; rheumatoid; lupus; tuberculous; esophageal rupture; malignant
- **pH <7.3:** Infectious/empyema; rheumatoid; lupus; tuberculous; esophageal rupture; high burden malignant
- **Elevated amylase (>serum):** Pancreatitis; esophageal rupture; malignancy
- **Adenosine deaminase >50 U/L:** Tuberculous (unlikely if level <40)
- **Triglycerides >110 mg/dL:** Chylothorax

LDH, lactate dehydrogenase; PE, pulmonary embolism.

- **Thoracic ultrasonography**
  - Accurate and practical in **detecting loculations**.
  - Provides **real-time guidance for thoracentesis or thoracostomy tube placement**, reducing complication rates.
- **Chest CT with contrast**
  - Helpful in distinguishing fluid from lung mass, atelectasis, pneumonia, or suggesting hemothorax.
  - Defines and characterizes pleural loculations, thickening, nodularity, or other abnormalities.

Diagnostic Procedures

- **Thoracentesis:** Can be performed safely at the bedside on effusions layering >1 cm on lateral decubitus CXR.
  - **Complicated/organized effusions should be accessed using real-time ultrasound or CT guidance.**

- ○ **Optimize hemostasis:** PT/PTT $<2\times$ normal, platelets $>25k$, creatinine <6 (*Transfusion 1991;31:164*).
- ○ **Microbiologic studies** of a parapneumonic effusion may be falsely negative after antibiotic administration.
- ○ Repeat thoracentesis increases diagnostic yield.
- ○ **Cytology for malignancy positive up to 60%** but probably not dependent on fluid volume obtained (*Chest 2002;122:1913*).
- ○ **Acid-fast bacteria (AFB) stain and culture sensitivity <30%** (*Chest 2007; 131:880*).
- **Closed pleural biopsy:** Performed by transthoracic needle approach.
- ○ **Indicated for the undiagnosed, suspected tuberculous or rheumatoid effusion. Sensitivity >80% when combined with pleural fluid AFB stain and culture** since tuberculous pleuritis is usually diffuse (*Chest 1997;112:702*).
- ○ **Consider for the undiagnosed, suspected malignant effusion.** Obtaining four to six consecutive samples from a locally thickened pleura (as seen on chest CT), may offer diagnostic yields $>50\%$, and $>70\%$ when combined with fluid cytology (*J Bronchol 1998;5:327*; *Chest 2006;129:1549*).
- **Thoracoscopic pleural biopsy:** Performed under direct pleural visualization.
- ○ **Indicated for the undiagnosed suspected malignant effusion.**
- ○ **Diagnostic yield is >70% to 90%** (*Ann Intern Med 1991;114:271*; *ANZ J Surg 2006;76:722*).

TREATMENT

- **Transudates: Usually resolve with treatment of the underlying cause** (heart failure, hepatic disease, nephrotic syndrome).
- ○ Therapeutic thoracentesis as indicated for persistent larger effusions.
- ○ Uncommonly, more aggressive measures including pleurodesis, shunts, or placement of a chronic indwelling pleural catheter are indicated for comfort or palliation.
- **Simple/uncomplicated parapneumonic effusion:** Antibiotics and close observation.
- **Complicated parapneumonic effusion and empyema** (Figure 10-4): Antibiotics and **early thoracostomy tube drainage** to avoid inflammatory adhesion and organization (*Chest 2000;118:1158*).
- ○ **Antibiotics should also target anaerobic organisms** as they often complicate empyema (*Lancet 1974;1:338*; *Chest 1993;103:1502*).
- ○ **Intrapleural fibrinolysis for loculated effusions is controversial**, but may improve drainage and decrease the need for surgical intervention (*Chest 2006;129:783*). There is a possible **risk of pleural hemorrhage** in patients undergoing concomitant systemic anticoagulation (*Radiology 2008;246:956*).
- ○ Chest tube can be removed when adequate drainage is accomplished (<50 to 100 mL output per day AND resolution documented on follow-up imaging).
- ○ **Surgical decortication (thoracoscopic vs. open) may be required for effusions exhibiting complex anatomy** (extensive pleural thickening, fibrous organization, and/or multiple loculations), or for those unresponsive to tube drainage.
- **Malignant pleural effusion** (Figure 10-5): recur in approximately 95% of cases, usually within a week.
- ○ Observation is appropriate in cases of small, asymptomatic, stable effusions.
- ○ **Therapeutic (large volume) thoracentesis** (LVT) for comfort.
  - ▪ Repeat thoracentesis is reasonable if effusion reaccumulates slowly.

Figure 10-4. Suggested general approach to managing complicated parapneumonic effusions and empyema.

- **Reexpansion pulmonary edema is very rare**, and is unlikely related to rate or volume of fluid removed (*Ann Thorac Surg 2007;84:1656*).
- **Removal of at least 1.5 L at a time is safe.** However, **LVT should be discontinued with development of chest discomfort**, which may be a surrogate marker for unsafe drop in pleural pressures (*Chest 2006;129:1556*).
- **Chemical pleurodesis:** Instillation of a pleural sclerosing agent such as talc or doxycycline (*Ann Intern Med 1994;120:56*).
  - Recommended when there is **rapid reaccumulation of fluid**.
  - **Talc**, instilled either as **"slurry"** through a thoracostomy tube, or through insufflation during thoracoscopy (**"poudrage"**), is very effective and more comfortable than doxycycline (*Chest 2005;127:909*).
  - Less effective if lung reexpansion is incomplete after drainage ("trapped lung").
  - Often requires hospitalization for approximately 3 to 5 days.
- **Chronic indwelling pleural catheter:** Practical, can be performed in the outpatient setting, and maintained easily by the patient and caregiver.
  - Similar indication as chemical pleurodesis, and preferred if there is "trapped lung."

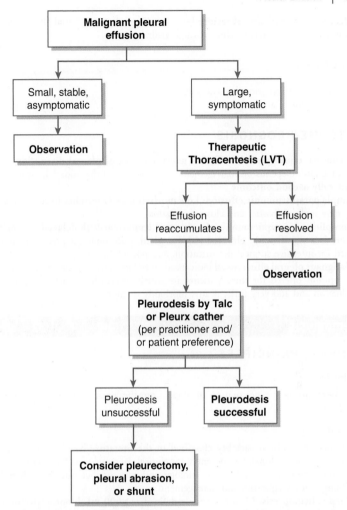

Figure 10-5. Suggested general approach to managing malignant pleural effusions. LVT, large-volume thoracentesis.

- There is a 50% pleurodesis rate with repeated drainage, allowing for removal.
- More successful at palliation than doxycycline pleurodesis (*Cancer 1999;86: 1992*).
- Pleurectomy, pleuroperitoneal shunt, chemo/radiation therapy.

Surgical Management

- **Thoracic decortication:** In cases of complicated parapneumonic effusions that have complex pleural anatomy due to fibrous organization and/or not amenable or responsive to pleural drainage.

- **Pleurectomy or pleural abrasion:** For recurring malignant pleural effusion unresponsive to pleurodesis or chronic catheter drainage.

REFERRAL

- Pulmonary (interventional if available)
- Thoracic surgery as needed

OUTCOME/PROGNOSIS

Depends on etiology of the effusion and the extent of pleural disruption.
- **Transudate:** Depends on management and prognosis of the underlying cause but **generally a good outcome**.
- **Simple parapneumonic effusion: Low morbidity and mortality** if treated appropriately with antibiotics and close observation.
- **Complicated parapneumonic effusion and empyema:With delayed treatment, there is a significantly elevated risk for pleuropulmonary sequelae,** including need for intensive surgical decortication, and possibly death.
- **Malignant pleural effusions** all indicate advanced malignant spread. The therapeutic options offered for these patients are usually successful in achieving desired palliation and add very little, if any, morbidity or mortality risk.

Hemoptysis

GENERAL PRINCIPLES

Definition

True hemoptysis is expectoration of blood from the lower respiratory tree (below the glottis).

Classification

- Hemoptysis has been **variably classified in the literature** based on appearance, frequency, rate, volume, and potential for clinical consequences. These characteristics often suggest an underlying etiology and may predict outcome, therefore helping guide diagnostics and management.
- **Massive hemoptysis:** Most commonly defined as **>600 mL blood expectorated per 24 hours** (*Flexible Bronchoscopy. 2nd ed. Hoboken: Wiley-Blackwell, 2004*).

Epidemiology

Depends on the underlying cause.

Etiology

- According to acuity:
  - **Acute/single or few episodes: bronchitis, pneumonia**, trauma, pulmonary embolism (PE), left heart failure
  - **Subacute/recurrent: malignancy, cavitary lung disease** (TB, aspergilloma, lung abscess), arteriovenous malformation (AVM), pulmonary endometriosis
- According to volume:
  - **Nonmassive hemoptysis: bronchitis, malignancy**, bronchiectasis, pneumonias

- **Massive hemoptysis: bronchiectasis, cavitary lung disease** (TB, aspergilloma, lung abscess), AVM, malignancy
- According to **anatomic location**:
  - **Airway: bronchitis/bronchiectasis, malignancy**, foreign body, trauma
  - **Parenchyma/alveoli: pneumonia, rheumatologic vasculitides, and pulmonary hemorrhage syndromes** (ANCA+ vasculitis, Goodpasture syndrome, SLE)
  - **Vascular: elevated pulmonary venous pressure** (LV failure, mitral stenosis), PE, AVM, varices/aneurysms, rheumatologic vasculitides, and pulmonary hemorrhage syndromes
- Coagulopathy: thrombocytopenia, disseminated intravascular coagulation (DIC)
- Meds, drugs: Anticoagulants, aspirin, cocaine
- Iatrogenic: lung biopsy, pulmonary arterial trauma (i.e., PA catheter)
- Rare causes: Broncholithiasis, pulmonary endometriosis, bronchovascular fistula, bronchopulmonary sequestration, Dieulafoy disease
- **Idiopathic/undiagnosed up to 25%:** Prognosis usually favorable (*Ann Intern Med 1985;102:829*)

Pathophysiology

- Specific pathogenesis depends on etiology and location of disease.
- Generally due to **inflammation/irritation of local respiratory tissue and its associated hyperplastic or otherwise abnormal vascular supply**.
- **Bronchial arterial circulation** (branching from the aorta) supplies high pressure blood to the airways and any associated pathology.
- **Pulmonary circulation** supplies the lung parenchyma and is under low pressure but receives all of cardiac output. Vascular causes, vascular malformations, Rasmussen's aneurysm (pulmonary artery aneurysm associated with TB).

DIAGNOSIS

Screening for the underlying disease is the basis for diagnosing the cause of hemoptysis and helps guide management.

Clinical Presentation

Hemoptysis may be the only presenting sign or may accompany other manifestations of an underlying disorder (Table 10-14).

History

- Most important: Age, smoking history, prior lung disease, previous malignancy, risk for coagulopathy.
- Review of systems should focus on symptoms suggesting cardiopulmonary disease, active infection, underlying malignancy, and systemic inflammatory disorders.

Physical Examination

- Most important: Vital signs including oxygen saturation, general state of health, lung exam noting focal or diffuse abnormal sounds.
- A thorough exam should always be performed, noting any manifestations suggesting underlying cardiopulmonary, infectious, immunologic, or malignant disease.

Differential Diagnosis

Pseudohemoptysis: Upper airway or gastrointestinal (GI) blood that is expectorated with or without aspiration.

Table 10-14	Clues to Diagnosing the Cause of Hemoptysis from the History and Physical Exam	
Cause of Hemoptysis	Historical Clue	Physical Exam Finding
Bronchogenic carcinoma	Smoker, age >40 yr; recurrent nonmassive hemoptysis, weight loss	Local chest wheezing
Chronic bronchitis/ bronchiectasis	Frequent, copious sputum production; frequent "pneumonias"	Scattered, bilateral coarse chest crackles, wheezes; clubbing
TB, fungal lung disease, lung abscess	Subacute constitutional symptoms; travel and exposure history	Fever, focal coarse chest crackles, cachexia
Acute pneumonia	Acute fever, productive cough, pleurisy, rusty brown hemoptysis	Fever, focal coarse chest crackles, bronchial breath sounds
Vasculitis, hemorrhage syndrome	Subacute constitutional symptoms; hematuria, rash, arthralgias	Diffuse chest crackles, mucosal ulcers, rash
Heart failure	Orthopnea, lower extremity edema, history of valvular disease	Murmurs, diastolic rumble, S_3, loud S_1 or P_2, lower extremity edema
AVM/hereditary hemorrhagic telangiectasia	Platypnea, epistaxis; family history of similar signs and symptoms	Mucosal telangiectasias, orthodeoxia
Pulmonary embolus	Acute dyspnea, pleurisy	Hypoxemia, pleural rub, unilateral lower extremity edema

AVM, arteriovenous malformation; TB, tuberculosis.

Diagnostic Testing

- Evaluate for adequacy of oxygenation, extent of blood loss, evidence of infection, and other underlying systemic disease.
- Localize the source of hemoptysis.

Laboratories
- CBC, CMP, coagulation studies, urinalysis with microscopy.
- Type and cross-match blood if hemoptysis massive.
- ABG if indicated.
- Sputum studies: Routine gram stain and culture. Fungal, AFB, cytology studies as indicated.
- Specialized studies as suggested by clinical suspicion.
  - CHF: BNP
  - Immunologic disease: ANA/ANCA screen, anti-GBM antibodies, complement levels, cryoglobulins, etc.

Figure 10-6. Suggested general approach to diagnosing the cause of nonmassive hemoptysis. *RFBC, risk factors for bronchogenic carcinoma (as outlined in the text). **Consider chest computed tomography (CT) if not yet done, as indicated by clinical history.

Electrocardiography

Assess for underlying structural cardiac disease; otherwise, usually noncontributory.

Imaging

- **PA/lateral CXR** should be performed in all cases of hemoptysis.
  - **Normal or nonlocalizing in up to 50% of all cases** (*Chest 1988;92:70; Clin Radiol 1996;51:391*).
  - **Normal in up to 10% of cases caused by bronchogenic carcinoma** (*Chest 1988;92:70*).
- **Chest CT:** Indication often depends on clinical suspicion but should be performed if the diagnosis remains in doubt after initial clinical evaluation, or if bronchoscopy is unrevealing (Figure 10-6).
  - Advantages:
    - Can visualize parenchyma, vasculature, and airways to varying extent.
    - **Especially useful for bronchiectasis, cavitary lung disease, masses, and vascular malformations** (*Chest 1994;105:1155*).
    - High-resolution CT may visualize tumors with efficacy comparable to bronchoscopy (*Radiology 1993;189:677*).
  - Disadvantages:
    - Less efficacious in recognizing subtle bronchial and mucosal lesions (*Chest 1994;105:1155*).

- Nonspecific in cases of pulmonary hemorrhage.
- High risk in an unstable patient.
- **Echocardiography** if suspect structural or valvular cardiac disease.

Diagnostic Procedures
- **Fiber optic (flexible) bronchoscopy:** Generally **localizes/lateralizes bleeding source** in over two-thirds of cases, depending on the setting (*Ann Thorac Surg 1989;48:272*).
  - Useful in order to **inspect airways** for mucosal and vascular abnormalities; perform segmental **lavage** for cell count, gram stain, cultures, cytology; assess for alveolar hemorrhage; and obtain brushings and/or biopsy.
  - **Indications** (see Figure 10-6):
    - Unclear source after initial evaluation and imaging, or if hemoptysis persists/recurs.
    - Clinical presentation suggests airway abnormality.
    - CXR/imaging suggests malignancy.
    - CXR/imaging normal or nonlocalizing but with **presence of at least two risk factors for bronchogenic carcinoma:** male sex, age >40 years, >40 pack-year smoking, duration of hemoptysis >1 week, volume expectorated >30 mL (*Chest 1985;87:142*; *Chest 1988;92:70*; *Ann Intern Med 1991;151:171*).
    - Potential for arterial embolization.
  - Timing: Controversial, although increased yield when performed during or within 48 hours of bleeding (*Am Rev Resp Dis 1981;124:221*).
- **Bronchial and pulmonary arteriography:** Perform in **persistent or recurring massive hemoptysis**.
  - Advantage: **Embolization** of the culprit vessel can be simultaneously performed if localized.
  - Disadvantage: **Variable and inexact localization** of bleeding depending on clinical setting (*Ann Thorac Surg 1989;48:272*).
    - Anatomic variability.
    - Bleeding usually insufficient for contrast extravasation.
    - Diffuse lung diseases often have associated diffuse vascular abnormalities, making localization difficult (i.e., bronchiectasis).

TREATMENT

- **General approach**
  - **Distinguish massive from nonmassive hemoptysis.**
  - Three main goals: (1) stabilize, (2) diagnose and localize, (3) decide on need and type of therapy.
- **Nonmassive hemoptysis:** usually treated conservatively and based on underlying disorder (see Figure 10-6).
  - Reverse coagulopathy
  - Antitussives and mild sedatives
  - Bronchoscopy if recurrent
- **Massive hemoptysis:** Requires urgent action, intensive monitoring, and an early multidisciplinary approach including a pulmonologist and/or thoracic surgeon and an interventional radiologist (Figure 10-7).

Figure 10-7. Suggested general approach to managing massive hemoptysis. *Consider BAE in all cases of massive hemoptysis regardless of recurrence.

- **Initial stabilization:**
  - Ensure **airway patency**: Very low threshold for intubation, with a large endotracheal tube.
  - **Lateral decubitus positioning** (affected lung down) to minimize aspiration into unaffected lung.
  - Single-lumen main stem intubation for selective ventilation of unaffected lung.
  - Double-lumen endotracheal intubation for selective ventilation of unaffected lung. Should be performed and managed only under appropriately skilled supervision.
- **Bronchoscopy** with directed airway therapy:
  - **Rigid bronchoscopy** favored if available: Provides better airway access and ventilatory control with easier suctioning and manipulation of instruments.
  - Direct bronchoscopic tamponade.
  - **Balloon tamponade**, left in place for 1 to 2 days. Fogarty, bronchial blocker, PA catheter balloons have all been described. Watch for ischemic mucosal injury or postobstructive pneumonitis (*Thorax 2003;58:814*).

- **Endobronchial electrocautery, Argon-Plasma coagulation** (*Chest 2001;119: 781*; *Can Respir J 2004;11:305*).
    - **Topical hemostatic agents:** Epinephrine, vasopressin, thrombin, cold saline (*Am Rev Respir Dis 1987;135:A108*; *Chest 1989;96:473*; *Thorax 1980;35:901*).
- **Bronchial arteriography and embolization should be performed early** in massive or recurrent hemoptysis.
    - **Successful embolization (>85%)** with careful localization (*Chest 2002;121: 789*; *Radiology 2004;233:741*).
    - Particularly useful in cystic fibrosis (CF) patients (*Am J Respir Crit Care Med 1998;157:1951*; *Chest 2002;121:796*).
    - **Early failure usually due to inadequate or incomplete source vessel identification.** Postembolization arteriography may identify additional systemic culprit vessels, most commonly from the intercostal and phrenic arteries (*Am J Roent 2003;180:1577*).
    - **Rebleeding common** (up to 20%) over 1 year (*Chest 1999;115:912*; *Respiration 2000;67:412*).
    - **Risks** include bronchial or partial pulmonary infarct/necrosis and, rarely, ischemic myelopathy due to inadvertent embolization of a spinal artery.

Medications

Systemic procoagulants: Use only in unstable massive hemoptysis as a temporizing measure, or when conventional bronchoscopic, interventional, or surgical therapies are contraindicated and/or unavailable. Some examples are Factor VII, vasopressin, and aminocaproic acid.

Surgical Management

- **Lobectomy/pneumonectomy offers definitive cure.**
- **Indications: persistent focal/unilateral massive hemoptysis despite other therapy**; particularly useful for stable patients with hemoptysis due to cavitary lung disease (i.e., aspergilloma), localized bronchogenic carcinoma, AVM, traumatic injuries (*Crit Care Med 2000;28:1642*).
- **Contraindications:** Poor pulmonary reserve, advanced malignancy, active TB, diffuse lung disease, diffuse alveolar hemorrhage.
- Emergent surgery has high morbidity and mortality compared to elective surgery after stabilization.

REFERRAL

- Pulmonary (interventional for massive hemoptysis, if available)
- Thoracic surgery
- Interventional radiology

OUTCOME/PROGNOSIS

Mortality depends on etiology and amount (*Arch Intern Med 1983;143:1343*; *Am J Med Sci 1987;294:301*).
- Up to 80% with massive hemoptysis due to malignancy
- Less than 10% with nonmassive hemoptysis
- Less than 1% in bronchiectasis and lung infections

Cystic Fibrosis

GENERAL PRINCIPLES

Definition

CF is an **autosomal recessive disorder** caused by mutations of the cystic fibrosis transmembrane conductance regulator gene (*CFTR*), located on chromosome 7, that results in multisystem exocrine organ dysfunction.

Epidemiology

- In the United States, approximately 30,000 people are affected by CF with an incidence of 1 in 3,500 live births (*Clin Chest Med 2007;28:279*).
- CF is the most common lethal genetic disease in Caucasians, but the diagnosis needs to be considered in patients of diverse ethnic backgrounds as well.
- Patients are typically diagnosed during childhood, but there is increasing recognition of milder variants that may not present until later in life.

Etiology

- CF is caused by **mutations in the *CFTR* gene**, a cyclic AMP-regulated chloride channel (*Science 1989;245:1073*).
- CFTR normally maintains hydration of exocrine organ secretions.
- Abnormal CFTR ultimately results in decreased chloride secretion and increased sodium absorption on the surface of epithelial cells with resulting thickened secretions in the airways, sinuses, pancreatic ducts, biliary tree, intestines, sweat ducts, and reproductive tract.

Pathophysiology

- CFTR normally regulates transport of electrolytes across the epithelium (*Curr Opin Pulm Med 2003;9:486*).
- The primary pulmonary manifestations of disease are thought to be related to abnormal electrolyte transport in the airway, which results in diminished airway surface liquid and impaired mucociliary clearance.
- The airways enter a vicious cycle of infection, inflammation, and chronic airway obstruction. This results in bronchiectasis, chronic infection, and ultimately, premature death (*N Engl J Med 2005;352:1992*).
- Similarly, thickened secretions in the pancreatic and biliary ducts lead to maldigestion, malabsorption, and occasionally, liver disease and diabetes.

DIAGNOSIS

- The diagnosis of CF is typically made during childhood, but approximately 10% of patients are diagnosed after age 10 (*CFF Patient Registry, 2011*).
- Newborn screening leads to increased frequency of early diagnosis (*J Pediatr 2002;141:804*). In 2010, over half of new diagnoses were the result of newborn screening (*CFF Patient Registry, 2011*).
- **At least one criterion** from each set of features must be met to diagnose CF (*J Pediatr 2008;153:S1*):
  - Compatible clinical feature of CF (see clinical features), or
  - A positive family history, or

- A positive newborn screening test, *and*
- Elevated sweat chloride >60 mmol/L on two occasions, or
- Presence of two disease causing mutations in *CFTR*, or
- Abnormal nasal transepithelial potential difference test
- Atypical patients may lack classic symptoms and signs or have normal sweat tests (*Curr Opin Pulm Med 2003;9:498*).
- Although genotyping may assist in the diagnosis, it alone cannot establish or rule out the diagnosis of CF, and the initial test of choice remains the sweat test.

Clinical Presentation

- **Pulmonary manifestations**
  - Cough with purulent sputum production
  - Sinopulmonary infection with pathogens typical of CF
  - Progressive dyspnea
  - Acute pulmonary disease exacerbations
  - Recurrent infection and inflammation
  - Bronchiectasis
  - Airflow obstruction
- **Extrapulmonary manifestations**
  - Chronic sinusitis
  - Nasal polyposis
  - Nutritional failure
  - Pancreatic insufficiency (PI)—vitamin A, D, E, and K deficiency
  - Meconium ileus
  - Distal intestinal obstruction syndrome
  - Volvulus, intussusception, and rectal prolapse
  - Diabetes mellitus
  - Liver cirrhosis and portal hypertension
  - Cholelithiasis and cholecystitis
  - Nephrolithiasis
  - Male infertility (bilateral absence of the vas deferens) and epididymitis
  - Growth retardation, osteoarthropathy, and osteopenia

History

Presenting symptoms may include (*J Pediatr 1993;122:1*):
- Cough with purulent sputum production (40%)
- Failure to thrive (29%)
- Steatorrhea
- Meconium ileus

Physical Examination

- Malnourished, underweight
- Inspiratory crackles on lung exam typically anterior and in the apices
- Digital clubbing

Differential Diagnosis

- **Primary ciliary dyskinesia:** Bronchiectasis, sinusitis, and infertility, but limited GI symptoms and normal sweat chloride levels, occasionally seen with dextrocardia or *situs inversus totalis* (Kartagener syndrome).

- **Shwachman-Diamond syndrome:** PI, cyclic neutropenia, and short stature, which may lead to lung disease, but normal sweat chloride levels (*Hematol Oncol Clin North Am 2009;23:233*).
- **Young's syndrome:** Bronchiectasis, sinusitis, and azoospermia, but mild respiratory symptoms, lack of GI symptoms, and normal sweat chloride levels (*Thorax 1987;42:815*).
- **Immunoglobulin deficiency:** Recurrent sinus and pulmonary infections but typically no GI symptoms and normal sweat chloride levels.
- **Idiopathic bronchiectasis**
- **Chronic rhinosinusitis:** Recurrent sinus infections but limited GI symptoms and normal sweat chloride levels.
- **Chronic idiopathic pancreatitis:** Recurrent pancreatitis but limited sinopulmonary disease and normal sweat chloride levels.

Diagnostic Testing

- **Skin sweat testing** with a standardized quantitative pilocarpine iontophoresis method remains the **gold standard for the diagnosis of CF** (*Am J Respir Crit Care Med 2006;173:475*).
  - A sweat chloride concentration of ≥60 mmol/L on two separate occasions is consistent with the diagnosis of CF.
  - Borderline sweat test results (40 to 59 mmol/L sweat chloride) or nondiagnostic results in the setting of high clinical suspicion should also lead to repeat sweat testing, nasal potential difference testing, genetic testing, or additional clinical evaluation.
  - Sweat testing should be performed at a CF care center to ensure reliability of results.
  - Abnormal sweat chloride concentrations are rarely detected in non-CF patients.
- **Genetic tests** have detected more than 1,800 putative CF mutations.
  - Two recessive mutations on different alleles must be present to cause CF.
  - The most commonly encountered CF mutation is a deletion of the three nucleotides that code for phenylalanine (F) at amino acid 508 (F508del or ΔF508) of the CFTR protein, which is present in approximately 70% of alleles in affected individuals (*Am J Respir Crit Care Med 2006;173:475*).
  - Commercially available probes identify more than 90% of the abnormal genes in a Caucasian Northern European population, although they test for only a minority of the known CF genes. Full gene sequencing is commercially available but interpretation may be complex. Information about specific mutations and reported clinical phenotype may be found at *http://www.cftr2.org/*.
- **Transepithelial nasal potential difference.**
  - A test in which the voltage across the epithelium lining the nose is measured at baseline, after inhibiting sodium channels, and after stimulating CFTR (*J Pediatr 1986;108:517; Chest 2010;138:919*).
  - The test should be repeated on 2 separate days to confirm diagnosis and should be performed at specialized centers.

Laboratories

- Sputum cultures typically identify multiple organisms, including *Pseudomonas aeruginosa*, *Staphylococcus aureus*, nontypable *Haemophilus influenzae*, *Stenotrophomonas maltophilia*, and *Burkholderia cepacia*. Isolation of mucoid variants of *P. aeruginosa* from the respiratory tract occurs frequently. Use of special culture media to fastidious organisms is recommended. Nontuberculous mycobacteria are frequently isolated from the airways of persons with CF and may be pathogenic in some.

- **Testing for malabsorption** due to pancreatic exocrine insufficiency is often not formally performed because clinical evidence (the presence of foul-smelling, bulky, and loose stools; low fat-soluble vitamin levels [vitamins A, D, and E]; and a prolonged prothrombin time [vitamin K dependent]) and a clear response to pancreatic enzyme treatment are usually considered sufficient for the diagnosis. In atypical cases, low fecal elastase level or coefficient of fat absorption <85% on a formal 72-hour fecal fat collection may confirm PI.
- Tests that identify chronic sinusitis or infertility, especially obstructive azoospermia in men, would also support the diagnosis of CF.
- Monitoring of electrolytes is indicated in patients with a history of electrolyte abnormalities or renal insufficiency.

Imaging
- Chest radiography ultimately shows enlarged lung volumes with cystic lung disease, bronchiectasis, and mucous plugging, especially in the upper lobes.
- High-resolution CT scan may be helpful in evaluating patients with early or mild disease by detecting early airway changes.
- Pulmonary function tests eventually show expiratory airflow obstruction with increased residual volume and total lung capacity.
- Impairment of alveolar gas exchange may be present as well, progressing to hypoxemia and hypercapnia.

TREATMENT

- CF therapy aims to improve quality of life and functioning, decrease the number of exacerbations and hospitalizations, avoid complications associated with therapy, reduce the rate of decline in lung function, and decrease mortality.
- A comprehensive program addressing multiple organ system derangements, as provided at CF care centers, is recommended.
- Most adults with CF have significant lung disease, and a large portion of therapy is focused on clearing pulmonary secretions and controlling infection (*N Engl J Med 1996;335:179*).
- **Pulmonary therapy** (*Am J Respir Crit Care Med 2007;176:957*)
  - **Inhaled bronchodilators:** β-adrenergic agonists (albuterol MDI, 2 to 4 puffs bid–qid; salmeterol or formoterol, one dry powder inhalation bid)
    - Used to treat the reversible components of airflow obstruction and facilitate mucus clearance.
    - Contraindicated in the rare patient with associated paradoxical deterioration of airflow after their use.
  - **Recombinant human deoxyribonuclease:** DNase, dornase-α, Pulmozyme (2.5 mg or one ampule per day inhaled using a jet nebulizer)
    - Digests extracellular DNA, decreasing the viscoelasticity of the sputum.
    - It improves pulmonary function and decreases the incidence of respiratory tract infections that require parenteral antibiotics (*N Engl J Med 1992;326:812; Am Rev Respir Dis 1993;148:145*).
    - Adverse effects may include pharyngitis, laryngitis, rash, chest pain, and conjunctivitis.

- ○ **Hypertonic saline:** (4 mL of inhaled 7% saline twice daily)
  - A recent study showed fewer exacerbations and possible improvement in lung function in patients treated with hypertonic saline (*N Engl J Med 2006;354:229*).
  - Inhaled bronchodilators should be administered prior to treatments to avoid treatment-induced bronchospasm.
- ○ **Antibiotics**
  - A combination of an IV semisynthetic penicillin, a third- or fourth-generation cephalosporin, or a quinolone and an aminoglycoside is typically recommended during acute exacerbations (*Am J Respir Crit Care Med 2009;180:802*).
  - Sputum culture and sensitivities should guide therapy. *P. aeruginosa* is the most frequent pulmonary pathogen.
  - The duration of antibiotic therapy is dictated by the clinical response. At least 14 days of antibiotics is typically given to treat an exacerbation.
  - Home IV antibiotic therapy is common, but hospitalization may allow better access to comprehensive therapy and diagnostic testing. Oral antibiotics are recommended only for mild exacerbations.
  - The use of chronic or intermittent prophylactic antibiotics can be considered, especially in patients with frequent recurrent exacerbations, but antimicrobial resistance may develop.
  - Inhaled aerosolized antibiotics tobramycin (300 mg nebulized bid, or aztreonam lysinate 75 mg nebulized tid, 28 days on alternating with 28 days off using appropriate nebulizer and compressor) improves pulmonary function, decreases the density of *P. aeruginosa*, and decreases the risk of hospitalization. Voice alteration (13%) and tinnitus (3%) are potential adverse events associated with long-term inhaled tobramycin (*N Engl J Med 1999;340:23*), and pyrexia and airway irritation have been reported with inhaled aztreonam (*Chest 2009;135: 1223*).
  - Patients with CF have atypical pharmacokinetics and often require higher drug doses at more frequent intervals. In adult patients with CF, for example, cefepime is often dosed at 2 g IV q8h, and gentamicin or tobramycin is often dosed at 3 mg/kg IV q8h (aiming for peak levels of 10 mg/mL and trough levels of <2 mg/mL).
  - Once-daily aminoglycoside dosing is preferred and should be guided by pharmacokinetic testing. Monitoring levels (peaks and troughs) of drugs such as aminoglycosides helps to ensure therapeutic levels and to decrease the risk of toxicity.
- ○ **Anti-inflammatory therapy**
  - **Azithromycin** (500 mg oral 3×/wk) used chronically shows mild improvement in lung function and reduces days in the hospital for treatment of respiratory exacerbations in patients who are chronically infected with *P. aeruginosa* (*JAMA 2003;290:1749*).
  - **Glucocorticoids** used in short courses may be helpful to some patients, but long-term therapy should be avoided to minimize the side effects that include glucose intolerance, osteopenia, and growth retardation.
  - **Ibuprofen** used in high doses has been used as a chronic anti-inflammatory agent in children with mild impairment of lung function (*Chest 1999;124:689*).
- ○ **Restoration of CFTR function**
  - **Ivacaftor** (150 mg oral twice daily) is a CFTR potentiator that improves lung function and decreases the risk of pulmonary exacerbations in patients with the **missense G551D mutation** (*N Engl J Med 2011;365:1663*). It is not effective in patients homozygous for the F508del mutation. Only about 4%

of the U.S. CF population carries a G551D mutation. Efficacy studies in patients with non-G551D gating mutations are underway.

- CFTR corrector molecules, and molecules that suppress CFTR nonsense mutations (premature stop codons) are in various phases of clinical development and testing.

○ **Mechanical airway clearance devices:** Flutter valve, acapella device, high-frequency chest oscillation vests, low- and high-pressure positive expiratory pressure devices

- Can be used in combination with medical therapy to promote airway clearance.
- Other alternatives include postural drainage with chest percussion and vibration, and breathing and coughing exercises.

○ **Pulmonary rehabilitation**

- When done with exercise rehabilitation may improve functional status and promote clearance of airway secretions.

○ **Oxygen therapy**

- May be indicated based on standard recommendations used for the treatment of chronic obstructive pulmonary disease (COPD).
- Rest and exercise oxygen assessments should be performed as clinically indicated.

○ **Noninvasive ventilation**

- Used for chronic respiratory failure due to CF-related bronchiectasis.
- Has not been clearly demonstrated to provide a survival benefit, although it may provide symptomatic relief or may be used as a bridge to transplantation.

• **Extrapulmonary therapy**

○ **Pancreatic insufficiency**

- PI is managed with **pancreatic enzyme supplementation**.
- Enzyme dose should be titrated to achieve one to two semisolid stools per day and to maintain adequate growth and nutrition.
- Enzymes are taken immediately before meals and snacks.
- Dosing of pancreatic enzymes should be initiated at 500 U lipase/kg/meal and should not exceed 2,500 U lipase/kg/meal.
- **High doses** (6,000 U lipase/kg/meal) have been associated with **chronic intestinal strictures** (*N Engl J Med 1997;336:1283*).
- Gastric acid suppression may enhance enzyme activity.

○ **Vitamin deficiency**

- Vitamin supplementation is recommended in extrapulmonary disease, especially with fat-soluble vitamins that are not well absorbed in the setting of PI. Vitamins should be taken with meals/enzymes.
- **Vitamins A, D, E, and K** can all be taken orally on a regular basis.
- Iron-deficiency anemia requires iron supplementation.

○ **CF-related diabetes mellitus (CFRD)**

- CFRD is usually managed with **insulin**.
- Typical diabetic dietary restrictions are liberalized (high-calorie diet with unrestricted fat) to meet the increased energy requirements of patients with CF and to encourage appropriate growth and weight maintenance.

○ **Bowel impaction**

- **Laxatives** such as senna, magnesium citrate, or polyethylene glycol can be tried initially.
- Refractory cases may require a Hypaque enema.
- Can be mistaken for appendicitis or gall bladder disease as the appendix can be enlarged in CF due to mucus inspissation and white blood cell counts and/or alkaline phosphatase elevations, which are common in CF.

- Narcotic use and/or significant dehydration can precipitate severe bowel obstruction, so prophylactic laxatives like daily polyethylene glycol (e.g., MiraLAX 17 g in 8 oz water) in postsurgical patients is often indicated.
  - **Osteopenia**
    - **Screening** should be routinely performed on patients with CF, and if present may be managed with calcium, vitamin D supplementation, and bisphosphonate therapy as clinically indicated (*Am J Respir Crit Care Med 2004;169:77*).
  - **Chronic sinusitis**
    - Many patients will benefit from chronic **nasal steroid** administration.
    - Nasal saline washes may also be helpful.
    - Patients whose symptoms cannot be controlled with medical management may benefit from functional endoscopic sinus surgery and nasal polypectomy.

Surgical Management

- **Massive hemoptysis:** This is usually controlled with antibiotics and bronchial artery embolization. Surgical lung resection is rarely needed (*Am J Respir Crit Care Med 2010;182:298*).
- **Pneumothorax**
  - Unless small, pneumothoraces are treated with chest tube placements. Surgical pleurodesis should be considered in cases of recurrent pneumothorax (*Am J Respir Crit Care Med 2010;182:298*).
- **Lung transplantation**
  - The majority of patients with CF die from pulmonary disease.
  - FEV_1 is a strong predictor of mortality and has been helpful in deciding when to refer patients for lung transplantation (*N Engl J Med 1992;326:1187*).
  - However, other factors such as marked alveolar gas exchange abnormalities (resting hypoxemia or hypercapnia), evidence of PH, or increased frequency or severity of pulmonary exacerbations should also be considered when deciding on referral for transplantation.

Lifestyle/Risk Modification

- **Avoidance of irritating inhaled fumes, dusts, or chemicals**, including second-hand smoke, is recommended.
- **Yearly influenza vaccination** (0.5 mL intramuscularly [IM]) decreases the incidence of infection and subsequent deterioration (*N Engl J Med 1984;311:1653*).
- **Pneumovax** (0.5 mL IM) may also provide benefit.

Diet

A high-calorie diet with vitamin supplementation is typically recommended.

Activity

- CF patients should maintain as much activity as possible.
- Exercise is an excellent form of airway clearance.

SPECIAL CONSIDERATIONS

- Although fertility may be decreased in women with CF secondary to thickened cervical mucus, many women with CF have tolerated pregnancy well (*N Engl J Med 1984;311:1653*).

- Maternal and fetal outcomes are good for women with adequate pulmonary reserve (FEV_1 >50% predicted) and good nutritional status, and pregnancy does not appear to affect their survival (*Chest 2000;118:85*).
- Pregnancies should be planned to optimize patient status and coordinate care with obstetrics. CF genetic screening should be offered to partners of patients with CF.

COMPLICATIONS

Other pulmonary complications of CF may include allergic bronchopulmonary aspergillosis, massive hemoptysis, acquisition of atypical mycobacterium, and pneumothorax.

REFERRAL

- CF patients or suspected CF patients should be referred to a national CFF-accredited care center.
- Tests such as sweat chloride testing and nasal potential difference are best done at specialized CF care centers.
- A team of CF specialists, including physicians, nutritionists, respiratory therapists, and social workers, aid in the routine care of these patients.

PATIENT EDUCATION

Information can be found at the CF Foundation Web site (*www.cff.org*).

MONITORING/FOLLOW-UP

All persons with CF should be followed in an accredited CF Care Center. Recommendations are to follow patients every 3 months with pulmonary function tests (PFTs) and yearly lab work including vitamin levels and screening for CFRD.

OUTCOME/PROGNOSIS

- Predictors of increased mortality include age, female gender, low weight, low FEV_1, PI, diabetes mellitus, infection with *B. cepacia*, and the number of acute exacerbations (*JAMA 2001;286:2683*).
- With improved therapy, the median survival has been extended to approximately 38 years (CF Foundation, *www.cff.org*).

11 Allergy and Immunology

Sarena Sawlani, Jennifer M. Welch, and Andrew L. Kau

Adverse Drug Reactions

GENERAL PRINCIPLES

Definition

- An **adverse drug reaction** (ADR) is an undesired or unintended response that occurs when a drug is given for the appropriate purpose.
- The etiology of a drug reaction can be immunologic, toxic, or idiosyncratic in nature.
- An allergic drug reaction is due to an immune response that is mediated by immunoglobulin E (IgE) or T cells.

Classification

- ADRs can be divided into two groups: Type A and Type B.
- *Type A* reactions are more commonly seen and are predictable. They are often dose dependent and related to the pharmacokinetics of the drug.
- *Type B* reactions are unpredictable and are not related to the dose or the drug's pharmacokinetics. They account for 10% to 15% of all ADRs.
  - ○ Immune-mediated adverse reactions can be from a variety of mechanisms (see in the following text). They usually occur upon reexposure to the offending drug.
  - ○ **Pseudoallergic reactions**, formerly called anaphylactoid reactions, are caused by IgE-independent degranulation of mast cells.

Epidemiology

- From 1966 to 1996, 15.1% of hospitalized U.S. patients experienced an ADR with an incidence of 3.1% to 6.2% of hospital admissions due to ADRs (*JAMA 1998;279:1200*).
- Mortality incidence from ADRs are significant and ranges from 0.14% to 0.32% (*Curr Opin Allergy Clin Immunol 2005;5(4):309*).

Etiology

- **β-Lactam** antibiotics are most commonly associated with immunologically mediated drug reactions.
  - ○ Anaphylaxis has been reported to occur in 1:100,000 with serious allergic reactions in 4.6 per 10,000 dispenses (*Drug Saf 2007;30(8):705*).
  - ○ Typical reactions include rash, urticaria, fever, and bronchospasm.
  - ○ The chemical structure of penicillins results in their high immunogenicity.

- The core structure is composed of a reactive β-lactam ring that covalently binds with carrier proteins to form a hapten, which creates an immune response. The major determinant of immunogenicity of penicillin is the benzylpenicilloyl form seen in 93% of tissue-bound penicillin.
- The minor antigenic determinants are all remaining penicillin conjugates. It is comprised of benzylpenicillin, benzylpenicilloate, and benzylpenilloate.
- Most immediate reactions to penicillins are related to the major determinant. In other penicillins such as ampicillin, the side chain is the antigenic determinant.

○ Cross-reactivity of β-lactams
  - The cross-reactivity between β-lactam antibiotics is variable and largely determined by their side-chain structure attached to the β-lactam ring.
  - Prior to the 1980s, cephalosporins had a higher cross reactivity to penicillin as they were contaminated with a small amount of penicillin (*J Allergy Clin Immunol 2010;125(2 suppl 2):S126*). Risk of a cross-reaction with a first-generation cephalosporins is 5.0% to 16.5%, second generation is 4%, and third or fourth generation is 1% to 3% (*J Allergy Clin Immunol 2006;117(2 suppl mini-primer):S464*).
    □ Although many of the reactions to second- and third-generation cephalosporins are directed at the side chains, skin testing to penicillin in these patients can be helpful because most severe anaphylactic reactions are directed against the reactive bicyclic core.
    □ Patients with a history of a severe reaction to penicillin should be considered sensitive to cephalosporin unless they are skin test negative. Although patients with a history of a nonanaphylactic reaction to penicillin can often be given a second- or third-generation cephalosporin safely, it is advisable to precede the dose with an oral provocation challenge.
  - Skin test cross-reactivity has been documented in carbapenems. Patient undergoing a graded carbapenem challenge with a positive penicillin skin test and a negative carbapenem skin test did not have any hypersensitivity reactions (*J Allergy Clin Immunol 2010;125(2 suppl 2):S126*).
  - The monobactam aztreonam rarely cross-reacts with penicillins. Ceftazidime does share an identical side chain to aztreonam and is highly reactive (*Ann Pharmacother 2009;43(2):304*).

- **Sulfonamide allergy**
  ○ There is an increase in allergy to sulfonamides in patients with HIV compared to the general population. Trimethoprim–sulfamethoxazole hypersensitivity occurs in 60% of HIV patient compared to 5% of HIV-negative patients (*Curr Opin Allergy Clin Immunol 2007;7(4):324*).
  ○ Most frequently seen reaction is a maculopapular rash that develops 7 to 12 days after initiating drug. Other reactions include urticaria and, less commonly, anaphylaxis, Stevens-Johnson syndrome (SJS), and toxic epidermal necrolysis (TEN).

- **NSAIDs** (including aspirin) can induce pseudoallergic reactions through shunting of prostaglandin production to leukotriene synthesis in susceptible individuals. **Samter's triad** is the combination of asthma, nonsteroidal anti-inflammatory drug (NSAID) sensitivity, and nasal polyposis.

Pathophysiology

The immunologic mechanisms for a drug allergy are demonstrated in the Gell and Coomb's classification of hypersensitivity (Table 11-1).

Table 11-1	Immunologically Mediated Drug Reactions	
Type of Reaction	Representative Examples	Mechanism
Anaphylactic (Type 1)	Anaphylaxis Urticaria Angioedema	IgE-mediated degranulation of mast cell with resultant mediator release
Cytotoxic (Type 2)	Autoimmune hemolytic anemia Interstitial nephritis	IgG or IgM antibodies against cell antigens and complement activation
Immune complex (Type 3)	Serum sickness Vasculitis	Immune complex deposition and subsequent complement activation
Cell mediated (Type 4)	Contact dermatitis Photosensitivity dermatitis	Activated T cells against cell surface–bound antigens

Ig, immunoglobulin.

Risk Factors

Factors that increase a patient's risk of an ADR include size and structure of drug, route of exposure (cutaneous most immunogenic), dose, duration, frequency, gender (women > men), genetic factors (HLA type, history of atopy), prior drug reaction, coexisting medical illnesses, and concurrent medical therapy.

DIAGNOSIS

Clinical Presentation

- A history is essential for making the diagnosis of an allergic drug reaction. Questions should be directed at establishing the following information: sign and symptoms, timing of the reaction, purpose of the drug, other medications patient is receiving, prior exposure to drug or related drug, and history of other allergic drug reactions.
- Urticaria, angioedema, wheezing, and anaphylaxis are all characteristics of IgE-mediated (Type 1) reactions.
  - Symptoms do not typically occur on the first exposure to the medication unless the patient has been exposed to structurally related medication. On reexposure, however, symptoms tend to manifest acutely (often <1 hour).
  - IgE-mediated reactions tend to worsen with repeated exposure to offending medication.
  - Pseudoallergic reactions (non-IgE mediated) can be clinically indistinguishable from IgE-mediated reactions because the final common pathway for their reaction is mast cell degranulation.
- **Maculopapular exanthemas** are the most common cutaneous manifestation of drug allergy.
  - These reactions are mediated by T cells and typically delayed in onset, first occurring between 2 and 14 days of exposure to culprit medications. Lesions typically begin on the trunk, especially in dependent areas, and spread to the extremities.

- ○ Rarely, these rashes can progress to DRESS (**d**rug **r**eaction with **e**osinophilia and **s**ystemic **s**ymptoms) or SJS.
- **DRESS** or hypersensitivity syndrome is a serious ADR, often presenting with rash and fever (*Expert Opin Drug Saf 2005;4(3):571*).
  - ○ Systemic involvement can manifest as hepatitis, eosinophilia, pneumonitis, lymphadenopathy, and nephritis.
  - ○ Symptoms tend to present 2 to 6 weeks after introduction of medication.
  - ○ First described with antiepileptic (carbamazepine) agents but has also been reported to occur with allopurinol, NSAIDs, some antibiotics and β-blockers.
- **Erythema multiforme (EM), SJS, and TEN** are all serious drug reactions primarily involving the skin.
  - ○ EM is characterized most typically by target lesions.
  - ○ SJS and TEN manifest with varying degrees of sloughing of the skin and mucous membranes (<10% of the epidermis in SJS and >30% in TEN).
- Readministration or future skin testing with the offending drug is absolutely contraindicated.

TREATMENT

- **Discontinuation** of the suspected drug or drugs is the most important initial approach in managing an allergic drug reaction.
- Other therapeutic maneuvers are directed at limiting further exacerbation of ADR and may include management of anaphylaxis (see earlier) as well as other supportive measures. Care in intensive care unit (ICU) may be required for severe adverse reactions.
- Future use of the drug in question should **always be avoided** unless there is no therapeutic alternative available.
- If use of the drug must be considered, a careful history of the reaction is helpful in defining the potential risk. Patient may lose their sensitivity to a drug over time and determining date of reaction is useful. Symptoms that occurred with the start of a drug course are more likely to be IgE-mediated than symptoms that develop several days after the completion of a course.
- On occasion, a patient may be inadvertently reexposed to a drug that had previously caused a reaction. If this reexposure was not associated with any reaction, it is due to lack of true IgE-mediated hypersensitivity or potentially a loss of sensitivity that may have developed.
- The types of symptoms are also important. Toxic reactions (e.g., nausea secondary to macrolide antibiotics or codeine) are not immunologic reactions and do not necessarily predict problems with other members in their respective class.
- If the patient is taking the drug for a life-threatening illness (e.g., meningitis with penicillin allergy) and the reaction is a mild skin reaction, it may be reasonable to continue the medication and treat the reaction symptomatically. **If the rash is progressive, however, the drug must be discontinued to avoid a desquamative process such as SJS.**

REFERRAL

- If no alternative drug is available and the patient has a history of an IgE-mediated reaction, the patient should be referred to an allergist for further evaluation.
- The allergist may perform one of several procedures if indicated depending on the medication, type of reaction, and availability of testing reagents.

- **Skin testing** may be performed to assess for the presence of IgE to the medication.
  - While skin testing may be performed to nearly any medication, sensitivity and specificity of the skin test results have only been established for penicillin. No case of penicillin-induced anaphylaxis has been reported in a patient who is skin test negative.
  - Results of testing to drugs other than penicillin must be interpreted within the clinical context of the case.
- **Graded dose challenge** assesses how the patient tolerates progressively larger doses of medication (e.g., 1/1,000, 1/10, and full dose given 20 minutes apart).
- **Drug desensitization** is performed when patient has an identified IgE-mediated reaction but still requires the medications.
  - The exact mechanism by which desensitization prevents anaphylaxis is unclear.
  - The drug must be taken daily at a specified dose to maintain the "desensitized state."
  - If a dose of drug is missed for >48-hour period following a desensitization procedure, the patient will often need to undergo a repeat desensitization.
- Successful desensitization or graded challenge does not preclude the development of a non–IgE-mediated, delayed reaction (e.g., rash).

Anaphylaxis

GENERAL PRINCIPLES

Definition

Anaphylaxis is a rapidly developing, life-threatening systemic reaction mediated by the release of mast cell – and basophil-derived mediators in the circulation. The peak severity is seen usually within 5 to 30 minutes.

Classification

- **Immunologic anaphylaxis:**
  - Allergic IgE-mediated anaphylaxis (Type I hypersensitivity)
  - Immune complex–complement-mediated anaphylaxis
  - Cytotoxic-mediated anaphylaxis
- **Nonimmunologic anaphylaxis**
  - **Nonallergic anaphylaxis (used to be called anaphylactoid)**
  - Idiopathic

Epidemiology

Incidence of anaphylaxis is approximately 50 to 2,000 episodes per 100,000 person-years with a lifetime prevalence of 0.05% to 2%. Fatality is estimated at 0.7% to 2% per case of anaphylaxis.

Etiology

- **Immunologic causes**
  - Foods
  - Hymenoptera stings (bees, wasps, and fire ants)
  - Medications (i.e., antibiotics and muscle relaxants)
  - Latex rubber
  - Blood products

- **Nonimmunologic causes**
  - Radiocontrast media
  - Medications (i.e., Vancomycin, opiates, muscle relaxants, NSAIDs, rarely angiotensin-converting enzyme inhibitors [ACE-Is], and sulfating agents)
  - Hemodialysis
  - Physical factors (cold temperature or exercise)
  - Idiopathic

Pathophysiology

- Immunologic
  - Anaphylaxis is due to sensitization to an antigen and formation of specific IgE to that antigen. On reexposure, the IgE on mast cells and basophils binds the antigen and cross-links the IgE receptor, which causes activation of the cells with subsequent release of preformed mediators, such as histamine.
  - The release of mediators ultimately causes capillary leakage, cellular edema, and smooth muscle contractions resulting in the constellation of physical symptoms.
- Nonimmunologic
  Non–IgE-mediated anaphylaxis is also mediated by direct degranulation of mast cells and basophils in the absence of immunoglobulins.

Risk Factors

- Immunologic anaphylaxis: IgE-mediated reactions.
  Previous sensitization and formation of antigen-specific IgE with history of anaphylaxis.
- Nonimmunologic anaphylaxis:
  - Mastocytosis patients are at higher risk for future episodes if not recognized or not premedicated.
  - Radiocontrast sensitivity reactions
    - Age >50 years
    - Preexisting cardiovascular or renal disease
    - History of allergy
    - History of previous reaction to radiocontrast media
    - **Sensitivity to seafood or iodine does not predispose to radiocontrast media reactions**

Prevention

- **For all types of anaphylaxis, recognition of potential triggers and avoidance is the best prevention.**
- **Self-injectable epinephrine and patient education for all patients with a history of anaphylaxis.**
- Radiocontrast sensitivity reactions.
  - Use of low-ionic contrast media is strongly suggested.
  - Premedication before procedure.
    - Prednisone 50 mg PO given 13, 7, and 1 hour prior to procedure
    - Diphenhydramine 50 mg PO given 1 hour before procedure
    - H2 blocker may also be given 1 hour before procedure
  - **Premedication is not 100% effective and appropriate precautions for handling a reaction should be taken.**
  - Anaphylaxis can be a presenting sign of underlying mastocytosis.

- Red man's syndrome from vancomycin
  Symptoms can usually be prevented by slowing the rate of infusion and premedicating with diphenhydramine (50 mg PO) 30 minutes prior to start of the infusion.

DIAGNOSIS

Diagnosis is based primarily on history and physical examination with confirmation in some cases provided by the laboratory finding of an elevated serum β-tryptase level. However, the absence of an elevated β-tryptase level does not exclude anaphylaxis.

Clinical Presentation

- The clinical manifestations of allergic and nonallergic anaphylaxis are the same. Most serious reactions occur within minutes after exposure to the antigen. However, the reaction may be delayed for hours. Some patients experience a biphasic reaction characterized by a recurrence of symptoms after 4 to 8 hours. A few patients have a protracted course that requires several hours of continuous supportive treatment.
- Manifestations include pruritus, urticaria, angioedema, respiratory distress (due to laryngeal edema, laryngospasm, or bronchospasm), hypotension, abdominal cramping, and diarrhea.

History
History is taken to help identify the potential trigger, such as new foods, medications, or other commonly known allergens. Also documenting the time of onset of symptoms—that is, minutes to hours or days after a suspected exposure—can help to classify the type of anaphylaxis.

Physical Examination
- Pay special attention to vital signs: Blood pressure, respiratory rate, and oxygen saturation.
- Airway and pulmonary: Assess for any evidence of laryngeal edema or angioedema. Auscultate lung fields to listen for evidence of wheezing. Continue to assess for need to protect the airway.
- Perform a focused cardiovascular exam.
- Skin: Urticaria or erythema.

Diagnostic Criteria
See Table 11-2 **for diagnostic criteria for anaphylaxis.**
Severity of anaphylactic reactions can be judged by the following:
- **Mild anaphylactic reactions:** Generalized erythema, urticaria, angioedema, or pruritus.
- **Moderate anaphylactic reaction:** (features suggesting respiratory, cardiovascular, or gastrointestinal involvement): Dyspnea, stridor, wheezing, nausea, vomiting, dizziness (presyncope), diaphoresis, chest or throat tightness, and abdominal pain in addition to cutaneous symptoms.
- **Severe anaphylactic reaction:** (hypoxia, hypotension, or neurologic compromise): May have cyanosis or PaO_2 ≤92% at any stage, hypotension (systolic blood pressure <90 mm Hg), confusion, loss of consciousness, or neurologic compromise. In severe anaphylaxis, there is concern of respiratory and/or cardiac arrest leading to demise.

Table 11-2	Anaphylaxis

Anaphylaxis is likely when one of the three criteria occurs:

1. Acute skin and/or mucosal symptoms (e.g., hives, pruritus, flushing, lip/tongue/uvula swelling)

   AND ONE OF THE FOLLOWING:

   • Respiratory symptoms (e.g., wheezing, stridor, shortness of breath, hypoxia)
   • Hypotension or associated end-organ dysfunction (e.g., hypotonia, syncope, incontinence)
2. Exposure to probable allergen for the patient and two or more of the following:
   • Skin-mucosal tissue involvement
   • Respiratory symptoms
   • Hypotension or end-organ dysfunction
   • Persistent gastrointestinal symptoms (e.g., emesis, abdominal pain)
3. Decreased blood pressure after exposure to known allergen for the patient:
   • Adults: Systolic blood pressure <90 mm Hg or >30% decrease
   • Infants and children: Hypotension for age or >30% decrease in systolic blood pressure.

Adapted from Sampson HA, Munoz-Furlong A, Campbell RL, et al. Second symposium on the definition and management of anaphylaxis: summary report–Second National Institute of Allergy and Infectious Disease/Food Allergy and Anaphylaxis Network symposium. *J Allergy Clin Immunol.* 2006;117:391–397.

Differential Diagnosis

• Anaphylaxis due to **preformed IgE and reexposure**: Medications, Hymenoptera sting, and foods are the most common causes of anaphylaxis.
• Causes of **nonallergic anaphylaxis**:
  ○ **Radiocontrast sensitivity reactions** are thought to be from direct degranulation of mast cells in susceptible patients due to osmotic shifts. Reactions can occur in 5% to 10% of patients, with fatal reactions occurring in 1 in 40,000 procedures.
  ○ **Red man's syndrome** from vancomycin consists of pruritus and flushing of the face and neck.
  ○ **Mastocytosis** should be considered in patients with recurrent unexplained anaphylaxis or flushing, especially with previous reactions to nonspecific mast cell degranulators such as opiates and radiocontrast media.
  ○ **Ingestant-related reactions** can mimic anaphylaxis. This is usually due to sulfites or the presence of a histamine-like substance in spoiled fish (scombroidosis).
  ○ **Flushing syndromes** include flushing due to red man's syndrome, carcinoid, vasointestinal peptide (and other vasoactive intestinal peptide-secreting tumors), postmenopausal symptoms, and alcohol use.
• Other forms of shock such as hypoglycemic, cardiogenic, septic, and hemorrhagic
• Miscellaneous syndromes such as C1 esterase (C1 INH) deficiency syndrome, pheochromocytoma, neurologic (seizure, stroke), and capillary leak syndrome
• Idiopathic

Diagnostic Testing

- Serum β-tryptase peaks at 1 hour after symptoms begin and may be present up to 6 hours.
- Epicutaneous skin testing, ImmunoCAP, and RAST (radioallergosorbent test) testing when available to identify trigger allergens.

TREATMENT

- Early recognition of signs and symptoms of anaphylaxis is a critical first step in treatment.
- **Maintain recumbent position while assessing and starting therapy.**
- **Airway management is a priority.** Supplemental 100% oxygen therapy should be administered. Endotracheal intubation may be necessary. If laryngeal edema is not rapidly responsive to epinephrine, cricothyroidotomy or tracheotomy may be required.
- **Volume expansion with intravenous (IV) fluids may** be necessary. An initial bolus of 500 to 1,000 mL normal saline should be followed by an infusion at a rate that is titrated to blood pressure (BP) and urine output.
- *α-Adrenergic or mixed adrenergic agonist vasopressors must be avoided in this setting due to resultant unopposed α-mediated vasoconstriction.*

Medications

- **Epinephrine** should be administered immediately.
  - Adult: 0.3 to 0.5 mg (0.3 to 0.5 mL of a 1:1,000 solution) intramuscularly (IM) in the lateral thigh, repeated at 10- to 15-minute intervals if necessary.
  - Child: 1:1,000 dilution at 0.01 mg/kg or 0.1 to 0.3 mL administered IM in the lateral thigh, repeated at 10- to 15-minute intervals if necessary.
  - 0.5 mL of 1:1,000 solution sublingually in cases of major airway compromise or hypotension.
  - 3 to 5 mL of 1:10,000 solution via central line.
  - 3 to 5 mL of 1:10,000 solution diluted with 10 mL of normal saline via endotracheal tube.
  - Protracted symptoms that require multiple doses of epinephrine, an IV epinephrine drip may be useful; the infusion is titrated to maintain adequate BP.
- **Glucagon**, given as a 1-mg (1 ampule) bolus and followed by a drip of up to 1 mg/hr can be used to provide inotropic support for patients who are taking β-adrenergic antagonists.
  β-Adrenergic antagonists therapy increases the risk of anaphylaxis and renders the reaction more difficult to treat (*Ann Intern Med 1991;115:270*).
- **Inhaled β-adrenergic agonists** should be used to treat resistant bronchospasm. Albuterol 0.5 mL (2.5 mg) or metaproterenol 0.3 mL (15 mg) in 2.5 mL of normal saline.
- **Glucocorticoids** have no significant immediate effect. However, they may prevent relapse of severe reactions.
  - Adult: Hydrocortisone 100 mg to 1 g IV or IM.
  - Child: Hydrocortisone 10 to 100 mg IV.
- **Antihistamines** relieve skin symptoms but have no immediate effect on the reaction. They may shorten the duration of the reaction.
  - Adult: Diphenhydramine 25 to 50 mg IM or IV.
  - Child: Diphenhydramine 12.5 to 25.0 mg IM or IV.

REFERRAL

Referrals to an allergist for further evaluation should be offered to all patients with a history of anaphylaxis. More importantly, patients with Hymenoptera sensitivity should be evaluated to determine eligibility for venom immunotherapy.

Eosinophilia

GENERAL PRINCIPLES

- Eosinophils are a blood granulocyte that can be involved in a variety of infectious, allergic, neoplastic, and idiopathic diseases.
- Eosinophil maturation is promoted by GM-CSF, interleukin (IL)-3, and IL-5.
- Eosinophils are normally seen in peripheral tissue such as mucosal tissues in the gastrointestinal and respiratory tracts. They are recruited to sites of inflammation.

Definition
- The upper limit of normal varies for blood eosinophilia.
- A value >500 eosinophils/μL is abnormal in most cases.
- The extent of eosinophilia can be categorized as mild (500 to 1,500 cells/μL), moderate (1,500 to 5,000 cells/μL), or severe (>5,000 cells/μL).

Classification
- Peripheral eosinophilia can be divided into primary, secondary, or idiopathic.
  - Primary eosinophilia is seen with hematologic disorders where there may be a clonal expansion of eosinophils (chronic eosinophilic leukemia) or a clonal expansion of cells, which stimulate eosinophil production (chronic myeloid or lymphocytic disorders).
  - Secondary eosinophilia has numerous causes such as parasites, allergic diseases, autoimmune disorders, toxins, medications, and endocrine disorders such as Addison's disease.
  - Idiopathic eosinophilia is considered when primary and secondary causes are excluded.
- **Eosinophilia associated with atopic disease.**
  - In allergic rhinitis, increased nasal eosinophilia is more common than peripheral blood eosinophilia.
  - Nasal eosinophilia with or without blood eosinophilia may be seen in asthma, nasal polyposis, or nonallergic rhinitis with eosinophilia syndrome (NARES).
  - NARES is a syndrome of marked nasal eosinophilia and nasal polyps. These patients do not have a history of allergies, asthma, aspirin sensitivity, and have negative skin tests and IgE levels.
- **Eosinophilia associated with pulmonary infiltrates.** This classification is inclusive of the pulmonary infiltrates with eosinophilia (PIE) syndromes and the eosinophilic pneumonias.
  - Allergic bronchopulmonary aspergillosis (ABPA), an IgE-dependent immunologic reaction to *Aspergillus fumigatus* consisting of pulmonary infiltrates, proximal bronchiectasis, and asthma- and drug-induced pneumonitis.
  - **Eosinophilic pneumonias** consist of pulmonary infiltrates with lung eosinophilia and are only occasionally associated with blood eosinophilia.

- Acute eosinophilic pneumonia is an idiopathic disease that presents with fever, cough, and dyspnea occurring days to weeks, typically in males.
- Chronic eosinophilic pneumonia is an idiopathic disease that presents with fever, cough, dyspnea, and significant weight loss occurring weeks to months, typically in females. It is associated with peripheral blood eosinophilia.
- Loffler syndrome is combination of blood eosinophilia and transient pulmonary infiltrates due to passage of helminthic larvae, usually *Ascaris lumbricoides*, through the lungs.
- Tropical pulmonary eosinophilia is a hypersensitivity response in the lung to lymphatic filariae.

- **HIV.** Modest to marked eosinophilia of unknown cause can be seen occasionally in patients with HIV. The eosinophilia is usually due to reactions to medications, adrenal insufficiency due to cytomegalovirus with consequent eosinophilia, or eosinophilic folliculitis (common dermatologic disorder seen in HIV patients).
- **Eosinophilia associated with parasitic infection.** Various multicellular parasites or helminths such as *Ascaris*, hookworm, or *Strongyloides* can induce blood eosinophilia, whereas single-celled protozoan parasites such as *Giardia lamblia* do not. The level of eosinophilia reflects the degree of tissue invasion by the parasite.
  - In cases of blood eosinophilia, **Strongyloides stercoralis** infection **must be excluded** because this helminth can set up a cycle of autoinfection leading to chronic infection with intermittent, sometimes marked, eosinophilia.
  - Tissue eosinophilia may not be accompanied by blood eosinophilia when the organism is sequestered within tissues (e.g., intact echinococcal cysts) or is limited to the intestinal lumen (e.g., tapeworms).
  - Among the helminths, the principal parasites that need to be evaluated are *S. stercoralis*, hookworm, and *Toxocara canis*. The diagnostic consideration can also vary according to geographic region.
  - There are some important caveats that need to be considered when evaluating patients for parasitic diseases and eosinophilia: *Strongyloides* can persist for decades without causing major symptoms and can elicit varying degrees of eosinophilia ranging from minimal to marked eosinophilia.
  - *T. canis* (visceral larva migrans) should be considered in children with a propensity to eat dirt contaminated by dog ascaris eggs.
- **Eosinophilia associated with cutaneous disease.**
  - **Atopic dermatitis** is classically associated with blood and skin eosinophilia.
  - **Eosinophilic fasciitis (Shulman's syndrome)** is characterized by acute erythema, swelling, and induration of the extremities progressing to symmetric induration of the skin that spares the fingers, feet, and face. Can be precipitated by exercise.
  - **Eosinophilic cellulitis (Wells' syndrome)** presents with recurrent swelling of an extremity without tactile warmth and failure with antibiotic therapy.
  - Patients with HIV are at risk for **eosinophilic pustular folliculitis.**
  - **Episodic angioedema with eosinophilia** is a rare disease that leads to recurrent attacks of fever, angioedema, and blood eosinophilia without other organ damage.
- **Eosinophilia associated with multiorgan involvement**
  - **Drug-induced eosinophilia.** Numerous drugs can cause blood and/or tissue eosinophilia. Drug-induced eosinophilia typically responds to cessation of the culprit medication. Asymptomatic drug-induced eosinophilia does not necessitate cessation of therapy.
  - **Churg–Strauss syndrome** (CSS) is a small- and medium-vessel vasculitis with chronic rhinosinusitis, asthma, and peripheral blood eosinophilia. The onset of asthma and eosinophilia may precede the development of CSS by several years.

- Noted to have intravascular and extravascular eosinophilic granuloma formation and lung involvement with transient infiltrates on chest radiograph. Other manifestations include mononeuropathy or polyneuropathy, rash, gastroenteritis, renal insufficiency, cardiac arrhythmias, and heart failure.
- Half the patients have antineutrophil cytoplasmic antibodies directed against myeloperoxidase (p-ANCA). Biopsy of affected tissue reveals a necrotizing vasculitis with extravascular granulomas and tissue eosinophilia.
- Initial treatment involves high-dose glucocorticoids with the addition of cyclophosphamide if necessary. Leukotriene modifiers, like all systemic steroid-sparing agents (including inhaled steroids), have been associated with unmasking of CSS due to a decrease in systemic steroid therapy; however, no evidence exists that these drugs *cause* CSS (*Chest 2000;117:708*).

- **Mastocytosis.** Systemic mastocytosis is characterized by infiltration of mast cells into various organs including the skin, liver, lymph nodes, bone marrow, and spleen. Peripheral eosinophilia can be seen in up to 20% of cases of systemic mastocytosis, and bone marrow biopsies often show an excess number of eosinophils.
- Idiopathic **hypereosinophilic syndrome** (HES) is a proliferative disorder of eosinophils characterized by infiltration of eosinophils in and consequent damage to organs such as the heart, gastrointestinal tract, kidneys, brain, and lung.
  - HES occurs predominantly in men between the ages of 20 and 50 years and presents with insidious onset of fatigue, cough, and dyspnea and an associated eosinophil count of >1,500 cells/μL documented on two occasions with organ involvement.
  - At presentation, patients typically are in the late thrombotic and fibrotic stages of eosinophil-mediated cardiac damage with signs of a restrictive cardiomyopathy and mitral regurgitation. An echocardiogram may detect intracardiac thrombi, endomyocardial fibrosis, or thickening of the posterior mitral valve leaflet. Neurologic manifestations range from peripheral neuropathy to stroke or encephalopathy. Bone marrow examination reveals increased eosinophil precursors.
- **Acute eosinophilic leukemia** is a rare myeloproliferative disorder that is distinguished from HES by several factors: an increased number of immature eosinophils in the blood and/or marrow, >10% blast forms in the marrow, as well as symptoms and signs compatible with an acute leukemia. Treatment is similar to other leukemias.
- **Lymphoma.** As many as 5% of patients with non-Hodgkin lymphoma and up to 15% of patients with Hodgkin lymphoma have modest peripheral blood eosinophilia. Eosinophilia in Hodgkin lymphoma has been correlated with IL-5 mRNA expression by Reed–Sternberg cells.
- **Atheroembolic disease.** Cholesterol embolization can lead to eosinophilia, eosinophiluria, renal dysfunction, livedo reticularis, increased erythrocyte sedimentation rate (ESR), and purple toes.
- **Immunodeficiency.** Hyper-IgE syndrome characterized by recurrent infections and dermatitis is often associated with eosinophilia as is Omenn syndrome (eosinophilia and combined variable immunodeficiency).

Epidemiology

In industrialized nations, peripheral blood eosinophilia is most often due to atopic disease, whereas helminthic infections are the most common cause of eosinophilia in the rest of the world.

Pathophysiology

Eosinophilic granules contain basic proteins, which bind to acidic dye. Once activated, eosinophils produce major basic protein, eosinophil cationic protein, and eosinophil peroxidase, which are toxic to bacteria, helminths, and normal tissue.

DIAGNOSIS

There are two approaches that are useful for evaluating eosinophilia, either by associated clinical context (Table 11-3) or by degree of eosinophilia (Table 11-4).

Table 11-3	Causes of Eosinophilia

Eosinophilia Associated with Atopic Disease

Allergic rhinitis
Asthma
Atopic dermatitis

Eosinophilia Associated with Pulmonary Infiltrates

Passage of larvae through the lung (Loffler syndrome)
Chronic eosinophilic pneumonia
Acute eosinophilic pneumonia
Tropical pulmonary eosinophilia
Allergic bronchopulmonary aspergillosis (ABPA)
Coccidiomycosis

Eosinophilia Associated with Parasitic Infection

Helminths (*Ascaris lumbricoides*, *Strongyloides stercoralis*, hookworm, *Toxocara canis or cati*, *Trichinella*)
Protozoa (only *Dientamoeba fragilis* and *Isospora belli*)

Eosinophilia Associated with Primary Cutaneous Disease

Atopic dermatitis
Eosinophilic fasciitis
Eosinophilic cellulitis
Eosinophilic folliculitis
Episodic angioedema with anaphylaxis

Eosinophilia Associated with Multiorgan Involvement

Drug-induced eosinophilia
Churg–Strauss syndrome
Idiopathic hypereosinophilic syndrome
Eosinophilic leukemia

Miscellaneous Causes

Eosinophilic gastroenteritis
Interstitial nephritis
HIV infection
Eosinophilia myalgia syndrome
Transplant rejection
Atheroembolic disease

Table 11-4	Classification of Eosinophilia Based on the Peripheral Blood Eosinophil Count	
Peripheral Blood Eosinophil Count (cells/μL)		
500–2,000	**2,000–5,000**	**>5,000**
Allergic rhinitis	Intrinsic asthma	Eosinophilia myalgia syndrome
Allergic asthma	Allergic bronchopulmonary aspergillosis	Idiopathic hypereosinophilic syndrome
Food allergy	Helminthiasis	Episodic angioedema with eosinophilia
Urticaria	Churg–Strauss syndrome	Leukemia
Addison disease	Drug reactions	
Pulmonary infiltrates with eosinophilia syndromes	Vascular neoplasms	
Solid neoplasms	Eosinophilic fasciitis	
Nasal polyposis	HIV	

Clinical Presentation

History

- The presence of cough, dyspnea, fever, or any symptoms of cancer should be determined, as should any history of rhinitis, wheezing, or rash.
- A history is important in narrowing the differential diagnosis of eosinophilia. It is important to determine if the patient has symptoms of atopic disease (rhinitis, wheezing, rash) or cancer (weight loss, fatigue, fever, night sweats) and to evaluate for other specific organ involvement such as lung, heart, or nerves.
- A complete medication list, including over-the-counter supplements, and a full travel history focused on countries where filariasis may be endemic (e.g., Southeast Asia, Africa, South America, or the Caribbean) should be obtained.
- Any pet contact should be ascertained for possible exposure to toxocariasis.

Physical Examination
Physical examination should be guided by the history, with a special focus on the skin, upper and lower respiratory tracts, as well as cardiovascular and neurologic systems.

Differential Diagnosis

- Various conditions can result in **eosinophilia associated with pulmonary infiltrates** (see Table 11-3). The presence of asthma should lead to consideration of ABPA, CSS, or tropical pulmonary eosinophilia.
- The etiology of **eosinophilia associated with cutaneous lesions** (see Table 11-3) pis guided by the appearance of the lesions and results of the skin biopsy. The diagnosis of CSS cannot be made without a tissue biopsy showing infiltrating eosinophils and granulomas.
- When eosinophilia is marked and all other causes have been ruled out, the diagnosis of **idiopathic HES** should be considered. Diagnosis requires a blood eosinophilia of >1,500/μL on two occasions with associated organ involvement. No specific test exists to identify these patients and, in general, this is a diagnosis of exclusion.

Diagnostic Testing

Laboratories

- The differential diagnosis can be narrowed based on the clinical findings and history. Depending on the travel history, stool exam for ova and parasites should be performed.
- Mild **eosinophilia associated with symptoms of rhinitis or asthma** is indicative of underlying atopic disease, which can be confirmed by skin testing.
- **Stool examination** for ova and parasites should be done on three separate occasions. Because only small numbers of helminths may pass in the stool and because tissue- or blood-dwelling helminths will not be found in the stool, **serologic tests** for antiparasite antibodies should also be sent. Such tests are available for strongyloidiasis, toxocariasis, and trichinellosis.
- Diagnosis at the time of presentation with Loffler syndrome can be made by detection of *Ascaris* larvae in respiratory secretions or gastric aspirates but not stool.
- A history of asthma, significant peripheral blood eosinophilia (>10% of the leukocyte count), and pulmonary infiltrates suggests CSS. In this case, sinus computed tomography, nerve conduction studies, and testing for p-ANCA may aid in diagnosis.
- Peripheral blood smear can aid in the diagnosis of malignancy. May require bone marrow biopsy and can obtain testing on bone marrow and/or peripheral blood for *FIP1L1/PDGFRA* mutation. Can also see an increase in vitamin B12 level.
- Evaluation for idiopathic HES should also consist of troponin, echocardiogram, and electrocardiogram (ECG).
- Immunoglobulin levels are helpful if concerned for an immunodeficiency.
- A tryptase level can exclude mastocytosis as a cause of eosinophilia.

Imaging

Chest X-ray findings may also help to narrow the differential diagnosis.

- Peripheral infiltrates with central clearing are indicative of chronic eosinophilic pneumonia.
- Diffuse infiltrates in an interstitial, alveolar, or mixed pattern may be seen in acute eosinophilic pneumonia as well as drug-induced eosinophilia with pulmonary involvement.
- Transient infiltrates may be seen in Loffler syndrome, CSS, or ABPA.
- Central bronchiectasis is a major criterion in the diagnosis of ABPA.
- A diffuse miliary or nodular pattern, consolidation, or cavitation may be found in cases of tropical pulmonary eosinophilia.

Diagnostic Procedures

- If no other cause of pulmonary infiltrates has been identified, a **bronchoscopy** may be necessary for analysis of bronchoalveolar lavage (BAL) fluid and lung tissue. The presence of eosinophils in BAL fluid or sputum with eosinophilic infiltration of the parenchyma is most typical of acute or chronic eosinophilic pneumonia.
- Skin biopsy will help to aid in diagnosing cutaneous eosinophilic disease CSS.

TREATMENT

- When a drug reaction is suspected, discontinuation of the drug is both diagnostic and therapeutic. Other treatment options depend on the exact cause of eosinophilia because, with the exception of idiopathic HES, eosinophilia itself is a manifestation of an underlying disease.

- **Hypereosinophilic syndrome:** Patients with marked eosinophilia with no organ involvement may have a benign course. In contrast, those with organ involvement and with FIP1L1/PDGFA-associated disease may have an extremely aggressive course without treatment.
  - Monitoring and early initiation of high-dose glucocorticoids should be pursued in all patients except those who have the FIP1L1/PDGFA fusion.
  - Patients with the FIP1L1/PDGFA fusion mutation should be started on imatinib mesylate (Gleevec), a tyrosine kinase inhibitor. Treatment should be initiated promptly in these patients to prevent progression of cardiac disease and other end-organ damage. Imatinib has been shown to induce disease remission and progression (*Blood 2003;101(12):4714*).
  - Hydroxyurea has been the most frequently used effective second-line agent and/ or steroid-sparing agent for HES. Interferon-α has been effective in a small number of case series (*Br J Haematol 1996;92:17*). Its mechanism of action is not completely understood but may involve inhibition of eosinophil proliferation and differentiation.
  - Mepolizumab, a humanized anti-IL-5 antibody, has shown promising results in patients who do not have the FIP1L1/PDGFA fusion protein (*N Engl J Med 2008;358(12):1215*).
  - Alemtuzumab, an anti-CD52 antibody (CD52 is expressed on the surface of eosinophils), has been shown in a clinical trial to decrease eosinophils counts (*Clin Cancer Res 2009;15:368*).
- Primary eosinophilia disorders should be followed by a specialist; any cases of unresolved or unexplained eosinophilia warrant evaluation by an allergist/immunologist.

Urticaria and Angioedema

GENERAL PRINCIPLES

Definition

- **Urticaria** (hives) are raised, flat-topped, well-demarcated pruritic skin lesions with surrounding erythema. Central clearing can cause an annular lesion and is often seen after antihistamine use. An individual lesion usually lasts minutes to hours.
- **Angioedema** is a deeper lesion causing painful areas of localized swelling. It can be found anywhere on the body but most often involves the tongue, lips, eyelids, and/or genitals. When angioedema occurs without urticaria, specific diagnoses must be entertained (see Differential Diagnosis section).

Classification

- **Acute urticaria (with or without angioedema)** is defined as an episode lasting <6 weeks. Usually, it is caused by an allergic reaction to a medication or food, but it may be related to underlying infection, recent insect sting, or exposure (contact or inhalation) to an allergen. Patients can develop a hypersensitivity to a food, medication, or self-care product that previously had been used without difficulty.
- **Chronic urticaria (with or without angioedema)** is defined as episodes that persist for >6 weeks. There are many possible causes of chronic urticaria and angioedema, including medications, autoimmunity, self-care products, and physical triggers. However, the etiology remains unidentified in >80% of cases.

Epidemiology

- Urticaria is a common condition that affects 15% to 24% of the U.S. population at some time in their life. Chronic idiopathic urticaria occurs in 0.1% of the U.S. population, and there does not appear to be an increased risk in persons with atopy.
- Angioedema generally lasts 12 to 48 hours and occurs in 40% to 50% of patients with urticaria.

Etiology

- IgE and non–IgE-mediated reactions: Drugs (ACE-Is and NSAIDs), foods, inhalant, or contact allergen
- Transfusion reactions
- Infections (i.e., viral, bacterial, parasitic)
- Insects
- Autoimmune diseases
- Malignancy
- Physical urticaria: Dermographism, cold, cholinergic, pressure, vibratory, solar, and aquagenic
- Mastocytosis
- Hereditary diseases
- Idiopathic

Pathophysiology

Mechanisms for initiation of urticaria and angioedema differ depending on the classification and are not fully understood. However, the final common pathway is the degranulation of mast cells or basophils and the release of inflammatory mediators. Histamine is the primary mediator and elicits edema (wheal) and erythema (flare).

DIAGNOSIS

Diagnosis is based upon complete history and physical examination, which should elicit identifiable triggers.

Clinical Presentation

- Patients with an acute urticaria episode present with history of pruritus, erythematous cutaneous lesions with less than 6 weeks duration, and usually after exposure to an antigen. Chronic patients will have relapsing symptoms interspersed with symptom-free periods.
- Angioedema patients usually present without symptoms of pruritus, and the lesions are described as swollen and painful.
- Urticaria and angioedema can occur together.

History
- A detailed history should elicit identifiable triggers and rule out any systemic causes. This also includes determining whether an individual lesion lasts >24 hours in which case the diagnosis of urticarial vasculitis must be investigated by a skin biopsy.
- Any changes in environmental exposures, foods, medications, personal care products, etc., should be determined.

Physical Examination
- Complete examination of the affected and nonaffected skin.
- Urticaria appears as erythematous, raised lesions that blanch with pressure.

- Angioedema often involves the face, tongue, extremities, or genitalia, and may be asymmetric.

Differential Diagnosis

- IgE-mediated allergic reaction to drugs, foods, insects, inhalant, or contact allergen
- Non–IgE-mediated reactions (i.e., medications including NSAIDs, vancomycin, radioactive iodine, opiates, muscle relaxants, foods including tomato and strawberries)
- Physical urticaria
- Mast cell release syndromes (i.e., systemic mastocytosis, cutaneous mastocytosis, including urticaria pigmentosa)
- Cutaneous small vessel vasculitis (i.e., urticarial vasculitis, systemic lupus erythematosus)
- Toxic drug eruptions
- EM
- Allergic contact dermatitis (i.e., poison ivy, poison oak)
- **Angioedema without urticaria** should lead to consideration of specific entities.
  - Use of ACE-Is or **angiotensin II receptor blockers** (ARBs) can be associated with angioedema at any point in the course of therapy.
  - **Hereditary angioedema (HAE), or C1 esterase inhibitor (C1 INH) deficiency**, is inherited in an autosomal dominant pattern.
  - **Acquired C1 INH deficiency** presents similarly to HAE but is typically associated with an underlying lymphoproliferative disorder or connective tissue disease.

Diagnostic Testing

Epicutaneous skin testing and patch testing is indicated when symptoms are associated with specific triggers.

Laboratories
- A complete blood count (CBC), ESR, urinalysis, and liver function tests should be obtained to screen for systemic etiologies of chronic urticaria, such as hematologic malignancies, autoimmune diseases, and occult infections, including hepatitis.
- All patients with **angioedema without urticaria** *should be screened with a C4 level, which is reduced during and between attacks of HAE.* If the C4 level is reduced, a quantitative and functional C1 INH assay should be performed. Measuring C1 INH levels alone is not sufficient because 15% of patients have normal levels of a dysfunctional C1 INH protein; therefore, it is important to also obtain the functional assay.
- Acquired C1 INH deficiency patients have reduced C1q, C1 INH, and C4 levels. Other patients with the acquired form have an autoantibody to C1 INH with low C4 and C1 INH levels but a normal C1 level.

Diagnostic Procedures
- A skin biopsy should be performed if individual lesions persist for >24 hours to rule out urticarial vasculitis.
- Biopsy of acute urticarial lesions reveals dilation of small venules and capillaries located in the superficial dermis with widening of the dermal papillae, flattening of the rete pegs, and swelling of collagen fibers.
- Chronic urticaria is characterized by a dense, nonnecrotizing, perivascular infiltrate consisting of T lymphocytes, mast cells, eosinophils, basophils, and neutrophils.

- Angioedema shows similar pathologic alterations in the deep, rather than superficial, dermis and subcutaneous tissue.

TREATMENT

- The ideal treatment of acute urticaria with or without angioedema is identification and avoidance of specific causes. **All potential causes should be eliminated.** Most cases resolve within 1 week. In some instances, it is possible to reintroduce an agent cautiously if it is believed not to be the etiologic agent. This trial should be done in the presence of a physician with epinephrine readily available.
- Careful consideration should be given to the **elimination or substitution of each prescription or over-the-counter medication** or supplement. If a patient reacts to one medication in a class, the reaction likely will be triggered by all medications in that class. Exacerbating agents (such as NSAIDs, including aspirin, opiates, vancomycin, and alcohol) should be avoided because they may induce nonspecific mast cell degranulation and exacerbate urticaria caused by other agents.
- **Elimination of all self-care products**, with the exception of those that contain no methylparaben, fragrance, or preservative, is useful when sensitivity to these products is a possibility.
- In patients presenting with hereditary and acquired angioedema, a prompt assessment of airway is critical in especially those presenting with a laryngeal attack.

Medications

In acute urticaria in the presence of anaphylaxis, which consists of systemic symptoms such as hypotension, laryngeal edema, or bronchospasm, treatment with epinephrine (0.3 to 0.5 mL of a 1:1,000 solution IM) should be administered immediately. See Anaphylaxis section for additional information.

First Line
- **Acute urticaria and/or isolated angioedema:**
  - **A second-generation oral antihistamine** such as cetirizine, levocetirizine, fexofenadine, desloratadine, or loratadine should be administered to patients until the hives have cleared. A first-generation antihistamine such as hydroxyzine may be added as an evening dose if needed to obtain control in refractory cases. H2 antihistamines, such as ranitidine, may also be added to the above treatment.
  - **Oral corticosteroids** should be reserved for patients with laryngeal edema or systemic symptoms of anaphylaxis after treatment with epinephrine. Corticosteroids will not have an immediate effect but may prevent relapse. They may also be helpful for patients with severe symptoms who have not responded to antihistamines.
  - If a patient presents with systemic symptoms, self-administered epinephrine should be prescribed for use in the case of accidental exposure to the same trigger in the future.
- **Chronic urticaria**
  - **Antihistamines** for symptom control are the mainstay of treatment. Treatment should be continued for a period of 6 months, and then lowered to the level needed to maintain symptom control.
  - Second-generation H_1 antihistamines, such as cetirizine, levocetirizine, fexofenadine, loratadine, and desloratadine, are well tolerated and should be used as first-line agents. Cetirizine, the breakdown product of hydroxyzine, is often used for

chronic urticaria treatment because it is thought to concentrate in the skin; however, it is minimally sedating. H_2 antihistamines, such as ranitidine, may also be added to the earlier discussed treatment. Several drugs in this class are now available over the counter.

○ Classic H_1 antihistamines, such as hydroxyzine or diphenhydramine, 25 mg PO q4–6h or prn, can be added for better control of lesions or for breakthrough lesions. The dose is usually limited by sedation.

• **Hereditary and acquired angioedema (disorder of C1 inhibitor)**
Laryngeal attacks or severe abdominal attacks: C1-inhibitor replacement (C1INHRP) is a first-line agent. Other options include fresh frozen plasma and tranexamic acid. Also pursue symptomatic therapy and rehydration.

Second Line
Chronic Urticaria

• Doxepin, an antidepressant with H_1- and H_2-blocking effects, is a useful addition and often is less sedating than hydroxyzine.

• H_2-blocking agents may be helpful in addition to H_1 antihistamines to control breakthrough hives.

• Leukotriene receptor antagonists may be helpful in combination with antihistamines in treatment of chronic urticaria.

• Oral corticosteroids should be reserved for those patients in whom adequate control cannot be achieved with a combination of the aforementioned agents. Steroids should be used only for short periods of time.

• Cyclosporine may be used in cases where patients have antihistamine refractory urticaria and require chronic systemic steroids for symptom control.

REFERRAL

All patients with chronic urticaria or a history of anaphylaxis should be referred to an allergy specialist for evaluation to identify potential allergic and autoimmune triggers, including the presence of antithyroid antibodies or antibodies against the Fc portion of the IgE receptor.

Immunodeficiency

GENERAL PRINCIPLES

Definition

• Primary immunodeficiencies (PIDs) are disorders of the immune system that result in an increased susceptibility to infection.

• Secondary immunodeficiencies are also disorders of increased susceptibility to infection but are attributable to an external source.

Classification

PIDs can be organized by the defective immune components.

• Humoral immunodeficiency: The defect is primarily in the ability to make antibodies.
  ○ Common variable immune deficiency
  ○ X-linked (Bruton's) agammaglobulinemia
  ○ IgG subclass deficiency
  ○ IgA deficiency
  ○ Hyper-IgE (Job) syndrome

- Cell-mediated immunodeficiency: The defect is primarily with cell-mediated (T-cell) immune response.
- Combined immunodeficiency: The defect results in deficiencies in both cellular and humoral immune responses.
- Innate immune system defects:
  - Chronic granulomatous disease (CGD)
  - Complement deficiencies
  - Mendelian susceptibility to mycobacterial diseases (MSMDs)

Epidemiology

- Secondary immunodeficiency syndromes, particularly HIV/AIDS, are the most common immunodeficiency disorders.
- Most PIDs presenting in adulthood are humoral immune defects.
- Common variable immunodeficiency (CVID) is the most common symptomatic PID, occurring with a frequency of 1/10,000.

Etiology

- CVID is largely idiopathic, though there are genetic mutations (such as TACI, ICOS, and CD19) with some forms of the disorder.
- Humoral immune deficiencies are generally thought to be caused by defects in B-cell maturation.
- A variety of genetic mutations have been associated with specific PID syndromes.
- Secondary immunodeficiencies can be caused by medications (chemotherapy, immunomodulatory agents, corticosteroids), infectious agents (e.g., HIV), malignancy, antibody loss (e.g., nephrotic syndrome, protein losing enteropathy, or consumption during a severe underlying infection), autoimmune disease (e.g., systemic lupus erythematosis [SLE], rheumatoid arthritis [RA]), malnutrition (vitamin D), and other underlying diseases (e.g., diabetes mellitus [DM], cirrhosis, uremia).

DIAGNOSIS

Clinical Presentation

- The hallmark of PID is recurrent infections. Clinical suspicion should be increased by recurrent sinopulmonary infection, deep-seated infections, or disseminated infections in an otherwise healthy patient.
- Specific PIDs are often associated with particular types of pathogens (e.g., catalase-positive infections in CGD or MSMD).
- Recurrent urinary tract infections are only rarely associated with PID.
- **IgA deficiency** is the most common immune deficiency, with a prevalence of 1 out of 500 people.
  - Patients may be asymptomatic or present with recurrent sinus and pulmonary infections. Therapy is directed at early treatment with antibiotics because IgA replacement is not available.
  - In 15% of cases, an associated IgG subclass deficiency is present.
  - Truly IgA-deficient patients (rather than those with very low levels) are at risk for developing a severe transfusion reaction because of the presence in some individuals of IgE anti-IgA antibodies; therefore, these patients should be transfused with washed red blood cells or receive blood products only from IgA-deficient donors.

- **CVID** includes a heterogeneous group of disorders in which most patients present in the second to fourth decade of life with recurrent sinus and pulmonary infections and are discovered to have *low and dysfunctional IgG, IgA, and IgM antibodies.*
  - Patients with CVID are particularly susceptible to infection with encapsulated organisms.
  - B-cell numbers are usually normal, but there is decreased ability to produce immunoglobulin after immunization. Some patients may also exhibit T-cell dysfunction and be anergic.
  - Patients may have associated gastrointestinal disease or autoimmune abnormalities (most commonly autoimmune hemolytic anemia, idiopathic thrombocytopenic purpura, pernicious anemia, and rheumatoid arthritis).
  - There is an increased incidence of malignancy, especially lymphoid and gastrointestinal malignancy.
  - Therapy consists of IV immunoglobulin (IVIG) replacement therapy as well as prompt treatment of infections with antibiotics.
- **X-linked (Bruton's) agammaglobulinemia** clinically manifests very similarly to severe CVID and is typically diagnosed in childhood but can present in adulthood.
  - Patients usually have low levels of all immunoglobulin types and very low levels of B cells.
  - Specific genetic defect is in Bruton's tyrosine kinase, which is involved in B-cell maturation.
- **Subclass deficiency.** Deficiencies of each of the IgG subclasses (IgG1, IgG2, IgG3, and IgG4) have been described.
  - These patients present with similar complaints as the CVID patients.
  - Total IgG levels may be normal. A strong association with IgA deficiency exists. There is disagreement as to whether this is a separate entity from CVID.
  - In most cases, there is no need to evaluate IgG subclass levels.
- **Hyper-IgE syndrome (Job syndrome)** is characterized by recurrent pyogenic infections of the skin and lower respiratory tract. This infection can result in severe abscess and empyema formation.
  - The most common organism involved is *Staphylococcus aureus*, but other bacteria and fungi have been reported.
  - Patients present with recurrent infections and have associated pruritic dermatitis, coarse (lion-like) facies, growth retardation, and hyperkeratotic nails. Laboratory data reveal the presence of normal levels of IgG, IgA, and IgM but markedly elevated levels of IgE. A marked increase in tissue and blood eosinophils may also be observed.
  - Mutations in *STAT3* have been linked to development of this disease (*N Engl J Med 2007;357(16):1608*).
  - No specific therapy exists except for early treatment of infection with antibiotics.
- **Complement deficiencies** are a broad category of PID characterized recurrent infections to a range of pathogens.
  - Recurrent disseminated neisserial infections are associated with a deficiency in the terminal complement system (C5–C9).
  - Systemic lupus-like disorders and recurrent infection with encapsulated organisms have been associated with deficiencies in other components of complement.
- **CGD** is characterized by defective killing of intracellular pathogens by neutrophils.
  - Patients usually present with frequent infection, often with abscesses, from *S. aureus* and other catalase-positive organisms. *Aspergillus* is a particularly troublesome pathogen for patients with CGD.

- ○ Diagnosis is made by demonstration of defective respiratory burst with nitroblue tetrazolium or using flow cytometry assay using dihydrorhodamine.
- **MSMD** is a relatively newly described PID caused by defects in Th1 immunity and is associated with mutations in genes involved in interferon gamma and IL-12 signaling. Characteristic infections include mycobacterial infections (including typical and atypical mycobacterium) and salmonella infections.

Diagnostic Testing

- Initial evaluation should focus on identifying possible secondary causes of recurrent infection such as allergy, medications, and anatomic abnormalities.
- Workup begins with a CBC with differential, HIV test, quantitative immunoglobulin levels, and complement levels. Often the evaluation will need to include enumeration of B and T cells in the peripheral blood.
- If clinical suspicion is high for an underlying humoral PID, B-cell function can be assessed by measuring immunoglobulin response to vaccinations. Preimmunization and postimmunization titers for both a protein antigen (i.e., tetanus) and a polysaccharide antigen (i.e., Pneumovax, the unconjugated 23-valent vaccine) are measured because proteins and polysaccharide antigens are handled differently by the immune system.
- Titers of specific antibodies are measured before and at least 4 weeks after immunization, with a good response defined as a fourfold increase in the antibody titer of at least 70% of the tested serotypes (*Ann Allergy Asthma Immunol 2005;94(5 suppl 1):S1*).
- A patient with normal or low IgG and a poor response to immunization is classified as having CVID.

TREATMENT

- IgA deficiency: No specific treatment is available. However, these patients should be promptly treated at the first sign of infection with an antibiotic that covers *Streptococcus pneumoniae* or *Haemophilus influenzae*.
- CVID should be treated with IVIG. Numerous preparations of IVIG are available, all of which undergo viral inactivation steps.
  - ○ Replacement should be initiated with 400 mg/kg and infused slowly according to the manufacturer's suggestions (for most preparations, begin at 30 mL/hr and increase by 30 mL/hr every 15 minutes as tolerated to a maximum rate of 210 mL/hr).
  - ○ Possible side effects include myalgias, vomiting, chills, and lingering headache (due to immune complex–mediated aseptic meningitis).
  - ○ Patients, especially those with no detectable IgA, need to have vital signs monitored q15min initially because anaphylaxis from IgE anti-IgA antibodies can develop in these patients. For these patients, it is best to use IVIG preparations that have very low IgA.

REFERRAL

- Patients in whom a PID is being seriously considered merit evaluation by an allergist/clinical immunologist with expertise in diagnosing and treating PID.

12 Fluid and Electrolyte Management

Judy L. Jang and Steven Cheng

FLUID MANAGEMENT AND PERTURBATIONS IN VOLUME STATUS

GENERAL PRINCIPLES

- **Total body water (TBW).** Water comprises approximately 60% of lean body weight in men and 50% in women. TBW is distributed in two major compartments: two-thirds is **intracellular fluid** (ICF) and one-third is **extracellular fluid** (ECF). The latter is further subdivided into intravascular and interstitial spaces in a ratio of 1:4. This proportional distribution of water enables us to approximate the amount of water in each compartment under normal circumstances.
  - **Example**: For a healthy 70-kg man,

$$TBW = 0.6 \times 70 = 42 \text{ L}$$

    - ICF = 2/3 TBW = $0.66 \times 42 = 28$ L
    - ECF = 1/3 TBW = $0.33 \times 42 = 14$ L
    - Intravascular compartment = $0.25 \times 14 = 3.5$ L
    - Interstitial compartment = $0.75 \times 14 = 10.5$ L
  - The distribution of water between intravascular and interstitial spaces can also be affected by changes to the Starling balance of forces. Low oncotic pressure (i.e., low albumin states) and high hydrostatic pressure (i.e., Na^+-retentive states) increase the movement of fluid from vascular to interstitial compartments. This is an important step in the development of edema.
  - Because the majority of water is contained in the intracellular space, the loss of water alone (without Na^+) does not typically result in the hemodynamic changes associated with volume depletion. Instead, disturbances in TBW change serum **osmolality** and electrolyte concentrations.
  - The intact kidney adapts to changes in TBW by increasing water excretion or reabsorption. This is mediated by the **antidiuretic hormone (ADH; vasopressin)**, which permits water movement across the distal nephron. Although vasopressin release is predominately responsive to osmotic cues, volume contraction can cause a nonosmotic release of vasopressin, resulting in a reduction of renal water excretion.
- **Total body Na^+.** Eighty-five percent to 90% of **total body Na^+** is extracellular and constitutes the predominate solute in the ECF. Changes to the body's total Na^+ content typically results from a loss or gain of this Na^+-rich fluid, leading

to contraction or expansion of the ECF space. Clinically, this manifests as volume depletion (hypotension, tachycardia) and volume expansion (peripheral or pulmonary edema), respectively.

○ Na^+ *concentration* is distinct from Na^+ *content*. Na^+ concentration reflects the amount of Na^+ distributed in a fixed quantity of water. As such, an increase in TBW can decrease the Na^+ concentration even if the body's total Na^+ content remains unchanged.

○ The intact kidney can respond to altered Na^+ content in the ECF space by increasing or decreasing Na^+ reabsorption. This response is mediated by cardiovascular, renal, hepatic, and central nervous system sensors of the effective circulating volume.

The Euvolemic Patient

GENERAL PRINCIPLES

Maintenance Fluids

- In the euvolemic patient, the goal of fluid and electrolyte administration is to maintain homeostasis. The best way to accomplish this is to allow free access to food and drink rather than providing intravenous (IV) therapy. However, patients who are unable to tolerate oral input require maintenance fluids to replace renal, gastrointestinal (GI), and insensible fluid losses.
- The decision to provide maintenance IV fluid (IVF) should be thoughtfully considered and not administered by rote. Fluid administration should therefore be reassessed *at least* daily, and patient weight, which can may indicate net fluid balance, should be monitored carefully.
- Consider the **water** and **electrolyte** needs of the patient separately when prescribing IVF therapy.
  ○ Minimum **water** requirements for daily fluid balance can be approximated from the sum of the required urine output, stool water loss, and insensible losses.
    ▪ The minimum urine output necessary to excrete the daily solute load is simply the amount of solute consumed each day (roughly 600 to 800 mOsm/d in the average individual) divided by the maximum amount of solute that can be excreted per liter of urine (maximum urine concentrating capacity is 1,200 mOsm/L in healthy kidneys). The result is an obligate urine output of *at least* 0.5 L/d.
    ▪ The water lost in stool is typically 200 mL/d.
    ▪ **Insensible water losses** from the skin and respiratory tract amount to roughly 400 to 500 mL/d. The volume of water produced from endogenous metabolism (~250 to 350 mL/d) should be considered as well. The degree of insensible loss may vary tremendously depending on respiratory rate, metabolic state, and temperature (water losses increase by 100 to 150 mL/d for each degree of body temperature over 37°C).
    ▪ Fluid from drain losses must be factored in as well.
    ▪ After adding each of these components, the minimum amount of water needed to maintain homeostasis is roughly 1400 mL/d or 60 mL/hr.
  ○ The **electrolytes** that are usually administered during maintenance fluid therapy are Na^+ and K^+ salts. Requirements depend on minimum obligatory and ongoing losses.

Table 12-1	Commonly Used Parenteral Solutions				
IV solution	Osmolality (mOsm/L)	[Glucose] (g/L)	[Na^+] (mEq/L)	[Cl^-] (mEq/L)	HCO_3^- Equivalents (mEq/L)
D_5W	278	50	0	0	0
0.45% NaCl[a]	154	—[b]	77	77	0
0.9% NaCl[a]	308	—[b]	154	154	0
3% NaCl	1,026	—	513	513	0
Lactated Ringer's[c]	274	—[b]	130	109	28

[a]NaCl 0.45% and 0.9% are half-normal and normal saline, respectively.
[b]Also available with 5% dextrose.
[c]Also contains 4 mEq/L K^+, 1.5 mEq/L Ca^{2+}, and 28 mEq/L lactate.
D_5W, 5% dextrose in water; $D_{50}W$, 50% dextrose in water; IV, intravenous.

- It is customary to provide **75 to 175 mEq Na^+/d** as NaCl. (A typical 2-g Na^+ diet provides 86 mEq Na^+/d.)
- Generally, **20 to 60 mEq K^+/d** is included if renal function is normal.
- Carbohydrate in the form of **dextrose**, **100 to 150 g/d**, is given to minimize protein catabolism and prevent starvation ketoacidosis.
○ Table 12-1 provides a list of common IV solutions and their contents. By combining the necessary components, one can derive an appropriate maintenance fluid regimen tailored for each patient.
○ **Example:** A patient is admitted for a procedure and is made nothing by mouth (NPO). To maintain homeostasis, you must replace 2 L of water, 154 mEq Na^+, 40 mEq K^+, and 100 g dextrose over the next 24 hours (values are within **water** and **electrolyte** requirements described earlier).
   - 2 L of water: Dose fluid at 85 mL/hr (2,000 mL ÷ 24 hours)
   - 154 mEq of Na^+: Use 0.45% normal saline (NS) (77 mEq Na^+/L)
   - 40 mEq of K^+: Add 20 mEq/L KCl to each liter of IVF
   - 100 g dextrose: Use D5 (50 g of dextrose/L)
   - Order: **D_5 0.45% NaCl with 20 mEq/L KCl at 85 mL/hr**

The Hypovolemic Patient

GENERAL PRINCIPLES

Etiology

- Volume depletion generally results from a deficit in **total body Na^+** content. This may result from **renal** or **extrarenal losses** of Na^+ from the ECF. **Water** losses alone can also cause volume depletion, but the quantity required to do so is large, as water is lost mainly from the ICF and not the ECF, where volume contraction can be assessed.
- **Renal losses** may be secondary to enhanced diuresis, salt-wasting nephropathies, mineralocorticoid deficiency, or the resolution of obstructive renal disease.

- **Extrarenal losses** include fluid loss from the GI tract (vomiting, nasogastric suction, fistula drainage, diarrhea), respiratory losses, skin losses (especially with burns), hemorrhage, and severe third spacing of fluid in critical illness.

Diagnosis

Clinical Presentation

- **Symptoms** include complaints of thirst, fatigue, weakness, muscle cramps, and postural dizziness. Sometimes, syncope and coma can result with severe volume depletion.
- **Signs** of hypovolemia include low jugular venous pressure, postural hypotension, postural tachycardia, and the absence of axillary sweat. Diminished skin turgor and dry mucous membranes are poor markers of decreased interstitial fluid. Mild degrees of volume depletion are often not clinically detectable, while larger fluid losses can lead to mental status changes, oliguria, and hypovolemic shock.

Diagnostic Testing

Laboratories

Laboratory studies are often helpful but must be used in conjunction with the clinical picture.

- **Urine sodium** is a marker for Na^+ avidity in the kidney.
  - Urine Na^+ <15 mEq is consistent with volume depletion, as is a fractional excretion of sodium (FeNa) <1%. The latter can be calculated as [(Urine Na^+ × Serum Cr) ÷ (Urine Cr × Serum Na^+)] × 100.
  - Concomitant metabolic alkalosis may increase urine Na^+ excretion despite volume depletion due to obligate excretion of Na^+ to accompany the bicarbonate anion. In such cases, a urine chloride of <20 mEq is often helpful to confirm volume contraction.
- **Urine osmolality** and **serum bicarbonate** levels may also be elevated.
- **Hematocrit** and **serum albumin** may be increased from hemoconcentration.

TREATMENT

- It is often difficult to estimate the **volume deficit** present, and therapy is thus largely empiric, requiring frequent reassessments of volume status while resuscitation is under way.
- Mild volume contraction can usually be corrected via the oral route. However, the presence of hemodynamic instability, symptomatic fluid loss, or intolerance to oral administration requires IV therapy.
- The primary therapeutic goal is to protect hemodynamic stability and replenish **intravascular volume** with fluid that will preferentially expand the ECF compartment. This can be accomplished with Na^+-based solutions, since the Na^+ will be retained in the ECF.
  - **Isotonic fluid**, such as NS (0.9% NaCl), contains a Na^+ content similar to that of plasma fluid in the ECF and thus remains entirely in the ECF space. It is the initial fluid of choice for replenishing **intravascular volume**.
    - The administration of solute-free water is largely ineffective, since the majority of water will distribute to the ICF space.
    - Half-normal saline (0.45% NS) has 77 mEq of Na^+ per liter, roughly half the Na^+ content of an equal volume in the ECF. Thus, half of this solution will stay in the ECF, and half will follow the predicted distribution of water.

○ Fluids can be administered as a bolus or at a steady maintenance rate. In patients with symptomatic volume depletion, a 1- to 2-L bolus is often preferable to acutely expand the intravascular space. This should be followed by a careful reassessment of the patient's volume status. The bolus can be repeated if necessary, although close attention should be directed toward possible signs of volume overload. Smaller boluses should be used for patients with poor cardiac reserve or significant edema. Once the patient is stable, fluids can be administered at a maintenance rate to replace ongoing losses. In patients with hemorrhage or GI bleeding, **blood transfusion** can accomplish both volume expansion and concomitant correction of anemia.

The Hypervolemic Patient

GENERAL PRINCIPLES

Etiology

The clinical manifestations of hypervolemia result from a surplus of **total body Na⁺**. Na⁺ retention can be caused by a primary disorder of renal Na⁺ retention. Alternatively, it may be secondary to decreased **effective circulating volume**, as in heart failure, cirrhosis, or profound hypoalbuminemia.

DIAGNOSIS

Clinical Presentation

- Expansion of the **interstitial compartment** may result in peripheral edema, ascites, and pleural effusions. Expansion of the **intravascular compartment** may result in pulmonary rales, elevated jugular venous pressure, hepatojugular reflux, an S_3 gallop, and elevated blood pressures.
- As overt signs of hypervolemia may not manifest until 3 to 4 L of fluid retention, a gradual rise in water weight is often the earliest indication of Na⁺ retention.
- **Symptoms** may include dyspnea, abdominal distention, or swelling of the extremities.

Diagnostic Testing

Laboratories
- Laboratory studies are generally not needed and hypervolemia is primarily a bedside diagnosis.
- **The urine [Na⁺]** may be low (<15 mEq/L) with decreased **effective circulating volume** reflecting renal sodium retention.

Imaging
A chest radiograph may show pulmonary edema or pleural effusions, but clear lung fields do not exclude volume overload.

TREATMENT

Treatment must address not only the ECF volume excess but also the underlying pathologic process. Alleviating the Na⁺ excess can be accomplished by the judicious use of diuretics and by limiting Na⁺ intake.

Medications

- Diuretics enhance the renal excretion of Na^+ by blocking the various sites of Na^+ reabsorption along the nephron.
  - Thiazide diuretics block the NaCl transporters in the distal convoluted tubule. They are often used for mild states of chronic Na^+ retention. Because of their specific site of action, thiazide diuretics impair urinary dilutional capacity (the ability to excrete water) and often stimulate a responsive increase in proximal tubule reabsorption.
  - Loop diuretics block the Na^+-K^+-$2Cl^-$ transporter in the ascending loop of Henle. They are often used in circumstances requiring a brisk and immediate diuresis, such as acute volume overload. Loop diuretics impair urinary concentration (increase renal free water excretion) and enhance the excretion of divalent cations (Ca^{2+} and Mg^{2+}).
  - Potassium-sparing diuretics act by decreasing Na^+ reabsorption in the collecting duct. While the overall diuretic of these agents is comparatively small, they serve as useful adjunctive agents. Furthermore, as aldosterone antagonists do not require tubular secretion, they can be particularly useful in those with decreased renal perfusion or impaired tubular function.
- Treatment of the underlying disease process is critical to prevent continued Na^+ reabsorption in the kidney. Nephrotic syndrome is discussed in Chapter 13, Renal Diseases. Treatment of heart failure is discussed in Chapter 5, Heart Failure and Cardiomyopathy, and cirrhosis are addressed in Chapter 19, Liver Diseases.

Disorders of Sodium Concentration

GENERAL PRINCIPLES

Hypernatremia and **hyponatremia** are primarily disorders of *water balance* or *water distribution*. The body is designed to withstand both drought and deluge with adaptations to renal water handling and the thirst mechanism. A persistent abnormality in [Na^+] thus requires both an initial challenge to water balance as well as a disturbance of the adaptive response.

Hyponatremia

GENERAL PRINCIPLES

Definition
Hyponatremia is defined as a plasma [Na^+] **<135 mEq/L**.

Etiology
- To maintain a normal [Na^+], the ingestion of water must be matched with an equal volume of water excretion. Any process that limits the elimination of water or expands the volume around a fixed Na^+ content may lead to a decrease in Na^+ concentration.
- Expansion of the space surrounding the Na^+ content can occur in a variety of ways:
  - **Pseudohyponatremia** refers to a laboratory phenomena by which a high content of plasma proteins and lipids expands the nonaqueous portion of the plasma

sample, leading to an errant report of a low ECF [Na$^+$]. This can be averted with Na$^+$-sensitive electrodes, and the normal ECF [Na$^+$] can be confirmed with a normal serum osmolality.

○ **Hyperosmolar hyponatremia** refers to circumstances in which an osmotically active solute other than Na$^+$ accumulates in the ECF, drawing water into the ECF and diluting the Na$^+$ content. This is most commonly caused by **hyperglycemia**, resulting in a fall in plasma [Na$^+$] of 1.6 to 2.4 mEq/L for every 100 mg/dL rise in plasma glucose (*Am J Med 1999;106:399*). Other solutes, such as glycine, mannitol, or sorbitol, can be absorbed into the ECF during bladder irrigation, leading to the transient hyponatremia seen in **posttransurethral resection of the prostate (post-TURP) syndrome**. Prompt renal excretion and metabolism of the absorbed fluid usually corrects the hyponatremia rapidly, although symptomatic hyponatremia can occasionally be seen in the setting of renal insufficiency.

○ Rarely, the ECF water content rises simply because the ingested quantity of water exceeds the physiologic capacity of water excretion in the kidney. This is seen in psychogenic polydipsia, water intoxication from poorly conceived drinking games, beer potomania, and the so-called "tea and toast" diet. Underlying each of these circumstances is the fact that there is a limit to renal water clearance. Urine cannot be diluted to an osmolality less than ~50 mOsm/L, meaning that a small amount of solute is required in even the most dilute urine. Ingestion of a high volume of water can thus exceed the capacity for excretion, particularly in those with a solute-poor diet, since the solute load required to generate urinary water loss is quickly depleted. The excess water is retained, Na$^+$ concentrations falls, and hyponatremia results.

• Decreased clearance of water from the kidney can also occur through a variety of processes. As mentioned previously, renal water handling is largely controlled by ADH (or vasopressin). Nonosmotic stimulation of this hormone occurs with volume contraction. Although this seems counterintuitive from an osmotic standpoint (it further reduces renal water clearance and increases water retention), it is an "appropriate" adaptive response to the threat of volume loss, tissue hypoperfusion, and impending hemodynamic collapse. Other conditions are characterized by secretion of ADH, which is "inappropriate," stimulated by neither osmotic nor volume related changes.

• **"Appropriate"** ADH secretion occurs with a fall in effective circulating volume. In these conditions, thirst and water retention is stimulated, protecting volume status at the cost of the osmolar status. This category is classically subdivided based on the associated assessment of ECF status.

○ **Hypovolemic hyponatremia** may result from **any** cause of net Na$^+$ loss, such as in thiazide use and cerebral salt wasting.

○ **Hypervolemic hyponatremia** occurs in edematous states such as congestive heart failure (CHF), hepatic cirrhosis, and severe nephrotic syndrome. Despite the expanded interstitial space, the circulating volume is reduced. Alterations in Starling forces contribute to this apparent paradox, shifting fluid from the intravascular to interstitial space.

• **"Inappropriate"** secretion of ADH is characterized by the activation of water-conserving mechanisms despite the absence of osmotic- or volume-related stimuli. Because the renal response to volume expansion remains intact, these patients are typically **euvolemic**. However, because of the rise in TBW, serum concentrations of Na$^+$ are decreased.

- ○ The most common form of this is the well-named **syndrome of inappropriate ADH (SIADH)**. This disorder is caused by the nonphysiologic release of vasopressin from the posterior pituitary or an ectopic source. Common causes of SIADH include neuropsychiatric disorders (e.g., meningitis, encephalitis, acute psychosis, cerebrovascular accident, head trauma), pulmonary diseases (e.g., pneumonia, tuberculosis, positive-pressure ventilation, acute respiratory failure), and malignant tumors (most commonly, small cell lung cancer).
  - **SIADH** is diagnosed by the following:
    - □ Hypoosmotic hyponatremia
    - □ Urine osmolality >100 mOsm/L
    - □ Euvolemia
    - □ The absence of conditions, which stimulate ADH secretion, including volume contraction, nausea, adrenal dysfunction, and hypothyroidism
  - **Pharmacologic agents** may also stimulate inappropriate ADH secretion. Common culprits include antidepressants (particularly selective serotonin reuptake inhibitors [SSRIs]), narcotics, antipsychotic agents, chlorpropamide, and nonsteroidal anti-inflammatory drugs (NSAIDs).
- ○ **Reset osmostat** is a phenomenon in which the set point for plasma osmolality is reduced. Thus, ADH and thirst responses, although functional, maintain plasma osmolality at this new, lower level. This phenomenon occurs in almost all pregnant women (perhaps in response to changes in the hormonal milieu) and occasionally in those with a chronic decreased effective circulating volume.

DIAGNOSIS

Clinical Presentation

- The clinical features of hyponatremia are related to the osmotic intracellular water shift leading to cerebral edema. Therefore, the symptoms are primarily neurologic, and their severity is dependent on both the magnitude of the fall in plasma $[Na^+]$ and the rapidity of the decrease. In **acute hyponatremia** (i.e., developing in <2 days), patients may complain of nausea and malaise with $[Na^+]$ ~125 mEq/L. As the plasma $[Na^+]$ falls further, symptoms may progress to include headache, lethargy, confusion, and obtundation. Stupor, seizures, and coma do not usually occur unless the plasma $[Na^+]$ falls acutely below 115 mEq/L. In **chronic hyponatremia** (>3 days' duration), adaptive mechanisms designed to defend cell volume occur and tend to minimize the increase in ICF volume and its symptoms.
- The underlying cause of hyponatremia can often be ascertained from an accurate history and physical examination, including an assessment of **ECF volume status** and the **effective circulating volume**.

Diagnostic Testing

Laboratories

Three laboratory analyses, when used with a clinical assessment of volume status, can narrow the differential diagnosis of hyponatremia: (a) the **plasma osmolality**, (b) the **urine osmolality**, and (c) the **urine $[Na^+]$** (Figure 12-1).

- **Plasma osmolality.** Most patients with hyponatremia have a low plasma osmolality (<275 mOsm/L). If the plasma osmolality is not low, **pseudohyponatremia** and **hyperosmolar hyponatremia** must be ruled out.

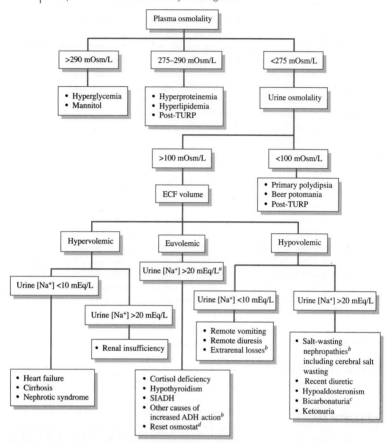

Figure 12-1. Algorithm depicting the diagnostic approach to hyponatremia. ADH, antidiuretic hormone; ECF, extracellular fluid; SIADH, syndrome of inappropriate antidiuretic hormone; post-TURP, posttransurethral resection of the prostate syndrome. [a]Urine [Na^+] may be <20 mEq/L with low Na^+ intake. [b]See text for details. [c]From vomiting-induced contraction alkalosis or proximal renal tubular acidosis. [d]Urine osmolality may be <100 mOsm/L after a water load.

- **Urine osmolality.** The appropriate renal response to hypoosmolality is to excrete a maximally dilute urine (urine osmolality <100 mOsm/L and specific gravity of <1.003). A urine sample that is not dilute suggests impaired free water excretion due to appropriate or inappropriate secretion of the ADH.
- **Urine [Na^+]** adds laboratory corroboration to the bedside assessment of effective circulating volume and can discriminate between **extrarenal** and **renal losses** of Na^+. The appropriate response to decreased effective circulating volume is to enhance tubular Na^+ reabsorption such that urine [Na^+] is <10 mEq/L. A urine [Na^+] of >20 mEq/L suggests a normal effective circulating volume or a Na^+-wasting defect. Occasionally, the excretion of a nonreabsorbed anion obligates loss of the Na^+ cation despite volume depletion (ketonuria, bicarbonaturia).

TREATMENT

- Management requires one to determine **the rate of correction**, **the appropriate intervention**, and **the presence of other underlying disorders**.
- The **rate of correction** of hyponatremia depends on the acuity of its development and the presence of neurologic dysfunction.
- **Acute symptomatic hyponatremia.** Severe symptomatic hyponatremia, with evidence of neurologic dysfunction, should generally be treated promptly with hypertonic saline; however, any saline solution that is hypertonic to the urine (if the urine osmolality is known at the start of therapy) can increase the [Na^+] when oral water intake is restricted.
  - The risks of correcting hyponatremia too rapidly are volume overload and the development of **central pontine myelinolysis** (CPM). CPM is thought to result from damage to neurons resulting from rapid osmotic shifts. In its most overt form, it is characterized by flaccid paralysis, dysarthria, and dysphagia, and in more subtle presentations, it can be confirmed by computed tomography (CT) scan or magnetic resonance imaging (MRI) of the brain. The risk of precipitating CPM is increased with correction of the [Na^+] by >12 mEq/L in a 24-hour period (*J Am Soc Nephrol 1994;4:1522*). In addition to overaggressive correction, other risk factors for developing CPM include preexisting hypokalemia, malnutrition, and alcoholism.
  - In patients with severe hyponatremia, in which an immediate rise in [Na^+] is necessary, [Na^+] should be corrected 1 to 2 mEq/L/hr for 3 to 4 hours. However, this initial rate of correction should be tapered off once the patient is safe, such that the rise in [Na^+] does not exceed 10 to 12 mEq/L over the 24-hour period.
- **Chronic asymptomatic hyponatremia.** The risks of iatrogenic injury is actually increased in patients with chronic hyponatremia. Because cells gradually adapt to the hypo-osmolar state, an abrupt normalization presents a dramatic change from the accommodated osmotic milieu. As such, we suggest a more modest rate of correction on the order of 5 to 8 mEq/L over a 24-hour period.
- **Severe, symptomatic hyponatremia.** In patients with symptomatic hyponatremia, hypertonic saline provides an immediate and titratable intervention necessary to acutely raise serum Na^+ levels while avoiding the disastrous complications of over correction.
  - The most accurate way to correct hyponatremia entails a detailed registry matching total solute and water output with desired input. In clinical practice, this is often impractical.
  - In lieu of this, the following equation is often used to approximate the change in [Na^+] in mEq/L from the infusion of 1 L of fluid:

$$\Delta[Na^+] = \{[Na^+_i] + [K^+_i] - [Na^+_s]\} \div \{TBW + 1\}$$

  [Na^+_i] and [K^+_i] are the sodium and potassium concentrations in the infused fluid, and [Na^+_s] is the starting serum sodium (*Intensive Care Med 1997;23:309*). Recall that TBW is estimated by multiplying the lean weight (in kilograms) by 0.6 in men (and 0.5 in women). This formula does not account for ongoing electrolyte or water losses and is only a rough guide.
  - Dividing the desired rate of correction (mEq/L/hr) by $\Delta[Na^+]$ (mEq/L/L of fluid) gives you the appropriate **rate of administration (liter of fluid per hour)**.
  - Because this equation does not account for ongoing losses, one **must recheck laboratory data and adjust fluid rates** to make sure the patient is improving appropriately.

○ **Example:** An 80-kg woman is seizing. Her [Na^+] is 103 mEq/L.
   ▪ **Rate of correction:** She has symptomatic hyponatremia requiring an acute correction (1 to 2 mEq/L/hr for the first 3 to 4 hours) but no more than 12 mEq/L corrected over 24 hours.
   ▪ **Means of correction:**
      □ Given the acuity, the patient should be given hypertonic saline, which has 513 mEq of Na^+ per liter.
      □ One liter of this fluid would increase [Na^+] by 10 mEq/L.

$$\Delta[Na^+] = \{513 - 108\} \div \{80 \times 0.5 + 1\} = 10 \text{ mEq/L}$$

      □ Dose hypertonic saline at 200 mL/hr until symptoms improve.

$$\text{Rate} = [2 \text{ mEq/L/hr}] \div [10 \text{ mEq/L per 1 L of saline}]$$

   ▪ To prevent a change of >10 to 12 mEq/L over 24 hours, no more than 1 L of fluid should be given.
• **Asymptomatic hyponatremia**
   ○ **Hypovolemic hyponatremia.** In patients with asymptomatic hypovolemic hyponatremia, **isotonic** saline can be used to restore the intravascular volume. Restoration of a euvolemic state will reduce the impetus toward renal water retention, leading to normalization of [Na^+]. If the duration of hyponatremia is unknown, the process described earlier can be used to calculate the expected change from 1 L of 0.9% NS, the rate of administration, and the maximal amount that can be given to avoid overcorrection.
   ○ **Hypervolemic hyponatremia.** Hyponatremia in CHF and cirrhosis often reflects the severity of the underlying disease. However, the hyponatremia itself is typically asymptomatic. Although *effective* circulating volume is decreased, the administration of fluid may worsen the volume-overloaded state. Definitive treatment requires management of the underlying condition, although restriction of water intake and increasing water diuresis may help to attenuate the degree of hyponatremia.
      ▪ Oral fluid intake should be less than daily urine output.
      ▪ Urinary excretion of water can be promoted through the use of loop diuretics, which reduce the concentration gradient necessary to reabsorb water in the distal nephron. Vasopressin antagonists may also be helpful in both euvolemic (SIADH) and hypervolemic hyponatremia (particularly CHF). When using medications to promote water loss, laboratory data and volume status must be followed extremely closely, as the effect on water and electrolyte loss cannot be accurately predicted.
      ▪ **SIADH** should first be distinguished from the previously listed conditions that stimulate vasopressin secretion. The standard first-line therapy is water restriction and correction of any contributing factors (nausea, pneumonia, drugs, etc). If this fails or if the patient is symptomatic, the following can be attempted to promote water excretion.
      ▪ **Water restriction.** The amount of fluid restriction necessary depends on the extent of water elimination. A useful guide to the necessary degree of fluid restriction is as follows:
         □ If (Urine Na^+ + Urine K^+)/Serum Na^+ <0.5, restrict to 1 L/d.
         □ If (Urine Na^+ + Urine K^+)/Serum Na^+ is 0.5 to 1.0, restrict to 500 mL/d.

- If (Urine Na^+ + Urine K^+)/Serum Na^+ is >1, the patient has a negative renal free water clearance and is actively reabsorbing water. Any amount of water given may be retained and clinicians should consider the following options to enhance free water excretion.
  - **High dietary solute load.** The volume of water excreted as urine is governed by a relatively fixed urine osmolality. Thus, increasing solute intake with a high-salt, high-protein diet or administration of oral urea (30 to 60 g) may increase the capacity for water excretion and improve the hyponatremia.

Medications

- Loop diuretics impair the urinary concentrating mechanism and can enhance free water excretion.
- Vasopressin antagonists promote a water diuresis and may be useful in the therapy of SIADH. Both IV (conivaptan) and oral (tolvaptan) preparations are approved for the treatment of euvolemic hyponatremia. However, given the risks of overcorrection, these agents should be initiated in a closely monitored inpatient setting.
- Lithium and demeclocycline interfere with the collecting tubule's ability to respond to ADH but are rarely used because of significant side effects. They should only be considered in severe hyponatremia that is unresponsive to more conservative measures.

Hypernatremia

GENERAL PRINCIPLES

Definition

Hypernatremia is defined as a plasma $[Na^+]$ **>145 mEq/L** and represents a state of **hyperosmolality** (see Disorders of Sodium Concentration, General Principles section).

Etiology

- Hypernatremia may be caused by a primary **Na^+ gain** or a **water deficit**, the latter being much more common. Normally, this hyperosmolar state stimulates thirst and the excretion of a maximally concentrated urine. For hypernatremia to persist, one or both of these compensatory mechanisms must also be impaired.
- **Impaired thirst response** may occur in situations where access to water is limited, often due to physical restrictions (institutionalized, handicapped, postoperative, or intubated patients) or the mentally impaired (delirium, dementia).
- **Hypernatremia due to water loss.** The loss of water must occur in excess of electrolyte losses in order to raise $[Na^+]$.
  - **Nonrenal water loss** may be due to evaporation from the skin and respiratory tract (insensible losses) or loss from the GI tract. Diarrhea is the most common GI cause of hypernatremia. Osmotic diarrhea (induced by lactulose, sorbitol, or malabsorption of carbohydrate) and viral gastroenteritis, in particular, result in disproportional water loss.
  - **Renal water loss** results from either **osmotic diuresis** or **diabetes insipidus (DI)**.
    - **Osmotic diuresis** is frequently associated with glycosuria and high osmolar feeds. In addition, increased urea generation from accelerated catabolism, high-protein feeds, and stress-dose steroids can also result in an osmotic diuresis.

- Hypernatremia secondary to nonosmotic urinary water loss is usually caused by (a) impaired vasopressin secretion (**central diabetes insipidus [CDI]**) or (b) resistance to the actions of vasopressin (**nephrogenic diabetes insipidus [NDI]**). Partial defects occur more commonly than complete defects in both types.
  - The most common cause of CDI is destruction of the neurohypophysis from trauma, neurosurgery, granulomatous disease, neoplasms, vascular accidents, or infection. In many cases, CDI is idiopathic.
  - NDI may either be inherited or acquired. The latter often results from a disruption to the renal concentrating mechanism due to drugs (lithium, demeclocycline, amphotericin), electrolyte disorders (hypercalcemia, hypokalemia), medullary washout (loop diuretics), and intrinsic renal diseases.
- **Hypernatremia due to primary Na^+ gain** occurs infrequently due to the kidney's capacity to excrete the retained Na^+. However, it can rarely occur after repetitive **hypertonic saline** administration or chronic **mineralocorticoid excess**.
- **Transcellular water shift** from ECF to ICF can occur in circumstances of transient intracellular hyperosmolality, as in seizures or rhabdomyolysis.

DIAGNOSIS

Clinical Presentation

- Hypernatremia results in contraction of brain cells as water shifts to attenuate the rising ECF osmolality. Thus, the most severe symptoms of hypernatremia are neurologic, including altered mental status, weakness, neuromuscular irritability, focal neurologic deficits, and, occasionally, coma or seizures. As with hyponatremia, the severity of the clinical manifestations is related to the *acuity* and *magnitude* of the rise in plasma [Na^+]. **Chronic hypernatremia** is generally less symptomatic as a result of adaptive mechanisms designed to defend cell volume.
- **CDI** and **NDI** generally present with complaints of polyuria and thirst. Signs of volume depletion or neurologic dysfunction are generally absent unless the patient has an associated thirst abnormality.

DIAGNOSTIC TESTING

Laboratories

Urine osmolality and the **response to desmopressin acetate (DDAVP)** can help narrow the differential diagnosis for hypernatremia (Figure 12-2).
- The appropriate renal response to hypernatremia is a small volume of concentrated (urine osmolality >800 mOsm/L) urine. Submaximal **urine osmolality** (<800 mOsm/L) suggests a defect in renal water conservation.
  - A urine osmolality <300 mOsm/L in the setting of hypernatremia suggests complete forms of CDI and NDI.
  - Urine osmolality between 300 and 800 mOsm/L can occur from partial forms of diabetes insipidus (DI) as well as osmotic diuresis. The two can be differentiated by quantifying the daily solute excretion (estimated by the urine osmolality multiplied by urine volume in 24 hours). A daily solute excretion >900 mOsm/L defines an osmotic diuresis.
- **Response to DDAVP.** Complete forms of CDI and NDI can be distinguished by administering the vasopressin analog DDAVP (10 mcg intranasally) after careful water restriction. The urine osmolality should increase by at least 50% in complete CDI and does not change in NDI. The diagnosis is sometimes difficult when partial defects are present.

Figure 12-2. Algorithm depicting the diagnostic approach to hypernatremia. BUN, blood urea nitrogen; ↑Ca$^+$, hypercalcemia; CDI, central diabetes insipidus; DDAVP, desmopressin acetate; ECF, extracellular fluid; GI, gastrointestinal; NDI, nephrogenic diabetes insipidus; ↓K$^+$, hypokalemia; (+), conditions with increase in urine osmolality in response to desmopressin acetate; (−), conditions with little increase in urine osmolality in response to desmopressin acetate.

TREATMENT

- Management requires one to determine **the rate of correction**, **the appropriate intervention**, and **the presence of other underlying disorders**.
- **The rate of correction** of hypernatremia depends on the acuity of its development and the presence of neurologic dysfunction.
- **Symptomatic hypernatremia.** As in hyponatremia, aggressive correction of hypernatremia is potentially dangerous. The rapid shift of water into brain cells increases the risk of seizures or permanent neurologic damage. Therefore, the water deficit should be reduced gradually by roughly **10 to 12 mEq/L/d**.
- In **chronic asymptomatic hypernatremia**, the risk of treatment-related complication is increased due to the cerebral adaptation to the chronic hyperosmolar state, and the plasma [Na^+] should be lowered at a more moderate rate (between 5 and 8 mEq/L/d).
- **Intervention**
  - The mainstay of management is the administration of water, preferably by mouth or nasogastric tube. Alternatively, 5% dextrose in water (D_5W) or quarter NS can be given intravenously.
  - Traditionally, correction of hypernatremia has been accomplished by calculating **free water deficit** by the equation:

$$\text{Free water deficit} = \{([Na^+] - 140)/140\} \times (\text{TBW})$$

While this is helpful in approximating the total water deficit, it does not provide sufficient guidance regarding the rate and content of infusate. Alternatively, we suggest approaching treatment in a manner similar to that used in the treatment of hyponatremia. The change in [Na^+] from the administration of fluids can be estimated as follows:

$$\Delta[Na^+] = \{[Na^+_i] + [K^+_i] - [Na^+_s]\} \div \{\text{TBW} + 1\}$$

[Na^+_i] and [K^+_i] are the sodium and potassium concentrations in the infused fluid and [Na^+_s] is the starting serum sodium (*Intensive Care Med 1997;23:309*). Because hypernatremia suggests a contraction in water content, TBW is estimated by multiplying lean weight (in kilograms) by 0.5 in men (rather than 0.6) and 0.4 in women.

  - **An example:** A 70-kg man with diarrhea (2 L/d) from laxative abuse presents with obtundation and [Na^+] = 164 mEq/L, [K^+] = 3.0. A replacement fluid of D_5W with 20 mEq KCl/L is chosen.
    - The $\Delta[Na^+]$ with 1 L of this fluid would be $^-$4 mEq/L

$$\{0 + 20 - 164\} \div \{(70 \times 0.5) + 1\}$$

3 L are necessary for a $\Delta[Na^+]$ $-$ 12 mEq/L/24 hours

$$(-12 \text{ mEq/L/day}) \div (-4 \text{ mEq/L/L of solution})$$

    - The hourly rate of infusion is 125 mL/hr (3 L/day ÷ 24 hours/day = 0.125 L/hour). However, this should be followed closely as it does not account for ongoing GI or insensible losses, which may account for another 1.4 L/d of water required to keep [Na^+] stable.

- **Specific therapies for the underlying cause**
  - ○ **Hypovolemic hypernatremia.** In patients with mild volume depletion, Na^+-containing solutions, such as 0.45% NS, can be used to replenish the ECF as well as the water deficit. If patients have severe or symptomatic volume depletion, correction of volume status with **isotonic fluid** should take precedence over correction of the hyperosmolar state. Once the patient is hemodynamically stable, administration of hypotonic fluid can be given to replace the free water deficit.
  - ○ **Hypernatremia from primary Na^+ gain** is unusual. Cessation of iatrogenic Na^+ is typically sufficient.
  - ○ **DI without hypernatremia.** DI is best treated by removing the underlying cause. Despite the renal water loss, DI should not result in hypernatremia if the thirst mechanism remains intact. Therefore, therapy, if required at all, is directed toward symptomatic polyuria.
    - ▪ **CDI.** Because the polyuria is the result of impaired secretion of vasopressin, treatment is best accomplished with the administration of DDAVP, a vasopressin analog.
    - ▪ **NDI.** A low-Na^+ diet combined with *thiazide* diuretics will decrease polyuria through inducing mild volume depletion. This enhances proximal reabsorption of salt and water, thus decreasing urinary free water loss. Decreasing protein intake will further decrease urine output by minimizing the solute load that must be excreted.

POTASSIUM

GENERAL PRINCIPLES

- Potassium is the major **intracellular** cation. Of the 3,000 to 4,000 mEq of K^+ found in the average human, 98% is sequestered within cells. Thus, while ECF $[K^+]$ is normally 3.5 to 5.0 mEq/L, the intracellular concentration is roughly 150 mEq/L. This difference in ICF and ECF K^+ content is maintained by the **Na^+/K^+-adenosine triphosphatase pump**.
- The K^+ intake of individuals on an average Western diet is approximately 1 mEq/kg/d, 90% of which is absorbed by the GI tract. Maintenance of the steady state necessitates matching K^+ excretion with ingestion.
- The elimination of potassium occurs predominately through **renal excretion** at the distal nephron. K^+ secretion is enhanced by distal Na^+ reabsorption, which generates a **lumen-negative gradient**, and **distal urine flow rate**.
- Renal potassium handling is responsive to **aldosterone**, which stimulates the expression of distal luminal Na^+ channels, and the **serum potassium concentration**. Aldosterone secretion is, in turn, responsive to angiotensin II and hyperkalemia.

Hypokalemia

GENERAL PRINCIPLES

Definition

Hypokalemia is defined as a plasma $[K^+]$ <3.5 mEq/L.

Etiology

- **Spurious hypokalemia** may be seen in situations in which high numbers of metabolically active cells present in the blood sample absorb the ECF potassium.
- True hypokalemia may result from one or more of the following: (a) **decreased net intake,** (b) **shift into cells,** or (c) **increased net loss.**
  - ○ **Diminished intake** is seldom the sole cause of K^+ depletion because urinary excretion can be effectively decreased to <15 mEq/d. However, dietary K^+ restriction may exacerbate the hypokalemia from GI or renal loss.
  - ○ **Transcellular shift.** Movement of K^+ into cells may transiently decrease the plasma $[K^+]$ without altering total body K^+ content. These shifts can result from alkalemia, insulin, and catecholamine release. **Periodic paralysis** is a rare disorder that predisposes patients to transcellular K^+ shifts that result in episodic muscle weakness. Both hypokalemic and hyperkalemic forms have been described.
  - ○ **Nonrenal K^+ loss.** Hypokalemia may result from the loss of potassium-rich fluids from the lower GI tract. Hypokalemia from the loss of upper GI contents is typically more attributable to renal K^+ secretion from secondary hyperaldosteronism. Rarely, in excessive sweating, loss of K^+ through the integument can provoke hypokalemia.
  - ○ **Renal K^+ loss** accounts for most cases of *chronic* hypokalemia. This may be caused by factors that increase the lumen-negative gradient, thus enhancing K^+ secretion, or that augment distal urine flow rate.
    - ▪ **Augmented distal urine flow** occurs commonly with diuretic use and osmotic diuresis (e.g., glycosuria). Bartter's and Gitelman's syndromes mimic diuretic use and promote renal K^+ loss by the same mechanism.
    - ▪ A variety of disorders promote K^+ loss by increasing the **lumen-negative gradient,** which drives K^+ secretion. This can be achieved with the reabsorption of a cation (Na^+) or presence of a nonreabsorbed anion.
      - □ Distal Na^+ reabsorption is largely influenced by mineralocorticoid activity.
      - □ **Primary mineralocorticoid excess** can be seen in primary hyperaldosteronism due to an adrenal adenoma or adrenocortical hyperplasia.
      - □ Cortisol also has an affinity for mineralocorticoid receptors but is typically converted quickly to cortisone, which has markedly less mineralocorticoid activity. Still, if cortisol is present in abundance (Cushing's syndrome) or fails to be converted to cortisone (syndrome of mineralocorticoid excess), it may mimic hyperaldosteronism.
      - □ **Secondary hyperaldosteronism** can be seen in any situation with a decreased effective circulating volume.
      - □ Constitutive activation of the distal renal epithelial Na^+ channel, independent of aldosterone, occurs in **Liddle's syndrome.**
    - ▪ Increased distal delivery of a nonreabsorbable anion can also potentiate the lumen-negative gradient that drives K^+ secretion. Examples include bicarbonate (metabolic alkalosis or type 2 renal tubular acidosis [RTA]), ketones, and hippurate (from toluene intoxication or glue sniffing).

DIAGNOSIS

Clinical Presentation

- The clinical features of K^+ depletion vary greatly, and their severity depends in part on the degree of hypokalemia. Symptoms seldom occur unless the plasma $[K^+]$ is <3.0 mEq/L.

- Fatigue, myalgias, and muscular weakness or cramps of the lower extremities are common. Smooth muscle function may also be affected and may manifest with complaints of constipation or frank paralytic ileus. Severe hypokalemia may lead to complete paralysis, hypoventilation, or rhabdomyolysis.

Diagnostic Testing

Laboratories

When the etiology is not immediately apparent, **renal K⁺ excretion** and the **acid–base status** can help identify the cause (Table 12-2).

- **Urine K⁺**. The appropriate response to hypokalemia is to excrete <25 mEq/d of K⁺ in the urine. The patient's urinary K⁺ excretion can be measured with a 24-hour urine collection or estimated by multiplying the spot urine $[K^+]$ by the total daily urine output. A spot urine $[K^+]$ may be helpful (urine $[K^+]$ <15 mEq/L suggests appropriate K⁺ conservation), but the results can be confounded by a variety of factors. Alternatively, a transtubular potassium gradient (TTKG) can be calculated as follows:

$$TTKG = (Urine\ K^+/Serum\ K^+) \div (Urine\ Osmolality/Serum\ Osmolality)$$

A TTKG <2 suggests a nonrenal source, while a TTKG >4 suggests inappropriate renal K⁺ secretion.

- **Acid–base status.** Intracellular shifting and renal excretion of K⁺ are often closely linked with the acid–base status. Hypokalemia is generally associated with metabolic alkalosis and can play a critical role in the maintenance of metabolic alkalosis. The finding of metabolic acidosis in a patient with hypokalemia thus narrows the differential significantly, implying lower GI loss, distal RTA, or the excretion of a nonreabsorbable anion from an organic acid (diabetic ketoacidosis [DKA], hippurate from toluene intoxication).

Table 12-2	Approach to Dyskalemias	
	Hypokalemia	**Hyperkalemia**
Transcellular shift	Insulin, alkalemia, catecholamines, hypokalemic periodic paralysis	Cell lysis, ↓insulin, metabolic acidosis, β-blockers, hyperkalemic periodic paralysis
Change in K⁺ content (nonrenal causes)	Dx: [K⁺] <25 mEq/d or TTKG <2 Examples: Poor intake or GI loss	Dx: TTKG >10 Examples: Salt substitutes, tomatoes, potatoes, bananas, oranges
Change in K⁺ content (renal causes)	Dx: TTKG >4 Examples: Enhanced diuresis, increased luminal gradient (hyperaldosteronism, Liddle's syndrome, nonreabsorbed anion)	Dx: TTKG <7 Examples: Acute/chronic kidney disease, hypoaldosteronism, type 4 RTA

Dx, diagnosis; GI, gastrointestinal; RTA, renal tubular acidosis; TTKG, transtubular potassium gradient.

Electrocardiography

Electrocardiogram (ECG) changes associated with hypokalemia include flattening or inversion of the T wave, a prominent U wave, ST-segment depression, and a prolonged QU interval. Severe K^+ depletion may result in a prolonged PR interval, decreased voltage, and widening of the QRS complex.

TREATMENT

The **therapeutic goals** are to safely correct the K^+ deficit and to minimize ongoing losses through treatment of the underlying cause. Hypomagnesemia should also be sought in all hypokalemic patients and corrected to allow effective K^+ repletion.

Medications

- Correction of the K^+ deficit can be accomplished with either oral or IV therapy.
  - **Oral therapy.** It is generally safer to correct the K^+ deficit via the oral route when hypokalemia is mild and the patient can tolerate oral administration. Oral doses of 40 mEq are generally well tolerated and can be given as often as every 4 hours. Traditionally, 10 mEq of potassium salts are given for each 0.10 mEq/L decrement in serum $[K^+]$. However, with increasing severity of hypokalemia, this grossly underestimates the K^+ necessary to normalize *total* K^+ content. Furthermore, as the K^+ shifts back to the intracellular space, it may appear as though K^+ supplementation is doing very little to correct ECF $[K^+]$. Although this may appear discouraging, it simply reflects the true extent of hypokalemia. In such cases, potassium supplementation should be increased and continued until serum levels rise.
  - **IV therapy.** Patients with imminently life-threatening hypokalemia and those who are unable to take anything by mouth require IV replacement therapy with KCl. The maximum concentration of administered K^+ should be no more than 40 mEq/L via a peripheral vein or 100 mEq/L via a central vein. The rate of infusion should not exceed 20 mEq/hr unless paralysis or malignant ventricular arrhythmias are present. Ideally, KCl should be mixed in NS because dextrose solutions may initially exacerbate hypokalemia (as a result of insulin-mediated movement of K^+). Rapid IV administration of K^+ should be used judiciously and requires close observation.

Hyperkalemia

GENERAL PRINCIPLES

Definition

Hyperkalemia is defined as a plasma $[K^+]$ **>5.0 mEq/L**.

Etiology

- **Pseudohyperkalemia** represents an artificially elevated plasma $[K^+]$ due to K^+ movement out of cells immediately before or following venipuncture. Contributing factors include repeated fist clenching, hemolysis, and marked leukocytosis or thrombocytosis.

- True hyperkalemia occurs as a result of (a) **transcellular shift**, (b) **increased exposure to K⁺**, and most commonly, (c) **decreased renal K⁺ excretion**. Combinations of these mechanisms often underlie cases of hyperkalemia in clinical practice, and decreased renal excretion is nearly always some component of the pathophysiology.
  - ○ **Transcellular shift.** Insulin deficiency, hyperosmolality, nonselective β-blockers, digitalis, metabolic acidosis (excluding those from organic acids), and depolarizing muscle relaxants, such as succinylcholine, release K⁺ from predominate ICF stores into the ECF compartment. Exercise-induced hyperkalemia results from release of K⁺ from muscles. Familial periodic paralysis, mentioned previously, is a rare cause of hyperkalemia. Massive cellular destruction, as seen in tumor lysis syndrome, also liberates cellular K⁺ stores and releases them into the ECF.
  - ○ **Increased exposure to K⁺** is rarely the sole cause of hyperkalemia unless there is an impairment in renal excretion. Foods with a high content of K⁺ include salt substitutes, dried fruits, nuts, tomatoes, potatoes, spinach, bananas, and oranges. Juices derived from these foods may be especially rich sources.
  - ○ **Decreased renal K⁺ excretion.** In the setting of hyperkalemia, the kidney is capable of generating a significant urinary excretion of K⁺. This process can be impaired by a number of processes, including intrinsic renal disease, decreased delivery of filtrate to the distal nephron, adrenal insufficiency, and hyporeninemic hypoaldosteronism (type 4 RTA).
- **Drugs** may also be implicated in the genesis of hyperkalemia through a variety of mechanisms. Common culprits include angiotensin-converting enzyme inhibitors and angiotensin receptor blockers, potassium-sparing diuretics, NSAIDs, and cyclosporine. Heparin and ketoconazole can also contribute to hyperkalemia through the decreased production of aldosterone, although these agents alone are typically insufficient to sustain a clinically significant hyperkalemia.

DIAGNOSIS

Clinical Presentation

- The most serious effect of hyperkalemia is cardiac arrhythmogenesis secondary to potassium's pivotal role in membrane potentials. Patients may present with palpitations, syncope, or even sudden cardiac death.
- Severe hyperkalemia causes partial depolarization of the skeletal muscle cell membrane and may manifest as weakness, potentially progressing to flaccid paralysis and hypoventilation if the respiratory muscles are involved.

Diagnostic Testing

Laboratories

- If the etiology is not readily apparent and the patient is asymptomatic, **pseudohyperkalemia** should be excluded by rechecking laboratory data.
- An assessment of **renal [K⁺]** excretion and the **renin-angiotensin-aldosterone axis** can help narrow the differential diagnosis when the etiology is not immediately apparent.
  - ○ Renal [K⁺] excretion can be assessed using the TTKG previously described.
    - ▪ A TTKG >10 suggests that renal tubular mechanisms for K⁺ secretion are intact. The persistence of hyperkalemia despite an intact renal response suggests poor filtrate delivery to the distal mechanisms of K⁺ regulation, as occurs with a decreased effective circulating volume.

- A TTKG <7 implies impaired K^+ secretion caused by hypoaldosteronism, aldosterone resistance, or hyporeninemic hypoaldosteronism. An evaluation of the renin–aldosterone axis may help to differentiate these entities.
  □ Low aldosterone levels suggest either adrenal disease (renin levels elevated; TTKG improves with fludrocortisone) or hyporeninemic hypoaldosteronism (renin levels low; occurs with type 4 RTA as well as chloride shunting, or Gordon's syndrome).
  □ High aldosterone levels, typically accompanied by high renin levels, suggest aldosterone resistance (pseudohypoaldosteronism) but can also be seen in K^+-sparing diuretics.

Electrocardiography

ECG changes include increased T-wave amplitude, or peaked T waves. More severe degrees of hyperkalemia result in a prolonged PR interval and QRS duration, atrioventricular conduction delay, and loss of P waves. Progressive widening of the QRS complex and its merging with the T wave produce a sine wave pattern. The terminal event is usually ventricular fibrillation or asystole.

TREATMENT

Severe hyperkalemia with ECG changes is a medical emergency and requires immediate treatment directed at minimizing membrane depolarization and acutely reducing the ECF $[K^+]$. **Acute therapy** may consist of some or all of the following (the hypokalemic effect is additive):

Medications

- Administration of **calcium gluconate** decreases membrane excitability but does not lower $[K^+]$. The usual dose is 10 mL of a 10% solution infused over 2 to 3 minutes. The effect begins within minutes but is short lived (30 to 60 minutes), and the dose can be repeated if no improvement in the ECG is seen after 5 to 10 minutes.
- **Insulin** causes K^+ to shift into cells and temporarily lowers the plasma $[K^+]$. A commonly used combination is 10 to 20 U of regular insulin and 25 to 50 g glucose administered intravenously. Hyperglycemic patients should be given the insulin alone.
- **NaHCO$_3$** is effective for severe hyperkalemia associated with metabolic acidosis. In the acute setting, it can be given as an IV isotonic solution (three ampules of $NaHCO_3$ in 1 L of 5% dextrose).
- **β$_2$-Adrenergic agonists** promote cellular uptake of K^+. The onset of action is 30 minutes, lowering the plasma $[K^+]$ by 0.5 to 1.5 mEq/L, and the effect lasts for 2 to 4 hours. Albuterol can be administered in a dose of 10 to 20 mg as a continuous nebulized treatment over 30 to 60 minutes.
- **Longer term** means for $[K^+]$ removal.
  ○ Increasing distal Na^+ delivery in the kidney enhances renal K^+ clearance. This can be achieved with the administration of saline in patients who appear volume depleted. Otherwise, diuretics can be used if renal function is adequate.
  ○ **Cation exchange resins**, such as sodium polystyrene sulfonate (Kayexalate), promote the exchange of Na^+ for K^+ in the GI tract. When given by mouth, the usual dose is 25 to 50 g mixed with 100 mL 20% sorbitol to prevent constipation. This generally lowers the plasma $[K^+]$ by 0.5 to 1.0 mEq/L within

1 to 2 hours and lasts for 4 to 6 hours. Sodium polystyrene sulfonate can also be administered as a retention enema consisting of 50 g resin in 150 mL tap water. Enemas should be avoided in postoperative patients because of the increased incidence of colonic necrosis, especially following renal transplantation.

- **Dialysis** should be reserved for patients with renal failure and those with severe life-threatening hyperkalemia who are unresponsive to more conservative measures.
- **Chronic therapy** may involve dietary modifications to avoid high K^+ foods (see Potassium, Hyperkalemia, General Principles, Etiology section), correction of metabolic acidosis with oral alkali, promoting kaliuresis with diuretics, and/or administration of exogenous mineralocorticoid in states of hypoaldosteronism.

CALCIUM

GENERAL PRINCIPLES

- Calcium is essential for bone formation and neuromuscular function.
- Approximately 99% of body calcium is in bone; most of the remaining 1% is in the ECF. Nearly 50% of serum calcium is ionized (free), whereas the remainder is complexed to albumin (40%) and anions such as phosphate (10%).
- **Calcium balance** is regulated by **parathyroid hormone** (PTH) and **calcitriol**.
  - ○ **PTH** increases serum calcium by stimulating bone resorption, increasing calcium reclamation in the kidney, and promoting renal conversion of vitamin D to calcitriol. Serum calcium regulates PTH secretion by a negative feedback mechanism: Hypocalcemia stimulates and hypercalcemia suppresses PTH release.
  - ○ **Calcitriol** (1,25-dihydroxycholecalciferol, 1,25-dihydroxyvitamin D_3, or 1,25 $(OH)_2D_3$) is the active form of vitamin D. It stimulates intestinal absorption of calcium and is one of many factors that provide feedback to the parathyroid gland.

Hypercalcemia

GENERAL PRINCIPLES

Definition
A serum calcium **>10.3 mg/dL** with a normal serum albumin or an ionized calcium **>5.2 mg/dL** defines hypercalcemia.

Etiology
- Clinically significant hypercalcemia typically requires both an increase in ECF calcium and a decrease in renal calcium clearance. Underlying disturbances to calcium metabolism are thus often masked by compensatory mechanisms until the patient develops a concomitant disorder, such as decreased renal clearance from volume depletion. More than 90% of cases are due to **primary hyperparathyroidism** or **malignancy**.
- **Primary hyperparathyroidism** causes most cases of hypercalcemia in *ambulatory* patients. It is a common disorder, especially in elderly women, in whom the annual incidence is approximately 2 in 1,000. Nearly 85% of cases are due to an **adenoma** of a single gland, 15% to **hyperplasia** of all four glands, and 1% to **parathyroid carcinoma**.

- **Malignancy** is responsible for most cases of hypercalcemia among *hospitalized* patients. Patients usually have advanced, clinically obvious disease. In these patients, hypercalcemia may develop from stimulation of osteoclast bone resorption from tumor cell products, tumor derived **PTH-related peptides** (PTHrPs), and tumor calcitriol production.
- Less common causes account for about 10% of cases of hypercalcemia:
  - **Increased vitamin D activity** occurs with exogenous exposure to vitamin D or increased generation of calcitriol in chronic granulomatous diseases (e.g., sarcoidosis, tuberculosis).
  - The **milk-alkali syndrome** describes the acute or chronic development of hypercalcemia, alkalosis, and renal failure that may result from the ingestion of large quantities of calcium-containing antacids.
  - **Other.** Hyperthyroidism, adrenal insufficiency, prolonged immobilization, Paget's disease, and acromegaly may be associated with hypercalcemia. **Familial hypocalciuric hypercalcemia** is a rare, autosomal-dominant disorder of the calcium-sensing receptor, which is characterized by asymptomatic hypercalcemia from childhood and a family history of hypercalcemia.

DIAGNOSIS

Clinical Presentation

Clinical manifestations generally are present only if serum calcium exceeds 12 mg/dL and tend to be more severe if hypercalcemia develops rapidly. Most patients with **primary hyperparathyroidism** have asymptomatic hypercalcemia that is found incidentally.

- Renal manifestations include polyuria and nephrolithiasis. If serum calcium rises above 13 mg/dL, renal failure with nephrocalcinosis and ectopic soft tissue calcifications are possible.
- GI symptoms include anorexia, vomiting, constipation, and, rarely, signs of pancreatitis.
- Neurologic findings include weakness, fatigue, confusion, stupor, and coma.
- Osteopenia and frequent fractures may occur from the disproportional resorption of bone in hyperparathyroidism. Rarely, **osteitis fibrosa cystica** can develop when hyperparathyroidism is profound and prolonged, resulting in "brown tumors" and marrow replacement.
- The history and physical examination should focus on (a) the duration of symptoms of hypercalcemia, (b) clinical evidence of any of the unusual causes of hypercalcemia, and (c) symptoms and signs of malignancy (which almost always precede **malignant hypercalcemia**). If hypercalcemia has been present for more than 6 months without an obvious etiology, primary hyperparathyroidism is almost certainly the cause.

Diagnostic Testing

Laboratories

- In most patients, the diagnosis can be made with the history and physical and a limited laboratory workup.
- The **serum calcium** should be interpreted with knowledge of the serum albumin, or an ionized calcium should be measured. **Corrected $[Ca^{++}]$** $= [Ca^{++}] + \{0.8 \times (4.0 - [Albumin])\}$. Many patients with primary hyperparathyroidism will have a calcium level that is chronically within the high-normal range.

- The **serum PTH** level is mandatory for the evaluation of hypercalcemia. Assays measuring intact PTH should be used, as these are independent of renal function.
  - ○ Elevations in ECF calcium typically result in suppression of PTH. Thus, the finding of a normal or elevated intact PTH in the setting of hypercalcemia is suggestive of primary hyperparathyroidism.
  - ○ When the intact PTH is appropriately suppressed, **PTHrP** can be measured to investigate possible humoral hypercalcemia of malignancy. Causes of vitamin D disorders should also be considered. The $1,25(OH)_2D_3$ levels are elevated in granulomatous disorders, primary hyperparathyroidism, calcitriol overdose, and acromegaly. The $25(OH)D_3$ levels are elevated with noncalcitriol vitamin D intoxication.
- The **serum phosphorus** may help to identify the underlying disturbance in calcium homeostasis. Hyperparathyroidism often decreases phosphorus levels by stimulating phosphaturia, while Paget's disease and vitamin D intoxication both tend to increase phosphorus levels.
- **Urine calcium** may be elevated in primary hyperparathyroidism due to a filtered load of calcium that exceeds the capacity for renal reabsorption. If the family history and clinical picture is suggestive, patients with **familial hypocalciuric hypercalcemia** can be distinguished from primary hyperparathyroidism by documenting a low calcium clearance by 24-hour urine collection (<200 mg calcium per day) or fractional excretion of calcium (<1%).

Electrocardiography
The **ECG** may reveal a shortened QT interval and, with very severe hypercalcemia, variable degrees of atrioventricular block.

TREATMENT

- **Acute management** of hypercalcemia is warranted if severe symptoms are present or with serum calcium >12 mg/dL. The following regimen is presented in the order that therapy should be given.
- **Correction of hypovolemia** with 0.9% saline fluid is mandatory in patients who demonstrate volume depletion, since hypovolemia prevents effective calciuresis. Maintenance fluids can be continued after achieving euvolemia to sustain a urine output of 100 to 150 mL/hr. The patient should be monitored closely for signs of volume overload.

Medications

- **Loop diuretics** can be used if signs of volume overload limit further saline administration while hypercalcemia persists. These agents reduce paracellular reabsorption of calcium in the loop of Henle and thus may slightly enhance calcium excretion. However, they should not be used in euvolemic or hypovolemic patients as they may further contract the ECF volume and prevent adequate restoration of the volume status.
- **IV bisphosphonates** can be used to decrease the liberation of calcium from bone in persistent hypercalcemia. Pamidronate 60 mg is infused over 2 to 4 hours; for severe hypercalcemia (>13.5 mg/dL), 90 mg can be given over the same duration. A hypocalcemic response is typically seen within 2 days and may persist for 2 weeks or longer. Treatment can be repeated after 7 days if hypercalcemia recurs. Zoledronate is a more potent bisphosphonate that is given as a 4-mg dose infused

over at least 15 minutes. Hydration should precede bisphosphonate use. Renal insufficiency is a relative contraindication.

- Other options
  - **Calcitonin** inhibits bone resorption and increases renal calcium excretion. Salmon calcitonin, 4 to 8 IU/kg intramuscularly (IM) or SC q6–12h, lowers serum calcium 1 to 2 mg/dL within several hours in 60% to 70% of patients. Although it is less potent than other inhibitors of bone resorption, it has no serious toxicity, is safe in renal failure, and may have an analgesic effect in patients with skeletal metastases.
  - **Glucocorticoids** are effective in hypercalcemia due to hematologic malignancies and granulomatous production of calcitriol. The initial dose is 20 to 60 mg/d of prednisone or its equivalent. After serum calcium stabilizes, the dose should be gradually reduced to the minimum needed to control symptoms of hypercalcemia. Toxicity (see Chapter 25, Arthritis and Rheumatologic Diseases) limits the usefulness of glucocorticoids for long-term therapy.
  - **Gallium nitrate** inhibits bone resorption as effectively as the IV bisphosphonates and has a similar delayed onset of 2 days. It is given as a 100- to 200-mg/m^2/d continuous infusion for up to 5 days, unless normocalcemia is achieved sooner. There is, however, a significant risk of nephrotoxicity and it is contraindicated if the serum creatinine is >2.5 mg/dL.
  - **Dialysis.** Hemodialysis and peritoneal dialysis using low calcium dialysate are effective for patients with very severe hypercalcemia (>16 mg/dL) and CHF or renal insufficiency.
- **Chronic management** of hypercalcemia
  - **Primary hyperparathyroidism.** In many patients, this disorder has a benign course, with minimal fluctuation in serum calcium concentration and no obvious clinical sequelae. Parathyroidectomy is indicated in patients with (a) corrected serum calcium >1 mg/dL over the upper limit of normal, (b) calciuria >400 mg/d, (c) renal insufficiency, (d) reduced bone mass (T score ≤2.5 by dual-energy absorptiometry), (e) age <50 years, and (f) unfeasibility of long-term follow-up (*J Bone Miner Res 2002;17(suppl 2):N2*). Surgical intervention typically has a high success rate (95%) with low morbidity and mortality.
  - **Medical therapy** may be a reasonable option in asymptomatic patients who are not surgical candidates. Management consists of liberal oral hydration with a high-salt diet, daily physical activity to lessen bone resorption, and avoidance of thiazide diuretics. Oral bisphosphonates and estrogen replacement therapy or raloxifene in postmenopausal women can be considered in the appropriate clinical context. Cinacalcet, an activator of the calcium-sensing receptor, has also been shown to reduce PTH secretion and serum calcium levels.
  - **Malignant hypercalcemia.** Bisphosphonate and glucocorticoid therapy with a calcium-restricted diet (<400 mg/d) can be tried, although these maneuvers rarely yield long-term success unless the malignancy responds to treatment.

Hypocalcemia

GENERAL PRINCIPLES

Definition

A serum calcium **<8.4 mg/dL** with a normal serum albumin or an ionized calcium **<4.2 mg/dL** defines hypocalcemia.

Etiology

- **Pseudohypocalcemia** describes the situation in which the total calcium is reduced due to hypoalbuminemia, but the **corrected [Ca^{2+}]** (see Calcium, Hypercalcemia, Diagnosis, Laboratory Studies section) and ionized calcium remain within the normal ranges.
- **Effective hypoparathyroidism.** Reduced PTH activity can result from decreased PTH release from autoimmune, infiltrative, or iatrogenic (e.g., postthyroidectomy) destruction of parathyroid tissue. In rare patients, the hypoparathyroidism is congenital, as in DiGeorge syndrome or **familial hypocalcemia**. Release of PTH is also impaired with both hypomagnesemia ($<$1 mg/dL) and severe hypermagnesemia ($>$6 mg/dL).
- **Vitamin D deficiency** lowers total body calcium but does not usually affect serum calcium levels unless the deficiency is severe, since the resultant secondary hyperparathyroidism often corrects serum calcium levels. Significant vitamin D deficiency can occur in the elderly or those with limited sun exposure, in advanced liver disease (due to decreased synthesis of precursors), and in nephrotic syndrome. Reduced activity in vitamin D activation via 1-α-hydroxylase activity can be seen with vitamin D–dependent rickets and chronic renal insufficiency.
- Serum calcium levels may also be reduced by profound elevations in serum phosphorus, which binds with the calcium and deposits in a variety of tissues. Calcium can also be bound by citrate (during transfusion of citrate-containing blood products or with continual renal replacement using citrate anticoagulation) as well as by drugs such as foscarnet and fluoroquinolones. Increased binding to albumin can also be seen in the context of alkalemia, which increases the exposure of negatively charged binding sites on albumin.
- **Other.** A low serum free calcium level is common in critically ill patients perhaps due to a cytokine-mediated decrease in PTH and calcitriol release with target organ resistance to their effects.

DIAGNOSIS

Clinical Presentation

- Clinical manifestations vary with the *degree of hypocalcemia* and *rate of onset.*
- Acute, moderate hypocalcemia may cause increased excitability of nerves and muscles, leading to circumoral or distal paresthesias and tetany.
- **Trousseau's sign** is the development of carpal spasm when a blood pressure cuff is inflated above systolic pressure for 3 minutes. **Chvostek sign** refers to twitching of the facial muscles when the facial nerve is tapped anterior to the ear. The presence of these signs is known as **latent tetany**.
- Acute, severe hypocalcemia may cause laryngospasm, confusion, seizures, or vascular collapse with bradycardia and decompensated heart failure.
- Clues to the diagnosis may be provided by a bedside evaluation for (a) previous neck surgery (postoperative hypoparathyroidism), (b) systemic diseases (autoimmune, infiltrative disorders), (c) family history of hypocalcemia, (d) drug induced hypocalcemia, and (e) conditions associated with vitamin D deficiency (e.g., uremia).

Diagnostic Testing

Laboratories

- Laboratory data should be used to evaluate the calcium–PTH axis as well as concurrent mineral abnormalities.

- **Albumin** should be measured anytime there is an abnormality in serum calcium levels to rule out pseudohypocalcemia. As mentioned previously, calcium can be corrected by adding $\{0.8 \times (4 - [\text{albumin}])\}$ to the total serum calcium level.
- **Serum PTH** that is low or inappropriately normal in the setting of hypocalcemia is indicative of hypoparathyroidism. A high PTH is often found with vitamin D deficiency, PTH resistance, and hyperphosphatemia.
- **Serum phosphorus** is often helpful in identifying vitamin D deficiency (low calcium, low phosphorus) or intravascular chelation of calcium (low calcium, high phosphorus).
- **Vitamin D** stores are usually assessed by measuring only $25(\text{OH})\text{D}_3$ since calcitriol $(1,25(\text{OH})_2\text{D}_3)$ levels can be normalized through the compensatory increase of 1-α-hydroxylase activity.
- **Magnesium** deficiency should always be ruled out during management of hypocalcemia.

Electrocardiography
The **ECG** may show a prolonged QT interval and bradycardia.

TREATMENT

Acute management of symptomatic hypocalcemia requires prompt and aggressive therapy.

Medications
- **Phosphorus** must first be checked. In severe hyperphosphatemia, administration of calcium will increase the calcium–phosphorus product and may exacerbate the formation of ectopic calcifications. In acute, symptomatic hypocalcemia with severe hyperphosphatemia, dialysis may be needed to acutely manage the mineral abnormalities. If the hypocalcemia is asymptomatic, a reduction of phosphorus should precede aggressive calcium supplementation.
- **Hypomagnesemia**, if present, must be treated first in order to effectively correct the hypocalcemia. Two grams of magnesium sulfate can be given IV over 15 minutes followed by an infusion (see Magnesium, Hypomagnesemia, Treatment section) and may even be given empirically if renal failure is not present.
- **Calcium supplementation.** IV calcium should be reserved for severe or symptomatic hypocalcemia and can be administered as calcium chloride or calcium gluconate. Calcium gluconate is typically favored due to reduced risk of tissue toxicity with extravasation. Calcium gluconate is often prepared as a 10% solution (100 mg of calcium gluconate per mL). One ampule (10 mL) of calcium gluconate thus contains 1,000 mg of calcium gluconate and ~90 mg of elemental calcium.
  ○ When necessary to treat severe or symptomatic hypocalcemia, an initial dose of 90 to 180 mg of elemental calcium can be achieved with 1 to 2 g of **calcium gluconate** (equal to 10 to 20 mL or one to two ampules of 10% calcium gluconate) mixed in 50 to 100 mL of D_5W administered over 10 to 20 minutes.
  ○ The effect of initial treatment is only transient, and maintenance of calcium levels typically requires a continuous infusion of 0.5 to 1.5 mg/kg/hr of elemental calcium. A solution comprised of 1 L D_5W with 100 mL of 10% calcium gluconate contains ~900 mg of elemental calcium per liter, approximating 1 mg of elemental calcium per mL of fluid. Infusion is typically begun at a rate of 50 mL/hr (~50 mg of elemental calcium per hour) and titrated up as needed.

- **Chronic management.** Treatment requires calcium supplements and vitamin D or its active metabolite to increase intestinal calcium absorption.
  - ○ **Oral calcium supplements.** Calcium carbonate (40% elemental calcium) or calcium acetate (25% elemental calcium) can be given with the goal administration of 1 to 2 g of *elemental* calcium PO tid. Calcium supplementation should be given apart from meals to minimize binding with phosphorus and maximize enteric absorption. Serum levels should be checked once to twice per week to guide ongoing therapy.
  - ○ **Vitamin D.** Simple dietary deficiency can be corrected by the use of ergocalciferol 400 to 1,000 IU/d. However, in conjunction with other hypocalcemic disorders, larger doses may be required. A 6- to 8-week regimen of 50,000 IU should be dosed weekly in those with underlying impairments in vitamin D metabolism (i.e., renal insufficiency) and daily in patients with severe malnutrition or malabsorption.
  - ○ In comparison, **calcitriol** has a much more rapid onset of action. The initial dosage is 0.25 mcg daily, and most patients are maintained on 0.5 to 2.0 mcg daily. The dose can be increased at 2- to 4-week intervals. Because calcitriol increases enteric absorption of phosphorus as well as calcium, phosphorus levels should be monitored and oral phosphate binders initiated if phosphorus exceeds the normal range.

Complications

Development of hypercalcemia. In the event that hypercalcemia develops, vitamin D and calcium supplements should be stopped. Once serum calcium falls to normal, both forms of supplementation should be restarted at lower doses. Hypercalcemia due to calcitriol usually resolves within 1 week.

PHOSPHORUS

GENERAL PRINCIPLES

- Phosphorus is critical for bone formation and cellular energy metabolism.
- Approximately 85% of **total body phosphorus** is in bone, and most of the remainder is within cells. Thus, serum phosphorus levels may not reflect total body phosphorus stores.
- **Phosphorus balance** is determined primarily by four factors:
  - ○ **PTH** regulates the incorporation and release of minerals from bone stores and decreases proximal tubular reabsorption of phosphate, causing urinary wasting.
  - ○ The **phosphate concentration** itself regulates renal proximal reabsorption.
  - ○ **Insulin** lowers serum levels by shifting phosphate into cells.
  - ○ **Calcitriol** $(1,25[OH]_2D_3)$ increases serum phosphate by enhancing intestinal phosphorus absorption.

Hyperphosphatemia

GENERAL PRINCIPLES

Definition

A serum phosphate **>4.5 mg/dL** defines hyperphosphatemia.

Etiology

- **Hyperphosphatemia** is caused by (a) **transcellular shift**, (b) **increased intake**, and most commonly, (c) **decreased renal excretion**. In clinical practice, renal insufficiency is usually present and serves as the major predisposing factor toward the development of hyperphosphatemia.
- **Transcellular shift** occurs in rhabdomyolysis, tumor lysis syndrome, and massive hemolysis as phosphorus is released from cells into the ECF. Metabolic acidosis and hypoinsulinemia reduce phosphorus flux into cells and contribute to the hyperphosphatemia sometimes seen in DKA.
- **Increased intake** leading to hyperphosphatemia usually occurs in the setting of renal insufficiency, either with dietary indiscretion in chronic kidney disease or as an iatrogenic complication. The latter can be seen when Phospho-Soda enemas (e.g., Fleet) or active vitamin D analogs are given to patients with renal insufficiency.
- **Decreased renal excretion** occurs most commonly in the setting of renal failure. Occasionally, hypoparathyroidism and pseudohypoparathyroidism reduce renal phosphorus clearance as well.

DIAGNOSIS

Clinical Presentation

- Signs and symptoms are typically attributable to hypocalcemia and the metastatic calcification of soft tissues. Occasionally, skin deposition can result in severe pruritus. **Calciphylaxis** describes the tissue ischemia that may result from the calcification of smaller blood vessels and their subsequent thrombosis.
- Chronic hyperphosphatemia contributes to the development of renal osteodystrophy (see Chapter 13, Renal Diseases).

Diagnostic Testing

The elevated serum phosphorus can be accompanied by hypocalcemia as a result of **intravascular chelation** of calcium by phosphorus.

TREATMENT

- **Acute hyperphosphatemia** is treated by increasing renal excretion of phosphorus and, as such, is limited when renal insufficiency is present.
  - **Recovery of renal function** will often correct the hyperphosphatemia in the patient within 12 hours. Saline and/or acetazolamide (15 mg/kg q4h) can be given to further encourage phosphaturia, if needed.
  - **Hemodialysis** may be required, especially if irreversible renal insufficiency or symptomatic hypocalcemia is present.
- **Chronic hyperphosphatemia** is almost always associated with chronic renal insufficiency. Its management consists of reducing phosphorus intake through dietary modification and the use of phosphate binders. This is discussed more fully in Chapter 13, Renal Diseases.

Hypophosphatemia

GENERAL PRINCIPLES

Definition

A serum phosphate **<2.8 mg/dL** defines hypophosphatemia.

Etiology

Hypophosphatemia may be caused by (a) **impaired intestinal absorption**, (b) **increased renal excretion**, or (c) **transcellular shift** into cells. Often, there are several mechanisms that work in concert to lower serum phosphate.

- **Impaired intestinal absorption** occurs with the malabsorption syndromes, the use of oral phosphate binders, or vitamin D deficiency from any cause (see Calcium, Hypocalcemia, General Principles, Etiology section). *Chronic alcoholism* is often associated with poor intake of both phosphate and vitamin D, resulting in total body phosphorus depletion.
- **Increased renal excretion** occurs with high levels of PTH, as seen in hyperparathyroidism. This can be particularly pronounced in patients with secondary or tertiary hyperparathyroidism who undergo renal transplantation, as the high PTH causes a profound phosphaturic effect on the functional allograft. Hypophosphatemia may also occur from osmotic diuresis and disorders of proximal tubular transport such as familial X-linked hypophosphatemic rickets and Fanconi syndrome.
- **Transcellular shift** is stimulated by respiratory alkalosis as well as insulin. The latter is responsible for the paradoxical reduction in phosphorus during treatment of malnutrition with hyperalimentation (the refeeding syndrome). The endogenous increase in insulin during treatment shifts phosphorus intracellularly, further reducing serum phosphorus in the malnourished individual. Phosphorus can also be rapidly absorbed into bone following parathyroidectomy for severe hyperparathyroidism (hungry bone syndrome).

DIAGNOSIS

Clinical Presentation

Signs and symptoms typically occur only if total body phosphate depletion is present and the serum phosphorus level is <1 mg/dL. These end-organ effects are due to the inability to form ATP and the impaired tissue oxygen delivery that occurs with a decrease in red blood cell 2,3-diphosphoglycerate. These include muscle injury (rhabdomyolysis, impaired diaphragmatic function, and heart failure), neurologic abnormalities (paresthesias, dysarthria, confusion, stupor, seizures, and coma), and, rarely, hemolysis and platelet dysfunction.

Diagnostic Testing

- The cause is usually apparent from the clinical situation in which the hypophosphatemia occurs. If not, measurement of **urine phosphorus excretion** helps define the mechanism. Renal excretion of >100 mg by 24-hour urine collection or a fractional excretion of phosphate >5% during hypophosphatemia indicates excessive renal loss.

- Low serum **25(OH)D$_3$** suggests dietary vitamin D deficiency or malabsorption. An elevated **intact PTH** may occur in primary or secondary hyperparathyroidism.

TREATMENT

- **Acute moderate hypophosphatemia** (1.0 to 2.5 mg/dL) is common in the hospitalized patient and is often due simply to **transcellular shifts**, requiring no treatment if asymptomatic, except correction of the underlying cause.
- **Acute severe hypophosphatemia** (<1.0 mg/dL) may require IV phosphate therapy when associated with serious clinical manifestations. IV preparations include potassium phosphate (1.5 mEq potassium/mmol phosphate) and sodium phosphate (1.3 mEq sodium/mmol phosphate).
  ○ An infusion of phosphate, 0.08 to 0.16 mmol/kg in 500 mL 0.45% saline, is given intravenously over 6 hours (1 mmol phosphate = 31 mg phosphorus). IV repletion should be stopped when the serum phosphorus level is >1.5 mg/dL and when oral therapy (see the following text) is possible. Because of the need to replenish intracellular stores, 24 to 36 hours of phosphate administration may be required.
  ○ Extreme care must be used to avoid hyperphosphatemia, which may lead to hypocalcemia. If hypotension occurs, acute hypocalcemia should be suspected, and the infusion should be stopped or slowed. Further doses should be based on symptoms and on the serum calcium and phosphorus levels, which should be measured every 8 hours.
- **Chronic hypophosphatemia.** Vitamin D deficiency, if present, should be treated first (see Calcium, Hypocalcemia, Treatment section) followed by oral supplementation of 0.5 to 1.0 g elemental phosphorus PO bid to tid. Preparations include Neutra-Phos (250 mg elemental phosphorus and 7 mEq of Na$^+$ and K$^+$ per capsule) and Neutra-Phos K$^+$ (250 mg elemental phosphorus and 14 mEq K$^+$ per capsule). Contents of the capsules should be dissolved in water. Fleet Phospho-Soda (815 mg phosphorus and 33 mEq sodium per 5 mL) is an alternative oral agent. Limiting side effects include nausea and diarrhea.

MAGNESIUM

- **Magnesium** plays an important role in neuromuscular function.
- Approximately 60% of body magnesium is stored in bone, and most of the remainder is found in cells. Only 1% is in the ECF. As a result, the serum magnesium is a poor predictor of intracellular and total body stores and may grossly underestimate total magnesium deficits.
- The main determinant of magnesium balance is the **magnesium concentration** itself, which directly influences renal excretion. Hypomagnesemia stimulates tubular reabsorption of magnesium, whereas hypermagnesemia inhibits it.

Hypermagnesemia

GENERAL PRINCIPLES

Definition

A serum magnesium **>2.2 mEq/L** defines hypermagnesemia.

Etiology

- Most cases of clinically significant hypermagnesemia are **iatrogenic**, occurring with large doses of magnesium-containing antacids or laxatives and during treatment of preeclampsia with IV magnesium. Since renal excretion is the only means of lowering serum magnesium levels, the presence of significant renal insufficiency can lead to magnesium toxicity even with therapeutic doses of these antacids and laxatives.
- Mild, insignificant elevations in magnesium can occur in end-stage renal disease patients, theophylline intoxication, DKA, and tumor lysis syndrome.

DIAGNOSIS

Clinical Presentation

- Signs and symptoms are seen only if the serum magnesium level is >4 mEq/L.
- Neuromuscular abnormalities usually include hyporeflexia (usually the first sign of magnesium toxicity), lethargy, and weakness that can progress to somnolence and paralysis. With diaphragmatic involvement, this can lead to respiratory failure.
- Cardiac findings include hypotension, bradycardia, and cardiac arrest.

Diagnostic Testing

The **ECG** may reveal bradycardia and prolonged PR, QRS, and QT intervals with magnesium levels of 5 to 10 mEq/L. Complete heart block or asystole may eventually ensue with levels >15 mEq/L.

TREATMENT

- **Prevention.** In the setting of significant renal insufficiency, the inadvertent administration of magnesium-containing medications (e.g., Maalox, magnesium citrate) should be avoided.
- **Asymptomatic hypermagnesemia.** In the setting of normal renal function, normal magnesium levels will quickly be attained with removal of the magnesium load.
- **Symptomatic hypermagnesemia**
  - Prompt supportive therapy is critical, including mechanical ventilation for respiratory failure and a temporary pacemaker for significant bradyarrhythmias.
  - The effects of hypermagnesemia can be antagonized quickly by the administration of 10% calcium gluconate 10 to 20 mL IV (1 to 2 g) over 10 minutes.
  - Renal excretion can be encouraged with saline administration.
  - With significant renal insufficiency, hemodialysis is required for definitive therapy.

Hypomagnesemia

GENERAL PRINCIPLES

Definition

A serum magnesium **<1.3 mEq/L** defines hypomagnesemia.

Etiology

- Hypomagnesemia is most commonly caused by impaired intestinal absorption and increased renal excretion.

- **Decreased intestinal absorption** occurs in malnutrition, as is common in chronic alcoholics or any malabsorption syndrome. Magnesium can also be lost through prolonged diarrhea and nasogastric aspiration.
- **Increased renal excretion** of magnesium can occur from increased renal tubular flow (as occurs with osmotic diuresis) as well as impaired tubular function (as seen with resolving acute tubular necrosis [ATN], loop diuretics, and Bartter's and Gitelman's syndromes).
- **Drugs.** Several medications similarly induce defects in tubular magnesium transport including aminoglycosides, amphotericin B, cisplatin, pentamidine, and cyclosporine.

DIAGNOSIS

Clinical Presentation

- Neurologic manifestations include lethargy, confusion, tremor, fasciculations, ataxia, nystagmus, tetany, and seizures.
- Atrial and ventricular arrhythmias may occur, especially in patients treated with digoxin.

Diagnostic Testing

Laboratories

- Low serum [Mg^{2+}] in conjunction with an appropriate clinical scenario is sufficient to establish the diagnosis of **magnesium deficiency**. However, due to the slow exchange of magnesium between the bone and intracellular pools (see Magnesium, General Principles section), a normal serum level does not exclude total body **magnesium deficiency**.
- The etiology of hypomagnesemia usually is evident from the clinical context, but if there is uncertainty, measurement of **urine magnesium excretion** is helpful. A 24-hour urine magnesium of >2 mEq (or >24 mg), or a fractional excretion of magnesium of >2% during hypomagnesemia suggests **increased renal excretion**. The fractional excretion of magnesium is calculated by

$$(\text{Urine } Mg^{2+}/\text{Urine Cr}) \div \{(\text{Serum } Mg^{2+} \times 0.7)/\text{Serum Cr}\} \times 100$$

- Hypocalcemia (see Calcium, Hypocalcemia, General Principles, Etiology section) and/or hypokalemia (see Potassium, Hypokalemia, General Principles, Etiology section) can often be found as a result of hypomagnesemia-induced derangements in mineral homeostasis.
- **ECG** abnormalities may include a prolonged PR and QT interval with a widened QRS. **Torsades de pointes** is the classically associated arrhythmia.

TREATMENT

- In patients with normal renal function, excess magnesium is readily excreted, and there is little risk of causing hypermagnesemia with recommended doses. However, *magnesium must be given with extreme care in the presence of renal insufficiency.*
- The route of magnesia administration depends on whether clinical manifestations from magnesium deficiency are present.
  - **Asymptomatic hypomagnesemia** can be treated orally. Numerous preparations exist, including Mag-Ox 400 (240 mg elemental magnesium per 400-mg tablet),

UroMag (84 mg per 140-mg tablet), and sustained-release Slow-Mag (64 mg per tablet). Typically, ~240 mg of elemental magnesium is administered daily for mild deficiency, while more severe hypomagnesemia may require up to 720 mg/d of elemental magnesium. The major side effect is diarrhea. Normalization of serum magnesium levels can be deceiving, since the administered magnesium slowly shifts to replete intracellular and bone stores. Furthermore, abrupt increases in serum levels stimulate renal excretion. Thus, serum levels should be followed closely, and replacement should be maintained until patients demonstrate stable normalization of serum magnesium concentrations.

○ **Severe symptomatic hypomagnesemia** should be treated with 1 to 2 g magnesium sulfate (1 g magnesium sulfate = 96 mg elemental magnesium) IV over 15 minutes. Again, to account for gradual redistribution to severely depleted intracellular stores, replacement therapy may need to be maintained, often for 3 to 7 days. Serum magnesium should be measured q24h and the infusion rate adjusted to maintain a serum magnesium level of <2.5 mEq/L. Tendon reflexes should be tested frequently, as hyporeflexia suggests hypermagnesemia. Reduced doses and more frequent monitoring must be used even in mild renal insufficiency.

ACID–BASE DISTURBANCES

GENERAL PRINCIPLES

- The normal ECF **pH is 7.40 ± 0.03**. Perturbations in pH can occur with changes in the ratio of $[HCO_3^-]$ to pCO_2 as described by the **Henderson-Hasselbalch equation**:

$$pH = 6.1 + \log\{[HCO_3^-] \div (pCO_2 \times 0.3)\}$$

- Maintenance of pH is essential for normal cellular function. Three general mechanisms exist to keep it within a narrow window:
  - ○ **Chemical buffering** is mediated by HCO_3^- in the ECF and by protein and phosphate buffers in the ICF. The normal $[HCO_3^-]$ is 24 ± 2 mEq/L.
  - ○ **Alveolar ventilation** minimizes variations in the pH by altering the partial pressure of carbon dioxide (pCO_2). The normal pCO_2 is 40 ± 5 mm Hg.
  - ○ **Renal H^+ handling** allows the kidney to adapt to changes in acid–base status via HCO_3^- reabsorption and excretion of titratable acid (e.g., $H_2PO_4^-$) and NH_4^+.

Definition

Acidemia and **alkalemia** refer to processes that lower and raise pH regardless of mechanism. They can be caused by metabolic or respiratory disturbances.
- **Metabolic acidosis** is characterized by a decrease in the plasma $[HCO_3^-]$ due to either HCO_3^- loss or the accumulation of acid.
- **Metabolic alkalosis** is characterized by an elevation in the plasma $[HCO_3^-]$ due to either H^+ loss or HCO_3^- gain.
- **Respiratory acidosis** is characterized by an elevation in pCO_2 resulting from alveolar hypoventilation.
- **Respiratory alkalosis** is characterized by a decrease in pCO_2 resulting from hyperventilation.

DIAGNOSIS

Differential Diagnosis

Analysis should be systematic so that accurate conclusions are drawn and appropriate therapy initiated. Once the acid–base process is correctly identified, further diagnostic studies may be undertaken to determine the precise etiologies at play. The systematic approach to acid–base conditions follows five steps: checking an arterial blood gas (ABG), establishing a primary disorder, assessing compensation, calculating an anion gap (AG), and evaluating the delta gap.

- **Step 1.** Check ABG. Acidemia is present when pH is <7.37 and alkalemia when pH >7.43.
- **Step 2.** Establish the primary disturbance by determining whether the change in $[HCO_3^-]$ or pCO_2 can account for the observed deflection in pH.
  - In acidemia, a decreased $[HCO_3^-]$ suggests metabolic acidosis, and an elevated pCO_2 suggests respiratory acidosis. In alkalemia, an elevated $[HCO_3^-]$ suggests metabolic alkalosis while a decreased pCO_2 suggests respiratory alkalosis.
  - A **combined disorder** is present when pH is normal but the pCO_2 and $[HCO_3^-]$ are both abnormal. Changes in both pCO_2 and $[HCO_3^-]$ can cause the change in pH.
- **Step 3.** Determine whether compensation is appropriate.
  - The **compensatory mechanism** is an adaptation to the primary acid–base disturbance intended to stabilize the changing pH. A respiratory process that shifts the pH in one direction will be compensated by a metabolic process that shifts the pH in the other and vice versa.
  - The effect of compensation is to attenuate, but not completely correct, the primary change in pH.
  - The expected compensations for the various primary acid–base derangements are given in Table 12-3.
  - An inappropriate compensatory response suggests the presence of a combined disorder.
  - Example: In a patient with metabolic acidosis, respiratory compensation attenuates the metabolic disturbance to pH by lowering pCO_2. However, if the pCO_2 is higher than expected, respiratory compensation is insufficient, revealing a respiratory acidosis with the primary metabolic acidosis. If pCO_2 is lower than expected, compensation is excessive, revealing a concomitant respiratory alkalosis.
- **Step 4.** Determine the **anion gap**.
  - In normal individuals, the total serum cations are balanced with the total serum anions. Total cations are comprised of measured cations (MCs) and unmeasured cations (UCs), while total anions are comprised of measured anions (MAs) and unmeasured anions (UAs). Certain forms of acidosis are characterized by an increase in the pool of UAs. The **anion gap** is merely a way of demonstrating the accumulation of this UA.
  - $AG = [Na^+] - ([Cl^-] + [HCO_3^-])$. The normal AG is 10 ± 2 mEq/L.

$$AG = \text{the excess of unmeasured anions (vs. unmeasured cations)}$$
$$= UA - UC$$

Since total cations = total anions:

$$MC + UC = MA + UA$$

Table 12-3	Expected Compensatory Responses to Primary Acid–Base Disorders	
Disorder	**Primary Change**	**Compensatory Response**
Metabolic acidosis	$\downarrow [HCO_3^-]$	$\downarrow pCO_2$ 1.2 mm Hg for every 1 mEq/L $\downarrow [HCO_3^-]$ OR pCO_2 = last two digits of pH
Metabolic alkalosis	$\uparrow [HCO_3^-]$	$\uparrow pCO_2$ 0.7 mm Hg for every 1 mEq/L $\uparrow [HCO_3^-]$
Respiratory acidosis	$\uparrow pCO_2$	
Acute		$\uparrow [HCO_3^-]$ 1.0 mEq/L for every 10 mm Hg $\uparrow pCO_2$
Chronic		$\uparrow [HCO_3^-]$ 3.5 mEq/L for every 10 mm Hg $\uparrow pCO_2$
Respiratory alkalosis	$\downarrow pCO_2$	
Acute		$\downarrow [HCO_3^-]$ 2.0 mEq/L for every 10 mm Hg $\downarrow pCO_2$
Chronic		$\downarrow [HCO_3^-]$ 5.0 mEq/L for every 10 mm Hg $\downarrow pCO_2$

Rearranging the equation:

$$UA - UC = MC - MA$$

MCs are Na^+; MAs are Cl^- and HCO_3^-.

○ Since albumin is the principle UA, the AG should be corrected if there are gross changes in serum albumin levels.

$$AG_{correct} = AG + \{(4 - [albumin]) \times 2.5\}$$

○ An elevated AG suggests the presence of metabolic acidosis with a circulating anion (Table 12-4).

- **Step 5.** Assess the delta gap.
  ○ To maintain a stable total anion content, every increase in a UA should be met with a decrease in $[HCO_3^-]$. Comparing the change in the AG (ΔAG) with the change in the $[HCO_3^-]$ ($\Delta[HCO_3^-]$) is a simple way of making sure that each change in the AG is accounted for.
  ○ If the $\Delta AG = \Delta[HCO_3^-]$, this is a simple AG metabolic acidosis.
  ○ If the $\Delta AG > \Delta[HCO_3^-]$,
    ▪ The $[HCO_3^-]$ did not decrease as much as expected.
    ▪ This is a metabolic alkalosis **and** AG metabolic acidosis.
    ▪ **Example:** A patient with DKA has been vomiting prior to admission. He has an AG of 20 and a $[HCO_3^-]$ of 20. His $\Delta AG = 10$ and $\Delta[HCO_3^-] = 4$, revealing an AG metabolic acidosis (DKA) with a metabolic alkalosis (vomiting).
      □ If the $\Delta AG < \Delta[HCO_3^-]$,
      □ The $[HCO_3^-]$ decreased more than expected.
      □ This is a nongap metabolic acidosis **and** AG metabolic acidosis.

Table 12-4	The Four Primary Acid–Base Disorders and Their Common Etiologies	

	Acidosis	Alkalosis
Metabolic	Gap: • Ketoacids (starvation, alcoholic, diabetic) • Exposures (methanol, ethylene glycol, salicylates) • Lactic acid (shock, drug related) • Profound uremia	Generation: • Loss of H^+-rich fluids (GI loss) • Contraction alkalosis • Alkali administration
	Nongap: • Nonrenal HCO_3^- loss (diarrhea) • Renal HCO_3^- loss/RTA2 • ↓ H^+ secretion/RTA1 • Hypoaldosterone related/RTA4	Maintenance: • Volume contraction • Chloride depletion • Hypokalemia

	RTA1	RTA2	RTA4
Serum [K^+]	↓ or nl	↓ or nl	↑
Serum [HCO_3]	<10	15–20	>15
U pH	>5.3	Varies	<5.3

	Acidosis	Alkalosis
Respiratory	Depression of respiratory center Neuromuscular failure Lung disease	CNS stimulation Hypoxemia Anxiety

CNS, central nervous system; GI, gastrointestinal; RTA, renal tubular acidosis; U, urine.

- **Example:** A patient is admitted with fevers and hypotension after a prolonged course of diarrhea. She has an AG of 15 and a [HCO_3^-] of 12. Her ΔAG is 5 and her Δ[HCO_3^-] is 12, revealing a nongap metabolic acidosis (diarrhea) and an AG metabolic acidosis (lactic acidosis).

Metabolic Acidosis

GENERAL PRINCIPLES

Etiology

- The causes of a metabolic acidosis can be divided into those that cause an **elevated anion gap** and those with a **normal anion gap**. Many of the causes seen in clinical practice can be found in Table 12-4.
- AG acidosis results from exposure to acids, which contribute an unmeasured anion to the ECF. Common causes are diabetic ketoacidosis, lactic acidosis, and toxic alcohol ingestions.

- Nonanion gap acidosis can result from the loss of $[HCO_3^-]$ from the GI tract. Renal causes due to renal excretion of $[HCO_3^-]$ or disorders of renal acid handling are referred to collectively as **renal tubular acidoses (RTAs)**.
- Enteric $[HCO_3^-]$ loss occurs most commonly in the setting of severe diarrhea.
- The three forms of RTA correlate with the three mechanisms that facilitate renal acid handling: proximal bicarbonate reabsorption, distal H^+ secretion, and generation of NH_3, the principle urinary buffer. Urinary buffers reduce the concentration of free H^+ in the filtrate, thus attenuating the back leak of H^+, which occurs at low urinary pH.
  - **Proximal (type 2) RTA** is caused by impaired proximal tubular HCO_3^- reabsorption. Causes include inherited disorders (Wilson's disease), toxins (heavy metals, ifosfamide), multiple myeloma, autoimmune diseases (Sjögren syndrome), and acetazolamide use.
  - **Distal (type 1) RTA** results from impaired distal H^+ secretion. This may occur due to impairment in H^+ secretion, as seen with a variety of autoimmune (Sjögren syndrome, lupus, rheumatoid arthritis) or renal disorders. It can also be caused by a back leak of H^+ due to increased membrane permeability, as seen with amphotericin B.
  - **Distal hyperkalemic (type 4) RTA** may result from either low aldosterone levels or from aldosterone resistance. The resulting hyperkalemia reduces the availability of NH_3 to buffer urinary H^+. Hyporeninemic hypoaldosteronism is seen with some frequency in patients with diabetes. Certain drugs including NSAIDs, β-blockers, and cyclosporine have also been implicated.
  - Occasionally, the kidney is unable to secrete sufficient H^+ due to an impaired luminal gradient. In these situations, poor filtrate delivery or impaired Na^+ reabsorption in the distal nephron are responsible for decreasing the voltage gradient, which augments H^+ secretion. This can be seen with marked volume depletion, urinary tract obstruction, sickle cell nephropathy, and amiloride or triamterene use.

DIAGNOSIS

Diagnostic Testing

- The first step in narrowing the differential diagnosis for a metabolic acidosis is to calculate the **anion gap**.
  - The specific cause of an **elevated anion gap** can usually be determined by clinical history. However, specific laboratory studies are available to identify certain anions such as lactate, acetoacetate, acetone, and β-hydroxybutyrate. (It should be noted that the use of nitroprusside to detect ketones may fail to identify ketoacidosis due to β-hydroxybutyrate.) The presence of an alcohol (methanol, ethanol, ethylene glycol) can also be determined with laboratory assays. Clinical suspicion for toxic alcohol ingestion is corroborated by an increased **osmolal gap**. This gap is the difference between measured and calculated serum osmolality:

$$[Osm]_{meas} - \{([Na^+] \times 2) + ([glucose] \div 18) + ([BUN] \div 2.8)\}$$

  - If a **normal anion gap** is present, the GI HCO_3^- losses can be differentiated from RTAs via the **urine anion gap** (UAG). The **UAG** is the difference between the major measured anions and cations in urine: $[Na^+]_u + [K^+]_u - [Cl^-]_u$. Because NH_4^+ is the major unmeasured urinary cation, a negative UAG reflects high NH_4^+ excretion, an appropriate response to a metabolic acidosis. Conversely, a positive UAG signifies low NH_4^+ excretion, which in the face of a metabolic acidosis, suggests a renal tubular defect.

∘ Serum $[K^+]$ and urine pH can be helpful in distinguishing between the RTAs.
  ▪ Types 1 and 2 are typically associated with hypokalemia, while type 4 is characterized by hyperkalemia.
  ▪ Urine pH is low (usually <5.3) in type 4 RTA since the defect is in the generation of the NH_3 buffer, and the mechanism for H^+ secretion is intact. In contrast, urine pH is inappropriately high in type 1 RTA (urine pH >5.3). In type 2 RTA, the urine pH is variable. It is elevated during the initial bicarbonaturia, when filtered bicarbonate exceeds the threshold for reabsorption, and low when the filtered load is below this threshold.

TREATMENT

- **Ketoacidosis** attributable to ethanol abuse and starvation can be corrected with the resumption of caloric intake through PO intake or dextrose-containing fluids and by correction of any volume depletion that may be present. The treatment of diabetic ketoacidosis is described in Chapter 23, Diabetes Mellitus and Related Disorders.
- **Lactic acidosis** will resolve once the underlying cause is treated and tissue perfusion is restored. Often, this involves aggressive therapeutic maneuvers for the treatment of shock as described in Chapter 8, Critical Care. The administration of alkali does not appear to have clear benefit in lactic acidosis, and it may lead to a rebound metabolic alkalosis once the underlying cause is managed. Its use in dire circumstances or severe acidosis remains controversial.
- Management of toxic ingestions is described in Chapter 28, Toxicology.
- **Normal AG metabolic acidosis.** Treatment with $NaHCO_3$ is appropriate for patients with a normal AG metabolic acidosis. The HCO_3^- deficit can be calculated in mEq:

$$HCO_3^- \text{ deficit} = (0.5 \times \text{lean weight} \times [24 - (HCO_3^-)])$$

However, this assumes a volume of distribution equal to 50% of total body weight. In reality, the distribution of HCO_3^- increases with the severity of the acidosis and may exceed 100% of total body weight in very severe acidosis. It should be noted that the standard 650-mg tablet of oral $NaHCO_3$ provides only 7 mEq of HCO_3-, while one ampule of IV $NaHCO_3$ contains 50 mEq. Still, parenteral $NaHCO_3$ should always be prescribed with caution because of the potential adverse effects, including pulmonary edema, hypokalemia, and hypocalcemia.
- **Treatment of the RTAs.** Correction of the chronic acidemia with alkali administration is warranted in order to prevent its catabolic effect on bone and muscle.
  ∘ In *distal (type 1) RTA*, correction of the metabolic acidosis requires oral HCO_3^- replacement on the order of 1 to 2 mEq/kg/d with $NaHCO_3$ or sodium citrate. Potassium citrate replacement may be necessary for patients with hypokalemia, nephrolithiasis, or nephrocalcinosis. Underlying conditions should be sought and treated.
  ∘ In *proximal (type 2) RTA*, much larger amounts of alkali (10 to 15 mEq/kg/d) are required to reverse the acidosis. Administration of potassium salts minimizes the degree of hypokalemia associated with alkali therapy.

○ Management of *type 4 RTA* requires correction of the underlying hyperkalemia. This consists of dietary K^+ restriction (40 to 60 mEq/d) and possibly a loop diuretic with or without oral $NaHCO_3$ (0.5 to 1 mEq/kg/d). Mineralocorticoid administration (fludrocortisone, 50 to 200 mcmg PO daily) should be used in patients with primary adrenal insufficiency and may be considered in other causes of hypoaldosteronism.

Metabolic Alkalosis

GENERAL PRINCIPLES

Etiology

• Development of a persistent metabolic alkalosis requires both generation (an inciting cause) and maintenance (a persistent impairment of the corrective renal response).

• Generation often occurs with a primary increase in the plasma $[HCO_3^-]$ and may be due to either HCO_3^- **gain** from alkali administration or, more commonly, **excessive H^+ loss**. The latter results may result from the loss of H^+ rich fluids, including upper GI secretions. **Contraction alkalosis** refers to the contraction of volume around a fixed content of bicarbonate.

• Maintenance requires a concomitant impairment in renal HCO_3^- excretion, since the kidney normally has a large capacity to excrete HCO_3^-. This occurs as a result of a **decreased glomerular filtration rate (GFR)** or enhanced tubular HCO_3^- reabsorption from **chloride depletion**, **volume contraction**, and **hypokalemia**. A decrease in filtered chloride is sensed by the macula densa and, as a result of tubuloglomerular feedback, reduces filtered HCO_3^- and stimulates aldosterone release. It also limits adaptive distal HCO_3^- secretion. Metabolic alkalosis is often described as being **chloride responsive** or **chloride unresponsive**.

DIAGNOSIS

Clinical Presentation

• The generation of metabolic acidosis is often obvious from the history. Common causes include loss of upper GI secretions through vomiting or excessive urinary H^+ loss from diuretics.

• As key causes of metabolic alkalosis are related to volume contraction (vomiting and diuretic use), patients may present with signs of volume depletion. Occasionally, patients demonstrate hypertension or mild ECF expansion as a result of mineralocorticoid excess.

Diagnostic Testing

• Urine electrolytes are generally useful in identifying the etiology of a metabolic alkalosis when the history and physical is unrevealing.

○ A **urine $[Cl^-]$** <20 mEq/L is consistent with **chloride-responsive** metabolic alkalosis and usually indicates volume depletion. A urine $[Cl^-]$ >20 mEq/L indicates a chloride-unresponsive cause (see Table 12-4).

○ Urine $[Na^+]$ is not reliable in predicting the effective circulating volume in these conditions, since bicarbonaturia obligates renal Na^+ loss even in volume depletion.

- **Serum potassium** levels are often low in metabolic alkalosis. Hypokalemia contributes to alkalosis by increasing tubular H^+ secretion and Cl^- wasting. Hypokalemia is also a result of alkalosis due to transcellular shifts.

TREATMENT

- **Chloride-responsive** metabolic alkaloses are most effectively treated with saline resuscitation until euvolemia is achieved. The increase in filtered chloride leads to improved renal handling of the bicarbonate load.
- **Chloride-unresponsive** metabolic alkaloses do not respond to saline administration and are often associated with a normal or expanded ECF volume.
  - Mineralocorticoid excess can be managed with a K^+-sparing diuretic (amiloride or spironolactone) and repletion of the K^+ deficit.
  - The alkalosis from excessive alkali administration will quickly resolve once the HCO_3^- load is withdrawn, assuming normal renal function.
- Presence of hypokalemia will continue to perpetuate some degree of alkalosis regardless of other interventions. Potassium must therefore be repleted in all cases of metabolic alkalosis.
- Acetazolamide may be useful if the alkalosis persists despite the above interventions, or if saline administration is limited by a patient's volume overload. This therapy promotes bicarbonaturia, although renal K^+ loss is enhanced as well. Acetazolamide can be dosed at 250 mg q6h × 4, or with a single dose of 500 mg.
- Severe alkalemia (pH >7.70) with ECF volume excess and/or renal failure can be treated with isotonic (150 mEq/L) HCl administered via a central vein. The amount of HCl required can be calculated as $\{(0.5 \times \text{lean weight in kg}) \times ([HCO_3^-] - 24)\}$. Correction should occur over 8 to 24 hours.

Respiratory Acidosis

GENERAL PRINCIPLES

The causes of respiratory acidosis can be divided into hypoventilation from (a) **respiratory center depression**, (b) **neuromuscular failure**, (c) **decreased respiratory system compliance**, (d) **increased airway resistance**, and (e) **increased dead space** (see Table 12-3).

DIAGNOSIS

- Symptoms of respiratory acidosis result from changes in the cerebrospinal fluid (CSF) pH. A very severe hypercapnia may be well tolerated if it is accompanied by renal compensation and a relatively normal pH. Conversely, a modest rise in pCO_2 can be very symptomatic if acute.
- Initial symptoms and signs may include headache and restlessness, which may progress to generalized hyperreflexia/asterixis and coma.

TREATMENT

- Treatment is directed at correcting the underlying disorder and improving ventilation (see Chapter 10, Pulmonary Diseases).
- Administration of $NaHCO_3$ in order to improve the acidemia may paradoxically worsen the pH in situations of limited ventilation. The administered HCO_3^- will combine with H^+ in the tissues and form pCO_2 and water. If ventilation is fixed, this extra CO_2 generated cannot be blown off and worsening hypercapnia will result. Therefore, HCO_3^- should, in general, be avoided in *pure* respiratory acidoses.

Respiratory Alkalosis

GENERAL PRINCIPLES

The common causes of hyperventilation resulting in respiratory alkalosis are given in Table 12-3.

Diagnosis
Clinical Presentation
- The rise in CSF pH that occurs with **acute respiratory alkalosis** is associated with a significant reduction in cerebral blood flow that may lead to light-headedness and impaired consciousness. Generalized membrane excitability can result in seizures and arrhythmias. Symptoms and signs of acute hypocalcemia (see Calcium, Hypocalcemia, Diagnosis, Clinical Presentation section) may be evident from the abrupt fall in ionized calcium that can occur.
- **Chronic respiratory alkalosis** is usually asymptomatic since a normal pH is well defended by compensation.

Diagnostic Testing
The rise in pH from **acute respiratory alkalosis** can cause a reduced ionized calcium (see Calcium, Hypocalcemia, General Principles, Etiology section), a profound hypophosphatemia (see Phosphorus, Hypophosphatemia, General Principles, Etiology section), and hypokalemia (see Potassium, Hypokalemia, General Principles, Etiology section).

TREATMENT

- Treatment of respiratory alkalosis should focus on identifying and treating the underlying disease.
- In intensive care unit patients, this may involve changing the ventilator settings to decrease ventilation (see Chapter 8, Critical Care).

13 Renal Diseases

Seth Goldberg and Daniel Coyne

Evaluation of the Patient with Renal Disease

DIAGNOSIS

Clinical Presentation

- Renal disease is often asymptomatic or presents with nonspecific complaints. Its presence is frequently first noted on abnormal routine laboratory data, generally as an elevated serum creatinine (Cr) level. An abnormal urinalysis or sediment, with proteinuria, hematuria, or pyuria, may also indicate renal disease.
- When the decline in renal function is acute or advanced, a variety of nonspecific symptoms may be present. Generalized malaise, worsening hypertension, dependent or generalized edema, or decreasing urine output may accompany more severe renal insufficiency.
- The focus of the initial evaluation of the patient with renal disease is to determine the need for emergent dialysis. Then, investigations to identify the etiology are undertaken, while differentiating components of acute and chronic disease.

Diagnostic Testing

Laboratories
- **Serum chemistries**
  - A basic evaluation includes electrolytes (with calcium and phosphorus), Cr, blood urea nitrogen (BUN), and albumin. When at a stable baseline, the Cr is a serviceable marker of the glomerular filtration rate (GFR), which can be calculated by the Cockcroft–Gault formula for Cr clearance:

    [(140–age) × (ideal body weight in kg) (× 0.85 for women)]/[72 × Cr in mg/dL]
  - However, as Cr is secreted by the tubules, particularly as renal function worsens, this formula has the tendency to overestimate the GFR.
  - The Modification of Diet in Renal Disease (MDRD) formulas can calculate the GFR and takes into account BUN, albumin, and race in addition to age and gender (*http://mdrd.com*). When the MDRD GFR is >60 mL/min/1.73 m^2, chronic kidney disease (CKD) should not be diagnosed unless other evidence of renal damage (e.g., proteinuria) is present.
  - When a glomerular process is suspected, it may be useful to check for antinuclear antibodies (ANA), antiglomerular basement membrane (anti-GBM) antibodies, antineutrophil cytoplasmic antibodies (ANCA), complement levels (C3, C4), cryoglobulins, antistreptolysin-O (ASO) titers, and viral (HIV, hepatitis B and C) serologies. A serum protein electrophoresis (SPEP) can be performed in proteinuric patients to evaluate for monoclonal gammopathy, and may be suspected by a large protein–albumin gap.

- **Urine studies**
  - Routine urine studies include a urine dipstick (for protein, blood, glucose, leukocyte esterase, nitrites, pH, and specific gravity) as well as a freshly voided specimen for microscopic examination (looking for cells, casts, and crystals). The urine sample is centrifuged at 2,100 rpm for 5 minutes, and then most of the supernatant is poured off. The pellet is resuspended by gently tapping the side of the tube.
    - **Proteinuria** can be estimated from a spot urine protein-to-creatinine ratio, where the serum Cr must be stable to ensure a steady state in the urine. A normal ratio is <250 mg of protein per gram of Cr. A 24-hour urine collection for protein can be obtained when the serum Cr is not at a stable baseline.
    - **Hematuria** (>3 red blood cells [RBCs] per high-power field) can represent an infectious, inflammatory, or malignant process anywhere along the urinary tract. Dysmorphic RBCs (with rounded protuberances) suggest a glomerular source of bleeding and can be accompanied by RBC casts formed within the tubules. The absence of RBCs in a patient with a positive dipstick for blood suggests hemolysis or rhabdomyolysis (forms of pigment nephropathy).
    - **White blood cells** (WBCs) in the urine represent an infectious or inflammatory process. This may be seen with a urinary tract infection (UTI), parenchymal infections such as pyelonephritis or abscess, or acute interstitial nephritis (AIN). Urine eosinophils can be identified with the Giemsa stain when evaluating for AIN, atheroembolic disease, or prostatitis, although the sensitivity of this test is low. WBC casts are consistent with AIN and pyelonephritis but can also be seen as part of an active sediment in glomerulonephritic diseases.
  - Supplemental urine studies can be ordered in specific circumstances. When differentiating between oliguric prerenal azotemia and acute tubular necrosis (ATN), a urine sodium, urea, and Cr can be obtained with simultaneous serum measurements to calculate the fractional excretions of sodium and urea (see the following text). Urine sodium, potassium, and chloride can be helpful in evaluating acid–base disturbances for calculating a urine anion gap, while a urine osmolality can be useful in disorders of water handling (hyponatremia and hypernatremia) (see Chapter 12, Fluid and Electrolyte Management). A urine protein electrophoresis (UPEP) can help identify dysproteinemic disorders. Routine dipstick is less sensitive to nonalbumin proteins and may not detect heavy and light immunoglobulin (Ig) chains.

Imaging
- **Renal ultrasonography** can document the presence of two kidneys, assess size, and identify hydronephrosis or renal cysts. Small kidneys (<9 cm) generally reflect chronic disease, although kidneys may be large in diabetes, HIV, deposition disorders, and polycystic kidney disease. A discrepancy in kidney size of >2 cm suggests unilateral renal artery stenosis with atrophy of the affected kidney. The presence of hydronephrosis suggests obstructive nephropathy. Retroperitoneal fibrosis can encase the ureters and prevent dilation despite the presence of an obstruction.
- **Intravenous urography** is useful in the evaluation of nonglomerular hematuria, stone disease, and voiding disorders. It should be reserved for patients with normal renal function as the iodinated contrast dye has the potential to adversely affect kidney function.
- **Radionuclide scanning** uses technetium isotopes to assess the contribution of each kidney to the overall renal function, providing important information if unilateral nephrectomy is being considered for malignancy or for living donation. Renal scanning is also useful in transplantation, where renal perfusion and excretion of the tracer can be followed.

- **Magnetic resonance imaging** (MRI) and magnetic resonance angiography (MRA) can be helpful in evaluating renal masses, detecting renal artery stenosis, and diagnosing renal vein thrombosis. Unlike standard arteriography, MRA does not require the administration of nephrotoxic contrast agents, but does employ gadolinium-based contrast agents, which are associated with the development of **nephrogenic systemic fibrosis** (NSF) in patients with advanced renal failure or dialysis dependence (*Am J Kidney Dis 2008;51:966*). The U.S. Food and Drug Administration (FDA) has stated that three of the five available gadolinium-contrast agents are inappropriate for use in patients with acute kidney injury (AKI) or severe CKD due to a higher incidence of NSF, while the remaining two agents should be used with caution when necessary.
- **Computed tomography** (CT) has less utility in the evaluation of kidney disease as the iodinated contrast dye can be nephrotoxic and may cause worsening renal function. However, noncontrast helical CT scanning has become the test of choice in evaluating nephrolithiasis.

Diagnostic Procedures
- **Kidney biopsy** can determine diagnosis, guide therapy, and provide prognostic information in many settings, particularly in the evaluation of glomerular or deposition diseases. Biopsy of a renal transplant allograft may be necessary to distinguish acute rejection from medication toxicity and other causes of renal dysfunction.
- Biopsy of a native kidney may be indicated in adults with unexplained proteinuria, hematuria, or renal dysfunction. In systemic lupus erythematosus (SLE) with renal involvement, biopsy results may help classify disease and guide therapy. Shrunken fibrotic kidneys are unlikely to yield useful diagnostic information; they also have an increased risk of postprocedural bleeding and biopsy should generally be avoided in these cases.
- Preparative measures for native kidney biopsy include avoiding aspirin, antiplatelet agents, and anticoagulants for several days before and after the procedure, ultrasonography (to document the presence of two kidneys, assess size, and location), urinalysis or urine culture to exclude infection, blood pressure control, and correction of coagulation parameters. If uremic platelet dysfunction is suspected by an elevated bleeding time (>10 minutes) or abnormal platelet function assays, intravenous desmopressin acetate (DDAVP at 0.3 mcg/kg) can be infused 30 minutes prior to biopsy. Patients on dialysis should not receive heparin immediately after the biopsy. In patients at high risk for bleeding, a transjugular renal biopsy can be performed.
- Serial blood counts should be obtained at 6-hour intervals overnight. A hemoglobin drop of approximately 10% is common postprocedurally. Difficulty voiding after the procedure may represent urethral clot obstructing the flow of urine.

Acute Kidney Injury

GENERAL PRINCIPLES

Definition

There is no precise definition for AKI. It may be characterized by an abrupt increase in serum Cr ≥ 0.3 mg/dL within 48 hours, or a similar increase over a few weeks or months. AKI has multiple etiologies, which are usually revealed by careful history, physical exam, and laboratory testing.

Table 13-1	Causes of Acute Renal Failure

Prerenal

Hypovolemia
Hypotension (including sepsis)
Loss of autoregulation (NSAIDs, RAAS blockers)
Abdominal compartment syndrome
Heart failure
Hepatic cirrhosis

Intrinsic renal

Tubular: Ischemic ATN, toxic ATN (contrast, pigment, uric acid)
Vascular: Glomerulonephritis, dysproteinemia, thrombotic microangiopathy
　(HUS, TTP), atheroembolic disease
Interstitial: Acute interstitial nephritis, pyelonephritis

Postrenal

Urethral obstruction
Ureteral obstruction (bilateral, or unilateral if solitary kidney)

ATN, acute tubular necrosis; HUS, hemolytic–uremic syndrome; NSAIDs, nonsteroidal anti-inflammatory drugs; RAAS, renin–angiotensin–aldosterone system; TTP, thrombotic thrombocytopenic purpura.

Classification

Renal failure can be classified as oliguric or nonoliguric based on the amount of urine output. Cutoffs of approximately 500 mL/d or 25 mL/hr for 4 hours are frequently used in clinical practice.

Etiology

Etiologies of AKI are classically divided according to the anatomic location of the physiologic defect. **Prerenal** disease involves a disturbance of renal perfusion, while **postrenal** disease involves obstruction of the urinary collecting system. **Intrinsic** renal disease involves the glomeruli, microvasculature, tubules, or interstitium of the kidneys. Table 13-1 lists some of the common causes of AKI.

DIAGNOSIS

- Uncovering the cause of AKI requires careful attention to the events preceding the rise in Cr. In the hospitalized patient, blood pressure patterns, hydration status, medications, and radiocontrast use must be investigated. Antibiotic dose and duration as well as PRN medications should not be overlooked.
- Evidence of ongoing hypovolemia or hypoperfusion is suggestive of prerenal disease. Most causes of postrenal disease are identified on ultrasound by dilation of the collecting system or by massive urine output on placement of a bladder catheter. When promptly corrected, prerenal and postrenal disorders can show a rapid decrease in the serum Cr and failure of this to occur can suggest an alternative diagnosis.
- **Urinary casts** point toward an intrinsic cause of AKI. Granular casts ("muddy brown") suggest ATN, WBC casts suggest an inflammatory or infectious interstitial

| Table 13-2 | Laboratory Findings in Oliguric Acute Kidney Injury | | | | | |

Diagnosis	BUN:Cr	FE$_{Na}$ (%)	Urine Osmolality (mOsm/kg)	Urine Na	Urine SG	Sediment
Prerenal azotemia	>20:1	<1%	>500	<20	>1.020	Bland
Oliguric ATN	<20:1	>1%	<350	>40	Variable	Granular casts

ATN, acute tubular necrosis; BUN, blood urea nitrogen; Cr, creatinine; FE$_{Na}$, fractional excretion of sodium; SG, specific gravity.

process, and RBC casts strongly suggest glomerular disease. This underscores the importance of examining a urinary sediment in the evaluation of AKI.

- Various laboratory parameters can be used to differentiate prerenal states from ATN in oliguric patients and are summarized in Table 13-2. The basis for these tests is to evaluate tubular integrity, which is preserved in prerenal disease and lost in ATN. In states of hypoperfusion, the kidneys should avidly reabsorb sodium, resulting in a low fractional excretion of sodium (FE$_{Na}$): FE$_{Na}$ = [(U$_{Na}$ × P$_{Cr}$)/(P$_{Na}$ × U$_{Cr}$)] × 100, where U is urine and P is plasma.
  - ○ **A value <1% suggests renal hypoperfusion with intact tubular function.** Loop diuretics and metabolic alkalosis can induce natriuresis, increase the FE$_{Na}$, and mask the presence of renal hypoperfusion. The fractional excretion of urea (FE$_{Urea}$) can instead be calculated in these settings, where a value of <35% suggests a prerenal process.
  - ○ Contrast and pigment nephropathy can result in a low FE$_{Na}$ due to early vasoconstriction ("prerenal" drop in glomerular perfusion), as can glomerular diseases due to intact tubular function. The FE$_{Na}$ also has limited utility when AKI is superimposed on CKD as the underlying tubular dysfunction makes the test difficult to interpret.
  - ○ With hypoperfusion, the urine is typically concentrated, containing an osmolality >500 mOsm/kg and a high specific gravity (>1.020). In ATN, concentrating ability is lost and the urine is usually isosmolar to the serum (isosthenuria). In the blood, the ratio of BUN to Cr is normally <20:1 and an elevation is consistent with hypovolemia.

Differential Diagnosis

Identifying whether the defect is prerenal, postrenal, or intrinsic to the kidney is useful in arriving at the diagnosis.

Prerenal
- The term **prerenal azotemia** implies preserved intrinsic renal function in the setting of renal hypoperfusion and reduced GFR. The effective circulating volume is decreased, resulting from intravascular volume depletion, low cardiac output, or disordered vasodilation (hepatic cirrhosis).
- When the cause is true volume depletion, presentation involves a history of excessive fluid loss, reduced intake, or orthostatic symptoms. The physical exam may reveal dry mucous membranes, poor skin turgor, and orthostatic vital signs (drop in

blood pressure by at least 20/10 mm Hg or an increase in heart rate by 10 bpm after standing from a seated or lying position). The central venous pressure is typically <8 cm H_2O.

- Low cardiac output causes prerenal azotemia via a drop in the effective circulating volume, despite total body volume overload. In heart failure, diuresis may paradoxically improve the prerenal azotemia by unloading the ventricles and improving cardiac function (see Chapter 5, Heart Failure and Cardiomyopathy).
- Hepatic failure leads to splanchnic vasodilation and venous pooling, which diminishes the effective circulating volume despite total body volume overload. This can progress to the **hepatorenal syndrome** (HRS), which is characterized by a rising Cr in the setting of low systolic blood pressures (90 to 100 mm Hg), mild to moderate hyponatremia (120 to 130 mEq/L), and very low urine sodium excretion (<10 mEq/L). Spontaneous bacterial peritonitis, overdiuresis, gastrointestinal bleeding, or large-volume paracentesis can precipitate HRS in a cirrhotic patient. Management of the renal disease is supportive, and if definitive treatment of the liver disorder (either through recovery or via transplantation) can occur, renal recovery is common. Temporizing measures include treatment of the underlying precipitating factor (e.g., peritonitis, gastrointestinal bleeding) and withholding diuretics. Dialytic support can be used as a bridge to transplantation in appropriate candidates. Additional treatment options are discussed further in Chapter 19, Liver Diseases.
- In the volume-depleted patient, certain medications can block the ability of the kidney to autoregulate blood flow and GFR. Nonsteroidal anti-inflammatory drugs (NSAIDs) inhibit the counterbalancing vasodilatory effects of prostaglandins and can induce AKI in volume-depleted patients. Angiotensin-converting enzyme (ACE) inhibitors and angiotensin receptor blockers (ARBs) can cause efferent arteriolar vasodilation and a drop in the GFR.
- Abdominal compartment syndrome, from intestinal ischemia, obstruction, or massive ascites, can compromise flow through the renal vasculature via increased intraabdominal pressure (IAP). An IAP >20 mm Hg, measured via a pressure transducer attached to the bladder catheter, suggests the diagnosis.

Postrenal

- Postrenal failure occurs when the flow of urine is obstructed anywhere within the urinary collecting system. Common causes include **prostatic enlargement, bilateral kidney stones, or malignancy**. The increased intratubular hydrostatic pressure leads to the diminished GFR. Bilateral involvement (or unilateral obstruction to a solitary kidney) is required to produce a significant change in the Cr level. When the diagnosis is suspected, a renal ultrasound should be performed early to evaluate for hydronephrosis. However, hydronephrosis may be less pronounced when there is concomitant volume depletion or if retroperitoneal fibrosis has encased the ureters, preventing their expansion.
- Treatment depends on the level of obstruction. When urethral flow is impeded (usually by prostatic enlargement in men), placement of a bladder catheter can be both diagnostic and therapeutic; **a postvoid residual urine volume >300 mL** strongly suggests the diagnosis. When the upper urinary tract is involved, urologic or radiologic decompression is necessary, with stenting or placement of percutaneous nephrostomy tubes.
- Relief of bilateral obstruction is frequently followed by a **postobstructive diuresis**. Serum electrolytes need to be closely monitored if polyuria ensues, and replacement of approximately half of the urinary volume with 0.45% saline is recommended.

- Crystals may cause micro-obstructive uropathy within the tubules. Intravenous acyclovir and the protease inhibitor indinavir can induce AKI by this mechanism. The urine may show evidence of crystals, although sometimes not until urine flow is reestablished. Treatment is typically supportive after the offending agent is discontinued. As with relief of other forms of obstructive uropathy, a polyuric phase may occur.

Intrinsic Renal

Causes of intrinsic renal failure can be divided anatomically into tubular, glomerular/vascular, and interstitial categories. Disease can be primarily renal in nature, or part of a systemic process.

- **Tubular**
  - **Ischemic ATN** is the most common cause of renal failure in the intensive care setting, and is the end result of any process that leads to significant hypoperfusion of the kidneys, including sepsis, hemorrhage, or any prolonged prerenal insult.
    - The injury results in the sloughing of renal tubular cells, which can congeal with cellular debris in a matrix of Tamm–Horsfall protein to form granular casts. These have a "muddy brown" appearance and are strongly suggestive of ATN in the proper context. The FE_{Na} ($>1\%$) and FE_{Urea} ($>50\%$) are typically elevated as the tubules lose their ability to concentrate the urine.
    - Management of ATN is supportive, with avoidance of further nephrotoxic insults. Fluid management is aimed at maintaining euvolemia. Volume deficits, if present, should be corrected. If volume overload and oliguria become evident, a diuretic challenge is reasonable, typically with intravenous furosemide (40 to 120 mg boluses or a continuous drip at 10 to 20 mg/hr). This has not been shown to hasten recovery but can simplify overall management.
    - Recovery from ATN may take days to weeks to occur but can be expected in over 85% of patients with a previously normal Cr. Dialysis may be necessary to bridge the time to recovery.
  - Toxic ATN can result from endogenous chemicals (e.g., hemoglobin, myoglobin) or exogenous medications (e.g., iodinated contrast, aminoglycosides). These forms share many of the diagnostic features of ischemic ATN.
    - **Iodinated contrast** is a potent renal vasoconstrictor and is toxic to renal tubules. When renal injury occurs, the Cr typically rises 24 hours after exposure and peaks in 3 to 5 days. Risk factors for contrast nephropathy include CKD, diabetes, volume depletion, heart failure, higher contrast volumes, and use of hyperosmolar contrast. Preventative measures include periprocedure hydration and discontinuation of diuretics. Sodium bicarbonate at 154 mEq/L (three ampules in D5 Water [D5W]) can be given at 3 mL/kg/hr for 1 hour prior to exposure, then at 1 mL/kg/hr for 6 hours after the procedure (*JAMA 2004;291:2328*). Acetylcysteine may reduce the incidence of contrast nephropathy and is given as four oral doses of 1,200 mg 12 hours apart, with two doses given prior to the contrast study.
    - **Aminoglycoside nephrotoxicity** is typically nonoliguric, occurs from direct toxicity to the proximal tubules, and results in the renal wasting of potassium and magnesium. Replacement of these electrolytes may become necessary. A similar pattern of potassium and magnesium loss is seen in cisplatin toxicity. A prolonged exposure to the aminoglycoside of at least 5 days is required. Peak and trough levels correlate poorly with the risk of developing renal injury. Risk may be minimized by avoiding volume depletion and by using the extended-interval dosing method (see Chapter 15, Antimicrobials).

- **Pigment nephropathy** results from direct tubular toxicity by hemoglobin and myoglobin. Vasoconstriction may also play a role. The diagnosis may be suspected by a positive urine dipstick test for blood but an absence of RBCs on microscopic examination. In **rhabdomyolysis**, the creatine kinase (CK) level is elevated to at least 10 times the upper limit of normal with a disproportionate rise in Cr, potassium, and phosphorus. Aggressive intravenous fluid administration should be initiated immediately, and large quantities are generally required to replace the fluid lost into necrotic muscle tissue. If urine flow is established, alkalinization with sodium bicarbonate (154 mEq/L, approximately three ampules) can increase the solubility of these pigments, although this maneuver may worsen the hypocalcemia and is of limited benefit.
  - In the treatment of hematologic malignancies, acute uric acid nephropathy can result as part of the **tumor lysis syndrome**. In addition to the elevated Cr, there is typically hyperuricemia, hyperphosphatemia, and hypocalcemia. A ratio of urine uric acid to urine Cr that is >1 is consistent with this diagnosis. Prophylaxis with allopurinol 600 mg can decrease uric acid production. Rasburicase (15 mg/kg intravenously) is highly effective at depleting uric acid levels and can be given as prophylaxis or as treatment. Alkalinization of the urine should be avoided if hyperphosphatemia is present as this could increase the risk of calcium phosphate precipitation in the urine.
- **Glomerular/vascular**
  - The finding of **dysmorphic urinary RBCs, RBC casts, or proteinuria in the nephrotic range (>3.5 g/d)** strongly suggests the presence of a glomerular disease. This group encompasses a large variety of primary renal or systemic disorders. Glomerular diseases are described individually in further detail later in this chapter.
  - A small subgroup of glomerular diseases can present with rapidly deteriorating renal function, termed **rapidly progressive glomerulonephritis** (RPGN). A nephritic picture is common, with RBC casts, edema, and hypertension. A renal biopsy may reveal the specific underlying disease, but crescent formation in >50% of glomeruli is usually present. For those deemed to have salvageable renal function, management is with high-dose pulse glucocorticoid therapy (intravenous methylprednisolone 7 to 15 mg/kg/d for 3 days) followed by a course of oral prednisone (1 mg/kg/d for 1 month, then tapered over the next 6 to 12 months). Cyclophosphamide is typically added to this regimen, with monthly intravenous doses ($1 g/m^2$) having less cumulative toxicity than the daily oral dosing strategy (2 mg/kg/d).
  - Thrombotic microangiopathy (TMA) includes both **hemolytic–uremic syndrome (HUS) and thrombotic thrombocytopenic purpura (TTP)**. These diseases share many of the same characteristics. Causes include bacterial toxins (diarrheal forms), medications (mitomycin-C, clopidogrel, cyclosporine, tacrolimus), and may be associated with pregnancy or malignancies of the gastrointestinal tract. Diagnosis and therapy are discussed in Chapter 20, Disorders of Hemostasis and Thrombosis.
  - **Atheroembolic disease** can be seen in patients with diffuse atherosclerosis after undergoing an invasive aortic or other large artery manipulation, including cardiac catheterization, coronary bypass surgery, aortic aneurysm repair, and placement of an intra-aortic balloon pump. Physical findings may include retinal arteriolar plaques, lower extremity livedo reticularis, and areas of digital necrosis. Eosinophilia, eosinophiluria, and hypocomplementemia may be present, and WBC casts may be found in the urine sediment. However, in many cases, the only laboratory abnormality is a rising Cr that follows a stepwise progression.

Renal biopsy shows cholesterol clefts in the small arteries. Anticoagulation may worsen embolic disease and should be avoided if possible. No specific treatment is available. Many patients progress to CKD, and even to end-stage renal disease (ESRD).

- **Interstitial**
  - **AIN** involves inflammation of the renal parenchyma, typically caused by medications or infections. The classic triad of **fever, rash, and eosinophilia** is seen in less than one-third of patients and their absence does not exclude the diagnosis. Pyuria, WBC casts, and eosinophiluria are all also suggestive of AIN. Beta-lactam antibiotics are the most frequently cited causative agents, but nearly all antibiotics can be implicated. The time course typically requires exposure for at least 5 to 10 days before renal impairment occurs. Other medications, such as proton pump inhibitors and allopurinol, have been associated with AIN. NSAIDs can produce AIN with nephrotic range proteinuria. Streptococcal infections, leptospirosis, and sarcoidosis have all been implicated in AIN.
  - Treatment is principally the withdrawal of the offending agent. Renal recovery typically ensues, although the time course is variable, and temporary dialytic support may be necessary in severe cases. A short course of prednisone at 1 mg/kg/d may hasten recovery.
  - Parenchymal infections with **pyelonephritis or renal abscesses** are uncommon causes of AKI. Bilateral involvement is usually necessary to induce a rise in Cr. Urine findings include pyuria and WBC casts, and antibiotic therapy is guided by culture results.

TREATMENT

- Disease-specific therapies are covered earlier. With advanced renal failure, general complications can be anticipated and addressed.
- **Hyperkalemia**, when mild (<6 mEq/L), can be treated with dietary potassium restriction and potassium-binding resins (e.g., sodium polystyrene sulfonate). When further elevated or accompanied by electrocardiogram abnormalities, immediate medical therapy is indicated, with calcium gluconate, insulin and glucose, inhaled beta-agonist, and possibly bicarbonate (see Chapter 12, Fluid and Electrolyte Management). Severe hyperkalemia that is refractory to medical management is an indication for urgent dialysis.
- Mild **metabolic acidosis** can be treated with oral sodium bicarbonate, 650 to 1,300 mg thrice daily. Severe acidosis (pH <7.2) can be temporized with intravenous sodium bicarbonate but requires monitoring for volume overload, rebound alkalosis, and hypocalcemia. Acidosis that is refractory to medical management is an indication for urgent dialysis.
- **Volume overload** can complicate AKI. After volume deficits are corrected, the goal of fluid management should be to keep input equal to output. In the oliguric setting, a trial of diuretics (usually high-dose loop diuretics in a bolus or as a continuous drip) may simplify management. Volume overload causing respiratory compromise that is refractory to medical management is an indication for urgent dialysis.
- **Anemia** is common in AKI and is usually caused by decreased RBC production and increased blood loss. Gastrointestinal bleeding may be exacerbated by uremic platelet dysfunction and may respond to DDAVP 0.3 mcg/kg. Transfusion is

appropriate for patients with symptoms attributable to anemia. Erythropoiesis stimulating agents (e.g., epoetin) are not effective for short-term correction of anemia.

SPECIAL CONSIDERATIONS

- All patients with AKI require daily assessment to determine the need for renal replacement therapy. It is preferable to initiate dialytic support before significant uremia develops or a life-threatening complication becomes evident. Patients suffering from acute oliguric renal failure who are not expected to recover promptly likely benefit from earlier initiation of dialysis.
- Severe acidosis, hyperkalemia, or volume overload refractory to medical management mandates the initiation of dialysis. Certain drug and alcohol intoxications (methanol, ethylene glycol, or salicylates) should be treated with hemodialysis. Uremic pericarditis (with a friction rub) or encephalopathy should also be treated promptly with renal replacement therapy. Issues specific to dialysis techniques are discussed later in this chapter.

Glomerulopathies

GENERAL PRINCIPLES

Classification
- The presentation of glomerular diseases can be thought of as existing on a continuum. On one end is the nephrotic syndrome, characterized by proteinuria >3.5 g/d, and accompanied by hypoalbuminemia, hyperlipidemia, and edema. On the other end of the spectrum is the nephritic syndrome, characterized by hematuria, hypertension, edema, and renal insufficiency. Most specific disease entities present somewhere in between, with overlapping features, but with a tendency to produce one syndrome over the other.
- Biopsy findings also correlate with these syndromes. Nephrotic diseases typically show injury along the filtration barrier, with thickening of the glomerular basement membrane or fusion of the podocyte foot processes. By comparison, nephritic diseases generally show varying degrees of mesangial cell proliferation and mesangial deposition.

TREATMENT

- Specific therapies for individual glomerular diseases are discussed in the following text. However, many disorders share the same features and general therapeutic maneuvers can be addressed as a group.
- Glomerular disease presenting with proteinuria should rely on treatment with **ACE inhibitors or ARBs** to reduce the intraglomerular pressure. Efficacy can be monitored by serial urine protein-to-creatinine ratios. Electrolytes and Cr should be checked within 1 to 2 weeks of initiation of therapy or an increase in dose to document stability of renal function and potassium. Modest dietary protein restriction to 0.8 g/kg/d may slow progression, but this remains controversial.

- Edema and volume overload can usually be effectively managed with **diuretics** combined with **salt restriction**. Aggressive treatment of hypertension can also slow progression of renal disease.
- The hyperlipidemia associated with the nephrotic syndrome responds to dietary modification and **statins (HMG-CoA reductase inhibitors)**. They are effective at improving the lipoprotein profile and may slow renal decline.
- The nephrotic syndrome produces a hypercoagulable state and can predispose to thromboembolic complications. Deep venous thrombi and renal vein thrombosis may occur and should be treated with heparin anticoagulation followed by long-term warfarin therapy. Prophylactic anticoagulation is controversial and may be beneficial in severely nephrotic patients, particularly with membranous nephropathy (MN). Exact mechanism of thrombosis remain controversial but likely include urinary loss of anti-clotting proteins, increased synthesis of clotting factors, or by local activation of the glomerular hemostasis system.
- When **immunosuppression** is considered, the risk of therapy should always be weighed against the potential benefit. Renal salvageability should be addressed and patients with advanced disease on presentation who are unlikely to benefit from such treatment may be better served by avoiding the risks of high-dose immunosuppression. Cytotoxic agents (e.g., cyclophosphamide, chlorambucil) require close monitoring of WBC counts, checked at least weekly at the initiation of therapy. Dose adjustments may be needed to maintain the WBC count above 3,500 cells/μL. Rituximab, a monoclonal antibody directed against CD20, has shown promise in a variety of immune-mediated disorders, including severe lupus nephritis (LN), MN, and ANCA-positive vasculitis where it has been given intravenously as four weekly doses of 375 mg/m^2 (*N Engl J Med 2010;363:221*).

PRIMARY GLOMERULOPATHIES

Minimal Change Disease

GENERAL PRINCIPLES

Epidemiology

Minimal change disease (MCD) is the most common cause of the nephrotic syndrome in children but has a second peak in adults aged 50 to 60 years. Typically, there is sudden onset of proteinuria with hypertension and edema as well as the full nephrotic syndrome, although renal insufficiency is unusual.

Associated Conditions

Secondary forms of MCD may accompany certain malignancies (Hodgkin disease and solid tumors being the most common). A form of interstitial nephritis associated with NSAID use may also be associated with MCD.

DIAGNOSIS

The kidney biopsy reveals normal glomeruli on light microscopy and negative immunofluorescence. Electron microscopy shows effacement of the foot processes as the only histological abnormality.

TREATMENT

- In adults, treatment with oral prednisone at 1 mg/kg/d may induce remission (decrease in proteinuria) in 8 to 16 weeks. Once in remission, the steroids can be tapered over 3 months then discontinued. The urine protein excretion should be followed during this taper.
- Relapse may occur in up to 75% of adults. Reinstitution of prednisone is often effective. If the patient is steroid dependent or steroid resistant, cytotoxic agents may be needed, with cyclophosphamide 2 mg/kg/d or chlorambucil 0.2 mg/kg/d. Cyclosporine 5 mg/kg/d is an alternative therapy.

Focal Segmental Glomerulosclerosis

GENERAL PRINCIPLES

- Focal segmental glomerulosclerosis (FSGS) is not a single disease but rather a descriptive classification for diseases with shared histopathology. Presentation is with the nephrotic syndrome, hypertension, and renal insufficiency.
- Secondary forms of FSGS are associated with obesity, HIV (collapsing variant), and intravenous drug abuse.

DIAGNOSIS

The kidney biopsy reveals focal and segmental sclerosis of glomeruli under light microscopy. The degree of interstitial fibrosis and tubular atrophy (rather than glomerular scarring) correlates with prognosis. Immunofluorescence shows staining for C3 and IgM in areas of sclerosis, representing areas of trapped immune deposits. Electron microscopy shows effacement of the podocyte foot processes.

TREATMENT

For patients with nephrotic range proteinuria, a trial of prednisone 1 mg/kg/d can be attempted for 16 weeks. Patients who relapse after a period of apparent responsiveness may benefit from a repeat course of steroids. Nonresponders and relapsers may respond to treatment with cyclosporine 5 mg/kg/d. Cyclophosphamide and mycophenolate mofetil can also be used. Induction of a complete remission (<0.3 g/d) or a partial remission (50% reduction in proteinuria and <3.5 g/d) is associated with significantly slower loss of renal function.

Membranous Nephropathy

GENERAL PRINCIPLES

- MN usually presents with the nephrotic syndrome or heavy proteinuria, while renal function is often normal or near normal. Disease progression is variable, with one-third remitting spontaneously, one-third progressing to ESRD, and one-third with an intermediate course.

- Secondary forms of MN are associated with SLE (class V), viral hepatitis, syphilis, or solid organ malignancies. Medications such as gold and penicillamine can also induce this process.

DIAGNOSIS

Kidney biopsy shows thickening of the glomerular basement membrane on light microscopy, with "spikes" on silver stain, representing areas of normal basement membrane interposed between subepithelial deposits. These deposits correlate with IgG and C3 on immunofluorescence and are also seen on electron microscopy. Antibodies to the podocyte antigen phospholipase A_2 receptor have been implicated in 70% of adult idiopathic MN, although serologic testing is currently only used in the research setting.

TREATMENT

Because of the generally good prognosis, specific therapy should be reserved for patients at higher risk for progression (reduced GFR, male gender, age >50 years, hypertension), or nephrotic range proteinuria. Treatment options include regimens with prednisone 0.5 mg/kg/d and cytotoxic agents (chlorambucil 0.2 mg/kg/d or cyclophosphamide 2.5 mg/kg/d) on alternating months for 6 to 12 months.

Membranoproliferative Glomerulonephropathy

GENERAL PRINCIPLES

Primary idiopathic membranoproliferative glomerulonephropathy (MPGN) is uncommon. Hepatitis C accounts for most cases of secondary MPGN, frequently in association with cryoglobulinemia. Other secondary causes include SLE, chronic infections, and various malignancies.

DIAGNOSIS

Clinical Presentation

MPGN can present with the nephrotic syndrome, nephritic syndrome, or a combination of both. Classically, there are three defined subtypes of MPGN (I, II, and III). However, as the molecular basis for disease is elucidated, an alternate classification has been proposed (*N Engl J Med 2012;366:1119*). Types I and III are mediated through immune complex formation. Type II MPGN (also called dense-deposit disease) and the related disorder C3 glomerulonephritis (C3GN) depend on activation of the alternative complement pathway. Both C3 and C4 are usually low in the immune complex-mediated forms of MPGN while only C3 is low in Type II MPGN. The antibody "C3-nephritic factor" may be present in Type II MPGN, stabilizing the C3-convertase and promoting complement consumption. Deficiencies of or antibodies against the complement regulators (factors H and I) may also activate the complement cascade.

Diagnostic Testing

The kidney biopsy shows mesangial proliferation and hypercellularity on light microscopy, with "lobulization" of the glomerular tuft. Accumulation of debris along the filtration barrier may lead to a damage–repair cycle that results in duplication of the glomerular basement membrane giving a double-contour or "tram-track" appearance on silver stain. Immunofluorescence can show granular mesangial and capillary wall deposits of Ig in the immune complex-mediated forms while only the C3 staining is positive in Type II MPGN or C3GN. Electron microscopy can show subendothelial (Type I) or intramembranous (Type II) deposits. Type III disease has subendothelial and subepithelial deposits.

TREATMENT

In adult idiopathic MPGN, treatment with immunosuppression has not shown a consistent benefit, although this may have been a result of the lumping together of pathophysiologically dissimilar diseases under the older classification scheme. Treatment of the secondary forms is targeted at the underlying disease. If renal function is rapidly deteriorating in the presence of cryoglobulins, plasmapheresis may help stabilize disease. Case reports have demonstrated possible efficacy of eculizumab, an anti-C5 monoclonal antibody, in the treatment of Type II MPGN (*N Engl J Med 2012;366:1161*).

IgA Nephropathy/Henoch–Schönlein Purpura

DIAGNOSIS

Clinical Presentation

- IgA nephropathy is typically idiopathic, characterized by a nephritic picture with microscopic (and less commonly macroscopic) hematuria, and mild nonnephrotic range proteinuria. Presentation is most commonly in the second or third decade of life, generally following a slowly progressive course. However, some patients may exhibit a crescentic form with a rapid decline in renal function resulting in ESRD.
- Henoch–Schönlein purpura is a related disorder that may represent a systemic form of the same disease, with vasculitic involvement of the skin (palpable purpura of the lower trunk and extremities), gastrointestinal tract, and joints.

Diagnostic Testing

Kidney biopsy shows increased mesangial cellularity on light microscopy, with IgA and C3 deposition on immunofluorescence. Abnormally glycosylated IgA is thought to be responsible for immune complex formation and mesangial deposition. Although serum IgA levels do not correlate with disease activity, events that potentially lead to overproduction (concurrent upper respiratory infection) or decreased clearance (hepatic cirrhosis) may predispose to disease.

TREATMENT

Aggressiveness of therapy depends on severity of disease. For patients with a benign course, conservative management with ACE inhibitors, ARBs, or fish oil (omega-3 fatty acids) may prevent deterioration of renal function, although the benefit of fish oil remains controversial. Progressive disease may benefit from a course of prednisone 1 mg/kg/d with or without cytotoxic agents.

Pulmonary–Renal Syndromes

DIAGNOSIS

Clinical Presentation

Several distinct clinical entities make up the pulmonary–renal syndromes where there is vasculitic involvement of the alveolar and glomerular capillaries. Typically, this results in rapidly progressive renal failure often with concurrent pulmonary involvement in the form of alveolar hemorrhage. A nephritic picture predominates, with dysmorphic RBCs and RBC casts in the urine. Arthralgias and fever may represent other systemic manifestations.

Differential Diagnosis

- In **anti-GBM antibody disease**, circulating antibody to the alpha-3 chain of Type IV collagen is deposited in the basement membrane of alveoli and glomeruli, resulting in linear staining on immunofluorescence. Goodpasture's syndrome includes pulmonary involvement and can present with life-threatening alveolar hemorrhage. The presence of anti-GBM antibody in the serum supports the diagnosis, and 10% to 30% of patients will have a positive ANCA serology as well.
- In **granulomatosis with polyangiitis** (GPA, formerly known as Wegener's granulomatosis), vasculitic lesions involve the small vessels of the kidneys and may also involve the lungs, skin, and gastrointestinal tract. As in anti-GBM antibody disease, pulmonary hemorrhage may be life threatening. Biopsy findings include a small vessel vasculitis with noncaseating granuloma formation in the kidneys, lungs, or sinuses. GPA is part of a group of diseases known as pauci-immune glomerulonephritis (referring to the absence of immunostaining deposits), including Churg–Strauss syndrome (asthma and eosinophilia) and microscopic polyangiitis. In GPA, there is a positive cytoplasmic ANCA directed against serine proteinase-3, while in microscopic polyangiitis and Churg–Strauss syndrome, there is a positive perinuclear ANCA directed against myeloperoxidase.

TREATMENT

- In anti-GBM antibody disease, the goal of therapy is to clear the pathogenic antibody while suppressing new production. Treatment is with daily total volume plasmapheresis for approximately 14 days in conjunction with cyclophosphamide 2 mg/kg/d and glucocorticoids (intravenous methylprednisolone 7 to 15 mg/kg/d for 3 days, followed by oral prednisone 1 mg/kg/d). Immunosuppression is tapered over 8 weeks. Serial measurement of the anti-GBM antibody level is useful to monitor therapy with plasmapheresis and immunosuppression continuing until it is undetectable. Poor response to therapy is predicted by the presence of oliguria, Cr >5.7 mg/dL, or dialysis dependence on presentation. Even if the likelihood of renal recovery is low, evidence of pulmonary involvement warrants aggressive therapy.
- Treatment of GPA is with combined prednisone 1 mg/kg/d (with taper) and cyclophosphamide (intravenous at 1 g/m^2 or orally at 2 mg/kg/d) for at least

3 months to induce remission. Therapy should then continue with oral steroids for 1 year to prevent relapse. Double-strength sulfamethoxazole–trimethoprim given twice daily has been shown to reduce extrarenal relapses and to prevent *Pneumocystis (carinii) jiroveci* infection for patients on high-dose immunosuppression. More aggressive management with plasmapheresis and pulse intravenous steroids may be beneficial for patients presenting with pulmonary hemorrhage or dialysis dependence. Recently, rituximab given intravenously as four weekly doses of 375 mg/m^2, in combination with steroids, has been approved for treatment of GPA (*N Engl J Med 2010;363:221*).

SECONDARY GLOMERULOPATHIES

Diabetic Nephropathy

DIAGNOSIS

Diagnostic Criteria

Diabetic nephropathy (DN) is the most common cause of ESRD in the United States. Albuminuria is "microscopic" when levels are 30 to 300 mg/g Cr. Overt nephropathy is characterized by albuminuria >300 mg/g Cr. Early disease has glomerular hyperfiltration with an elevated GFR, followed by a linear decline that may progress to ESRD.

Diagnostic Testing

Kidney biopsy is not usually performed, unless the rate of renal decline is more rapid than would be anticipated, suggesting another possible diagnosis. Histology for DN shows glomerular sclerosis with nodular mesangial expansion (Kimmelstiel–Wilson nodules) on light microscopy. Immunofluorescence does not reveal immune deposition. Electron microscopy may show GBM thickening.

TREATMENT

Treatment is centered on aggressive control of glucose and blood pressure. Specific hyperglycemic therapy is discussed further in Chapter 23, Diabetes Mellitus and Related Disorders. An ACE inhibitor or ARB is considered the first-line agent in the treatment of hypertension in diabetic patients and can offer better control of proteinuria. Studies combining ACE inhibitors with an ARB or the direct renin inhibitor aliskiren have shown worse renal and cardiovascular outcomes (*N Engl J Med 2008;358:1547*).

Lupus Nephritis

DIAGNOSIS

Diagnostic Testing

Laboratories

LN can manifest as proteinuria of varying degrees with dysmorphic RBCs and RBC casts, and renal insufficiency. Positive lupus serology (e.g., ANA, anti-double-stranded DNA antibodies) and hypocomplementemia are often present during acute flares.

Diagnostic Procedures

Renal biopsy can provide useful information on disease activity and prognosis. The World Health Organization classification has five major categories based on histologic appearance. Class I has normal glomeruli, classes II to IV have increasing degrees of mesangial proliferation, and class V has an appearance similar to MN. Immunofluorescence is usually positive for IgG, IgA, IgM, C1q, C3, and C4, for the "full-house" fluorescence pattern.

TREATMENT

Aggressiveness of therapy considers the renal and extrarenal manifestations of the disease. Classes I and II LN rarely require specific treatment and therapy is directed at the extrarenal manifestations. Class III LN, when mild or moderate, can generally be treated with a short course of high-dose steroids (prednisone 1 mg/kg/d). Patients with more severe class III or class IV LN should undergo pulse intravenous methylprednisolone (7 to 15 mg/kg/d for 3 days) followed by oral prednisone at 0.5 to 1.0 mg/kg/d. A second agent should be used and can be monthly intravenous cyclophosphamide 0.5 to 1.0 g/m^2 or oral mycophenolate mofetil 1,000 mg thrice daily for a course of 6 months. Remission can be maintained for several years with mycophenolate mofetil 1,000 mg twice daily, which was shown to be superior to azathioprine 2 mg/kg/d in preventing relapse (*N Engl J Med 2011;365:1886*). As the prognosis of class V LN is better as compared to classes III or IV, treatment is reserved primarily for patients with severe nephrotic syndrome, with a short course of high-dose steroids (prednisone 1 mg/kg/d).

Postinfectious Glomerulonephropathy

DIAGNOSIS

Clinical Presentation

Postinfectious glomerulonephropathy (GN) classically presents with the nephritic syndrome of hematuria, hypertension, edema, and renal insufficiency. Proteinuria may be present and is usually in subnephrotic range. Streptococcal infection typically affects children under the age of 10 years, after a latent period of 2 to 4 weeks from onset of pharyngitis or skin infection. Bacterial endocarditis, visceral abscesses, and ventriculoperitoneal shunt infections can also lead to this immune complex–mediated disease. Low complement levels are usually seen. ASO titers may be elevated serially as may anti-DNaseB antibodies in streptococcal-associated disease.

Diagnostic Testing

Kidney biopsy reveals subepithelial humps on light and electron microscopy corresponding to the deposits on immunofluorescence (IgG, C3). There is widespread mesangial proliferation as well as an infiltration of polymorphonuclear cells.

TREATMENT

Treatment of the renal disease is primarily supportive. Resolution of the underlying infection typically leads to renal recovery in 2 to 4 weeks, even in cases where dialytic support was needed. A brisk diuresis should be anticipated in the recovery period.

Deposition Disorders/Dysproteinemias

DIAGNOSIS

Differential Diagnosis

Dysproteinemias include **amyloidosis, light chain deposition disease (LCDD), heavy chain deposition disease (HCDD), fibrillary glomerulopathy, and immunotactoid glomerulopathy**. Multiple myeloma may be associated with amyloidosis or LCDD. These disorders can affect the kidney in a variety of ways, including glomerular or tubular deposition, formation of insoluble protein casts in the tubules (micro-obstructive cast nephropathy), or through hypercalcemia and volume depletion. Glomerular deposition is typically associated with heavy proteinuria due to overflow as well as disruption of filtration barrier integrity.

Diagnostic Testing

Laboratories

Diagnosis is suggested by an abnormal monoclonal protein found in the SPEP or UPEP. Ig chains are not detected by routine urine dipstick and may be missed unless glomerular involvement has led to general protein leakage.

Diagnostic Procedures

- Biopsy of the kidney can show characteristic deposits. For amyloidosis, this appears as Congo Red–positive beta-pleated fibrils of 10 nm in diameter under electron microscopy. Immunofluorescence can identify the specific Ig chains for LCDD (more likely to occur with kappa light chains) and HCDD. Fibrillary and immunotactoid deposits are Congo Red negative. The fibrils of fibrillary glomerulopathy (12 to 20 nm) are typically thicker than those for amyloid while the microtubules of immunotactoid glomerulopathy are even wider (20 to 60 nm) with a visible lumen in cross-section, with a strong association with myelodysplastic disorders.
- When cast nephropathy is implicated in a dysproteinemic disorder, the biopsy shows enlarged tubules filled with proteinaceous material. Immunofluorescence can identify the specific components of these casts.

TREATMENT

Melphalan and prednisone are beneficial in the treatment of amyloidosis and LCDD. Chemotherapy aimed at the underlying disease can be effective in reversing renal disease. When cast nephropathy is present on biopsy, a course of plasmapheresis in conjunction with treatment of the myeloma may stabilize renal function. There is no specific treatment for fibrillary or immunotactoid glomerulopathy, although addressing an underlying malignancy, if present, may slow progression in the latter.

HIV-Associated Nephropathy

DIAGNOSIS

- HIV-associated nephropathy (HIVAN) is characterized by nephrotic range proteinuria, edema, and hypertension with or without an elevated Cr. Kidneys are typically enlarged (>12 cm) on ultrasonography.

- On biopsy, HIVAN has the appearance of the collapsing variant of FSGS, with proliferative podocytes. However, it should be mentioned that HIV can produce secondary forms of other glomerular diseases, including MPGN and MN.
- In the current era of antiretroviral therapy, HIVAN is less common. Renal dysfunction in patients with HIV is now more commonly due to the antiretroviral medications, with HIVAN generally limited to untreated or noncomplaint patients. Nucleotide reverse transcriptase inhibitor tenofovir is a notable cause of proximal tubular injury; protease inhibitor indinavir can cause nephrolithiasis, obstructive nephropathy, and can also result in interstitial nephritis from crystal deposits (*Adv Chronic Kidney Dis. 2010;17(1):72*).

TREATMENT

The widespread use of antiretroviral therapy has improved the overall outcomes of HIVAN, allowing stabilization of renal function and proteinuria. Use of ACE inhibitors and ARBs can also help reduce the degree of proteinuria.

Polycystic Kidney Disease

GENERAL PRINCIPLES

Epidemiology

Autosomal dominant polycystic kidney disease (ADPKD) is a hereditary disorder resulting in cystic enlargement of the kidney. Prevalence is approximately 1/1,000. There are two well-described mutations in the polycystin genes, with PKD1 being the most common (85%). PKD2 is associated with a later onset of disease.

Pathophysiology

The polycystin gene products primarily localize to the cilia of the tubular apical membrane where they are thought to sense flow. Disordered regulation of cell division may lead to overgrowth of the tubular segment, eventually pinching off from the rest of the collecting system. Cyst formation affects only a relatively small percentage of tubules, suggesting a "two-hit" hypothesis where a sporadic mutation of the wild-type allele results in local cystogenesis.

Associated Conditions

- Onset of kidney failure is highly variable, with half of patients reaching ESRD by the age of 60.
- Hypertension is an early feature of ADPKD. As the affected tubules enlarge, they impinge upon the blood flow to neighboring glomeruli, rendering them ischemic. This is turn activates the renin–angiotensin–aldosterone system leading to systemic hypertension.
- Cerebral aneurysms, hepatic cysts, mitral valve prolapse, and colonic diverticula are features found in association with ADPKD. Patients with a family history of cerebral aneurysms or with symptoms attributable to a cerebral aneurysm should undergo evaluation with brain MRI/MRA.
- As cysts enlarge, they may result in a palpable flank mass. Gross hematuria and pain may indicate cysts hemorrhage into the collecting system. Flank pain may also be caused by cyst infection or stretching of the renal capsule.

DIAGNOSIS

- Ultrasonography reveals multiple cysts. In the setting of a positive family history, a diagnosis of ADPKD can be made from ultrasound findings, with criteria differing according to age. At least three cysts are required in patients under the age of 40 years. In patients aged 40 to 59 years, at least two cysts in each kidney are needed. For patients 60 years and older, the diagnosis requires at least four cysts in each kidney.
- Approximately 20% of patients with ADPKD do not have a positive family history. Differentiation from other cystic diseases (acquired cystic disease, medullary sponge kidney, medullary cystic kidney disease) can be made by the presence of enlarged cystic kidneys rather than shrunken or normal-sized cystic kidneys.

TREATMENT

- There is currently no specific treatment to prevent cyst formation or slow cyst growth. Aggressive control of hypertension should be practiced and blockade of the renin–angiotensin–aldosterone system with an ACE inhibitor or ARB is recommended as first-line therapy.
- Gross hematuria from cyst hemorrhage can usually be managed with bed rest, hydration, and analgesia. Resolution may take 5 to 7 days.
- Cyst infections are generally treated with antibiotics that achieve good penetration into the cysts. Sulfamethoxazole-trimethoprim or ciprofloxacin are the antibiotics of choice. The absence of bacterial growth in the urine does not rule out infection since the cystic fluid does not generally communicate with the rest of the collecting system.
- Pain that persists without an obvious hemorrhagic or infectious cause may respond to cyst reduction surgery, particularly if there is a culprit cyst that can be identified and targeted.
- As the underlying mechanism for cyst growth is clarified, newer treatment options are emerging. Trials lasting 2 years for the antimetabolites sirolimus and everolimus have been disappointing, whereas trials using tolvaptan, octreotide, and water therapy are ongoing.

PROGRESSIVE LOSS OF RENAL FUNCTION

Chronic Kidney Disease

GENERAL PRINCIPLES

Classification

- CKD is divided into five stages based on the estimated GFR (Table 13-3). To be classified as stage 1 or stage 2, there must be an accompanying structural or functional defect (e.g., proteinuria, hematuria) as the GFR is normal or near normal in these stages. Treatment goals are frequently guided by CKD stage.
- Patients are usually asymptomatic until significant renal function is lost (late stage 4 and stage 5). However, complications including hypertension, anemia, and bone mineral disease (renal osteodystrophy [ROD] and secondary hyperparathyroidism)

Table 13-3	Stages of Chronic Kidney Disease
CKD Stage	**Glomerular Filtration Rate**
1	>90 mL/min
2	60–89 mL/min
3	30–59 mL/min
4	15–29 mL/min
5	<15 mL/min or dialysis

CKD, chronic kidney disease.

often develop during stage 3 and thus must be investigated and addressed before patients become symptomatic.

- The decline in GFR may be followed by plotting the reciprocal of Cr versus time; revealing a linear decrement. This can be useful in end-stage planning and in predicting when renal replacement therapy will be needed. Initiation of dialysis based solely on a target GFR has not shown a mortality benefit (*N Engl J Med 2010;363:609*). In CKD, dialysis should be started prior to the worsening of the patient's metabolic or nutritional status. A steeper than anticipated decline in GFR suggests a superimposed renal insult.

Risk Factors

- Decreased renal perfusion can lead to a decline in GFR. This can occur with true volume depletion or diminished effective circulating volume (e.g., congestive heart failure, hepatic cirrhosis). The use of **NSAIDs** can be particularly deleterious in this setting as they block the renal autoregulatory mechanisms to preserve GFR. ACE inhibitors or ARBs can also produce a reversible decrement in GFR.
- **Uncontrolled hypertension** can also be harmful to kidneys. Hyperfiltration may lead to worsening proteinuria and further damage to the glomeruli.
- **Nephrotoxic agents**, such as iodinated contrast agents and aminoglycosides, should be avoided when possible. Careful attention to drug dosing is mandatory, frequently guided by the estimated GFR or CKD stage. Drug levels should be monitored where appropriate.
- Patients undergoing coronary angiography are at particular risk for worsening CKD. **Contrast nephropathy and atheroembolic disease** are potential complications and the risks and benefits of the procedure must be weighed with the patient prior to proceeding.
- **UTI or obstruction** should be considered in all patients with an unexplained drop in renal function. Worsening renal artery stenosis may also lead to a more rapid decline in GFR as well as sudden worsening in previously controlled hypertension.
- **Renal vein thrombosis** may occur as a complication of the nephrotic syndrome and can exacerbate CKD. Hematuria and flank pain may occur.

TREATMENT

- Treatment of CKD is focused on avoidance of risk factors (listed earlier), dietary modification, blood pressure control, adequate treatment of the associated conditions (listed in the following text), and ultimately, preparation for renal replacement therapy.

- **Dietary restrictions**
  - **Sodium restriction** to less than 3 g/d is usually adequate for most CKD patients. Restriction to less than 2 g/d should be employed if heart failure or refractory hypertension is present. A 24-hour urine sodium level of 100 mEq roughly correlates with a 2 g/d diet.
  - Fluid restriction is generally not required in CKD patients and, if excessive, may lead to volume depletion and hypernatremia. Restriction is appropriate in patients with dilutional hyponatremia, or if AKI occurs.
  - **Potassium should be restricted** to 60 mEq/d in individuals with hyperkalemia. Tomato-based products, bananas, potatoes, and citrus drinks are high in potassium and should be avoided in these patients.
  - **Dietary phosphate restriction** should be to 800 to 1,000 mg/d. Dairy products, dark colas, and nuts should be avoided in hyperphosphatemia. Oral binders (calcium carbonate or acetate, lanthanum carbonate, sevelamer carbonate) can be used if dietary restrictions are unable to control phosphate levels.
- **Hypertension**
  - Uncontrolled hypertension accelerates the rate of decline of renal function. Intensive control of blood pressure in patients with CKD to <130/80 may have benefit in patients with baseline proteinuria (*N Engl J Med 2010;363:918*).
  - **ACE inhibitors and ARBs** should be used preferentially in the CKD population. They lower intraglomerular pressure and possess renoprotective properties beyond the antihypertensive effect, particularly in proteinuric states. Due to their effects on intrarenal hemodynamics, a 30% rise in serum Cr should be anticipated and tolerated; a further rise should prompt a search for possible renal artery stenosis. The Cr and serum potassium should be checked approximately 1 to 2 weeks after a dose adjustment.
  - **Diuretics** are also beneficial in achieving euvolemia in hypertensive CKD patients. Thiazide diuretics become less effective as the GFR falls below 30 mL/min, while loop diuretics retain their efficacy although higher doses may be required for the desired effect.
- **Anemia**
  - A normocytic anemia is common in CKD, and should be searched for once the GFR falls below 60 mL/min (stage 3).
  - Alternate causes for an anemia should be entertained in the appropriate setting and iron stores assessed. If the transferrin saturation is <25% and there is no evidence of iron overload (ferritin <1000 ng/mL), consideration should be given to iron repletion with 1 g of an intravenous preparation of iron dextran (1,000 mg, once with test dose of 25 mg), ferric gluconate (125 mg, 8 doses), or iron sucrose (100 mg, 10 doses).
  - Erythropoiesis-stimulating agents (ESA) such as epoetin and darbepoetin can effectively reduce but do not prevent the need for RBC transfusions. ESA therapy increases the risk of stroke, thrombotic and cardiovascular events, and worsens outcomes in patients with cancer. These agents should not be started in CKD unless the hemoglobin is <10 g/dL, other causes of anemia such as iron deficiency are addressed, and reduction in transfusions is a goal. The minimum dose that maintains the hemoglobin above the need for transfusion and below 11 g/dL should be used. Correction of iron deficiency frequently decreases the ESA dose requirement and may defer the need for ESA. Targeting the hemoglobin to higher levels has been associated with increased cardiovascular mortality, and this risk may be related to the higher doses of ESA (*N Engl J Med 2010;363:1146*).

- **Renal osteodystrophy and secondary hyperparathyroidism**
  - ROD refers to a variety of bone mineral disorders encountered in CKD and ESRD. Prevalence increases as the GFR declines, through stage 3 and more advanced disease.
  - **Osteitis fibrosa cystica** is commonly associated with secondary hyperparathyroidism and increased bone turnover, resulting in bone pain and fractures. Adynamic bone disease is a low-turnover state with suppressed parathyroid hormone (PTH) levels. Osteomalacia can involve deposition of aluminum into bone and is less commonly seen today with the decreased use of aluminum-based phosphate binders.
  - In CKD, starting in stage 3, vitamin D deficiency, low calcium, and elevated phosphate can all contribute to **secondary hyperparathyroidism**. The general goal of therapy is to suppress PTH toward normal while maintaining normal serum calcium and phosphate. This can be addressed in three steps: repletion of vitamin D stores (25-OH vitamin D), control of dietary phosphate with binders, and administration of active vitamin D (1,25-dihydroxyvitamin D or an analog).
    - Deficient stores (25-OH vitamin D <30 ng/mL) should be corrected with oral ergocalciferol 50,000 IU capsule weekly or every other week, or cholecalciferol 2,000 to 4,000 IU daily. The duration of treatment depends on severity of the deficiency, with levels <5 ng/dL warranting at least 12 weeks of treatment. Once at goal, maintenance therapy can rely on either monthly ergocalciferol 50,000 IU or daily cholecalciferol 1,000 to 2,000 IU.
    - Phosphate control can be difficult as GFR declines, even with appropriate dietary restriction. Phosphate binders inhibit gastrointestinal absorption. Calcium-based binders are effective when given with meals, as calcium carbonate (200 mg of elemental calcium per 500 mg tablet) or calcium acetate (169 mg of elemental calcium per 667 mg tablet). In general, the total daily elemental calcium administered should be <1,500 mg. Lanthanum carbonate and sevelamer carbonate are non–calcium-based alternatives.
    - Active vitamin D (1,25-dihydroxyvitamin D) and its synthetic analogs are potent suppressors of PTH, and can be administered if serum PTH remains elevated. Options include daily calcitriol (0.25 to 1 mcg), paricalcitol (1 to 5 mcg), or doxercalciferol (1 to 5 mcg). Calcium levels need to be monitored regularly and doses adjusted to avoid hypercalcemia.
    - Cinacalcet is a calcimimetic that acts on the parathyroid gland to suppress PTH release. It should be used only in dialysis patients, and usually in conjunction with active vitamin D, as it may induce significant hypocalcemia and is relatively ineffective as monotherapy.
- **Metabolic acidosis.** As renal function deteriorates, the kidney is unable to appropriately excrete sufficient acid resulting in metabolic acidosis (mixed high and normal anion gap). To compensate, alkaline buffer is released from the skeleton but can ultimately worsen bone mineral disease.
  - Treatment with **sodium bicarbonate** 650 to 1,300 mg thrice daily can help maintain the serum bicarbonate level at 22 mEq/L. Such therapy, however, can increase the sodium load and contribute to edema or hypertension.
  - Citrate, another alkaline source, should not be used in the CKD or ESRD population as it can dramatically enhance gastrointestinal absorption of aluminum and lead to aluminum toxicity or osteomalacia.
- **Hyperlipidemia.** Therapy with statins combined with ezetimibe has shown improved cardiovascular outcomes with fewer major atherosclerotic events in

patients with moderate-to-severe CKD as well as in the dialysis population, although the benefit in patients on dialysis was less (*Lancet 2011;377:2181*). Use of lipid-lowering therapy is appropriate in patients with atherosclerotic disease at all stages of CKD.

- **Preparation for renal replacement therapy**
  - Patients should be counseled at an early stage to determine preferences for renal replacement therapies, including hemodialysis, peritoneal dialysis (PD), and eligibility for renal transplantation.
  - In stage 4 CKD, preparation for the creation of a permanent vascular access for hemodialysis should be initiated by protecting the nondominant forearm from intravenous catheters and blood draws. Timely referral for vein mapping and to an access surgeon can facilitate the creation and maturation of an arteriovenous (AV) access.

RENAL REPLACEMENT THERAPIES

Approach to Dialysis

TREATMENT

- **Modalities**
  - Renal replacement therapy is indicated when conservative medical management is unable to control the metabolic derangements of kidney disease. This applies to the acute and chronic settings. Common acute indications include **hyperkalemia**, **metabolic acidosis**, and **volume overload** that are refractory to medical management. Uremic **encephalopathy** or **pericarditis**, as well as certain **intoxications** (methanol, ethylene glycol, or salicylates), can all be indications to initiate dialytic therapy acutely. In the chronic setting, renal replacement therapy is typically begun prior to the worsening of the metabolic or nutrition status of the patient, and basing the decision solely on a target GFR has not shown a mortality advantage. A deteriorating nutritional status is also an indication to start dialytic therapy in advanced CKD.
  - Dialysis modalities work by solute diffusion and water transport across a selectively permeable membrane. In hemodialysis, blood is pumped counter-currently to a dialysis solution within an extracorporeal membrane. This can be performed intermittently (3 to 4 hours during the day) or in a continuous 24-hour fashion depending on hemodynamic stability or goals of therapy. PD utilizes the patient's peritoneal membrane as the selective filter and dialysis fluid is instilled into the peritoneal cavity. Transplantation offers the best long-term survival and most completely replaces the filtrative and endocrine functions of the native kidney. However, it carries the risks that accompany long-term immunosuppression.
- **Diffusion**
  The selectively permeable membrane contains pores that allow electrolytes and other small molecules to pass by diffusion while holding back larger molecules and cellular components of the blood. Movement relies on the molecular size and the concentration gradient, where Cr, urea, potassium, and other waste products of metabolism pass into the dialysis solution while alkaline buffers (bicarbonate or lactate) enter the blood from the dialysis solution.

- **Ultrafiltration/convection**
  - Removal of water is termed ultrafiltration (UF). It can be achieved in hemodialysis via a transmembrane hydrostatic pressure that removes excess fluid from the blood compartment. In PD, water follows its osmotic gradient into the relatively hyperosmolar dialysis solution (usually with dextrose providing the osmotic driving force).
  - As water is removed from the vascular compartment, it drags along solute. This is termed convective clearance. This usually accounts for only a small fraction of the total clearance but can be significantly increased if a physiologic "replacement fluid" is infused into the patient concurrently to prevent hypovolemia. This strategy is frequently employed by continuous hemodialysis modalities (see the following text).

Hemodialysis

GENERAL PRINCIPLES

- **Modalities**
  - Hemodialysis is by far the most commonly used form of renal replacement therapy in the United States. Intermittent hemodialysis (IHD) typically runs for 3 to 4 hours per session and is performed three times weekly. Outpatient, in-center hemodialysis for ESRD generally employs this modality, although variations are available for patients undergoing home treatments.
  - Continuous renal replacement therapy (CRRT) can be used in specialized circumstances, particularly when the patient's hemodynamic status would not tolerate the rapid fluid shifts of IHD. Although less efficient (with slower blood flows) and utilizing slower UF rates, CRRT can achieve equivalent clearances of both solute and fluid as compared to IHD due to its continuous, 24-hour nature. The slower blood flows necessitate anticoagulation (with systemic heparin or regional citrate) in order to prevent the filter from clotting. Continuous modalities generally require specialized nursing and an intensive care setting.
    - The most frequently employed form of CRRT is continuous veno-venous hemodiafiltration (CVVHDF).
    - In CVVHDF, blood is slowly pumped counter-currently to a dialysis solution (diffusion) and a replacement fluid (a "cleansed" physiologic solution devoid of uremic toxins) is infused into the circuit to balance most of the ultrafiltrate (convection).
  - Sustained low efficiency dialysis (SLED) is essentially a hybrid form of IHD and CRRT used in an intensive care setting. Intermediate blood flows lower the clotting risk if anticoagulation is not used, while intermediate treatment lengths (8 to 10 hours) still allow for adequate clearances. Patients also spend a significant portion of the day off the machine to allow for nonbedside testing, procedures, and physical therapy.
- **Prescription and adequacy**
  - IHD typically runs for 3 to 4 hours and can ultrafiltrate 3 to 4 L safely in hemodynamically stable patients. It can be used in ESRD as well as AKI. In the chronic setting, IHD is generally performed three times weekly, although the longer interdialytic interval on the weekend has been associated with a heightened mortality risk (*N Engl J Med 2011;365:1099*). In the acute setting, the appropriate interval is not clearly known, although a thrice-weekly schedule is likely adequate; daily assessment should be performed to reevaluate dialytic needs.

○ Adequacy is assessed by calculating the clearance of BUN, which serves as a surrogate marker of the "uremic factors." The urea reduction ratio (URR) can be calculated by the following:

$$URR = [(predialysis\ BUN-postdialysis\ BUN)/(predialysis\ BUN)] \times 100$$

- A reduction rate of >65% is considered adequate in the chronic setting (*N Engl J Med 2002;347:2010*). An adequacy target is less well defined for AKI.
- Intensive daily hemodialysis was not shown to be superior to standard thrice-weekly treatments (*N Engl J Med 2008;359:7*).

○ Clearance is measured differently in CRRT where dialytic therapy is taking place around the clock, effectively serving as an extracorporeal "GFR." Drug dosing needs to be adjusted accordingly. An estimate of this clearance can be calculated by the sum of the dialysis fluid, replacement fluid, and net UF rates are expressed in the number of milliliters per minute. For most circumstances, this approximates a clearance of 20 to 50 mL/min.

- With CRRT, the net UF rate can be adjusted as needed, according to the patient's hemodynamic status. One must be vigilant in checking electrolyte levels (particularly ionized calcium and phosphorus) to ensure they remain within the desired ranges. Calcium levels are especially important to follow when regional citrate anticoagulation is being used.
- Phosphate, which is predominantly intracellular, is generally poorly removed by IHD; however, in CRRT, there is continuous efflux of this anion and significant hypophosphatemia can occur and lead to muscle weakness if not corrected.

COMPLICATIONS

- Nontunneled catheters are typically placed in the internal jugular or femoral vein and carry the same risks as other central venous catheters (infection, bleeding, pneumothorax). They are almost exclusively used in the inpatient setting and are generally used for 1 to 2 weeks. Tunneled catheters have lower rates of infection and can be used for 6 months while a more definitive access is maturing (AV fistula or graft).
  ○ Fevers and rigors, particularly during dialysis, should prompt a search for an infectious cause and empiric antibiotic coverage for *Staphylococci* and gram-negative bacteria should be administered.
  ○ The catheter should then be replaced after a period of defervescence and sterilization of the blood (at least 48 hours). Documented bacteremia should be treated with antibiotics for at least 3 weeks.
- Thrombosis of an AV fistula or graft can frequently be recanalized by thrombolysis or thrombectomy. Stenotic regions can be evaluated by a fistulogram, and treatment may encompass angioplasty or stent deployment.
- Intradialytic hypotension is most commonly due to intravascular volume depletion from rapid UF. Antihypertensive medications may also contribute. Infectious causes should be sought in the appropriate setting. Acute treatment of the drop in blood pressure includes infusion of normal saline (as 200 mL boluses) and reduction of the UF rate.
- Dialysis disequilibrium is an uncommon syndrome that may occur in severely uremic patients undergoing their first few treatments. Rapid clearance of toxins is thought to

induce cerebral edema by osmolar shifts and can present as nausea, emesis, headache, confusion, or seizures. Occurrence can be prevented or ameliorated by initiating patients on dialysis with slower blood flows and shorter treatments.

Peritoneal Dialysis

GENERAL PRINCIPLES

- **Modalities**
  - Historically, PD has been used in the acute setting for hemodynamically unstable patients. However, with the development and availability of safe and effective continuous hemodialysis, use of PD in the treatment of AKI in adults has been mostly abandoned in the United States. Currently, its use is primarily in the treatment of ESRD.
  - There are two modalities in use: manual exchanges and automated cycler exchanges.
    - The manual modality, also called continuous ambulatory peritoneal dialysis (CAPD), has the patient instill dialysis fluid into the peritoneum for a specified length of time after which the dialysate is drained and replaced by another dwell.
    - The automated modality, also called continuous cycling peritoneal dialysis (CCPD), typically operates overnight where a machine runs a preprogrammed set of exchanges while the patient sleeps. A final fill usually remains in the peritoneum and is carried during the daytime for continued solute exchange.
  - Either PD modality requires strict adherence to sterile technique and careful patient selection is necessary. Generally, PD should not be used if there is a history of recent abdominal surgery or if multiple peritoneal adhesions are present.
- **Prescription and adequacy**
  - The choice between CAPD and CCPD usually depends on patient preference and on the transport characteristics of the peritoneal membrane. Manual exchanges (i.e., CAPD) can be used as a backup modality, particularly in the hospital where nurse staffing or machine availability may be limited.
  - In writing PD orders, the following variables must be specified: dwell volume, dwell time, number of exchanges, and dextrose concentration of the dialysis solution. The dwell volume is typically between 2 and 3 L. The dextrose concentration can be 1.50%, 2.50%, or 4.25%, providing the osmotic gradient for fluid removal. Higher concentrations not only allow for greater UF but also lead to more glucose absorption and worsening control of diabetes. Icodextrin is a glucose polymer preparation that can be used in longer dwell as it is minimally absorbed and thus maintains an effective osmotic gradient up to 18 hours. Commercially available PD solutions may have color-coded tabs and patients may know these better than the actual concentrations (yellow for 1.50%, green for 2.50%, red for 4.25%). A sample order set for manual CAPD would be 2.5 L, four exchanges, 6 hours each, with 2.5% dextrose.
  - PD is less efficient than conventional hemodialysis. However, given its continuous nature, solute clearance and UF can approximate that of other modalities. Larger volumes and more frequent exchanges can assist with solute exchange. Increasing the concentration of dextrose can promote greater UF in volume overloaded patients. Residual renal function is very important in the PD population and avoidance of nephrotoxins should be practiced (*J Am Soc Nephrol 2002;13:1307*).

COMPLICATIONS

- **Peritonitis** typically presents with diffuse abdominal pain and cloudy peritoneal fluid. A sample should be sent for cell count, differential, Gram stain, and culture. A WBC count of >100 cells/mm^3, of which at least 50% are neutrophils, supports the diagnosis.
  - Empiric therapy should cover for both gram-positive and gram-negative organisms, with a first-generation cephalosporin (cefazolin or cephalothin) and ceftazidime at 15 to 20 mg/kg of each in the longest dwell of the day (*Perit Dial Int 2005;25:107*). If methicillin-resistant organism is suspected, use vancomycin (30 mg/kg every 5–7 days) for gram-positive coverage and third-generation cephalosporin for gram-negative coverage, including *Pseudomonas*, should be used.
  - The intraperitoneal route is the preferred method of administration, unless the patient is overtly septic in which case intravenous antibiotics should be employed. Antibiotics can be tailored once culture results are known and should be continued for 2 to 3 weeks. Multiple organisms, particularly if gram negative, should prompt a search for intestinal perforation.
- Tunnel or exit site infections may present with local erythema, tenderness, or purulent drainage, although crusting at the exit site alone does not necessarily indicate infection. Treatment can be with oral cephalosporins (gram positive) or fluoroquinolones (gram negative). However, infections can be difficult to eradicate and catheter removal may be required with a temporary transition to hemodialysis.
- Failure of PD fluid to drain is termed outflow failure. This may result from kinking of the catheter, constipation, or plugging of the catheter with fibrin strands. Conservative treatment should aim at resolving constipation if present and instilling heparin into the PD fluid at 500 U/L.
- Small hernias are at particularly high risk for incarceration and should be corrected surgically while the patient is temporarily treated with hemodialysis. Fluid leaks can lead to abdominal wall and genital edema and typically result from anatomic defects. Hydrothorax usually occurs on the right side, and can be diagnosed by a markedly elevated glucose concentration in the pleural fluid. Pleurodesis can eliminate the potential space and permit continuation of PD.
- **Sclerosing encapsulating peritonitis** is a complication of long-term PD. The peritoneal membrane becomes thickened and entraps loops of bowel leading to symptoms of bowel obstruction. A bloody drainage may be present. Treatment is supportive with the focus on bowel rest and surgical lysis of adhesions. A trial of immunosuppression with prednisone 10 to 40 mg/d may have limited benefit.
- Hyperglycemia results from the systemic absorption of glucose from the dialysis fluid. Since peritoneal uptake of insulin is unpredictable, treatment with subcutaneous insulin is preferred. Hyperlipidemia is common in the PD population and treatment should be for a goal LDL of <100 mg/dL, with statins (HMG-CoA reductase inhibitors) as the first-line agents.
- Unlike hemodialysis, patients on PD tend to experience hypokalemia, likely due to a continuous potassium exodus in the dialysate as well as from an intracellular shift from the increased endogenous insulin production. Oral replacement is usually sufficient, either with relaxation of prior dietary restrictions or with low-dose supplementation (10 to 20 mEq/d of potassium chloride).
- Protein loss can be high and the dietary protein intake should be 1.2 to 1.3 g/kg/d. Episodes of peritonitis can make the membrane even more susceptible to protein losses.

Transplantation

GENERAL PRINCIPLES

- Renal transplantation offers patients an improved quality of life and survival as compared to other renal replacement modalities.
- The pretransplant evaluation focuses on cardiopulmonary status, vascular sufficiency, and human lymphocyte antigen typing. Structural abnormalities of the urinary tract need to be addressed. Contraindications include most malignancies, active infection, or significant cardiopulmonary disease.
- In adult recipients, the renal allograft is placed in the extraperitoneal space, in the anterior lower abdomen. Vascular anastomosis is typically to the iliac vessels while the ureter is attached to the bladder through a muscular tunnel to approximate sphincter function.
- Immunosuppression protocols vary among institutions. A typical regimen would include prednisone along with a combination of a calcineurin inhibitor (cyclosporine or tacrolimus) and an antimetabolite (mycophenolate derivative, azathioprine, or rapamycin).
- Evaluation of allograft dysfunction frequently requires kidney biopsy. Current laboratory and radiologic tests cannot reliably distinguish acute rejection from drug toxicity, the two most common causes of a rising Cr in the transplant population.
- Complications and long-term management of transplant recipients are discussed further in Chapter 17, Solid Organ Transplant Medicine.

NEPHROLITHIASIS

Approach to Kidney Stones

GENERAL PRINCIPLES

Classification

- Overall, **calcium-based stones** are the most common and appear predominantly as calcium oxalate or calcium phosphate salts. These stones are radiopaque. Calcium phosphate stones can appear as elongated, blunt crystals and form in alkaline urine. Calcium oxalate stones can be found in acidic urine and can be dumbbell shaped or appear as paired pyramids (giving them an envelope appearance when viewed on end).
- **Uric acid stones** can be idiopathic or develop as part of hyperuricosuric states such as gout and myeloproliferative disorders. These stones are radiolucent and are found in acidic urine. Uric acid crystals exhibit a variety of shapes, with needles and rhomboid forms being the most common.
- **Struvite stones** contain magnesium, ammonium, and phosphate. They develop in alkaline urine associated with urea-splitting organisms (e.g., *Proteus*, *Klebsiella*). They are radiopaque and can extend to fill the renal pelvis, taking on a staghorn configuration. On microscopy, struvite crystals have a characteristic coffin-lid shape.
- **Cystine stones** are uncommon and can form as the result of an autosomal recessive disorder. These stones have an intermediate radiolucency and appear as hexagonal crystals in the urine.

DIAGNOSIS

Clinical Presentation

Clinical presentation is with costovertebral angle or flank pain which can radiate to the scrotum or labia. Hematuria with nondysmorphic RBCs may be noted. Oliguria and AKI are uncommon but can result if there is bilateral obstruction or if a solitary functioning kidney is affected.

Diagnostic Testing

Laboratories

- Metabolic evaluation should include urine culture, pH, and microscopy. Serum calcium, phosphate, parathyroid hormone, and uric acid levels complement routine studies. Urine should be strained and passed stones analyzed for composition.
- Recurrent stone formers should undergo a more extensive evaluation, with 24-hour urine collections for calcium, phosphate, uric acid, citrate, oxalate, and cystine. This collection should not be done during an acute episode in a hospitalized patient but rather reserved for when the patient is on his or her normal outpatient diet.

Imaging

A plain abdominal film may reveal the radiopaque stones composed of calcium salts, struvite, or cystine. However, noncontrast CT scanning has replaced other imaging modalities as the study of choice for suspected nephrolithiasis.

TREATMENT

- General treatment of nephrolithiasis is with **hydration** to increase urine output and with analgesia. If the stone is obstructing outflow or is accompanied by infection, removal is indicated with urgent urologic or radiologic intervention.
- After passage of a stone, treatment is directed at **prevention of recurrent stone formation**. Regardless of stone type, the foundation of therapy is maintenance of high urine output (2 to 3 L/d) with oral hydration and a low-salt diet (<2 g/d).
- For calcium oxalate stones, a low-calcium diet is no longer recommended given the risks of osteoporosis. A normal-calcium diet with no added calcium supplements is now in favor. Patients should avoid oxalate-rich foods (e.g., spinach, rhubarb). Thiazide diuretics may reduce calciuria, and potassium citrate may be added in patients with hypocitraturia.
- Uric acid stones can be prevented or reduced in size by allopurinol. A low-protein diet may be helpful as can urinary alkalinization with citrate, bicarbonate, or acetazolamide.
- Struvite calculi frequently require surgical intervention for their removal. Extracorporeal shock-wave lithotripsy can be used as adjunctive therapy. Aggressive antibiotic treatment is indicated if monthly urine cultures become positive.
- Cystine stones require extensive urinary alkalinization to a pH of 7.0 to 7.5 to induce solubility. D-penicillamine and mercaptopropionylglycine can further increase solubility through breakage and exchange of disulfide bonds.

14 Treatment of Infectious Diseases

Stephen Y. Liang, Sara L. Cross, and Nigar Kirmani

Principles of Therapy

GENERAL PRINCIPLES

The decision to initiate, continue, and stop antimicrobial therapy should be made carefully. Indiscriminate use of antibiotics is associated with adverse effects, mounting drug resistance, and excess costs. When antimicrobial therapy is indicated, a number of factors reviewed in this chapter must be considered. In the case of industry-related antibiotic shortages, consultation with an infectious disease specialist for alternative options is recommended.

DIAGNOSIS

- **During the initial evaluation**, a Gram stain of the potentially infected tissue or material often permits a rapid presumptive diagnosis and informs antibiotic selection.
- **Local susceptibility patterns** must be considered in selecting empiric therapy because patterns vary widely among communities and individual hospitals.
- **Cultures** are usually necessary for precise diagnosis and are required for susceptibility testing. Whenever organisms with special growth requirements are suspected, the microbiology laboratory should be consulted to ensure appropriate transport and processing of cultures.
- **Susceptibility testing** facilitates rational selection of antimicrobial agents for targeted therapy and should be performed on all positive bacterial cultures.
- **Rapid diagnostic testing**, such as polymerase chain reaction (PCR) and antigen detection, may also provide early confirmation of an infectious etiologic agent.

TREATMENT

- **Choice of initial antimicrobial therapy**
  - Empiric therapy should be directed against the most likely pathogens and possess the narrowest spectrum.
  - Therapy should be modified in accordance with the patient's clinical course and culture results.
  - Thorough review of the patient's drug allergies and prior antibiotic treatment is essential.
- **Timing for the initiation of antimicrobial therapy**
  - In acute clinical scenarios, empiric therapy is usually begun immediately after appropriate cultures have been obtained. However, if the patient's condition is

stable, delaying the empiric use of antimicrobials allows for more targeted therapy based on initial testing and avoids the use of unnecessary drugs.
- ○ Urgent therapy is indicated in febrile patients who are neutropenic or asplenic. Sepsis, meningitis, and rapidly progressive anaerobic or necrotizing infections should also be treated promptly with antimicrobials.
- **Route of administration**
  Patients with serious infections should be given antimicrobial agents intravenously (IV). In less urgent circumstances, intramuscular (IM) or oral (PO) therapy is often sufficient. Oral therapy is acceptable if adequate drug concentrations can be achieved at the site of infection.
- **Type of therapy**
  - ○ Bactericidal therapy is preferred over bacteriostatic regimens for patients with immunologic compromise or life-threatening infection. It is also preferred for infections characterized by impaired regional host defenses, such as endocarditis, meningitis, and osteomyelitis.
  - ○ Renal and hepatic function determine antimicrobial dosing regimens.
  - ○ Drug interactions impact effectiveness of therapy and should always be assessed before starting treatment.
- **Assessment of outcomes on antimicrobial therapy**
  If there is concern for potential treatment failure, consider the following questions:
  - ○ Is the isolated organism the etiologic agent?
  - ○ Has an appropriate antimicrobial regimen been selected to cover the organism?
  - ○ Is the concentration of antimicrobial agent adequate at the site of infection?
  - ○ Have resistant pathogens emerged?
  - ○ Is a persistent fever due to underlying disease, abscess formation, an iatrogenic complication, a drug reaction, or another process?
- **Duration of therapy**
  - ○ The duration of treatment depends on the nature and severity of infection.
  - ○ Treatment of acute uncomplicated infections should be continued until the patient has been afebrile and clinically well, usually for a minimum of 72 hours.
  - ○ Infections at certain sites (e.g., endocarditis, septic arthritis, osteomyelitis) require prolonged therapy.

SPECIAL CONSIDERATIONS

- **Status of the host**
  - ○ The clinical status of the patient guides the speed with which therapy must be instituted, the route of administration, and the type of therapy.
  - ○ Patients should be evaluated promptly for hemodynamic instability, rapidly progressive or life-threatening infections, and immune defects.
- **Pregnancy and the postpartum patient**
  - ○ Although no antimicrobial agent is known to be completely safe in pregnancy, the penicillins and cephalosporins are most often used. **Tetracyclines and fluoroquinolones are contraindicated**. Sulfonamides and aminoglycosides should not be used if alternative agents are available.
  - ○ Many antibiotics appear in breast milk and should be used with caution in mothers who are nursing.

TOXIN-MEDIATED INFECTIONS

Clostridium Difficile Infection

GENERAL PRINCIPLES

Frequently seen after systemic antimicrobial therapy.

DIAGNOSIS

Clinical Presentation

Symptoms may range from mild or moderate watery diarrhea to severe and potentially fatal pseudomembranous colitis. Abdominal pain, cramping, low-grade fever, and leukocytosis are often present. Fulminant disease can manifest as colonic ileus or toxic megacolon leading to bowel perforation.

Differential Diagnosis

Diarrhea directly related to antibiotic use without *C. difficile* infection should be considered, which will resolve after withdrawal of the antibiotic.

Diagnostic Testing

Diagnosis is made by detection of *C. difficile* toxin in stool or by colonoscopic visualization of pseudomembranes.

TREATMENT

- For **mild-to-moderate disease**, treatment should consist of metronidazole 500 mg PO (preferred over IV) tid for 10 to 14 days, and discontinuation of the offending antibiotic if possible (*Infect Control Hosp Epidemiol 2010;31:431*). In **severe disease**, vancomycin 125 to 500 mg PO qid (IV is not effective) is preferred (*Clin Infect Dis 2007;45:302*). For infections complicated by ileus, toxic megacolon, or shock, the addition of IV metronidazole and intracolonic vancomycin is recommended (*Clin Infect Dis 2002;35:690*). In some cases, colectomy may be necessary.
- Endpoint of therapy is cessation of diarrhea; **do not retest stool for toxin clearance**.
- Avoid antimotility agents in severe disease.
- Recurrence is common and is treated with metronidazole or vancomycin in extended duration, pulsed, or tapered regimens. Adjunctive therapy with oral rifaximin is sometimes used (*Clin Infect Dis 2007;44:846*).
- Fidaxomicin may have an evolving role in the treatment and prevention of recurrent *C. difficile* infection (*N Engl J Med 2011;364:422*).

Tetanus

GENERAL PRINCIPLES

Caused by intoxication with *Clostridium tetani* toxin from wound contamination with spores.

Prevention

Tetanus is best prevented by immunization (*MMWR 2012;61(4):1*). For high-risk wounds, human tetanus immunoglobulin 250 U IM is used (*MMWR 2006;55 (No. RR-17):1*).

DIAGNOSIS

Clinical Presentation

Classically presents with intensely painful muscle spasms and rigidity, followed by autonomic dysfunction. Symptoms often begin in the face (trismus, risus sardonicus) and neck muscles. Delirium and high fever are usually absent. Diagnosis is clinical.

TREATMENT

Passive immunization with human tetanus immunoglobulin 3,000 to 5,000 U IM (in divided doses) to neutralize unbound toxin is warranted. Active immunization with tetanus toxoid should be given at a separate site. Benzodiazepines or neuromuscular blocking agents may be used to control spasms. Surgical debridement of the wound is critical. Antibiotics, usually metronidazole 500 mg IV every 6 to 8 hours for 7 to 10 days, are controversial. Care is otherwise supportive.

TOXIC SHOCK SYNDROME

Toxic shock syndrome (TSS) is a life-threatening systemic disease caused by exotoxin superantigens produced by *Staphylococcus aureus* or group A β-hemolytic *Streptococcus* (GABHS) tissue infections (Table 14-1).

Staphylococcal Toxic Shock Syndrome

GENERAL PRINCIPLES

Most often associated with colonization of surgical wounds, burns, vaginitis, or tampon use in young women. Cases are also seen after nasal packing for epistaxis.

DIAGNOSIS

Clinical Presentation

Typical findings are fever, hypotension, and a macular desquamating erythroderma of the palms and soles. Vomiting, diarrhea, myalgias, weakness, shortness of breath, and altered mental status may be early signs of multiorgan failure.

Diagnostic Testing

Blood cultures are usually negative. Creatine phosphokinase (CPK) is often elevated. Detection of antibodies against toxic shock syndrome toxin-1 (TSST-1) is helpful in that it indicates protection against recurrence.

OUTCOME/PROGNOSIS

Mortality is relatively low.

Table 14-1	Treatment of Toxic Shock Syndromes		
Etiology	Antibiotic Therapy	Adjunctive Therapy	Notes
Group A β-hemolytic Streptococcus (GABHS)	Penicillin G 4 million U IV q4h + Clindamycin 900 mg IV q8h for 10–14 d	IVIG 1 g/kg on day 1, then 0.5 g/kg on days 2 and 3 (*Clin Infect Dis 2003;37:333*)	Surgical intervention almost always indicated for necrotizing infections. Clindamycin is added to decrease toxin production.
Staphylococcus	Oxacillin 2 g IV q4h or vancomycin 1 g IV q12h for 10–14 d	IVIG as per GABHS may be useful in severe cases, but higher doses may be needed (*Clin Infect Dis 2004;38:836*)	Treatment is primarily supportive. Tampons must be removed and avoided in future, especially if TSST-1 antibody titers are negative. Antibiotics decrease the risk of relapse.

IVIG, intravenous immunoglobulin; TSST-1, toxic shock syndrome toxin-1.

Streptococcal Toxic Shock Syndrome

GENERAL PRINCIPLES

Associated with invasive GABHS infections, particularly necrotizing fasciitis or myositis (80% of cases). Mortality is much higher than in staphylococcal TSS.

DIAGNOSIS

Clinical Presentation

Initial presentation is typically abrupt onset of severe diffuse or localized pain. The systemic manifestations are otherwise similar to staphylococcal TSS, but the desquamating erythroderma is much less common.

Diagnostic Testing

Blood cultures are usually positive and antistreptolysin O (ASO) titers are elevated.

TREATMENT

See Table 14-1.

SKIN, SOFT TISSUE, AND BONE INFECTIONS

The increased incidence of community-associated methicillin-resistant *Staphylococcus aureus* (CA-MRSA) has altered the approach to management of skin and soft tissue infections (SSTIs) (*Clin Infect Dis 2011;52:1*).

Abscesses, Furuncles and Carbuncles

GENERAL PRINCIPLES

MRSA and methicillin-sensitive *S. aureus* (MSSA) accounts for 25% to 50% of cases.

TREATMENT

- Incision and drainage (I&D) alone is usually adequate, especially for abscesses <5 cm.
- Antibiotic therapy is needed for extensive disease; systemic illness; rapid progression with associated cellulitis; comorbid diseases (diabetes mellitus); immunosuppression; location on face, hand, or genitalia; or lack of response to I&D.
- Empiric antibiotic therapy should cover CA-MRSA (see the following text).
- Duration of antibiotic therapy is usually 5 to 7 days.

Cellulitis

TREATMENT

- **Purulent cellulitis** (exudate or purulent drainage without a drainable abscess) is caused predominantly by CA-MRSA (59%) or MSSA (17%) and requires empiric coverage for CA-MRSA (*N Engl J Med 2006;355:666*). Oral antibiotic options are clindamycin 300 to 450 mg thrice daily; trimethoprim-sulfamethoxazole (TMP-SMX) 1 to 2 double strength (DS) tablets twice daily; doxycycline 100 mg twice daily; minocycline 200 mg once, then 100 mg twice daily; and linezolid 600 mg twice daily.
- **Nonpurulent cellulitis** (no purulent drainage or associated abscess) may be caused by β-hemolytic streptococci (73%) and *S. aureus* (*Medicine 2010;89:217*). A β-lactam antibiotic (cephalexin or dicloxacillin 500 mg PO four times daily) can be used. CA-MRSA coverage should be added if there is no response. Clindamycin or linezolid are also options for monotherapy. TMP-SMX can be used if combined with a β-lactam antibiotic (e.g., amoxicillin 500 mg PO thrice daily) to cover streptococci.
- **Waterborne pathogens:** Severe cellulitis is sometimes seen after exposure to fresh (*Aeromonas hydrophila*) or salt water (*Vibrio vulnificus*). Initial therapy should consist of ceftazidime 2 g IV q8h, cefepime 2 g IV q8h, or ciprofloxacin 750 mg

PO bid. Doxycycline 100 mg IV/PO q12h should be added for *Vibrio* infections, which have a strong predilection for patients with cirrhosis.

Erysipelas

GENERAL PRINCIPLES

Erysipelas appears as painful, superficial, erythematous, sharply demarcated lesion that is usually found on lower extremities. In normal hosts, GABHS are responsible for this infection.

TREATMENT

Penicillin V 250 to 1,000 mg PO qid or penicillin G 1.0 to 2.0 million U IV q6h, depending on the severity of illness. In patients who are penicillin allergic, macrolides or clindamycin are alternatives.

Complicated Skin and Soft Tissue Infections

GENERAL PRINCIPLES

Deep soft-tissue infections, surgical and traumatic wound infections, large abscesses, complicated cellulitis, and infected ulcers and burns fall under this classification.

DIAGNOSIS

Cultures of abscesses and surgical debridement specimens should be obtained in hospitalized patients.

TREATMENT

- Patients should be hospitalized to receive intravenous antibiotics and undergo surgical intervention as necessary. Vancomycin 15 to 20 mg/kg IV twice daily, linezolid 600 mg PO/IV twice daily, daptomycin 4 mg/kg daily, telavancin 10 mg/kg once daily, clindamycin 600 mg thrice daily, and ceftaroline 600 mg twice daily are all acceptable antibiotic options.
- Rifampin is not recommended as a single agent or in combination with other antibiotics.

Infected Decubitus Ulcers and Limb-Threatening Diabetic Foot Ulcers

GENERAL PRINCIPLES

Usually polymicrobial; *superficial swab cultures are unreliable*. Osteomyelitis is a frequent complication and should be excluded.

TREATMENT

- Wound care and debridement are important first-line therapies.
- **Moderate-to-severe infections** require systemic antibiotics covering *S. aureus*, anaerobes, and enteric gram-negative organisms. Options include vancomycin plus a β-lactam/β-lactamase inhibitor combination, a carbapenem (ertapenem, doripenem or meropenem), or vancomycin with metronidazole combined with either ciprofloxacin or a third-generation cephalosporin.
- **Less severe diabetic foot infections** are usually due to *S. aureus* and *Streptococci* and can be treated with clindamycin plus ciprofloxacin or TMP-SMX plus amoxicillin-clavulanate. Clindamycin or linezolid alone can be used for mild infections (*Clin Infect Dis 2004;39:885*).

Necrotizing Fasciitis

GENERAL PRINCIPLES

This is an infectious disease emergency with high mortality manifested by extensive soft-tissue infection and thrombosis of the microcirculation with resulting necrosis (*Clin Infect Dis 2007;44:705*). Infection spreads quickly along fascial planes and may be associated with sepsis or TSS. Fournier's gangrene is necrotizing fasciitis of the perineum. Bacterial etiology is either mixed (aerobic and anaerobic organisms) or monomicrobial (GABHS or *S. aureus*, including CA-MRSA).

DIAGNOSIS

Clinical Presentation

May present initially like simple cellulitis rapidly progressing to necrosis with dusky, hypoesthetic skin and bulla formation in association with severe pain.

Diagnostic Testing

- Diagnosis is clinical. High suspicion should prompt *immediate surgical exploration* where lack of resistance to probing is diagnostic.
- Cultures of operative specimens and blood should be obtained. CPK may be elevated.
- Computed tomography (CT) and plain films may demonstrate gas and fascial edema early in the disease process.

TREATMENT

- Aggressive surgical debridement is critical, along with IV antibiotics and volume support. Initial empiric antibiotic therapy should be broad spectrum and consist of a β-lactam/β-lactamase inhibitor, high-dose penicillin, carbapenem, or fluoroquinolone in combination with clindamycin. Vancomycin should also be added until MRSA can be excluded.
- Adjunctive hyperbaric oxygen may be useful.

Anaerobic Myonecrosis (Gas Gangrene)

GENERAL PRINCIPLES

Usually due to *Clostridium perfringens*, *Clostridium septicum*, *S. aureus*, GABHS, or other anaerobes. Distinguishing this condition from necrotizing fasciitis requires gross inspection of the involved muscle at the time of surgery.

TREATMENT

Treatment requires prompt surgical debridement and combination antimicrobial therapy with intravenous penicillin plus clindamycin. A third-generation cephalosporin, ciprofloxacin, or an aminoglycoside should be added until the Gram stain excludes gram-negative involvement.

Osteomyelitis

GENERAL PRINCIPLES

Osteomyelitis is an inflammatory process caused by an infecting organism that can lead to bone destruction. It should be considered when skin or soft-tissue infections overlie bone and when localized bone pain accompanies fever or sepsis (*Lancet 2004;364:369*).

Etiology
- **Acute hematogenous osteomyelitis** is most frequently caused by *S. aureus*.
- **Vertebral osteomyelitis** may be due to *S. aureus*, gram-negative bacilli, or *Mycobacterium tuberculosis*.
- **Osteomyelitis associated with a contiguous focus of infection** may be due to *S. aureus*, gram-negative bacilli, coagulase-negative staphylococci (surgical site infections), or anaerobes (infected sacral decubitus ulcers).
- **Osteomyelitis in the presence of an orthopedic device** is most often caused by *S. aureus* or coagulase-negative *Staphylococcus* species.
- **Osteomyelitis associated with hemoglobinopathies** is caused by *S. aureus* or *Salmonella* species.
- **Chronic osteomyelitis** is usually associated with a sequestrum of necrotic bone and may involve gram-negative pathogens as well as *S. aureus*.

DIAGNOSIS

- Diagnosis is made by detection of exposed bone through a skin ulcer or by imaging with plain films, bone scintigraphy, or magnetic resonance imaging (MRI) (*Clin Infect Dis 2008;47:519*).
- Biopsy and cultures of the affected bone should be performed (prior to initiation of antimicrobials when possible) for pathogen-directed therapy.
- Erythrocyte sedimentation rate and C-reactive protein are usually markedly elevated and can be used to monitor the response to therapy.

TREATMENT

- If a causative organism is not identified, empiric therapy should cover *S. aureus* and all other likely pathogens (as listed earlier).
- Parenteral β-lactam antibiotics (oxacillin, cefazolin) are effective against MSSA. Vancomycin, daptomycin, and linezolid are used to treat MRSA osteomyelitis. Oral agents capable of achieving reasonable bone levels include trimethoprim-sulfamethoxazole, clindamycin, and doxycycline.
- Gram-negative osteomyelitis can be treated with parenteral or oral fluoroquinolones, which have excellent bone penetration and bioavailability, or with a third-generation cephalosporin.
- Cure typically requires at least 4 to 6 weeks of high-dose antimicrobial therapy. Parenteral therapy should be given initially; oral regimens may be considered after 2 to 3 weeks if the pathogen is susceptible and adequate bactericidal levels can be achieved. (*Clin Infect Dis 2012;54:403*).
- **Acute hematogenous osteomyelitis.** In the absence of vascular insufficiency or a foreign body, this disease can be treated with antimicrobial therapy alone.
- **Osteomyelitis associated with vascular insufficiency** (e.g., in diabetic patients) is seldom cured by drug therapy alone; revascularization, debridement, or amputation is often required. Infections are generally polymicrobial, including anaerobes.
- **Osteomyelitis in the presence of an orthopedic device** is rarely eradicated by antimicrobials alone, and typically requires removal of the device. When removal is impossible, the addition of rifampin 300 mg PO three times daily is recommended. Long-term, suppressive antimicrobial therapy may be needed.
- **Chronic osteomyelitis.** Eradication requires a combination of medical and surgical treatment to remove the persistent nidus of infection. Long-term, suppressive antimicrobial therapy can be used if surgery is not feasible. Hyperbaric oxygen may be a useful adjunctive therapy.

CENTRAL NERVOUS SYSTEM INFECTIONS

Meningitis

GENERAL PRINCIPLES

Meningitis is the inflammation of the meninges around the brain and/or spinal cord. It can be caused by bacterial or viral infections, or by noninfectious causes such as medications.

DIAGNOSIS

Clinical Presentation

- Meningitis should be considered in any patient with fever and stiff neck or neurologic symptoms, especially if another concurrent infection or head trauma is present.
- **Bacterial meningitis** is a medical emergency. Therapy should not be delayed for diagnostic measures because prognosis hinges on rapid initiation of antimicrobial treatment.

- **Aseptic meningitis** is usually milder than bacterial meningitis and may be preceded by upper respiratory symptoms or pharyngitis. Viruses are common causes, as is drug-induced inflammation (e.g., nonsteroidal anti-inflammatory drugs [NSAIDs], TMP-SMX).
- Distinction between bacterial, viral, and noninfectious etiologies cannot be made clinically.

Diagnostic Testing

Diagnosis requires a lumbar puncture with measurement of opening pressure, examination of cerebrospinal fluid (CSF) protein, glucose, and cell count with differential, and Gram stain with culture. Blood cultures should always be obtained. A head CT scan before lumbar puncture is controversial but is generally not required for nonelderly, immunocompetent patients who present without focal neurologic abnormalities, seizures, or diminished level of consciousness (*Clin Infect Dis 2004;39:1267*).

- Typical CSF findings in **bacterial meningitis** include a neutrophilic pleocytosis, markedly elevated CSF protein, and decreased glucose level.
- In **aseptic meningitis**, a lymphocytic CSF pleocytosis is common (although neutrophils may predominate very early in the disease course). CSF PCR can detect enteroviruses, herpes simplex virus (HSV), and HIV.
- Depending on the clinical scenario, other potentially useful CSF studies include rapid plasma reagin (RPR), acid-fast stain, latex agglutination antigen detection, cryptococcal antigen, and arbovirus antibodies.

TREATMENT

Treatment consists of supportive measures and antimicrobial therapy (*Clin Infect Dis 2004;39:1267*). Whenever acute bacterial meningitis is suspected, high-dose parenteral antimicrobial therapy should be started as soon as possible. Until the etiology of the meningitis is known, an empiric regimen should be based on patient risk factors and Gram stain of the CSF:

- **If no organisms are seen**, high-dose third-generation cephalosporins (ceftriaxone 2 g IV q12h) and vancomycin 1 g IV q8–12h are recommended while culture results are pending.
- Ampicillin 2 g IV q4h should be added for **immunocompromised and older patients (>50 years of age)** to cover *Listeria monocytogenes*.
- In the **postneurosurgic setting, or after head or spinal trauma**, broad-spectrum coverage with high-dose vancomycin and ceftazidime or cefepime 2 g IV q8h is indicated. Empiric regimens should be altered once culture and sensitivity data are known.
- **Dexamethasone** 10 mg IV q6h started just prior to or with initial antibiotics and continued for 4 days reduces the risk of a poor neurologic outcome in patients with meningitis caused by *Streptococcus pneumoniae*. Steroids have not proven to be of benefit for bacterial meningitis caused by other organisms, and should be discontinued if a different pathogen is isolated (*N Engl J Med 2002;347:1549*).
- **Therapy for specific infections**
  ○ For *S. pneumoniae*, IV penicillin G 4 million U q4h for 14 days, is appropriate when the isolate is fully susceptible to penicillin. High-dose ceftriaxone or cefotaxime (as described earlier) is used for susceptible or intermediate penicillin-resistant isolates, and vancomycin is added if there is ceftriaxone resistance or high-level penicillin resistance. Options for severely penicillin-allergic patients are vancomycin plus rifampin 300 mg PO tid, or chloramphenicol 1 g IV q6h.

Vancomycin should not be used alone. Dexamethasone, as described earlier, can be a valuable adjunct if given early in treatment.

o For ***N. meningitidis***, high-dose ceftriaxone or cefotaxime is continued for at least 5 days after the patient has become afebrile, usually a 7-day total course. Chloramphenicol is an option for the penicillin-allergic patient. Patients should be placed in a private room on respiratory isolation for at least the first 24 hours of treatment. Close contacts (e.g., persons living in the same household and health care workers having close contact with secretions, such as intubation) should receive prophylaxis with either ciprofloxacin 500 mg PO once; rifampin, 600 mg PO bid for 2 days; or ceftriaxone 250 mg IM. Terminal component complement deficiency (C5 through C9) should be ruled out in patients with recurrent meningococcal infections.

o ***Listeria monocytogenes*** meningitis is seen in immunosuppressed adults and the elderly. Treatment is with ampicillin 2 g IV q4h in combination with a systemically administered aminoglycoside for at least 3 to 4 weeks. Trimethoprim-sulfamethoxazole (TMP-SMX; TMP 5 mg/kg IV q6h) or meropenem (2 g IV q8h) is an alternative for the penicillin-allergic patient.

o **Gram-negative bacillary meningitis** is usually a complication of head trauma or neurosurgical procedures. High-dose ceftazidime or cefepime 2 g IV q8h is used for most pathogens, including *Pseudomonas aeruginosa*. High-dose ceftriaxone or cefotaxime may be used for susceptible pathogens. Alternatives include meropenem and ciprofloxacin.

o ***S. aureus*** **meningitis** is usually a result of high-grade bacteremia, direct extension from a parameningeal focus, or recent neurosurgical procedure. Oxacillin and nafcillin 2 g IV q4h are the drugs of choice. First-generation cephalosporins do not reliably penetrate into the CSF. Vancomycin should be used for penicillin-allergic patients and when methicillin resistance is likely or confirmed. Rifampin may also be necessary.

o For **enteroviral** meningitis, the treatment is supportive care. Acyclovir, 10 mg/kg IV q8h, is used for moderate-to-severe **HSV meningitis**.

Ventriculitis and Ventriculoperitoneal Shunt Infections

GENERAL PRINCIPLES

Typically seen in neurosurgical patients. Caused by coagulase-negative staphylococci, *S. aureus*, and *Propionibacterium* species.

TREATMENT

Treated with IV vancomycin with or without rifampin or intraventricular vancomycin. Removal of the infected shunt is often necessary for cure.

Encephalitis

GENERAL PRINCIPLES

Encephalitis is inflammation of the brain parenchyma, usually associated with viral infections.

HSV-1 is the most common and most important cause of sporadic infectious encephalitis. Other important causes include **Dengue** and the arboviral meningoencephalitides such as **West Nile virus (WNV)** (see the Mosquito-Borne Infections section).

DIAGNOSIS

Clinical Presentation
Presenting complaints include fever and neurologic abnormalities, particularly with personality change or seizures, usually without meningeal signs.

Diagnostic Testing
Diagnosis is confirmed by detection of HSV-1 in the CSF by PCR. However, a negative PCR does not rule out HSV encephalitis. Temporal lobe enhancement is typically seen on brain MRI.

TREATMENT

Treatment is acyclovir 10 mg/kg IV q8h infused over 1 hour with adequate hydration, which should be initiated at first suspicion and continued for 14 to 21 days, unless diagnosis is ruled out. Delayed initiation of therapy greatly increases the risk of poor neurologic outcomes (*Clin Infect Dis 2008;47:303*).

Brain Abscess

GENERAL PRINCIPLES

Brain abscess in the immunocompetent host is usually bacterial in origin and a result of spread from a contiguous focus or from septic emboli from endocarditis. Infection is often mixed, with oral streptococci, *S. aureus*, and anaerobes being the most common pathogens.

DIAGNOSIS

- Diagnosis is radiographic, with ring-enhancing lesions seen on MRI or contrast-enhanced CT scan.
- A microbiologic etiology must be determined by aspiration, biopsy, or at the time of surgery.

TREATMENT

Empiric therapy should cover the most likely pathogens based on the primary infection site.

When no preceding infection can be found, a third-generation cephalosporin combined with metronidazole and vancomycin is a reasonable regimen until culture data are available (*Int J Surg 2011;9:136*). Therapy is often surgical with the addition of systemic antimicrobials.

Neurocysticercosis

GENERAL PRINCIPLES

This disease is caused by cyst forms of *Taenia solium* in the brain. Infection is acquired from eating undercooked pork containing the eggs of *T. solium*, which is endemic in Mexico and Central America. Diagnoses of neurocysticercosis in developed countries have recently increased due to immigration of carriers from endemic areas.

DIAGNOSIS

Clinical Presentation

Can present as new-onset seizures, hydrocephalus, or focal neurologic abnormalities.

Diagnostic testing

Neurocysticercosis should be suspected in patients with new-onset seizures of unknown etiology and exposure to endemic areas. Brain imaging reveals characteristic multiple unilocular cysts that may or may not enhance. A finding of eosinophils in the CSF is suggestive of the diagnosis. Serologic tests are available at the Centers for Disease Control (CDC).

TREATMENT

Treatment may require surgery and/or high-dose albendazole or praziquantel, depending on the location of cysts and severity. Anticonvulsants, intracranial pressure monitoring, and steroids may be needed to control symptoms (*Lancet 2003;362:547*).

CARDIOVASCULAR INFECTIONS

Infective Endocarditis

GENERAL PRINCIPLES

Epidemiology
- The incidence of acute bacterial endocarditis (ABE) and health care–associated endocarditis (related to IV catheters and invasive procedures) is rising (*Arch Intern Med 2009;109:463*).
- **Prosthetic valve endocarditis (PVE)** occurs in 1% to 4% of patients with prosthetic heart valves.

Etiology
- **Infective endocarditis (IE)** is usually caused by gram-positive cocci. *S. aureus* is the most common pathogen followed by viridans streptococci, enterococci, and coagulase-negative staphylococci.
- Gram-negative and fungal IE occur infrequently and are usually associated with injection drug use or prosthetic heart valves.
- Dental procedures and bacteremia from distant foci of infection are frequent seeding events.
- **PVE.** Early infections (within 2 months of surgery) are caused by *S. aureus*, coagulase-negative staphylococci, gram-negative bacilli, and *Candida* species. *S. aureus*,

coagulase-negative staphylococci, enterococci, and viridans streptococci are the most common causes of late-onset PVE.

Risk Factors

Structural heart disease, IV drug use, prosthetic heart valve, and a prior history of endocarditis are important predisposing factors for endocarditis.

DIAGNOSIS

The modified Duke criteria (Table 14-2a and b) for diagnosis of IE, incorporating microbiologic, pathologic, echocardiographic, and clinical findings, are widely used (*Clin Infect Dis 2000;30:633*).

Table 14-2a	Modified Duke Criteria for the Diagnosis of Infective Endocarditis

Major Criteria

I. Positive blood cultures for IE

1. Two separate blood cultures with viridans streptococci, *Streptococcus bovis, Staphylococcus aureus*, HACEK group, or community-acquired enterococci (no primary focus)
2. Persistently positive blood cultures drawn more than 12 hours apart **OR** all of three or a majority of four separate blood cultures, drawn 1 hour apart
3. Single positive blood culture for *Coxiella burnetii*

II. Evidence of endocardial involvement

1. Positive echocardiogram for IE
2. Oscillating intracardiac mass on a valve or supporting structure, in the path of regurgitant jets, or on implanted materials in the absence of another anatomic explanation
3. Abscess
4. New partial dehiscence of a prosthetic valve
5. New valvular regurgitation (change in preexisting murmur not sufficient)

Minor Criteria

1. Predisposing heart condition or intravenous drug use
2. Fever ≥38°C (100.4°F)
3. Vascular phenomena: Arterial emboli, septic pulmonary infarcts, mycotic aneurysm, intracranial hemorrhage, Janeway lesions
4. Immunologic phenomena: Glomerulonephritis, Osler's nodes, Roth spots, rheumatoid factor
5. Microbiologic evidence: Positive blood culture but not meeting major criteria or serologic evidence of infection with an organism consistent with IE

HACEK, *Haemophilus, Actinobacillus, Cardiobacterium, Eikenella, Kingella*; IE, infective endocarditis.

Table 14-2b	Classification of Infective Endocarditis by Modified Duke Criteria

Definite IE

Pathologic Criteria:

Vegetation or intracardiac abscess confirmed by histology showing active endocarditis **AND** an associated microorganism demonstrated by culture or histology

Clinical Criteria:

2 major criteria **OR**
1 major and 3 minor criteria **OR**
5 minor criteria

Possible IE

1 major and 1 minor criteria **OR**
3 minor criteria

Rejected IE

Firm alternative diagnosis **OR**
Resolution of manifestations with therapy for ≤4 days **OR**
No pathologic evidence at surgery or autopsy after antibiotic therapy ≤4 days

IE, infective endocarditis.
Adapted from Li JS, Sexton DJ, Mick N, et al. Proposed Modifications to the Duke Criteria for the Diagnosis of Infective Endocarditis. *Clin Infect Dis* 2000;30:633–638.

Clinical Presentation

- Patients with **ABE** may present within 3 to 10 days of onset of infection with critical illness.
- **Subacute bacterial endocarditis (SBE)** may present over weeks to months with constitutional symptoms (fever, malaise, anorexia), immune complex disease (nephritis, arthralgias, Osler nodes), and embolic phenomenon (renal, splenic, and cerebral infarcts; petechiae; Janeway lesions).
- **PVE** must be considered in any patient with persistent bacteremia after heart valve surgery.

Diagnostic Testing

- The most reliable diagnostic criterion for IE is persistent bacteremia in a compatible clinical setting. Three blood cultures should be taken from separate sites over at least a 1-hour period prior to empiric antimicrobial therapy. Blood cultures are positive in at least 90% of patients but can be negative if the patient has already received antibiotics.
- Echocardiography plays an important role in establishing the diagnosis of IE and determining the need for surgical intervention.
  - Patients with IE and vegetations seen by transthoracic echocardiography (TTE) are at higher risk of embolism, heart failure, and valvular disruption. However, a negative TTE cannot rule out IE.
  - When clinical evidence of IE exists, **transesophageal echocardiography (TEE)** improves the sensitivity of the Duke criteria, especially in patients with prosthetic heart valves.

TREATMENT

- *High doses of intravenous antimicrobials for extended periods (generally, 4 to 6 weeks) are required.*
- Quantitative antimicrobial susceptibility testing of the causative organism is essential to optimal treatment.
- **ABE** often requires empiric antimicrobial treatment before culture results become available. Initial treatment for *S. aureus* should consist of vancomycin 15 mg/kg IV q12h. Therapy should then be modified on the basis of culture and susceptibility data. For methicillin-sensitive isolates, oxacillin 2 g IV q4h is superior to vancomycin.
- **SBE** caused by susceptible organisms should be treated with penicillin, as this typically results in cure rates of >90%. Therapy can usually be delayed until culture data can confirm a specific organism and its susceptibilities.
- **PVE** should be treated aggressively for extended periods because of the increased risk for treatment failure and relapse. Indications for valve replacement are detailed in the following text.
- Baseline audiometry is recommended for patients who will receive 7 or more days of aminoglycoside therapy, with repeat testing weekly while on treatment or if symptoms develop.
- **Antibiotic therapy for specific organisms** (Table 14-3)
  - For **viridans streptococci** that are penicillin-susceptible, penicillin G, or ceftriaxone for 4 weeks should be given. An abbreviated 2-week course in combination with gentamicin can also be considered but carries the risk of nephrotoxicity and ototoxicity and should not be used for PVE or serious disease. Streptococci with intermediate or high resistance to penicillin should receive combination and often extended therapy. Penicillin desensitization is preferable to vancomycin for penicillin-allergic patients.
  - *S. pyogenes* and *S. pneumoniae* should be treated with penicillin G 2 to 4 million U IV q4h for 4 to 6 weeks. Penicillin-resistant pneumococci should be treated with ceftriaxone 2 g IV q24h for 4 to 6 weeks. *Streptococcus bovis* bacteremia and endocarditis are associated with lower gastrointestinal (GI) tract disease, including neoplasms. Groups B and G streptococcal endocarditis may also be associated with lower intestinal pathology.
  - *Enterococcus* **species** cause 5% to 20% of cases of SBE. Isolates from patients with enterococcal endocarditis should be screened for β-lactamase production and susceptibility to vancomycin, quinupristin/dalfopristin, linezolid, and gentamicin. Vancomycin-resistant enterococcus (VRE) IE is difficult to treat; infectious disease consultation is recommended.
  - *S. aureus* (MSSA) should be treated with oxacillin. Penicillins are superior to vancomycin, and desensitization is preferred when possible (*Medicine (Baltimore) 2003;82:333*). Cefazolin can be substituted in penicillin-allergic patients with no history of anaphylaxis. Right-sided IE in IV drug users can be treated with 2 weeks of oxacillin plus an aminoglycoside. Vancomycin, linezolid, and daptomycin can be used for MRSA. Initial low-dose gentamicin for synergy in native valve IE risks renal impairment without demonstrated benefit (*Clin Infect Dis 2009;48:713*).
  - *Coagulase-negative staphylococcus* (*e.g.,* **Staphylococcus epidermidis**) IE primarily occurs in patients with prosthetic heart valves, although native valve endocarditis is increasing, particularly in health care settings. *Staphylococcus lugdunensis* IE is associated with a high rate of perivalvular extension and

Table 14-3 Treatment of Endocarditis Caused by Specific Organisms[a]

Organism	Antibiotic Regimen	Duration	Notes
Viridans streptococci			
MIC <0.12 mcg/mL	• [Penicillin G 12–18 million U IV q24h or ceftriaxone] + gentamicin (low dose) • Vancomycin if PCN allergic	• 4 wk (2 wk total if used in combination with gentamicin)	• 2-wk course not indicated for prosthetic valves, major embolic or extended symptoms
MIC 0.12–0.5 mcg/mL	• [Penicillin G 4 million U IV q4h or ceftriaxone] + gentamicin • Vancomycin if PCN allergic	• 4 wk total with 2 wk of gentamicin	• Vancomycin monotherapy in allergic patients
MIC >0.5 mcg/mL	• Ampicillin/sulbactam ± gentamicin (if β-lactamase producing) • Vancomycin ± gentamicin	• 4–6 wk	
Enterococcus species			
Penicillin susceptible	• Ampicillin ± gentamicin • Vancomycin	• 4–6 wk	• High-level gentamicin resistance, substitute streptomycin or ceftriaxone

(continued)

Table 14-3 Treatment of Endocarditis Caused by Specific Organisms[a] (*Continued*)

Organism	Antibiotic Regimen	Duration	Notes
Penicillin resistant	• *β-lactamase:* Ampicillin/ sulbactam + gentamicin • *Intrinsically resistant:* Vancomycin + gentamicin	• 6 wk	
Vancomycin and ampicillin resistant	• Linezolid or daptomycin • Quinupristin/dalfopristin ± doxycycline	• ≥8 wk	• Consult infectious diseases specialist
Staphylococcus species			
Native valve, MSSA	• Oxacillin • Cefazolin if penicillin allergy without anaphylaxis	• 6 wk	• Initial 3–5 d gentamicin for synergy may not be beneficial
Tricuspid valve, MSSA (IV drug user)	• Oxacillin + gentamicin	• 2 wk	
Native valve, MRSA	• Vancomycin or daptomycin or linezolid (also for MSSA if anaphylactic allergy)	• 6 wk	

Staphylococcus species (prosthetic valve)

MSSA/MSSE	• Oxacillin + rifampin + gentamicin	• ≥6 wk total (2 wk of gentamicin)
MRSA/MRSE	• Vancomycin + rifampin + gentamicin	
HACEK organisms and culture-negative IE	• Ceftriaxone or ampicillin-sulbactam or ciprofloxacin	• 4 wk • HACEK stands for *Haemophilus, Actinobacillus, Cardiobacterium, Eikenella, Kingella.*

Dosing: Ceftriaxone 2 g IV q24h; gentamicin 2 g g qd or 1 mg/kg q8h; vancomycin 15 mg/kg q12h; ampicillin-sulbactam 3 g IV q6h; ampicillin 2 g IV q4h; oxacillin 2 g IV q4h; rifampin 300 mg PO q8h; cefazolin 2 g IV q8h; daptomycin 6 mg/kg/d; linezolid 600 mg IV q12h; ciprofloxacin 400 mg IV q12h. Baseline and weekly audiometry recommended for patients receiving aminoglycosides for >7 days. Monitor aminoglycoside and vancomycin levels. Goal vancomycin trough levels are near 15–20 μg/mL.

[a]See Circulation 2005;111:e393.

IE, infective endocarditis; IV, intravenous; MIC, minimum inhibitory concentration; MRSA, methicillin-resistant *Staphylococcus aureus*; MRSE, methicillin-resistant *Staphylococcus epidermidis*; MSSA, methicillin-sensitive *Staphylococcus aureus*; MSSE, methicillin-sensitive *Staphylococcus epidermidis*; PCN, penicillin.

metastatic spread. These organisms have become increasingly resistant to β-lactam antibiotics.

○ **PVE** requires aggressive combination therapy for at least 6 weeks. Initial empiric therapy pending culture data includes the addition of rifampin to vancomycin and gentamicin to improve biofilm penetration. Oxacillin should be substituted for vancomycin if supported by culture and sensitivity data. Treatment failure or relapse is common.

○ **HACEK** is an acronym for a group of fastidious, slow-growing gram-negative bacteria (*Haemophilus, Actinobacillus, Cardiobacterium, Eikenella*, and *Kingella* species) that have a predilection for infecting heart valves.

○ **Culture-negative IE** is usually encountered when prior antimicrobial therapy has been given, or rarely, with fastidious pathogens, such as nutritionally deficient streptococci, HACEK organisms, *Coxiella burnetii* (Q fever), *Bartonella, Brucella, Tropheryma whippelii* (Whipple's disease), and fungi. Empiric therapy can be initiated despite negative cultures (see Table 14-3).

• **Response to antimicrobial therapy**
○ Clinical improvement is frequently seen within 3 to 10 days of initiating therapy.
○ Blood cultures should be obtained daily until clearance of bacteremia has been documented.
○ Persistent or recurrent fever usually represents extensive cardiac infection but also may be due to septic emboli, drug hypersensitivity, or subsequent nosocomial infection (*Circulation 2005;111:e393*).

Surgical Management

• For native valve endocarditis, indications for surgery include refractory heart failure, aortic or mitral regurgitation with hemodynamic evidence of elevated left ventricular end-diastolic pressure; complications such as heart block, annular or aortic abscess, fistula, or perforation; and infection with fungi or other highly resistant organisms. Recurrent emboli and sustained bacteremia on appropriate therapy are other indications.

• For PVE, indications include heart failure, valve dehiscence, increasing valve obstruction or worsening regurgitation, complications such as abscess formation, persistent bacteremia or recurrent emboli, and relapsing infection (*J Am Coll Cardiol 2006;48:e1*).

SPECIAL CONSIDERATIONS

The American Heart Association recommendations for prophylaxis for IE have been revised and are outlined in Table 14-4.

Myocarditis

GENERAL PRINCIPLES

• When the heart is involved in an inflammatory process, the cause is often an infectious agent. Myocarditis may occur during and after viral, rickettsial, bacterial, fungal, and parasitic infections.

• Viruses are the most frequent cause, and include enteroviruses (Coxsackie B and echovirus), adenovirus, human herpes virus 6, parvovirus B-19, and many others. Myocarditis can also be a rare complication of smallpox vaccination.

Table 14-4	Endocarditis Prophylaxis[a]

Clinical Scenario	Drug and Dosage

I. Endocarditis prophylaxis is recommended for the following cardiac conditions: prosthetic valves; previous endocarditis; unrepaired congenital heart disease, including palliative shunts or conduits, repaired congenital heart disease with prosthetic material during the first 6 months after procedure, or with residual defects at or adjacent to the site of the prosthetic device; and cardiac valvulopathy in transplant recipients.

II. Regimens for dental, oral, or respiratory tract procedures (including dental extractions, periodontal or endodontic procedures, professional teeth cleaning, bronchoscopy with biopsy, rigid bronchoscopy, surgery on respiratory mucosa, tonsillectomy).

Standard prophylaxis	Amoxicillin 2 g PO 1 h before procedure
Unable to take PO	Ampicillin 2 g IM or IV, or cefazolin or ceftriaxone 1 g IM or IV within 30 min before procedure
Penicillin-allergic patient	Clindamycin 600 mg PO, or cephalexin 2 g PO, or clarithromycin or azithromycin 500 mg PO 1 h before procedure
Penicillin allergic and unable to take PO	Clindamycin 600 mg IV, or cefazolin or ceftriaxone 1 g IV within 30 min before procedure

III. Gastrointestinal and genitourinary procedures do not require routine use of prophylaxis. High-risk patients infected or colonized with enterococci should receive amoxicillin, ampicillin, or vancomycin to eradicate the organism prior to urinary tract manipulation.

IV. Prophylaxis is recommended for procedures on infected skin, skin structures, or musculoskeletal tissue ONLY for patients with cardiac conditions outlined above. An antistaphylococcal penicillin or cephalosporin should be used.

[a]See *Circulation* 2007;116:1736.
IM, intramuscular; IV, intravenous; PO, by mouth.

DIAGNOSIS

- Nasopharyngeal swab testing and serology may be performed to detect viral infections.
- Endomyocardial biopsy for histopathology and viral PCR may also be helpful.

TREATMENT

Therapeutic regimens should be targeted to the identified agent. The role of IV immunoglobulin and antiviral agents in viral-mediated myocarditis remains anecdotal.

Pericarditis

GENERAL PRINCIPLES

Acute pericarditis is a syndrome caused by inflammation of the pericardium and characterized by chest pain, a pericardial friction rub, and diffuse ST-segment elevations on electrocardiogram (ECG). Viruses are the most common infectious etiology. Bacterial causes include staphylococci and *Streptococcus pneumoniae*. Tuberculosis (TB) or histoplasmosis are occasional causes (see the Tuberculosis section).

TREATMENT

The role of antiviral therapies in viral pericarditis remains unclear. NSAIDs may be used for pain.

UPPER RESPIRATORY TRACT INFECTIONS

Pharyngitis

GENERAL PRINCIPLES

Pharyngitis is commonly caused by viruses, with infections due to GABHS and other bacteria responsible to a lesser extent.

DIAGNOSIS

Clinical Presentation
Fever, cervical lymphadenopathy, tonsillar exudates, and the absence of a cough may or may not be present in addition to throat pain. Distinguishing bacterial from viral pharyngitis based on clinical grounds alone can be challenging.

Differential Diagnosis
- **Acute HIV infection** should be considered in the setting of pharyngitis with atypical lymphocytosis and negative streptococcus and Epstein–Barr virus testing.
- **Epiglottitis** should be considered in the febrile patient with severe throat pain, odynophagia, new-onset drooling, and dysphagia, but in whom minimal findings are noted on inspection of the pharynx.
- Suppurative complications including **peritonsillar or retropharyngeal abscess** should be considered in the patient with severe unilateral pain, muffled voice, trismus, and dysphagia.

Diagnostic Testing
- Diagnostic testing is usually reserved for symptomatic patients with exposure to a documented case of streptococcal pharyngitis, individuals with signs of significant infection (i.e., fever, tonsillar exudates, and cervical adenopathy), patients whose symptoms fail to clear despite symptomatic therapy, and patients with a history of rheumatic fever.

- Rapid antigen detection testing (RADT) is useful for identifying **GABHS**, which requires therapy to prevent suppurative complications and rheumatic fever. A negative test does not reliably exclude GABHS, making throat culture necessary when RADT is negative.
- Serology for **Epstein–Barr virus** (e.g., heterophile agglutinin or monospot) and examination of a peripheral blood smear for atypical lymphocytes should be performed when infectious mononucleosis is suspected.

TREATMENT

- Most cases of pharyngitis are self-limited and do not require antimicrobial therapy.
- Treatment for **GABHS** is indicated with a positive culture or RADT, if the patient is at high risk for development of rheumatic fever, or if the diagnosis is strongly suspected, pending the results of culture. Treatment options include penicillin V 250 mg PO qid or 500 mg PO bid for 10 days, clindamycin 300 to 450 mg PO q6–8h for 5 days, azithromycin 500 mg PO on day 1 followed by 250 mg on days 2 to 5, or benzathine penicillin G 1.2 million U IM as a one-time dose (*Clin Infect Dis 2002;35:113*; *Circulation 2009;119:1541*).
- Gonococcal pharyngitis is treated with ceftriaxone 250 mg IM as a single dose.

Epiglottitis

GENERAL PRINCIPLES

Haemophilus influenzae type B, *Streptococcus pneumoniae*, *S. aureus*, and GABHS are common bacterial causes of epiglottitis, although viral and fungal pathogens may also be implicated.

DIAGNOSIS

Clinical Presentation

Fever, sore throat, odynophagia, drooling, muffled voice, and dysphagia in a patient a normal oropharyngeal examination should prompt a clinical diagnosis of epiglottitis.

Diagnostic Testing

- Throat and blood cultures are useful in determining the etiology.
- Soft-tissue lateral radiographs of the neck may aid in establishing the diagnosis.
- Definitive diagnosis is made by visualization of the epiglottis.

TREATMENT

Prompt treatment including hospitalization and otolaryngologic consultation for airway management is suggested in all suspected cases. Antimicrobial therapy should include an agent that is active against *H. influenzae*, such as ceftriaxone 2 g IV q24h or cefotaxime 2 g IV q6–8h.

Sinusitis

GENERAL PRINCIPLES

- Sinusitis is caused by obstruction of the osteomeatal complex.
- **Acute rhinosinusitis** is usually caused by upper respiratory viruses. Bacterial pathogens, such as *S. pneumoniae*, *H. influenzae*, *Moraxella catarrhalis*, and anaerobes are involved in less than 2% of cases and should be considered only if symptoms are severe or if they persist for more than 10 days.
- **Chronic rhinosinusitis** may be caused by any of the etiologic agents responsible for acute sinusitis, as well as *S. aureus*, *Corynebacterium diphtheriae*, and many anaerobes (e.g., *Prevotella* spp., *Veillonella* spp.). Possible contributing factors include asthma, nasal polyps, allergies, or immunodeficiency.

DIAGNOSIS

Clinical Presentation

- **Acute rhinosinusitis** is a clinical diagnosis that presents with purulent nasal discharge, nasal obstruction, and sinus tenderness with or without fever, lasting less than 4 weeks.
- **Chronic rhinosinusitis** is defined by symptoms lasting more than 12 weeks including mucopurulent drainage, nasal obstruction, facial pain or pressure, and decreased sense of smell with documented signs of inflammation.

Diagnostic Testing

- Diagnosis requires objective evidence of mucosal disease, usually with rhinoscopy and nasal endoscopy or a sinus CT. Plain films are not recommended.
- Sinus cultures can be obtained from nasal endoscopy or sinus puncture. Nasal swabs are not helpful.

TREATMENT

The goals of medical therapy for acute and chronic rhinosinusitis are to control infection, reduce tissue edema, facilitate drainage, maintain patency of the sinus ostia, and break the pathologic cycle that leads to chronic sinusitis.

- **Acute rhinosinusitis**
  - ○ **Symptomatic treatment** is the mainstay of therapy, including oral decongestants and analgesics with or without a short course of topical decongestant or intranasal glucocorticoid (*Otolaryngol Head Neck Surg 2007;137:S1*).
  - ○ **Empiric antibiotic therapy** is indicated only for severe persistent symptoms ($\geq$10 days) or failure of symptomatic therapy. First-line therapy should consist of a 5 to 7 day course of amoxicillin-clavulanate 875 mg/125 mg PO bid. Doxycycline or a respiratory fluoroquinolone (e.g., moxifloxacin, levofloxacin) may be used as a second-line agent in case of β-lactam allergy or primary treatment failure. TMP-SMX and macrolides are not recommended for empiric therapy due to high rates of resistance (*Clin Infect Dis 2012;54:e72*).
- **Chronic rhinosinusitis.** Treatment usually includes topical and/or systemic glucocorticoids; the role of antimicrobial agents is unclear. If they are used, amoxicillin-

clavulanate is the first-line treatment, with clindamycin for penicillin-allergic patients. Some chronic cases may require endoscopic surgery.

Influenza Virus Infection

GENERAL PRINCIPLES

Influenza is readily transmissible and associated with outbreaks of varying severity during the winter months.

DIAGNOSIS

Clinical Presentation

Influenza virus infection causes an acute, self-limited febrile illness marked with headache, myalgias, cough, and malaise.

Diagnostic Testing

Diagnosis is usually made clinically during influenza season, with confirmation by nasopharyngeal swab for rapid antigen testing, PCR, or direct fluorescent antibody test and culture.

TREATMENT

- Treatment is usually symptomatic.
- Antiviral medications may shorten the duration of illness but must be initiated within 24 to 48 hours of the onset of symptoms to be effective in immunocompetent patients (*MMWR 2011;60(1):1*). That being said, antiviral therapy should not be withheld from patients presenting more than 48 hours after symptom onset requiring hospitalization or at high risk for complications (see Complications).
  - The **neuraminidase inhibitors** (oseltamivir 75 mg PO bid or zanamivir 10 mg inhaled twice a day; each for 5 days) are used in treatment and prophylaxis of influenza A and B.
  - **Adamantanes** (amantadine and rimantadine, each 100 mg PO bid) are *not* effective against influenza B.
  - Circulating strains change annually with varying resistance patterns to both classes of antivirals. *Treatment decisions must be based on annual resistance data*, available from the CDC at *http://www.cdc.gov*.
- **Vaccination** is the most reliable prevention strategy. Annual vaccination is recommended for all individuals 6 months of age and older (*MMWR 2011;60(33):1128*).

COMPLICATIONS

- Adults over 65 years of age, residents of nursing homes and other long-term care facilities, pregnant women (and those up to 2 weeks' postpartum), and patients with chronic medical conditions (e.g., pulmonary disease, cardiovascular disease, active malignancy, diabetes mellitus, chronic renal insufficiency, chronic liver disease, immunosuppression including HIV and transplantation, morbid obesity) are at greater risk of complications.

- Influenza pneumonia and secondary bacterial pneumonia are the most common complications of influenza infection.
- Viral antigenic drift and shift can cause emergence of strains with enhanced virulence or the potential for pandemic spread, requiring modified therapy or heightened infection control measures.

LOWER RESPIRATORY TRACT INFECTIONS

Acute Bronchitis

GENERAL PRINCIPLES

Acute bronchitis involves inflammation of the bronchi. The usual etiologies are viral agents, such as coronavirus, rhinovirus, influenza, or parainfluenza. Uncommon causes include *Mycoplasma pneumoniae*, *Chlamydophila pneumoniae*, and *Bordetella pertussis*.

DIAGNOSIS

Clinical Presentation

Symptoms include cough with or without sputum production lasting more than 5 days and may be indistinguishable from an upper respiratory tract infection early on. Fever is uncommon.

Diagnostic Testing

- Diagnosis is made clinically. Sputum cultures are not recommended.
- In febrile, systemically ill, or older patients, pneumonia should be ruled out clinically or radiographically, and diagnostic tests for influenza should be performed depending on the season and local disease trends.
- Cough lasting >2 weeks in an adult should be evaluated for pertussis with a nasopharyngeal swab for culture or PCR.

TREATMENT

- Treatment is symptomatic and should be directed toward controlling cough (dextromethorphan 15 mg PO q6h).
- Routine antimicrobial use is not recommended unless pertussis has been diagnosed (*Ann Intern Med 2001;134:521*).
- **Pertussis** treatment consists of clarithromycin 500 mg PO bid for 14 days or azithromycin 500 mg PO single dose followed by 250 mg PO daily for 4 more days.
- Pertussis cases should be reported to the local health department for contact tracing and administration of postexposure prophylaxis with azithromycin when indicated.

Community-Acquired Pneumonia

GENERAL PRINCIPLES

The predominant etiologic agent is *S. pneumoniae* in which multidrug resistance is rapidly increasing. Pneumonia caused by atypical agents, such as *Legionella pneumophila, C. pneumoniae,* or *M. pneumoniae* cannot be reliably determined clinically. Influenza and other respiratory viruses may also cause pneumonia in adults. MRSA is an important cause of severe, necrotizing pneumonia.

DIAGNOSIS

Clinical Presentation

Fever and respiratory symptoms, including cough with sputum production, dyspnea, and pleuritic chest pain, are common presenting features in immunocompetent patients. Signs include tachypnea, rales, or consolidation on auscultation.

Diagnostic Testing

- Assessment of etiologic agents in all hospitalized patients should include sputum Gram stain and culture and blood cultures prior to antibiotic therapy.
- If an atypical agent is suspected, urine *Legionella* antigen should be obtained. Respiratory specimens may be sent for enzyme immunoassay (EIA), immunofluorescence, or PCR to detect other atypical or viral pathogens (including influenza). Acute and convalescent serologic testing can retrospectively identify several atypical pathogens including *C. pneumoniae, C. burnetii* (Q fever), and *Hantavirus.*
- Chest radiography should be performed and may reveal lobar consolidation, interstitial infiltrates, or cavitary lesions, confirming the diagnosis.
- Fiber optic bronchoscopy is used for detection of less common organisms, especially in immunocompromised patients, as well as to identify associated anatomic lesions, perform tissue biopsy for histopathology, and obtain quantitative cultures.

TREATMENT

- Most patients can be treated as outpatients, although all should be evaluated for severity of illness, comorbid factors, and oxygenation. Guidelines giving detailed empiric treatment regimens have been published, with an emphasis on targeting the most likely pathogens within specific risk groups (*Clin Infect Dis 2007;44:S27*). Antibiotic therapy should be narrowed once a specific microbiologic etiology has been identified.
- **Immunocompetent outpatients** with no recent antibiotic exposure and no comorbidities should receive a macrolide, such as azithromycin 500 mg PO single dose followed by 250 mg PO daily for 4 more days, or doxycycline 100 mg PO for at least 5 days.
- **Outpatients with recent antibiotic exposure or comorbidities** should receive a respiratory fluoroquinolone (e.g., moxifloxacin) monotherapy or macrolide (azithromycin or clarithromycin) with or without high-dose amoxicillin 1 g PO tid for at least 5 days.
- **Hospitalized patients** should be treated with ceftriaxone 1 g IV daily or cefotaxime 1 g IV q8h plus a macrolide (azithromycin or clarithromycin), or monotherapy

with a respiratory fluoroquinolone. Minimum duration of therapy should be at least 5 days but is typically longer, as the patient should be afebrile for 48 to 72 hours with signs of clinical improvement on therapy prior to discontinuation.

- In **critically ill patients**, the addition of azithromycin or a respiratory fluoroquinolone to a β-lactam (ceftriaxone, cefotaxime, ampicillin-sulbactam) is necessary to provide coverage for *L. pneumophila*. MRSA coverage with vancomycin or linezolid should also be considered. Intravenously administered penicillin G, which reaches high concentrations in lung tissue, remains an effective treatment for sensitive *S. pneumoniae* isolates (*Clin Infect Dis 2003;37:230*). For coverage of *Pseudomonas aeruginosa*, an antipseudomonal β-lactam (cefepime, piperacillin-tazobactam, meropenem, imipenem) in combination with an antipseudomonal fluoroquinolone (ciprofloxacin, levofloxacin) is recommended.
- **Thoracentesis** of pleural effusions should be performed, with analysis of pH, cell count, Gram stain and bacterial culture, protein, and lactate dehydrogenase (see Chapter 10, Pulmonary Diseases). Empyemas should be drained.

Lung Abscess

GENERAL PRINCIPLES

Lung abscess typically results from aspiration of oral flora. Polymicrobial infections are common, and may involve oral anaerobes (*Prevotella* spp., *Fusobacterium nucleatum*, *Actinomyces* spp., and anaerobic and microaerophilic streptococci), enteric gramnegative bacilli (*K. pneumoniae*), and *S. aureus*. Risk factors include periodontal disease and conditions that predispose patients to aspiration of oropharyngeal contents.

DIAGNOSIS

Clinical Presentation

Infections are indolent and may be reminiscent of pulmonary TB, with dyspnea, fever, chills, night sweats, weight loss, and cough productive of putrid or blood-streaked sputum for several weeks.

Diagnostic Testing

Chest radiography is sensitive and typically reveals infiltrates with cavitation and air–fluid levels in dependent areas of the lung, such as the lower lobes or the posterior segments of the upper lobes. CT can provide additional anatomic detail.

TREATMENT

- Antibiotic therapy should consist of an antipneumococcal fluoroquinolone (moxifloxacin, levofloxacin) plus clindamycin, or monotherapy with a β-lactam/β-lactamase inhibitor (ampicillin-sulbactam, piperacillin-tazobactam, amoxicillin-clavulanate) or a carbapenem (meropenem, imipenem). MRSA can cause cavitary lung lesions similar to abscesses, in which case vancomycin or linezolid should be used.
- Percutaneous drainage or surgical resection is reserved for antibiotic-refractory disease, usually involving large abscesses (>8 cm) or infections with resistant organisms.

Tuberculosis

GENERAL PRINCIPLES

TB is a systemic disease caused by *M. tuberculosis*. Most cases result from reactivation of prior infection. The prevalence of TB, particularly multidrug-resistant forms (MDR-TB), has increased among immigrants from Southeast Asia, Sub-Saharan Africa, the Indian subcontinent, and Central America. Extensively drug resistant TB (XDR-TB) is becoming increasingly prevalent in Sub-Saharan Africa. Persons at highest risk include those with HIV infection, silicosis, diabetes mellitus, chronic renal insufficiency, malignancy, malnutrition, and other forms of immunosuppression, including therapy with tumor necrosis factor (TNF) antagonists such as infliximab and etanercept (*Clin Infect Dis 2004;39:300*).

DIAGNOSIS

Clinical Presentation
- The most frequent clinical presentation is pulmonary disease. Symptoms are often indolent and may include cough, hemoptysis, dyspnea, fever, night sweats, weight loss, or fatigue.
- Extrapulmonary disease can present as cervical lymphadenitis, genitourinary disease, osteomyelitis, miliary dissemination, meningitis, peritonitis, or pericarditis.

Diagnostic Testing
- Chest radiography may reveal focal infiltrates, nodules, cavitary lesions, miliary disease, pleural effusions, or hilar lymphadenopathy. In primary infection, middle and lower lobe infiltrates are more common. Reactivation disease classically involves the upper lobes.
- A presumptive diagnosis of active TB is usually made with positive fluorochrome or acid-fast bacteria (AFB) smears of sputum. However, nontuberculous mycobacteria (NTM) and some *Nocardia* species may also yield positive results with these techniques.
- TB can take several weeks to grow in culture so if the clinical suspicion is high, presumptive therapy even with negative smears may be indicated until cultures are negative. Use of radiometric culture systems and species-specific DNA probes can provide results faster than traditional methods.
- Drug susceptibility testing should be performed on all initial isolates as well as on subsequent isolates obtained from patients who do not respond to standard therapy.

TREATMENT

- Treatment (*MMWR 2003;52(RR-11):1*; *Clin Infect Dis 2000;31(3):633*) does not have to take place in a hospital setting, but hospitalization to initiate therapy provides an opportunity for intensive patient education. If a patient is hospitalized, proper isolation in a **negative-pressure room** is essential.
- The local health department should be notified of all cases of TB so that contacts can be identified and adherence to medical treatment ensured through directly observed therapy (DOT).

- **Antituberculosis treatment regimens** should include at least two drugs to which the organism is susceptible given the high frequency with which primary drug resistance develops when a single drug is administered. Extended therapy is necessary because of the prolonged generation time of mycobacteria. Because adherence to multidrug regimens for prolonged periods is difficult, DOT should be used for all patients.
- **Initial therapy** (the first 8 weeks) of uncomplicated pulmonary TB should consist of four drugs: **isoniazid** (**INH** 5 mg/kg; maximum, 300 mg PO daily), **rifampin** (**RIF**, 10 mg/kg; maximum, 600 mg PO daily), **pyrazinamide** (**PZA**, 15 to 30 mg/kg; maximum, 2 g PO daily), and either **ethambutol** (**EMB**, 15 to 25 mg/kg PO daily) or **streptomycin** (**SM**, 15 mg/kg; maximum, 1 g IM daily). Pyridoxine (vitamin B_6) 25 to 50 mg PO daily should be used with INH to prevent neuropathy. If the isolate proves to be **fully susceptible** to INH and RIF, then EMB (or streptomycin) can be dropped and INH, RIF, and PZA continued to complete this initial phase.
- **Continuation therapy** most commonly consists of an additional 16 weeks of INH and RIF, to reach a standard total of 6 months of therapy for pulmonary TB. Patients at high risk for relapse (cavitary pulmonary disease or positive TB cultures after 2 months of therapy) should be treated for a total of 9 months.
- After at least 2 weeks of daily therapy, intermittent drug administration (two or three times per week at adjusted doses) can be considered as part of DOT supervised by public health departments.
- If **INH resistance** is documented at any point, INH should be discontinued, and RIF, PZA, and EMB continued for the remaining duration of therapy. Organisms resistant only to INH can be effectively treated with a 6-month regimen if a standard four-drug regimen consisting of INH, RIF, PZA, and EMB or streptomycin was started initially.
- Therapy for **multidrug-resistant TB** has been less well studied, and consultation with an expert in the treatment of TB is strongly recommended.
- **Extrapulmonary disease** in adults can be treated in the same manner as pulmonary disease, with 6- to 9-month regimens. TB meningitis should be treated for 9 to 12 months.
- **Pregnant women** should not receive PZA or streptomycin, and should be treated with a 9-month regimen. INH, RIF, and EMB, with pyridoxine, should be administered during the initial 8 week phase. If the isolate proves to be INH sensitive, EMB can be stopped with continuation of INH and RIF for the remainder of therapy.
- **Glucocorticoids** remain controversial in the management of TB but have been used in combination with antituberculous drugs to treat life-threatening complications such as pericarditis (*Circulation 2005;112:3608*) and meningitis (*N Engl J Med 2004;351:1741*). Regimens have included prednisone 1 mg/kg (maximum, 60 mg) PO daily or dexamethasone 12 mg IV daily tapering over several weeks.
- **Monitoring response to therapy.** Patients with initial positive sputum AFB smears prior to treatment should submit sputum for AFB smear and culture every 1 to 2 weeks until AFB smears become negative. Sputum should then be obtained monthly until two consecutive negative cultures are documented. Conversion of cultures from positive to negative is the most reliable indicator of response to treatment. Continued symptoms or persistently positive AFB smears or cultures after 3 months of treatment should raise the suspicion of drug resistance or nonadherence and prompt referral to an expert in the treatment of TB.

- **Monitoring for adverse reactions.** Most patients should have a baseline laboratory evaluation at the start of therapy that includes hepatic enzymes, bilirubin, complete blood count (CBC), and serum creatinine. Routine laboratory monitoring for patients with normal baseline values is probably unnecessary except in the setting of HIV (particularly if receiving concurrent antiretroviral therapy), alcohol abuse, chronic liver disease, or pregnancy. Monthly clinical evaluations with specific inquiries about symptoms of drug toxicity are essential. Patients taking EMB should be tested monthly for visual acuity and red–green color perception.
- **Latent tuberculosis infection**
  Latent TB infection (LTBI) occurs when someone has been exposed to TB, as demonstrated by a positive tuberculin skin test (TST) or interferon gamma release assay (IGRA), but has no signs or symptoms of current active disease.
  Criteria for a **positive TST** are based on the **maximum diameter of induration** (not erythema):
  - A **5-mm induration** is considered positive in patients with HIV infection or another defect in cell-mediated immunity, close contacts of a known case of TB, patients with chest radiographs indicative of healed TB, and individuals with organ transplantation or other immunosuppression.
  - A **10-mm induration** is considered positive in immigrants from high-prevalence areas (Asia, Africa, Latin America, Eastern Europe), prisoners, the homeless, IV drug users, nursing home residents, low-income populations, patients with chronic medical illnesses or health and economic disparities, and those people who have frequent contact with these groups (e.g., health care workers, prison guards).
  - A **15-mm induration** is considered positive TST for otherwise healthy individuals not in a high-prevalence group.
  - Untreated, approximately 5% of persons with LTBI develop active TB disease within 2 years of infection. TB disease develops in an additional 5% of persons with LTBI over their remaining life span. Adequate prophylactic treatment can substantially reduce the risk of disease.
- **Chemoprophylaxis for latent tuberculosis infection**
  Chemoprophylaxis for LTBI should be administered only after active disease has been ruled out by a proper evaluation (chest radiography, sputum collection, or both). **INH** 300 mg PO daily for 9 months should be administered to persons with LTBI who have risk factors for progression to active TB disease, regardless of age.
  - Risk factors for progression include a TST conversion within 2 years of a previously negative TST; a history of untreated TB or chest radiographic evidence of previous disease; HIV infection, diabetes mellitus, end-stage renal disease, hematologic or lymphoreticular malignancy, conditions associated with rapid weight loss, chronic malnutrition, silicosis, or patients who are receiving immunosuppressive therapy; and household members and other close contacts of patients with active disease who have a reactive TST.
  - Persons with **HIV** infection or other severely immunocompromised states (e.g., transplant) who have had known contact with a patient with active TB should be treated for LTBI regardless of the TST.
  - Newer alternative regimens of shorter duration but potentially higher toxicity can be considered in consultation with a TB expert (*N Engl J Med 2011;365:2155*).
  - Referral to the public health department for LTBI chemoprophylaxis is recommended to ensure adherence and to monitor for medication-related complications.

GASTROINTESTINAL AND ABDOMINAL INFECTIONS

Peritonitis

GENERAL PRINCIPLES

- **Primary** or **spontaneous bacterial peritonitis (SBP)** is a common complication of cirrhosis and ascites and should be ruled out in any patients with ascites and fever or other clinical decompensation including encephalopathy, renal failure, and GI bleed. *M. tuberculosis* and *Neisseria gonorrhoeae* (Fitz-Hugh–Curtis syndrome in women) also occasionally cause primary peritonitis in patients at risk.
- **Secondary peritonitis** is caused by a perforated viscus in the GI or genitourinary tract, or contiguous spread from a visceral infection, usually resulting in an *acute* surgical abdomen. Pathogens are virtually always mixed.
- Peritonitis related to **peritoneal dialysis** is addressed in Chapter 13, Renal Diseases.

DIAGNOSIS

Clinical Presentation

Signs and symptoms can be absent in patients with SBP; therefore, a diagnostic paracentesis should be performed in all patients at hospital admission with cirrhosis and ascites, or with GI bleeding, encephalopathy, or declining liver/renal function (*Gut 2012;61:297*).

Diagnostic Testing

- Diagnosis of **SBP** is made by sending ascites fluid for culture (directly inoculate culture bottles at bedside), cell count, and differential. SBP is diagnosed when ascites fluid has >250 neutrophils.
- Diagnosis of **secondary peritonitis** is made clinically, supplemented by blood culture (positive 20% to 30%) and imaging to evaluate for free air (perforation) or other source of infection.

TREATMENT

- Initial broad spectrum antibiotic coverage for SBP, culture-negative neutrophilic ascites (CNNA), and *symptomatic* nonneutrophilic bacterascites (culture-positive ascites with <250 polymorphonuclear neutrophils [PMNs]) should be narrowed if a causative organism is isolated. Treatment duration is 7 days but should be extended to 2 weeks if bacteremia is present. Administration of IV albumin on days 1 and 3 of treatment may improve survival (*N Engl J Med 1999;341(6):403*). If a repeat paracentesis reveals <250 PMNs and cultures remain negative, treatment may be shortened to 5 days. **SBP prophylaxis** should be initiated after the first episode of SBP or after variceal bleeding.

* **Secondary peritonitis** primarily requires surgical intervention. Empiric antimicrobial therapy must be broad spectrum and tailored for severity and the presumed source while awaiting cultures. Empiric antifungal coverage is usually not indicated. Intra-abdominal abscess formation is a complication of secondary peritonitis that usually requires drainage. Antibiotics are often continued until imaging demonstrates resolution of the abscess (Table 14-5).

Table 14-5	Empiric Therapy for Peritonitis		
Disease	**Common Pathogens**	**Empiric IV Therapy**	**Notes**
Secondary peritonitis (acute abdomen)	Mixed gut flora (enteric gram negatives, gram positives, anaerobes)	β-lactam/β-lactamase inhibitor[a] or third-/fourth-generation cephalosporin + metronidazole/clindamycin[b] or carbapenem[c]	Always look for and address source of infection; treat for 5–7 d postoperatively
Fungal peritonitis or abscess	*Candida* spp.	Anidulafungin or voriconazole or itraconazole[d]	Treat for 2 wk
Chronic TB peritonitis	*Mycobacterium tuberculosis*	Treat the same as pulmonary TB	
Primary or spontaneous bacterial peritonitis	See Chapter 19, Liver diseases		
Peritoneal dialysis-related peritonitis	See Chapter 13, Renal Diseases		
Fitz-Hugh–Curtis	See Sexually Transmitted Diseases section for treatment of disseminated *Neisseria gonorrhea*		

[a]Ticarcillin-clavulanate 3.1 g q6h; piperacillin-tazobactam 3.375 g q6h or 4.5 g q8h; ampicillin-sulbactam 3 g q6h.
[b]For example, ceftriaxone 1 g q24h plus either metronidazole 500 mg q8h or clindamycin 600 to 900 mg q8h.
[c]Ertapenem 1 g q24h; imipenem 500 mg q6h; meropenem 1 g q8h; doripenem 500 mg q8h.
[d]Anidulafungin 200 mg × 1, then 100 mg IV q24h; voriconazole 6 mg/kg IV q12h × 1 d, then 4 mg/kg IV q12h; itraconazole 200 mg PO q12h.
TB, tuberculosis.

Hepatobiliary Infections

GENERAL PRINCIPLES

- **Acute cholecystitis** is typically preceded by biliary colic associated with cholelithiasis and characteristically presents with fever, right upper quadrant (RUQ) tenderness with Murphy's sign, and vomiting. Acalculous cholecystitis occurs in 5% to 10% of cases. Organisms usually consist of normal gut flora. Leukocytosis and mild elevations of bilirubin, transaminases, and alkaline phosphatase are possible.
- **Ascending cholangitis** is a sometimes fulminant infectious complication of an obstructed common bile duct, often following pancreatitis or cholecystitis.

DIAGNOSIS

Clinical Presentation

- The classic presentation is the Charcot triad of fever, RUQ pain, and jaundice; the additional symptoms of confusion and hypotension (Reynolds' pentad) warrant rapid intervention. Bacteremia and shock are common.
- Tenderness and guarding of the RUQ is a common sign. Murphy's sign can be useful if tenderness on exam is absent.

Diagnostic Testing

- Liver function test (LFT) abnormalities are often severe.
- Diagnosis of biliary tract infections is usually made by imaging, with ultrasonography being the primary modality. Technetium-99m-hydroxy iminodiacetic acid scanning and CT scanning may also be useful (*N Engl J Med 2008; 358(26):2804*).
- Endoscopic retrograde cholangiopancreatography (ERCP) allows for diagnosis as well as therapeutic intervention in the case of common bile duct obstruction and should be considered in patients with common bile duct dilation, jaundice, or LFT abnormalities.

TREATMENT

- Management of **acute cholecystitis** includes parenteral fluids, restricted PO intake, analgesia, and surgery. Consider perioperative antibiotics in mild disease as they may reduce the risk of postsurgical infections, but advanced age, severe disease, or complications such as gallbladder ischemia or perforation, peritonitis, or bacteremia mandated broad-spectrum antibiotics. Immediate surgery is usually necessary for severe disease, but surgery can be otherwise delayed up to 6 weeks if there is an initial response to medical therapy.
- The mainstay of therapy for **ascending cholangitis** is aggressive supportive care and surgical or endoscopic decompression and drainage. Broad-spectrum antibiotics

Table 14-6	Empiric Therapy for Cholangitis and Cholecystitis[a]		
Disease	Common Pathogens	Empiric IV Therapy	Notes
Cholecystitis	*Escherichia coli* *Klebsiella* *Enterococcus* *Enterobacter*	β-lactam/β-lactamase inhibitor[b] or fluoroquinolone[c] or third-generation cephalosporin + metronidazole/clindamycin[d] or carbapenem[e] if severe or risk of resistant organisms	Treat for 3–4 d postop or 5–7 d if no cholecystectomy
Cholangitis	*E. coli* *Klebsiella* *Enterococcus* *Enterobacter*	β-lactam/β-lactamase inhibitor or carbapenem or tigecycline (100 mg × 1, then 50 mg q12h)	Requires biliary decompression Treat 4–7 d after relief of obstruction

[a]*Clin Infect Dis* 2003;37:997.
[b]Ticarcillin-clavulanate 3.1 g q6h; piperacillin-tazobactam 3.375 g q6h or 4.5 g q8h; ampicillin-sulbactam 3 g q6h.
[c]Ciprofloxacin 400 mg q12h; levofloxacin 500 mg q24h; moxifloxacin 400 mg q24h.
[d]For example, ceftriaxone 1 g q24h plus either metronidazole 500 mg q8h or clindamycin 600 to 900 mg q8h.
[e]Ertapenem 1 g q24h; imipenem 500 mg q6h; meropenem 1 g q8h; doripenem 500 mg q8h.

are mandatory. Development of an abscess is a complication requiring surgical drainage (Table 14-6).

OTHER INFECTIONS

- **Infectious diarrhea** (see Chapter 18, Gastrointestinal Diseases).
- **Viral hepatitis** (see Chapter 19, Liver Diseases).
- *Helicobacter pylori*–associated disease (see Chapter 18, Gastrointestinal Diseases).

Diverticulitis

GENERAL PRINCIPLES

Enteric gram-negative bacilli and gut anaerobes are the causative organisms.

DIAGNOSIS

- Diverticulitis presents initially with left lower quadrant abdominal pain and fever. Obstipation is also commonly seen.
- Diagnosis is frequently clinical, but abdominal/pelvic CT scan can be helpful to rule out pericolic abscess and is recommended as the initial radiologic exam.

TREATMENT

The standard treatment regimen for mild diverticulitis is TMP-SMX 160 mg/800 mg (DS) PO bid or ciprofloxacin 500 mg PO bid combined with metronidazole 500 mg PO bid for 7 to 10 days. Broader antimicrobial coverage (as for secondary peritonitis), which could consist of a β-lactam/β-lactamase inhibitor, and surgical intervention are warranted for more severe cases (*N Engl J Med 2007;357(20):2057*).

Appendicitis

DIAGNOSIS

- Presents classically with vague abdominal pain followed by more localizing right lower quadrant (RLQ) pain and signs and symptoms of secondary peritonitis.
- As with diverticulitis, diagnosis is frequently clinical.

TREATMENT

Treatment is surgical, usually with adjuvant antimicrobial therapy as for secondary peritonitis.

GENITOURINARY INFECTIONS

Diagnostic and therapeutic approaches to adult genitourinary infections are determined by gender-specific anatomic differences, prior antimicrobial exposures, and the presence of medical devices.

Lower Urinary Tract Infections

DIAGNOSIS

Clinical Presentation

- Lower urinary tract infections (UTIs) are characterized by pyuria and bacteriuria, often with dysuria, urgency, or frequency. Fever is usually absent unless pyelonephritis is present.
- Dysuria without pyuria in sexually active patients warrants consideration of sexually transmitted infection.

Diagnostic Testing

- A rapid presumptive diagnosis can be made by urinalysis (UA) or microscopic examination of a fresh, unspun, clean-voided urine specimen suggesting pyuria (positive leukocyte esterase or >8 leukocytes per high-power field) or bacteriuria (positive nitrites or >1 organism per oil-immersion field). A urine Gram stain can be helpful in guiding initial antimicrobial choices. Quantitative culture often yields >10^5 bacteria/mL, but colony counts as low as 10^2 to 10^4 bacteria/mL may indicate infection in women with acute dysuria.

- An incidental finding of **asymptomatic bacteriuria** is of limited clinical significance except in pregnant women or patients undergoing urologic surgery (*Clin Infect Dis 2005;40:643*).

- **Acute uncomplicated cystitis in women.** A pretreatment urine culture is recommended for diabetics, patients who are symptomatic for >7 days, individuals with recurrent UTI, women who use a contraceptive diaphragm, and individuals older than 65 years. Therapy should be extended to 7 days in this subset of patients. Infections are primarily caused by *E. coli* (80%) and *Staphylococcus saprophyticus* (5% to 15%).

- **Recurrent cystitis in women.** Repeat infections are usually reinfections rather than recurrences, due to host–dependent risk factors, which vary for young women, healthy postmenopausal women, and older women who are institutionalized.

- **Complicated UTIs.** UTIs associated with anatomic abnormalities; functional, metabolic, or immunologic abnormalities; pregnancy; indwelling catheters; or unusual pathogens are termed "complicated." Pretreatment and posttreatment urine cultures are needed, and initial broad coverage pending culture data for 10 to 14 days of therapy is appropriate. Foreign bodies must be removed.

- **UTIs in men.** Cystitis is uncommon in young men. It may not necessarily indicate a urologic abnormality, and sexually transmitted infections should be considered as an alternate diagnosis. Risk factors include anal intercourse and lack of circumcision. Chronic prostatitis is a frequent cause of recurrent UTI in men.

- **Catheter-associated bacteriuria.** Catheter-associated bacteriuria is a common source of gram-negative bacteremia in hospitalized patients and is often polymicrobial. Duration of catheterization is the biggest risk factor.

- **Acute urethral syndrome** is a condition occurring in women who have lower UTI symptoms and pyuria with <10^5 bacteria/mL urine. These patients may have bacterial cystitis or urethritis caused by *Chlamydia trachomatis*, *Ureaplasma urealyticum*, or less frequently, *N. gonorrhoeae*. Specific cultures of the endocervix for sexually transmitted diseases should be performed (see the Sexually Transmitted Diseases section). If no specific etiology is found, **empiric treatment** with doxycycline 100 mg PO bid for 7 days or azithromycin 1 g PO in a single dose is recommended.

- **Acute prostatitis** is often a severe systemic illness characterized by fever, chills, dysuria, and a boggy, tender prostate on examination. Diagnosis is usually obvious by physical exam and urine Gram stain and culture. Prostatic massage is not necessary or recommended to diagnose acute prostatitis. Enteric gram negatives are the usual causative organisms.

- **Chronic prostatitis** can manifest vaguely as low back pain; perineal, testicular, or penile pain; dysuria; ejaculatory pain; recurrent UTIs with the same organism; or hematospermia. Physical exam is usually unrevealing. Prostatitis is frequently abacterial; diagnosis requires identification of organisms by quantitative urine cultures before and after prostatic massage (*Tech Urol 1997;3:38*). Causative organisms are the same as for acute prostatitis. Transrectal ultrasound is only helpful if abscess is suspected.

- **Epididymitis** presents as a unilateral scrotal ache with swollen and tender epididymis on exam. Causative organisms are usually *N. gonorrhoeae* or *C. trachomatis* in sexually active young men and gram-negative enteric organisms in older men. Diagnosis and therapy should be directed according to this epidemiology, with ceftriaxone and doxycycline in young men and TMP-SMX or ciprofloxacin in men older than 35 years.

TREATMENT

See Table 14-7 for details.
- **Acute uncomplicated cystitis in women.** A 3-day course of empiric antibiotic therapy is recommended for symptomatic women with pyuria.
- **Recurrent cystitis in women**
  - Treatment regimens for simple cystitis are successful for most recurrences. Relapses with the original infecting organism that occur within 2 weeks of cessation of therapy should be treated for 2 weeks and may indicate a urologic abnormality.
  - **Prophylactic therapy** for patients with frequent reinfection should be initiated only after sterilization of the urine with a standard treatment regimen. An alternative method of contraception might decrease the frequency of reinfection in women who use a diaphragm and/or spermicide. Prophylaxis regimens can be continuous, postcoital, or self-initiated.
- **UTIs in men.** Treatment with a typical antibiotic regimen as for cystitis in women should be continued for a full 7-day course. If the response to therapy is prompt, a urologic evaluation is unlikely to be useful. Urologic studies are appropriate when no underlying risk factor is identified, when treatment fails, in the event of recurrent infections, or when pyelonephritis occurs.
- **Catheter-associated bacteriuria**
  - Treatment is generally not indicated for asymptomatic bacteriuria in the absence of pregnancy, immunocompromise, or planned urologic procedure.
  - Symptomatic catheter-associated UTIs should prompt removal or exchange of the catheter, collection of blood and urine cultures, and treatment with 7 to 10 days of antibiotic therapy appropriate for complicated UTI.
  - Candiduria should not be treated unless the patient is immunocompromised and at high risk for candidemia, or there are symptoms and pyuria with no bacterial source. Otherwise, host status optimization (e.g., glucose control in diabetics, removal or exchange of Foley catheter) is sufficient.
  - **Prevention** measures include employing aseptic technique during urinary catheter insertion, use of a closed drainage system, and timely removal of the catheter when no longer needed.
  - In patients with chronic indwelling catheters, the development of bacteriuria is inevitable, and long-term antimicrobial suppression simply selects for multidrug-resistant bacteria. Such patients should only be treated with systemic antimicrobials when symptomatic infection with pyuria is evident.
- Treatment of **acute bacterial prostatitis** is a 2- to 4-week course of either ciprofloxacin 500 mg PO bid or TMP-SMX 160 mg/800 mg (DS) PO bid. Culture-positive chronic bacterial prostatitis should receive prolonged therapy (for at least 6 weeks with a fluoroquinolone or 3 months with TMP-SMX).

Table 14-7	Empiric Therapy for Urinary Tract Infections

Disease	Empiric Therapy	Notes
Simple cystitis (*Clin Infect Dis* 2011;52:e103)	*First line*: TMP-SMX DS PO bid or TMP (if sulfa-allergic) 100 mg PO bid; nitrofurantoin sustained release 100 mg PO bid (× 3–7 d therapy only); or fosfomycin 3 g PO single dose *Alternate*: Ciprofloxacin 250 mg PO bid or norfloxacin 400 mg PO bid for *severe symptoms* or based on local resistance patterns.	Choose antibiotics based on local susceptibility patterns. Usually treat for 3 d. Extend therapy to 7 d for diabetics and older patients, avoid TMP-SMX in older women. Fosfomycin has lower efficacy than other recommended agents; avoid if early pyelonephritis suspected.
Cystitis in men (*J Antimicrob Chemother* 2000;46(suppl 1): 23–27)	As per simple cystitis in women with the exception of nitrofurantoin, which should not be used (does not achieve reliable tissue concentrations). Treat × 7 d.	Consider urologic evaluation for recurrent disease or pyelonephritis.
Recurrent cystitis (*N Engl J Med* 2003;349:259)	*Postcoital prophylaxis*: TMP-SMX SS × 1 or ciprofloxacin 250 mg × 1 or nitrofurantoin 100 mg × 1. *Continuous prophylaxis*: TMP-SMX 0.5 SS qd or qod × 6 mos or nitrofurantoin 50–100 mg qhs × 6 mos. *Intermittent self-treatment*: TMP-SMX DS PO bid × 3 d or ciprofloxacin 250 mg PO bid × 3 d.	Cranberry juice, topical vaginal estrogen in postmenopausal women, and voiding after intercourse may have a role in preventing recurrent UTI.
Pregnancy (*Cochrane Database Syst Rev 2011; 19:CD002256*)	Nitrofurantoin 100 mg PO qid × 7 d or cephalexin 200–500 mg PO qid × 7 d or cefuroxime axetil 250 mg PO qid × 7 d.	Treat all asymptomatic bacteriuria in pregnancy. Screen pregnant women near end of first trimester with urine culture (*Clin Infect Dis 2005;40: 643–654*).

(continued)

Table 14-7	Empiric Therapy for Urinary Tract Infections (*Continued*)	
Disease	**Empiric Therapy**	**Notes**
Complicated UTI (*N Engl J Med 31993; 329:1328*)	*Mild-to-moderate illness*: Second-generation FQ.[a] *Severe illness, recent FQ, or institutionalized*: Cefepime 2 g IV q12h or third-generation cephalosporin[b] or carbapenem[c] or piperacillin-tazobactam 3.375–4.5 g IV q6h. Consider adding vancomycin empirically for gram-positive cocci on urine Gram stain.	Base empiric coverage on local sensitivity patterns, and narrow therapy when organism identified. Continue therapy for 10–14 d but can consider shortening if complicating factor is resolved (i.e., removal of indwelling device or stone).
Candiduria (*Clin Infect Dis 2004;38:161*)	*Candida albicans*: Fluconazole 100–200 mg PO qd × 7–14 d. *Critically ill or nonalbicans species*: amphotericin B × 5–10 d.	Remove catheter if present. *Indications to treat*: Symptoms with pyuria, hardware, pregnancy, neutropenia, renal allografts, prior to GU surgery, or risk of dissemination.
Pyelonephritis (*Clin Infect Dis 2011;52:e103*)	*Outpatient*: Second-generation FQ[a]. *Inpatient*: Second-generation FQ[a] or aminoglycoside[d] or ampicillin-sulbactam 1–2 g IV q6h or third-generation cephalosporin.[b] *Pregnancy*: Cefazolin 1 g IV q8h or ceftriaxone 1 g IV or IM q24h or piperacillin 4 g IV q8h.	Treat IV until afebrile × 48 h, then change to PO to complete 14 d. Consider single dose IV followed by outpatient oral therapy in stable patients. Do not use fluoroquinolones in pregnancy.

[a]Oral: Ciprofloxacin 500 mg PO bid; ofloxacin 200 mg PO bid; levofloxacin 500 mg PO qd; norfloxacin 400 mg PO bid. Parenteral: Levofloxacin 500 mg IV qd; ciprofloxacin 400 mg IV q12h.
[b]Cefotaxime 1 or 2 g IV q8h; ceftriaxone 1 g IV qd; ceftazidime 1 to 2 g IV q8–12h.
[c]Imipenem 500 mg IV q6h; meropenem 1 g IV q8h.
[d]Gentamicin or tobramycin 2 mg/kg loading dose IV, then 1.5 to 3.0 mg/kg/d or divided dose.
DS, double strength; FQ, fluoroquinolone; GU, genitourinary; IM, intramuscular; IV, intravenous; PO, by mouth; SS, single strength; TMP, trimethoprim; TMP-SMX, trimethoprim-sulfamethoxazole; UTI, urinary tract infection.

Pyelonephritis

DIAGNOSIS

Clinical Presentation
- Patients present with fever, flank pain, and lower UTI symptoms due to ascending infection from the lower urinary tract.
- Dysuria without pyuria in sexually active patients warrants consideration of sexually transmitted infection.

Diagnostic Testing
- Urine specimens characteristically demonstrate significant bacteriuria, pyuria, red blood cells (RBCs), and occasional leukocyte casts.
- Diagnosis should include urine culture in all patients. Blood cultures should be obtained in those who are hospitalized as bacteremia may be present in 15% to 20% of cases. The causative agents are *E. coli*, *S. saprophyticus*, and rarely, *Proteus* sp. No further tests are usually needed for initial workup, but the presence of other organisms may suggest an anatomic abnormality or immune compromise.

TREATMENT

- See Table 14-7 for details.
- Treatment of patients with **mild-to-moderate illness** who are able to take oral medication can be safely initiated in the outpatient setting. Patients with more **severe illness**, those who are nauseated and vomiting, and pregnant patients should be treated initially with parenteral therapy.

SPECIAL CONSIDERATIONS

Evaluation for anatomic abnormalities should be done for patients who do not respond to initial empiric treatment within 48 hours. Presence of an anatomic abnormality such as a renal abscess or renal calculi should be evaluated by ultrasonography, CT scan, or intravenous pyelogram (IVP) (Table 14-7).

SEXUALLY TRANSMITTED INFECTIONS, ULCERATIVE DISEASES

Genital Herpes

GENERAL PRINCIPLES

Genital herpes is caused by **HSV**, usually type 2, but genital HSV-1 is increasing in incidence.

DIAGNOSIS

- Infection is characterized by painful grouped vesicles in the genital and perianal regions that rapidly ulcerate and form shallow tender lesions.
- The initial episode may be associated with inguinal adenopathy, fever, headache, myalgias, and aseptic meningitis; recurrences are usually less severe. Asymptomatic shedding of virus is frequent and leads to transmission.
- Confirmation of HSV infection requires culture or PCR; however, clinical presentation is often adequate for diagnosis.

TREATMENT

For treatment options, see Table 14-8.

Syphilis

GENERAL PRINCIPLES

Syphilis is caused by the spirochete *Treponema pallidum*. There is a high degree of HIV coinfection in patients with syphilis, and HIV infection should be excluded with appropriate testing (*JAMA 2003;290(11):1510*).

DIAGNOSIS

Clinical Presentation

- **Primary syphilis** develops within several weeks of exposure and manifests as one or more painless, indurated, superficial ulcerations (chancre).
- **Secondary syphilis** develops 4 to 10 weeks after the chancre resolves and may produce a rash, mucocutaneous lesions, adenopathy, and constitutional symptoms.
- **Tertiary syphilis** follows between 1 and 20 years after infection, and includes cardiovascular, gummatous, and neurologic disease (general paresis, tabes dorsalis, or meningovascular syphilis).

Diagnostic Testing

- In **primary syphilis**, dark-field microscopy of lesion exudates, when available, may reveal spirochetes. A nontreponemal serologic test (e.g., RPR or venereal disease research laboratory [VDRL]) should be confirmed with a treponemal-specific test (e.g., fluorescent treponemal antibody absorption or *T. pallidum* particle agglutination).
- Diagnosis of **secondary syphilis** is made on the basis of positive serologic studies and the presence of a compatible clinical illness.
- **Latent syphilis** is a serologic diagnosis in the absence of symptoms—early latent syphilis is serologically positive for <1 year, and late latent syphilis is serologically positive for >1 year.
- To exclude **neurosyphilis**, a lumbar puncture (LP) should be performed in the presence of neurologic or ophthalmic or auditory signs or symptoms, evidence of tertiary disease, or treatment failure. Some experts recommend LP in HIV-infected patients with serum RPR or VDRL of ≥1:32 or with CD4 <350 mm^3 (*Clin Infect Dis 2009;48:816*). VDRL should be performed on CSF.

Table 14-8	Treatment of Sexually Transmitted Diseases	
Disease	**Recommended Regimen**	**Alternative Regimen**
Genital ulcer disease		
Herpes simplex		
First episode	• Acyclovir 400 mg PO thrice daily × 7–10 d or 200 mg PO five times daily × 7–10 d • Valacyclovir 1 g PO twice daily × 7–10 d • Famciclovir 250 mg PO thrice daily × 7–10 d	
Recurrent episodes	• Acyclovir 400 mg PO thrice daily × 5 d or 800 mg PO thrice daily × 2 d • Valacyclovir 1 g PO once daily × 5 d or 500 mg PO twice daily × 3 d • Famciclovir 1 g PO twice daily × 1 d or 125 mg PO twice daily × 5 d	
Suppressive therapy	• Acyclovir 400 mg PO twice daily • Valacyclovir 500 mg or 1 g PO once daily • Famciclovir 250 mg PO twice daily	
Syphilis		
Primary, secondary, or early latent <1 yr	• Benzathine penicillin G 2.4 million U IM single dose	Penicillin-allergic: • Doxycycline 100 mg PO twice daily × 14 d • Tetracycline 500 mg PO four times daily × 14 d
Latent >1 yr, latent unknown duration	• Benzathine penicillin G 2.4 million U IM once weekly × 3 doses	• Doxycycline 100 mg PO twice daily × 28 d • Tetracycline 500 mg PO four times daily × 28 d

(continued)

Table 14-8	Treatment of Sexually Transmitted Diseases[a] (Continued)

Disease	Empiric Therapy	Notes
Neurosyphilis	• Aqueous crystalline penicillin G 18–24 million U/d × 10–14 d	• Procaine penicillin 2.4 million U IM once daily + probenecid 500 mg PO four times daily × 10–14 d
Pregnancy	• Penicillin is the recommended treatment—desensitize if necessary	
Chancroid	• Azithromycin 1 g PO single dose • Ceftriaxone 250 mg IM single dose	• Ciprofloxacin 500 mg PO twice daily × 3 d • Erythromycin base 500 mg PO twice daily × 7 d
Lymphogranuloma venereum	• Doxycycline 100 mg PO twice daily × 21 d	• Erythromycin 500 mg PO four times a day × 21 d
Urethritis/cervicitis		
Gonorrhea (GC)	• (Ceftriaxone 125 mg IM once or cefixime 400 mg PO once) + (azithromycin or doxycycline to treat chlamydia)	• If allergy and not pharyngeal GC, may use spectinomycin 2 g IM once (not available in United States) • Fluoroquinolones are not recommended
Disseminated gonococcal infection	• Ceftriaxone 1 g IV daily or cefotaxime 1 g IV every 8 h × 7 d	
Chlamydia	• Azithromycin 1 g PO single dose • Doxycycline 100 mg PO twice daily × 7 d	• Erythromycin base 500 mg PO four times a day × 7 d
Pelvic inflammatory disease		
Outpatient	• Ceftriaxone 250 mg IM once + doxycycline 100 mg PO twice daily × 14 d + metronidazole 500 mg orally twice daily × 14 d	Cefoxitin 2 g IM + probenecid 1 g PO once can be substituted for ceftriaxone

(continued)

Table 14-8	Treatment of Sexually Transmitted Diseases[a] (Continued)	
Disease	**Empiric Therapy**	**Notes**
Inpatient	• (Cefoxitin 2 g IV every 6 h or cefotetan 2 g IV every 12 h) + doxycycline 100 mg PO twice daily × 14 d + metronidazole 500 mg PO twice daily × 14 d	• Clindamycin 900 mg IV every 8 h + gentamicin 2 mg/kg loading dose, then 1.5 mg/kg every 8 h + doxycycline 100 mg PO twice daily × 14 d • Ampicillin-sulbactam 3 g IV every 6 h + doxycycline 100 mg PO twice daily × 14 d
Vaginitis/vaginosis		
Trichomonas	• Metronidazole 2 g PO single dose • Tinidazole 2 g PO single dose	• Metronidazole 500 mg PO twice daily × 7 d
Pregnancy	• Metronidazole 2 g PO × 1 (not teratogenic)	
Bacterial vaginosis	• Metronidazole 500 mg PO twice daily × 7 d • Clindamycin cream 2% intravaginal at bedtime × 7 d • Metronidazole gel 0.75% intravaginal once a day for 5 d	• Clindamycin 300 mg PO twice daily × 7 d • Clindamycin ovules 100 mg intravaginal × 3 d • Tinidazole 2 g PO once daily × 2 d or 1 g PO once daily × 5 d
Candidiasis	• Fluconazole 150 mg PO × 1	• Intravaginal azoles in variety of strengths for 1–7 d
Severe candidiasis	• Fluconazole 150 mg PO every 72 h × 2–3 doses	• Intravaginal azoles for 7–14 d
Recurrent candidiasis	• Fluconazole 100, 150, or 200 mg PO once weekly × 6 mo	

IM, intramuscular; IV, intravenous; PO, by mouth.
MMWR 2010;59 (RR-12).

TREATMENT

For treatment options, see Table 14-8.

Chancroid

GENERAL PRINCIPLES

Chancroid is caused by *Haemophilus ducreyi*.

DIAGNOSIS

- Chancroid produces a painful genital ulcer and tender suppurative inguinal lymphadenopathy.
- Identification of the organism is difficult and requires special culture media.

TREATMENT

For treatment options, see Table 14-8.

Lymphogranuloma Venereum

GENERAL PRINCIPLES

Lymphogranuloma venereum (LGV) is caused by *C. trachomatis* (serovars L_1, L_2, or L_3).

DIAGNOSIS

- Manifests as a painless genital ulcer, followed by heaped up, matted inguinal lymphadenopathy. Proctocolitis with pain and discharge can occur with anal intercourse (*Clin Infect Dis 2007;44:26*).
- Diagnosis is based on clinical suspicion and *C. trachomatis* antibody testing, if available.

TREATMENT

For treatment options, see Table 14-8.

SEXUALLY TRANSMITTED INFECTIONS, VAGINITIS AND VAGINOSIS

Trichomoniasis

DIAGNOSIS

Clinical Presentation

- Clinical symptoms of infection by *Trichomonas vaginalis* include malodorous purulent vaginal discharge, dysuria, and genital inflammation.
- Examination reveals profuse frothy discharge and cervical petechiae.

Diagnostic Testing

Diagnosis requires visualization of motile trichomonads on a saline wet mount of vaginal discharge. Elevated vaginal pH ($\geq$4.5) may be seen.

TREATMENT

For treatment options, see Table 14-8.

Bacterial Vaginosis

GENERAL PRINCIPLES

The replacement of normal lactobacilli with high concentrations of anaerobic bacteria in the vagina leads to bacterial vaginosis.

DIAGNOSIS

Three of the following criteria are needed to make the diagnosis:
• Homogenous, thin, white discharge
• Presence of clue cells on microscopic examination
• Elevated vaginal pH ($\geq$4.5)
• Fishy odor associated with vaginal discharge before or after addition of 10% potassium hydroxide (KOH) (whiff test)

TREATMENT

For treatment options, see Table 14-8.

Vulvovaginal Candidiasis

GENERAL PRINCIPLES

Vulvovaginal candidiasis (VVC) is not generally considered a sexually transmitted disease but commonly develops in the setting of oral contraceptive use or antibiotic therapy. Recurrent infections may be a presenting manifestation of unrecognized HIV infection.

DIAGNOSIS

• Thick, cottage cheese–like vaginal discharge in conjunction with intense vulvar inflammation, pruritus, and dysuria is often present.
• Definitive diagnosis requires visualization of fungal elements on a potassium hydroxide preparation of the vaginal discharge.

TREATMENT

• Therapy is often initiated on the basis of the clinical presentation (Table 14-8).
• Fluconazole failure may indicate the presence of a **non–*C. albicans* species**.

Cervicitis/Urethritis

GENERAL PRINCIPLES

Cervicitis and urethritis are frequent presentations of infection with *N. gonorrhoeae* or *C. trachomatis*, and occasionally *Mycoplasma hominis, U. urealyticum,* and *T. vaginalis*. These infections often coexist, and clinical presentations can be identical.

DIAGNOSIS

Clinical Presentation

- Women with urethritis, cervicitis, or both, complain of mucopurulent vaginal discharge, dyspareunia, and dysuria.
- Men with urethritis may have dysuria and purulent penile discharge.
- Disseminated gonococcal infection (DGI) can present with fever, tenosynovitis, vesicopustular skin lesions, and polyarthralgias. DGI may also manifest solely as septic arthritis of the knee, wrist, or ankle (see Chapter 25, Arthritis and Rheumatologic Diseases).

Diagnostic Testing

- A positive nucleic acid amplification test performed on endocervical, vaginal, urethral (men), or urine samples is recommended to make the diagnosis of *C. trachomatis* or *N. gonorrhoeae* infection. In the case of *N. gonorrhoeae*, a Gram stain of endocervical or urethral discharge with gram-negative intracellular diplococci can rapidly establish the diagnosis. Culture can be performed on urethral or endocervical swab specimens.
- In addition to studies earlier, patients with suspected DGI should have blood cultures drawn. In the setting of septic arthritis, synovial fluid analysis and culture is indicated.

TREATMENT

Because of increasing resistance, fluoroquinolones *should not be used* to treat *N. gonorrhoeae* infection (*MMWR 2010;59(RR-12):1*) (see Table 14-8 for treatment options).

Pelvic Inflammatory Disease

GENERAL PRINCIPLES

Pelvic inflammatory disease (PID) is an upper genital tract infection in women, usually preceded by cervicitis. Long-term consequences of untreated PID include chronic pain, increased risk of ectopic pregnancy, and infertility.

DIAGNOSIS

Clinical Presentation

Symptoms can range from mild pelvic discomfort and dyspareunia to severe abdominal pain with fever, which may signal complicating perihepatitis (Fitz-Hugh-Curtis syndrome) or tubo-ovarian abscess.

Diagnostic Testing

- Cervical motion tenderness or uterine or adnexal tenderness and the presence of at least 10 white blood cells per low-power field on a saline preparation of vaginal or endocervical fluid are consistent with a diagnosis of PID.
- Nucleic acid amplification tests or culture of endocervical specimens should be obtained to identify *C. trachomatis* or *N. gonorrhoeae* infection.
- All women diagnosed with PID should be screened for HIV infection.

TREATMENT

- See Table 14-8 for treatment options.
- Severely ill, pregnant, and HIV-infected women with PID should be hospitalized. Patients unable to tolerate oral antibiotics also warrant admission.

SYSTEMIC MYCOSES AND ATYPICALS

Clinical presentations are protean and not pathogen specific. The systemic mycoses should be considered in normal hosts with unexplained chronic pulmonary pathology, chronic meningitis, lytic bone lesions, chronic skin lesions, fever of unknown origin (FUO), or cytopenias. In immunocompromised patients, the development of new pulmonary, cutaneous, funduscopic, or head-and-neck signs and symptoms, or persistent unexplained fever should prompt consideration of these pathogens.

The mycoses can often be identified by taking into account epidemiological clues (many are geographically restricted), site of infection, inflammatory response, and microscopic fungal appearance. These infections can be complex and difficult to treat, and infectious disease consultation is recommended. For details on treatment of fungal pathogens, Nocardia, and Actinomyces, see Table 14-9.

Candidiasis

GENERAL PRINCIPLES

Candida species are the most common cause of invasive fungal infections in humans. Infections ranging from uncomplicated mucosal disease to life-threatening invasive disease affecting any organ can occur (*Clin Infect Dis 2009;48:503*). Infections are often associated with concurrent antibiotic use, contraceptive use, immunosuppressant and cytotoxic therapy, and indwelling foreign bodies. Mucocutaneous disease may resolve after elimination of the causative condition (e.g., antibiotic therapy) or may persist and progress in the setting of immunosuppressive conditions. Serious complications, such as candidemia leading to skin lesions, ocular disease, endocarditis, and osteomyelitis, can occur.

DIAGNOSIS

Diagnostic Testing

Diagnosis of **mucocutaneous candidiasis** is usually based on clinical findings but can be confirmed by a potassium hydroxide preparation of exudates. Cultures can

Table 14-9 Treatment of Fungal Infections, *Nocardia*, and *Actinomyces*

Pathogen	Primary Therapy	Suppressive Rx	Notes
Candida spp.			
Mucosal (*Clin Infect Dis 2009; 48:503*)	Topical clotrimazole troches, 10 mg dissolved PO 5 ×/d × 14 d. *Esophageal:* Fluconazole 100–200 mg PO qd × 14 d. *Vaginal:* Topical azole × 1–14 d or fluconazole 150 mg PO × 1.	Generally not indicated in *HIV* unless frequent severe recurrences. *Neutropenia:* Fluconazole 400 mg PO qd, posaconazole 200 mg tid, or itraconazole 200 mg PO daily. Continue prophylaxis until ANC >500 or 3 mo post–solid organ transplant.	
Invasive (*Clin Infect Dis 2009; 48:503*)	Fluconazole 800 mg loading dose, then 400 mg IV/PO qd × 7 d, then PO × 14 d. Severe dz, recent azole exposure, suspicion of nonalbicans species (e.g., echinocandin, anidulafungin 200 mg IV × 1, then 100 mg qd, or amphotericin B*).		Treat all positive blood cultures as invasive disease, with at least 14-d therapy. Catheters must be removed. Treat for 14 d beyond last positive blood Cx. *C. parapsilosis* should not be initially treated with an echinocandin.
Catheter associated	See Nosocomial Infections section.		

Cryptococcus neoformans

Nonmeningeal disease (Clin Infect Dis 2010; 50:291)	Fluconazole 400 mg PO or IV qd × 6–12 mos.	Immunosuppressed: Fluconazole 200 mg PO qd.	Isolated pulmonary disease in immunocompetent patients can be followed expectantly.

C. neoformans
Meningitis (Clin Infect Dis 2010;50:291)

Immunocompetent	Amphotericin B* + flucytosine 25 mg/kg q6h IV × 2 wks, then fluconazole 400 mg PO qd × 8 wk.	Not indicated.	Always check opening pressure, and reduce by 50% if elevated above 25 cm H_2O by removing up to 30 mL CSF. Serial LPs to reduce pressure are required as long as CSF is elevated.
Immunosuppressed	Amphotericin B* + flucytosine 25 mg/kg q6h IV × 2 wks, then fluconazole 400 mg PO qd × 8 wk.	Fluconazole 200 mg PO qd.	Continue prophylaxis until immunocompetent or CD4 count sustained >200 for 6 mos.

Histoplasma capsulatum
(Clin Infect Dis 2007;45:807)

Chronic forms, mild disease, immunocompetent	Itraconazole 200–400 mg/d PO for ≥6 mo.	Not indicated.	Goal serum itraconazole level >1 µg/mL.
Acute dissemination; severe disease; immunocompromised	Amphotericin B* for 2 wks or until clinically improved, then itraconazole 200 mg PO bid >12 mo.	Itraconazole 200 mg PO qd.	Continue prophylaxis until sustained CD4 count >200 for 6 mo.

(continued)

Table 14-9 Treatment of Fungal Infections, Nocardia, and Actinomyces (Continued)

Pathogen	Primary Therapy	Suppressive Rx	Notes
Blastomyces dermatitidis (Clin Infect Dis 2008;46:1801)			
Nonmeningeal disease; mild-to-moderate disease; immunocompetent	Itraconazole 200–400 mg/d PO for 6 mos.	Not indicated.	
Acute dissemination; severe disease; immunocompromised	Amphotericin B* for 2 wk or until clinically improved, then itraconazole 200–400 mg PO qd × 6 mo.	Itraconazole 200–400 mg PO qd.	
CNS infection	Amphotericin B* for 4–6 wk, then itraconazole 200 mg bid or voriconazole 200–400 mg bid for at least 12 mo or until resolution of CNS abnormalities.	Not indicated.	
Coccidioides immitis (Clin Infect Dis 2005;41:1217)			
Nonmeningeal disease	Itraconazole 200 mg PO bid or fluconazole 400 mg PO qd × 12 mo.	Fluconazole 400 mg PO qd (lifelong suppression required if disseminated).	Follow serum CF titers after treatment. Rising titers suggest recurrence. For pulmonary nodules and asymptomatic cavitary disease, no therapy indicated. Consider surgery if cavitary disease persists >2 yr, progresses >1 yr, or is located near pleura.
Meningitis	Fluconazole 400–800 mg IV/PO q24h. Intrathecal amphotericin B deoxycholate 0.1–1.5 mg qd to qwk may be added to azole therapy for severe meningeal disease.	Fluconazole 400 mg PO qd indefinitely.	

Aspergillus

Aspergilloma

Surgical resection in case of severe hemoptysis.

Not indicated.

Use liposomal

Invasive aspergillosis (*Clin Infect Dis 2008;46:327*)

Voriconazole 6 mg/kg q12h PO/IV × 2 doses, then 4 mg/kg q12h, then 200 mg bid. Continue for at least 6–12 wk, as long as immunosuppression continues, and until lesions resolve.

Continue or restart therapy if immunosuppression recurs.

Amphotericin B* to cover mucormycosis as initial therapy for sinus disease pending confirmation of diagnosis.

Sporothrix (*Clin Infect Dis 2007;45:1255*)

Itraconazole, 200 mg PO qd × 3–6 mos.
Alt: Saturated solution of K Iodide, 5 drops PO tid, increased to 40 drops tid as tolerated.

Not indicated.

Severe and meningeal disease: Amphotericin B* for initial 6 wk of therapy, then itraconazole 200 mg bid to complete at least 12 mo.
Follow levels of itraconazole.

Mucormycosis

Amphotericin B* at upper dose range × 6 mos.

Not indicated.

(continued)

Table 14-9 Treatment of Fungal Infections, *Nocardia*, and *Actinomyces* (Continued)

Pathogen	Primary Therapy	Suppressive Rx	Notes
Nocardia *(Clin Infect Dis 2007;44:1307)*			
Pulmonary	TMP-SMX 15 mg/kg/d IV (TMP) in div. doses + imipenem 500 mg IV q6h × 3–4 wk, then 1–2 DS PO bid. *Less serious:* TMP-SMX 1–2 DS bid up to 2 DS tid or minocycline 100 mg PO bid.	TMP-SMX 1–2 DS bid or dapsone 100 mg PO qd or minocycline 100 mg PO bid.	Treat initially for 6 mo if immunocompetent or ≥12 mo if immunocompromised.
CNS	TMP-SMX 15 mg/kg/d IV (TMP) + imipenem 500 mg IV q6h × 3–6 wk, then TMP-SMX 3 DS PO bid. If immunocompromised consider treating with two drugs for 1 yr.		
Actinomyces	(Penicillin G 18–24 million U IV/d or clindamycin 600 mg IV q8h) × 2–6 wk, then penicillin V 2–4 g PO/d in four divided doses OR doxycycline 100 mg PO bid OR oral clindamycin for 6–12 mo.	Not indicated.	

*Amphotericin dosing: Amphotericin B deoxycholate 0.7–1.0 mg/kg. Liposomal amphotericin B 3–5 mg/kg.
ANC, absolute neutrophil count; CF, complement fixation; CNS, central nervous system; CSF, cerebrospinal fluid; Cx, culture; DS, double strength; dz, disease; IV, intravenous; LP, lumbar puncture; PO, by mouth; TMP-SMX, trimethoprim-sulfamethoxazole.

be obtained in refractory cases to exclude the presence of non–*C. albicans* species. **Invasive candidiasis** is diagnosed by positive cultures of blood or tissue.

TREATMENT

Mucocutaneous candidiasis usually responds to topical therapy but oral and even parenteral therapy may be required depending on severity and other host factors (see Table 14-9). **Candidemia and other invasive candidiasis** necessitate prolonged therapy. **Isolated catheter-related candidemia** (see the Health Care–Associated Infections section).

Cryptococcosis

GENERAL PRINCIPLES

Cryptococcus neoformans is a ubiquitous yeast associated with soil and pigeon excrement. Disease is principally meningeal (headache and mental status changes) and pulmonary (ranging from asymptomatic nodular disease to fulminant respiratory failure). Skin lesions can also be seen. Significant infections are usually opportunistic.

DIAGNOSIS

Diagnosis requires detection of encapsulated yeast in tissue or body fluids (India ink stain) with confirmation by culture. The latex agglutination test for cryptococcal antigen in serum or CSF is helpful, and a positive serum antigen titer is highly suggestive of disseminated disease. Lumbar puncture is necessary in persons with systemic disease to exclude coexistent central nervous system (CNS) involvement. Always measure opening pressure, as elevated opening pressure (>25 cm H_2O) has poor prognostic implications and must be managed, usually with serial LPs, or with a lumbar drain.

TREATMENT

Treatment is dependent on the patient's immune function and site of infection (Table 14-9). **Management of elevated intracranial pressure is critical**. CSF opening pressure above 25 cm H_2O should be reduced by 50% if possible by removal of up to 30 mL of fluid, repeated daily as needed. If the initial opening pressure is not elevated, repeat LP is only needed if new symptoms arise (*Clin Infect Dis 2010;50:291*). **HIV patients** need suppressive therapy until immune function is improved by antiretrovirals.

Histoplasmosis

GENERAL PRINCIPLES

Histoplasma capsulatum is more prevalent in the Ohio and Mississippi River Valleys of the United States and in Latin America, and grows in soil contaminated by bat or bird droppings.

DIAGNOSIS

Clinical manifestations are extremely varied, including acute flu-like or chronic granulomatous pulmonary disease or fulminant multiorgan failure in the immunocompromised patient.

Diagnosis is based on culture or histopathology, antigen assay (urine, blood, or CSF), or complement fixation (CF) assay ($\geq$1:16 or fourfold rise). Urine antigen assay is good for detecting disseminated disease and is helpful in following response to therapy.

TREATMENT

Treatment for most symptomatic infections is an extended course of itraconazole. Mild pulmonary disease can be observed without specific therapy (Table 14-9).

Blastomycosis

GENERAL PRINCIPLES

Blastomyces dermatitidis is endemic in the upper Midwestern, South Central, and Southeastern United States. This organism commonly disseminates, even in immunocompetent patients, and tends to affect the lungs, skin, bone, and genitourinary tract. Aggressive pulmonary and CNS disease can occur in both immunocompromised and immunocompetent patients.

DIAGNOSIS

Diagnosis requires isolation of the organism by culture or histopathology. Serologic studies cross-react with tests for *Histoplasma* and *Cryptococcus* species and are unreliable for diagnosis but can be used to assess early response to therapy when positive.

TREATMENT

Treatment is usually a 6-month course of itraconazole but requires an initial course of amphotericin B for life-threatening or CNS disease (see Table 14-9).

Coccidioidomycosis

GENERAL PRINCIPLES

Coccidioides immitis is endemic to the Southwestern United States and Central America.

Disease is usually a self-limited pulmonary syndrome. Less common are chronic pulmonary illness and disseminated disease, which can affect the meninges, bones, joints, and skin.

DIAGNOSIS

• Diagnosis requires culture or histopathology, or positive CF serology.

- Serum CF titer of 1:16 or greater suggests extrathoracic dissemination.
- **Lumbar puncture** should be performed for culture and CF to rule out CNS involvement in persons with severe, rapidly progressive, or disseminated disease.
- **Skin testing** should only be used for epidemiologic purposes to evaluate exposure.

TREATMENT

Treatment can be avoided for most forms of **acute pulmonary disease**, as it resolves spontaneously. For **disseminated disease**, immunocompromised patients, or pulmonary disease that persists beyond 6 weeks, treatment is typically 1 year of oral azole therapy. CF titers can be followed after therapy, as rising titers suggest recurrence (see Table 14-9).

Aspergillosis

GENERAL PRINCIPLES

- *Aspergillus* species are ubiquitous environmental fungi that cause a broad spectrum of disease, usually affecting the respiratory system and sinuses.
- **Pulmonary aspergilloma.** Pulmonary aspergilloma occurs in the setting of preexisting bullous lung disease and can be easily recognized by characteristic radiographic presentation and *Aspergillus* serology.
- **Invasive aspergillosis (IA).** IA is a serious condition associated with vascular invasion, thrombosis, and ischemic infarction of involved tissues and progressive disease after hematogenous dissemination. IA is usually seen in severely immunocompromised patients and clinical features vary by predisposing host characteristics.
- **Allergic bronchopulmonary aspergillosis (ABPA).** ABPA is a chronic relapsing and remitting respiratory syndrome associated with colonization with *Aspergillus*.

DIAGNOSIS

- Diagnosis can be very difficult given the varied manifestations of IA, and a high index of suspicion should be applied to patients with prolonged severe immunosuppression.
- Radiographic findings can be highly suggestive, if not diagnostic of pulmonary IA, particularly the halo-crescent sign on CT in immunosuppressed patients.
- The diagnosis can be confirmed with characteristic histologic evidence of involved tissue. Fungal culture has a low yield.
- The galactomannan assay can support a diagnosis of IA and can be followed prospectively in at risk patients (*Clin Infect Dis 2004;39:797*). Sensitivity is higher when performed on respiratory secretions as compared to serum (*Am J Respir Crit Care Med 2008;177:27*).

TREATMENT

- **Pulmonary aspergilloma.** Treatment by surgical resection or arterial embolization is indicated only in the setting of severe hemoptysis (see Table 14-9).

- **Invasive aspergillosis.** Treatment of locally IA requires surgical excision of affected tissue. Empiric therapy of head and neck disease should include amphotericin B in order to also cover the zygomycoses, while awaiting final speciation (*N Engl J Med 2009;360:1870*).
- **Allergic bronchopulmonary aspergillosis.** Intermittent steroids are the primary therapy; a course of itraconazole may decrease exacerbations.

Sporotrichosis

GENERAL PRINCIPLES

Sporothrix schenckii is a globally endemic fungus and causes disease following traumatic inoculation with soil or plant material; most cases are vocational. Infection can also be associated with spread from infected cats or other digging animals (*Clin Infect Dis 2007;45:1255*).

DIAGNOSIS

Clinical Presentation

Lymphocutaneous disease is the usual manifestation with localization to skin and soft tissues.
Pulmonary and disseminated forms of the infection are rarely seen from inhalation of the fungus.

Diagnostic Testing

Diagnosis requires culture or histopathologic demonstration of yeast in tissue or body fluids.

TREATMENT

Treatment for lymphocutaneous disease is itraconazole elixir or saturated solution of potassium iodide. Severe and meningeal disease should be treated with amphotericin B (see Table 14-9).

Mucormycosis

GENERAL PRINCIPLES

Caused by class of fungi called Zygomycetes that includes *Mucor*, though most disease is caused by others in the class, such as *Rhizopus*. This group causes head and neck, pulmonary, GI, cutaneous, and disseminated disease with angioinvasion and multiorgan infarction. Risk factors include immunosuppression, iron overload, high-dose glucocorticoid therapy, and diabetes with or without ketoacidosis.

DIAGNOSIS

- Clinical manifestations vary depending on which organ is affected. Invasive mucormycosis is devastating with rapid development of tissue necrosis from vascular invasion and thrombosis (*Lancet Infect Dis 2011;11:301*).

- Diagnosis requires tissue culture and silver stain with care to avoid disrupting fungal architecture. MRI with contrast is helpful in head and neck disease to identify involved structures.

TREATMENT

Treatment requires aggressive surgical resection and debridement with clean margins, followed by liposomal amphotericin B 5 mg/kg qd for 6 months. Nondesferrioxamine iron chelators can be tried as salvage adjuncts (see Table 14-9) (*Antimicrob Agents Chemother 2006;50:3768*).

PROGNOSIS

Mortality is very high in immunosuppressed patients and disseminated disease.

Nocardiosis

GENERAL PRINCIPLES

Nocardia is a ubiquitous group of aerobic gram-positive branching filamentous bacteria that causes severe local and disseminated disease in the setting of impaired cell-mediated immunity (*Clin Infect Dis 2007;44:1307*). Typical infection tends to be pulmonary infiltrate, abscess, or empyema, but dissemination is common and tends to favor CNS infection, causing abscess.

DIAGNOSIS

- Clinical presentation can be acute, subacute, or chronic pneumonia.
- Chest imaging can reveal a variety of findings such as infiltrates, nodules, pleural effusions, or cavities (*Infection 2010;38:89*).
- Diagnosis requires sputum or tissue Gram stain and culture (including AFB), often needing multiple samples as yields are low.
- Look for CNS disease with brain MRI in patients with pulmonary disease.

TREATMENT

Treatment with combination therapy, consisting of a high-dose sulfonamide and imipenem, is preferred. Duration of therapy can range from 6 to 12 months, depending on immune status. Long-term suppressive therapy is necessary for immunocompromised patients (see Table 14-9).

Actinomycosis

GENERAL PRINCIPLES

Actinomyces is a microaerophilic gram-positive bacillus that usually causes oropharyngeal, pulmonary, and GI disease. Classic infections are chronic, indurated soft-tissue lesions associated with draining fistulae that pass through tissue planes, and microscopic "sulfur granules." Unlike *Nocardia*, infection is not limited to immuno-compromised hosts.

DIAGNOSIS

Clinical presentation varies depending on what site is affected. Orocervicofacial infection is the most common form. Rare sites include the CNS and bones. Diagnosis is made by histopathology or observation of "sulfur granules" in drainage (*BMJ 2011;343:d6099*).

TREATMENT

Treatment requires an extended course of amoxicillin, doxycycline, or clindamycin, with an initial 2- to 6-week course of high-dose IV penicillin or clindamycin. Surgery is occasionally required (see Table 14-9).

Atypical (Nontuberculous) Mycobacteria

GENERAL PRINCIPLES

- NTM are ubiquitous environmental organisms that cause a spectrum of disease involving the lungs, skin, soft tissue, and lymph nodes. Susceptibility testing and infectious disease consultation is recommended to guide treatment.
- *M. avium* (*MAI*), *M. kansasii* (see Chapter 16, HIV Infection and AIDS)
- *M. fortuitum, M. marinum, M. ulcerans, M. haemophilum,* and *M. scrofulaceum* cause a spectrum of chronic progressive disease of soft tissue and bone. *M. leprae* is typically classified separately from the other NTM because of its potential for human-to-human transmission.

TICK-BORNE INFECTIONS

Tick-borne infections (TBIs) are common during the summer months in many areas of the United States; prevalence of specific diseases depends on the local population of vector ticks and animal reservoirs. Coinfection with multiple TBIs can occur and should be considered when patients present with overlapping syndromes. Risk should be assessed by outdoor activity in endemic regions rather than the report of a tick bite, which often goes unnoticed.

Lyme Borreliosis (Lyme Disease)

GENERAL PRINCIPLES

Lyme borreliosis is the most common vector-borne disease in the United States and is a systemic illness of variable severity caused by the spirochete *Borrelia burgdorferi*. It is seen in endemic regions, including northeastern coastal states, the upper Midwest, and northern California. Prophylactic doxycycline 200 mg PO (single dose) may reduce the risk of Lyme disease in endemic areas following a bite by a nymph-stage deer tick (*N Engl J Med 2001;345:79*).

DIAGNOSIS

Clinical Presentation

Lyme disease has three distinct clinical stages, which start after an incubation period of 7 to 10 days:
* Stage 1 (early local disease) is characterized by erythema migrans, a slowly expanding macular rash >5 cm in diameter, often with central clearing, and by mild constitutional symptoms.
* Stage 2 (early disseminated disease) occurs within several weeks to months and includes multiple erythema migrans lesions, neurologic symptoms (e.g., seventh cranial nerve palsy, meningoencephalitis), cardiac symptoms (atrioventricular block, myopericarditis), and asymmetric oligoarticular arthritis.
* Stage 3 (late disease) occurs after months to years and includes chronic dermatitis, neurologic disease, and asymmetric monoarticular or oligoarticular arthritis. Chronic fatigue is not seen more frequently in patients with Lyme borreliosis than in control subjects.

Diagnostic Testing

Diagnosis rests on clinical suspicion in the appropriate setting but can be supported by two-tiered serologic testing (screening enzyme-linked immunosorbent assay [ELISA] followed by Western blot) with acute and convalescent serologies.

TREATMENT

* Treatment depends on stage and severity of disease (*Clin Infect Dis 2006;43:1089*). Oral therapy (doxycycline 100 mg PO bid, amoxicillin 500 mg PO tid, or cefuroxime axetil 500 mg PO bid for 10 to 21 days) is used for early localized or disseminated disease without neurologic or cardiac involvement. The same agents, given for 28 days, are recommended for late Lyme disease. Doxycycline has the added benefit of covering potential coinfection with ehrlichiosis.
* Parenteral therapy (ceftriaxone 2 g IV daily, cefotaxime 2 g IV q8h, penicillin G 3 to 4 million U IV q4h) for 14 to 28 days should be used for severe neurologic or cardiac disease, regardless of stage.

Rocky Mountain Spotted Fever

GENERAL PRINCIPLES

Rocky Mountain spotted fever (RMSF) is caused by *Rickettsia rickettsii* after a tick bite, which may go unrecognized. Endemic regions are east of the Rocky Mountains.

DIAGNOSIS

Clinical signs include fever, headache, and myalgias, followed 1 to 5 days later by a petechial rash starting on the distal extremities that may be faint and difficult to detect. Initial diagnosis leading to presumptive treatment should be based on the clinical syndrome, but skin biopsy and acute and convalescent serologies can provide additional support.

TREATMENT

Antibiotic treatment of choice is doxycycline 100 mg q12h IV or PO for 7 days, or until afebrile for 2 days. Chloramphenicol is an alternative (*Lancet Infect Dis 2007;7:724*).

OUTCOME/PROGNOSIS

Death can occur when treatment is delayed.

Ehrlichiosis and Anaplasmosis

GENERAL PRINCIPLES

Ehrlichiosis and anaplasmosis are systemic TBIs caused by intracellular pathogens of the closely related *Ehrlichia* and *Anaplasma* genera. Two similar syndromes are recognized:
• **Human monocytic ehrlichiosis** (HME), caused by *Ehrlichia chaffeensis*, is endemic in the south and south central United States.
• **Human granulocytic anaplasmosis** (HGA, formerly HGE), caused by *Anaplasma phagocytophilum*, is found in the same regions as Lyme borreliosis due to a shared tick vector.

DIAGNOSIS

Clinical Presentation
Clinical onset of illness usually occurs 1 week after tick exposure with fever, headache, and myalgias. Rash is only occasionally seen. Severe disease can result in respiratory failure, renal insufficiency, and neurologic decompensation. Leukopenia, thrombocytopenia, and elevated liver transaminases are the hallmarks of moderately severe disease.

Diagnostic Testing
• Diagnosis can be made by identification of morulae in circulating monocytes (HME) or granulocytes (HGA), which is uncommon but diagnostic in the appropriate clinical setting. Confirmation is by acute and convalescent serologies.
• PCR of blood or other fluids is rapidly becoming the test of choice (*Clin Infect Dis 2007;45:S45*).

TREATMENT

Prompt initiation of treatment with antimicrobials is likely to improve prognosis in severe disease. The drugs of choice are doxycycline 100 mg PO or IV q12h or tetracycline 25 mg/kg/d PO divided qid for 7 to 14 days. RIF dosed at 300 mg PO q12h × 7 to 10 days is an alternative treatment and is recommended only for patients with contraindications to doxycycline or tetracycline therapy (*Clin Infect Dis 2007;45:S45*).

Tularemia

GENERAL PRINCIPLES

Tularemia is caused by the gram-negative bacteria *Francisella tularensis* and is endemic to the south central United States. It is transmitted by tick bite, by exposure to infected animals (particularly rabbits), or by exposure to infectious aerosol. *F. tularensis* is one of the most infectious pathogenic bacteria known. Inoculation or inhalation of as little as 10 organisms is adequate to cause disease. It is considered to be a dangerous potential biologic weapon due to its extreme infectivity, ease of dissemination, and capacity to cause illness and subsequent death (*JAMA 2001;285:2763*).

DIAGNOSIS

Clinical Presentation

Fever and malaise occurs 2 to 5 days after exposure. The clinical presentation depends on the inoculation site and route of exposure. Painful regional lymphadenitis with (ulceroglandular) or without (glandular) a skin ulcer is the most common finding. Oculoglandular disease can occur. Systemic (typhoidal) and pneumonic diseases are more likely to be severe, with high mortality if not treated promptly.

Diagnostic Testing

Diagnosis can be confirmed by culture of blood, sputum, or pleural fluid but can lack sensitivity. The microbiology laboratory must be alerted promptly of culture specimens from patients with suspected tularemia to allow for use of advanced biohazard precautions. Acute and convalescent serologic studies provide a retrospective diagnosis.

TREATMENT

Treatment of choice is streptomycin 1 g IM q12h for 10 days; however, gentamicin 5 mg/kg IV divided q8h, is nearly as effective and easier to administer. Doxycycline 100 mg PO/IV q12h for 14 to 21 days is an oral alternative but is more likely to result in relapse. Ciprofloxacin 500 to 750 mg PO bid for 14 to 21 days may also be effective (*JAMA 2001;285:2763*).

Babesiosis

GENERAL PRINCIPLES

Babesiosis is a malaria-like illness and is caused by the intraerythrocytic parasite *Babesia microti* after a tick bite. It is endemic in the same regions as Lyme borreliosis, with which patients may be coinfected.

DIAGNOSIS

Clinical disease ranges from subclinical to severe, with fever, chills, myalgias, and headache. Hemolytic anemia may also be present. Diagnosis is made by visualization of the parasite in erythrocytes on thin blood smears. A serologic test is also available at the CDC.

TREATMENT

Treatment may be necessary for moderate or severe disease, especially in asplenic patients. Atovaquone 750 mg PO bid plus azithromycin 600 mg PO daily for 7 to 10 days is the first choice. Clindamycin 600 mg IV q8h plus quinine 650 mg PO tid for 7 to 10 days should be considered for life-threatening disease. Exchange transfusions may also be needed. Longer duration of therapy may be necessary in patients with persistent symptoms until parasitemia has cleared (*Clin Infect Dis 2006;43:1089*).

MOSQUITO-BORNE INFECTIONS

Arboviral Meningoencephalitis

GENERAL PRINCIPLES

Arboviral meningoencephalitis can be caused by multiple viral agents, which vary by geographic area (e.g., WNV, Eastern and Western equine encephalitis, La Crosse encephalitis, St. Louis encephalitis). In addition to mosquitoes, transmission can occur from blood transfusion, organ transplant, and breast feeding. Infections usually occur in the summer months, and most are subclinical.

DIAGNOSIS

Clinical Presentation

Symptomatic cases of WNV infection range from a mild febrile illness to aseptic meningitis, fulminant encephalitis, or a poliomyelitis-like presentation with flaccid paralysis. Long-term neurologic sequelae are common with severe disease.

Diagnostic Testing

Diagnosis is usually clinical or by acute and convalescent serologic studies. Specific IgM antibody detection in CSF is diagnostic for acute WNV.

TREATMENT

Treatment for all arboviral meningoencephalitides is supportive.

Malaria

GENERAL PRINCIPLES

Malaria is a systemic parasitic disease that is endemic to most of the tropical and subtropical world. Several species of the parasite exist.

Prevention

Travel advice and appropriate chemoprophylaxis regimens are available from the CDC at *http://www.cdc.gov/travel/*.

DIAGNOSIS

Clinical Presentation

The onset of illness occurs within weeks or up to 6 to 12 months after infection with fever, headache, myalgias, and fatigue. Malaria is sometimes characterized by triphasic, periodic (every 48 hours for *Plasmodium ovale* and *Plasmodium vivax*) paroxysms of rigors followed by high fever with headache, cough, and nausea, then culminating in profuse sweating. *Plasmodium falciparum* malaria, the most severe form of the disease, is a potential medical emergency. Complicated, or severe, falciparum malaria is diagnosed in the setting of hyperparasitemia (>5%), cerebral malaria, hypoglycemia, lactic acidosis, renal failure, acute respiratory distress syndrome, or coagulopathy.

Diagnostic Testing

- Malaria should be suspected and excluded in all persons with fever who have traveled to an endemic area within the previous year.
- Diagnosis is made by visualization of parasites on Giemsa-stained thick blood smears. Smears should be obtained during febrile episodes to maximize parasite yield.
- Rapid diagnostic tests targeting antigens common to all *Plasmodium* species as well those specific to *P. falciparum* are available but should be confirmed with microscopy.

TREATMENT

- Treatment is dependent on the type of malaria, severity, and risk of chloroquine resistance where the infection was acquired. Updated information on geographic locations of chloroquine resistance and recommended treatment regimens from the CDC can be found at *http://www.cdc.gov/travel/* and *http://www.cdc.gov/malaria*.
- **Uncomplicated *P. falciparum*** from **chloroquine-sensitive areas** and *P. malariae*: chloroquine 600 mg base (1,000 mg chloroquine phosphate) PO single dose followed by 300 mg base PO 6, 24, and 48 hours later.
- *P. ovale* **and most *P. vivax*** from **chloroquine-sensitive areas:** Same as above, plus primaquine phosphate 15.3-mg base (26.5 mg salt) PO daily for 14 days to prevent relapse. Glucose 6-phosphate dehydrogenase deficiency must be ruled out before primaquine is initiated.
- **Uncomplicated *P. falciparum*** from **chloroquine-resistant areas** and *P. vivax from Australia, Indonesia, or South America*: Quinine sulfate 650 mg PO tid plus doxycycline 100 mg PO bid for 7 days. Alternatives are atovaquone 1 g PO daily plus proguanil 400 mg PO daily both for 3 days, or mefloquine.
- **Complicated or severe P. falciparum:** Quinidine gluconate 10 mg salt/kg (maximum, 600 mg) IV over 1 to 2 hours followed by 0.02 mg/kg/min as a continuous infusion for 72 hours or until parasitemia is <1%, at which time the 72-hour course can be completed with oral quinine sulfate as previously described. Already in use worldwide, intravenous artesunate is available in the United States on

emergency request through the CDC Malaria Branch (*http://www.cdc.gov/malaria/*). Exchange transfusion may also be considered when *P. falciparum* parasitemia exceeds 15%, although the benefit has not been proven.

ZOONOSES

Avian and Swine Influenza (see the Emerging Infections and Bioterrorism section).
Anthrax (see the Emerging Infections and Bioterrorism section).
Plague (see the Emerging Infections and Bioterrorism section).

Cat-Scratch Disease (Bartonellosis)

GENERAL PRINCIPLES

Bartonellosis is caused by the bacterium *Bartonella henselae*. It is usually self-limiting.

DIAGNOSIS

Clinical presentation usually consists of a few papulopustular lesions appearing 3 to 10 days after a cat bite or scratch, followed by regional lymphadenitis (usually cervical or axillary) and mild constitutional symptoms. Atypical presentations include oculoglandular disease, encephalopathy, arthritis, and severe systemic disease. Diagnosis is made by exclusion of other causes of lymphadenitis and by detection of antibodies to *B. henselae* or PCR of infected tissue, skin, or pus.

TREATMENT

Treatment of localized disease is usually unnecessary because spontaneous resolution usually occurs in 2 to 4 months. If antimicrobial therapy is prescribed, azithromycin 500 mg PO single dose followed by 250 mg PO for 4 more days is recommended. Needle aspiration of suppurative lymph nodes may provide symptomatic relief (*Clin Infect Dis 2005;41:1373*).

Leptospirosis

GENERAL PRINCIPLES

- Leptospirosis is an acute febrile illness with varying presentations caused by *Leptospira interrogans*, a ubiquitous pathogen of wild and domestic mammals, reptiles, and amphibians. Symptom onset is 5 to 14 days after contact with infected animals or water contaminated with their urine.
- **Anicteric leptospirosis**, which accounts for most cases, is a biphasic illness that starts with influenza-like symptoms and proceeds to conjunctival suffusion and aseptic meningitis after a brief defervescent period.
- A minority of cases progress directly to **Weil's disease (icteric leptospirosis)**, with multiorgan failure manifested by severe jaundice, uremia, and hemorrhagic pneumonitis.

DIAGNOSIS

Diagnosis is confirmed by specific cultures of urine or blood, PCR, or paired serologic studies.

TREATMENT

Therapy for anicteric disease, which can shorten the duration of illness, is doxycycline 100 mg PO bid or amoxicillin 500 mg PO q6h for 7 days. Penicillin G 1.5 million U IV q4–6h or a third-generation cephalosporin is used for treatment of severe disease, during which a Jarisch–Herxheimer reaction is possible (*Clin Microbiol Rev 2001;14:296*).

Brucellosis

GENERAL PRINCIPLES

Brucellosis is a protean systemic infection caused by members of the *Brucella* genus of gram-negative coccobacilli. Infection is usually preceded by direct contact with body fluids of livestock animals, by eating unpasteurized dairy foods, or by inhalation of infected aerosolized particles.

DIAGNOSIS

Clinical Presentation

Symptoms are initially nonspecific but usually include constitutional symptoms such as fever and perspiration. Fever can be spiking and accompanied by rigors but can also be relapsing and protracted. Malodorous perspiration is almost pathognomonic. Physical exam can be nonrevealing, although lymphadenopathy, hepatomegaly, or splenomegaly may often be present. Complications within every organ system can occur (e.g., diarrhea, arthritis, meningitis, endocarditis, pneumonia, hepatitis).

Diagnostic Testing

Diagnosis is confirmed by isolation of the organism from blood or tissue culture.

TREATMENT

Antimicrobial treatment with doxycycline 100 mg PO bid for 6 weeks with or without gentamicin for 2 to 3 weeks, or RIF for 6 weeks, reduces duration and complications of the disease. Audiometry should be performed weekly while gentamicin therapy is administered (*N Engl J Med 2005;352:2325*).

BITE WOUNDS

Animal Bites

GENERAL PRINCIPLES

Management includes copious irrigation, culturing visibly infected wounds, and obtaining imaging to exclude fracture, foreign body, or joint space involvement.

Most wounds should not be sutured unless they are on the face and have been thoroughly irrigated. Wound elevation should be encouraged.

TREATMENT

- Antimicrobial therapy is given to treat overt infection and as prophylaxis for high-risk bite wounds based on severity (e.g., moderate to severe), location (e.g., hands, genitalia, near joints), bite source (e.g., cats), immune status (e.g., diabetes mellitus, asplenia, immunosuppression), and type of injury (e.g., puncture, crush injury). Tetanus toxoid should be administered if the patient has been previously vaccinated but has not received a booster in the last 5 years.
- Prophylactic antibiotic therapy with amoxicillin-clavulanate 875 mg/125 mg PO bid for 3 to 5 days should usually be administered, unless the bite is trivial. Antibiotics are most effective for patients presenting >8 hours after the injury (*Arch Emerg Med 1989;6:251*).

SPECIAL CONSIDERATIONS

- **Dog bites:** Normal oral flora includes *Pasteurella multocida*, streptococci, staphylococci, and *Capnocytophaga canimorsus*. Dog bites comprise 80% of animal bites, but only 5% of such bites become infected. For infected dog bite wounds, amoxicillin-clavulanate, or clindamycin plus ciprofloxacin, is effective.
- **Cat bites:** Normal oral flora includes *P. multocida* and *S. aureus*. Because more than 80% of cat bites become infected, prophylaxis with amoxicillin-clavulanate should be routinely provided. Cephalosporins should not be used. Bartonellosis can also develop after a cat bite.
- **Wild animal bites:** The need for rabies vaccination should be determined (see the following text). For most animal bites, amoxicillin-clavulanate is a good choice for prophylaxis and empiric treatment. Monkey bites should be treated with acyclovir because of the risk of *Herpesvirus simiae* (B virus).
- **Rabies**
  ○ Rabies causes an invariably fatal neurologic disease classically manifesting with hydrophobia, aerophobia, pharyngeal spasm, seizures, and coma.
  ○ The need for rabies vaccination and immunoglobulin prophylaxis (see Appendix A, Immunizations and Postexposure Therapies) should be determined after any animal bite. Risk of rabies depends on the animal species and geographic location. In the United States, most recent indigenous cases have been associated with bats, while dog bites account for the vast majority of human cases in the developing world.
  ○ Regardless of species, if the animal is rabid or suspected to be rabid, the human diploid vaccine and rabies immunoglobulin should be administered immediately. Bites by domestic animals rarely require prophylaxis unless the animal's condition is unknown. Public health authorities should be consulted to determine whether prophylaxis is recommended for other types of animal bites.
  ○ A single case of survival after symptom onset by an aggressive coma-inducing regimen has been reported (*N Engl J Med 2005;352:2508*).

Human Bites

GENERAL PRINCIPLES

- Human bites, particularly clenched-fist injuries, are prone to infection and other complications. The normal oral flora of humans includes viridans streptococci, staphylococci, *Bacteroides* spp., *Fusobacterium* spp., peptostreptococci, and *Eikenella corrodens*.
- **Prophylaxis** with amoxicillin-clavulanate 875 mg/125 mg PO bid for 5 days is recommended for uninfected wounds.
- Infected wounds may require **parenteral therapy**, such as ampicillin-sulbactam 1.5 g IV q6h; cefoxitin, 2 g IV q8h; or ticarcillin-clavulanate 3.1 g IV q6h for 1 to 2 weeks. Therapy should be extended to 4 to 6 weeks if osteomyelitis is present.

HEALTH CARE–ASSOCIATED INFECTIONS

Health care–associated infections (HAIs) substantially contribute to morbidity, mortality, and excess health care costs. Efforts to control and prevent the spread of HAIs require an institutional assessment of resources, priorities, and commitment to infection control practices (see Appendix B, Infection Control and Isolation Recommendations).

Catheter-Related Bloodstream Infections

GENERAL PRINCIPLES

- *S. aureus, S. epidermidis* (coagulase-negative staphylococci), aerobic gram-negative species, and *Candida* species are the most common organisms associated with catheter-related bloodstream infections (CRBSIs) (*Clin Infect Dis 2001;32:1249*).
- Subclavian central venous catheters (CVCs) are associated with lower CRBSI rates than internal jugular CVCs, while femoral CVCs have the highest rates and should be removed within 72 hours of placement.
- Strategies for decreasing the incidence of CRBSIs include proper hand hygiene, skin antisepsis using an alcohol-based chlorhexidine solution, maximal sterile barrier precautions during insertion, strict adherence to aseptic technique, and removal of nonessential CVCs as soon as possible (*Infect Control Hosp Epidemiol 2008;29(suppl 1):S22*). Subcutaneous tunneling and use of antiseptic-impregnated CVCs may further reduce the incidence of CRBSIs. Routine exchange of CVCs over guide wire is not recommended.

DIAGNOSIS

Clinical Presentation

CRBSIs should be suspected in any febrile patient with a CVC. Clinical findings that increase the suspicion of CRBSIs include local inflammation or phlebitis at the CVC insertion site, sepsis, endophthalmitis, lack of another source of bacteremia, and resolution of fever after catheter removal.

Diagnostic Testing

- Diagnosis is established by obtaining ≥2 blood cultures from both the CVC and a peripheral vein prior to initiation of antibiotics.
- Repeat blood cultures should be obtained after starting antibiotic therapy to demonstrate clearance of bacteremia.
- TEE is recommended to rule out endocarditis if the patient has an implantable cardiac pacemaker or defibrillator, a prosthetic heart valve, persistent bacteremia or fungemia, persistent fever more than 3 days after initiation of appropriate antibiotic therapy and catheter removal, or if *S. aureus* is involved and <4 weeks of therapy is being considered.

TREATMENT

- Host factors, including comorbidities, severity of illness, multidrug-resistant colonization, prior infections, and current antimicrobial agents, are important considerations when selecting an antimicrobial regimen. Management guidelines are available from the Infectious Diseases Society of America (*Clin Infect Dis 2009;49:1*).
- **Empiric therapy**
  - Vancomycin 15 to 20 mg/kg IV q12h is appropriate for empiric therapy as a majority of CRBSIs are caused by staphylococci. The dose should be adjusted to achieve a vancomycin trough between 15 and 20 μg/mL.
  - Gram-negative bacilli, including *Pseudomonas*, should be covered broadly until species identification and susceptibilities are known. Fourth-generation cephalosporins (e.g., cefepime), carbapenems, or a β-lactam/β-lactamase inhibitor combined with or without an aminoglycoside are potential options.
  - The recommended duration of therapy depends on whether the infection is complicated or uncomplicated, beginning from the date of the first negative blood culture or removal of the infected CVC, whichever came later.
- **Pathogen-specific therapy:** Once the pathogen has been identified, antimicrobial therapy should be narrowed to the most effective regimen.
  - *S. aureus*: **Methicillin-sensitive** *S. aureus* CRBSI should be treated with oxacillin 2 g IV q4h or alternatively with cefazolin 1 to 2 g IV q8h. First-line therapy for **MRSA** is vancomycin 15 to 20 mg/kg IV q12h with a target vancomycin trough between 15 and 20 μg/mL. Linezolid 600 mg PO or IV q12h or daptomycin 6 mg/kg IV daily are alternatives. Routine use of gentamicin for synergy in *S. aureus* bacteremia is not recommended (*Clin Infect Dis 2009;48:722*). TEE should be considered to evaluate for endocarditis. The recommended duration of therapy is generally 4 to 6 weeks. A 2-week course is acceptable for uncomplicated MRSA bacteremia, as defined by a negative TEE, negative blood cultures and defervescence within 72 hours of starting effective therapy, absence of prosthetic material (e.g., pacemaker, valve), and no evidence of metastatic infection (*Clin Infect Dis 2011;52:1*).
  - *S. epidermidis* (**coagulase-negative staphylococci**) CRBSI is treated similarly to MRSA, with vancomycin being the drug of choice in most cases. Duration of therapy is 7 days after CVC removal or 14 days if the CVC is retained.
  - Sensitive **enterococcus** CRBSI should be treated with ampicillin. Vancomycin should be used in the setting of ampicillin resistance. Vancomycin-resistant enterococci may require therapy with daptomycin or linezolid. Duration of treatment should be 7 to 14 days.

- Therapy against **gram-negative bacilli** should be guided by antibiotic susceptibility testing. Duration may range from 7 to 14 days.
- **Candidemia** should be treated with an echinocandin (e.g., caspofungin 70 mg IV single dose followed by 50 mg IV daily) in cases of moderate-to-severe illness pending species identification, after which therapy can be tailored. Fluconazole 400 mg IV or PO daily may be appropriate for stable patients who have not had any recent azole exposure. Duration of antifungal treatment should be for 14 days after the last positive blood culture (*Clin Infect Dis 2009;48:503*). A dilated ophthalmologic examination is advised to look for Candida endophthalmitis.
- **CVC removal** is always preferable. At a minimum, it is recommended that CVCs be removed in the following situations:
  - Any CRBSI involving *S. aureus*, most gram-negative bacilli, or *Candida* spp.
  - Insertion-site or tunnel-site infection (pus or significant inflammation at the site)
  - Immunocompromised patients with fever, neutropenia, and hemodynamic instability (e.g., sepsis)
- Antibiotic lock therapy in combination with an extended course of antibiotics may be an option in certain situations where CVC salvage is absolutely necessary.

Hospital- and Ventilator-Associated Pneumonia

GENERAL PRINCIPLES

The most frequent pathogens are gram-negative bacilli and *S. aureus*.

DIAGNOSIS

Clinical Presentation

The clinical presentation includes a new pulmonary infiltrate or increasing oxygen requirement in patients with fever, with or without cough, occurring >48 hours after admission.

Diagnostic Testing

Diagnosis is made by clinical criteria as well as microbiologic testing. Optimal specimens are uncontaminated sterile body fluids (pleural or blood), bronchoscopy aspirates (cultured quantitatively), or aspirates from endotracheal tubes. Fiber optic bronchoscopy may be diagnostic (quantitative cultures) and therapeutic (reexpansion of lung segment).

TREATMENT

Initial empiric antimicrobial therapy should cover common health care–acquired pathogens, particularly *P. aeruginosa* and MRSA. Targeted therapy should be based on culture results and in vitro sensitivity testing. Empyemas require drainage.

Methicillin-Resistant *Staphylococcus aureus* Infections

GENERAL PRINCIPLES

MRSA infection should be distinguished from MRSA colonization, especially when isolated from nonsterile sites such as sputum. Contact precautions are indicated.

TREATMENT

- First-line therapy for most MRSA infections is vancomycin (dosed to therapeutic trough levels). Alternative agents include linezolid 600 mg IV or PO q12h, daptomycin 6 mg/kg IV q24h, ceftaroline, and telavancin. Daptomycin should not be used to treat pneumonia due to inactivation by pulmonary surfactant.
- Eradication of MRSA nasal carriage can sometimes be achieved with a 5-day course of twice-daily intranasal mupirocin. Other regimens include chlorhexidine soap products, bleach baths, and oral antibiotic treatment with TMP-SMX with or without rifampin. However, mupirocin resistance can develop and carriage often recurs. Eradication efforts should target patients with recurrent MRSA infections.

Vancomycin-Resistant Enterococcus Infections

GENERAL PRINCIPLES

VRE infection should be distinguished from VRE colonization. Most VRE-related lower UTIs can be treated with nitrofurantoin, ampicillin, ciprofloxacin, or other agents that achieve high urinary concentrations. Contact precautions are indicated. Eradication of enteric VRE colonization has been attempted without success.

TREATMENT

The majority of patients with VRE bloodstream infections are treated with linezolid, daptomycin, or quinupristin/dalfopristin.

Multidrug-Resistant Gram-Negative Infections

GENERAL PRINCIPLES

Highly resistant gram-negative organisms (e.g., *Acinetobacter*, *Klebsiella*, and *Pseudomonas* species) have become increasingly common causes of HAI. Contact precautions are indicated.

TREATMENT

Antimicrobial choices are often limited. In addition to broad-spectrum agents such as β-lactam/β-lactamase inhibitor combinations and carbapenems, tigecycline, and colistin may occasionally be useful. Infectious disease consultation is recommended for complicated multidrug-resistant infections.

EMERGING INFECTIONS AND BIOTERRORISM

Changing patterns in human behavior and demographics, natural phenomena, and microbial evolution continually introduce new pathogens to human contact, leading to the introduction and spread of new or previously rare diseases. Included in this category are several highly fatal and easily produced microorganisms, which have the potential to be used as agents of bioterrorism and produce substantial illness in large populations via an aerosol route of exposure. Most of the likely diseases are rare, so a high index of suspicion is necessary to identify the first few cases. A bioterrorism-related outbreak should be considered if an unusually large number of patients present simultaneously with a respiratory, GI, or febrile rash syndrome; if several otherwise healthy patients present with unusually severe disease; or if an unusual pathogen for the region is isolated.

Anthrax

GENERAL PRINCIPLES

Spores from the gram-positive *Bacillus anthracis* germinate at the site of entry into the body, causing cutaneous, GI, or inhalational anthrax.

DIAGNOSIS

Clinical Presentation

Natural transmission can occur through butchering and eating infected animals, usually resulting in cutaneous or GI disease.

- **Cutaneous anthrax** ("Woolsorter's disease") is characterized by a painless black eschar with surrounding tissue edema.
- **Gastrointestinal anthrax** can present with nausea, vomiting, abdominal pain, ascites, and hemorrhage related to necrotic mucosal ulcers.
- **Inhalational anthrax** (45% case-fatality rate) may result from inadvertent aerosolization of spores from contaminated animal products (e.g., wool or animal hides) or an intentional release (*JAMA 2001;286:2549*). Infection presents initially with an influenza-like illness, GI symptoms, or both, followed by fulminant respiratory distress and multiorgan failure.

Diagnostic Testing

Diagnosis of inhalational disease is suggested by a widened mediastinum without infiltrates on chest radiography and confirmed by blood culture and PCR. Notify local infection control and public health department immediately for confirmed cases.

TREATMENT

Treatment with immediate antibiotic initiation on first suspicion of inhalational anthrax reduces mortality. Empiric therapy is ciprofloxacin 400 mg IV q12h *or* doxycycline 100 mg IV q12h *and* one or two other antibiotics that are active against *B. anthracis* (e.g., penicillin, clindamycin, vancomycin) (*JAMA 2002;287:2236*). Oral therapy with ciprofloxacin 500 mg PO bid *or* doxycycline 100 mg PO bid *and* one other active agent should be started after improvement and continued for 60 days to reduce the risk of delayed spore germination.

- Uncomplicated cutaneous anthrax can be treated with oral ciprofloxacin 500 mg bid *or* doxycycline 100 mg bid for the same duration. GI anthrax should be treated the same as inhalational disease.

- Postexposure prophylaxis for individuals at risk for inhalational anthrax consists of oral ciprofloxacin 500 mg bid for 60 days after exposure. Doxycycline or amoxicillin are alternatives if the strain proves susceptible.

Smallpox

GENERAL PRINCIPLES

The variola virus that causes smallpox is easily transmitted person to person through respiratory droplets and carries a case-fatality ratio of 25% to 30%. Smallpox, as a naturally occurring disease, was declared eradicated in 1979. However, remaining viral stocks pose a potential bioterrorism threat to unimmunized populations.

DIAGNOSIS

Clinical Presentation

High fever, myalgias, low back pain, and headache appear 7 to 17 days after exposure, followed by a distinctive rash 3 to 5 days later. Lesions progress through stages of macules, deep vesicles, pustules, scabs, and permanent pitting scars. The rash starts on the face and distal extremities, including palms and soles, with relative sparing of the trunk, and all lesions in one area are in the same stage of development. These features help to distinguish smallpox from chickenpox (varicella).

Diagnostic Testing

Diagnosis is primarily clinical but can be confirmed by electron microscopy and PCR of pustule fluid at reference laboratories. Notify local infection control, public health departments, and the CDC immediately. Treat all diagnostic samples as highly infectious.

TREATMENT

- Treatment consists of supportive care. No specific antiviral treatment is currently available, although several investigational drugs are in development.
- All suspected cases must be placed in contact and airborne isolation; patients remain infectious until all scabs have separated from the skin.
- Postexposure prophylaxis with live vaccinia virus vaccine within 3 days of exposure offers near-complete protection for responders but is associated with uncommon severe adverse reactions. Progressive vaccinia, eczema vaccinatum, and severe cases of generalized vaccinia can be treated with vaccinia immunoglobulin.

Plague

GENERAL PRINCIPLES

Plague is caused by the gram-negative bacillus *Yersinia pestis*. Naturally acquired plague occurs rarely in the Southwestern United States after exposure to infected animals (e.g., through scratches, bites, direct handling, inhalation of aerosolized respiratory secretions) and via rodent flea bites.

DIAGNOSIS

Clinical Presentation

There are three forms of plague

- **Bubonic:** Local painful lymphadenitis (bubo) and fever (14% case-fatality ratio).
- **Septicemic:** Can cause peripheral necrosis and disseminated intravascular coagulation (DIC) ("black death"). Usually from progression of bubonic disease (30% to 50% case-fatality ratio).
- **Pneumonic:** Severe pneumonia with hemoptysis preceded by initial influenza-like illness (57% case-fatality ratio, nearing 100% when treatment is delayed). Pneumonic disease can be transmitted from person to person and would be expected after inhalation of aerosolized *Y. pestis*.

Diagnostic Testing

Diagnosis is confirmed by isolation of *Y. pestis* from blood, sputum, or CSF. Treat all diagnostic samples as highly infectious. Notify local infection control and public health departments immediately.

TREATMENT

- Treatment should start at first suspicion of plague because rapid initiation of antibiotics improves survival. Agents of choice are streptomycin 1 g IM q12h; gentamicin 5 mg/kg IV/IM q24h *or* a 2 mg/kg loading dose then 1.7 mg/kg IV/IM q8h, with appropriate monitoring of drug levels; or doxycycline 100 mg PO/IV bid. Alternatives include ciprofloxacin and chloramphenicol. Oral therapy can be started after clinical improvement, for a total course of 10 to 14 days.
- Postexposure prophylaxis is indicated after unprotected face-to-face contact with patients with known or suspected pneumonic plague, and consists of doxycycline 100 mg PO bid or ciprofloxacin 500 mg PO bid for 7 days.

Botulism

GENERAL PRINCIPLES

Botulism results from intoxication with botulinum toxin, produced by the anaerobic gram-positive bacillus *Clostridium botulinum*. Modes of acquisition include ingestion of the neurotoxin from improperly canned food and contamination of wounds with *C. botulinum* from the soil. Inhalational botulism could result from an intentional release of aerosolized toxin. Mortality is low when botulism is recognized early but may be very high in the setting of mass exposure and limited access to mechanical ventilation equipment.

DIAGNOSIS

The classic triad consists of an absence of fever, clear sensorium, and symmetric descending flaccid paralysis with cranial nerve involvement, beginning with ptosis, diplopia, and dysarthria, and progressing to loss of gag reflex and diaphragmatic function with respiratory failure, followed by diffuse skeletal muscle paralysis. Sensation remains intact. Paralysis can last from weeks to months. Diagnosis is confirmed by detection of toxin in serum. Notify local infection control and public health departments.

TREATMENT

- Treatment is primarily supportive, and may require mechanical ventilation in the setting of respiratory failure. Wound botulism requires extensive surgical debridement.
- Further progression of paralysis can be halted by early administration of botulinum antitoxin, available through the state public health department or the CDC. Antitoxin is reserved only for cases where there is a high suspicion for botulism based on clinical presentation and exposure history. Routine postexposure prophylaxis with antitoxin is not recommended because of the high incidence (10%) of hypersensitivity reactions and limited supply.

Viral Hemorrhagic Fever

GENERAL PRINCIPLES

This syndrome is caused by many different RNA viruses, including filoviruses (Ebola and Marburg), flaviviruses (dengue, yellow fever), bunyaviruses (hantaviruses, Congo-Crimean hemorrhagic fever [CCHF], Rift Valley Fever [RVF]), and arenaviruses (South American hemorrhagic fevers, Lassa fever). All cause sporadic disease in endemic areas, and most can be transmitted as an aerosol or contact with infected body fluids. Case-fatality ratios are variable but can be as high as 90% for severe cases of Ebola.

DIAGNOSIS

Clinical Presentation
Early symptoms include fevers, myalgias, and malaise, with varying severity and symptomatology depending on the virus, but all can severely disrupt vascular permeability and cause DIC. Thrombocytopenia, leukopenia, and hepatitis are common.

Diagnostic Testing
Diagnosis requires consideration of epidemiology and patient risk factors, especially travel to endemic areas. Serology performed by reference laboratories can confirm diagnosis. Notify local infection control and public health departments immediately.

TREATMENT

- Treatment is primarily supportive with attention to infection control. Ribavirin (2 g IV × 1, then 1 g q6h × 4 d, then 500 mg q8h × 6 d) has been used for CCHF, Lassa, and RVF (*JAMA 2002;287:2391*; *J Antimicrob Chemother 2011;66:1215*).
- Exposed contacts should monitor temperature twice daily for 3 weeks. Postexposure prophylaxis with oral ribavirin can be administered to febrile CCHF, Lassa, and RVF contacts.

Severe Acute Respiratory Syndrome

GENERAL PRINCIPLES

Severe acute respiratory syndrome (SARS) is a fulminant febrile influenza-like respiratory illness that progresses to pneumonia and acute respiratory distress syndrome (ARDS) (*JAMA 2003;290:374*), caused by SARS-associated coronavirus (SARS-CoV). SARS should be considered in clusters of cases of undiagnosed febrile illness, particularly in the setting of travel to mainland China, Hong Kong, or Taiwan within 10 days of symptom onset.

DIAGNOSIS

Diagnosis is confirmed by acute or convalescent SARS-CoV antibodies or PCR by the CDC.

TREATMENT

Treatment is primarily supportive. Interferon and high-dose steroids have been used.

Pandemic, Avian, and Swine Influenza

GENERAL PRINCIPLES

Genetic reassortment can result in influenza strains that were previously confined to avian and swine hosts gaining human infectivity, causing severe disease and/or rapid spread through human populations. Infection control measures and close communication with public health authorities are critical when pandemic strains are circulating. Each new strain may have different virulence, affected age ranges, clinical presentation, and antiviral susceptibilities. Following updated, local data during an outbreak is essential.

15 Antimicrobials

Bernard C. Camins and David J. Ritchie

Empiric antimicrobial therapy should be initiated based on expected pathogens for a given infection. As microbial resistance is increasing among many pathogens, a review of institutional as well as local, regional, national, and global susceptibility trends can assist in the development of empiric therapy regimens. In addition, an accurate allergy history and pregnancy/lactation status should be elicited from patients. Antimicrobial therapy should be modified, if possible, based on results of culture and sensitivity testing to agent(s) that have the narrowest spectrum possible. Shorter courses have been shown to be as effective as longer courses in some indications without emergence of resistance. Attention should be paid to the possibility of switching from parenteral to oral therapy where possible, as many oral agents have excellent bioavailability. Several antibiotics have major drug interactions or require alternate dosing in renal or hepatic insufficiency, or both. For antiretroviral and antiparasitic agents, see Chapter 16, Human Immunodeficiency Virus and Acquired Immunodeficiency Syndrome, and Chapter 14, Treatment of Infectious Diseases, respectively.

ANTIBACTERIAL AGENTS

Penicillins

GENERAL PRINCIPLES

- Penicillins (PCNs) irreversibly bind PCN-binding proteins in the bacterial cell wall, causing osmotic rupture and death. These agents have a diminished role today because of acquired resistance in many bacterial species through alterations in PCN-binding proteins or expression of hydrolytic enzymes.
- PCNs remain among the drugs of choice for syphilis, group A streptococci, *Listeria monocytogenes*, *Pasteurella multocida*, *Actinomyces*, and some anaerobic infections.

TREATMENT

Medications

- **Aqueous penicillin G** (2 to 5 million U intravenous [IV] q4h or 12 to 30 million U daily by continuous infusion) is the IV preparation of PCN and the drug of choice for most PCN-susceptible streptococcal infections and neurosyphilis.
- **Procaine penicillin G** is an intramuscular (IM) repository form of penicillin G that can be used as an alternative treatment for neurosyphilis at a dose of 2.4 million U IM daily in combination with probenecid, 500 mg by mouth (PO) qid for 10 to 14 days.
- **Benzathine PCN** is a long-acting IM repository form of penicillin G that is commonly used for treating early latent syphilis (<1 year duration [one dose,

2.4 million U IM]) and late latent syphilis (unknown duration or >1 year [2.4 million U IM weekly for three doses]). It is occasionally given for group A strepto-coccal pharyngitis and prophylaxis after acute rheumatic fever.

- **Penicillin V** (250 to 500 mg PO q6h) is an oral formulation of PCN that is typically used to treat group A streptococcal pharyngitis.
- **Ampicillin** (1 to 3 g IV q4–6h) is the drug of choice for treatment of infections caused by susceptible enterococcus species or *L. monocytogenes*. Oral ampicillin (250 to 500 mg PO q6h) may be used for uncomplicated sinusitis, pharyngitis, otitis media, and urinary tract infections (UTIs), but amoxicillin is generally preferred.
- **Ampicillin/sulbactam** (1.5 to 3.0 g IV q6h) combines ampicillin with the β-lactamase inhibitor sulbactam, thereby extending its spectrum to include methicillin-sensitive *Staphylococcus aureus* (MSSA), anaerobes, and many Enterobac-teriaceae. The sulbactam component also has unique activity against some strains of *Acinetobacter*. The agent is effective for infections of the upper and lower respiratory tract; genitourinary tract; and abdominal, pelvic, and polymicrobial soft tissue infections, including those due to human or animal bites.
- **Amoxicillin** (250 to 1,000 mg PO q8h or 775 mg extended-release q24h) is an oral antibiotic similar to ampicillin that is commonly used for uncomplicated sinusitis, pharyngitis, otitis media, community-acquired pneumonia, and UTIs.
- **Amoxicillin/clavulanic acid** (875 mg PO q12h, or 500 mg PO q8h, or 90 mg/kg/d divided q12h [Augmentin ES-600 suspension], or 2,000 mg PO q12h [Augmentin XR]) is an oral antibiotic similar to ampicillin/sulbactam that combines amoxicillin with the β-lactamase inhibitor clavulanate. It is useful for treating complicated sinusitis and otitis media and for prophylaxis of human or animal bites after appropriate local treatment.
- **Nafcillin and oxacillin** (1 to 2 g IV q4–6h) are penicillinase-resistant synthetic PCNs that are the drugs of choice for treating MSSA infections. Dose reduction should be considered in decompensated liver disease.
- **Dicloxacillin and cloxacillin** (250 to 500 mg PO q6h) are oral antibiotics with a spectrum of activity similar to that of nafcillin and oxacillin, which are typically used to treat localized skin infections.
- **Piperacillin** (3 g IV q4h or 4 g IV q6h) is an extended-spectrum PCN with enhanced gram-negative activity as well as enterococcal activity. This agent has reasonable antipseudomonal activity but generally requires coadministration of an aminoglycoside for treatment of serious infections.
- **Ticarcillin/clavulanic acid** (3.1 g IV q4–6h) combines ticarcillin with the β-lactamase inhibitor clavulanic acid. This combination extends the spectrum to include most Enterobacteriaceae, MSSA, and anaerobes, making it useful for intra-abdominal and complicated soft tissue infections. Ticarcillin/clavulanic acid also has a unique role in treatment of *Stenotrophomonas* infections. This agent has a high sodium content and should be used cautiously in patients at risk for fluid overload.
- **Piperacillin/tazobactam** (3.375 g IV q6h or the higher dose of 4.5 g IV q6h for *Pseudomonas*) combines piperacillin with the β-lactamase inhibitor tazobactam. It has a similar spectrum and indications as ticarcillin/clavulanic acid but has enhanced activity against ampicillin-sensitive enterococci. The addition of an aminoglycoside should be considered for treatment of serious infections caused by *Pseudomonas aeruginosa* or for nosocomial pneumonia. Interestingly, the tazobactam component is superfluous in treating *Pseudomonas* infections, but in most situations, this is the only piperacillin formulation available.

SPECIAL CONSIDERATIONS

All PCN derivatives have been rarely associated with anaphylaxis, interstitial nephritis, anemia, and leukopenia. Prolonged high-dose therapy (>2 weeks) is typically monitored with weekly serum creatinine and complete blood count (CBC). Liver function tests (LFTs) are also monitored with oxacillin/nafcillin, as these agents can cause hepatitis. Ticarcillin/clavulanic acid can aggravate bleeding by interfering with platelet adenosine diphosphate receptors. All patients should be asked about PCN, cephalosporin, or carbapenem allergies. These agents should not be used in patients with a reported serious PCN allergy without prior skin testing or desensitization, or both.

Cephalosporins

GENERAL PRINCIPLES

- Cephalosporins exert their bactericidal effect by interfering with cell wall synthesis by the same mechanism as PCNs.
- They are clinically useful because of their low toxicity and broad spectrum of activity. All cephalosporins are devoid of activity against enterococci and until recently, all were inactive against methicillin-resistant *S. aureus* (MRSA), but there are now cephalosporins that have bactericidal activity against MRSA.

TREATMENT

Medications

- **First-generation cephalosporins** have activity against staphylococci, streptococci, and most *Escherichia coli*, *Klebsiella*, and *Proteus* species. These agents have limited activity against other enteric gram-negative bacilli and anaerobes. **Cefazolin** (1 to 2 g IV/IM q8h) is the most commonly used parenteral preparation, and **cephalexin** (250 to 500 mg PO q6h) and **cefadroxil** (500 mg to 1 g PO q12h) are oral preparations. These limited-activity agents are commonly used for treating skin/ soft tissue infections, UTIs, minor MSSA infections, and for surgical prophylaxis (cefazolin).
- **Second-generation cephalosporins** have expanded coverage against enteric gram-negative rods and can be divided into above-the-diaphragm and below-the-diaphragm agents.
- **Cefuroxime** (1.5 g IV/IM q8h) is useful for treatment of infections above the diaphragm. This agent has reasonable antistaphylococcal and antistreptococcal activity in addition to an extended spectrum against gram-negative aerobes and can be used for skin/soft tissue infections, complicated UTIs, and some community-acquired respiratory tract infections. It does not reliably cover *Bacteroides fragilis*.
- **Cefuroxime axetil** (250 to 500 mg PO q12h), **cefprozil** (250 to 500 mg PO q12h), and **cefaclor** (250 to 500 mg PO q12h) are oral second-generation cephalosporins typically used for bronchitis, sinusitis, otitis media, UTIs, local soft tissue infections, and oral step-down therapy for pneumonia or cellulitis responsive to parenteral cephalosporins.
- **Cefoxitin** (1 to 2 g IV q4–8h) and **cefotetan** (1 to 2 g IV q12h) are useful for treatment of infections below the diaphragm. These agents have reasonable activity

against gram negatives and aerobes, including *B. fragilis*, and are commonly used for intra-abdominal or gynecologic surgical prophylaxis and infections, including diverticulitis and pelvic inflammatory disease.

- **Third-generation cephalosporins** have broad coverage against aerobic gram-negative bacilli and retain significant activity against streptococci and MSSA. They have moderate anaerobic activity but generally not against *B. fragilis*. Ceftazidime is the only third-generation cephalosporin that is useful for treating serious *P. aeruginosa* infections. Some of these agents have substantial central nervous system (CNS) penetration and are useful in treating meningitis (see Chapter 14, Treatment of Infectious Diseases). Third-generation cephalosporins are not reliable for the treatment of serious infections caused by organisms producing AmpC β-lactamases regardless of the results of susceptibility testing. These pathogens should be treated empirically with carbapenems, cefepime, or fluoroquinolones.
- **Ceftriaxone** (1 to 2 g IV/IM q12–24h) and **cefotaxime** (1 to 2 g IV/IM q4–12h) are very similar to one another in spectrum and efficacy. They can be used as empiric therapy for pyelonephritis, urosepsis, pneumonia, intra-abdominal infections (combined with metronidazole), gonorrhea, and meningitis. They can also be used for osteomyelitis, septic arthritis, endocarditis, and soft tissue infections caused by susceptible organisms.
- **Cefpodoxime proxetil** (100 to 400 mg PO q12h), **cefdinir** (300 mg PO q12h), **ceftibuten** (400 mg PO q24h), and **cefditoren pivoxil** (200 to 400 mg PO q12h) are oral third-generation cephalosporins useful for the treatment of bronchitis and complicated sinusitis, otitis media, and UTIs. These agents can also be used as step-down therapy for community-acquired pneumonia. Cefpodoxime can be used as single-dose therapy for uncomplicated gonorrhea.
- **Ceftazidime** (1 to 2 g IV/IM q8h) may be used for treatment of infections caused by susceptible strains of *P. aeruginosa*.
- **The fourth-generation cephalosporin cefepime** (500 mg to 2 g IV/IM q8–12h) has excellent aerobic gram-negative coverage, including *P. aeruginosa* and other bacteria producing AmpC β-lactamases. Its gram-positive activity is similar to that of the ceftriaxone and cefotaxime. **Cefepime** is routinely used for empiric therapy in febrile neutropenic patients. It also has a prominent role in treating infections caused by antibiotic-resistant gram-negative bacteria and some infections involving both gram-negative and gram-positive aerobes in most sites, although clinical experience in the treatment of meningitis is more limited. Anti-anaerobic coverage should be added where anaerobes are suspected.
- Broad-spectrum cephalosporins that have activity against MRSA are now available. Ceftobiprole is not available for use in the United States, but **ceftaroline** (usual U.S. Food and Drug Administration [FDA]–approved dose is 600 mg IV q12h; 600mg IV q8h is an alternative dose for more serious infections) is indicated for acute bacterial skin and skin structure infections and community-acquired bacterial pneumonia. **Ceftaroline** has similar activity to ceftriaxone against gram-negative pathogens, with virtually no activity against *Pseudomonas* spp., *Acinetobacter*, and AmpC β-lactamase; extended-spectrum β-lactamase (ESBL); and *Klebsiella pneumoniae* carbapenemase (KPC)–producing gram-negative pathogens. What distinguishes ceftaroline from the earlier cephaloporins is its affinity for penicillin binding protein 2a (PBP2a)—the same cell wall component that renders MRSA resistant to all other β-lactams. By binding to this cell wall component, ceftaroline interferes with cell wall synthesis and causes cell rupture in MRSA, vancomycin-intermediate

S. aureus (VISA), or vancomycin-resistant *S. aureus* (VRSA) isolates. Like all cephalosporins, though, it has no activity against *Enterococcus* spp.

SPECIAL CONSIDERATIONS

All cephalosporins have been rarely associated with anaphylaxis, interstitial nephritis, anemia, and leukopenia. **PCN-allergic patients have a 5% to 10% incidence of a cross-hypersensitivity reaction to cephalosporins.** These agents should not be used in a patient with a reported severe PCN allergy (i.e., anaphylaxis, hives) without prior skin testing or desensitization, or both. Prolonged therapy (>2 weeks) is typically monitored with a weekly serum creatinine and complete blood count. Ceftriaxone can cause biliary sludging, requiring discontinuation of the medication.

Monobactams

GENERAL PRINCIPLES

Definition

- **Aztreonam** (1 to 2 g IV/IM q6–12h) is a monobactam that is active only against aerobic gram-negative bacteria, including *P. aeruginosa*.
- It is useful in patients with known β-lactam allergy as there is no apparent cross-reactivity.

Carbapenems

GENERAL PRINCIPLES

- **Imipenem** (500 mg to 1 g IV/IM q6–8h), **meropenem** (1 to 2 g IV q8h or 500 mg IV q6h), **doripenem** (500 mg IV q8h), and **ertapenem** (1 g IV q24h) are the currently available carbapenems.
- Carbapenems exert their bactericidal effect by interfering with cell wall synthesis, similar to PCNs and cephalosporins, and are active against most gram-positive and gram-negative bacteria, including anaerobes. They are among the antibiotics of choice for infections caused by organisms producing AmpC or ESBLs.

TREATMENT

- Carbapenems are important agents for treatment of many antibiotic-resistant bacterial infections at most body sites. These agents are commonly used for severe polymicrobial infections, including Fournier's gangrene, intra-abdominal catastrophes, and sepsis in immunocompromised hosts.
- Notable bacteria that are **resistant** to carbapenems include ampicillin-resistant enterococci, MRSA, *Stenotrophomonas*, *Burkholderia*, and KPC-producing gram-negative organisms. In addition, ertapenem does not provide reliable coverage against *P. aeruginosa*, *Acinetobacter*, or enterococci; therefore, imipenem, doripenem, or meropenem would be preferred for empiric treatment of nosocomial infections when these pathogens are suspected. **Meropenem** is the preferred carbapenem for treatment of CNS infections.

SPECIAL CONSIDERATIONS

- Carbapenems can precipitate seizure activity, especially in older patients, individuals with renal insufficiency, and patients with preexisting seizure disorders or CNS pathology. Carbapenems should be avoided in these patients unless no reasonable alternative therapy is available. Like cephalosporins, carbapenems have been rarely associated with anaphylaxis, interstitial nephritis, anemia, and leukopenia.
- **Patients who are allergic to PCNs/cephalosporins may have a cross-hypersensitivity reaction to carbapenems**, and these agents should not be used in a patient with a reported severe PCN allergy without prior skin testing, desensitization, or both. Prolonged therapy (>2 weeks) is typically monitored with a weekly serum creatinine, LFTs, and CBC.

Aminoglycosides

GENERAL PRINCIPLES

- Aminoglycosides exert their bactericidal effect by binding to the bacterial ribosome, causing misreading during translation of bacterial messenger RNA into proteins. These drugs are often used in combination with cell wall–active agents (i.e., β-lactams and vancomycin) for treatment of severe infections caused by gram-positive and gram-negative aerobes.
- Aminoglycosides tend to be synergistic with cell wall–active antibiotics such as PCNs, cephalosporins, and vancomycin. However, they do not have activity against anaerobes, and their activity is impaired in the low pH/low oxygen environment of abscesses. Cross-resistance among aminoglycosides is common, and in cases of serious infections, susceptibility testing with each aminoglycoside is recommended. Use of these antibiotics is limited by significant nephrotoxicity and ototoxicity.

TREATMENT

Medications
- Traditional dosing of aminoglycosides involves daily divided dosing with the upper end of the dosing range reserved for life-threatening infections. Peak and trough concentrations should be obtained with the third or fourth dose and then every 3 to 4 days, along with regular serum creatinine monitoring. **Increasing serum creatinine or peak/troughs out of the acceptable range requires immediate attention.**
- **Extended-interval dosing of aminoglycosides** is an alternative method of administration and is more convenient than traditional dosing for most indications. Extended-interval doses are provided in the following specific drug sections. A drug concentration is obtained 6 to 14 hours after the first dose, and a nomogram (Figure 15-1) is consulted to determine the subsequent dosing interval. Monitoring includes obtaining a drug concentration 6 to 14 hours after the dosage at least every week and a serum creatinine at least three times a week. In patients who are not responding to therapy, a 12-hour concentration should be checked, and if that concentration is undetectable, extended-interval dosing should be abandoned in favor of traditional dosing.

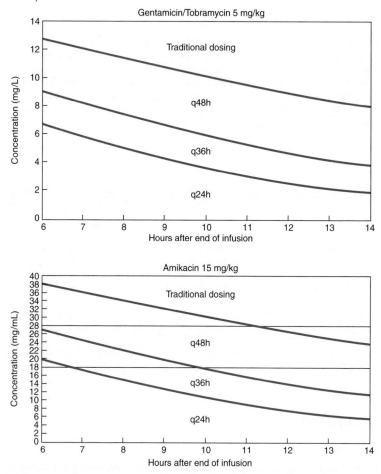

Figure 15-1. Nomograms for extended-interval aminoglycoside dosing. (Adapted from Bailey TC, Little JR, Littenberg B, et al. A meta-analysis of extended-interval dosing versus multiple daily dosing of aminoglycosides. *Clin Infect Dis* 1997;24:786–795).

- For **obese patients** (actual weight >20% above ideal body weight [IBW]), an obese dosing weight (IBW + 0.4 × [actual body weight − IBW]) should be used for determining doses for both traditional and extended-interval methods. Traditional dosing, rather than extended-interval dosing, should be used for pregnant patients, patients with endocarditis, burns that cover more than 20% of the body, cystic fibrosis, anasarca, and creatinine clearance (CrCl) of <20 mL/min.
- **Specific agents**
  - **Gentamicin and tobramycin** traditional dosing is administered with an initial loading dose of 2 mg/kg IV (2 to 3 mg/kg in the critically ill), followed by 1.0 to 1.7 mg/kg IV q8h (peak, 4 to 10 μg/mL; trough, <1 to 2 μg/mL). Extended-interval dosing is administered with an initial loading dose of 5 mg/kg, with

the subsequent dosing interval determined by a nomogram (see Figure 15-1). Tobramycin is also available as an inhaled agent for adjunctive therapy for patients with cystic fibrosis or bronchiectasis complicated by *P. aeruginosa* infection (300 mg inhalation q12h).

○ **Amikacin** has an additional unique role for mycobacterial and *Nocardia* infections. Traditional dosing is an initial loading dose of 5.0 to 7.5 mg/kg IV (7.5 to 9.0 mg/kg in the critically ill), followed by 5 mg/kg IV q8h or 7.5 mg/kg IV q12h (peak, 20 to 35 μg/mL; trough, <10 μg/mL). Extended-interval dosing is 15 mg/kg, with the subsequent dosing interval determined by a nomogram (see Figure 15-1).

SPECIAL CONSIDERATIONS

- **Nephrotoxicity** is the major adverse effect of aminoglycosides. Nephrotoxicity is reversible when detected early but can be permanent, especially in patients with tenuous renal function due to other medical conditions. Aminoglycosides should be used cautiously or avoided, if possible, in patients with decompensated kidney disease.
- **Ototoxicity** (vestibular or cochlear) is another possible adverse event that necessitates baseline and weekly hearing tests with extended therapy (>14 days). Concomitant administration of aminoglycosides with other known nephrotoxic agents (i.e., amphotericin B formulations, foscarnet, nonsteroidal anti-inflammatory drugs, pentamidine, polymyxins, cidofovir, and cisplatin) should be avoided if possible.

Vancomycin

GENERAL PRINCIPLES

- Vancomycin (15 mg/kg IV q12h; up to 30 mg/kg IV q12h for meningitis) is a glycopeptide antibiotic that interferes with cell wall synthesis by binding to D-alanyl-D-alanine precursors that are critical for peptidoglycan cross-linking in most gram-positive bacterial cell walls. Vancomycin is bactericidal for staphylococci but bacteriostatic for enterococci.
- Today, most hospitals have serious problems with vancomycin-resistant *Enterococcus faecium* (VRE), and there are now reports of clinical isolates of *S. aureus* that are intermediately resistant (VISA) and resistant to vancomycin (VRSA).

TREATMENT

- Indications for use are listed in Table 15-1.
- The **goal trough** concentration is 10 to 20 μg/mL and perhaps up to 15 to 20 μg/mL or higher for other serious infections. Patients with severe renal insufficiency should receive a single 15 mg/kg dose and then be redosed when the concentration drops below 10 to 20 μg/mL.

SPECIAL CONSIDERATIONS

Vancomycin is typically administered by slow IV infusion over at least 1 hour per gram dose. More rapid infusion rates can cause the **red man syndrome**, which is a

Table 15-1	Indications for Vancomycin Use

Treatment of serious infections caused by methicillin-resistant *Staphylococcus aureus* (MRSA)

Treatment of serious infections caused by ampicillin-resistant, vancomycin-sensitive enterococci

Treatment of serious infections caused by gram-positive bacteria in patients who are allergic to other appropriate therapies

Oral treatment of severe *Clostridium difficile* colitis

Surgical prophylaxis for placement of prosthetic devices at institutions with known high rates of MRSA or in patients who are known to be colonized with MRSA

Empiric use in suspected gram-positive meningitis until an organism has been identified and sensitivities confirmed

Life-threatening sepsis syndrome in patients with known MRSA colonization or extended hospitalization until pathogen(s) are identified

Documented coagulase-negative staphylococcal endocarditis or catheter-related bloodstream infection

Empiric use for serious dialysis catheter–related bloodstream infections until the results of blood culture data are available

histamine-mediated reaction that is typically manifested by flushing and redness of the upper body. Nephrotoxicity, ototoxicity, neutropenia, thrombocytopenia, and rash may also occur.

Fluoroquinolones

GENERAL PRINCIPLES

- Fluoroquinolones exert their bactericidal effect by inhibiting bacterial DNA gyrase and topoisomerase function, which are critical for DNA replication. In general, these antibiotics are well absorbed orally, with serum concentrations that approach those of parenteral administration.
- These agents typically have poor activity against enterococci, although they may have some efficacy if susceptible for enterococcal UTIs when other agents are inactive or contraindicated. Concomitant administration with aluminum- or magnesium-containing antacids, sucralfate, bismuth, oral iron, oral calcium, and oral zinc preparations can markedly impair absorption of all orally administered fluoroquinolones.

TREATMENT

- **Norfloxacin** (400 mg PO q12h) is useful for the treatment of UTIs caused by gram-negative bacilli; however, other fluoroquinolones are preferred in this setting. This agent should not be used to treat systemic infections.
- **Ciprofloxacin** (250 to 750 mg PO q12h or 500 mg PO q24h [Cipro XR] or 200 to 400 mg IV q8–12h) and **ofloxacin** (200 to 400 mg IV or PO q12h) are active against gram-negative aerobes including many AmpC β-lactamase–producing pathogens.

These agents are commonly used for UTIs, pyelonephritis, infectious diarrhea, prostatitis, and intra-abdominal infections (with metronidazole). Ciprofloxacin is the most active quinolone against *P. aeruginosa* and is the quinolone of choice for serious infections with that pathogen. However, ciprofloxacin has relatively poor activity against gram-positive pathogens and anaerobes and should not be used as empiric monotherapy for community-acquired pneumonia, skin and soft tissue infections, or intra-abdominal infections. Oral and IV ciprofloxacin give similar maximum serum levels; thus, oral therapy is appropriate unless contraindicated. If given orally, fluoroquinolones should not be taken with milk products, multivitamins, antacids, liquid nutritional supplements, or any other product with polyvalent metallic cations (e.g., iron).

- **Levofloxacin** (250 to 750 mg PO or IV q24h), **moxifloxacin** (400 mg PO/IV q24h daily), and **gemifloxacin** (320 mg PO q24h daily) are newer fluoroquinolones with improved coverage of streptococci but less gram-negative activity (especially against *P. aeruginosa*) than ciprofloxacin. Moxifloxacin may be used as monotherapy of complicated intra-abdominal or skin and soft tissue infections due to its anti-anaerobic activity. Each of these agents is useful for treatment of sinusitis, bronchitis, community-acquired pneumonia, and UTIs (except moxifloxacin, which is only minimally eliminated in the urine). Some of these agents have activity against mycobacteria and have a potential role in treating drug-resistant tuberculosis (TB) and atypical mycobacterial infections. Levofloxacin may be used as an alternative for treatment of chlamydial urethritis.

SPECIAL CONSIDERATIONS

- Adverse reactions include nausea, CNS disturbances (headache, restlessness, and dizziness, especially in the elderly), rash, and phototoxicity. These agents can cause prolongation of the QT_c interval and should not be used in patients who are receiving class I or class III antiarrhythmics, in patients with known electrolyte or conduction abnormalities, or in those who are taking other medications that prolong the QT_c interval or induce bradycardia. These agents should also be used with caution in the elderly, in whom asymptomatic conduction disturbances are more common. Fluoroquinolones should not be routinely used in patients younger than 18 years or in pregnant or lactating women due to the risk of arthropathy in pediatric patients. They may also cause tendinitis or tendon rupture, especially the Achilles tendon, particularly in elderly. A common drug interaction is an increase in the international normalized ratio (INR) when used concurrently with warfarin.
- **This class of antimicrobials has major drug interactions.** Before initiating its use, it is necessary to review concomitant medications taken by patients.

Macrolide and Lincosamide Antibiotics

GENERAL PRINCIPLES

- Macrolide and lincosamide antibiotics are bacteriostatic agents that block protein synthesis in bacteria by binding to the 50S subunit of the bacterial ribosome.
- This class of antibiotics has activity against gram-positive cocci, including streptococci and staphylococci, and some upper respiratory gram-negative bacteria, but minimal activity against enteric gram-negative rods.

TREATMENT

- Macrolides are commonly used to treat pharyngitis, otitis media, sinusitis, and bronchitis, especially in PCN-allergic patients, and are among the drugs of choice for treating *Legionella*, *Chlamydia*, and *Mycoplasma* infections. Azithromycin and clarithromycin can be used as monotherapy for outpatient community-acquired pneumonia and have a unique role in the treatment and prophylaxis against *Mycobacterium avium* complex (MAC) infections in AIDS patients. Many PCN-resistant strains of pneumococci are also resistant to macrolides.

- **Erythromycin** (250 to 500 mg PO q6h or 0.5 to 1.0 g IV q6h) possesses activity against gram-positive cocci (except enterococci) and can be used to treat bronchitis, pharyngitis, sinusitis, otitis media, and soft tissue infections in PCN-allergic patients. It is effective for treatment of atypical respiratory tract infections due to *Legionella pneumophila* (1 g IV q6h), *Chlamydophila pneumoniae*, and *Mycoplasma pneumoniae*. However, there is significant resistance to erythromycin among *Haemophilus influenzae* species and, therefore, efficacy of this drug for upper and lower respiratory tract infections is limited. It can also be used for treatment of *Chlamydia trachomatis* infections (500 mg PO q6h for 7 days) and as an alternate therapy for syphilis in PCN-allergic patients. Use is limited by poor tolerability and drug interactions.

- **Clarithromycin** (250 to 500 mg PO q12h or 1,000 mg XL PO q24h) has a spectrum of activity similar to that of erythromycin but with enhanced activity against some respiratory pathogens (especially *Haemophilus*). It is commonly used to treat bronchitis, sinusitis, otitis media, pharyngitis, soft tissue infections, and community-acquired pneumonia. It has a prominent role in treating MAC infection in HIV patients and is an important component of regimens used to eradicate *Helicobacter pylori* (see Chapter 18, Gastrointestinal Diseases).

- **Azithromycin** (500 mg PO for 1 day, then 250 mg PO q24h for 4 days; 500 mg PO q24h for 3 days; 2,000 mg microspheres PO for one dose; 500 mg IV q24h) has a similar spectrum of activity to clarithromycin and is commonly used to treat bronchitis, sinusitis, otitis media, pharyngitis, soft tissue infections, and community-acquired pneumonia. It has a prominent role in MAC prophylaxis (1,200 mg PO every week) and treatment (500 to 600 mg PO q24h) in HIV patients. It is also commonly used to treat *C. trachomatis* infections (1 g PO single dose). A major advantage of azithromycin is that it does not have the numerous drug interactions seen with erythromycin and clarithromycin.

- **Clindamycin** (150 to 450 mg PO q6–8h or 600 to 900 mg IV q8h) is chemically classified as a lincosamide (related to macrolides), with a predominantly gram-positive spectrum similar to that of erythromycin with additional activity against most anaerobes, including *B. fragilis*. It has excellent oral bioavailability (90%) and penetrates well into the bone and abscess cavities. It is also used for treatment of aspiration pneumonia and lung abscesses. Clindamycin is often active against community-associated strains of MRSA, and the agent has emerged as a treatment option for skin and soft tissue infections caused by this organism. Clindamycin may be used as a second agent in combination therapy for invasive streptococcal and clostridial infections to decrease toxin production. The agent may also be used for treatment of suspected anaerobic infections (peritonsillar/retropharyngeal abscesses, necrotizing fasciitis), although metronidazole is used more commonly for intra-abdominal infections (clindamycin has less reliable activity against *B. fragilis*). Clindamycin has additional uses, including treatment of babesiosis (in combination with quinine), toxoplasmosis (in combination with pyrimethamine), and *Pneumocystis jiroveci* pneumonia (in combination with primaquine).

SPECIAL CONSIDERATIONS

Macrolides and clindamycin are associated with nausea, abdominal cramping, and LFT abnormalities (particularly erythromycin). Liver function profiles should be checked intermittently during extended therapy. Hypersensitivity reactions with prominent skin rash are more common with clindamycin, as is pseudomembranous colitis secondary to *Clostridium difficile*. **Erythromycin and clarithromycin have major drug interactions** caused by inhibition of the cytochrome P450 system.

Sulfonamides and Trimethoprim

GENERAL PRINCIPLES

Sulfadiazine, sulfamethoxazole, and trimethoprim slowly kill bacteria by inhibiting folic acid metabolism. This class of antibiotics is most commonly used for uncomplicated UTIs, sinusitis, and otitis media. Some sulfonamide-containing agents also have unique roles in the treatment of *P. jiroveci*, *Nocardia*, *Toxoplasma*, and *Stenotrophomonas* infections.

TREATMENT

- **Trimethoprim** (100 mg PO q12h) is occasionally used as monotherapy for treatment of UTIs. Trimethoprim is more often used in the combination preparations/regimens outlined in the following sections. Trimethoprim in combination with dapsone is an alternate therapy for mild *P. jiroveci* pneumonia.
- **Trimethoprim/sulfamethoxazole** is a combination antibiotic (IV or PO) with a 1:5 ratio of trimethoprim to sulfamethoxazole. The IV preparation is dosed at 5 mg/kg IV q8h (based on the trimethoprim component) for serious infections. The oral preparations (160 mg trimethoprim/800 mg sulfamethoxazole per double-strength [DS] tablet) are extensively bioavailable, with similar drug concentrations obtained with IV and PO formulations. Both components have excellent tissue penetration, including bone, prostate, and CNS. The combination has a broad spectrum of activity but typically does not inhibit *P. aeruginosa*, anaerobes, or group A streptococci. It is the therapy of choice for *P. jiroveci* pneumonia, *Stenotrophomonas maltophilia*, *Tropheryma whippelii*, and *Nocardia* infections. It is commonly used for treating sinusitis, otitis media, bronchitis, prostatitis, and UTIs (1 DS PO q12h). Trimethoprim/sulfamethoxazole is active against the majority of community-associated strains of MRSA, and the agent has emerged as a viable treatment for uncomplicated cases of skin and soft tissue infections caused by this organism (2 to 3 DS tabs PO q12h). It is used as *P. jiroveci* pneumonia prophylaxis (1 DS PO twice a week, three times a week, or single strength or DS daily) in HIV-infected patients, solid organ transplant patients, bone marrow transplant

patients, and patients receiving fludarabine. IV therapy is routinely converted to the PO equivalent for patients who require prolonged therapy.
- For serious infections, such as *Nocardia* brain abscesses, it may be useful to monitor drug levels with sulfamethoxazole peaks (100 to 150 μg/mL) and troughs (50 to 100 μg/mL) occasionally during the course of therapy and adjust the dose accordingly. In patients with renal insufficiency, doses can be adjusted by following trimethoprim peaks (5 to 10 μg/mL). Prolonged therapy can cause bone marrow suppression, possibly requiring treatment with leucovorin (5 to 10 mg PO q24h) until cell counts normalize.
- **Sulfadiazine** (1.0 to 1.5 g PO q6h) in combination with pyrimethamine (200 mg PO followed by 50 to 75 mg PO q24h) and leucovorin (10 to 20 mg PO q24h) is the regimen of choice for toxoplasmosis. Sulfadiazine is also occasionally used to treat *Nocardia* infections.

SPECIAL CONSIDERATIONS

These drugs are associated with cholestatic jaundice, bone marrow suppression, hyperkalemia (with trimethoprim/sulfamethoxazole), interstitial nephritis, "false" elevations in serum creatinine, and severe hypersensitivity reactions (Stevens–Johnson syndrome/erythema multiforme). Nausea is common with higher doses. **All patients should be asked whether they are allergic to "sulfa drugs,"** and specific commercial names should be mentioned (i.e., Bactrim or Septra).

Tetracyclines

GENERAL PRINCIPLES

- Tetracyclines are bacteriostatic antibiotics that bind to the 30S ribosomal subunit and block protein synthesis.
- These agents have unique roles in the treatment of *Rickettsia*, *Ehrlichia*, *Chlamydia*, and *Mycoplasma* infections. They are used as therapy for most tick-borne infections, Lyme disease–related arthritis, alternate therapy for syphilis, and for *P. multocida* infections in PCN-allergic patients. Their general use is limited because of widespread resistance among more common bacterial pathogens.

TREATMENT

- **Tetracycline** (250 to 500 mg PO q6h) is commonly used for severe acne and in some *H. pylori* eradication regimens. It can also be used for treatment of acute Lyme borreliosis, Rocky Mountain spotted fever, ehrlichiosis, psittacosis, *Mycoplasma* pneumonia, *Chlamydia* pneumonia, and chlamydial infections of the eye or genitourinary tract, but these infections are generally treated with doxycycline or other antibiotics. Aluminum- and magnesium-containing antacids and preparations that contain oral calcium, oral iron, or other cations can significantly impair oral absorption of tetracycline and should be avoided within 2 hours of each dose.
- **Doxycycline** (100 mg PO/IV q12h) is the most commonly used tetracycline and is standard therapy for *C. trachomatis*, Rocky Mountain spotted fever, ehrlichiosis,

and psittacosis. This agent also has a role for malaria prophylaxis and for treatment of community-acquired pneumonia. It also has utility in the treatment of uncomplicated skin and skin structure infections caused by community-associated MRSA.

- **Minocycline** (200 mg IV/PO, then 100 mg IV/PO q12h) is similar to doxycycline in its spectrum of activity and clinical indications. It is second-line therapy for pulmonary nocardiosis and cervicofacial actinomycosis. Both minocycline and doxycycline also have activity against some multidrug-resistant gram-negative pathogens and may be used as adjunctive agents in this setting based on results of susceptibility testing.

SPECIAL CONSIDERATIONS

Nausea and photosensitivity are common side effects so patients should be warned about direct sun exposure. Rarely, these medications are associated with pseudotumor cerebri. **They should not routinely be given to children or to pregnant or lactating women** because they can cause tooth enamel discoloration in the developing fetus and young children. Minocycline is associated with vestibular disturbances.

ANTIMICROBIAL AGENTS, MISCELLANEOUS

Chloramphenicol

GENERAL PRINCIPLES

Chloramphenicol (12.5 to 25 mg/kg IV q6h; maximum, 1 g IV q6h) is a bacteriostatic antibiotic that binds to the 50S ribosomal subunit, blocking protein synthesis in susceptible bacteria. It has broad-spectrum activity against aerobic and anaerobic gram-positive and gram-negative bacteria, including *S. aureus*, enterococci, and enteric gram-negative rods. It is also active against spirochetes, *Rickettsia*, *Mycoplasma*, and *Chlamydia*. The drug may also be used for some serious VRE infections and for treatment of meningitis caused by *Francisella tularensis* or *Yersinia pestis*.

SPECIAL CONSIDERATIONS

Adverse events include idiosyncratic aplastic anemia ($-1/30,000$) and dose-related bone marrow suppression. Peak drug levels (1 hour postinfusion) should be checked every 3 to 4 days (goal peak <25 μg/mL) and doses adjusted accordingly. Dosage adjustment is necessary in the presence of significant liver disease. **This class of antibiotics has major drug interactions.**

Colistin and Polymyxin B

GENERAL PRINCIPLES

- Colistimethate sodium (2.5 to 5 mg/kg/d IV divided q12h) and polymyxin B (15,000 to 25,000 U/kg/d IV divided q12 hours) are bactericidal polypeptide antibiotics that kill gram-negative bacteria by disrupting the cell membrane. These drugs have roles in the treatment of multiple drug–resistant gram-negative bacilli but are inactive against *Proteus*, *Providencia*, and *Serratia*.

- **These medications should only be given under the guidance of an experienced clinician**, as parenteral therapy has significant CNS side effects and potential nephrotoxicity. Inhaled colistin (75 to 150 mg q12h given by nebulizer) is better tolerated, with only mild upper airway irritation and has some efficacy as adjunctive therapy for *P. aeruginosa* or *Acinetobacter* pulmonary infections.

SPECIAL CONSIDERATIONS

Adverse events with parenteral therapy include paresthesias, slurred speech, peripheral numbness, tingling, and significant dose-dependent nephrotoxicity. The dosage should be carefully reduced in patients with renal insufficiency, as overdosage in this setting can result in neuromuscular blockade and apnea. Serum creatinine should be monitored daily early in therapy and then at a regular interval for the duration of therapy. **Concomitant use with aminoglycosides, other known nephrotoxins, or neuromuscular blockers should be avoided if at all possible.**

Daptomycin

GENERAL PRINCIPLES

Daptomycin (4 mg/kg IV q24h for skin and skin structure infections; 6 mg/kg IV q24h for bloodstream infections) is a cyclic lipopeptide. The drug exhibits rapid bactericidal activity against a wide variety of gram-positive bacteria, including enterococci, staphylococci, and streptococci. Daptomycin also maintains activity against many antibiotic-resistant gram-positive bacteria and is currently FDA approved for treatment of complicated skin and skin structure infections as well as *S. aureus* bacteremia and right-sided endocarditis. The drug should not be used to treat primary lung infections due to its decreased activity in the presence of pulmonary surfactant. Resistance can develop and it is imperative that the susceptibility of the isolate be verified.

SPECIAL CONSIDERATIONS

Adverse events include gastrointestinal (GI) disturbances, injection site reactions, elevated LFTs, and elevated creatine phosphokinase. Serum creatine phosphokinase should be monitored at baseline and weekly, as daptomycin has been associated with skeletal muscle effects, including rhabdomyolysis; patients should also be monitored for signs of muscle weakness and pain, and the drug should be discontinued if these symptoms develop in conjunction with marked creatine phosphokinase elevations (5 to 10 times the upper limit of normal with symptoms or 10 times the upper limit of normal without symptoms). Consideration should also be given to avoiding concomitant use of daptomycin and 5-hydroxy-3-methylglutaryl-coenzyme A (HMG-CoA) reductase inhibitors due to the potential increased risk of myopathy.

Fosfomycin

GENERAL PRINCIPLES

- **Fosfomycin** (3-g sachet dissolved in cold water PO once) is a bactericidal oral antibiotic that kills bacteria by inhibiting an early step in cell wall synthesis. It has a spectrum of activity that includes most urinary tract pathogens, including *P. aeruginosa*, *Enterobacter* species, and enterococci (including VRE), and some multidrug-resistant gram-negative bacteria.
- It is most useful for treating uncomplicated UTIs in women with susceptible strains of *E. coli* or *Enterococcus faecalis*. It should not be used to treat pyelonephritis or systemic infections.

SPECIAL CONSIDERATIONS

Adverse events include diarrhea. It should not be taken with metoclopramide, as that drug interferes with fosfomycin absorption.

Linezolid

GENERAL PRINCIPLES

- Oxazolidinones are a newer class of antibiotics that block assembly of bacterial ribosomes and inhibit protein synthesis. **Linezolid** (600 mg IV/PO q12h) is the first FDA-approved drug in this class. IV and oral formulations produce equivalent serum concentrations, and the drug has potent activity against gram-positive bacteria, including drug-resistant enterococci, staphylococci, and streptococci. However, it has no meaningful activity against Enterobacteriaceae and borderline activity against *Moraxella* and *H. influenzae*.
- Linezolid is useful for serious infections with VRE, as an alternative to vancomycin for treatment of MRSA infections, for patients with an indication for vancomycin therapy who are intolerant of that medication, and as oral therapy of MRSA infections when IV access is unavailable. Limited data support use for treatment of osteomyelitis, endocarditis, and meningitis, and routine use for these infections should be carefully undertaken. In addition, linezolid is not FDA approved for catheter-related bloodstream or catheter-site infections. Resistance can develop to this antibiotic, and it is imperative that organism susceptibility is verified.

SPECIAL CONSIDERATIONS

- **Adverse events** include diarrhea, nausea, and headache. Thrombocytopenia occurs frequently in patients who receive more than 2 weeks of therapy, and serial platelet count monitoring is indicated. A CBC should be checked every week during prolonged therapy with this agent. Extremely prolonged therapy (typically longer than 6 months) has been associated with peripheral and optic neuropathy. Lactic acidosis may also rarely occur.
- Linezolid has **several important drug interactions**. It is a mild monoamine oxidase inhibitor, and patients should be advised not to take selective serotonin reuptake inhibitors (SSRIs), triptans, or meperidine while on linezolid to avoid the serotonin

syndrome. Ideally, patients should be off the SSRI for at least a week before initiating linezolid. Over-the-counter cold remedies that contain pseudoephedrine or phenylpropanolamine should also be avoided, as coadministration with linezolid can elevate blood pressure. Linezolid does not require dose adjustments for renal or hepatic dysfunction.

Methenamine

GENERAL PRINCIPLES

- Methenamine hippurate or methenamine mandelate (one or two tablets [depending on the specific preparation] PO q6–12h) is a urine/bladder antiseptic that is converted into formaldehyde in the urine when the pH is <6.0.
- This agent has a limited role in treating uncomplicated UTIs caused by multiple drug-resistant bacteria or yeast.

SPECIAL CONSIDERATIONS

Adverse events include bladder irritation, dysuria, and hematuria with prolonged use. Therapy should be limited to a maximum of 3 weeks at a time, and urine pH should be obtained once early during therapy to ensure an appropriately acidic pH. Vitamin C can be used to assist in urine acidification. It is contraindicated in the setting of glaucoma, significant renal insufficiency, and acidosis. It should not be given concomitantly with sulfonamides, as these drugs form an insoluble precipitate in the urine.

Metronidazole

GENERAL PRINCIPLES

- Metronidazole (250 to 750 mg PO/IV q6–12h) is only active against anaerobic bacteria and some protozoa. The drug exerts its bactericidal effect through accumulation of toxic metabolites that interfere with multiple biologic processes. It has excellent tissue penetration, including abscess cavities, bone, and CNS.
- It has greater activity against gram-negative than gram-positive anaerobes but is active against *Clostridium perfringens* and *C. difficile*. It is the treatment of choice as monotherapy for mild-to-moderate *C. difficile* colitis as well as bacterial vaginosis and can be used in combination with other antibiotics to treat intra-abdominal infections and brain abscesses. Protozoal infections that are routinely treated with metronidazole include *Giardia*, *Entamoeba histolytica*, and *Trichomonas vaginalis*. A dose reduction may be warranted for patients with decompensated liver disease.

SPECIAL CONSIDERATIONS

Adverse events include nausea, dysgeusia, disulfiram-like reactions to alcohol, and mild CNS disturbances (headache, restlessness). Rarely, metronidazole causes peripheral neuropathy and seizures.

Nitrofurantoin

GENERAL PRINCIPLES

- **Nitrofurantoin** (50 to 100 mg PO macrocrystals q6h or 100 mg PO dual-release formulation q12h for 5 to 7 days) is a bactericidal oral antibiotic that is useful for uncomplicated UTIs except those caused by *Proteus*, *P. aeruginosa*, or *Serratia*. The drug is metabolized by bacteria into toxic intermediates that inhibit multiple bacterial processes. It has had a modest resurgence in use, as it is frequently effective for uncomplicated VRE UTIs.
- Although it was commonly used in the past for UTI prophylaxis, this practice should be avoided, as prolonged therapy is associated with chronic pulmonary syndromes that can be fatal. Nitrofurantoin should not be used for pyelonephritis or any other systemic infections and should be avoided in patients with renal dysfunction.

SPECIAL CONSIDERATIONS

Adverse events. Nausea is the most common adverse effect, and the drug should be taken with food to minimize this problem. Patients should be warned that their urine may become brown secondary to the medication. Neurotoxicity, hepatotoxicity, and pulmonary fibrosis may also rarely occur with nitrofurantion. Furthermore, it should not be used in patients with CrCl <60 mL/min as the risk for development of treatment-associated adverse effects is increased. It should not be given with probenecid, as this combination decreases the concentration of nitrofurantoin in the urine.

Quinupristin/Dalfopristin

GENERAL PRINCIPLES

- **Quinupristin/dalfopristin** (7.5 mg/kg IV q8h) is the first FDA-approved drug in the streptogramin class.
- This agent has activity against antibiotic-resistant gram-positive organisms, especially VRE, MRSA, VISA, VRSA, and antibiotic-resistant strains of *Streptococcus pneumoniae*. It has some activity against gram-negative upper respiratory pathogens (*Haemophilus* and *Moraxella*) and anaerobes, but more appropriate antibiotics are available to treat these infections. Quinupristin/dalfopristin is bacteriostatic for enterococci and can be used for treatment of serious infections with VRE (only *E. faecium* as it is inactive against all *E. faecalis* isolates). It can also be used for treatment of serious infections with MRSA or *S. pneumoniae* when other agents are not feasible.

SPECIAL CONSIDERATIONS

Adverse events include arthralgias and myalgias, which occur frequently and can necessitate discontinuation of therapy. IV site pain and thrombophlebitis are common when the drug is administered through a peripheral vein. It has also been associated with elevated LFTs and, as it is primarily cleared by hepatic metabolism, patients with significant hepatic impairment require a dose adjustment. Quinupristin/dalfopristin is similar to erythromycin with regard to drug interactions.

Telavancin

GENERAL PRINCIPLES

Telavancin (7.5 to 10 mg/kg q24–48h, based on CrCl) is a new lipoglycopeptide antibiotic that is FDA approved for treatment of complicated skin and skin structure infections. Telavancin is broadly active against gram-positive bacteria, including MRSA, VISA, heteroresistant vancomycin-intermediate *S. aureus* (hVISA), daptomycin- and linezolid-resistant *S. aureus*, streptococci, vancomycin-sensitive enterococci, and some gram-positive anaerobes. The agent is not active against gram-negative bacteria, VRSA, and VRE.

Adverse effects include nausea, vomiting, metallic or soapy taste, foamy urine, and nephrotoxicity (which necessitates serial monitoring of serum creatinine). Prehydration with normal saline may mitigate the nephrotoxicity observed with the use of this drug. Telavancin can also cause a minor (4.1 to 4.6 ms) prolongation of the QT_c interval and should be avoided in patients with underlying cardiac conditions associated with QT_c prolongation. Women of childbearing potential require a negative serum pregnancy test prior to receiving telavancin due to teratogenic effects noted in animals.

Tigecycline

GENERAL PRINCIPLES

Tigecycline (100 mg IV loading dose, then 50 mg IV q12h) is the only FDA-approved antibiotic in the class of glycylcyclines. Its mechanism of action is similar to that of tetracyclines by inhibiting the translation of bacterial proteins through binding to the 30S ribosome. The addition of the glycyl side chain expands its activity against bacterial pathogens that are normally resistant to tetracycline and minocycline. It has a broad spectrum of bactericidal activity against gram-positive, gram-negative, and anaerobic bacteria except *P. aeruginosa* and some *Proteus* isolates. It is currently FDA approved for treatment of complicated skin and skin structure infections, complicated intra-abdominal infections, and community-acquired pneumonia. Additionally, it may be used for treatment of some other tissue infections due to susceptible strains of VRE and some multidrug-resistant gram-negative bacteria. Until more data are available, it should not be used to treat primary bacteremia.

SPECIAL CONSIDERATIONS

Adverse events. Nausea and vomiting are the most common adverse events. Tigecycline has not been studied in patients younger than 18 years and is contraindicated in pregnant and lactating women. Since it has a similar structure to tetracyclines, photosensitivity, tooth discoloration, and, rarely, pseudotumor cerebri may occur.

ANTIMYCOBACTERIAL AGENTS

Effective therapy of *Mycobacterium tuberculosis* (MTB) infections requires combination chemotherapy designed to prevent the emergence of resistant organisms and maximize efficacy. Increased resistance to conventional antituberculous agents has led to the use of more complex regimens and has made susceptibility testing an integral part of TB management (see Chapter 14, Treatment of Infectious Diseases).

Isoniazid

GENERAL PRINCIPLES

Isoniazid (INH, 300 mg PO q24h) exerts bactericidal effects on susceptible mycobacteria by interfering with the synthesis of lipid components of the mycobacterial cell wall. INH is a component of nearly all treatment regimens and can be given twice a week in directly observed therapy (15 mg/kg/dose; 900 mg maximum). INH remains the drug of choice for treatment of latent TB infection (300 mg PO q24h for 9 months).

SPECIAL CONSIDERATIONS

Adverse events include elevations in liver transaminases (20%). This effect can be idiosyncratic but is usually seen in the setting of advanced age, underlying liver disease, or concomitant consumption of alcohol, and may be potentiated by rifampin. Transaminase elevations to greater than threefold the upper limit of the normal range necessitate holding therapy. Patients with known liver dysfunction should have weekly LFTs during the initial stage of therapy. INH also antagonizes vitamin B_6 metabolism and potentially can cause a peripheral neuropathy. This can be avoided or minimized by coadministration of pyridoxine, 25 to 50 mg PO daily, especially in the elderly, in pregnant women, and in patients with diabetes, renal failure, alcoholism, and seizure disorders.

Rifamycins

GENERAL PRINCIPLES

Rifamycins exert bactericidal activity on susceptible mycobacteria by inhibiting DNA-dependent RNA polymerase, thereby halting transcription.
- **Rifampin** (600 mg PO q24h or twice a week) is an integral component of most TB treatment regimens. It is also active against many gram-positive and gram-negative bacteria. Rifampin is used as adjunctive therapy in staphylococcal prosthetic valve endocarditis (300 mg PO q8h), for prophylaxis of close contacts of patients with infection caused by *Neisseria meningitidis* (600 mg PO q12h), and as adjunctive treatment of bone and joint infections associated with prosthetic material or devices. The drug is well absorbed orally and is widely distributed throughout the body including the cerebrospinal fluid (CSF).
- **Rifabutin** (300 mg PO q24h) is primarily used to treat TB and MAC infections in HIV-positive patients who are receiving highly active antiretroviral therapy, as it has less deleterious effects on protease inhibitor metabolism than does rifampin

(see Chapter 16, Human Immunodeficiency Virus and Acquired Immunodeficiency Syndrome).

SPECIAL CONSIDERATIONS

Adverse events. Patients should be warned about reddish-orange discoloration of body fluids, and contact lenses should not be worn during treatment. Rash, GI disturbances, hematologic disturbances, hepatitis, and interstitial nephritis can occur. Uveitis has also been associated with rifabutin. **This class of antibiotics has major drug interactions.**

Pyrazinamide

GENERAL PRINCIPLES

- **Pyrazinamide** (15 to 30 mg/kg PO q24h; maximum, 2 g or 50 to 75 mg/kg PO twice a week; maximum, 4 g/dose) kills mycobacteria replicating in macrophages by an unknown mechanism.
- It is well absorbed orally and widely distributed throughout the body, including the CSF. Pyrazinamide is typically used for the first 2 months of therapy.

SPECIAL CONSIDERATIONS

Adverse events include hyperuricemia and hepatitis.

Ethambutol

GENERAL PRINCIPLES

- **Ethambutol** (15 to 25 mg/kg PO q24h or 50 to 75 mg/kg PO twice a week; maximum, 2.4 g/dose) is bacteriostatic with an unknown mechanism of action.
- Doses should be reduced in the presence of renal dysfunction.

SPECIAL CONSIDERATIONS

Adverse events. These may include optic neuritis, which manifests as decreased red-green color perception, decreased visual acuity, or visual field deficits. Baseline and monthly visual examinations should be performed during therapy. Renal function should also be carefully monitored as drug accumulation in the setting of renal insufficiency can increase risk of ocular effects.

Streptomycin

GENERAL PRINCIPLES

Streptomycin is an aminoglycoside that can be used as a substitute for ethambutol and for drug-resistant MTB. It does not adequately penetrate the CNS and should not be used for TB meningitis.

ANTIVIRAL AGENTS

Current antiviral agents only suppress viral replication. Viral containment or elimination requires an intact host immune response. Anti-HIV agents will be discussed in Chapter 16, Human Immunodeficiency Virus and Acquired Immunodeficiency Syndrome.

Anti-Influenza Agents

GENERAL PRINCIPLES

Anti-influenza drugs include not only **amantadine** and **rimantadine** but also two newer drugs, **zanamivir** and **oseltamivir**, that block influenza A and B neuraminidases. Neuraminidase activity is necessary for successful viral egress and release from infected cells. These drugs have shown modest activity in clinical trials, with a 1- to 2-day improvement in symptoms in patients who are treated within 48 hours of the onset of influenza symptoms. At the onset of each influenza season, a consultation with the local health department officials is recommended to determine the most effective antiviral agent. Although there are data showing that these agents are effective for prophylaxis of influenza, annual influenza vaccination remains the most effective method for prophylaxis in all high-risk patients and health care workers (see Appendix A, Immunizations and Postexposure Therapies).

- **Amantadine and rimantadine** (100 mg PO q12h for both; 100 mg PO q24h in elderly patients, dialysis patients, or those with decompensated liver disease) prevent influenza A entry into cells by blocking endosomal acidification, which is necessary for fusion of the viral envelope with the host cell membrane. **These agents have no activity against influenza B.** They are effective when therapy is initiated within 48 hours of initial symptoms and continued for 7 to 10 days. These drugs can also be used for influenza prophylaxis in nonimmune individuals who have been exposed to the virus and in patients and staff members of nursing homes or hospitals during an epidemic.
  - **Adverse events.** GI disturbances and CNS dysfunction, including dizziness, nervousness, confusion, slurring of speech, blurred vision, and sleep disturbances, may be experienced with use of these antivirals. Rimantadine has fewer side effects than amantadine.
- **Zanamivir** (10 mg [two inhalations] q12h for 5 days, started within 48 hours of the onset of symptoms) is an inhaled neuraminidase inhibitor that is active against influenza A and B. It is indicated for treatment of uncomplicated acute influenza infection in adults and children 7 years of age or older who have been symptomatic for <48 hours. The drug is also indicated for influenza prophylaxis in patients age 5 years and older.
  - **Adverse events.** Headache, GI disturbances, dizziness, and upper respiratory symptoms are sometimes reported. Bronchospasms or declines in lung function, or both, may occur in patients with underlying respiratory disorders and may require a rapid-acting bronchodilator for control.
- **Oseltamivir** (75 mg PO q12h for 5 days) is an orally administered neuraminidase inhibitor that is active against influenza A and B.
  - It is indicated for treatment of uncomplicated acute influenza in adults and children 1 year of age or older who have been symptomatic for up to 2 days.

This agent is also indicated for prophylaxis of influenza A and B in adults and children 1 year of age or older.

○ **Adverse events** include nausea, vomiting, and diarrhea. Dizziness and headache may also occur.

Antiherpetic Agents

GENERAL PRINCIPLES

Antiherpetic agents are nucleotide analogs that inhibit viral DNA synthesis.

- **Acyclovir** is active against herpes simplex virus (HSV) and varicella-zoster virus (VZV) (400 mg PO q8h for HSV, 800 mg PO five times a day for localized VZV infections, 5 mg/kg IV q8h for severe HSV infections, and 10 mg/kg IV q8h for severe VZV infections and HSV encephalitis).
  ○ It is indicated for treatment of primary and recurrent genital herpes, severe herpetic stomatitis, and herpes simplex encephalitis. It can be used as prophylaxis in patients who have frequent HSV recurrences (400 mg PO q12h). It is also used for herpes zoster ophthalmicus, disseminated primary VZV in adults (significant morbidity compared to the childhood illness), and severe disseminated primary VZV in children.
  ○ **Adverse events.** Reversible crystalline nephropathy may occur; preexisting renal failure, dehydration, and IV bolus dosing increase the risk of this effect. Rare cases of CNS disturbances, including delirium, tremors, and seizures, may also occur, particularly with high doses, in patients with renal failure and in the elderly.
- **Valacyclovir** (1,000 mg PO q8h for herpes zoster, 1,000 mg PO q12h for initial episode of genital HSV infection, and 500 mg PO q12h or 1,000 mg PO q24h for recurrent episodes of HSV) is an orally administered prodrug of acyclovir used for the treatment of acute herpes zoster infections and for treatment or suppression of genital HSV infection.
  ○ The most common **adverse effect** is nausea. Valacyclovir can rarely cause CNS disturbances, and high doses (8 g/d) have been associated with development of hemolytic–uremic syndrome/thrombotic thrombocytopenic purpura in immunocompromised patients, including those with HIV and bone marrow and solid organ transplants.
- **Famciclovir** (500 mg PO q8h for herpes zoster, 250 mg PO q8h for the initial episode of genital HSV infection, and 125 mg PO q12h for recurrent episodes of genital HSV infection) is an orally administered antiviral agent used for the treatment of acute herpes zoster reactivation and for treatment or suppression of genital HSV infections.
  ○ **Adverse events** include headache, nausea, and diarrhea.

Anticytomegalovirus Agents

- **Ganciclovir** (5 mg/kg IV q12h for 14 to 21 days for induction therapy of cytomegalovirus [CMV] retinitis, followed by 6 mg/kg IV for 5 days every week or 5 mg/kg IV q24h; the oral dose is 1,000 mg PO q8h with food) is used to treat CMV.
  ○ It has activity against HSV and VZV, but safer drugs are available to treat those infections. The drug is widely distributed in the body, including the CSF.

○ It is indicated for treatment of CMV retinitis and other serious CMV infections in immunocompromised patients (e.g., transplant and AIDS patients). Chronic maintenance therapy is generally required to suppress CMV disease in patients with AIDS.

○ **Adverse events.** Neutropenia, which may require treatment with granulocyte colony-stimulating factor for management (300 μg SC daily to weekly), is the main therapy-limiting adverse effect. Thrombocytopenia, rash, confusion, headache, nephrotoxicity, and GI disturbances may also occur. Blood counts and electrolytes should be monitored weekly while the patient is receiving therapy. Other agents with nephrotoxic or bone marrow suppressive effects may enhance the adverse effects of ganciclovir.

• **Valganciclovir** (900 mg PO q12–24h) is the oral prodrug of ganciclovir. This agent has excellent bioavailability and can be used for treatment of CMV retinitis and, thus, has supplanted the use of oral ganciclovir, which has poor oral bioavailability. Adverse events are the same as those for ganciclovir.

• **Foscarnet** (60 mg/kg IV q8h or 90 mg/kg IV q12h for 14 to 21 days as induction therapy, followed by 90 to 120 mg/kg IV q24h as maintenance therapy for CMV; 40 mg/kg IV q8h for acyclovir-resistant HSV and VZV) is used to treat CMV retinitis in patients with AIDS. It is typically considered for use in patients who are not tolerating or not responding to ganciclovir.

○ It is occasionally used for CMV disease in bone marrow transplant patients to avoid the bone marrow–suppressive effects of ganciclovir. It also has a role in treatment of acyclovir-resistant HSV/VZV infections or ganciclovir-resistant CMV infections.

○ **Adverse events.** Risk for nephrotoxicity is a major concern. CrCl should be determined at baseline and electrolytes (PO_4, Ca^{2+}, Mg^{2+}, K^+) and serum creatinine checked at least twice a week. Normal saline (500 to 1,000 mL) should be given before and during infusions to minimize nephrotoxicity. Foscarnet should be avoided in patients with a serum creatinine of >2.8 mg/dL or baseline CrCl of <50 mL/min. Concomitant use of other nephrotoxins (e.g., amphotericin, aminoglycosides, pentamidine, nonsteroidal anti-inflammatory drugs, cisplatin, or cidofovir) should also be avoided. Foscarnet chelates divalent cations and can cause tetany even with normal serum calcium levels. Use of foscarnet with pentamidine can cause severe hypocalcemia. Other side effects include seizures, phlebitis, rash, and genital ulcers. **Prolonged therapy with foscarnet should be monitored by physicians who are experienced with administration of home IV therapy and can systematically monitor patients' laboratory results.**

• **Cidofovir** (5 mg/kg IV qwk for 2 weeks as induction therapy, followed by 5 mg/kg IV q14d chronically as maintenance therapy) is used primarily to treat CMV retinitis in patients with AIDS. It can be administered through a peripheral IV line.

○ **Adverse events.** The most common is nephrotoxicity. It should be avoided in patients with a CrCl of <55 mL/min, a serum creatinine >1.5 mg/dL, significant proteinuria, or a recent history of receipt of other nephrotoxic medications.

○ **Each cidofovir dose should be administered with probenecid** (2 g PO 3 hours before the infusion and then 1 g at 2 and 8 hours after the infusion) along with 1 L normal saline IV 1 to 2 hours before the infusion to minimize nephrotoxicity. Patients should have a serum creatinine and urine protein check before each dose of cidofovir is given. These patients should be followed by a physician regularly, as administration of this drug requires systematic monitoring of laboratory studies.

ANTIFUNGAL AGENTS

Amphotericin B

GENERAL PRINCIPLES

Amphotericin B is fungicidal by interacting with ergosterol and disrupting the fungal cell membrane. Reformulation of this agent in various lipid vehicles has decreased some of its adverse side effects.

- **Amphotericin B deoxycholate** (0.3 to 1.5 mg/kg q24h as a single infusion over 2 to 6 hours) was once the mainstay of antifungal therapy but has now been supplanted by lipid-based formulations of the drug as a result of their improved tolerability. It is not effective for *Pseudallescheria boydii* or *Candida lusitaniae* infections.
- **Lipid complexed preparations** of amphotericin B, including amphotericin B lipid complex (5 mg/kg IV q24h), liposomal amphotericin B (3 to 6 mg/kg IV q24h), and amphotericin B colloidal dispersion (3 to 4 mg/kg IV q24h), have decreased nephrotoxicity and are generally associated with fewer infusion-related reactions than amphotericin B deoxycholate. Liposomal amphotericin B has the most FDA-approved uses and also appears to be the best tolerated lipid formulation.

SPECIAL CONSIDERATIONS

- The major **adverse event** of all amphotericin B formulations, including the lipid formulations, is **nephrotoxicity.** Patients should receive 500 mL of normal saline before and after each infusion to minimize nephrotoxicity. Irreversible renal failure appears to be related to cumulative doses. Therefore, concomitant administration of other known nephrotoxins should be avoided if possible.
- Common **infusion-related effects** include fever/chills, nausea, headache, and myalgias. Premedication with 500 to 1,000 mg of acetaminophen and 50 mg of diphenhydramine may control many of these symptoms. More severe reactions may be prevented by premedication with hydrocortisone, 25 to 50 mg IV. Intolerable infusion-related chills can be managed with meperidine, 25 to 50 mg IV.
- Amphotericin B therapy is associated with **potassium and magnesium wasting** that generally requires supplementation. Serum creatinine and electrolytes (including Mg^{2+} and K^+) should be monitored at least two to three times a week.

Azoles

GENERAL PRINCIPLES

Azoles are fungistatic agents that inhibit ergosterol synthesis.

- **Fluconazole** (100 to 800 mg PO/IV q24h) is the drug of choice for many localized candidal infections, such as UTIs, thrush, vaginal candidiasis (150-mg single dose), esophagitis, peritonitis, and hepatosplenic infection. It is also a viable agent for severe disseminated candidal infections (e.g., candidemia) and the treatment of choice for consolidation therapy of cryptococcal meningitis following an initial

14-day course of an amphotericin B product, or as a second-line agent for primary treatment of cryptococcal meningitis (400 to 800 mg PO q24h for 8 weeks, followed by 200 mg PO q24h thereafter for chronic maintenance treatment).

○ Fluconazole does not have activity against *Aspergillus* species or *Candida krusei* and therefore should not be used for treatment of those infections. *Candida glabrata* may also be resistant to fluconazole. Its absorption is not dependent on gastric acid.

• **Itraconazole** (200 to 400 mg PO q24h) is a triazole with broad-spectrum antifungal activity.

○ It is commonly used to treat the endemic mycoses like coccidioidomycosis, histoplasmosis, blastomycosis, and sporotrichosis.

○ It is an alternative therapy for *Aspergillus* and can also be used to treat infections caused by dermatophytes, including onychomycosis of the toenails (200 mg PO q24h for 12 weeks) and fingernails (200 mg PO q12h for 1 week, with a 3-week interruption, and then a second course of 200 mg PO q12h for 1 week).

○ The capsules require adequate gastric acidity for absorption and, therefore, should be taken with food or carbonated beverage, whereas the liquid formulation is not significantly affected by gastric acidity and is better absorbed on an empty stomach.

• **Posaconazole** (200 mg PO q8h for prophylaxis of invasive fungal infections; 100 to 400 mg PO q12–24 for oropharyngeal candidiasis, 200 mg PO q6 or 400 mg PO q12 for mucormycosis) is an oral azole agent that is FDA approved for prophylaxis of invasive aspergillosis and candidiasis in hematopoietic stem cell transplant patients with graft-versus-host disease or in patients with hematologic malignancies experiencing prolonged neutropenia from chemotherapy as well as oropharyngeal candidiasis. This drug has also been shown to be a useful agent for treatment of mucormycosis.

○ Each dose should be administered with a full meal, liquid supplement, or acidic carbonated beverage (e.g., ginger ale).

○ Rifabutin, phenytoin, and cimetidine significantly reduce posaconazole concentrations and should not routinely be used concomitantly.

○ Posaconazole significantly increases bioavailability of cyclosporine, tacrolimus, and midazolam necessitating dosage reductions of these agents when used with posaconazole. Dosage reduction of vinca alkaloids, statins, and calcium channel blockers should also be considered.

○ Terfenadine, astemizole, pimozide, cisapride, quinidine, and ergot alkaloids are contraindicated with posaconazole.

• **Voriconazole** (loading dose of 6 mg/kg IV [two doses 12 hours apart], followed by a maintenance dose of 4 mg/kg IV q12h or 200 mg PO q12h [100 mg PO q12h if <40 kg]) is a triazole antifungal with a spectrum of activity against a wide range of pathogenic fungi. It has enhanced in vitro activity against all clinically important species of *Aspergillus*, as well as *Candida* (including most nonalbicans), *Scedosporium apiospermum*, and *Fusarium* species.

○ It is the treatment of choice for most forms of invasive aspergillosis, for which it demonstrates typical response rates of 40% to 50% and superiority over conventional amphotericin B. It is also effective in treating candidemia, esophageal candidiasis, and *Scedosporium* and *Fusarium* infections.

○ An advantage of voriconazole is the easy transition from IV to PO therapy because of excellent bioavailability. For refractory fungal infections, a dose increase of

50% may be useful. The maintenance dose is reduced by 50% for patients with moderate hepatic failure.
- Because of its metabolism through the **cytochrome P450 system** (enzymes 2C19, 2C9, and 3A4), there are several **clinically significant drug interactions** that must be considered. Rifampin, rifabutin, carbamazepine (markedly reduced voriconazole levels), sirolimus (increased drug concentrations), and astemizole (prolonged QT_c) are contraindicated with voriconazole. Concomitantly administered cyclosporine, tacrolimus, and warfarin require more careful monitoring.

SPECIAL CONSIDERATIONS

Nausea, diarrhea, and rash are mild side effects of the azoles. Hepatitis is a rare but serious complication. Therapy must be monitored closely in the setting of compromised liver function, and LFTs should be monitored regularly with chronic use. Itraconazole levels should be checked after 1 week of therapy to confirm absorption. The IV formulation of voriconazole should not be used in patients with a CrCl of <50 mL/min because of the potential for accumulation and toxicity from the cyclodextrin vehicle. Transient visual disturbance is a common adverse effect (30%) of voriconazole. **This class of antibiotics has major drug interactions.**

Echinocandins

This class of antifungals inhibit the enzyme $(1,3)$-β-D-glucan synthase that is essential in fungal cell wall synthesis.
- **Caspofungin acetate** (70 mg IV loading dose, followed by 50 mg IV q24h) has fungicidal activity against most *Aspergillus* and *Candida* species, including azole-resistant *Candida* strains. However, *Candida guilliermondii* and *Candida parapsilosis* may be relatively resistant. Caspofungin does not have appreciable activity against *Cryptococcus*, *Histoplasma*, *Blastomyces*, *Coccidioides*, or *Mucor* species. It is FDA approved for treatment of candidemia, refractory invasive aspergillosis, and as empiric therapy in febrile neutropenic.
  - Metabolism is primarily hepatic, although the cytochrome P450 system is not significantly involved. An increased maintenance dosage is necessary with the use of drugs that induce hepatic metabolism (e.g., efavirenz, nelfinavir, phenytoin, rifampin, carbamazepine, dexamethasone). The maintenance dose should be reduced to 35 mg for patients with moderate hepatic impairment; however, no dose adjustment is necessary for renal failure.
  - In vitro and limited clinical data suggest a synergistic effect when caspofungin is given in conjunction with itraconazole, voriconazole, or amphotericin B for *Aspergillus* infections.
  - **Adverse events.** Fever, rash, nausea, and phlebitis at the injection site are infrequent.
- **Micafungin sodium** is used for candidemia (100 mg IV daily), esophageal candidiasis (150 mg IV q24h), and as fungal prophylaxis for patients undergoing hematopoietic stem cell transplantation (50 mg IV q24h). The spectrum of activity is similar to that of anidulafungin and caspofungin. Although micafungin increases serum concentrations of sirolimus and nifedipine, these increases may not be clinically significant. Micafungin may increase cyclosporine concentrations in about 20% of patients. No change in dosing is necessary in renal or hepatic dysfunction.

○ **Adverse events** include rash and delirium. Some patients may have elevated LFTs while on therapy.

- **Anidulafungin** (200-mg IV loading dose, followed by 100 mg IV q24h) is useful for treatment of candidemia and other systemic *Candida* infections (intra-abdominal abscess and peritonitis) as well as esophageal candidiasis (100-mg loading dose, followed by 50 mg daily). The spectrum of activity is similar to that of caspofungin and micafungin. Anidulafungin is not a substrate inhibitor or inducer of cytochrome P450 isoenzymes and does not have clinically relevant drug interactions. No dosage change is necessary in renal or hepatic insufficiency.
  ○ **Adverse events** include possible histamine-mediated reactions, elevations in LFTs, and, rarely, hypokalemia.

Miscellaneous

- **Flucytosine** (25 mg/kg PO q6h) exerts its fungicidal effects on susceptible *Candida* and *Cryptococcus* species by interfering with DNA synthesis.
  ○ Main clinical uses are in the treatment of cryptococcal meningitis and severe *Candida* infections in combination with amphotericin B.
  ○ **Adverse events** include dose-related bone marrow suppression and bloody diarrhea due to intestinal flora conversion of flucytosine to 5-fluorouracil.
  ○ Peak drug concentrations should be kept between 50 and 100 μg/mL. Close monitoring of serum concentrations and dose adjustments are critical in the setting of renal insufficiency. LFTs should be obtained at least once a week.
- **Terbinafine** (250 mg PO q24h for 6 to 12 weeks) is an allylamine antifungal agent that kills fungi by inhibiting ergosterol synthesis. It is FDA approved for the treatment of onychomycosis of the fingernail (6 weeks of treatment) or toenail (12 weeks of treatment). It is not generally used for systemic infections.
  ○ **Adverse events** include headache, GI disturbances, rash, LFT abnormalities, and taste disturbances. This drug should not be used in patients with hepatic cirrhosis or a CrCl of <50 mL/min because of inadequate data. It has only moderate affinity for cytochrome P450 hepatic enzymes and does not significantly inhibit the metabolism of cyclosporine (15% decrease) or warfarin.

16 Human Immunodeficiency Virus and Acquired Immunodeficiency Syndrome

Sara L. Cross and E. Turner Overton

HIV Type 1

GENERAL PRINCIPLES

Definition

Human immunodeficiency virus (HIV) type 1 is a retrovirus that predominantly infects lymphocytes that bear the CD4 surface protein, as well as coreceptors belonging to the chemokine receptor family (CCR5 or CXCR4), and causes acquired immunodeficiency syndrome (AIDS).

Classification

The Centers for Disease Control (CDC) classification is based on the CD4 count and presence of AIDS-associated conditions. Diagnosis of AIDS is made on the basis of CD4 cell count <200, CD4 percentage <14%, or development of one of the 25 AIDS-defining conditions (*MMWR 1992;41(RR-17)*).

Epidemiology

- HIV type 1 is common throughout the world. By the most recent estimates, over 34 million people worldwide are living with HIV or AIDS with a significant burden of disease in Sub-Saharan Africa (*http://www.who.int/hiv/data/en/index.html*).
- In the United States, 1.3 million people are estimated to be infected with HIV with one-fourth of these persons unaware of their infection. The CDC estimates that as many as 70% of the 50,000 new annual infections in the United States are transmitted by persons who are unaware of their HIV status.
- Despite comprising only 14% of the population in the United States, African Americans are disproportionately affected by HIV, accounting for nearly 44% of all new cases of HIV in this country. Hispanics are also disproportionately affected by HIV. Women comprise approximately 24% of the U.S. epidemic (*http://www.cdc.gov/hiv/topics/women*).
  Men who have sex with men (MSM) remain the population most heavily affected by HIV in the United States. Of all new HIV infections in 2009, 61% were MSM (*http://www.cdc.gov/nchhstp/newsroom/docs/HIV-Infections-2006-2009.pdf*).
- **HIV type 2** is endemic to regions in West Africa. It is characterized by much slower progression to AIDS and resistance to nonnucleoside reverse transcriptase inhibitors (NNRTIs).

Etiology

After entering the host cell, HIV utilizes **reverse transcriptase**, transcribing viral RNA into DNA, which integrates into the host DNA. The host cell machinery is then used to produce the relevant viral proteins, which are appropriately truncated by a viral protease. Infectious viral particles bud away to infect other CD4 lymphocytes before the infected cell is destroyed by the immune system. Infection usually leads to CD4 T-cell depletion, and **impaired cell-mediated immunity**.

Pathophysiology

Without highly active antiretroviral therapy (HAART), the immune dysfunction progresses to AIDS, which is characterized by development of opportunistic infections (OIs), malignancies, and wasting. The time from acute HIV infection to development of AIDS varies from months to years (depending on host and viral factors), with a median **latency period** of 10 years.

Risk Factors

The virus is primarily transmitted sexually but also parenterally and perinatally.

DIAGNOSIS

Clinical Presentation

- Acute retroviral syndrome is experienced by up to 75% of patients and is similar to other acute viral illnesses such as infectious mononucleosis due to Epstein–Barr virus (EBV) or cytomegalovirus (CMV) infection. As the acute illness resolves spontaneously, many people do not present for evaluation unless diagnosed by subsequent routine screening. A significant proportion of persons present to care late (CD4 count <200 cells/mm^3) at the time of diagnosis.
- Common presenting symptoms of acute retroviral syndrome are sore throat, nonspecific rash, myalgias, headache, and fatigue.

History

Initial evaluation of persons with a confirmed HIV infection should include the following measures:

- Complete history with emphasis on previous OIs, viral coinfections, and other complications.
- Psychological and psychiatric history. Depression and substance use are common and should be identified and treated as necessary.
- Family and social support assessment.
- Assessment of knowledge and perceptions regarding HIV is also crucial to initiate ongoing education regarding the nature and ramifications of HIV infection.

Physical Examination

Complete physical exam is important to evaluate for manifestations of immune compromise. Initial findings may include the following:

- Oral findings: hairy leukoplakia, aphthous ulcers, thrush (oral candidiasis)
- Lymphatic system: generalized lymphadenopathy
- Skin: *molluscum contagiosum*, *Cryptococcus*, psoriasis, eosinophilic folliculitis, Kaposi sarcoma
- Abdominal exam: evidence of hepatosplenomegaly

- Genital exam: presence of ulcers, genital warts, vaginal discharge, and rectal discharge
- Neurologic exam: Note presence of sensory deficits and cognitive testing.

Diagnostic Criteria

The CDC recommends that **all persons aged 13 to 64 years be offered HIV testing in all health care settings using an opt-out format** (*MMWR Recomm Rep 2006;55:1–17*). These recommendations are based on the following considerations: significant individual health benefits if HAART is initiated earlier in the course of illness, significant public health benefits with knowledge of HIV status leading to changes in risk behaviors, and the availability of inexpensive, reliable, and rapid testing technology. Barriers, however, still exist in certain settings and include inadequate infrastructure to provide testing and linkage to care, legally mandated counseling, and the requirement for a separate, signed informed consent.

Diagnostic Testing

Serology: Current guidelines recommend performing routine HIV serology in all persons regardless of risk using an opt-out testing format (assent is inferred unless the patient declines testing).
- **Persons at high risk should be screened for HIV infection at least annually. High-risk groups include** intravenous (IV) drug users, homosexual and bisexual men, hemophiliacs, sexual partners of the aforementioned persons, sexual partners of a known HIV patient, persons involved in sex trading and their sexual partners, persons with sexually transmitted diseases, persons who received blood products between 1977 and 1985, persons who have multiple sexual partners or who engage in unprotected intercourse, persons who consider themselves at risk, and persons with findings that are suggestive of HIV infection.
- Other groups for whom HIV testing is indicated:
  - Pregnant women (opt-out screening)
  - Patients with active tuberculosis (TB)
  - Donors of blood, semen, and organs
  - Health care workers who perform invasive procedures (depending on the policy of the institution in which they work)
  - Persons with occupational exposures (e.g., needle sticks) and source patients of the exposures
- Screening is performed with an **enzyme-linked immunosorbent assay (ELISA) or rapid HIV test**. The current HIV ELISA used in the United States is a combination HIV-1/HIV-2 enzyme immunoassay test kit that is also sensitive to antibodies to HIV-2.
- A positive screening test is confirmed by a repeat positive ELISA and a positive **Western blot** (presence of at least two of the following bands: p24, gp41, gp120/160).
- **An isolated positive ELISA result should not be reported to the patient until this result is confirmed by a Western blot.** In settings where the rapid HIV test is used for screening, preliminary positive results may be given to the patient with scheduled follow-up to give the results of the confirmatory Western Blot testing. An indeterminate test is one for which the ELISA is positive but the criteria for a positive Western blot are not fulfilled. Repeat testing should be considered for these patients to confirm whether they have a false-positive ELISA or have recent/ acute HIV infection.

- **If acute retroviral syndrome is suspected, a nucleic acid test such as plasma HIV RNA should be obtained in conjunction with HIV ELISA.** Low-level polymerase chain reaction (PCR) results, such as <5,000 copies/mL, are not diagnostic of acute infection. The plasma HIV RNA should be repeated to exclude a false-positive result (*http://guidelines.gov/content.aspx?id=15715*).

Laboratories
- Complete blood cell (CBC) count and comprehensive metabolic panel with assessment of liver and kidney parameters including urinalysis to evaluate for proteinuria and glycosuria.
- **CD4 cell count** (normal range, 600 to 1,500 cells/mm^3) and CD4 percentage. CD4 cell count should be assessed periodically (three to four times a year) to assess the immune status of the patient and to determine the need for OI prophylaxis.
- **Virologic markers:** Plasma HIV RNA is used for monitoring of HAART efficacy. The goal is to achieve maximal virologic suppression, that is, to reduce the viral load level to undetectable by available assays. Several quantitative HIV RNA viral load assays are currently in use, including a branched DNA assay and a nucleic acid sequence amplification assay. The reverse transcriptase PCR assay is the most widely used with a lower limit of detection of 40 to 50 copies/mL.
- **Fasting lipid panel.**
- **Tuberculin skin test.**
- **Rapid plasma reagin (RPR) test.**
- **Toxoplasma immunoglobulin (Ig)G and hepatitis A, B (HBsAg, HBsAb, HBcAb), and C serologies.**
- **Chlamydia/gonococcal urine/cervical probe** for all patients. If patients report receptive anal sex, **rectal probes for gonorrhea and Chlamydia** are recommended. For those reporting receptive oral sex, **pharyngeal sample for gonorrhea** should be obtained (*Clin Infect Dis 2009;49:651*).
- **Cervical Papanicolaou smear** (most commonly using the thin prep method)
- **HIV resistance testing** at baseline, with treatment failure, and particularly for pregnant women.
- **HLA B5701** for patients in whom one is considering the use of abacavir.
- **CCR5** tropism testing for patients in whom one is considering the use of maraviroc.
- **Glucose-6 phosphate dehydrogenase (G6PD) level** on initiation of care or prior to starting therapy with an oxidant drug in those with a predisposing ethnic background.

TREATMENT

Immunizations
- **Pneumoccal vaccine:** HIV infection is an indication for polysaccharide pneumococcal vaccination. Some experts recommend deferring the vaccine until the CD4 cell counts are >200 cells/mm^3, as responses are poor when vaccination occurs with low CD4 cell counts. Revaccination after 5 years is recommended (*http://www.cdc.gov/vaccines/recs/schedules/downloads/adult/06-07/adult-schedule.pdf*).
- **Hepatitis A and B virus (HAV and HBV):** Vaccination for HAV is recommended for certain high-risk HIV-positive subjects without HAV antibodies, although some experts recommend HAV vaccination for all. HIV-positive patients are at higher risk of becoming chronic carriers of HBV after having an acute HBV infection. Therefore, if serologies for hepatitis B are negative, HBV vaccination

is indicated. While there is no effective vaccine for hepatitis C, coinfection with HCV is very prevalent in this population (especially among IV drug abusers) and a clear indication for hepatitis A and B vaccination. Antibody response to these vaccines is improved with undetectable HIV viral load and higher CD4 count.

- **Influenza:** Annual inactivated influenza vaccination is recommended for all HIV-infected patients regardless of CD4 cell count. Use of the intranasally administered, live, attenuated vaccine is not currently recommended for HIV-infected persons.
- **Varicella:** The live, attenuated varicella vaccine can be safely given to persons with CD4 cell counts >200 cells/mm^3 but is contraindicated for persons with CD4 counts <200 cells/mm^3. Recently presented data demonstrated that the zoster vaccine was safe and induces effective immune responses in HIV-infected adults with CD4 counts >200 cells/mm^3. The Advisory Committee on Immunization Practices (ACIP) is expected to revise recommendations based on these study findings.
- **Measles/mumps/rubella (MMR):** MMR is a vaccine that can be safely given to persons with CD4 cell counts >200 cells/mm^3 but is contraindicated for persons with CD4 counts <200 cells/mm^3.
- **Tetanus/diphtheria/pertussis:** All adults should receive tetanus/diphtheria (Td) booster every 10 years with a one-time substitution with tetanus/diphtheria/acellular pertussis vaccine (Tdap).
- **Human papilloma virus (HPV) vaccine:** There are ongoing studies evaluating the safety and efficacy of HPV vaccination in HIV-infected men and women. The three dose vaccine series is currently recommended for females aged 11 to 26 years and males aged 12 to 26 years. Specifically, the ACIP recommends it be given for HIV-infected males in this age range.

Medications

Antiretroviral therapy

- Treatment decisions should be individualized by patient readiness, drug interactions, adherence issues, drug toxicities, comorbidities, and the level of risk indicated by CD4 T-cell counts.
- Maximal and durable suppression of HIV replications is the goal of therapy once it is initiated. **HAART** should be individualized and closely monitored by measuring plasma HIV viral load. Reductions in plasma viremia correlate with increased CD4 cell counts and prolonged AIDS-free survival. Isolated viral "blips" are not indicative of virologic failure, but confirmed virologic rebound should trigger an evaluation of adherence, drug interactions, and viral resistance.
- Women, especially if pregnant, should receive optimal antiretroviral therapy (ART) to reduce the risk of vertical transmission.
- Any change in ART increases future therapeutic constraints and potential drug resistance.
- **Current recommendations from the International AIDS Society-USA (IAS-USA)** (*http://www.iasusa.org/guidelines/*) for the initiation of ART include the following:
  - All patients with clinical AIDS or immunologic AIDS (CD4 count <200 cells/mm^3) to prevent progression of disease and incident or recurrent opportunistic disease.
  - Patients with symptomatic HIV disease, regardless of CD4 cell count.

- ○ Patients with CD4 cell count $\leq$500 cells/mm^3 with asymptomatic disease.
- ○ Other indications include the presence of HIV-associated nephropathy, hepatitis B virus coinfection, and pregnancy.
- ○ **In the asymptomatic patient, with the CD4 count >500 cells/mm^3**, the decision regarding treatment initiation should be determined on case-by-case basis.
- **Antiretroviral drugs:** (Tables 16-1 to 16-5) Approved antiretroviral drugs are grouped into five categories. Experts currently recommend using three active drugs from two different classes to maximally and durably suppress HIV viremia.
  - ○ **Nucleotide and nucleoside reverse transcriptase inhibitors (NRTIs)** constrain HIV replication by incorporating into the elongating strand of DNA, causing chain termination. All nucleoside analogs have been associated with **lactic acidosis**, presumably related to mitochondrial toxicity.
  - ○ **Nonnucleoside reverse transcriptase inhibitors (NNRTIs)** inhibit HIV by binding noncompetitively to the reverse transcriptase. A single dosage of nevirapine at the time of labor has been shown to decrease perinatal transmission of the virus. Side effects of NNRTIs include rash, hepatotoxicity, and Stevens–Johnson syndrome (more likely with nevirapine). Central nervous system (CNS) side effects are commonly experienced with the use of efavirenz.
  - ○ **Protease inhibitors (PIs)** block the action of the viral protease required for protein processing late in the viral cycle. Gastrointestinal (GI) intolerance is one of the most commonly encountered adverse effects. All PIs can produce increased bleeding in hemophiliacs. These agents have also been associated with metabolic abnormalities such as glucose intolerance, increased cholesterol and triglycerides, and body fat redistribution. Due to their metabolism via cytochrome P450, **PIs have important drug interactions**, and concomitant medications should be reviewed carefully (Table 16-6). Boosting with ritonavir is a common practice to achieve better therapeutic concentrations.
  - ○ **HIV entry inhibitors** target different stages of the HIV entry process. Two drugs are available in this class. **Enfuvirtide (T-20)** is a fusion inhibitor that prevents the fusion of the virus into the host cell. **Maraviroc** is a CCR5 receptor blocker. T-20 is only available for use as a subcutaneous injection, 90 mg bid. The most frequent side effect for T-20 is a significant local site reaction after the injection. Initiation of CCR5 inhibitor requires baseline determination of HIV coreceptor tropism (CCR5 or CXCR4). Both of these medications are indicated for treatment-experienced individuals.
  - ○ **Integrase inhibitors** are a new class of antiretroviral agents that target DNA strand transfer and integration into a human genome. There is one drug currently available for use, **raltegravir**, which demonstrates excellent potency and a low side effect profile.
- **Initial therapy:** ART should be started in an outpatient setting by a physician with expertise in the management of HIV infection. Adherence is the key factor for success. Treatment should be individualized and adapted to the patient's lifestyle and comorbidities. Any treatment decision influences future therapeutic options because of the possibility of drug cross-resistance. **Potent initial ART generally consists of a combination of two NRTIs plus one or two PIs or an NNRTI.**
- **Treatment monitoring:** After starting or changing ART, the viral load should be checked at 4 to 6 weeks with an expected 10-fold reduction (1.0 log$_{10}$) and suppression to <50 copies/mL by 24 weeks of therapy. The regimen should be then reassessed if response to treatment is inadequate. When the HIV RNA becomes

Table 16-1	Nucleoside Analog Reverse Transcriptase Inhibitors		
NRTIs	Dosage[a]	Food Restrictions	Common Side Effects
Abacavir (ABC) baseline testing for HLA B5701 is needed prior to initiating ABC	300 mg PO bid or combination tablets: ABC 300 mg + 3TC 150 mg + AZT 300 mg (Trizivir) one tablet bid or ABC 600 mg + 3TC 300 mg (Epzicom) one tablet daily	No	Hypersensitivity reaction; rechallenge in the setting of hypersensitivity can be fatal[b]
Didanosine (ddI)	Preferred as an enteric-coated formula (Videx EC); >60 kg: 400 mg PO daily, <60 kg: 250 mg PO daily When coadministered with TDF decrease ddI dose to 250 mg	On empty stomach	Pancreatitis, peripheral neuropathy, diarrhea
Emtricitabine (FTC)[c]	Closely related to 3TC (cross-resistance possible); 200 mg PO daily	No	No common severe side effects; may have gastrointestinal (GI) intolerance
Lamivudine (3TC)	150 mg PO bid 300 mg PO daily	No	Rare
Stavudine (d4T)	>60 kg: 40 mg PO bid, <60 kg: 30 mg PO bid; extended-release form: >60 kg: 100 mg PO daily, <60 kg: 75 mg PO daily	No	Peripheral neuropathy, pancreatitis, lipoatrophy

(continued)

Table 16-1	Nucleoside Analog Reverse Transcriptase Inhibitors (*Continued*)		
NRTIs	**Dosage**[a]	**Food Restrictions**	**Common Side Effects**
Zidovudine (ZDV, AZT)	300 mg PO bid or combination tablet AZT + 3TC (Combivir) one tablet bid or AZT + 3TC + ABC (Trizivir) one tablet bid	No	Bone marrow suppression, GI intolerance
Tenofovir (TDF)[d]	300 mg PO daily or combination tablet TDF 300 mg + FTC 200 mg one tablet daily or combination tablet TDF 300 mg + FTC 200 mg + Efavirenz 600 mg one tablet daily	No	Rare cases of renal toxicity, rare GI intolerance

[a]Dose adjustment required in patients with renal failure for most nucleoside reverse transcriptase inhibitors (NRTIs).
[b]ABC-related hypersensitivity reaction: flu-like symptoms, fever, rash, upper respiratory symptoms, GI intolerance.
[c]Zalcitabine (ddC) belongs to this class of NRTIs; however, it is rarely used in clinical practice.
[d]Tenofovir is a nucleotide that is available as tenofovir disoproxil fumarate.

undetectable and the patient is on a stable regimen, monitoring can be done every 3 months.

- **Treatment failure** is defined as less than a log (10-fold) reduction of the viral load 4 to 6 weeks after starting a new antiretroviral regimen, failure to reach an undetectable viral load after 6 months of treatment, detection of the virus after initial complete suppression of viral load, which suggests development of resistance, or persistent decline of CD4 cell count or clinical deterioration. Confirmed treatment failure should prompt changes in HAART based on results of genotype testing. In this situation, at least two of the drugs should be substituted with other drugs that have no expected cross-resistance.

  HIV resistance testing at this stage may help determine a salvage regimen in the patients with prior ART. The importance of adherence should be stressed. Referral to an HIV specialist is highly recommended in this situation.

- **Drug interactions:** (Table 16-6) Antiretroviral medications, especially PIs, have multiple drug interactions. **PIs both inhibit and induce the P450 system,**

Table 16-2	Nonnucleoside Reverse Transcriptase Inhibitors		
NNRTI[a]	**Dosage**	**Food Restrictions**	**Side Effects**
Efavirenz (EFV)	600 mg PO daily	On empty stomach; avoid taking after high-fat meals because of increased peak concentration	Central nervous system symptoms (dizziness, somnolence, insomnia, abnormal dreams), teratogenicity; false-positive urine cannabinoid test[b]
Nevirapine (NVP)[c]	200 mg PO daily for 2 wk, then 200 mg PO bid or 400 mg daily	No	Skin rash; hepatitis; severe life-threatening hepatotoxicity observed when used with initial CD4 count >250 cells/mm^3 in women and >400 cells/mm^3 in men
Etravirine (ETV)	100 mg PO bid	Take with food	Skin rash
Rilpivirine	25 mg PO daily	Take with food	Skin rash, insomnia, headache

[a]See Table 16-6 for interactions with other antiretrovirals.
[b]Use of gas chromatography or mass spectroscopy is recommended if screening for cannabis is desired.
[c]Delavirdine is rarely used in clinical practice in the United States.

and thus interactions are frequent with other inhibitors of the P450 system, including macrolides (erythromycin, clarithromycin) and antifungals (ketoconazole, itraconazole), as well as other inducers such as rifamycins (rifampin, rifabutin) and anticonvulsants (phenobarbital, phenytoin, carbamazepine). **Drugs with narrow therapeutic indices that should be avoided or used with extreme caution** include antihistamines (although loratadine is safe), antiarrhythmics (flecainide, encainide, quinidine), long-acting opiates (fentanyl, meperidine), long-acting benzodiazepines (midazolam, triazolam), warfarin, 3-hydroxy-3-methylglutaryl coenzyme A (HMG-CoA) reductase inhibitors (pravastatin is the safest), and oral contraceptives. Sildenafil concentrations are increased, while methadone and theophylline concentrations are decreased with concomitant administration of certain PIs and NNRTIs. Grapefruit juice can increase levels of saquinavir and decrease levels of indinavir.

Table 16-3	Protease Inhibitors		

Protease Inhibitor	Dosage[a]	Food Restrictions	Side Effects
Fosamprenavir (fAPV)[b]	1,400 mg PO bid; combined with RTV(r): fAPV/r, 700/100 mg bid or fAPV/r, 1,400/200 mg daily	No	Rash, diarrhea, nausea
Atazanavir (ATV)	400 mg PO daily; combined with RTV(r): ATZ/r, 300/100 mg daily if prior experience with PIs or taken with tenofovir (TDF)	Take with food	Increased indirect bilirubin, fewer metabolic effects
Indinavir (IDV)	800 mg PO tid usually with RTV(r): IDV/r, 800/100 mg bid; IDV/r, 800/200 mg bid	No food if taken alone, can be taken with or without food if combined with RTV(r)	Nephrolithiasis, increased indirect bilirubin, headache
Lopinavir (LPV)	Available only in fixed combination with RTV(r): LPV/r, 400/100 mg PO bid (Kaletra) 200/50 mg tablet, four tablets qd may be used in treatment-naïve patients only	Take with food; new formulation can be taken with or without food	Diarrhea, hyperlipidemia, hyperglycemia
Nelfinavir (NFV)	750 mg PO tid or 1,250 mg PO bid	Take with food	Diarrhea, nausea
Ritonavir (RTV)[c]	Usually added to achieve booster effect in combination with other PIs; not longer used in full dose	Take with food	Nausea and vomiting, paresthesias, hepatitis, taste perversion
Saquinavir (SQV)	SQV/r, 1,000/100 mg PO bid or used only with RTV boosting	Take with food	Headache, diarrhea
Tipranavir (TPV)	Used only with RTV boosting: TPV/r, 500/200 mg PO bid	Take with food	Hepatitis, skin rash, hyperlipidemia, hyperglycemia

(continued)

Table 16-3	Protease Inhibitors (*Continued*)		
Protease Inhibitor	Dosage	Food Restrictions	Side Effects
Darunavir (DRV)	DRV/r 800 mg PO qd with 100 mg RTV boosting may be used in treatment-naïve patients only or 600 mg po bid with RTV boosting	Take with food	Diarrhea, nausea, headache

[a]See Tables 16-5 and 16-6 for interactions with antiretrovirals and other medications.
[b]fAPV is the prodrug of amprenavir; amprenavir is no longer available in the United States.
[c]RTV is usually added using a lower dose to achieve a booster effect, especially with LPV, SQV, fAPV, and IDV.
ATZ/r, atazanavir/ritonavir; DRV/r, daranavir/ritonavir; IDV/r, indinavir/ritonavir; fAPV/r, fasamprenavir/ritonavir; LPV/r, lobinavir/ritonavir; PI, protease inhibitor; PO, by mouth; RTV(r), ritonavir; SQV/r, saquinavir/ritonavir.

Table 16-4	Entry Inhibitors		
Entry Inhibitor	Dosage	Food Restrictions	Side Effects
Enfuvirtide (T-20)	90 mg SQ bid	No	Injection site reactions
Maraviroc (MVC)[a]	300 mg po bid 150 mg po bid with all protease inhibitors except TPV/r 600 mg po bid if used with EFV	No	Abnormal liver function tests

[a]MVC is a CCR5 receptor antagonist; it is indicated for use only if evidence of CCR5 tropic virus.
EFV, enfuvirtide; SQ, subcutaneous; TPV/r, tipranavir/ritonavir.

Table 16-5	Integrase Inhibitors		
Integrase Inhibitor	Dosage	Food Restrictions	Side Effects
Raltegravir	400 mg PO bid	No	Rare, headache, depression

PO, by mouth.

Table 16-6	Selected Interactions between Antiretrovirals and Other Medications

Antiretrovirals	Interactions

Protease inhibitors (PIs)

Do not coadminister with simvastatin, lovastatin: levels increased; can cause myopathy and rhabdomyolysis. Atorvastatin or pravastatin can be administered with PIs with close monitoring.

Rifampin and rifapentine cannot be coadministered with PIs due to decreased plasma concentrations.

St. John's wort should not be used with any PIs: reduces PI plasma concentration.

Decrease in methadone levels observed with most of the PIs.

Caution when coadministered with sildenafil: increased concentration with all PIs.

Antiretrovirals	Interactions
Lopinavir/ritonavir (LPV/r)	Inhibitor of P450 system
	Fluticasone use can result in suppressed adrenal function
	Decrease rifabutin to 150 mg every other day or three times per week
Atazanavir (ATV)	Decreases clarithromycin dose by 50%
	PPIs significantly decrease ATV concentration; should not be coadministered
	When coadministered with H_2 blockers, should be given 12 hours apart
	Caution due to increased levels of antiarrhythmics
	Decrease rifabutin to 150 mg every other day or three times per week
	Monitor anticonvulsant levels
Nelfinavir (NFV)	Monitor anticonvulsant levels
	Decrease rifabutin to 150 mg every other day or three times per week
Tipranavir (TPV)	Inhibitor of P450 system
	Fluticasone use can result in suppressed adrenal function
	Do not coadminister with amiodarone, quinidine, flecainide
	Do not coadminister with oral contraceptives
	Decrease rifabutin to 150 mg every other day or three times per week
Darunavir (DRV)	Use the lowest dose of pravastatin with close monitoring

Nonnucleoside reverse transcriptase inhibitors (NNRTIs)

St. John's wort should not be coadministered due to suboptimal levels of NNRTIs.

Decreased levels of oral contraceptives when coadministered.

(continued)

Table 16-6	Selected Interactions between Antiretrovirals and Other Medications (*Continued*)

Antiretrovirals	Interactions
Efavirenz (EFV)	Inducer/inhibitor of the P450 system
	Do not coadminister with voriconazole: decreases voriconazole levels
	Decreases methadone levels; can cause opiate withdrawal
Nevirapine (NVP)	Inducer of the P450 system
	Rifabutin lowers NVP levels; do not coadminister with rifampin
Rilpivirine	Decreases methadone levels; can cause opiate withdrawal
	Substrate of cytochrome P450
	Requires an acidic environment for absorption; do not coadminister with PPIs
	When coadministered with H_2 blockers, should be given 12 hours apart
	Do not coadminister with rifamycins, certain anticonvulsants including phenytoin and carbamazepine, and St. John's wort as these decrease rilpivirine levels
	Macrolides and azole antifungals may increase rilpivirine levels

Nucleoside reverse transcriptase inhibitors (NRTIs)

Tenofovir (TDF)	Coadministration with cidofovir, acyclovir, valacyclovir, ganciclovir, and valganciclovir may increase serum concentrations of either tenofovir or the coadministered drug
Didanosine (ddI)	Do not coadminister with allopurinol (decreased didanosine concentrations), ribavirin (hepatic failure)
	Monitor for didanosine toxicity when coadministered with ganciclovir or valganciclovir
Zidovudine (AZT)	Avoid concomitant ribavirin and interferon use
	Increased hematologic toxicity with ganciclovir, valganciclovir, cidofovir

PPI, proton pump inhibitors.
Complete updated HIV clinical guidelines available at *http://www.aidsinfo.nih.gov/Guidelines/Default.aspx?Menuitem=Guidelines.*
From U.S. Food and Drug Administration. *http://www.fda.gov/cder/drug/default.htm.* National Institutes of Health. *http://www.aidsinfo.nih.gov/.*

SPECIAL CONSIDERATIONS

With the success of ART, HIV-related mortality is decreasing and HIV-infected persons are experiencing prolonged survival. The CDC estimates that in 2015, one-half of all HIV-infected persons will be over the age of 50 years. With the recognition that HIV induces premature end-organ disease, many of the comorbidities associated with aging may be exacerbated in this growing population, including cardiovascular disease, insulin resistance and diabetes, osteoporosis, neurocognitive impairment, and physical frailty.

COMPLICATIONS

Complications of ART: The long-term use of antiretrovirals has been associated with toxicity, the pathogenesis of which is only partially understood at this time.

- **Lipodystrophy syndrome** is an alteration in body fat distribution and can be stigmatizing to individuals. Changes consist of the accumulation of visceral fat in the abdomen, neck (buffalo hump), and pelvic areas, and/or the depletion of subcutaneous fat, causing facial or peripheral wasting. Lipodystrophy has been associated in particular with PIs and NRTIs, but other factors may also be important. Changes in the patient's ART regimen and lifestyle modifications such as exercise may improve morphologic changes. Other supplemental therapies such as rosiglitazone and cosmetic surgery are currently under investigation.
- **Hyperlipidemia**, especially hypertriglyceridemia, is associated mainly with PIs (especially ritonavir). Improvement has been seen after treatment with atorvastatin, pravastatin, and/or gemfibrozil.
- **Peripheral insulin resistance, impaired glucose tolerance, and hyperglycemia** have been associated with the use of PI-based regimens, mainly indinavir and ritonavir. Lifestyle changes or changing ART can be considered in these cases.
- **Lactic acidosis** with liver steatosis is a rare but sometimes fatal complication associated with NRTIs. The mechanism appears to be part of mitochondrial toxicity. Higher rates of lactic acidosis have been reported with the use of stavudine and didanosine. The clinical picture can range from asymptomatic hyperlactatemia to severe lactic acidosis with hepatomegaly and steatosis. Suspected drugs should be discontinued and supportive care given as needed.
- **Osteopenia and osteoporosis** are well described in HIV-infected individuals. The pathogenic mechanism of this problem is likely related to the inflammatory milieu of HIV itself. The role of ART is being further studied.
- **Osteonecrosis**, particularly of the hip, has been increasingly associated with HIV disease.

REFERRAL

- To HIV specialist
- **Contraception**, **safer sex practices**, counseling on medication adherence, and proper health maintenance
- **Social worker referral** to ensure adequate social support system including housing, mental health assistance, and substance abuse treatment

MONITORING/FOLLOW-UP

- Plasma HIV RNA is used for monitoring ART efficacy. The goal is to reduce the viral load levels to undetectable. CD4 cell count should be checked periodically (three to four times a year) to assess the immune status of the patient and to determine the need for OI prophylaxis. After starting or changing ART, the viral load should be checked at 4 to 6 weeks, and the regimen should be then reassessed if response to treatment is inadequate. When the HIV RNA becomes undetectable and the patient is on a stable regimen, monitoring can be done every 4 to 6 months.

- **HIV resistance testing** is done using two different types of assays: genotypic (in which the reverse transcriptase and the polymerase genes are sequenced using different techniques) and phenotypic (in which the HIV replication in vitro in the presence of antiretroviral drugs is examined). Results of resistance testing should be used to guide ART.

OUTCOME/PROGNOSIS

With the advent of potent HAART, which causes durable virologic suppression and reconstitution of the immune system, the mortality among HIV-infected persons continues to decline. In the modern era of HAART, the noninfectious conditions start to play a much more important role in the mortality among persons with HIV (*AIDS 2007;21(15):2093*).

Opportunistic Infections

GENERAL PRINCIPLES

- Potent ART has decreased the incidence, changed the manifestations, and improved the outcome of OIs.
- A clinical syndrome associated with the immune enhancement induced by potent ART, **immune reconstitution syndrome (IRIS)**, has been described and generally presents as local inflammatory reactions. Examples include paradoxical reactions with TB reactivation, localized *Mycobacterium avium* complex (MAC) adenitis, and CMV vitreitis immediately after the initiation of potent ART. Hepatitis virus infections can be aggravated with the immune reconstitution associated with ART.
  ○ In the case of IRIS, ART is usually continued, and the addition of low-dose steroids might decrease the degree of inflammation.

TREATMENT

- **Prophylaxis for OIs** can be divided into primary and secondary prophylaxis.
- **Primary prophylaxis** is established before an episode of OI occurs. Institution of primary prophylaxis depends on the level of immunosuppression as judged by the patient's CD4 cell count and percentage (Table 16-7).
  Primary prophylaxis is not routinely recommended for the following OIs: recurrent bacterial pneumonia, mucosal candidiasis, CMV retinitis, cryptococcosis, and endemic fungal infections such as histoplasmosis and coccidioidomycosis.
- **Secondary prophylaxis** is instituted after an episode of infection has been adequately treated. Most OIs will require extended therapy.
- **Withdrawal of prophylaxis:** Recommendations suggest withdrawing primary and secondary prophylaxis for most OIs if sustained immunologic recovery has occurred (CD4 cell counts consistently above 150 to 200 cells/mm^3) (*MMWR Recomm Rep 2009;58(RR-4):1*).

Table 16-7	Opportunistic Infection Prophylaxis	
Opportunistic Infection	**Indications for Prophylaxis**	**Medications**
PCP	Primary: CD4 <200 cells/mm^3	TMP-SMX DS PO daily or three times per week Alternatives: dapsone,[a] atovaquone, aerosolized pentamidine
Tuberculosis	PPD test >5 mm or a history of a previous untreated PPD test, or recent contact with an individual with active TB	Isoniazid (INH) + pyridoxine, for 9 months. Alternatives: rifampin or rifabutin for 4 months[b]
Toxoplasmosis[c]	CD4 <100 cells/mm^3, one tablet daily, is the preferred regimen	TMP-SMX DS PO daily Alternatives: combination of dapsone + pyrimethamine and leucovorin; atovaquone
Mycobacterium avium complex prophylaxis	CD4 cell count <50 cells/mm^3	Azithromycin 1,200 mg PO weekly Alternatives: clarithromycin or rifabutin

[a]Glucose-6 phosphate dehydrogenase (G6PD) testing should be done for dapsone.
[b]Potential for drug interactions.
[c]If toxoplasmosis immunoglobulin (Ig)G is positive.
DS, double strength; PCP, Pneumocystis jiroveci pneumonia; PO, by mouth; PPD, purified protein derivative; TB, tuberculosis; TMP-SMX, trimethoprim-sulfamethoxazole.

Cytomegalovirus Infection

GENERAL PRINCIPLES

CMV retinitis accounts for 85% of CMV disease in patients with AIDS. It commonly develops in a setting of profound CD4 depletions (CD4 cell count <50 cells/mm^3).

DIAGNOSIS

• CMV viremia can be detected by PCR and is usually present in end-organ disease but can also be seen in the absence of end-organ disease.
• The diagnosis of CMV retinitis is made based on characteristic findings during ophthalmoscopic exam.

TREATMENT

- Treatment of CMV retinitis can be local or systemic and is administered in two phases, induction and maintenance.
- **Ganciclovir** is given at an induction dosage of 5 mg/kg IV bid for 14 to 21 days and a maintenance dosage of 5 mg/kg IV daily indefinitely (unless immune reconstitution occurs). The most common side effect of ganciclovir is **myelotoxicity**, resulting in neutropenia. The neutropenia may respond to granulocyte colony-stimulating factor therapy. An intraocular ganciclovir implant is effective but does not provide systemic CMV therapy.
- **Valganciclovir**, a ganciclovir prodrug, has been approved for use in CMV retinitis. Drug levels are equivalent to those of IV ganciclovir. For induction, 900 mg PO bid for 21 days is given, followed by 900 mg once a day. **Treatment is indefinite unless immunologic recovery occurs.** Adverse effects are similar to those of ganciclovir.
- Alternatives include **IV foscarnet, IV cidofovir, and intraocular fomivirsen** (which does not provide systemic therapy). Both IV foscarnet and cidofovir administrations carry a significant risk of **nephrotoxicity**; therefore, adequate hydration and electrolyte monitoring (including calcium) are required.
- For other **invasive CMV disease**, the optimal therapy is with IV ganciclovir, PO valganciclovir, IV foscarnet, or a combination of two drugs (in persons with prior anti-CMV therapy), for at least 3 to 6 weeks. Foscarnet has the best cerebrospinal fluid (CSF) penetration and is the drug of choice for CMV encephalitis and myelopathy. Long-term maintenance therapy is indicated.

Mycobacterium Tuberculosis

GENERAL PRINCIPLES

M. tuberculosis is more frequent among HIV-infected patients, particularly IV drug abusers. Primary or reactivated disease is common (*MMWR Recomm Rep 2009;58(RR-4):1*).

DIAGNOSIS

- Clinical manifestations depend on the level of immunosuppression. Patients with higher CD4 cell counts tend to exhibit classic presentations with **apical cavitary disease**.
- Profoundly immunosuppressed patients may demonstrate atypical presentations that can resemble disseminated primary infection, with diffuse or localized pulmonary infiltrates and hilar lymphadenopathy.
- Extrapulmonary dissemination is common.

TREATMENT

For treatment recommendations, see Chapter 14, Treatment of Infectious Diseases.
- Current recommendations suggest the **substitution of rifabutin for rifampin** in patients who are receiving concomitant ART, especially PIs.
- The dosage for rifabutin needs readjustment due to many significant interactions (*http://www.hivmedicationguide.com/*). It should be reduced to 150 mg daily if the

patient is receiving ritonavir, indinavir, nelfinavir, or fosamprenavir, whereas it should be increased to 450 mg daily when combined with nevirapine or efavirenz.
- In subjects who are ART naïve, ART can be delayed for a few weeks after TB-specific therapy is started.

M. Avium Complex Infection

GENERAL PRINCIPLES

MAC infection is the most commonly occurring mycobacterial infection in AIDS patients and is responsible for significant morbidity in patients with advanced disease (CD4 cell count <100 cells/mm³).

DIAGNOSIS

Clinical Presentation
- Disseminated infection with fever, weight loss, and night sweats is the most frequent presentation.
- MAC infection can result in bacteremia in AIDS patients.

Diagnostic Testing
- Anemia and an elevated alkaline phosphatase level are the usual laboratory abnormalities.
- Mycobacterial blood cultures should be sent in suspected cases.

TREATMENT

- Initial therapy should include a **macrolide** (i.e., clarithromycin, 500 mg PO bid) and **ethambutol**, 15 mg/kg PO daily.
- Rifabutin, 300 mg PO daily, or ciprofloxacin, 500 mg PO bid, can be added in severe cases.
- Secondary prophylaxis for disseminated MAC can be discontinued if the CD count has a sustained increase >100 cells/mm³ for 6 months or longer in response to ART, and if 12 months of therapy for MAC is completed and there are no symptoms or signs attributable to MAC.

Pneumocystis Jiroveci Pneumonia

GENERAL PRINCIPLES

Pneumocystis jiroveci pneumonia (PCP) is the most common infection in patients with AIDS and is the leading cause of death in this population.

DIAGNOSIS

Positive direct immunoflourescent stain from induced sputum samples or bronchoalveolar lavage fluid. Alternatively, histopathologic demonstration of organisms in tissue is also adequate for diagnosis.

TREATMENT

- **Trimethoprim-sulfamethoxazole (TMP-SMX)** is the treatment of choice. The dosage is 5 mg/kg of the TMP component IV q6–8h for severe cases, with a switch to oral therapy when the patient's condition improves. Total duration of therapy is 21 days. **Prednisone** should be added if the patient has an arterial oxygen tension (PaO_2) of <70 mm Hg or an alveolar arterial oxygen gradient ($P[A - a]O_2$) in excess of 35 mm Hg. The most frequently prescribed prednisone regimen is 40 mg PO bid on days 1 to 5 and 20 mg bid on days 6 to 10, followed by 10 mg on days 11 to 21. For patients who cannot receive TMP-SMX, the following alternatives are available:
  - For mild to moderately severe disease (PaO_2 >70 mm Hg or $P[A - a]O_2$ <35 mm Hg):
    - TMP, 20 mg/kg/d PO, and dapsone, 100 mg PO daily. G6PD deficiency should be ruled out before dapsone is used.
    - Clindamycin, 600 mg IV or PO tid, plus Primaquine, 15 mg PO daily. G6PD deficiency should be ruled out before Primaquine is used.
    - Atovaquone, 750 mg PO tid. This drug should be administered with meals to increase absorption.
  - For severe disease (PaO_2 <70 mm Hg or $P[A - a]O_2$ >35 mm Hg):
    - Prednisone taper should be added.
    - IV pentamidine or trimetrexate are used in cases when all other options are exhausted. Both drugs require close monitoring for side effects.
- Primary prophylaxis is indicated (see Table 16-7). Secondary PCP prophylaxis can be discontinued if the CD4 count is >200 cells/mm³ for more than 3 months as a result of ART treatment.

Candidiasis

GENERAL PRINCIPLES

- The severity of infection depends on the degree of the patient's immunosuppression.
- Candidiasis is common in the HIV-infected host.

DIAGNOSIS

Location of infection can be oral, esophageal, or vaginal.

TREATMENT

- Oral and vaginal candidiasis usually respond to local therapy with troches or creams (**nystatin** or **clotrimazole**).
- For patients who do not respond or who have esophageal candidiasis, **fluconazole**, 100 to 200 mg PO daily, is the treatment of choice.

SPECIAL CONSIDERATIONS

- **Fluconazole-resistant candidiasis** is increasing, especially in patients with advanced disease who have been receiving antifungal agents for prolonged periods.

○ **Caspofungin**, an echinocandin, can be considered for refractory cases using an induction dose of 70 mg IV the first day and then 50 mg IV daily for maintenance.

○ **Itraconazole** oral suspension (200 mg bid) is occasionally effective, as is **posaconazole** oral solution and is generally better tolerated than itraconazole. Many patients require **amphotericin B**, either as an oral suspension (100 mg/mL swish and swallow qid) or parenterally. **Voriconazole** may also be useful.

Cryptococcus Neoformans

GENERAL PRINCIPLES

- The severity of infection depends on the degree of the patient's immunosuppression.
- **Cryptococcal meningitis** is the most frequent CNS fungal infection in AIDS patients.

DIAGNOSIS

- Patients with CNS infection usually present with headaches, fever, and possibly mental status changes, but presentation can be more subtle.
- Cryptococcal infection can also present as pulmonary or cutaneous disease.
- Diagnosis is based on **lumbar puncture** results and on the determination of latex cryptococcal antigen, which is usually positive in the serum and in the CSF.
- **CSF opening pressure** should always be measured to assess the possibility of elevated intracranial pressure.

TREATMENT

- Initial treatment is with **amphotericin B**, 0.7 mg/kg/d IV, and **5-flucytosine**, 25 mg/kg PO q6h for 2 to 3 weeks, followed by **fluconazole**, 400 mg PO daily for 8 to 10 weeks and then 200 mg PO daily, either lifelong or until immune reconstitution occurs. Fluconazole can be discontinued in those who are asymptomatic with regard to signs and symptoms of cryptococcosis, and have a sustained increase (>6 months) in their CD4+ counts to ≥200 cells/μL.
- The 5-flucytosine level should be monitored during therapy to avoid toxicity. A lipid preparation of amphotericin dosed at 4 to 6 mg/kg/d IV can be used in patients with renal insufficiency.
- Repeat lumbar punctures (removing up to 30 mL CSF until the pressure is below 20 to 25 cm H_2O) may be required to relieve elevated intracranial pressure.
- In persons who have persistent elevation of intracranial pressure, a temporary lumbar drain is indicated.

Histoplasma Capsulatum Infections

GENERAL PRINCIPLES

- The severity of infection depends on the degree of the patient's immunosuppression.
- Histoplasmosis often occurs in AIDS patients who live in endemic areas such as the Mississippi and Ohio River Valleys.
- Such infections are usually disseminated at the time of diagnosis.

DIAGNOSIS

- Suspect histoplasmosis in patients with fever, hepatosplenomegaly, and weight loss.
- Pancytopenia develops due to bone marrow involvement.
- Diagnosis is made by a positive culture or biopsy demonstrating 2 to 4 μm budding yeast, but the urine and serum *Histoplasma* antigens can also be used for diagnosis and to monitor treatment.

TREATMENT

- Treatment is with **liposomal amphotericin B**, 3 mg/kg daily for ≥2 weeks or until they clinically improve, followed by **itraconazole**, 300 mg PO bid for 3 days for induction therapy, followed by 200 mg PO bid indefinitely.
- Itraconazole absorption should be documented by a serum drug level.
- Discontinuation of itraconazole is possible if sustained increase in CD4 count is observed >100 to 200 cells/mm^3 for more than 6 months.

PROTOZOAL INFECTIONS

Toxoplasma Gondii

DIAGNOSIS

Toxoplasmosis typically causes multiple CNS lesions and presents with encephalopathy and focal neurologic findings.

Diagnostic Testing

Laboratories

Disease represents reactivation of a previous infection, and the serologic workup is usually positive.

Imaging

- Magnetic resonance imaging (MRI) of the brain is the best radiographic technique for diagnosis.
- Often the diagnosis relies on response to empiric treatment, as seen by a reduction in the size of the mass lesions.

TREATMENT

- **Sulfadiazine**, 25 mg/kg PO q6h, plus **pyrimethamine**, 100 mg PO on day 1, followed by 75 mg PO daily, is the therapy of choice.
- **Leucovorin**, 5 to 10 mg PO daily, should be added to prevent hematologic toxicity. For patients who are allergic to sulfonamides, clindamycin, 600 mg IV or PO q8h, can be used instead of sulfadiazine.
- Doses are reduced after 3 to 6 weeks of therapy.
- Secondary prophylaxis can be discontinued among patients with a sustained increase in CD4 count >200 cells/mm^3 for more than 6 months as a result of response to ART, and if the initial therapy is complete and there are no symptoms or signs attributable to toxoplasmosis.

Cryptosporidium

DIAGNOSIS

- *Cryptosporidium* causes chronic watery diarrhea with malabsorption in HIV-infected patients.
- Diagnosis is based on the visualization of the parasite in an acid-fast stain of stool.

TREATMENT

- No effective specific therapy has been developed.
- **Nitazoxanide**, 500 mg PO bid, may be effective.
- Potent ART also has been reported to be effective.

Cyclospora

DIAGNOSIS

Cyclospora causes chronic diarrhea.

TREATMENT

TMP-SMX, one DS tablet PO bid for 7 to 10 days, is usually effective.

Isospora Belli

DIAGNOSIS

Isospora causes chronic diarrhea.

TREATMENT

Treatment with **TMP-SMX**, one DS tablet PO qid for 10 days, followed by chronic suppression with TMP-SMX, one DS tablet PO daily, is effective.

Microsporidia

DIAGNOSIS

- Microsporidia can produce diarrhea and biliary tree disease in patients with advanced infection.
- Diagnosis is difficult and requires special staining of the stool. *Enterocytozoon bieneusi* and *Encephalitozoon intestinalis* are the microsporidia most commonly found. *E. intestinalis* can cause disseminated disease.

TREATMENT

Conventional therapy is with **albendazole**, 400 mg PO bid, but this regimen has only modest success for *E. bieneusi* infections. Relapses are common when therapy is stopped.

ASSOCIATED NEOPLASMS

Kaposi Sarcoma

GENERAL PRINCIPLES

Kaposi sarcoma is caused by coinfection with human herpes virus 8 (HHV8), also called Kaposi sarcoma–associated herpesvirus (KSHV).

DIAGNOSIS

In AIDS patients, it commonly presents as cutaneous lesions, but can be disseminated. The GI tract and lungs are the usual visceral organs involved.

TREATMENT

* Local therapy with **liquid nitrogen** or intralesional injection with alitretinoin or vinblastine has been used. Cryotherapy or radiation may be useful as well.
* Systemic therapy involves chemotherapy (e.g., liposomal doxorubicin, paclitaxel, liposomal daunorubicin, thalidomide, retinoids), radiation, and interferon-α.

Lymphoma

GENERAL PRINCIPLES

* Lymphomas commonly associated with AIDS are non-Hodgkin lymphoma, CNS and systemic lymphoma, and lymphomas of B-cell origin.
* **EBV** appears to be the associated pathogen.

DIAGNOSIS

* Primary CNS lymphomas are common and can be multicentric.
* Diagnosis is based on clinical symptoms, the presence of enhancing brain lesions, brain biopsy, and a positive EBV-PCR of the CSF.
* Other OIs need to be ruled out.
* Other potential extranodal sites of involvement including bone marrow, GI tract, and liver require tissue biopsy to confirm the diagnosis.

TREATMENT

Treatment involves **chemotherapy** and **radiation**.

Cervical and Perianal Neoplasias

GENERAL PRINCIPLES

* Both HIV-infected men and women are at high risk for HPV-related disease.
* Certain HPV subtypes such as 16 and 18 are oncogenic.
* Cancer can also arise from perianal condyloma acuminata.

DIAGNOSIS

- Screening for vaginal dysplasia with a Papanicolaou smear is indicated every 6 months during the first year and, if results are normal, annually afterward.
- Screening for anal intraepithelial neoplasms is currently under evaluation and is recommended by some experts in populations such as MSM, any patient with a history of anogenital condylomas, and women with abnormal vulvar or cervical histology (*http://hivguidelines.org/Content.aspx.*)

TREATMENT

Refer to Chapter 22, Medical Management of Malignant Disease, for specific treatments of these neoplasias.

SEXUALLY TRANSMITTED DISEASES

Genital Herpes

GENERAL PRINCIPLES

Herpes simplex virus 2 (HSV-2) (less frequently herpes simplex virus 1 [HSV-1]) causes recurrent genital and perirectal lesions. HIV-infected individuals are more likely to have prolonged and severe disease as well as treatment failures due to the development of resistance.

DIAGNOSIS

Type-specific HSV serology, HSV-PCR from the genital fluid, and viral culture are all useful tests in the diagnostic workup.

TREATMENT

- **Acyclovir**, 400 mg PO tid; **famciclovir**, 250 mg PO tid; or **valacyclovir**, 500 mg PO tid, for 1 week is usually effective. For more severe disease, IV acyclovir, 5 mg/kg q8h, is recommended.
- Relapses are frequent, and prophylactic acyclovir, 400 mg PO bid, may prevent recurrence as a part of a suppressive or episodic treatment strategy.
- **If resistant HSV, foscarnet, 40 mg/kg IV q8h for 10 to 14 days, or one dose of cidofovir, 5 mg/kg IV, should be used.** Alternatives to this include topical formulations of cidofovir, trifluridine, or imiquimod.

Genital Warts

GENERAL PRINCIPLES

Genital warts are caused by HPV. Different serotypes have been associated with the lesions, notably types 6 and 11. Other common HPV types (16, 18, 31, and 33)

Table 16-8 HIV-Associated Conditions

Disease	Definitions	Treatment Strategy	Medications
Viral infections			
Varicella–Zoster virus (VZV)	VZV may cause typical dermatomal lesions or disseminated infection.	May cause encephalitis, which is more common with ophthalmic distribution of facial nerve.	Acyclovir, 10 mg/kg IV q8h for 7 to 14 days, is the recommended therapy. For milder cases, administration of acyclovir (800 mg PO five times a day), famciclovir (500 mg PO tid), or valacyclovir (1 g PO tid) for 1 week is usually effective.
JC virus	Associated with progressive multifocal leukoencephalopathy. Symptoms include mental status changes, weakness, and disorders of gait.	Characteristic periventricular and subcortical white matter lesions are seen on MRI.	Potent ART has improved the survival of patients with progressive multifocal leukoencephalopathy.
Parvovirus B19	Chronic parvovirus infections can cause pure RBC aplasia.	Relapses are frequent.	Treatment is with IV immunoglobulin, 0.4 g/kg IV daily for 10 days.

Chronic hepatitis C	Chronic hepatitis C has a significant impact on morbidity and mortality in HIV-infected patients.	Sustained virologic response rates are lower, specifically in genotype 1.	Combination of pegylated interferon-α and ribavirin. New antiviral drugs against the hepatitis C virus have been developed and are currently in clinical trials in HIV-infected patients.
Chronic hepatitis B	Chronic hepatitis B has a significant impact on morbidity and mortality in HIV infection.	Determine the need for HIV treatment.	Antiretroviral combination of TDF/FTC (or 3TC) as part of a HAART. If HIV does not require treatment can use pegylated interferon-α, adefovir, or telbivudine.
Bacterial infections			
Bacillary angiomatosis	Rare condition caused by *Bartonella henselae*.	Characterized by multiple nodular, purplish lesions on the skin and other organs.	Erythromycin, 500 mg PO q6h. Alternatives: doxycycline, 100 mg PO bid; other macrolides and ciprofloxacin, 500 mg PO bid.
Campylobacter jejuni	C. jejuni can cause GI or disseminated infections.		Either erythromycin, 500 mg PO qid, or ciprofloxacin, 500 mg PO bid, can be used.

(continued)

Table 16-8	HIV-Associated Conditions *(Continued)*		
Disease	**Definitions**	**Treatment Strategy**	**Medications**
Rhodococcus equi	*R. equi* can cause necrotizing cavitary pneumonia.		Vancomycin, 1 g IV q12h following troughs to reach goal of 15–20 µg/mL, followed by chronic suppression with erythromycin, 500 mg PO qid, plus rifampin, 600 mg PO daily, or with ciprofloxacin, 500 mg PO bid.
Salmonella species	Can result in recurrent bacteremia in AIDS. It occurs more commonly in MSM.	Antibacterial therapy should be based on susceptibility pattern.	Ceftriaxone, 1 g IV daily; or ampicillin, 1 g IV q6h; or TMP-SMX, 1 DS tablet PO bid; or ciprofloxacin, 500 mg PO bid.
Bacterial pneumonias	Risk for bacterial pneumonia is several times higher in HIV-infected individuals.	*Streptococcus pneumoniae* or *Haemophilus influenzae*. Gram-negative rods (especially *Pseudomonas aeruginosa*).	Third-generation cephalosporin, oral fluoroquinolones, or antipseudomonal agent if indicated.
Mycobacterial			
Mycobacterium kansasii	Frequently occurs in HIV; should always be considered when identified in clinical samples.	Clinically, the infection appears similar to TB.	A combination of rifampin, 600 mg PO daily; ethambutol, 15 mg/kg/d PO; and INH, 300 mg PO daily, is the recommended therapy.
Mycobacterium haemophilum infection	*M. haemophilum* causes ulcerative skin lesions.		It requires treatment with a macrolide, rifampin, and two other drugs active against the organism.

Fungal

Coccidioides immitis

Frequent in AIDS patients in endemic areas of the Southwestern United States. Extensive disease with extrapulmonary spread is common.

Diagnosis is made by a positive culture, serum detection of IgM and IgG by immunodiffusion, and complement fixation.

Amphotericin B therapy initially, followed by lifelong suppression with fluconazole, 400 mg PO daily, or itraconazole, 200 mg PO bid. Coccidioidal meningitis requires intracisternal or intraventricular therapy with amphotericin B. Fluconazole may also be effective.

ART, antiretroviral therapy; DS, double strength; GI, gastrointestinal; HAART, highly active antiretroviral therapy; IG, immunoglobulin; INH, isoniazid; IV, intravenous; JC, John Cunningham; MRI, magnetic resonance imaging; MSM, men who have sex with men; PO, by mouth; RBC, red blood cell; TB, tuberculosis; TDF/FTC, tenofovir/emtricitabine; TMP-SMX, trimethoprim-sulfamethoxazole.

Data from Soriano V, Puoti M, Peters M, et al. Care of HIV patients with chronic hepatitis B: updated recommendations from the HIV-Hepatitis B Virus International Panel. AIDS. 2008;22(12):1399–1410.

are associated with malignant transformation in different anatomic sites. Genital warts in HIV-infected persons are typically more resistant to treatment in addition to a higher chance of recurrence (*http://www.cdc.gov/STD/treatment/2006/genital-warts.htm*).

DIAGNOSIS

Diagnosis is made on the basis of physical exam and history. In some situations, biopsy of the lesions may be necessary.

TREATMENT

Local therapy aimed at the removal of the warts.

Syphilis

GENERAL PRINCIPLES

Syphilis can have an atypical course in HIV-infected patients, and treatment failures are more frequent in this population.

DIAGNOSIS

A lumbar puncture should be performed in HIV-infected patients with latent syphilis to rule out neurosyphilis.

TREATMENT

- **Benzathine penicillin**, 2.4 million U intramuscular (IM) one time for primary syphilis or weekly for 3 weeks for secondary or latent syphilis (of >1 year in duration), is the regimen of choice.
- **Doxycycline**, 100 mg PO bid for 14 days, is an alternative.
- If neurosyphilis is present, **penicillin G**, 12 to 24 million U IV daily for 14 days, is the only approved treatment of choice. Patients who are allergic to penicillin should be desensitized. Data regarding the use of ceftriaxone, 1 to 2 g IV daily for 14 days, are limited.

MONITORING/FOLLOW-UP

- Close monitoring and follow-up using the nontreponemal test at 3, 6, and 12 months are necessary in all cases.
- Persons with a sustained positive nontreponemal titer should receive retreatment and be considered for CSF evaluation to rule out neurosyphilis (*MMWR Recomm Rep 2006;55(RR-11)*).

SPECIAL CONSIDERATIONS

Other sexually transmitted diseases are treated as they would be in non–HIV-infected patients (see Chapter 14, Treatment of Infectious Diseases). **Other commonly encountered conditions** in HIV-infected persons are listed in Table 16-8.

ADDITIONAL RESOURCES

- *www.aifsinfo.org*
- *www.aidsmeds.com*
- *www.thebody.com*
- *www.hivmedicine.com*
- *www.hivinsite.ucsf.edu*

17 Solid Organ Transplant Medicine

Christina L. Klein and Brent W. Miller

Solid Organ Transplant Basics

GENERAL PRINCIPLES

- Solid organ transplantation is a **treatment**, **not a cure**, for end-stage organ failure of the kidney, liver, pancreas, heart, and lung. The benefits of organ replacement coexist with the risks of chronic immunosuppression. Thus, not all patients with organ failure are transplant candidates.
- All organs remain in short supply with increasing waiting times for potential recipients. **Living-donor transplants** are increasingly common in kidney transplantation and are being evaluated in liver and lung transplantation as a partial solution to this shortage. Xenotransplantation is **not** a viable option in the near future.
- **Immunologic considerations** prior to the transplant must be fully evaluated, including ABO compatibility with the donor, human leukocyte antigen (HLA) typing, and some degree of immune response testing to the proposed donor. Newer protocols using desensitization techniques have had some success in overcoming these immunologic barriers.

DIAGNOSIS

- For indications and contraindications of heart, lung, kidney, and liver transplantations, see sections devoted to cardiology, pulmonology, nephrology, and hepatology.
- **Evaluation of the transplant patient.** The evaluation of the transplant recipient with general medical or surgical problems should always encompass the details of the patient's organ transplant and treatment. Thus, the following should always be reviewed when taking a history from an organ transplant recipient:
  - Cause of organ failure
  - Treatment for organ failure prior to transplantation
  - Type and date of transplant
  - Cytomegalovirus (CMV) serology of donor and recipient
  - Initial immunosuppression, particularly use of antibody-based induction therapy
  - Initial allograft function (e.g., nadir creatinine, forced ejection fraction volume in 1 second [FEV_1], ejection fraction, synthetic function and transaminases)
  - Current allograft function
  - Complications of transplantation (e.g., surgical problems, acute rejection, infections, chronic organ dysfunction)
  - Current immunosuppression regimen and recent drug levels

TREATMENT

- **Immunosuppression.** Immunosuppressive medications are used to promote acceptance of a graft (induction therapy), to reverse episodes of acute rejection (rejection therapy), and to prevent rejection (maintenance therapy). These agents are associated with immunosuppressive effects, immunodeficiency toxicity (e.g., infection and malignancy), and nonimmune toxicity (e.g., nephrotoxicity, diabetes mellitus, bone disease, gout, hyperlipidemia, cardiovascular disease, or neurotoxicity) (*N Engl J Med 2004;351:2715*). Immunosuppressive medications should only be prescribed and administered by physicians and nurses who have appropriate knowledge and expertise. Many variables factor into the choice and dose of drug, and the guidelines for each specific organ are different.
- **Glucocorticoids.** Glucocorticoids are immunosuppressive and anti-inflammatory. Their mechanisms of action include inhibition of cytokine transcription, induction of lymphocyte apoptosis, downregulation of adhesion molecule and major histocompatibility complex expression, and modification of leukocyte trafficking (*N Engl J Med 2005;353:1711*).
  - Side effects of chronic glucocorticoid therapy are well known.
  - As a result of the associated morbidity, steroids are tapered rapidly in the immediate posttransplant period to achieve maintenance doses of 0.1 mg/kg or less.
  - Four further strategies are developing to minimize side effects: steroid-free immunosuppression, steroid avoidance, rapid steroid tapering, and steroid withdrawal.
  - Although most long-term transplant recipients have abnormalities in the adrenal axis, increases in glucocorticoid therapy are not indicated for routine surgery or illness (*Arch Surg 2008;143:1222*).
- **Antiproliferative agents**
  - **Azathioprine** is a purine analog that is metabolized by the liver to 6-mercaptopurine (active drug), which in turn is catabolized by xanthine oxidase. Azathioprine inhibits the synthesis of DNA and thereby suppresses the proliferation of activated lymphocytes. The major dose-limiting toxicity of this agent is myelosuppression, which is usually reversible after dose reduction or discontinuation of the drug. The usual maintenance dose is 1.5 to 2.5 mg/kg/d in a single dose. Drug levels are generally not obtained.
  - **Mycophenolic acid (MPA)** is available in two forms: mycophenolic acid or its precursor, mycophenolate mofetil (which is converted to the active metabolite, MPA). MPA inhibits the rate-limiting step in de novo purine synthesis. Because lymphocytes are relatively dependent on the de novo pathway for purine synthesis, lymphocyte proliferation is selectively inhibited by MPA.
    - **Major adverse effects** of MPA are gastrointestinal disturbances (including nausea, diarrhea, and abdominal pain) and hematologic disturbances (leukopenia and thrombocytopenia).
    - Antacids that contain magnesium and aluminum interfere with the absorption of MPA and should not be given concurrently.
    - Proton pump inhibitors can also interfere with the bioavailability of mycophenolate mofetil, but not enteric-coated MPA, which is absorbed in the small intestine.
    - The usual dose is 1 to 2 g daily in divided doses, although lesser doses may be used with concomitant tacrolimus than cyclosporine (CsA), because of enterohepatic circulation affecting MPA levels. Additionally, the dosage of MPA should be reduced in the presence of renal impairment. Drug levels can be

obtained to verify absorption or compliance, but the clinical utility of MPA levels has not been determined.

- Mammalian target of rapamycin (mTOR) inhibitors: **Sirolimus** and everolimus inhibit the activation of a regulatory kinase, mTOR, and thus prohibit T-cell progression from the G1 to the S phase of the cell cycle. Unlike the calcineurin inhibitors, mTOR inhibitors do not affect cytokine transcription but inhibit cytokine and growth factor–induced cell proliferation.
  - The major adverse effects include hyperlipidemia, anemia, proteinuria, difficulty with wound healing, cytopenias, peripheral edema, oral ulcers, and gastrointestinal symptoms, although other less common side effects are present.
  - Although not directly nephrotoxic, mTOR inhibitors may compound the vasoconstriction of calcineurin inhibitors and potentiate their nephrotoxicity. Thus, mTOR inhibitors are best utilized alone or with steroids and/or other antiproliferative agents.
  - Sirolimus interacts with CsA metabolism, making monitoring of both drugs difficult.
  - The typical dose of sirolimus is 2 to 5 mg daily in a single dose. Everolimus is administered 0.75 to 1.50 mg twice daily. Therapeutic drug monitoring is being perfected, with current trough levels between 5 and 15 ng/mL for sirolimus and 3 to 8 ng/mL for everolimus most commonly being used.
  - Sirolimus should be avoided in moderate-to-advanced chronic kidney disease and immediately postoperatively as it is associated with poorer wound healing, delayed graft function (kidney transplant), anastomotic bronchial dehiscence (lung transplant), and hepatic artery thrombosis (liver transplant); limited data are available regarding use of everolimus in the immediate postoperative period.
- **Calcineurin inhibitors**
  - Calcineurin inhibitors inhibit T-lymphocyte activation and proliferation. Current strategies are being developed for calcineurin withdrawal and avoidance in solid organ transplantation because of nephrotoxicity. Intravenous (IV) calcineurin inhibitors should be avoided because of their extreme toxicity and must never be given as a bolus under any circumstance.
  - **Cyclosporine** is a cyclic 11-amino acid peptide derived from a fungus. Its major nonimmune side effect is nephrotoxicity due to glomerular afferent arteriolar vasoconstriction. This action leads to an immediate decline in glomerular filtration rate of up to 30% and a long-term vaso-occlusive fibrotic renal disease that often results in chronic kidney disease in recipients of all organ transplants. Angiotensin-converting enzyme inhibitors, mTOR inhibitors, volume depletion, and other nephrotoxins may potentiate this toxicity. Acute nephrotoxicity is reversible with dose reduction; chronic nephrotoxicity is generally irreversible and nearly universally present in all patients after 8 to 10 years of therapy.
  - Other **adverse effects** include gingival hyperplasia, hirsutism, tremor, hypertension, glucose intolerance, hyperlipidemia, hyperkalemia, and rarely, thrombotic microangiopathy. CsA has a narrow therapeutic window, and doses are adjusted based on blood levels (recommended maintenance trough levels of 100 to 300 ng/mL and 2-hour levels <800 to 1,200 ng/mL). Usual doses are 6 to 8 mg/kg/d in divided doses, with careful attention to levels and toxicities.
  - **Tacrolimus** is a macrolide antibiotic and, like CsA, is nephrotoxic. Tacrolimus is more neurotoxic and diabetogenic than CsA, but it is associated with less hirsutism, hypertension, and gingival hyperplasia. Tacrolimus dosing is based on

trough blood levels (recommended maintenance levels of 5 to 10 ng/mL). Usual starting dose is 0.15 mg/kg/d in divided doses.

- **Biologic agents**
  - ○ **Polyclonal antibodies**
    - ▪ Antithymocyte globulin is produced by injecting human thymocytes into animals and collecting sera. This process generates antibodies against a wide variety of human immune system antigens. When subsequently infused into human patients, T lymphocytes are depleted as a result of complement-mediated lysis and clearance of antibody-coated cells by the reticuloendothelial system. Lymphocyte function is also disrupted by blocking and modulating the expression of cell surface molecules by the antibodies. Infusion is through a central vein over 4 to 6 hours. The most common side effects are fever, chills, and arthralgias.
    - ▪ Other important **adverse effects** include myelosuppression, serum sickness, and rarely, anaphylaxis. Two preparations are available: horse antithymocyte globulin (ATGAM) and rabbit antithymocyte globulin (Thymoglobulin). Current literature suggests that rabbit antithymocyte globulin is more efficacious. These drugs can be utilized at the time of transplantation to promote engraftment ("induction") or as a subsequent treatment for acute rejection. The long-term risk of increased malignancy, particularly lymphoma, remains a concern with these agents.
  - ○ **Monoclonal antibodies**
    - ▪ **Anti–interleukin-2 receptor monoclonal antibodies.** Daclizumab (humanized) and basiliximab (chimeric) are monoclonal antibodies that competitively inhibit the interleukin-2 receptor (CD25) and thereby inhibit activation of T cells. Humanization and chimerization result in antibodies with an extended half-life and minimize the chance of developing antimurine antibodies. These drugs are administered by a peripheral vein perioperatively at the time of transplantation and are associated with few side effects.
    - ▪ **Belatacept.** Approved by the U.S. Food and Drug Administration (FDA) in 2011 for use in kidney transplants, belatacept is a fusion protein, which blocks T-cell costimulation and subsequent activation. It is contraindicated for use in nonrenal transplantation and additionally in patients seronegative for Epstein–Barr virus (EBV) as increased rates of posttransplant lymphoproliferative disease were reported in EBV-seronegative recipients.
    - ▪ Other biologic agents used off-label in transplantation include **alemtuzumab**, a monoclonal antibody against CD52, a molecule present on B and T cells; **eculizumab**, a humanized monoclonal antibody blocking activation of complement protein C5; and **rituximab**, a chimeric monoclonal antibody against the B-cell protein CD20.
- **Infection prophylaxis**
  - ○ **Immunization.** Pneumococcal and hepatitis B vaccination should be given at the time of pretransplant evaluation. Influenza A vaccination should be administered yearly. Live vaccines should be avoided after transplantation and if transplant is imminent (e.g., living donor kidney transplant) (*Am J Transplant 2004;4(suppl 10):160*). Varicella vaccination in seronegative patients and hepatitis A vaccination (particularly in liver transplant candidates) should be considered (*Clin Infect Dis 2009;49:1550*).
  - ○ **Trimethoprim/sulfamethoxazole** prevents urinary tract infections, *Pneumocystis jiroveci* pneumonia, and *Nocardia* infections. The optimal dose and duration of prophylaxis have not been determined though a minimum of 1 year is recom-

mended. In sulfa allergic patients, dapsone, aerosolized pentamidine, or atovaquone are alternatives.

○ **Acyclovir** prevents reactivation of herpes simplex virus (HSV) and varicella–zoster but is ineffective in CMV prophylaxis. HSV can be a serious infection in immunosuppressed individuals, and some form of prophylaxis should be utilized during the first year. Patients with recurrent HSV infections (oral or genital) should be considered candidates for long-term prophylaxis. Lifetime acyclovir should also be used in EBV-seronegative patients who receive an EBV-positive organ.

○ **Ganciclovir** or **valganciclovir** prevents reactivation of CMV infection when administered to patients who were previously CMV seropositive, received a CMV-positive organ, or both. Typically, they are administered from 3 to 12 months following transplantation. CMV hyperimmune globulin or IV ganciclovir can also be used for this purpose. Alternatively, patients can be monitored for the presence of CMV replication in the bloodstream by polymerase chain reaction before symptoms develop and can be treated preemptively.

○ **Fluconazole** or **ketoconazole** can be given to patients with a high risk of systemic fungal infections or recurrent localized fungal infections. Both medications increase CsA and tacrolimus levels (see Treatment under Solid Organ Transplant Basics section). **Nystatin suspension**, **clotrimazole** troches, or weekly fluconazole are used to prevent oropharyngeal candidiasis (thrush).

GRAFT REJECTION

Acute Rejection, Kidney

GENERAL PRINCIPLES

Most episodes of acute rejection occur in the first year after transplantation. The low incidence of acute rejection today usually entails a careful search for inadequate drug levels, noncompliance, or less common forms of rejection (such as antibody-mediated rejection or plasma cell rejection). Late acute rejection (>1 year after transplantation) usually results from inadequate immunosuppression or patient nonadherence.

Definition

An immunologically mediated, acute deterioration in renal function associated with specific pathologic changes on renal biopsy including lymphocytic interstitial infiltrates, tubulitis, and arteritis (cellular rejection) and/or glomerulitis, capillaritis, and positive staining of the peritubular capillaries for the complement component C4d (antibody-mediated rejection).

Epidemiology

Kidney allograft rejection currently occurs in only 10% of patients. Patients who do not receive induction therapy have a 20% to 30% incidence of acute rejection.

Associated Conditions

Diagnosis of acute renal allograft rejection is made by percutaneous renal biopsy after excluding prerenal azotemia via hydration and repeating laboratory tests. Further workup includes evaluation for calcineurin inhibitor nephrotoxicity (trough and/or

Table 17-1	Differential Diagnosis of Renal Allograft Dysfunction	
<1 Wk Posttransplant	<3 Mo Posttransplant	>3 Mo Posttransplant
Acute tubular necrosis	Acute rejection	Prerenal azotemia
Hyperacute rejection	Calcineurin inhibitor toxicity	Calcineurin inhibitor toxicity
Accelerated rejection	Prerenal azotemia	Acute rejection (nonadherence, low levels)
Obstruction	Obstruction	Obstruction
Urine leak (ureteral necrosis)	Infection	Recurrent renal disease
Arterial or venous thrombosis	Interstitial nephritis	De novo renal disease
Atheroemboli	Recurrent renal disease	Renal artery stenosis (anastomotic or atherosclerotic)
	BK virus nephropathy	BK virus nephropathy

peak levels and associated signs), infection (urinalysis and culture), obstruction (renal ultrasound), and surgical complications such as urine leak (renal scan). Newer techniques evaluating early markers of acute rejection in the blood and urine are being developed.

DIAGNOSIS

Clinical Presentation

Manifestations include an elevated serum creatinine, decreased urine output, increased edema, or worsening hypertension. Initial symptoms are often absent except for the rise in creatinine. Constitutional symptoms (fever, malaise, arthralgia, painful or swollen allograft) are uncommon in current practice.

Differential Diagnosis

Differential diagnosis varies with duration after transplantation (Table 17-1).

Acute Rejection, Lung

GENERAL PRINCIPLES

- Of the solid organ transplants, the lung is the most immunogenic organ. The majority of patients have at least one episode of acute rejection. Multiple episodes of acute rejection predispose to the development of chronic rejection (bronchiolitis obliterans syndrome).
- **Lung transplant rejection** occurs frequently and most commonly in the first few months after transplantation.

DIAGNOSIS

Diagnosis is generally made by fiberoptic bronchoscopy with bronchoalveolar lavage and transbronchial biopsies.

Clinical Presentation

Manifestations are nonspecific and include fever, dyspnea, and a nonproductive cough. The chest radiograph is usually unchanged, and is generally nondiagnostic even when abnormal (perihilar infiltrates, interstitial edema, pleural effusions). Change in pulmonary function testing is not specific for rejection, but a 10% or greater decline in forced vital capacity or FEV_1, or both, is usually clinically significant.

Differential Diagnosis

It is important to attempt to distinguish rejection from infection, because although the symptoms are similar, the treatments are markedly different.

Acute Rejection, Heart

GENERAL PRINCIPLES

Heart transplant recipients typically have two to three episodes of acute rejection in the first year after transplantation with a 50% to 80% chance of having at least one rejection episode, most commonly in the first 6 months.

DIAGNOSIS

- **Diagnosis** is established by endomyocardial biopsy performed during routine surveillance or as prompted by symptoms. None of the noninvasive techniques has demonstrated sufficient sensitivity and specificity to replace the endomyocardial biopsy. Repeated endomyocardial biopsies predispose to severe tricuspid regurgitation.
- **Manifestations** may include symptoms and signs of left ventricular dysfunction, such as dyspnea, paroxysmal nocturnal dyspnea, orthopnea, syncope, palpitations, new gallops, and elevated jugular venous pressure. Many patients are asymptomatic. Acute rejection may also be associated with a variety of tachyarrhythmias, atrial more often than ventricular.

Acute Rejection, Liver

GENERAL PRINCIPLES

- Many **liver transplant recipients** may be maintained on minimal immunosuppression. Acute rejection typically occurs within the first 3 months after transplant and often in the first 2 weeks after the operation. Acute rejection in the liver is generally reversible and does not portend a potentially serious adverse outcome

as in other organs. Recurrent viral hepatitis is a much more frequent and morbid problem.
- **Liver transplant recipients** commonly experience acute allograft rejection, with at least 60% having one episode.

DIAGNOSIS

Diagnosis is made by liver biopsy after technical complications are excluded.

Clinical Presentation
Manifestations may be absent with only a slight elevation in transaminases, or the patients may have signs and symptoms of liver failure including fever, malaise, anorexia, abdominal pain, ascites, decreased bile output, elevated bilirubin, and elevated transaminases.

Differential Diagnosis
Differential diagnosis of early liver allograft dysfunction includes primary graft nonfunction, preservation injury, vascular thrombosis, biliary anastomotic leak, or stenosis. These disorders should be excluded clinically or by Doppler ultrasonography. Late allograft dysfunction may be due to rejection, recurrent hepatitis B or C, CMV infection, EBV infection, cholestasis, or drug toxicity.

Acute Rejection, Pancreas

GENERAL PRINCIPLES

- The majority of rejection episodes occur within the first 6 months posttransplant. Unlike other organs, clinical findings and biochemical markers correlate poorly with rejection; in particular, if hyperglycemia occurs due to rejection it is often late, severe, and irreversible. Since 80% of pancreas transplants are performed with a simultaneous kidney transplant with the same immunologic status, renal allograft function and histopathology can be a valuable surrogate for diagnosis of pancreas allograft rejection.
- Most pancreas transplants are done with quadruple immunosuppression, consisting of an induction agent and triple maintenance immunosuppression, including corticosteroids. One year posttransplant acute rejection rates range between 25% and 40%; this contributes significantly to early and late graft loss.

DIAGNOSIS

At time of surgery, the exocrine (digestive enzymes) secretions of the pancreas can be drained into the recipients intestine (enteric drainage) or into the bladder (bladder drainage). Serum amylase and lipase are used in both the enteric and bladder drained recipient to monitor for rejection but lack specificity. For the bladder drained allograft, a fall in urinary amylase correlates with rejection. However, allograft biopsy remains the gold standard, demonstrating septal, ductal and acinar inflammation, and endotheliitis. If a recipient received a simultaneous kidney transplant from the same donor, the creatinine and renal biopsy may also be used to diagnose rejection, although isolated pancreas or kidney rejection may rarely occur.

Clinical Presentation

Manifestations may be absent with only a slight elevation in serum amylase and lipase, or fall in urinary amylase (bladder drained). **Hyperglycemia is a late manifestation of rejection.**

Differential Diagnosis

Differential diagnosis of hyperglycemia includes thrombosis (affecting 7% of recipients), islet cell drug toxicity, steroid effect, infection, development of insulin resistance, or recurrent autoimmune disease. Differential diagnosis of elevated serum lipase includes graft pancreatitis, peripancreatic fluid/infection, obstruction, dehydration, and posttransplant lymphoproliferative disorder (PTLD).

Chronic Allograft Dysfunction

GENERAL PRINCIPLES

- Chronic allograft dysfunction accounts for the vast majority of late graft losses and is the major obstacle to long-term graft survival.
- **Chronic allograft dysfunction** (formerly chronic rejection) is a slowly progressive, insidious decline in function of the allograft characterized by gradual vascular and ductal obliteration, parenchymal atrophy, and interstitial fibrosis.

DIAGNOSIS

- Diagnosis is often difficult and generally requires a biopsy. The process is mediated by immune and nonimmune factors.
- The manifestations of chronic rejection are unique to each organ system.

TREATMENT

To date, no effective therapy is available for established immune-mediated chronic allograft dysfunction. Some patients, particularly those with renal transplants, will require a second solid organ transplant. Current investigational strategies are aimed at prevention.

Complications

GENERAL PRINCIPLES

- **Infections**
  - **CMV infection** (*N Engl J Med 1998;338:1741*) from reactivation of CMV in a seropositive recipient or new infection from a CMV-positive organ can lead to a wide range of presentations from a mild viral syndrome to allograft dysfunction, invasive disease in multiple organ systems, and even death. CMV-seronegative patients who receive a CMV-seropositive organ are at substantial risk, particularly in the first year (Table 17-2).

Table 17-2	Timing and Etiology of Posttransplant Infections	
Time Period	**Infectious Complication**	**Etiology**
<1 mo posttransplant	Nosocomial pneumonia, wound infection, urinary tract infection, catheter-related sepsis, biliary, chest or other drainage catheter infection	Bacterial or fungal infections
1–6 mo posttransplant	Opportunistic infections	Cytomegalovirus *Pneumocystis jiroveci* *Aspergillus* spp. *Toxoplasma gondii* *Listeria monocytogenes* *Strongyloides stercoralis* West Nile virus Varicella–zoster virus (VZV)
	Reactivation of preexisting infections	*Mycobacteria* spp. Endemic mycoses Viral hepatitis
>6 mo posttransplant	Community-acquired infections	Bacterial Tick-borne disease Influenza Metapneumovirus Norovirus
	Chronic progressive infection	Reactivated VZV (Zoster) Hepatitis B Hepatitis C HIV Cytomegalovirus Epstein–Barr virus Papillomavirus Polyoma virus (BK)
	Opportunistic infections	*P. jiroveci* *L. monocytogenes* *Nocardia asteroides* *Cryptococcus neoformans* *Aspergillus* spp. West Nile virus

- Because of the potential progression and severity of untreated disease, treatment is usually indicated in the transplant patient without tissue diagnosis of invasive disease. Shell-vial culture of the buffy coat is accurate only when plated within 24 hours of sample collection. Seroconversion with a positive immunoglobulin (Ig)M titer or a fourfold increase in IgM or IgG titer suggests acute infection; however, many centers now use polymerase chain reaction–based diagnostic techniques from blood samples, and treatment is usually administered in the patient with evidence of viral replication (*J Am Soc Nephrol 2001;12:848*).
- Treatment is with oral valganciclovir, 450 to 900 mg by mouth (PO) bid (adjusted for renal function) or IV ganciclovir, 2.5 to 5.0 mg/kg bid (adjusted

for renal function), for 3 to 4 weeks. Hyperimmune globulin is often used in combination with ganciclovir for patients with organ involvement.

- Foscarnet and cidofovir are more toxic alternatives and should be reserved for ganciclovir-resistant cases.

o **Hepatitis B and C.** Patients with active hepatitis or cirrhosis are not considered for nonhepatic transplantation. Immunosuppression increases viral replication in organ transplant recipients with either hepatitis B or C.

- **Hepatitis B** can recur as fulminant hepatic failure even in patients with no evidence of viral DNA replication before transplantation. In liver transplantation, the risk of recurrent hepatitis B virus infection can be reduced by the administration of hepatitis B immunoglobulin during and after transplantation. Experience with lamivudine therapy initiated before transplantation to lower viral load has shown decreased likelihood of recurrent hepatitis B virus.

- **Hepatitis C** typically progresses slowly in nonhepatic transplants, and the effect of immunosuppression on mortality due to liver disease remains to be determined. Treatment protocols for hepatitis C in the nonhepatic transplant population are not yet established. Hepatitis C nearly always recurs in liver transplant recipients whose original disease was due to hepatitis C. Therapy for recurrent hepatitis C virus with a combination of ribavirin and interferon results in histopathologic improvement of disease, although dosage and duration of therapy remain controversial.

o **EBV** plays a role in the development of PTLD. This life-threatening lymphoma is treated by withdrawal or reduction in immunosuppression and often aggressive chemotherapy. The role of newly discovered viral agents such as human herpesvirus (HHV)-6, HHV-7, HHV-8, and polyoma (BK and JC) virus after transplantation remains to be established. BK virus is known to cause interstitial nephritis resulting in renal allograft loss and occasionally ureteral stricture resulting in obstruction. As BK virus nephropathy results primarily from reactivation of latent BK in the transplanted organ, this is rarely seen in nonrenal transplant recipients.

o **Fungal and parasitic infections**, such as *Cryptococcus*, *Mucor*, aspergillosis, and *Candida* species, result in increased mortality after transplantation and should be aggressively diagnosed and treated. The role of prophylaxis with oral fluconazole has not been established.

- **Renal disease.** Chronic allograft dysfunction is the leading cause of allograft loss in renal transplant recipients. Calcineurin inhibitor (CsA or tacrolimus) nephrotoxicity or recurrent native disease may also develop in these patients. Chronic calcineurin inhibitor nephrotoxicity may also lead to chronic renal insufficiency and end-stage renal disease (ESRD), requiring dialysis or transplantation in recipients of lung, heart, liver, or pancreas transplants. The incidence of ESRD secondary to calcineurin inhibitor toxicity in recipients of solid organ transplants is at least 10%, and the incidence of significant chronic kidney disease approaches 50% (*N Engl J Med 2003;349:931*).

- **Malignancy** occurs in transplant patients with an overall incidence that is three- to fourfold higher than that seen in the general population (age matched). Some cancers occur at the same rate, whereas other neoplasms have a much higher frequency than normal. Cancers with an increased risk of fivefold or greater compared to the general population are Kaposi sarcoma, non-Hodgkin lymphoma, skin, lip, vulvar, anal, and liver cancer, illustrating the oncogenic potential of associated viral infections (*JAMA 2011;306:1891*).

○ **Skin and lip cancers** are the most common malignancies (40% to 50%) seen in transplant recipients, with an incidence 10 to 250 times that of the general population. Risk factors include immunosuppression, ultraviolet radiation, and human papillomavirus infection. These cancers develop at a younger age, and they are more aggressive in transplant patients than in the general population. Using protective clothing and sunscreens and avoiding sun exposure are recommended. Examination of the skin is the principal screening test, and early diagnosis offers the best prognosis. The mTOR inhibitors may be better immunosuppressive choices in patients with recurrent skin cancer as long as no contraindications to use otherwise exist.

○ **Posttransplant lymphoproliferative disease** accounts for one-fifth of all malignancies after transplantation, with an incidence of approximately 1%. This is 30- to 50-fold higher than in the general population, and the risk increases with the use of antilymphocyte therapy for induction or rejection. The majority of these neoplasms are large-cell non-Hodgkin lymphomas of the B-cell type. Posttransplant lymphoproliferative disease results from EBV-induced B-cell proliferation in the setting of chronic immunosuppression. The EBV-seronegative recipient of a seropositive organ is at greatest risk. The presentation is often atypical and should always be considered in the patient with new symptoms. Diagnosis requires a high index of suspicion followed by a tissue biopsy. Treatment includes reduction or withdrawal of immunosuppression and chemotherapy.

SPECIAL CONSIDERATIONS

Important drug interactions are always a concern given the polypharmacy associated with transplant patients. Before prescribing a new medication to a transplant recipient, always investigate drug interactions.

• The combination of **allopurinol and azathioprine** should be avoided or used cautiously due to the risk of profound myelosuppression.

• CsA and tacrolimus are metabolized by cytochrome P450 (3A4). Therefore, CsA and tacrolimus levels are decreased by drugs that induce cytochrome P450 activity, such as rifampin, isoniazid, barbiturates, phenytoin, and carbamazepine. Conversely, CsA and tacrolimus levels are increased by drugs that compete for cytochrome P450, such as verapamil, diltiazem, nicardipine, azole antifungals, erythromycin, and clarithromycin. Similar effects are seen with tacrolimus and sirolimus.

• Tacrolimus and CsA should not be taken together because of the increased risk of severe nephrotoxicity.

• Lower doses of MPA should be used when either tacrolimus or sirolimus is taken concurrently.

• Concomitant administration of CsA and sirolimus may result in a twofold increase in sirolimus levels; to avoid this drug interaction, CsA and sirolimus should be dosed 4 hours apart.

18 Gastrointestinal Diseases

C. Prakash Gyawali and Amit Patel

Gastrointestinal Bleeding

GENERAL PRINCIPLES

Acute gastrointestinal (GI) bleeding results in substantial morbidity, mortality, and health care costs, especially when it develops after hospitalization, and in portal hypertension or neoplasia (*Gut 2011;60:1327*).

- GI bleeding may manifest as passage of bright or altered blood with emesis or bowel movements.
- **Overt GI bleeding** is the passage of fresh or altered blood in emesis or in the stool.
- **Occult bleeding** refers to a positive fecal occult blood test (stool guaiac) or iron-deficiency anemia without visible blood in the stool.
- **Obscure bleeding** consists of GI blood loss of unknown origin that persists or recurs after negative initial endoscopic evaluation (*Gastroenterology 2007;133: 1697*).

DIAGNOSIS

Clinical Presentation

History

- Hematemesis, coffee-ground emesis, and aspiration of blood or coffee-ground material from a nasogastric (NG) tube suggest an upper GI source of blood loss.
- **Melena**, black sticky stool with a characteristic odor, usually indicates an upper GI source, although small-bowel and right colonic bleeds can also result in melena.
- Various shades of **bloody stool (hematochezia)** are seen with distal small-bowel or colonic bleeding, depending on the rate of blood loss and colonic transit. Rapid upper GI bleeding can present with hematochezia, invariably associated with hemodynamic compromise or circulatory shock.
- **Bleeding from the anorectal area** typically results in bright blood coating the exterior of formed stool associated with distal colonic symptoms (e.g., rectal urgency, straining, or pain with defecation).
- **Anemia** from blood loss can cause fatigue, weakness, abdominal pain, pallor, or dyspnea.
- Estimation of **amount of blood lost** is often inaccurate. If the baseline hematocrit is known, the drop in hematocrit provides a rough estimate of blood loss. In general, lower GI bleeding causes less hemodynamic compromise compared to upper GI bleeding.
- **Coagulation abnormalities** can propagate bleeding from a preexisting lesion in the GI tract. Disorders of coagulation (e.g., liver disease, von Willebrand disease,

vitamin K deficiency, and disseminated intravascular coagulation) can influence the course of GI bleeding (see Chapter 20, Disorders of Hemostasis and Thrombosis).

- **Medications** known to affect the coagulation process or platelet function include warfarin, heparin, aspirin, nonsteroidal anti-inflammatory drugs (NSAIDs), clopidogrel (Plavix), thrombolytic agents, antithrombotic agents such as glycoprotein IIb/IIIa receptor antagonists (abciximab [ReoPro], eptifibatide [Integrilin], tirofiban [Aggrastat]), and direct thrombin inhibitors (argatroban, bivalirudin, dabigatran etexilate). NSAIDs and aspirin can result in mucosal damage anywhere in the GI tract.

Physical Examination

- **Color of stool.** Direct examination of spontaneously passed stool or that from a digital rectal examination can help localize the level of bleeding (*Dig Dis Sci 1995; 40:1614*). A **digital rectal examination** may identify anorectal abnormalities including anal fissures, which induce extreme discomfort during a rectal examination.
- Fresh blood on an **NG aspirate** may indicate ongoing upper GI bleeding requiring urgent endoscopic attention (*Gastrointest Endosc 2004;59:172*). The aspirate should be considered positive only if blood or dark particulate matter ("coffee grounds") is seen, and **hemoccult testing of NG aspirate has no clinical utility**. A bleeding source in the duodenum can result in a negative NG aspirate. Gastric lavage with water or saline may be useful in assessing the activity and severity of upper GI bleeding and in clearing the stomach of blood and clots before endoscopy (*N Engl J Med 2008;359:928*). After a diagnosis of upper GI bleeding is made, the NG tube can be removed in a stable patient.
- Constant **monitoring** or frequent assessment of vital signs is necessary early in the evaluation, as a sudden increase in pulse rate or decrease in blood pressure (BP) may be an early indicator of recurrent or ongoing blood loss.
- If the baseline BP and pulse are within normal limits, sitting the patient up or having the patient stand may result in **orthostatic hemodynamic changes** (drop in systolic BP of >10 mm Hg, rise in pulse rate of >15 bpm). Orthostatic changes in pulse and BP are seen with loss of 10% to 20% of the circulatory volume; supine hypotension suggests a >20% loss. Hypotension with a systolic BP of <100 mm Hg or baseline tachycardia >100 bpm suggests significant hemodynamic compromise that requires urgent volume resuscitation (*N Engl J Med 2008; 359:928*).

Diagnostic Testing

Laboratories

- Complete blood cell (CBC) count
- Coagulation parameters (international normalized ratio, partial thromboplastin time)
- Blood group, cross-matching of 2 to 4 units of blood
- Comprehensive chemical profile (including liver function tests, serum creatinine)

Diagnostic Procedures

- **Endoscopy**
  - **Esophagogastroduodenoscopy (EGD)** has high diagnostic accuracy, therapeutic capability, and low morbidity, and is the preferred investigative test in upper GI bleeding. Volume resuscitation or blood transfusion should precede endoscopy in hemodynamically unstable patients. Patients with ongoing bleeding or at risk

Table 18-1	Rockall Score for Risk Stratification of Acute Upper Gastrointestinal Bleeding	
	Variable	**Points**
Clinical Rockall Score	Age	
	<60 yrs	0
	60–79 yrs	1
	≥80 yrs	2
	Shock	
	Heart rate >100 bpm	1
	Systolic blood pressure <100 mm Hg	2
	Coexisting illness	
	Coronary artery disease, congestive heart failure, other major illness	2
	Renal failure, hepatic failure, metastatic cancer	3
	Endoscopic diagnosis	
	No finding, Mallory–Weiss tear	0
	Peptic ulcer, erosive disease, esophagitis	1
	Cancer of the upper GI tract	2
	Endoscopic stigmata of recent bleeding	
	Clean based ulcer, flat pigmented spot	0
	Blood in upper GI tract, active bleeding, visible vessel, clot	2

(Left bracket labels: "Complete Rockall Score" spans the Clinical Rockall Score and additional variables.)

A clinical score of 0 or a complete score of 2 or less indicate low risk for rebleeding or death.
GI, gastrointestinal.
Adapted from Gralnek IM, Barkun AN, Bardou M. Management of acute bleeding from a peptic ulcer. *N Engl J Med.* 2008;359:928, with permission.

for an adverse outcome (Table 18-1) benefit most from urgent EGD, while stable patients can be endoscoped electively during the hospitalization. Intravenous (IV) erythromycin (infusion of 125 to 250 mg completed 30 minutes before EGD) empties the stomach of blood and clots, and improves visibility for EGD (*Gastrointest Endosc 2011;73:245*). Second-look EGD after hemostasis has no proven benefit in reducing surgical intervention or overall mortality (*J Gastroenterol Hepatol 2010;25:8*).

○ **Colonoscopy** can be performed after a rapid bowel purge in clinically stable patients; the purge solution can be infused through an NG tube when not tolerated orally. While diagnostic yield is highest with colonoscopy performed within 24 hours of presentation, (*Am J Gastroenterol 2005;100:2395*), patient outcome does not necessarily improve during the initial 24 hours (*Am J Gastroenterol 2010;105:2636*). Therapeutic colonoscopy, however, may reduce transfusion requirements, need for surgery, and length of hospital stay. All patients with acute lower GI bleeding from an unknown source should eventually undergo colonoscopy during the initial hospitalization, regardless of the initial mode of investigation.

○ **Anoscopy** may be useful in the detection of internal hemorrhoids and anal fissures but does not replace need for colonoscopy.

○ **Push enteroscopy** allows evaluation of the proximal small bowel beyond reach of a standard EGD, especially if no source is found on careful colonoscopy.

○ **Capsule endoscopy** is most useful after the upper gut and the colon have been thoroughly examined and the bleeding source is expected in the small bowel (*Gastroenterology 2007;133:1697*). Capsule endoscopy has diagnostic value in acute obscure-overt GI bleeding. However, images cannot be viewed in real time, exact localization within the small bowel cannot be pinpointed, and therapy cannot be administered; consequently, improvements in diagnostic yield do not translate into better outcomes (*Gastroenterology 2010;138:1673*).

○ **Single- and double-balloon enteroscopy** allow visualization of most of the small bowel through either an oral or anal approach. Balloons at the endoscope tip and overtube can be consecutively inflated and deflated while inserting and pulling out the endoscope to allow bowel to pleat over the overtube, thus allowing deep endoscope insertion into the small bowel. Double-balloon enteroscopy affords valuable adjunctive insight and therapeutic potential, especially for lesions detected on capsule endoscopy (*Endoscopy 2009;41:587*).

○ **Intraoperative enteroscopy** may assist endoscopic therapy or surgical resection of an actively bleeding source in the small bowel. The surgeon, through an abdominal incision, advances the endoscope (inserted either through the mouth, the anus, or an enterotomy) by pleating bowel over the instrument.

○ **Spiral enteroscopy** and **power-driven enteroscopy** represent two new promising enteroscopy techniques for evaluating the small bowel (*Endoscopy 2011;43:477*).

• **Computed tomography (CT) enteroclysis** has value when both conventional endoscopy and capsule endoscopy are nondiagnostic in obscure-overt bleeding with prominent anemia (*Gastrointest Endosc 2011;73:1002*).

• **Tagged red blood cell (TRBC) scanning** involves labeling red blood cells (RBCs) with technetium-99m that may extravasate into the bowel lumen with active bleeding, detected as pooling of the radioactive tracer on gamma camera scanning. The pattern of peristaltic movement of the pooled tracer can help identify the potential site of bleeding (*Dis Colon Rectum 1997;40:471*). **CT angiography** may have similar benefit in localizing bleeding prior to catheter angiography (*J Vasc Interv Radiol 2010;21:848*). These tests are useful in unstable active bleeding precluding urgent colonoscopy.

• **Arteriography** demonstrates extravasation of the dye into the intestine when bleeding rates exceed 0.5 mL/min, thereby localizing bleeding. Arteriography is often performed after bleeding is initially localized by other means. Superselective cannulation and infusion of vasopressin vasoconstricts the bleeding vessel: alternatively, the vessel can be embolized (*Am J Gastroenterol 2005;100:2395*). Methylene blue staining of the bleeding bowel segment at arteriography helps the surgeon if resection is indicated. In upper GI bleeding, arteriography is reserved for situations where brisk bleeding makes endoscopy difficult.

TREATMENT

• **Restoration of intravascular volume.** Two large-bore (16- to 18-gauge) IV lines or a central venous line should be urgently placed. Isotonic saline, lactated Ringer solution, or 5% hetastarch can be initiated. Circulatory shock may require volume administration using pressure infusion devices or hand infused using large syringes and stopcocks, guided by the patient's condition and degree of volume loss (*N Engl J Med 2008;359:928*). **Packed RBC transfusion** should be used for volume replacement whenever possible; O-negative blood or simultaneous multiple-unit transfusions may be indicated if bleeding is massive. Transfusion should be continued until hemodynamic stability is achieved and the hematocrit reaches ≥25% to 30%. Overcorrection of volume and blood counts does not necessarily improve outcome, and may be detrimental in variceal bleeding (*Aliment Pharmacol Ther. 2010;32:215*). Vasopressors are generally not indicated, although transient IV pressor therapy is sometimes beneficial until enough volume is infused.

- **Oxygen administration.** Supplemental oxygen enhances the oxygen-carrying capacity of blood, and should be universally administered in acute GI bleeding.
- **Correction of coagulopathy.** Coagulopathy (INR ≥1.5) increases morbidity and mortality in acute GI bleeding (*Aliment Pharmacol Ther. 2011;33:1010*), and should be corrected. After discontinuation of warfarin, an initial infusion of 2 to 4 units of fresh frozen plasma (FFP) can be supplemented with further infusion after reassessment of INR. Parenteral vitamin K (10 mg SC or intramuscular [IM]) also corrects prolonged prothrombin time from warfarin therapy or hepatobiliary disease in several hours to days. Protamine infusion (1 mg antagonizes ~100 units of heparin) reverses anticoagulation from heparin infusion. Platelet infusion may be indicated when the platelet count is <50,000/mm^3.
- **Endotracheal intubation** protects the airway and prevents aspiration in obtunded patients (shock, hepatic encephalopathy) with massive hematemesis and in active variceal bleeding.
- **Risk stratification.** Validated risk stratification tools, such as the Rockall and Glasgow Blatchford Scores, are available to identify patients at highest risk for an adverse outcome (*Aliment Pharmacol Ther. 2011;34:470*). The Rockall score (see Table 18-1) has a *clinical* component that is rapidly calculated at presentation, and a *complete* final score that takes endoscopic findings into account (*Gut 1996;38:316*).

Medications

- **Nonvariceal upper GI bleeding.** IV **proton pump inhibitors** (PPIs) reduce the rate of recurrent bleeding, rebleeding after initial hemostasis, need for surgery and mortality in bleeding peptic ulcer disease (PUD) (*Am J Gastroenterol 2004;99:1238*; *Br J Surg 2011;98:640*). IV infusions of PPI (e.g., 80 mg IV bolus followed by 8 mg/h continuous infusion for 72 hours) may have value in ongoing PUD bleeding; however, meta-analysis does not demonstrate benefits in rates of rebleeding, surgical intervention, or mortality between IV infusions and IV bolus therapy in unselected cases (*Arch Intern Med 2010;170:751*). However, PPI therapy, IV or oral (e.g., omeprazole 40 mg PO bid or equivalent), is more effective than IV histamine-2 receptor antagonist (H$_2$RA) therapy. **Thalidomide** may be an effective approach for refractory chronic bleeding from GI vascular malformations (*Gastroenterology 2011;141:1629*).
- **Variceal bleeding. Octreotide** infusion acutely reduces portal pressures and controls variceal bleeding with very few side effects, improving the diagnostic yield and therapeutic success of subsequent endoscopy. Octreotide should be initiated immediately (50- to 100-μg bolus, followed by infusion at 25 to 50 μg/hr), and continued for 3 to 5 days (*Hepatology 2007;46:922*). **Vasopressin** (0.3 U/min IV, titrated by increments of 0.1 U/min q30 min until hemostasis is achieved, side effects develop, or the maximum dose of 0.9 U/min is reached) is an alternative agent, rarely used because of significant cardiovascular complications including

cardiac arrest and myocardial infarction. Concomitant infusion of **nitroglycerin** (10 μg/min IV, increased by 10 μg/min q10–15 min until the systolic BP falls to 100 mm Hg or a maximum dose of 400 μg/min is reached) may reduce undesirable cardiovascular side effects and provide more effective control of bleeding. May reduce undesirable cardiovascular side effects and provide more effective control of bleeding but can only be used if the systolic BP is >100 mm Hg. **Terlipressin** has been shown to be as effective as octreotide for controlling variceal bleeding (*Am J Gastroenterol 2009;104:617*). Antibiotic prophylaxis with a fluoroquinolone (**norfloxacin** or **ciprofloxacin**) is recommended in any patient with cirrhosis and variceal bleeding; **ceftriaxone** (1 g/d) is an alternative (*Hepatology 2007;46:922*).

Other Nonpharmacologic Therapies

- **Endoscopic therapy**
  - **Therapeutic endoscopy** offers the advantage of immediate treatment, and should be implemented early in acute upper GI bleeding (within 12 to 24 hours).
  - **Variceal ligation** or **banding** is the endoscopic therapy of choice for esophageal varices, in the emergency room or intensive care unit (ICU), and with endotracheal intubation if bleeding is massive or the patient is obtunded (*Hepatology 2007;46:922*). Variceal banding has value in both primary and secondary prophylaxis of variceal bleeding, with benefits similar to that from β-blocker therapy alone (*Gastroenterology 2010;139:1238*). Complications include superficial ulceration, dysphagia, and transient chest discomfort.
  - **Sclerotherapy** is also effective but is used mostly when variceal banding is not technically feasible because of complications (ulcerations, strictures, perforation, pleural effusions, adult respiratory distress syndrome, sepsis).
  - Endoscopic injection of **cyanoacrylate (glue)** is more effective than β-blocker therapy in primary and secondary prophylaxis of gastric variceal bleeding (*Gut 2010;59:729*) but not esophageal variceal bleeding.
  - Newer modalities of therapy include **hemosprays** of nanopowders with clotting properties during endoscopy, but further research is needed.
- **Transjugular intrahepatic portosystemic shunt (TIPS)** is a radiologic procedure wherein an expandable metal stent is deployed between the hepatic veins and the portal vein to reduce portal venous pressure in refractory esophageal and/or gastric variceal bleeding from portal hypertension (*Hepatology 2007;46:922*). Early TIPS may be of value in reducing treatment failure and mortality in acute variceal bleeding (*N Engl J Med 2010;362:2370*). Encephalopathy may occur in up to 25% of patients and is treated medically (see Chapter 19, Liver Diseases). TIPS stenosis responds to balloon dilation; screening with duplex Doppler ultrasound is recommended if variceal bleeding recurs, or if esophageal or gastric varices redevelop.
- **Balloon-occluded retrograde transvenous obliteration (BRTO)** is a new rescue treatment option for gastric variceal bleeding, wherein gastric varices are approached and obliterated through a gastrorenal shunt (*J Gastroenterol Hepatol 2009;24:372*).

Surgical Management

- **Emergent total colectomy** may rarely be required as a lifesaving maneuver for massive, unlocalized, colonic bleeding; this should be preceded by emergent EGD to rule out a rapidly bleeding upper source whenever possible. Certain lesions (e.g., neoplasia, Meckel's diverticulum) require surgical resection for a cure.
- **Total or partial colectomy** may be required for diverticular bleeding. Ongoing bleeding with transfusion requirements exceeding 4 to 6 units over 24 hours or

10 units overall, or more than two to three recurrent bleeding episodes from the same source are indications.
- **Splenectomy** is curative in bleeding gastric varices from splenic vein thrombosis.
- **Shunt surgery** (portacaval or distal splenorenal shunt) should be considered in patients with good hepatic reserve.

SPECIAL CONSIDERATIONS

Cardiac Patients and Gastrointestinal Bleeding

- In acute coronary syndromes (ACSs), GI bleeding increases 30-day all-cause mortality rates by a factor of almost 5, with significant increase in cardiac mortality and ischemic complications (*J Am Coll Cardiol 2009;29:1293*). Dual antiplatelet agents (e.g., aspirin plus clopidogrel) is the most important risk factor. Among patients on low-dose aspirin with history of PUD bleeding, continuous aspirin therapy increases the risk for recurrent PUD bleeding (*Ann Intern Med 2010;152:1*).
- **PPI prophylaxis** decreases the risk of GI bleeding, including settings of dual antiplatelet agents, without significant effects on the incidence of hospital-acquired pneumonia or 30-day mortality (*J Crit Care 2011;26:434*; *Aliment Pharmacol Ther. 2011;34:519*).
- Despite concerns that PPIs competitively inhibit the cytochrome P450 enzyme that activates clopidogrel, randomized controlled trials have not substantiated higher vascular events with concurrent use of clopidogrel and PPI (*N Engl J Med 2010;11:363*). Although conflicting data exist, genetic variations in enzyme expression may play an important role in clopidogrel failure. Among PPIs, pantoprazole may have the least pharmacodynamic interaction with clopidogrel (*Eur J Gastroenterol Hepatol 2011;23:396*).
- **Left ventricular assist devices (LVADs)**, used in end-stage heart failure, are associated with GI bleeding rates significantly higher than that seen with dual antiplatelet therapy or anticoagulation. Bleeding is predominantly overt and from an upper GI source (*Gastrointest Endosc 2012;75:973*; *J Card Surg 2010;25:352*), making EGD or push enteroscopy the investigation of choice. Sedation and endoscopy are safe in LVAD recipients.

Dysphagia and Odynophagia

GENERAL PRINCIPLES

Definition

- **Oropharyngeal dysphagia** consists of difficulty in transferring food from the mouth to the esophagus, often associated with nasopharyngeal regurgitation and aspiration.
- **Esophageal dysphagia** is the sensation of impairment in passage of food down the tubular esophagus.
- **Odynophagia** is pain on swallowing food and fluids, and may indicate the presence of esophagitis, particularly infectious esophagitis and pill esophagitis.

Etiology

- **Oropharyngeal dysphagia** is typically caused by neuromuscular or structural disorders involving the pharynx and proximal esophagus (*Gastroenterology 1999; 116:452*).

- **Esophageal dysphagia** can occur from an obstructive process in the esophagus (*Gastroenterology 1999;117:233*). Progressive dysphagia may be seen with neoplasia, while intermittent symptoms can result from webs or rings. Acute onset of dysphagia following a meal may suggest food impaction. In the absence of a structural obstructive process, an esophageal motility disorder may be responsible for dysphagia.

DIAGNOSIS

Oropharyngeal Dysphagia

- Assessment is initiated with a detailed neurologic exam. Barium videofluoroscopy (modified barium swallow) evaluates the oropharyngeal swallow mechanism and may identify laryngeal penetration.
- Ear, nose, and throat exam; flexible nasal endoscopy; and imaging studies may identify structural etiologies.
- Laboratory tests for polymyositis, myasthenia gravis, and other neuromuscular disorders can be considered in the absence of neurologic and structural etiologies.

Esophageal Dysphagia

- Endoscopy is the test of choice in almost all situations. Endoscopy provides information on mucosal abnormalities, allows tissue sampling, and offers the option of dilation if a stricture is identified (*Gastroenterology 1999;117:233*).
- Barium swallow has value in defining anatomy, especially subtle rings and strictures, which may only be seen with a barium pill or a solid barium bolus.
- Acute esophageal obstruction is best investigated with endoscopy. Barium studies should not be performed when esophageal obstruction is expected, as it may take several days for barium to clear, thereby delaying endoscopy.
- Esophageal manometry is indicated when other studies are normal or suggest a motility disorder. High resolution manometry (HRM), with spatiotemporal display of esophageal motor phenomena, has several benefits over conventional manometry, including easier analysis (*Gut 2012;61:798*) and accurate diagnosis of esophageal outflow obstruction (*Am J Physiol 2007;293:G878*).

TREATMENT

- Modification of diet and swallowing maneuvers may benefit patients with dysphagia, especially oropharyngeal dysphagia. Patients with dysphagia are typically advised to chew their food well and eat foods of soft consistencies.
- Enteral feeding through a gastrostomy tube is indicated in patients with frank tracheal aspiration on attempted swallowing.
- Endoscopic retrieval of an obstructing food bolus relieves acute dysphagia.
- Nutrition needs to be addressed in patients with prolonged dysphagia causing weight loss.

Medications

- Mucosal inflammation from reflux disease can be treated with acid suppression.
- Odynophagia generally responds to specific therapy when the cause is identified (e.g., PPIs for reflux disease, antimicrobial agents for infectious esophagitis). Viscous lidocaine swish-and-swallow solutions may afford symptomatic relief.

- Anticholinergic medication (e.g., transdermal scopolamine) helps drooling of saliva.
- **Glucagon** (2 to 4 mg IV bolus) or sublingual **nitroglycerin** can be attempted in acute food impaction, but meat tenderizer should not be administered.

Other Nonpharmacologic Therapies

Endoscopic Therapy

- Esophageal dilation is performed for anatomic narrowings. Empiric dilation performed when a defined narrowing is not identified may also provide symptomatic benefit.
- Aggressive pneumatic dilation of the lower esophageal sphincter (LES) is sometimes performed for achalasia (see Esophageal Motor Disorders section). Botulinum toxin injections into the LES provide temporary symptom relief in achalasia and in errors of LES relaxation.
- Esophageal stent placement can alleviate dysphagia in inoperable neoplasia.

Nausea and Vomiting

GENERAL PRINCIPLES

- Nausea and vomiting may result from side effects of medications, systemic illnesses, central nervous system (CNS) disorders, and primary GI disorders.
- Vomiting that occurs during or immediately after a meal can result from acute pyloric stenosis (e.g., pyloric channel ulcer) or from functional disorders, while vomiting within 30 to 60 minutes after a meal may suggest gastric or duodenal pathology. Delayed vomiting after a meal with undigested food from a previous meal can suggest gastric outlet obstruction or gastroparesis.

DIAGNOSIS

- **Bowel obstruction and pregnancy should be ruled out.**
- Medication lists should be scrutinized, and systemic illnesses (acute and chronic) should be evaluated as etiologies or contributing factors.

TREATMENT

- Correction of fluid and electrolyte imbalances is an important supportive measure.
- Oral intake should be withheld or limited to clear liquids. Many patients with self-limited illnesses require no further therapy.
- NG decompression may be required for patients with bowel obstruction or protracted nausea and vomiting of any etiology.
- Patients with protracted nausea and vomiting may sometimes require enteral feeding through jejunal tubes, or rarely even total parenteral nutrition (TPN).

Medications

Empiric pharmacotherapy is often initiated while investigation is in progress, or when the etiology is thought to be self-limited.

- **Phenothiazines and related agents.** Prochlorperazine (Compazine), 5 to 10 mg PO tid–qid, 10 mg IM or IV q6h, or 25 mg PR bid; promethazine (Phenergan),

12.5 to 25.0 mg PO, IM, or PR q4–6h; and trimethobenzamide (Tigan), 250 mg PO tid–qid, or 200 mg IM tid–qid are effective. Drowsiness is a common side effect, and acute dystonic reactions or other extrapyramidal effects may occur.

- **Dopamine antagonists** include metoclopramide (10 mg PO 30 minutes before meals and at bedtime, or 10 mg IV PRN), a prokinetic agent that also has central antiemetic effects. Drowsiness and extrapyramidal reactions may occur, and a warning has been issued by the U.S. Food and Drug Administration (FDA) regarding the risk of permanent **tardive dyskinesia** with high-dose or long-term use (*Aliment Pharmacol Ther. 2010;31:11*). Tachyphylaxis may limit long-term efficacy. Domperidone is an alternate agent that does not cross the blood–brain barrier and therefore has no CNS side effects; however, it is not uniformly available.
- **Antihistaminic agents** are most useful for nausea and vomiting related to motion sickness but may also be useful for other causes. Agents used include diphenhydramine (Benadryl, 25 to 50 mg PO q6–8h, or 10 to 50 mg IV q2–4h), dimenhydrinate (Dramamine, 50 to 100 mg PO or IV q4–6h), and meclizine (Antivert, 12.5 to 25.0 mg 1 hour before travel).
- **Serotonin 5-HT$_3$ receptor antagonists. Ondansetron** (Zofran, 0.15 mg/kg IV q4h for three doses or 32 mg IV infused over 15 minutes beginning 30 minutes before chemotherapy) is effective in chemotherapy-associated emesis. It can also be used in emesis that is refractory to other medications (4 to 8 mg PO or IV up to q8h), especially the sublingual formulation. **Granisetron** (Kytril, 10 μg/kg IV for one to three doses 10 minutes apart, or 1 mg PO bid) is also effective.
- **Neurokinin-1 (NK-1) receptor antagonist. Aprepitant** (Emend, 125 mg PO day 1, 80 mg PO days 2 and 3) is an alternative agent currently indicated **only for chemotherapy-induced nausea and vomiting**.

Diarrhea

GENERAL PRINCIPLES

- **Acute diarrhea** consists of abrupt onset of increased frequency and/or fluidity of bowel movements. Infectious agents, toxins, and drugs are the major causes of acute diarrhea. In hospitalized patients, pseudomembranous colitis, antibiotic- or drug-associated diarrhea, and fecal impaction should be considered (*Gastroenterology 2004;127:287*).
- **Chronic diarrhea** consists of passage of loose stools with or without increased stool frequency for more than 4 weeks.

DIAGNOSIS

- Most acute infectious diarrheal illnesses last less than 24 hours and could be viral in etiology; therefore, stool studies are unnecessary in short-lived episodes without fever, dehydration, or presence of blood or pus in the stool (*N Engl J Med 2004;350:38*).
- Stool cultures, *Clostridium difficile* toxin assay, ova and parasite examinations, and sigmoidoscopy may be warranted in patients with severe, prolonged, or atypical symptoms.

- The **fecal osmotic gap** can be calculated in patients with chronic diarrhea and voluminous watery stools as follows: $290 - 2(\text{stool } [Na^+] + \text{stool } [K^+])$. The osmotic gap is **<50 mOsm/kg in secretory diarrhea** but **>125 mOsm/kg in osmotic diarrhea**.
- A positive fecal occult blood test or fecal leukocyte test suggests inflammatory diarrhea.
- Steatorrhea is traditionally diagnosed by demonstration of fat excretion in stool of >7 g/d in a 72-hour stool collection while the patient is on a 100-g/d fat diet. Sudan staining of a stool specimen is an alternate test; >100 fat globules per high-power field (HPF) is abnormal.
- Laxative screening should be considered when chronic diarrhea remains undiagnosed.

Clinical Presentation

- **Acute diarrhea**
  - **Viral enteritis** and **bacterial infections** with *E. coli*, *Shigella*, *Salmonella*, *Campylobacter*, and *Yersinia* species constitute the most common causes.
  - **Pseudomembranous colitis** is usually seen in the setting of antimicrobial therapy and is caused by toxins produced by *C. difficile*.
  - **Giardiasis** is confirmed by identification of *Giardia lamblia* trophozoites in the stool, in duodenal aspirate, or in small-bowel biopsy specimens. A stool immunofluorescence assay is also available for rapid diagnosis.
  - **Amebiasis** may cause acute diarrhea, especially in travelers to areas with poor sanitation and in homosexual men. Stool examination for trophozoites or cysts of *Entamoeba histolytica* or a serum antibody test confirms the diagnosis.
  - **Medications** including laxatives, antacids, cardiac medications (e.g., digitalis, quinidine), colchicine, and antimicrobial agents. Symptoms usually respond to discontinuation of the offending agent.
  - **Graft-versus-host disease** needs to be considered when diarrhea develops after organ transplantation, especially bone marrow transplantation.
- **Chronic diarrhea.** After a careful history, a thorough physical examination, and routine laboratory tests, chronic diarrhea can typically be classified into one of the following categories: watery diarrhea (secretory or osmotic), inflammatory diarrhea, or fatty diarrhea (steatorrhea) (*Gastroenterology 2004;127:287*).

TREATMENT

- Adequate hydration is an essential initial step in the therapy of diarrheal disease. IV hydration is required in severe cases.
- Antibiotic-associated diarrhea and *C. difficile* infections can be prevented by restricting high-risk antibiotics and using antibiotics based on sensitivity analysis.
- Symptomatic therapy is useful in simple self-limiting GI infections where diarrhea is frequent or troublesome, while diagnostic workup is in progress, when specific management fails to improve symptoms, or when a specific etiology is not identified.
  - **Loperamide**, 2 to 4 mg up to four times a day, **opiates** (tincture of opium; belladonna; and opium capsules), and **anticholinergic agents** (diphenoxylate and atropine [Lomotil], 15 to 20 mg/d of diphenoxylate in divided doses) are the most effective nonspecific antidiarrheal agents.

- ○ **Pectin** and **kaolin** preparations (bind toxins) and **bismuth subsalicylate** (antibacterial properties) are also useful in symptomatic therapy of acute diarrhea.
- ○ **Bile acid–binding resins** (e.g., cholestyramine, 1 g up to qid) are beneficial in bile acid–induced diarrhea.
- ○ **Octreotide** (100 to 200 μg bid–qid PRN) is useful in hormone-mediated secretory diarrhea but can be of benefit in refractory diarrhea.

Medications

- **Empiric antibiotic therapy** is only recommended in patients with moderate-to-severe disease and associated systemic symptoms, while awaiting stool cultures. Antibiotics can increase the possibility of hemolytic–uremic syndrome associated with shiga toxin producing *Escherichia coli* infections (*E. coli* O157:H7), especially in children and the elderly (*N Engl J Med 2000;342:1930*). Useful agents include **fluoroquinolones** (ciprofloxacin, 500 mg PO bid for 3 days, or norfloxacin, 400 mg PO bid for 3 days) and **trimethoprim–sulfamethoxazole** (160 mg/800 mg PO bid for 5 days).
- Oral **metronidazole** is the treatment of choice for pseudomembranous colitis. Oral **vancomycin** is reserved for resistant cases or intolerance to metronidazole. **Fidaxomicin** and stool transplant are newer options being studied (see Chapter 14, Treatment of Infectious Diseases).
- Symptomatic amebiasis is treated with **metronidazole**, 750 mg PO tid or 500 mg IV q8h for 5 to 10 days. This should be followed by **paromomycin**, 500 mg PO tid for 7 days, or **iodoquinol**, 650 mg PO tid for 20 days, to eliminate cysts.
- Therapy for giardiasis consists of metronidazole, 250 mg PO tid for 5 to 7 days, or tinidazole, 2-g single dose. Quinacrine, 100 mg PO tid for 7 days, is an alternative agent.

SPECIAL CONSIDERATIONS

Diarrhea in HIV Disease

- Opportunistic agents, including *Cryptosporidium*, *Microsporidium*, cytomegalovirus (CMV), *Mycobacterium avium* complex, and *Mycobacterium tuberculosis*, may cause diarrhea in patients with advanced HIV (CD4 counts <50 cells/μL). However, *C. difficile* may be the most commonly identified bacterial pathogen (*Gut 2008;57:861*).
- Other causes of diarrhea in this population include venereal infections (syphilis, gonorrhea, chlamydiosis, herpes simplex virus [HSV]) as well as other nonvenereal infections (amebiasis, giardiasis, salmonellosis, shigellosis). Intestinal lymphoma and Kaposi sarcoma can also cause diarrhea.
- Stool studies (ova and parasites, culture), endoscopic biopsies, and serologic testing may assist diagnosis. Management consists of specific therapy if pathogens are identified; symptomatic measures may be of benefit in idiopathic cases.
- Missed pathogens are an important cause of undiagnosed diarrhea. Drugs, antibiotics, HIV as a pathogen, autonomic disturbance, and abnormal motility may contribute.

Constipation

GENERAL PRINCIPLES

Definition

Constipation consists of infrequent (and frequently incomplete) bowel movements, sometimes associated with straining and passage of pellet-like stools.

Etiology

- A recent change in bowel habits may indicate an organic cause, whereas long-standing constipation is more likely functional.
- Medication (e.g., calcium blockers, opiates, anticholinergics, iron supplements, barium sulfate) and systemic disease (e.g., diabetes mellitus, hypothyroidism, systemic sclerosis, myotonic dystrophy) may contribute.
- Female gender, older age, lack of exercise, low caloric intake, low-fiber diet, and disorders that cause pain on defecation (e.g., anal fissures, thrombosed external hemorrhoids) are other risk factors (*Am Fam Physician 2011;84:299*).

DIAGNOSIS

- Colonoscopy and barium studies help rule out structural disease and may be particularly important in individuals >50 years without prior colorectal cancer screening, or with other alarm situations such as anemia, blood in the stool, and new onset symptoms (*Gastroenterology 2000;119:1761*).
- Colonic transit studies, anorectal manometry, and defecography are reserved for resistant cases without a structural explanation after initial workup.

TREATMENT

- Regular exercise and adequate fluid intake are nonspecific measures.
- Increase in **dietary fiber** intake to 20 to 30 g/d may have value. Fecal impactions should be resolved before fiber supplementation is initiated. Wheat bran or psyllium two to four times a day can be initiated with increased fluid intake. Transient bloating often occurs.

Medications

- **Laxatives**
  - **Emollient laxatives** such as docusate sodium, 50 to 200 mg PO daily, and docusate calcium, 240 mg PO daily, allow water and fat to penetrate the fecal mass. Mineral oil (15 to 45 mL PO q6–8h) can be given orally or by enema. Tracheobronchial aspiration of mineral oil can result in lipoid pneumonia.
  - **Stimulant cathartics** such as castor oil, 15 mL PO, stimulate intestinal secretion and increase intestinal motility. Anthraquinones (cascara, 5 mL PO daily; senna, one tablet PO daily to qid) stimulate the colon by increasing fluid and water accumulation in the proximal colon. Bisacodyl (10 to 15 mg PO at bedtime, 10-mg rectal suppositories) is structurally similar to phenolphthalein and stimulates colonic peristalsis, resulting in effective and well-tolerated treatment for chronic constipation (*Clin Gastroenterol Hepatol 2011;9:577*).

○ **Osmotic cathartics** include nonabsorbable salts or carbohydrates that cause water retention in the lumen of the colon. Magnesium salts include milk of magnesia (15 to 30 mL q8–12h) and magnesium citrate (200 mL PO), to be avoided in renal failure. Lactulose (15 to 30 mL PO bid–qid) can cause bloating as a side effect.

○ **Lubiprostone** (8 to 24 mcg PO bid) is a selective intestinal chloride channel activator, causing movement of fluid into the bowel lumen and stimulating peristalsis (*Dig Dis Sci 2010;55:1090*).

○ **Linaclotide** (145 to 290 mcg PO qd) is an agonist of the guanylate cyclase C receptor and also causes movement of fluid into the intestinal lumen, thereby improving symptoms of constipation (*N Engl J Med 2011;365:567*).

• **Enemas.** Sodium biphosphate (Fleet) enemas (one to two rectally PRN) can be used for mild-to-moderate constipation and for bowel cleansing before sigmoidoscopy; these should be avoided in renal failure. Tap water enemas (1 L) are also useful. Oil-based enemas (cottonseed colace, hypaque) are used in refractory constipation.

• **Other agents.** Polyethylene glycol in powder form (MiraLax, 17 g PO daily to bid) can be used regularly or intermittently for the treatment of constipation. Subcutaneous methylnaltrexone, a selective peripherally acting μ-opioid receptor antagonist, is effective for rapid relief of opioid-induced constipation (*N Engl J Med 2008;358:2332*). Prucalopride is approved in Europe for chronic constipation (*Aliment Pharmacol Ther. 2010;32:1113*).

• **Bowel-cleansing agents.** Patients should be placed on a clear liquid diet the previous day and kept NPO for 6 hours or overnight prior to bowel examination (colonoscopy or barium enema). Dehydration is avoided. Patients may experience mild abdominal discomfort, nausea, and vomiting with the bowel preparation.

○ An iso-osmotic **polyethylene glycol solution** (PEG, GoLYTELY or NuLYTELY, 1 gallon, administered at a rate of 8 oz every 10 minutes) is commonly used as a bowel-cleansing agent before colonoscopy. Lower-volume preparations, such as PEG (2 liters or 0.5 gallon) with ascorbic acid or other laxatives are alternatives (*Aliment Pharmacol Ther. 2010;32:637*). When the preparation is inadequate, more of the iso-osmotic solution can be administered until the stool is clear.

▪ **Nonabsorbable phosphate** (Fleet phosphosoda, 20 to 45 mL with 10 to 24 oz liquid, taken the day before and morning of the procedure), a hyperosmotic solution, draws fluid into the gut lumen and produces bowel movements in 0.5 to 6.0 hours. It is also available in pill form (Visicol or OsmoPrep, 32 to 40 tablets, taken at the rate of 3 to 4 tablets every 15 min with 8 oz fluid). Phosphosoda can result in severe dehydration, hyperphosphatemia, hypocalcemia, hypokalemia, hypernatremia, and acidosis. A dreaded rare complication is **acute phosphate nephropathy**, where calcium phosphate deposits cause irreversible dysfunction of renal tubules resulting in renal failure. Consequently, phosphosoda is used in limited instances.

○ **Split preparations.** Proximity of bowel preparation to procedure time improves effectiveness of cleansing and visualization during the procedure. Therefore, splitting bowel preparation into two doses may be useful, one dose administered the evening prior, and the second dose the morning of the procedure (*Am J Gastroenterol 2010;105:1319*), especially for colonoscopy scheduled in the afternoon hours.

○ **Two-day bowel preparation** is sometimes indicated in elderly or debilitated individuals when conventional bowel preparation is contraindicated, not tolerated, or ineffective. This consists of magnesium citrate (120 to 300 mL PO) adminis-

tered on 2 consecutive days while the patient remains on a clear liquid diet; Bisacodyl (30 mg PO or 10-mg suppository) is administered on both days.
   ○ **Tap water enemas** (1-L volume, repeated one to two times) can cleanse the distal colon when colonoscopy is indicated in patients with proximal bowel obstruction.
 • Other options: **Biofeedback therapy** and **sacral nerve stimulation** can be effective for idiopathic constipation resistant to medical treatment (*Gut 2010;59:333, 1288*).

LUMINAL GASTROINTESTINAL DISORDERS

Gastroesophageal Reflux Disease

GENERAL PRINCIPLES

Definition

Gastroesophageal reflux disease (GERD) is defined as symptoms and/or complications resulting from reflux of gastric contents into the esophagus and more proximal structures.

DIAGNOSIS

Clinical Presentation

 • Typical **esophageal symptoms** of GERD include heartburn and regurgitation. GERD can also present as **atypical chest pain**, where an important priority is to first exclude a cardiac source (*Am J Gastroenterol 2006;101:1900*).
 • **Extraesophageal manifestations** include cough, laryngitis, asthma, and dental erosions. A GERD association has been proposed for sinusitis, pulmonary fibrosis, pharyngitis, and recurrent otitis media under certain circumstances (*Am J Gastroenterol 2006;101:1900*).
 • Symptom response to a therapeutic trial of PPIs can be diagnostic, but a negative response does not exclude GERD (*Gastroenterology 2008;135:1392*).

Differential Diagnosis

Other disorders that can result in esophagitis include:
 • **Eosinophilic esophagitis (EoE)** is characterized by eosinophilic infiltration of esophageal mucosa. Atopy (allergic rhinitis, eczema, asthma) is common, and food allergens may trigger the process. Transit symptoms (dysphagia) are prominent, but symptoms can also mimic GERD. Common endoscopic findings include furrows, luminal narrowing, corrugations, and whitish plaques in the esophageal mucosa. The diagnosis of EoE is a clinicopathologic one, consisting of (1) symptoms including food impaction and dysphagia, (2) ≥15 eosinophils per HPF on esophageal biopsies, and (3) exclusion of other disorders including GERD (*Gastroenterology 2007;133:1342*). Food allergen testing can be considered, but the yield is typically low. Regardless, elimination of dietary allergens is appropriate when identified. Concomitant GERD requires PPI therapy. Specific treatment options include topical (swallowed fluticasone, 880 to 1,760 µg/d in two to four divided doses) and less commonly systemic corticosteroids (budesonide 1 mg twice daily for

15 days) (*Gastroenterology 2010;139:1526*). Mepolizumab, a humanized anti-interleukin [IL]-5 monoclonal antibody, decreases esophageal eosinophilia in clinically refractory EoE (*Gut 2010;59:21*). Cautious dilation of strictures can be considered if steroid therapy is unsuccessful, as the risk of perforation in EoE may not be as high as previously thought (*Dig Dis Sci 2010;55:1512*).

- **Infectious esophagitis** is seen most often in immunocompromised states (AIDS, organ transplant recipients), esophageal stasis (abnormal motility [e.g., achalasia, scleroderma], mechanical obstruction [e.g., strictures]), malignancy, diabetes mellitus, and antibiotic use. However, HSV and varicella esophagitis can rarely occur in the normal healthy host. The presence of typical oral lesions (thrush, herpetic vesicles) may suggest an etiologic agent. The usual presenting symptoms are dysphagia and odynophagia.

  ○ *Candida* **esophagitis** is the most common esophageal infection, and typically occurs in the setting of esophageal stasis, impaired cell-mediated immunity from immunosuppressive therapy (e.g., with steroids or cytotoxic agents), malignancies, or AIDS. Endoscopic visualization of typical whitish plaques has near 100% sensitivity for diagnosis. Empiric antifungal agents are appropriate when concurrent oropharyngeal thrush is present, reserving endoscopy for nonresponse. **Fluconazole** 100 to 200 mg/d or **itraconazole** 200 mg/d for 14 to 21 days is recommended as initial therapy for *Candida* esophagitis; nystatin (100,000 U/mL, 5 mL tid for 3 weeks) and clotrimazole troches (10 mg four to five times a day for 2 weeks) are alternatives for oropharyngeal candidiasis. For infections refractory to azoles, a short course of parenteral **amphotericin B** (0.3 to 0.5 mg/kg/d) can be considered (*Best Pract Res Clin Gastroenterol 2008;22:639*).

  ○ **HSV esophagitis** is characterized by small vesicles and well-circumscribed ulcers on endoscopy, and typical giant cells on histopathology. Viral antigen or DNA can be identified by immunofluorescent antibodies. Treatment consists of **acyclovir** 400 to 800 mg PO five times a day for 14 to 21 days or 5 mg/kg IV q8h for 7 to 14 days. **Famciclovir** and **valacyclovir** are alternate agents. The condition is usually self-limited in immunocompetent hosts (*Curr Opin Gastroenterol 2008;24:496*).

  ○ **CMV esophagitis**, which occurs exclusively in immunocompromised hosts, can cause erosions or frank ulcerations. IV therapy with **ganciclovir**, **foscarnet**, or **cidofovir** is effective for a variety of GI CMV infections. **Ganciclovir** 5 mg/kg IV q12h or **foscarnet** 90 mg/kg IV q12h for 3 to 6 weeks can be used as initial therapy. Oral **valganciclovir** may also be effective.

  ○ Symptomatic relief can be achieved with 2% viscous **lidocaine** swish and swallow (15 mL PO q3–4h PRN) or **sucralfate** slurry (1 g PO qid). Concomitant acid suppression should also be administered.

- **Chemical esophagitis**

  ○ Ingestion of caustic agents (alkalis, acids) or medications such as oral potassium, doxycycline, quinidine, iron, NSAIDs, aspirin, and bisphosphonates can result in mucosal irritation and damage.

  ○ Cautious early endoscopy is recommended to evaluate the extent and degree of mucosal damage. With caustic ingestions, the optimal time to perform endoscopy is 24 to 72 hours from ingestion.

  ○ The offending medication should be discontinued if possible. Mucosal coating agents (sucralfate) and acid suppressive agents may help. A second caustic agent to neutralize the first is contraindicated.

- **Nonspecific ulceration** can be seen with medications, malignancy, or AIDS.
  - Endoscopic biopsies, brushings, and culture specimens are essential.
  - Idiopathic ulcer of AIDS may respond to oral steroid or thalidomide therapy.

Diagnostic Testing

- **Endoscopy** is primarily indicated for avoiding misdiagnosis of alternate causes of esophageal symptoms (e.g., EoE), identification of complications, and evaluation of treatment failures. **Warning symptoms** of dysphagia, odynophagia, early satiety, weight loss, or bleeding should prompt endoscopy (*N Engl J Med 2008;359:1700*).
- **Ambulatory pH or pH-impedance monitoring** is used to quantify esophageal acid exposure and reflux events, and for symptom–reflux correlation in patients with ongoing symptoms despite acid suppression (especially if endoscopy is negative) or those with atypical symptoms. pH impedance testing can also determine adequacy of acid suppression in patients with established GERD and ongoing symptoms.
- **Esophageal manometry**, particularly HRM, may identify motor processes contributing to refractory symptoms.

TREATMENT

Medications

- Intermittent or prophylactic over-the-counter **antacids**, **histamine-2 receptor antagonists (H_2RAs)**, and **PPIs** are effective with mild or intermittent symptoms.
- **PPIs** are more effective than standard-dose H_2RA and placebo in symptom relief and endoscopic healing of GERD. Modest gain is achieved by doubling the PPI dose in severe esophagitis or persistent symptoms. Continuous long-term PPI therapy is effective in maintaining remission of GERD symptoms, but the dose should be decreased after 8 to 12 weeks to the lowest dose that achieves symptom relief (*N Engl J Med 2008;359:1700*). Abdominal pain, headache, and diarrhea are common side effects. Long term PPI use has been associated with bone demineralization, enteric infections, community-acquired pneumonia, and reduced circulating levels of vitamin B_{12} in observational studies, but benefits of PPI therapy continue to outweigh risks.
- Standard doses of **H_2RAs** (Table 18-2) can result in symptomatic benefit and endoscopic healing in up to half of patients (*N Engl J Med 2008;359:1700*). Dosage adjustments are required in renal insufficiency.
- **Reflux inhibitors** consist of gamma-aminobutyric acid (GABA) type B receptor agonists that block transient LES relaxations. **Baclofen**, the prototype agent, reduces reflux events, but central side effects can be limiting (*Am J Gastroenterol 2009;104:1764*). Both **Lesogaberan**, a GABA-B receptor agonist, and **arbaclofen placarbil**, the prodrug of the active R-isomer of baclofen, can improve refractory symptoms when added to PPI therapy (*Gastroenterology 2010;139:409; Am J Gastroenterol 2010;105:1266*), but neither is clinically available yet.

Surgical Management

Indications for **fundoplication** include the need for continuous PPIs in patients who are good surgical candidates, noncompliance or intolerance to medical therapy, ongoing nonacid reflux despite adequate medical therapy, and patient preference for surgery. When symptoms are controlled on PPI therapy, medical therapy and fundoplication are equally effective. Although fundoplication could provide better

Table 18-2	Dosage of Acid-Suppressive Agents		
Medication Therapy	**Peptic Ulcer Disease**	**GERD**	**Parenteral**
Cimetidine[a]	300 mg qid 400 mg bid 800 mg at bedtime	400 mg qid 800 mg bid	300 mg q6h
Ranitidine[a]	150 mg bid 300 mg at bedtime	150–300 mg bid–qid	50 mg q8h
Famotidine[a]	20 mg bid 40 mg at bedtime	20–40 mg bid	20 mg q12h
Nizatidine[a]	150 mg bid 300 mg at bedtime	150 mg bid	
Omeprazole	20 mg daily	20–40 mg daily–bid	
Esomeprazole	40 mg daily	20–40 mg daily–bid	20–40 mg q24h
Lansoprazole	15–30 mg daily	15–30 mg daily–bid	30 mg q12–24h
Dexlansoprazole		30–60 mg daily	
Pantoprazole	20 mg daily	20–40 mg daily–bid	40 mg q12–24h or 80 mg IV, then 8 mg/hr infusion

[a]Dosage adjustment required in renal insufficiency.
GERD, gastroesophageal reflux disease.

symptom control and quality of life in the short term (*Surg Endosc 2011;25:2547*), postoperative symptoms and surgical failure can also occur.
- Elevated esophageal acid exposure and correlation of symptoms to reflux events on ambulatory pH monitoring predict a higher likelihood of a successful surgical outcome.
- Patients with medical treatment failures need careful evaluation to determine whether symptoms are indeed related to acid reflux before surgical options are considered; these patients often have other diagnoses including EoE, esophageal motor disorders, visceral hypersensitivity, and functional heartburn.
- Potential complications of surgery include dysphagia, inability to belch, gas-bloat syndrome, and bowel symptoms including flatulence, diarrhea, and abdominal pain.

Lifestyle/Risk Modification
- Patients with nocturnal GERD symptoms may benefit from elevating the head of the bed by 6 to 8 in. and avoiding eating within 2 to 3 hours before bedtime.
- Weight loss may benefit certain overweight patients with GERD.
- Avoiding foods that trigger reflux (fatty foods, chocolate, coffee, cola) or foods that result in heartburn (spicy foods, tomato, citrus, carbonated drinks) may be prudent in the appropriate setting. Smoking cessation is also thought to be beneficial.
- Lifestyle modifications alone are unlikely to resolve symptoms in the majority of GERD patients, and should be recommended in conjunction with medications.

COMPLICATIONS

- **Esophageal erosion and ulceration** (esophagitis) can rarely lead to overt bleeding and iron-deficiency anemia.
- **Strictures** can form when esophagitis heals, leading to dysphagia. Endoscopic dilation and maintenance PPI therapy typically resolve dysphagia from strictures.
- **Barrett's esophagus (BE)** is a reflux-triggered change from normal squamous esophageal epithelium to specialized intestinal metaplasia, and carries a 0.5% per year risk of progression to esophageal adenocarcinoma. Endoscopic screening for BE is performed in patients ≥50 years or with GERD history that exceeds 5 to 10 years (*Gastroenterology 2008;135:1392*). Low-grade dysplasia in BE has a low annual incidence of adenocarcinoma similar to nondysplastic BE (*Gastroenterology 2011;141:1179*). NSAID and statin use may decrease the risk of neoplastic progression (*Gastroenterology 2011;141:2000*). Radiofrequency ablation (RFA) offers safe, effective, and durable eradication of both dysplasia and intestinal metaplasia in dysplastic BE (*N Engl J Med 2009;28:360*; *Gastroenterology 2011;141:460*). However, this does not obviate the need for continued surveillance.

Esophageal Motor Disorders

GENERAL PRINCIPLES

Definition

- **Achalasia** is the most easily recognized motor disorder of the esophagus, characterized by failure of the LES to relax completely with swallowing and aperistalsis of the esophageal body (*Am J Gastroenterol 1999;94:3406*).
- **Diffuse esophageal spasm** is a spastic disorder characterized by simultaneous, nonperistaltic contractions in the esophageal body. Since concomitant incomplete LES relaxation may be present, this could represent a variant of achalasia in certain situations. Nonspecific spastic disorders have limited spastic features from esophageal inhibitory dysfunction (*Gastroenterologist 1997;5:112*).
- **Esophageal hypomotility disorders** are characterized by fragmented, weak, or absent esophageal peristalsis, sometimes with LES hypomotility, leading to reflux symptoms.

DIAGNOSIS

Clinical Presentation

- Presenting symptoms in achalasia can include dysphagia, regurgitation, chest pain, weight loss, and aspiration pneumonia.
- Diffuse esophageal spasm and other spastic disorders may have obstructive symptoms (dysphagia, regurgitation) but also perceptive symptoms (chest pain) from heightened esophageal sensitivity.
- LES hypomotility diminishes barrier function and esophageal body hypomotility affects esophageal clearance of refluxed material, which can lead to prolonged reflux exposure and reflux complications.

Diagnostic Testing

- **Esophageal manometry** is the gold standard for diagnosis of motor disorders. HRM yields more reproducible results, allows accurate recognition of diagnoses and facilitates specific classification of motor disorders compared to conventional manometry (*Neurogastroenterol Motil. 2011;23:271*; *Neurogastroenterol Motil. 2012;24:20*). HRM features categorize achalasia into three subtypes that have symptomatic and therapeutic implications (*Gastroenterology 2008;135:1526*).

- **Barium radiographs** may demonstrate a typical achalasia appearance of a dilated intrathoracic esophagus with impaired emptying, an air±fluid level, absence of gastric air bubble, and tapering of the distal esophagus with a **bird's beak** appearance. A beaded or corkscrew appearance may be seen with diffuse esophageal spasm, sometimes with epiphrenic diverticula. A dilated esophagus with an open LES and free gastroesophageal reflux may be seen with severe esophageal hypomotility.
- **Endoscopy** may help exclude a stricture or neoplasia of the distal esophagus in achalasia and spastic disorders; the esophageal body may be dilated and contain food debris, whereas the LES, although spastic, typically allows passage of the endoscope into the stomach with minimal resistance. Hypomotility disorders may also manifest a dilated esophagus but with a gaping gastroesophageal junction and evidence of reflux disease.

TREATMENT

Medications

- **Smooth muscle relaxants** such as nitrates or calcium channel blockers administered immediately before meals may afford short-lived symptom relief in spastic disorders and achalasia, but symptom response is suboptimal.
- **Botulinum toxin** injection at endoscopy can improve dysphagia symptoms for several weeks to months in achalasia and spastic disorders with incomplete LES relaxation (*Neurogastroenterol Motil. 2011;23:139*). This approach may be useful in elderly and frail patients who are poor surgical risks or as a bridge to more definitive therapy (*Ann Surg 2009;249:45*).
- **Neuromodulators** (e.g., low-dose tricyclic antidepressants [TCAs]) may improve perceptive symptoms (such as chest pain) associated with spastic motor disorders and achalasia.
- **Antisecretory therapy** with a PPI is recommended for reflux associated with esophageal hypomotility disorders. No specific promotility therapy exists. Antireflux surgery should be approached with caution in advanced hypomotility disorders.

Surgical Management

Disruption of the circular muscle of the LES using **pneumatic dilation** or surgical incision **(Heller myotomy)** can result in durable symptom relief in achalasia (*Ann Surg 2009;249:45*), with comparable symptom outcomes (*N Engl J Med 2011;364:1807*). Gastroesophageal reflux can result, treated with lifelong acid suppression or concurrent partial fundoplication at myotomy. Esophageal perforation occurs in 3% to 5% with pneumatic dilation, requiring prompt surgical repair. Surgical myotomy is rarely indicated for diffuse esophageal spasm when incomplete LES relaxation is thought to contribute significantly to dysphagia symptoms. Peroral endoscopic myotomy (POEM) is a promising technique with potential for excellent short-term outcomes in achalasia (*Endoscopy 2010;42:265*).

COMPLICATIONS

- Complications of achalasia include aspiration pneumonia and weight loss.
- Achalasia is associated with a 0.15% risk of squamous cell cancer of the distal esophagus, a 33-fold higher risk relative to the nonachalasic population.

Peptic Ulcer Disease

GENERAL PRINCIPLES

Definition

PUD consists of mucosal breaks in the stomach and duodenum when corrosive effects of acid and pepsin overwhelm mucosal defense mechanisms. Other locations include esophagus, small bowel adjacent to gastroenteric anastomoses, and within a Meckel's diverticulum.

Etiology

- *Helicobacter pylori*, a spiral, gram-negative, urease-producing bacillus, is responsible for at least half of all PUD, and the majority of ulcers that are not due to NSAIDs.
- PUD can develop in 15% to 25% of **chronic NSAID and aspirin** users. Past history of PUD, age >60 years, concomitant corticosteroid or anticoagulant therapy, high-dose or multiple NSAID therapy, and presence of serious comorbid medical illnesses including end-stage renal disease increase risk for PUD (*J Clin Gastroenterol. 1997;24:2*).
- A gastrin-secreting tumor or **gastrinoma** accounts for <1% of all peptic ulcers.
- Gastric cancer or lymphoma may manifest as a gastric ulcer.
- When none of these etiologies are evident, PUD is designated idiopathic. Most idiopathic PUD could be due to undiagnosed *H. pylori* or undetected NSAID use.
- Cigarette smoking doubles the risk for PUD; it delays healing and promotes recurrence.

DIAGNOSIS

Clinical Presentation

- Epigastric pain or dyspepsia may be presenting symptoms; however, symptoms are not always predictive of the presence of ulcers. Epigastric tenderness may be elicited on abdominal palpation. Ten percent may present with a complication (see the following text).
- In the presence of **alarm symptoms** (weight loss, early satiety, bleeding, anemia, persistent vomiting, epigastric mass, and lack of response to PPI), endoscopy is indicated to evaluate for a complication or an alternate diagnosis (*BMJ 2008;337:a1400*).

Diagnostic Testing

- **Endoscopy** is the gold standard for diagnosis of peptic ulcers. **Barium studies** also have good sensitivity for diagnosis of ulcers, but smaller ulcers and erosions may be missed, and tissue sampling for *H. pylori* or cancer cannot be performed.
- **Serum *H. pylori* antibody testing** is the cheapest noninvasive test with a sensitivity of 85% and a specificity of 79% for the diagnosis of *H. pylori* infection. The antibody remains detectable as long as 18 months after successful eradication, and cannot be used to document successful eradication of the organism (*BMJ 2008;337:a1400*).
- **Stool *H. pylori* antigen testing** has 91% sensitivity and 93% specificity for the diagnosis of *H. pylori* infection, and can confirm eradication of *H. pylori* after triple therapy.

- **Rapid urease assay** (e.g., *Campylobacter*-like organism [CLO] test) and histopathologic examination of endoscopic biopsy specimens are commonly used for diagnosis in patients undergoing endoscopy but may be falsely negative in patients on PPI therapy.
- **Carbon-labeled urea breath testing** is the most accurate noninvasive test for diagnosis, with sensitivity and specificity of 95%; often used to document successful eradication after therapy of *H. pylori* infection (*BMJ 2008;337:a1400*).

TREATMENT

Medications

- Regardless of etiology, **acid suppression** forms the mainstay of therapy of PUD. Gastric ulcers are typically treated for 12 weeks, and duodenal ulcers for 8 weeks.
- Oral PPI or H_2RA therapy will suffice in most instances; IV PPI therapy is necessary in the presence of GI bleeding or when oral administration is not tolerated or not possible (see Table 18-2). See the section on GERD for PPI side effects. Headache and mental status abnormalities (lethargy, confusion, depression, hallucinations) can result from H_2RAs while hepatotoxicity, thrombocytopenia, and leukopenia are rare. Dosage adjustment of H_2RAs is necessary in renal insufficiency. Cimetidine can impair metabolism of many drugs, including warfarin anticoagulants, theophylline, and phenytoin.
- Two antibiotics and a PPI (triple therapy) is standard for *H. pylori* **eradication**, which promotes healing and markedly reduces PUD recurrence. Several antimicrobial and antisecretory agent regimens are available (Table 18-3). Levofloxacin-based sequential or triple therapy may be superior to standard triple therapy (clarithromycin, amoxicillin, PPI) (*Hepatogastroenterology 2011;58:1148*). Newer regimens under study include LOAD (**l**evofloxacin, **o**meprazole, nit**a**zoxanide, and **d**oxycycline) for 7 to 10 days and ofloxacin, azithromycin, omeprazole, and bismuth for 14 days (*Am J Gastroenterol 2011;106:1970*). Patients previously exposed to a macrolide antibiotic should be treated with a regimen that does not include clarithromycin. Clarithromycin may be replaced with furazolidone for resistance and cost concerns (*Helicobacter 2010;15:497*). Primary clarithromycin resistance and poor compliance with therapy affect eradication rates; metronidazole resistance does not (*Gastroenterology 2007;133:985*).
- NSAIDs and aspirin should be avoided when possible; if continued, maintenance PPI therapy or a mucosal protective agent (misoprostol, 400 to 800 μg/d) are recommended.
- **Sucralfate** coats the eroded mucosal surface without blocking acid secretion and is often used in stress ulcer prophylaxis. Side effects include constipation and reduction of bioavailability of certain drugs (e.g., cimetidine, digoxin, fluoroquinolones, phenytoin, and tetracycline) when administered concomitantly.
- **Antacids** can be useful as supplemental therapy for pain relief in PUD.
- **Nonpharmacologic measures.** Cessation of cigarette smoking should be encouraged. Alcohol in high concentrations can damage the gastric mucosal barrier, but no evidence exists to link alcohol with ulcer recurrence.

Surgical Management

Surgery is still occasionally required for intractable symptoms, GI bleeding, Zollinger–Ellison syndrome, and complicated PUD. Surgical options vary depending on the location of the ulcer and the presence of complications.

Table 18-3	Examples of Regimens Used for Eradication of *Helicobacter pylori*	
Medications	**Dose**	**Comments**
Clarithromycin	500 mg bid	First line
Amoxicillin	1 g bid	
PPI[a]	bid	
Metronidazole	500 mg bid	First line with history of exposure to clarithromycin
Amoxicillin	1 g bid	
PPI	bid	
Pepto-Bismol	524 mg qid	First line in penicillin-allergic patients
Metronidazole	250 mg qid	Salvage regimen if three-drug regimen fails
Tetracycline	500 mg qid	
PPI[a] or H$_2$RA[b]	bid	
Clarithromycin	500 mg bid	Alternate regimen if four-drug therapy is not tolerated
Metronidazole	500 mg bid	
PPI[a]	bid	
Levofloxacin	250 mg bid	Alternate salvage regimen
Amoxicillin	1 g bid	
PPI[a]	bid	
Rifabutin	300 mg daily	Alternate salvage regimen
Amoxicillin	1 g bid	
PPI	bid	
Furazolidone	200–400 mg daily	Alternate salvage regimen
Amoxicillin	1 g bid	
PPI[a]	bid	

Duration of therapy: 10 to 14 days. When using salvage regimens after initial treatment failure, choose drugs that have not been used before.
[a]Standard doses for PPI: omeprazole 20 mg, lansoprazole 30 mg, pantoprazole 40 mg, rabeprazole 20 mg, all twice a day. Esomeprazole is used as a single 40-mg dose once a day.
[b]Standard doses for H$_2$RA: ranitidine 150 mg, famotidine 20 mg, nizatidine 150 mg, cimetidine 400 mg, all twice a day.
H$_2$RA, histamine-2 receptor antagonists; PPI, proton pump inhibitor.

SPECIAL CONSIDERATIONS

Zollinger–Ellison syndrome

- This syndrome is caused by a gastrin-secreting, non–β islet cell tumor of the pancreas or duodenum. Multiple endocrine neoplasia type I can be associated with this syndrome in 25% of patients. The resultant hypersecretion of gastric acid can cause multiple PUD in unusual locations, ulcers that fail to respond to standard medical therapy, or recurrent PUD after surgical therapy. Diarrhea and GERD symptoms are common.
- Gastric acid output is typically >15 mEq/L, and gastric pH is <1.0. A fasting serum gastrin level while off acid suppression for at least 5 days serves as a screening

test in patients who make gastric acid; a value >1,000 pg/mL is seen in 90% of patients with Zollinger–Ellison syndrome. When serum gastrin is elevated but <1,000 pg/mL, a secretin stimulation test may demonstrate a paradoxical 200-pg increment in serum gastrin level after IV secretin in patients with gastrinomas (*Aliment Pharmacol Ther. 2009;29:1055*). High-dose PPIs are used for medical management. Specialized nuclear medicine scans (octreotide scans) can be useful in localizing the neoplastic lesion for curative resection (*Expert Opin Pharmacother 2009;10:1145*). Long-term survival is principally related to underlying comorbidity rather than metastatic gastrinoma (*Dig Liver Dis 2011;43:439*).

COMPLICATIONS

- **GI bleeding** (see Gastrointestinal Bleeding section)
- **Gastric outlet obstruction** can occur with ulcers close to the pyloric channel and can manifest as nausea and vomiting, sometimes several hours after meals. Plain abdominal X-rays can show a dilated stomach with an air–fluid level. NG suction should be maintained for 2 to 3 days to decompress the stomach while repleting fluids and electrolytes intravenously.
  - Medical management may be temporarily effective. Recurrence is common, and endoscopic balloon dilation or surgery is often necessary for definitive correction.
- **Perforation** occurs infrequently and usually necessitates emergency surgery. Perforation may occur in the absence of previous symptoms of PUD and may be asymptomatic in patients who are receiving glucocorticoids. A plain upright X-ray of the abdomen may demonstrate free air under the diaphragm.
- **Pancreatitis** can result from penetration into the pancreas from ulcers in the posterior wall of the stomach or duodenal bulb. The pain becomes severe and continuous, radiates to the back, and is no longer relieved by antisecretory therapy. Serum amylase may be elevated. CT scanning may be diagnostic. Surgery is often required for therapy.

MONITORING/FOLLOW-UP

- EGD or upper GI series should be performed 8 to 12 weeks after initial diagnosis of all gastric ulcers to document healing; repeat endoscopic biopsy should be considered for nonhealing ulcers to exclude the possibility of a malignant ulcer.
- Duodenal ulcers are almost never malignant, and therefore, documentation of healing is unnecessary in the absence of symptoms.

Inflammatory Bowel Disease

GENERAL PRINCIPLES

Definition
- **Ulcerative colitis (UC)** is an idiopathic chronic inflammatory disease of the colon and rectum, characterized by mucosal inflammation and typically presenting with bloody diarrhea. Rectal involvement is almost universal.
- **Crohn's disease (CD)** is characterized by transmural inflammation of the gut wall and can affect any part of the tubular GI tract.

DIAGNOSIS

Clinical Presentation

- Both disorders can present with diarrhea, weight loss, and abdominal pain. UC typically presents with bloody diarrhea. CD can also present with fistula formation, strictures, abscesses, or bowel obstruction.
- **Extracolonic manifestations** of inflammatory bowel disease (IBD) include arthritis, primary sclerosing cholangitis, and ocular and skin lesions.

Diagnostic Testing

- **Endoscopy** remains the preferred method for diagnosis, especially for UC where contiguous inflammation is seen starting at the rectum and extending varying distances into the colon. Endoscopy may demonstrate colonic involvement in CD (erosions or ulcers with a patchy distribution and skip lesions); ileoscopy during colonoscopy may demonstrate terminal ileal involvement. **Histopathology** demonstrates chronic mucosal inflammation with crypt abscesses and cryptitis in UC, and may demonstrate multinucleated giant cells and noncaseating granulomas in CD.
- Cross-sectional **imaging studies** (CT and magnetic resonance imaging [MRI] scans) have value in the evaluation of CD, especially when luminal narrowing (stricture) or extraluminal complications (abscess, fistula) are suspected. While MR and CT enterography both adequately assess disease activity and bowel involvement in CD, MRI may be superior to CT in detecting intestinal strictures and ileal wall enhancement (*Inflamm Bowel Dis 2011;17:1073*). Contrast radiography (small bowel follow through series, barium enema) may also be useful, particularly in CD.
- **Serologic markers** play a limited role as adjuncts for diagnosis. Anti–*Saccharomyces cerevisiae* antibodies are typically seen in CD, and perinuclear antineutrophil cytoplasmic antibodies (p-ANCA) in UC; the finding of one antibody in the absence of the other may help differentiate indeterminate colitis (*Gastroenterology 2002;122:1242*). C-reactive protein and erythrocyte sedimentation rate (ESR) are correlates for disease activity.
- *C. difficile* **colitis** is more frequent in IBD patients compared to non-IBD populations; therefore, **stool studies** are warranted to look for this organism with disease flares (*Clin Gastroenterol Hepatol 2007;5:339*). **CMV superinfection** can occur in patients on immunosuppressive agents and can be diagnosed by histopathology during endoscopy (*Am J Gastroenterol 2006;101:2857*).

TREATMENT

Medications

Treatment is based on the severity of disease, location, and associated complications. Management aims are to resolve the acute presentation and reduce future recurrences. Both UC and CD can be categorized into three categories of severity for management purposes:

- **Mild-to-moderate disease.** Patients have little to no weight loss, good functional capacity, and are able to maintain adequate oral intake. UC patients have less than four bowel movements daily with no rectal bleeding or anemia, normal vital signs and normal ESR, while CD patients have little or no abdominal pain. Treatment typically begins with aminosalicylates but can include antibiotics and glucocorticoids.

○ **5-Aminosalicylates (5-ASA).** The mechanism of action remains unknown but involves decreasing the production of arachidonic acid metabolites, particularly leukotrienes. Various formulations are available, each targeting different parts of the tubular gut, and are useful for both inducing and maintaining remission in mild-to-moderate disease. Infrequent hypersensitivity reactions include pneumonitis, pancreatitis, hepatitis, and nephritis.

■ **Sulfasalazine** reaches the colon intact, where it is metabolized to 5-ASA and a sulfapyridine moiety. Benefit is therefore limited to UC or CD limited to the colon, either as initial therapy (0.5 g PO bid, increased as tolerated to 0.5 to 1.5 g PO qid) or to maintain remission (1 g PO bid–qid). The sulfapyridine moiety is responsible for side effects of headache, nausea, vomiting, and abdominal pain, treated with dose reduction. Skin rash, fever, agranulocytosis, hepatotoxicity, and paradoxical exacerbation of colitis are rare hypersensitivity reactions. Reversible reduction in sperm counts can be seen in males. Folic acid supplementation is recommended as sulfasalazine can impair folate absorption.

■ **Mesalamine.** Newer 5-ASA preparations lack the sulfa moiety of sulfasalazine and are associated with fewer side effects but are expensive.

 □ **Asacol** is an oral formulation of 5-ASA released at a pH of 7 in the distal ileum. It is useful in UC and ileocecal/colonic CD at doses of 800 to 1,600 mg PO tid.

 □ **Pentasa** has a time- and pH-dependent release mechanism that allows drug availability throughout the small bowel and colon. It is useful in diffuse small bowel involvement with CD but can also be used in UC in doses of 0.5 to 1.0 g PO qid.

 □ **Apriso** also has a pH-dependent release mechanism, and distributes mesalamine throughout the colon when administered in doses of 1.5 g PO once daily.

 □ **Balsalazide** (**Colazal**) is cleaved by colonic bacteria to mesalamine and an inert molecule. It is therefore only useful for colonic disease, at doses of 2.25 g PO tid for active disease and 1.5 g PO bid for maintenance.

 □ **Multimatrix delivery system mesalamine** (**Lialda**) uses a novel delivery system that allows sustained 5-ASA release throughout the colon while decreasing frequency of administration. It is useful in colonic disease at doses of 1.2 to 2.4 g PO qd–bid.

■ **Olsalazine** (**Dipentum**) is a 5-ASA dimer cleaved by colonic bacteria and is useful in colonic disease. Significant diarrhea limits its use.

○ **Antibiotics** are commonly used clinically in mild-to-moderate CD as well as perianal disease but not in UC where the role of bacteria has not been established. Despite frequent usage, controlled studies have failed to consistently show efficacy for luminal inflammation. Their role should be limited to colonic or ileocolonic CD, perianal disease, fistulas, and abscesses. Typical antibiotics used are **metronidazole** (250 to 500 mg PO tid) and **ciprofloxacin** (500 mg PO bid), usually concurrently, for 2 to 6 weeks.

○ **Budesonide** (6 to 9 mg PO qd) is a synthetic corticosteroid with first pass liver metabolism that limits systemic toxicity while retaining local efficacy from high affinity to the glucocorticoid receptor, similar to oral corticosteroids. It is effective and safe for short-term use in mild-to-moderate ileocolonic CD and can replace mesalamine in inducing remission (*Am J Gastroenterol 2009;104:465*; *Gastroenterology 2011;140:425*). Efficacy has not been reported in UC.

- ○ **Topical therapy** is useful in IBD limited to distal left colon. Topical mesalamine agents are superior to topical steroids or oral aminosalicylates for mild-to-moderate distal UC or ulcerative proctitis (*Am J Gastroenterol 2010;105:501*). However, concurrent systemic therapy is administered in severe cases (*Am J Gastroenterol 2004;99:1371*). Sitz baths, analgesics, hydrocortisone creams, and local heat may provide symptomatic benefit in perianal CD in conjunction with systemic therapy.
- • **Moderate-to-severe disease** refers to CD patients who fail to respond to treatment for mild-to-moderate disease, or those with significant weight loss, anemia, fever, abdominal pain or tenderness, and intermittent nausea and vomiting without bowel obstruction (*Am J Gastroenterol 2009;104:465*), or UC patients with more than six bloody bowel movements daily, fever, mild anemia, and elevated ESR. The goal of therapy is to induce remission rapidly with corticosteroids, and to maintain remission with immunosuppressive agents and/or biologic agents as appropriate. Treatment is typically continued until the patient fails to respond to a particular agent, or the agent is no longer tolerated.
  - ○ **Glucocorticoids** are effective in inducing remission in moderate-to-severe disease, especially with flare-ups of disease activity (*Gut 2011;60:571*). Extracolonic manifestations of IBD (ocular lesions, skin disease, and peripheral arthritis) also respond to glucocorticoids.
    - ▪ **Prednisone** is started orally (typically 40 to 60 mg PO qd, as high as 1 mg/kg PO qd) and continued until symptom improvement. The dose can then be reduced by 5 to 10 mg weekly until the dose of 20 mg, following which taper can be continued by 2.5 to 5.0 mg weekly. Glucocorticoids are not recommended for maintenance therapy, and alternatives should be sought for the patient who appears dependent on these medications.
    - ▪ **Oral or parenteral glucocorticoids should not be prescribed before ruling out an infectious process and should not be initiated for the first time over the telephone.**
    - ▪ Patients treated with at least 5 mg prednisone for >2 months need to be continually monitored for osteoporosis (*JAMA 2001;285:785*). Other risk factors for osteoporosis include smoking, low body mass, sedentary lifestyle, family history of osteoporosis, and nutritional deficiencies (*Gastroenterology 2003;124:791*).
  - ○ **Immunosuppressive agents**
    - ▪ **6-Mercaptopurine** (1.0 to 1.5 mg/kg/d PO), a purine analog, and **azathioprine** (1.5 to 2.5 mg/kg/d PO), its S-imidazole precursor, cause preferential suppression of T-cell activation and antigen recognition and are useful in maintaining a glucocorticoid-induced remission in both UC and CD. Both azathioprine and 6-mercaptopurine are effective for inducing remission in active CD (*Cochrane Database Sys Rev 2010;16:CD000545*). Both agents have more favorable side effect profiles than glucocorticoids and are used as steroid-sparing agents in severe or refractory IBD. Response may be delayed for up to 1 to 2 months, with optimal response occurring about 4 months after treatment initiation. Side effects include reversible bone marrow suppression, pancreatitis, and allergic reactions.
      - ▫ Determination of **thiopurine methyltransferase (TPMT)** enzyme activity prior to initiation of therapy will identify genetic polymorphisms that may predispose to toxicity with the use of these agents (*Gastroenterology 2006; 130:935*).
      - ▫ Routine blood cell counts should be performed, initially every 1 to 2 weeks to monitor for acute or delayed bone marrow suppression. On stable doses, testing can be performed every 3 months.

□ 6-Thioguanine (6-TG) metabolite levels assess adequacy of dosing, while high 6-methyl mercaptopurine (6-MMP) levels may predict hepatotoxicity. Addition of allopurinol to the regimen preferentially pushes metabolism toward the active metabolite (6-TG) rather than the toxic metabolite (6-MMP) (*Aliment Pharmacol Ther. 2010;31:640*).

- **Methotrexate** (15 to 25 mg IM or PO weekly) is effective as a steroid-sparing agent in CD but not UC. Side effects include hepatic fibrosis, bone marrow suppression, alopecia, pneumonitis, allergic reactions, and teratogenicity. In CD patients in remission, methotrexate is not as effective as azathioprine or infliximab for mucosal healing (*Aliment Pharmacol Ther. 2011;33:714*).
  □ Baseline chest X-ray (CXR), and monitoring of CBC and liver functions tests should be performed routinely.
  □ Patients with abnormal transaminases may require a liver biopsy to assess for hepatic fibrosis prior to treatment, and subsequent biopsies are performed for significant elevations thereafter.

○ **Antitumor necrosis factor alpha (anti–TNF-α) monoclonal antibodies** modify immune system function and are beneficial in moderate-to-severe CD refractory to other approaches including immunosuppressives, and indicated both for induction and maintenance of remission. Benefit has also been demonstrated in moderate-to-severe UC (*Gastroenterology 2009;136:1182*; *Gut 2011;60:780*). **Infliximab** (5 mg/kg IV infusions at weeks 0, 2, and 6, followed by maintenance infusions every 8 weeks), **adalimumab** (160 mg SQ at week 0, then 80 mg SQ at week 2, followed by 40 mg SQ every 2 weeks), and **certolizumab pegol** (400 mg SQ at weeks 0, 2, and 4, followed by maintenance doses every 4 weeks) are the available anti-TNF agents. In addition to its role as an option for first-line therapy, adalimumab is also safe and effective for CD patients who have failed infliximab therapy (*Aliment Pharmacol Ther. 2010;32:1228*). However, as elective switching from IV infliximab to subcutaneous adalimumab is associated with loss of tolerance and efficacy, adherence to the first anti-TNF agent is encouraged (*Gut 2012;61:229*). In moderate-to-severe CD, infliximab plus azathioprine or infliximab monotherapy are more likely to attain steroid-free clinical remission than azathioprine monotherapy (*N Engl J Med 2010;362:1383*). Patients in remission with a low risk of relapse may be potentially identified for discontinuation of infliximab therapy using a combination of clinical and biologic markers (*Gastroenterology 2012;142:63*). The usage of step-up infliximab therapy has not reduced surgical requirements or the development of complications (*Aliment Pharmacol Ther. 2010;31:233*).

- Anti–TNF-α therapy has been associated with reactivation of latent tuberculosis, hence placement of a PPD and CXR are essential prior to initiation of therapy (*Am J Gastroenterol 2010;105:501*). Hepatitis B status also needs to be assessed. Opportunistic infections as well as infectious complications can develop, and congestive heart failure may worsen during therapy.
- Acute and delayed hypersensitivity reactions, antibodies to infliximab and anti–double-stranded DNA antibodies can develop with infliximab infusions. Local injection site reactions have been reported with adalimumab and certolizumab pegol therapy.

○ **Natalizumab** (300-mg infusions at weeks 0, 4, and 8, followed by monthly infusions thereafter) is a humanized monoclonal antibody to alpha-4 integrin, a cellular adhesion molecule, used for moderate-to-severe CD refractory to all other approaches including anti–TNF-α antibodies. This agent may induce reactivation of human JC polyoma virus causing progressive multifocal leukoencephalopathy

(PML). Risk for PML can be minimized by avoiding concomitant immunosuppressive agents and close monitoring (*Am J Gastroenterol 2009;104:465*). Other infectious complications and acute hypersensitivity reactions are also possible.

- **Severe or fulminant disease** describes patients typically hospitalized due to the severity of their symptoms. Fulminant CD patients have persistent symptoms despite conventional glucocorticoids or anti–TNF-α therapy, or have high fevers, persistent vomiting, intestinal obstruction, intra-abdominal abscess, peritoneal signs, or cachexia (*Am J Gastroenterol 2009;104:465*). Fulminant colitis (both CD and UC) can present with profuse bloody bowel movements, significant anemia, systemic signs of toxicity (fever, sepsis, electrolyte disturbances, dehydration), and elevated laboratory markers of inflammation (*Arch Surg 2005;140:300*). **Toxic megacolon** occurs in 1% to 2% of UC patients, wherein the colon becomes atonic and modestly dilated, with significant systemic toxicity.
  - ○ Supportive therapy consists of nothing by mouth (NPO) status with NG suction if there is evidence of small-bowel ileus. Dehydration and electrolyte disturbances are treated vigorously, and blood is transfused for severe anemia. Anticholinergic and opioid medication should be discontinued in toxic megacolon.
  - ○ Initial investigation includes cross-sectional imaging (i.e., CT, MRI) to evaluate for intra-abdominal abscess. A cautious flexible sigmoidoscopy may determine severity of colonic inflammation and for biopsies to exclude CMV colitis. Blood cultures and stool studies to exclude *C. difficile* colitis are performed.
  - ○ Intensive medical therapy with IV **corticosteroids** (methylprednisolone 1 mg/kg body weight or equivalent to 40 to 60 mg of prednisone) and broad-spectrum antimicrobials should be initiated.
  - ○ If response is not seen, **cyclosporine** infusion (2 to 4 mg/kg/d, to achieve blood levels of 200 to 400 ng/mL) is an option in fulminant UC colitis. Tacrolimus infusions are also an option. Once improved, the patient can gradually be transitioned to an equivalent oral regimen, supplemented with immunosuppressive agents (*Arch Surg 2005;140:300*).
  - ○ Nutritional support is administered as appropriate after 5 to 7 days; TPN is often indicated if enteral nutrition is not tolerated.
  - ○ Clinical deterioration/lack of improvement despite 7 to 10 days of intensive medical management, evidence of bowel perforation, or peritoneal signs are indications for urgent total colectomy.
  - ○ Surgical evaluation should be pursued in those with concern for abscess formation or GI obstruction. When refractory to medical management, surgical excision of the affected area should be considered. Stricturoplasty is an option for focal tight strictures; biopsies should be obtained to rule out cancer at stricture sites.

Surgical Management

- Surgery is generally reserved for fistulas, obstruction, abscess, perforation, or bleeding, for medically refractory disease, and neoplastic transformation (*Gut 2011;60:571*).
- In CD, recurrence close to the resected margins is common after bowel resection. Efforts should be made to avoid multiple resections in CD because of the risk of short-bowel syndrome. Immunosuppressive agents should be discontinued before surgery and reinstituted if necessary during the postoperative period.
- In UC, total colectomy is curative, and for some patients is preferred over long-term immunosuppressive or biologic therapy.

Lifestyle/Risk Modification

- A low-roughage diet often provides symptomatic relief in patients with mild-to-moderate disease or in patients with strictures. Elemental diets have been used in acute phases of the diseases, especially CD, but are unpalatable and disliked by patients.
- Patients with Crohn's ileitis or ileocolonic resection may need vitamin B_{12} supplementation. Specific oral replacement of calcium, magnesium, folate, iron, vitamins A and D, and other micronutrients may be necessary in patients with small-bowel CD.
- Patients with intermittent obstructive symptoms should avoid highly indigestible foods such as nuts, pits, hulls, skins, seeds, and pulps that may precipitate obstruction.
- **TPN** can be administered in patients with food intolerance for greater than 4 or 5 days. Bowel rest has not been shown to reduce time to remission but can be used for nutritional maintenance and symptom relief while waiting for the effects of medical treatment, or as a bridge to surgery.

SPECIAL CONSIDERATIONS

- In patients with both UC and Crohn's colitis lasting longer than 8 to 10 years, annual **colonoscopic surveillance for neoplasia** with four-quadrant mucosal biopsies every 5 to 10 cm is recommended. Histopathologic evidence of any grade of dysplasia is an indication for total colectomy. Narrow-band imaging during colonoscopy may represent an alternative to chromoendoscopy for targeted biopsies in IBD (*Gastrointest Endosc 2011;74:840*).
- **Smoking cessation** is generally warranted for all patients with IBD. There is epidemiologic evidence of a protective effect on a limited number of patients with UC. However, nicotine has been shown to increase metabolism of many medications routinely used to treat IBD, decreasing their efficacy.
- **Venous thromboembolism.** Patients with IBD are at increased risk for both first and recurrent venous thromboembolism (*Gastroenterology 2011;139:779*).
- **Symptom control** is important as adjunct to therapy but must be used cautiously.
  - **Antidiarrheal agents** may be useful as an adjunctive therapy in selected patients with mild exacerbations or postresection diarrhea. They are contraindicated in severe exacerbations and toxic megacolon.
  - **Narcotics** should be used sparingly for pain control, as the chronicity of symptoms can lead to potential for dependence.

Functional Gastrointestinal Disorders

GENERAL PRINCIPLES

Definition

- Functional GI disorders are characterized by the presence of abdominal symptoms in the absence of a demonstrable organic disease process. Symptoms can arise from any part of the luminal gut.

- **Irritable bowel syndrome (IBS)**, primarily characterized by abdominal pain linked to altered bowel habits of at least 3 months duration, is the best-recognized functional bowel disease (*Gastroenterology 2006;130:1480*).

DIAGNOSIS

- Clinical evaluation and investigation should be directed toward prudently excluding organic processes in the involved area of the gut while initiating therapeutic trials when functional symptoms are suspected.
- In the absence of alarm features (anemia, weight loss, family history of colorectal cancer, IBD, or celiac sprue), symptom-based diagnosis of IBS is generally accurate (*Am J Gastroenterol 2009;104(suppl 1):S1*).
- **Serologic tests for celiac sprue** are recommended in IBS patients. The prevalence of celiac sprue in diarrhea predominant IBS patients is estimated at 3.6%, compared to 0.7% of the general population (*Am J Gastroenterol 2009;104(suppl 1):S1*).
- Patients >50 years with new-onset bowel symptoms, patients with alarm symptoms (GI bleeding, anemia, weight loss, early satiety), and patients with symptoms not responding to empiric treatment need further workup with endoscopy. Routine cross-sectional imaging is not recommended with typical functional symptoms without alarm features.
- In young individuals with short-lived symptoms and no other explanation for dyspepsia, noninvasive testing for *H. pylori* can be considered (*BMJ 2008;337:a1400*).

TREATMENT

Patient education, reassurance, and help with diet and lifestyle modification are key to an effective physician–patient relationship. The psychosocial contribution to symptom exacerbation should be determined, and its management may be sufficient for many patients.

Medications

- **Symptomatic management**
  - **Antiemetic agents** are useful in functional nausea and vomiting syndromes, in addition to neuromodulators.
  - When pain and bloating are the predominant symptoms, **antispasmodic** or **anticholinergic** medications (hyoscyamine, 0.125 to 0.25 mg PO/sublingual up to qid; dicyclomine, 10 to 20 mg PO qid) may provide short-term relief.
  - Stool frequency, but not abdominal pain, improves with increased dietary fiber (25 g/d) supplemented with PRN laxatives in constipation-predominant IBS.
  - **Loperamide** (2 to 4 mg, up to qid/PRN) can reduce stool frequency, urgency, and fecal incontinence.
  - Short-term nonabsorbable **antibiotic** therapy may improve bloating and diarrhea in IBS; long-term treatment has not been adequately studied. **Probiotics** (e.g., bifidobacteria) are sometimes beneficial (*Am J Gastroenterol 2009;104(suppl 1):S1*).
  - **Lubiprostone** (8 μg bid), a selective chloride channel activator, and **linaclotide** (290 μg qd), a guanylate cyclase C agonist, may improve constipation-predominant IBS symptoms in women.
  - **Alosetron** (Lotronex, 1 mg daily to bid), a 5-HT$_3$ antagonist, is useful in women with diarrhea-predominant IBS (*Am J Gastroenterol 2009;104:1831*). However,

its use is restricted to refractory diarrhea because of the rare potential for ischemic colitis.

- **Neuromodulators**
  - ○ Low-dose **TCAs** (e.g., amitriptyline, nortriptyline, imipramine, doxepin: 25 to 100 mg at bedtime) have neuromodulatory and analgesic properties that are independent of their psychotropic effects. These can be beneficial, especially in pain-predominant functional GI disorders.
  - ○ **Selective serotonin reuptake inhibitors (SSRIs)** (e.g., fluoxetine, 20 mg; paroxetine, 20 mg; sertraline, 50 mg; duloxetine 20 to 60 mg) may also have efficacy, sometimes with better side effect profiles.
  - ○ **Cyclic vomiting syndrome (CVS)**, is an increasingly recognized illness that consists of stereotypic episodes of vigorous vomiting with asymptomatic intervals between episodes (*Aliment Pharmacol Ther. 2011;34:263*). Treatment with low-dose TCAs or antiepileptic medications (zonisamide, levetiracetam) has prophylactic benefits (*Clin Gastroenterol Hepatol 2007;5:44*; *Am J Gastroenterol 1999;94:2855*). Sumatriptan (25 to 50 mg PO, 5 to 10 mg transnasally, or 6 mg SC) or other triptans may abort an episode, especially if administered during a prodrome or early in the episode (*Cephalalgia 2011;31:504*). Established episodes may require IV hydration, scheduled IV antiemetics (ondansetron, prochlorperazine) and benzodiazepines (lorazepam), and pain control with IV narcotics for 1 to 2 days.

Acute Intestinal Pseudo-Obstruction (Ileus)

GENERAL PRINCIPLES

Definition

- **Acute intestinal pseudo-obstruction or ileus** consists of impaired transit of intestinal contents and obstructive symptoms (nausea, vomiting, abdominal distension, lack of bowel movements) without a mechanical explanation (*Med Clin North Am 2008;92:649*).
- **Acute colonic pseudo-obstruction** or **Ogilvie syndrome** describes massive colonic dilation without mechanical obstruction in the presence of a competent ileocecal valve, resulting from impaired colonic peristalsis (*Br J Surg 2009;96:229*).

Etiology

Ileus is frequently seen in the postoperative period. Narcotic analgesics administered for postoperative pain control may contribute, as can other medications that slow intestinal peristalsis (calcium channel blockers, anticholinergic medications, TCAs, antihistamines). Other predisposing causes include virtually any medical insult, particularly life-threatening systemic diseases, infection, vascular insufficiency, and electrolyte abnormalities. Etiology is similar for acute colonic pseudo-obstruction.

DIAGNOSIS

- A careful history and physical exam is essential in the initial evaluation.
- Conventional laboratory studies (CBC, complete metabolic profile, amylase, lipase) help in assessing for a primary intra-abdominal inflammatory process.

- **Obstructive series** (supine and upright abdominal X-ray with a CXR) determines the distribution of intestinal gas and assesses for the presence of free intraperitoneal air.
- **Additional imaging studies** assess for mechanical obstruction and inflammatory processes and include **CT scanning, contrast enema, and small-bowel series**.

TREATMENT

- Basic **supportive measures** consist of NPO, fluid replacement, and correction of electrolyte imbalances. Prompt antimicrobial therapy is indicated if an infectious process is suspected. Medications that slow GI motility (adrenergic agonists, TCAs, sedatives, narcotic analgesics) should be withdrawn or doses reduced. The ambulatory patient is encouraged to remain active and to undertake short walks.
- **Intermittent NG suction** prevents swallowed air from passing distally. In protracted cases, gastric decompression, either using an NG tube or a percutaneous endoscopic gastrostomy tube, vents upper GI secretions and decreases vomiting and gastric distension.
- **Rectal tubes** help decompress the distal colon; more proximal colonic distension may necessitate **colonoscopic decompression**, especially when the cecal diameter approaches 9 to 10 cm. A flexible decompression tube can be left in the proximal colon during colonoscopy. Turning the patient from side to side may potentiate the benefit of colonoscopic decompression.
- Temporary TPN may be required in protracted cases.

Medications

- **Neostigmine** (2 mg IV administered slowly over 3 to 5 minutes) is beneficial in selected patients with acute colonic distension. This can induce rapid reestablishment of colonic tone and is contraindicated if mechanical obstruction remains in the differential diagnosis. Side effects include abdominal pain, excessive salivation, symptomatic bradycardia, and syncope. A trial of neostigmine may be warranted before colonoscopic decompression in patients without contraindications (*N Engl J Med 1999;341:137*).
- **Erythromycin** (200 mg IV) acts as a motilin agonist and stimulates upper gut motility; it has been used with some success in refractory postoperative ileus.
- **Alvimopan** is a peripherally acting μ-opioid receptor antagonist that enhances return of bowel function after abdominal surgery (*Am Surg 2011;77:1460*) but has not been shown to shorten hospital stay.
- **Mosapride citrate** (15 mg PO tid), a 5-HT4 receptor agonist, may reduce the duration of post-operative ileus when administered postoperatively (*J Gastrointest Surg 2011;15:1361*).

Surgical Management

- **Surgical consultation** is required when the clinical picture is suggestive of mechanical obstruction or if peritoneal signs are present.
- **Cecostomy** treats acute colonic distension when colonoscopic decompression fails.

- Surgical exploration is reserved for acute cases with peritoneal signs, ischemic bowel, or other evidence for perforation.

PANCREATOBILIARY DISORDERS

Acute Pancreatitis

GENERAL PRINCIPLES

Definition

Acute pancreatitis consists of inflammation of the pancreas and peripancreatic tissue from activation of potent pancreatic enzymes within the pancreas, particularly trypsin.

Etiology

The most common causes are alcohol and gallstone disease, accounting for 75% to 80% of all cases. Less common causes include abdominal trauma, hypercalcemia, hypertriglyceridemia, and a variety of drugs. In one series, over 40% of patients admitted with acute pancreatitis used pancreatitis-associated drugs, suggesting that drug-induced pancreatitis may be under-recognized (*Am J Gastroenterol 2011;106: 2183*). Post–endoscopic retrograde cholangiopancreatography (ERCP) pancreatitis occurs in 5% to 10% of patients undergoing ERCP.

DIAGNOSIS

Clinical Presentation

Typical symptoms consist of acute onset epigastric abdominal pain, nausea, and vomiting often exacerbated by food intake. Systemic manifestations can include fever, shortness of breath, altered mental status, anemia, and electrolyte imbalances, especially with severe episodes.

Diagnostic Testing

Laboratories
- Serum **lipase** is more specific and sensitive than serum **amylase**, though both are usually elevated to two to three times the upper limits of normal. These values do not correlate with severity or resolution of symptoms. Patients with renal insufficiency may have elevated enzymes at baseline from impaired clearance.
- A CBC may demonstrate elevated hemoglobin levels from hemoconcentration; blood urea nitrogen (BUN) and serum creatinine levels may be elevated.
- Hepatic function testing may identify biliary obstruction as a possible etiology, and a lipid panel may suggest hypertriglyceridemia as the cause of acute pancreatitis.

Imaging
- **Dual-phase (pancreatic protocol) CT scanning** is useful in the initial evaluation of severe acute pancreatitis, but recent evidence suggests that early CT use should be restricted (*Pancreatology 2010;10:222*). Specifically, CT should be reserved for patients with severe or prolonged symptoms or if the diagnosis is unclear (*Med Clin North Am 2008;92:889*).

- **MRI with gadolinium** can also be used with at least similar efficacy, especially when CT is contraindicated. It may not be appropriate for patients who are hemodynamically unstable. MRCP is useful to detect a biliary source for pancreatitis before ERCP is performed (*Med Clin North Am 2008;92:889*).

TREATMENT

- **Aggressive volume repletion** with IV fluids must be undertaken, with careful monitoring of fluid balance urine output, and awareness of the potential for significant fluid sequestration within the abdomen. ICU monitoring may be necessary. Serum electrolytes, calcium, and glucose levels should be monitored and supplemented as necessary.
- Patients should receive **nothing by mouth** until they are free of pain and nausea. NG suction is reserved for patients with ileus or protracted emesis. TPN may be necessary when inflammation is slow to resolve (around 7 days) or if an ileus is present. Enteral nutrition through a tube placed distal to the ligament of Treitz is usually tolerated and is safer and more cost-effective than TPN (*Surg Clin North Am 2007;87:1403*).
- **Acid suppression** may be necessary in severely ill patients with risk factors for stress ulcer bleeding (see Gastrointestinal Bleeding section), though has not been shown to decrease symptom duration or severity (*Gastroenterology 2007;132:2022*).

Medications
- **Narcotic analgesics** are usually necessary for pain relief.
  Dilaudid is often used initially, but other narcotic analgesics (e.g., **meperidine**) are alternatives. **Patient-controlled analgesia (PCA)** is frequently necessary for adequate relief of pain.
- Prophylactic antibiotics are not indicated in the absence of systemic infection.

Other Nonoperative Therapies
Urgent **ERCP and biliary sphincterotomy** within 72 hours of presentation can improve the outcome of severe gallstone pancreatitis in the presence of biliary obstruction and is associated with fewer complications (*Ann Surg 2009;250:68*). This is thought to result from reduced biliary sepsis rather than true improvement of pancreatic inflammation.

Surgical Management
Cholecystectomy. A delay in cholecystectomy after gallstone pancreatitis carries a substantial risk of recurrent biliary events (*Br J Surg 2011;98:1446*).

COMPLICATIONS

- **Necrotizing pancreatitis** represents a severe form of acute pancreatitis, usually identified on dynamic dual-phase CT scanning with IV contrast. The presence of radiologically identified pancreatic necrosis increases the morbidity and mortality of acute pancreatitis. Increasing abdominal pain, fever, marked leukocytosis, and bacteremia suggest infected pancreatic necrosis that requires broad-spectrum antibiotics and often surgical debridement. **Carbapenems** or a combination of a **fluoroquinolone** and **metronidazole** have good penetration into necrotic tissue, but prophylactic antibiotics do not reduce pancreatic infection or mortality (*J Gastroenterol Hepatol 2009;24:736*; *J Gastrointest Surg 2009;13:768*). CT-guided percutaneous aspiration for Gram stain and culture can confirm the diagnosis of infected necrosis. Surgical debridement is required in severe cases.

- The presence of **pseudocysts** is suggested by persistent pain or high amylase levels. Complications include infection, hemorrhage, rupture (pancreatic ascites), and obstruction of adjacent structures. Asymptomatic nonenlarging pseudocysts can be followed clinically with serial imaging studies to resolution. Decompression of symptomatic or infected pseudocysts can be performed by percutaneous, endoscopic, or surgical techniques (*Gastrointest Endosc Clin N Am 2007;17:559*).
- **Infection.** Potential sources of fever include pancreatic necrosis, abscess, infected pseudocyst, cholangitis, and aspiration pneumonia. Cultures should be obtained, and broad-spectrum antimicrobials appropriate for bowel flora should be administered. In the absence of fever or other clinical evidence for infection, prophylactic antimicrobial therapy has no clear role in acute pancreatitis.
- **Pulmonary complications.** Atelectasis, pleural effusion, pneumonia, and acute respiratory distress syndrome can develop in severely ill patients (see Chapter 10, Pulmonary Diseases).
- **Renal failure** can result from intravascular volume depletion or acute tubular necrosis.
- **Other complications.** Metabolic complications include hypocalcemia, hypomagnesemia, and hyperglycemia. GI bleeding can result from stress gastritis, pseudoaneurysm rupture, or gastric varices from splenic vein thrombosis.

Chronic Pancreatitis

GENERAL PRINCIPLES

Definition

- Chronic pancreatitis represents inflammation, fibrosis, and atrophy of acinar cells resulting from recurrent acute or chronic inflammation of the pancreas.
- Most commonly seen with chronic alcohol abuse, it can also result from dyslipidemia, hypercalcemia, autoimmune disease, and exposure to various toxins. An inherited form is rarely seen (*Gastroenterology 2007;132:1557*).
- **Autoimmune pancreatitis (AIP)** represents an increasingly recognized subtype of chronic pancreatitis characterized by infiltration of immunoglobulin (Ig)G4-positive plasma cells in the pancreas. AIP can be difficult to distinguish from pancreatic cancer on CT, but typically features diffuse irregular narrowing of the main pancreatic duct on ERCP. Initial treatment with prednisolone 0.6 mg/kg/day, followed by a maintenance dose over 3 to 6 months, is indicated in the presence of symptoms (*Gut 2009;58:1504*).

DIAGNOSIS

Clinical Presentation

Chronic abdominal pain, exocrine insufficiency from acinar cell injury and fibrosis (manifesting as weight loss, and steatorrhea), and **endocrine insufficiency**

from destruction of islet cells (manifesting as brittle diabetes) are the main clinical manifestations.

Diagnostic Testing

Laboratories

- Lipase and amylase may be elevated but are frequently normal and are nonspecific. Bilirubin, alkaline phosphatase, and transaminases may be elevated if there is concomitant biliary obstruction. A lipid panel and serum calcium should also be assessed.
- Pancreatic function testing (such as secretin stimulation, fecal fat, and fecal elastase) can be obtained but are not widely available and difficult to perform. In the presence of steatorrhea, a serum trypsinogen level of <20 ng/mL is diagnostic of chronic pancreatitis with exocrine insufficiency (*Am Fam Physician 2007;76:1679*).

Imaging

- Calcification of the pancreas can be seen on plain films and ultrasound. Contrast-enhanced CT has a sensitivity of 75% to 90% and a specificity of 85% for the diagnosis of chronic pancreatitis, while MRCP is equivalent and a suitable alternative (*Gastroenterology 2007;132:1557*). ERCP is comparatively sensitive and specific but is rarely used because of invasiveness and associated complications.
- **Endoscopic ultrasound (EUS)** has higher sensitivity (97%) at the cost of lower specificity (60%) for the diagnosis of chronic pancreatitis. It is useful for evaluating lesions concerning for neoplasia in the setting of chronic pancreatitis.

TREATMENT

Medications

- **Narcotic analgesics** are frequently required for control of pain, and narcotic dependence is common. **Neuromodulators** (TCAs, SSRIs) and **pregabalin** may improve symptoms and decrease reliance on narcotics (*Gastroenterology 2011;141:536*). In patients with mild-to-moderate exocrine insufficiency, the addition of oral pancreatic enzyme supplements may be beneficial for pain control.
- **Pancreatic enzyme supplements** are the mainstay of management of pancreatic exocrine insufficiency, in conjunction with a low-fat diet (<50 g fat per day), facilitating weight gain and reduced stool frequency (*Aliment Pharmacol Ther. 2011;33:1152*). Enteric-coated preparations (Pancrease or Creon, one to two capsules with meals) are stable at acid pH.
- **Fat-soluble vitamin** supplementation may be necessary.
- **Insulin** therapy is generally required for endocrine insufficiency, as the resultant diabetes mellitus is characteristically brittle and thus unresponsive to oral agents.
- When identified, treatment of the underlying disorder (e.g., hyperparathyroidism, dyslipidemia) is indicated. Alcohol cessation should be advised.

Other Nonoperative Therapies

- Patients with pancreatic duct obstruction from stones, strictures, or papillary stenosis may benefit from **ERCP and sphincterotomy**.
- Intractable pain may necessitate **celiac plexus block** (often EUS guided), or even surgery, such as a **Whipple's procedure** (*Aliment Pharmacol Ther. 2009;29:979*).

Gallstone Disease

GENERAL PRINCIPLES

- **Asymptomatic gallstones (cholelithiasis)** is a common incidental finding for which no specific therapy is generally necessary (*J Gastroenterol Hepatol 2010;25: 719*). Cholesterol stones are the most common type, but pigmented stones can be seen with hemolysis or infection. Risk factors include obesity, female gender, and family history.
- **Symptomatic cholelithiasis**, when upper abdominal symptoms are linked to gallstones, is typically treated surgically with cholecystectomy.
- **Acute cholecystitis** is caused most often by obstruction of the cystic duct by gallstones, but acalculous cholecystitis can occur in severely ill or hospitalized patients.

DIAGNOSIS

Clinical Presentation

- Cholelithiasis may present as **biliary colic**, a constant pain lasting for hours, located in the right upper quadrant, radiating to the back or right shoulder, and sometimes associated with nausea or vomiting.
- Other presentations of gallstone disease include acute cholecystitis, acute pancreatitis, and cholangitis. Gallstone disease may rarely be associated with gallbladder cancer.
- Patients with **acute ascending cholangitis** present with right upper quadrant pain, fever with chills, and jaundice (Charcot's triad), usually in the setting of biliary obstruction (choledocholithiasis, neoplasia, sclerosing cholangitis, biliary stent occlusion). Elderly patients may lack abdominal symptoms.

Diagnostic Testing

- **Ultrasound scans** have a high degree of accuracy in diagnosis (sensitivity and specificity >95%) and are the preferred initial test.
- **Hydroxy iminodiacetic acid (HIDA)** scan can demonstrate nonfilling of the gallbladder in patients with acute cholecystitis.

TREATMENT

Medications

- **Supportive measures** include IV fluid resuscitation and broad-spectrum antimicrobial agents, especially in the event of complications such as acute cholecystitis with sepsis, perforation, peritonitis, abscess, or empyema formation.
- **Ursodeoxycholic acid** (8 to 10 mg/kg/d PO in two to three divided doses for prolonged periods) might be prudent in a small select group of patients with small cholesterol stones in normally functioning gallbladders who are at high risk for complications from surgical therapy. Side effects include diarrhea and reversible elevation in serum transaminases.

Other Nonpharmacologic Therapies

Percutaneous cholecystostomy can be performed under fluoroscopy in severely ill patients with acute cholecystitis who are not surgical candidates.

Surgical Management

Cholecystectomy is the therapy of choice for symptomatic gallstone disease and acute cholecystitis. Laparoscopic cholecystectomy compares favorably with the open procedure, with lower morbidity, lower cost, shorter hospital stay, and better cosmetic results (*Lancet 2006;368:230*).

COMPLICATIONS

- **Acute pancreatitis.** See Acute Pancreatitis section.
- **Choledocholithiasis.** Common bile duct obstruction, jaundice, biliary colic, cholangitis, or pancreatitis can result from stones retained in the common bile duct. The diagnosis can be made on ultrasonography, CT scanning, or magnetic resonance cholangiography. ERCP with sphincterotomy and stone extraction is curative.
- **Acute ascending cholangitis** represents a medical emergency with high morbidity and mortality if biliary decompression is not performed urgently. The condition should be stabilized with IV fluids and broad-spectrum antibiotics. Drainage of the biliary tree can be performed through the endoscopic (ERCP with sphincterotomy) or percutaneous approach under fluoroscopic guidance.

OTHER GASTROINTESTINAL DISORDERS

Anorectal Disorders

- **Thrombosed external hemorrhoids** present as acutely painful, tense, bluish lumps covered with skin in the anal area. The thrombosed hemorrhoid can be surgically excised under local anesthesia for relief of severe pain. In less severe cases, oral analgesics, sitz baths (sitting in a tub of warm water), stool softeners, and topical ointments may provide symptomatic relief (*BMJ 2008;336:380*).
- **Internal hemorrhoids** commonly present with either bleeding or a prolapsing mass with straining. Bulk-forming agents such as fiber supplements are useful in preventing straining at defecation. Sitz baths and Tucks pads (cotton soaked in witch hazel) may provide symptomatic relief. Ointments and suppositories that contain topical analgesics, emollients, astringents, and hydrocortisone (e.g., Anusol-HC Suppositories, one per rectum bid for 7 to 10 days) may decrease edema but do not reduce bleeding. Hemorrhoidectomy or band ligation can be curative and is indicated in patients with recurrent or constant bleeding (*BMJ 2008;336:380*).
- **Anal fissures** present with acute onset of pain during defecation and are often caused by hard stool. Anoscopy reveals an elliptical tear in the skin of the anus, usually in the posterior midline. Acute fissures heal in 2 to 3 weeks with the use of stool softeners, oral or topical analgesics, and sitz baths. Topical nitroglycerin ointment, 0.2%, applied three times a day may be beneficial. Chronic fissures often require surgical therapy.
- **Perirectal abscess** commonly presents as a painful induration in the perianal area. Patients with IBD and immunocompromised states are particularly susceptible. Prompt drainage is essential to avoid the serious morbidity associated with delayed treatment. Antimicrobials directed against bowel flora (metronidazole, 500 mg

PO tid, and ciprofloxacin, 500 mg PO bid) should be administered in patients with significant inflammation, systemic toxicity, or immunocompromised states.

Celiac Sprue

GENERAL PRINCIPLES

- Celiac sprue is a sensitivity to gluten, the protein found in wheat, barley, and rye. The resulting chronic inflammation in the small-bowel mucosa causes malabsorption of dietary nutrients.
- Clinical presentation can vary greatly from asymptomatic iron-deficiency anemia to significant diarrhea and weight loss. Other presenting features can include osteoporosis, dermatitis herpetiformis, abnormal liver enzymes, and abdominal pain; incidental recognition at endoscopy can also occur (*N Engl J Med 2007;357:1731*).
- More than 7% of patients with nonconstipated IBS have celiac-associated antibodies, suggesting that gluten sensitivity may mediate IBS symptoms (*Gastroenterology 2011;141:1187*).

DIAGNOSIS

- Noninvasive serologic tests are highly sensitive and specific. Both IgA antiendomysial antibodies and antitissue transglutaminase antibodies have accuracies close to 100% (*N Engl J Med 2007;357:1731*). Quantitative IgA levels should be checked; IgG antibodies against tissue transglutaminase are checked if the patient is IgA deficient.
- Endoscopic biopsy confirmation of the diagnosis is recommended. Classic biopsy findings include blunting or absence of villi and prominent intraepithelial lymphocytosis.
- Almost all patients with celiac sprue carry HLA DQ2 and HLA DQ8 molecules, so absence of these alleles has high negative predictive value when the diagnosis is in question (*Gastroenterology 2006;131:1981*).

TREATMENT

Medications

- Patients may require iron, folate, calcium, and vitamin supplements.
- **Corticosteroids** (prednisone, 10 to 20 mg/d) may be required in refractory cases; immunosuppressive drugs and infliximab have also been used (*N Engl J Med 2007;357:1731*).

Lifestyle/Risk Modification

- A gluten-free diet results in prompt improvement in symptoms. Dietary nonadherence is the most frequent cause for persistent symptoms.
- If symptoms persist despite a strict gluten-free diet, radiologic and endoscopic evaluation of the small bowel should be performed to rule out complications including collagenous colitis and **small-bowel lymphoma**. However, the prognosis of adults with unrecognized celiac disease is good despite positive celiac antibodies; therefore, mass screening appears unnecessary (*Gut 2009;58:643*).

Diverticulosis and Diverticulitis

GENERAL PRINCIPLES

Definition

- **Diverticula** consist of outpouchings in the bowel, most commonly in the colon, but also rarely seen elsewhere in the gut.
- **Diverticular bleeding** can rarely occur from an artery at the mouth of the diverticulum. See segment on Gastrointestinal Bleeding section for further details.
- **Diverticulitis** results from microperforation of a diverticulum and resultant extracolonic or intramural inflammation.

DIAGNOSIS

Clinical Presentation

- Diverticulosis is most frequently asymptomatic. Though diverticulosis may be found in patients being investigated for symptoms of abdominal pain and altered bowel habits, a causal link is difficult to establish.
- Typical symptoms of diverticulitis include left lower quadrant abdominal pain, fevers and chills, and alteration of bowel habits. Localized left lower quadrant abdominal tenderness may be elicited on physical examination.

Diagnostic Testing

Laboratories

Diverticulitis may be associated with an elevated white blood cell (WBC) count with a left shift.

Imaging

- Diverticula are frequently seen on screening colonoscopy.
- Imaging studies, most commonly CT scans, are useful in the diagnosis of diverticulitis.
- Colonoscopy is contraindicated for 4 to 6 weeks after an episode of acute diverticulitis but should be performed after that interval to exclude a perforated neoplasm.

TREATMENT

- Increased dietary fiber is generally recommended in patients with diverticulosis, although no hard data exist to support its benefit. No data exist to support exclusion of nuts and popcorn from the diet to prevent acute diverticulitis.
- A low-residue diet is recommended for mild diverticulitis. Oral feedings are withheld in complicated diverticulitis, and parenteral nutrition may be necessary if protracted.

Medications

- Oral **antibiotics** (e.g., ciprofloxacin, 500 mg PO bid, and metronidazole, 500 mg PO tid for 10 to 14 days) may suffice for mild diverticulitis.
- Hospital admission, bowel rest, IV fluids, and broad-spectrum IV antimicrobial agents are typically required in moderate-to-severe cases.

Surgical Management

- Surgical consultation should be obtained early in moderate-to-severe diverticulitis, as operative intervention may be necessary should complications arise.

- Surgical resection may also be necessary in recurrent diverticulitis, typically after three or more recurrences at the same location.

Gastroparesis

GENERAL PRINCIPLES

Definition
Gastroparesis consists of abnormally delayed emptying of stomach contents into the small bowel in the absence of mechanical obstruction, usually as a result of damage to the nerves or smooth muscle involved in gastric emptying (*Am J Gastroenterol 2006;127:287*).

Etiology
- Gastroparesis can result from chronic disorders (diabetes mellitus, scleroderma, intestinal pseudo-obstruction, previous gastric surgery) or, less frequently, from acute metabolic derangements (hypokalemia, hypercalcemia, hypocalcemia, hyperglycemia) or medications (narcotic analgesics, anticholinergic agents, chemotherapy agents); it is designated idiopathic when a predisposing cause is not identified (*Gastroenterology 2004;127:1589*).
- Mechanical obstruction should always be excluded.

DIAGNOSIS

Clinical Presentation
Symptoms include nausea, bloating, and vomiting, usually hours after a meal.

Diagnostic Testing
Imaging
- A gastric-emptying study consisting of gamma camera scanning after a radiolabeled meal can help with the diagnosis.
- Endoscopic evidence of retained food debris in the stomach after an overnight fast may be an indirect indicator of delayed gastric emptying.

TREATMENT

- Underlying metabolic derangements should be corrected. In particular, precise glucose control using short-acting insulin preparations may improve emptying in early stages of diabetic gastroparesis (*Clin Gastroenterol Hepatol 2005;3:642*).
- Nutritional consultation can help address nutritional deficiencies and optimize diet (*Gastroenterology 2011;141:486*). High-fat and insoluble fiber in meals can further delay gastric emptying, and should be avoided. High-calorie liquid iso-osmotic meals may be beneficial in refractory situations.

Medications
- **Prokinetic agents** have been used with varying degrees of success.
- **Metoclopramide** (10 mg PO qid half an hour before meals) has variable efficacy, and side effects (drowsiness, tardive dyskinesia, parkinsonism) may be limiting.

- **Domperidone** (20 mg PO qid before meals and at bedtime) does not cross the blood–brain barrier, but hyperprolactinemia can result. This is not universally available.
- **Erythromycin** (125 to 250 mg PO tid or 200 mg IV) is a motilin receptor agonist and stimulates gastric motility, but tachyphylaxis, abdominal pain, and nausea limit long-term therapy.

Surgical Management

- **Enteral feeding** through a jejunostomy feeding tube may be required for supplemental nutrition and is favored over TPN.
- **Gastric electrical stimulation** using a surgically implanted stimulator may reduce symptoms of nausea and vomiting in half of medically refractory patients, but gastric emptying is typically not enhanced by this approach (*Gastroenterology 2008;134:665*; *Gastrointest Endosc 2011;74:496*).

Ischemic Intestinal Injury

GENERAL PRINCIPLES

- **Acute mesenteric ischemia** results from arterial (or rarely venous) compromise to the superior mesenteric circulation.
- Emboli and thrombus formation are the most common causes of acute mesenteric ischemia, although **nonocclusive mesenteric ischemia** from vasoconstriction can also give rise to the disorder.
- **Ischemic colitis** results from mucosal ischemia in the inferior mesenteric circulation during a low-flow state (hypotension, arrhythmias, sepsis, aortic vascular surgery) in patients with atherosclerotic disease (*Gastroenterology 2000;118:951*).
- Vasculitis, sickle cell disease, vasospasm, and marathon running can also predispose to ischemic colitis.

DIAGNOSIS

Clinical Presentation

- Patients with acute mesenteric ischemia may present with abdominal pain, but physical examination and imaging studies can be unremarkable until infarction has occurred. As a result, diagnosis is late and mortality is high.
- Ischemic colitis may manifest as transient bleeding or diarrhea; severe insults can lead to stricture formation, gangrene, and perforation. The heterogeneity of clinical presentation of ischemic colitis helps explain why clinical suspicion is often low (*Scand J Gastroenterol 2011;46:236*).

Diagnostic Testing

- Urgent angiography is indicated if the suspicion for acute mesenteric ischemia is high.
- CT with contrast has high sensitivity and specificity for the diagnosis of primary acute mesenteric ischemia (*Radiology 2010;256:93*), while Doppler EUS may help exclude chronic mesenteric ischemia (*Dig Liver Dis 2011;43:470*).
- In patients with ischemic colitis, characteristic "thumb-printing" of the involved colon may be seen on plain radiographs of the abdomen.

- Colonoscopy may reveal mucosal erythema, edema, and ulceration, sometimes in a linear configuration; evidence of gangrene or necrosis is an indication for surgical intervention.

TREATMENT

- Treatment of acute mesenteric ischemia is essentially surgical, while both arterial bypass and percutaneous angioplasty are options for chronic mesenteric ischemia (*Ann Vasc Surg 2010;24:935*).
- In patients with ischemic colitis, in the absence of peritoneal signs or evidence of gangrene or perforation, expectant management with fluid and electrolyte repletion, broad-spectrum antimicrobials, and maintenance of stable hemodynamics usually suffices.
- Evidence of gangrene or necrosis in the setting of ischemic colitis is an indication for surgery (*Gastroenterology 2000;118:951*).

19 Liver Diseases

M. Katherine Rude, Thomas Kerr, and
Mauricio Lisker-Melman

Evaluation of Liver Disease

GENERAL PRINCIPLES

- Liver disease can present as a spectrum of clinical conditions that ranges from asymptomatic disease to end-stage liver disease (ESLD).
- A comprehensive investigation combining thorough history and physical examination combined with diagnostic tests, liver histology, and imaging can often establish a precise diagnosis.

DIAGNOSIS

Clinical Presentation

History

History taking should be focused on the following:
- History of present illnesses
- Medicine usage and toxin exposure (including alcohol)
- Associated signs and symptoms—development of jaundice, edema, pruritus, encephalopathy, gastrointestinal (GI) bleeding
- Family history of liver disease
- Comorbid conditions: obesity, diabetes, hyperlipidemia, inflammatory bowel disease, systemic hypotension
- Risk factors for infection: intravenous (IV)/intranasal drug use, body piercings, tattooing, sexual history, travel to foreign countries, occupation

Physical Examination
- Detailed physical exam is necessary. Physical stigmata of acute and chronic liver disease may be subtle or absent.
  - Jaundice, with close attention to the conjunctiva and soft palate
  - Ascites, peripheral edema, and pleural effusions
  - Hepatomegaly and splenomegaly
  - Gynecomastia, testicular hypotrophy
  - Muscle wasting
  - Telangiectasias, palmar erythema, pubic hair changes
- Specific liver disorders may be associated with distinctive physical abnormalities: arthritis, acne, skin color changes, Kayser–Fleischer rings, clubbing, S3 gallop.

Diagnostic Testing

Laboratories
- **Serum enzymes.** Hepatic disorders associated predominantly with elevation in aminotransferases are referred to as hepatocellular; hepatic disorders with predominant elevation in alkaline phosphatase (ALP) are referred to as cholestatic.

○ Elevation of **aspartate transaminase and alanine aminotransferases** (AST and ALT, respectively) indicates hepatocellular injury and necrosis. Markedly elevated levels (>1,000 U/L) typically occur with acute hepatocellular injury (e.g., viral, drug induced, or ischemic), whereas mild-to-moderate elevations may be seen in a variety of conditions (e.g., acute or chronic hepatocellular injury, infiltrative diseases, biliary obstruction). The ratio of serum AST to ALT is typically >2 in alcoholic liver disease and <1 in viral hepatitis.

○ **ALP** is an enzyme that is present in a variety of tissues (bone, intestine, kidney, leukocytes, liver, and placenta). The concomitant elevation of other hepatic enzymes (e.g., γ-glutamyl transpeptidase [GGT] or 5'-nucleotidase) assists in establishing the hepatic origin of ALP. Serum ALP level is often elevated in biliary obstruction, space-occupying lesions or infiltrative disorders of the liver, and conditions that cause intrahepatic cholestasis (primary biliary cirrhosis [PBC], primary sclerosing cholangitis [PSC], drug-induced cholestasis). The degree of elevation of ALP does not differentiate the site or cause of cholestasis.

○ **GGT** is an enzyme that is present in a variety of tissues. Increases in GGT and ALP tend to occur in similar hepatic diseases. GGT may be elevated in individuals who ingest barbiturates, phenytoin, or alcohol even when other liver enzyme and bilirubin levels are normal.

○ **5'-Nucleotidase** is comparable to ALP in sensitivity in detecting biliary obstruction, cholestasis, and infiltrative hepatobiliary diseases.

• **Synthetic products**
  ○ Serum **albumin** concentration is frequently decreased in chronic liver disease. However, chronic inflammation, expanded plasma volume, and GI or renal losses can also lead to hypoalbuminemia. Because the half-life of albumin is relatively long (20 days), serum levels may be normal in acute liver disease.

  ○ Several important proteins involved in hemostasis and fibrinolysis (coagulation factors: α_2-antiplasmin, antithrombin, heparin cofactor II, high–molecular-weight kininogen, prekallikrein, protein C and S) are synthesized by the liver. The synthesis of factors II, VII, IX, and X and proteins C and S depends on the presence of vitamin K. The adequacy of hepatic synthetic function can be estimated by the prothrombin time (PT) and the international normalized ratio (INR). PT/INR prolongation may result from impaired coagulation factor synthesis or vitamin K deficiency. Normalization of PT/INR after administration of vitamin K indicates vitamin K deficiency.

  ○ **Cholesterol** is synthesized in the liver. Patients with advanced liver disease may have very low cholesterol levels. However, in PBC, levels of serum cholesterol may be markedly elevated.

  ○ Other synthetic products whose levels can be measured in specific liver diseases are α_1-antitrypsin and ceruloplasmin.

• **Excretory products**
  ○ **Bilirubin** is a degradation product of hemoglobin and nonerythroid hemoproteins (e.g., cytochromes, catalases). Total serum bilirubin is composed of conjugated (direct) and unconjugated (indirect) fractions. Unconjugated hyperbilirubinemia occurs as a result of excessive bilirubin production (neonatal or physiologic jaundice, hemolysis and hemolytic anemias, ineffective erythropoiesis, and resorption of hematomas), reduced hepatic bilirubin uptake (Gilbert's syndrome and drugs such as rifampin and probenecid), or impaired bilirubin conjugation (Gilbert's or Crigler–Najjar syndrome). Elevation of conjugated and unconjugated fractions occurs in Dubin–Johnson's and Rotor's syndromes and in conditions

associated with intrahepatic (from hepatocellular, canalicular, or ductular damage) and extrahepatic (from mechanical obstruction) cholestasis.

○ **Bile acids** are produced in the liver and are secreted into the intestine, where they are required for lipid digestion and absorption. Elevated levels of serum bile acids are specific but not sensitive markers of hepatobiliary disease. Levels of individual bile acids are not useful in the differential diagnosis of liver disorders. Bile acid determination is uncommon in the regular workup of patients with liver disease.

○ **α-Fetoprotein (AFP)** is normally produced by fetal liver cells. Its production falls to normal adult levels of <10 ng/mL within 1 year of life. AFP is an insensitive marker for hepatocellular carcinoma (HCC). For example, a cutoff level of 20 ng/mL has only a 60% sensitivity for detecting HCC (*Hepatology 2011;53:1020*). One-third of HCCs have no increase in AFP level and only 30% have an AFP level >50 ng/mL (*Aliment Pharmacol Ther 2007;26:1187*). Levels of >400 ng/mL or a rapid doubling time are suggestive of HCC; mild-to-moderate elevations can also be seen in acute and chronic liver inflammation.

Imaging

• **Ultrasonography** is used to screen for dilation of the biliary tree and to detect gall-stones and cholecystitis in patients with right-sided abdominal pain associated with abnormal liver blood tests. It can reveal and characterize liver masses, abscesses, and cysts. Color flow Doppler ultrasonography can assess patency and direction of blood flow in the portal and hepatic veins. Ultrasonography is a frequently used modality for screening of HCC; however, this modality is less sensitive (tumors with diameters <2 cm) for the detection of HCC compared with computed tomography (CT) or magnetic resonance imaging (MRI). This technique is very operator dependent.

• **Helical CT scan** with IV contrast is useful in the evaluation of parenchymal liver disease. It has the added feature of contrast enhancement to define space-occupying lesions (e.g., abscess and tumor) and allows calculation of liver volume. Triple-phase CT (arterial, venous, and delayed phases) is indicated for liver mass evaluation. A delayed phase is useful when cholangiocarcinoma is suspected.

• **MRI** offers information similar to that provided by CT scan with the additional advantage of better characterization of liver lesions, fatty infiltration, and iron deposition. It is the modality of choice in patients with an allergy to iodinated contrast. Of all the cross-sectional imaging techniques, MRI provides the highest tissue contrast. This, in conjunction with various contrast agents (especially hepatobiliary contrast agents), allows for definitive noninvasive characterization of liver lesions.

• **Magnetic resonance cholangiopancreatography (MRCP)** is a specialized version of MRI that provides an alternative noninvasive diagnostic modality for visualizing the intrahepatic and extrahepatic bile ducts.

• **Positron emission tomography (PET)** is a modality that uses differences in metabolism among normal, inflammatory, and malignant tissues. PET scans are helpful in assessing the presence of hepatic metastasis in colorectal cancer. PET scans may also be helpful in diagnosing cholangiocarcinoma.

Diagnostic Procedures

• **Percutaneous transhepatic cholangiography (PTC) and endoscopic retrograde cholangiopancreatography (ERCP)** involve the instillation of contrast into the biliary tree. They are most useful after the preliminary determination of abnormalities detected by ultrasonography, CT, or MRI/MRCP. These procedures allow for diagnostic and therapeutic maneuvers including biopsy, brushings, stenting, and placement of drains.

- **Percutaneous liver biopsy** is an invasive procedure that can be performed with or without radiographic (ultrasound or CT) guidance. Percutaneous liver biopsy is generally safe and is usually performed as an outpatient procedure. Bleeding, pain, infection, injury to adjacent organs, and (rarely) death are potential complications. In the presence of coagulopathy, thrombocytopenia, and/or ascites, a biopsy can be obtained by the transjugular route. Suspicious liver lesions are usually biopsied with ultrasonographic or CT guidance. Laparoscopy is an alternative method for obtaining liver tissue.
- Noninvasive testing to assess fibrosis/cirrhosis: aspartate aminotransferase to platelet ratio index (APRI), FibroScan, FibroTest, transient elastography, and MR spectroscopy are under investigation and at this point they should be viewed as complementary to liver biopsy.

VIRAL HEPATITIS

The hepatotropic viruses include hepatitis A virus (HAV), hepatitis B virus (HBV), hepatitis C virus (HCV), hepatitis D virus (HDV), and hepatitis E virus (HEV) (Tables 19-1 and 19-2). Nonhepatotropic viruses (viruses that indirectly affect the liver) include Epstein–Barr virus, cytomegalovirus, herpes virus, measles, Ebola, and others.

Acute viral hepatitis is defined by the sudden onset of significant aminotransferase elevation as a consequence of diffuse necroinflammatory liver injury. Symptoms may vary. This condition may resolve or progress to acute liver failure (ALF) or chronic hepatitis.

Chronic viral hepatitis is defined as the presence of persistent (at least 6 months) viral activity (serologic and molecular studies), with necroinflammatory and fibrotic injury. Symptoms may be variable and mild-to-moderate elevation of liver enzymes is classically detected. Histopathologic classification of chronic viral hepatitis is based on etiology, grade, and stage. Grading and staging are measures of the severity of the necroinflammatory process and fibrosis, respectively. Chronic viral hepatitis may lead to cirrhosis and HCC.

Hepatitis A Virus

GENERAL PRINCIPLES

Classification

HAV is an **RNA virus** that belongs to the **picornavirus family**.

Epidemiology

- HAV is the most common cause of acute viral hepatitis worldwide.
- Approximately 1.5 million cases of hepatitis A are detected worldwide annually; however, the rate of infection is thought to be as much as 10 times higher (*World J Hepatol 2012;4:68*).
- Approximately 30% of acute viral hepatitis in the United States is caused by HAV.

Table 19-1	Clinical and Epidemiologic Features of Hepatotropic Viruses				
Organism	Hepatitis A	Hepatitis B	Hepatitis C	Hepatitis D	Hepatitis E
Incubation	15–45 d	30–180 d	15–150 d	30–150 d	30–60 d
Transmission	Fecal–oral	Blood Sexual Perinatal	Blood Sexual (rare) Perinatal (rare)	Blood Sexual (rare)	Fecal–oral
Risk groups	Residents of and travelers to endemic regions Children and caregivers in daycare centers	Injection drug users Multiple sexual partners Men who have sex with men Infants born to infected mothers Health care workers Transfusion recipients	Injection drug users Transfusion recipients	Any person with hepatitis B virus Injection drug users	Residents of and travelers to endemic regions
Fatality rate	1.0%	1.0%	<0.1%	2%–10%	1%
Carrier state	No	Yes	Yes	Yes	No
Chronic hepatitis	None	2%–10% in adults; 90% in children <5 yrs	70%–85%	Variable	None
Cirrhosis	No	Yes	Yes	Yes	No

Table 19-2	Viral Hepatitis Serologies			
Hepatitis	Acute	Chronic	Recovered/ Latent	Vaccinated
HAV	IgM anti-HAV+	NA	IgG anti-HAV+	IgG anti-HAV+
HBV	IgM anti-HBc+	IgG anti-HBc+	IgG anti-HBc+	Anti-HBs+ only
	HBeAg+	HBeAg±	HBeAg−	
	HBsAg+	Anti-HBe±[a]	Anti-HBe±[a]	
	HBV DNA+	HBsAg+	HBsAg−	
		HBV DNA±[a]	Anti-HBs Ab+	
			HBV DNA−	
HCV	All tests possibly negative	Anti-HCV Ab+	Anti-HCV Ab+	NA
		HCV RNA+	HCV RNA−[b]	
	HCV RNA+			
	Anti-HCV Ab+ in 8–10 wk			
HDV	IgM anti-HDV+[c]	IgG anti-HDV+[c]	IgG anti-HDV+[c]	NA[d]
	HDV Ag+[c]			
HEV	Available from CDC and research specialty laboratories	NA	Available from CDC and research specialty laboratories	NA

[a]HBeAg is present during periods of high replication along with HBV DNA. Anti-HBe is present during periods of low replication when HBeAg and HBV DNA may be undetectable.
[b]Negative HCV RNA results should be interpreted with caution. Differences are found in thresholds for detection among assays and among laboratories.
[c]Markers of HBV infection are also present, because HDV cannot replicate in the absence of HBV.
[d]Although no vaccine is available for HDV, immunity to HBV protects against HDV infection.
Ab, antibody; CDC, Centers for Disease Control and Prevention; HAV, hepatitis A virus; HBc, hepatitis B core antigen; HBeAg, hepatitis B e antigen; HBsAg, hepatitis B surface antigen; HBV, hepatitis B virus; HCV, hepatitis C virus; HDV, hepatitis D virus; HEV, hepatitis E virus; Ig, immunoglobulin; NA, not applicable.

Pathophysiology
- HAV infection is usually transmitted via **the fecal–oral route**.
- Large-scale outbreaks due to contamination of food and drinking water can occur.
- The period of greatest infectivity is 2 weeks before the onset of clinical illness; fecal shedding continues for 2 to 3 weeks after the onset of symptoms.
- Although the period of viremia is brief, sexual transmission and parenteral transmission may occur.

Risk Factors
High-risk groups include people living in or traveling to developing countries due to food and water contamination, men who have sex with men, staff and attendees at daycare centers, and patients with chronic liver disease (increased risk for acute HAV).

Prevention

Immunization programs are available.

- **Preexposure prophylaxis**
  - **HAV vaccine.** Inactivated HAV vaccines (containing the single HAV antigen) and combination vaccines (containing both HAV and hepatitis B surface antigen) are available. Vaccinations should be administered intramuscularly into the deltoid muscle in a two-dose regimen (single-antigen HAV vaccine; first dose at time 0 and second dose at 6 to 18 months) or in a three-dose regimen (combination vaccine; first dose at time 0, second dose at 1 month, and third dose at 6 months).
  - Protective antibody levels are present in 94% to 100% of those immunized 1 month after the first dose (*MMWR Recomm Rep 2006;55(RR-7):1*).
  - Currently, there is no role for a hepatitis A vaccine booster after appropriate immunization.
- **Postexposure prophylaxis**
  - Immunoglobulin (Ig) is a sterile preparation of concentrated antibody made from pooled human plasma that allows for passive transfer of antibodies.
  - Ig (0.02 mL/kg intramuscular [IM]) should be given as soon as possible after known exposure to HAV. Efficacy beyond 2 weeks after exposure has not been established.
  - Hepatitis A vaccine is not licensed for use as postexposure prophylaxis; however, patients who have been administered one dose of vaccine at more than 1 month prior to exposure do not need Ig.
  - If HAV vaccine and Ig are recommended, they may be administered simultaneously at separate injection sites.

DIAGNOSIS

- The diagnosis of acute HAV is made by the detection of **IgM anti-HAV antibodies**.
- Aminotransferase elevations range from 10 to 100 times the upper limit of normal.
- The **recovery phase** and **immunity phase** are characterized by the presence **IgG anti-HAV antibodies and a slow decline in IgM anti-HAV antibodies**.
- Liver biopsy is rarely needed.

Clinical Presentation

- HAV can be silent (subclinical), especially in children and young adults. Symptoms vary from mild illness to ALF.
- Malaise, fatigue, pruritus, headache, abdominal pain, myalgias, arthralgias, nausea, vomiting, anorexia, and fever are common but nonspecific symptoms.
- **Physical examination** may reveal jaundice, hepatomegaly, and in rare cases, lymphadenopathy, splenomegaly, or a vascular rash.

TREATMENT

- No specific treatment is available.
- Supportive symptomatic treatment is recommended.
- Liver transplantation may be an option for ALF.

OUTCOME/PROGNOSIS

- Almost all cases of acute HAV hepatitis will resolve in 4 to 8 weeks. HAV does not induce chronic hepatitis or cirrhosis.
- Prolonged cholestatic disease, characterized by persistent jaundice and waxing and waning of liver enzymes, is more frequently seen in adults.
- **Fulminant hepatic failure** is relatively rare, but risk increases with age: 0.1% in patients younger than 15 years to >1% in patients older than 40 years.

Hepatitis B Virus

GENERAL PRINCIPLES

Classification

- **HBV** is a **DNA virus** that belongs to the **hepadnavirus family**.
- Eight genotypes of HBV have been identified and labeled A through H.

Epidemiology

- Two billion people worldwide have serologic evidence of past or present infection and approximately 400 million people are chronic carriers.
- HBV is unevenly distributed throughout the world. In endemic areas such as Asia and Sub-Saharan Africa, infection is usually acquired in childhood, while in Western countries where HBV is relatively rare, the infection is acquired in adulthood.
- The prevalence of HBV genotypes varies depending on the geographic location. All known HBV genotypes have been found in the United States, with genotypes A, B, and C being the most prevalent (*Hepatology 2007;45:507*).
- HBV (with or without cirrhosis) causes 60% to 80% of HCC worldwide.
- HBV-related mortality is estimated between 500,000 and 1,000,000 deaths worldwide per year.
- HBV is an indication for l5% to 10% of the cases of liver transplantation.

Pathophysiology

- HBV liver damage is immune mediated.
- Modes of transmission include:
  - Horizontal transmission
    - Parenteral or percutaneous routes (e.g., needlestick injury, injection drug use, hemodialysis, transfusions)
    - Sexual contact (e.g., men who have sex with men, sexual promiscuity, or intercourse with HBV-infected partners)
  - Vertical transmission: Mother to infant

Risk Factors

High-risk groups include individuals with a history of multiple blood transfusions, patients on hemodialysis, injection drug users, sexual promiscuity, men who have sex with men, household and heterosexual contacts of hepatitis B carriers, residents and employees of residential care facilities, travelers to endemic regions, and individuals born in areas of high or intermediate prevalence (e.g., Alaska, southern Asia, Africa, South Pacific Islands, and the Amazon).

Associated Conditions

Extrahepatic manifestations include polyarteritis nodosa, glomerulonephritis, cryoglobulinemia, serum sickness–like illness, papular acrodermatitis (predominantly in children), and aplastic anemia.

DIAGNOSIS

Clinical Presentation

- Incubation period ranges from 30 to 160 days.
- According to the natural history of infection, different **clinical phases** have been defined:
  - **Acute hepatitis B:** Can be silent (subclinical), especially in children and young adults. Symptoms vary from mild illness to ALF. Malaise, fatigue, pruritus, headache, abdominal pain, myalgias, arthralgias, nausea, vomiting, anorexia, and fever are common but nonspecific symptoms. Progression to chronicity depends on age at acquisition (approximately 90% of children infected before age 6 will progress to chronic hepatitis B). Most acute HBV infections are self-limited in adults (5% to 10% of adults will progress to chronic hepatitis B).
  - **Chronic hepatitis B** runs an indolent course, sometimes for decades. Fatigue is a common symptom but frequently overlooked because of its subjectivity. The disease may only become clinically apparent late in the natural course, with symptoms typically associated with ESLD. Chronic HBV infection is a dynamic process that occurs in different phases:
    - **Immune tolerant:** Characterized by active viral replication with high levels of HBV DNA, positive hepatitis B e antigen (HBeAg), yet normal liver enzymes and low levels of inflammation and fibrosis. This phase is frequently seen in children or those infected early in life. It may last for decades.
    - **Immune active:** Characterized by active viral replication with high levels of HBV DNA, positive HBeAg, and elevation of liver enzymes as a consequence of a vigorous immune response. Histologic activity is manifested by inflammation and fibrosis. This phase is frequently seen in adults and may last for years.
    - **Low replication:** Characterized by low or undetectable HBV DNA levels and negative HBeAg. Usually, these patients have normal liver enzymes and reduced liver inflammation. During this phase, the disease is not progressive and there is low risk for development of HCC. Reactivation to the immunoactive (see earlier discussion) or HBeAg negative (precore or basal core promoter mutation) phase is possible.
    - **HBeAg negative (precore or basal core promoter mutations):** These patients harbor HBV mutations in the C gene (precore or basal core promoter regions) that prevent the production of, or have low expression of HBeAg. Despite the absence of HBeAg, HBV DNA levels are high, liver enzymes are elevated, and there is histologic activity. This is a late phase in the natural history of chronic HBV. This phase is often seen in older patients with more advanced disease and is usually triggered by frequent periods of reactivation.
  - **Resolution:** Chronic hepatitis B patients may have viral clearance, characterized by undetectable HBV levels. The serologic hallmark for these patients is antigen loss with antibody serum conversion (HBsAg loss and anti-HBs production). Seroconversion may occur spontaneously or with treatment. Patients with resolved HBV have normal liver enzymes.

Diagnostic Testing

The diagnosis of HBV often requires the combination of data obtained from liver chemistries, serology, molecular biology, and histology.

Laboratories
- Liver chemistries that are usually abnormal in acute hepatitis include AST, ALT, ALP, and total bilirubin. In chronic HBV, the biochemical changes are variable and aminotransferases may fluctuate ranging from normal to increased levels. Studies have recommended newer upper limits of normal for ALT in men and women (30 and 19 U/L, respectively).
- Tests that measure cholestasis (ALP, GGT, and total bilirubin) or liver synthetic function (albumin and PT/INR) may be abnormal according to the disease stage.
- HBV antigens detected in serum and used for diagnostic purposes in clinical practice include **hepatitis B surface antigen (HBsAg) and HBeAg**.
- HBV antigens detected in liver biopsy by immunoperoxidase staining include **HBsAg** stained in the hepatocyte cytoplasm and **hepatitis B core antigen (HBcAg)** stained in hepatocyte nuclei.
- HBV antibodies are specific to their corresponding antigen and include antibody against HBsAg (anti-HBs), antibody against HBeAg (anti-HBe), and IgM and IgG antibodies against HBcAg (IgM and IgG anti-HBc).
- **HBV DNA** is the most accurate marker of viral replication. It is detected by polymerase chain reaction (PCR) and is commonly reported as International Units per milliliter. Large long-term population-based studies have demonstrated a close correlation between HBV DNA levels and disease progression to cirrhosis and development of HCC (*Gastroenterology 2006;130:678*; *JAMA 2006;295:65*).
- For use of HBV markers in clinical practice, see Table 19-3.
- Genotypic determination is growing in clinical significance as data are emerging with respect to response to antivirals, disease progression, and risk of HCC (*Gastroenterol Rep 2012;14(1):37*).
  - Genotypes A and B have been associated with higher rates of response to interferon (IFN) therapy and higher rates of spontaneous HBeAg seroconversion.
  - Genotypes A and D progress to chronic infection more frequently than other genotypes following acute infection.
  - Genotypes C and D are more likely to progress to advanced liver disease and HCC.

Diagnostic Procedures
Liver biopsy is useful to assess the degree of inflammation (grade) and fibrosis (stage) in patients with chronic hepatitis. Liver histology is an important adjuvant diagnostic test in guiding treatment decisions.

TREATMENT

The treatment goal is viral eradication or suppression to prevent progression of ESLD and HCC. End points of treatment include
- Clearance of HBV DNA
- HBeAg and HBsAg seroconversion (i.e., antigen loss and antibody production)
- Normalization of liver enzymes
- Normalization of histology

Table 19-3   Use of Hepatitis B Virus Markers in Clinical Practice

Test	Acute Hepatitis B	Resolved Acute Hepatitis B	High-Replication Chronic HBV	Low-Replication Chronic HBV	HBV Precore Mutant	Vaccination
HBsAg	+	–	+	+	+	–
HBeAg	+	–	+	+	–	–
Anti-HBs	–	+	–	–	–	+
Anti-HBe	–	+	–	+	+	–
IgM anti-HBc	+	–	+	–	–	–
IgG anti-HBc	–	+	+	+	+	–
HBV DNA	$>10^5$ copies/mL	Negative	$>10^5$ copies/mL	10^2–10^4 copies/mL	$>10^4$ copies/mL	Negative
ALT/AST	+++	Normal	+++	Normal	+/++	Normal

ALT, alanine transaminase; AST, aspartate transaminase; HBc, hepatitis B core antigen; HBeAg, hepatitis B e antigen; HBsAg, hepatitis B surface antigen; HBV, hepatitis B virus; Ig, immunoglobulin.

Medications

- Medications for the treatment of hepatitis B are divided into three main groups: IFNs, nucleoside analogs (entecavir), and nucleotide analogs (tenofovir).
- Current indications for treatment include chronic hepatitis B (both HBeAg positive and HBeAg negative) with HBV DNA >2,000 IU/mL and/or elevated ALT and severe necroinflammation/fibrosis on liver biopsy. Patients with compensated or decompensated cirrhosis should be treated even with normal ALT levels or HBV DNA levels <2,000 IU/mL (*J Hepatol 2009;50:227*).
- Chronic hepatitis B immune tolerant patients and chronic hepatitis B with low replication should not be treated.
- The optimal treatment duration has not yet been defined. The ideal treatment outcome is HBsAg loss with seroconversion, unfortunately this goal is rarely achieved. Therefore, in patients who are HBeAg positive at baseline, the expected outcome is loss of HBeAg with anti-e seroconversion, clearance of HBV DNA, and normalization of liver enzymes. In patients who are HBeAg negative at baseline, the expected outcome is clearance of HBV DNA and normalization of liver enzymes. In patients who are HBeAg positive at baseline, treatment should be prolonged at least 6 months after HBeAg loss/seroconversion. These patients should be monitored, given the possibility of reactivation. In patients who are HBeAg negative at baseline, treatment should be continued indefinitely or until HBsAg loss/seroconversion is achieved.
- Antiviral resistance is a phenomenon observed with the use of nucleoside and nucleotide analogs. Resistance should be considered in patients with an HBV DNA level increase (>1 $\log_{10}$) from the lowest level of suppression achieved while on therapy. Tenofovir and entacavir have a high genetic barrier for resistance (lowest susceptibility) when compared to other nucleoside and nucleotide analogs and are therefore the preferred oral therapeutic agents.

First Line

Entecavir, tenofovir, and pegylated interferon alpha (pIFN-α) are first-line agents in patients with chronic hepatitis B (*Expert Opin Pharmacother 2011;12(13):2025*).

- **Entecavir (ETV)** is a potent anti-HBV **oral nucleoside (guanosine) analog** and is well tolerated. Dose: 0.5 and 1.0 mg in naïve and lamivudine (LAM)-resistant patients. In patients with renal impairment, dose adjustment is needed. In patients who are HBeAg positive at baseline, HBV DNA clearance occurs in 94% of patients at 5 years (*Hepatology 2010;51:422*). In patients who are HBeAg negative at baseline, HBV DNA clearance occurs in 90% of patients after 48 weeks (*N Engl J Med 2006;354:1011*). Histologic evaluation after treatment with ETV for 6 years shows improvement in necroinflammation in 96% and fibrosis in 88% of patients (*Hepatology 2010;52:886*). Patients resistant to LAM are prone to develop rapid antiviral resistance to ETV. Entacavir is pregnancy category C.
- **Tenofovir (TDF)** is a potent anti-HBV oral nucleotide (acyclic) analog and is well tolerated. Dose: 300 mg daily. It is rarely reported to induce renal failure and Fanconi syndrome. In patients who are HBeAg positive at baseline, HBV DNA clearance occurs in 68% of patients after 4 years of treatment (*Hepatology 2010;52(suppl):556A*). In patients who are HBeAg negative at baseline, HBV DNA clearance occurs in 84% of patients after 4 years of treatment (*Hepatology 2010;52(suppl):555A*). No clinical resistance has been identified. TDF is pregnancy category B.

- **The interferons** are antiviral, immunomodulatory, and antiproliferative glycoproteins that have been used in the treatment of chronic HBV for several years. IFNs are parenteral agents, associated with a poor tolerability profile, in particular in patients with advanced liver disease. Long-term studies have shown a durable benefit in responders. Neither IFN nor pIFN-α induce antiviral resistance.
  - The IFNs are pregnancy category C.
    pIFN-α has replaced conventional interferon alpha (IFN-α) because of its more convenient once-weekly administration, longer half-life, and bioavailability given its attachment to a polyethylene glycol molecule. The best results obtained with pIFN-α have been seen in patients who are HBeAg positive, and those with genotype A or B. pIFN-α has shown long-term sustainability of HBeAg and HBsAg negativity (37% and 11%, respectively) in those patients who were initially HBeAg positive (*Gastroenterology 2008;135:459*). In a large multicenter study, HBsAg clearance was 11% in patients who were initially HBeAg negative (*J Hepatol 2008;48(suppl 2):S46*). Research trials combining pIFN-α with nucleoside and nucleotide analogs to improve the HBV treatment efficacy are under investigation.

Second Line
- **Telbivudine (LdT)** is an oral nucleoside (thymidine) analog and is well tolerated. Dose: 600 mg daily. In patients with renal impairment, dose adjustment is needed. Its resistance profile is worse than the first-line agents and it is not useful in patients with antiviral resistance to other nucleoside analogs. LdT is pregnancy category B.
- **Adefovir (ADV)** is an oral nucleotide (adenosine) analog and is well tolerated. Dose: 10 mg daily. In patients with renal impairment, dose adjustment is needed. Its resistance profile is worse than the first-line agents. This agent is potentially useful in patients with nucleoside analog resistance. ADV is pregnancy category C.
- **Lamivudine** is an oral nucleoside (dideoxy-3′-thiacytidine) analog and is well tolerated. Dose: 100 mg daily. In patients with renal impairment, dose adjustment is needed. Its current use is very limited given its high rate of resistant mutations (70% at 5 years of treatment). LAM is pregnancy category B.

PREVENTION

Preexposure prophylaxis
- **HBV vaccine** should be considered for everyone but particularly in individuals who belong to high-risk groups (see Risk Factors section). HBV vaccines have been demonstrated to be safe. HBsAg is used to prepare the HBV vaccine (single-antigen). The HBV vaccine is also available in combination for the prevention of hepatitis A, *Haemophilus influenza* type B, *Neisseria meningitidis*, diphtheria, tetanus, pertussis, and polio.
- HBV vaccination schedule includes three IM injections at 0, 1, and 6 months in infants or healthy adults. Protective antibody response is >90% after the third dose. The protective antibody response declines with age. Smoking, obesity, genetics, and immunosuppression can contribute to a decreased protective response from vaccination. Response to vaccination is measured by anti-HBs (≥10 mIU/mL).
- Prevaccination screening for previous exposure or infection is recommended in high-risk groups to avoid vaccinating recovered individuals or those with chronic

infection. Postvaccination screening (to evaluate vaccine response) is recommended for individuals who belong to high-risk groups.

- Additional doses, higher doses, or revaccination can be considered in nonresponders and hyporesponders to elicit protective levels of immunity. Booster doses may be needed in immunosuppressed individuals.

Postexposure prophylaxis

- **Infants born to HBsAg-positive mothers should receive HBV vaccine and hepatitis B immunoglobulin (HBIg), 0.5 mL, within 12 hours of birth.** Immunized infants should be tested at approximately 12 months of age for HBsAg, anti-HBs, and anti-HBc. The presence of HBsAg indicates that the infant is actively infected. The presence of both anti-HBs and anti-HBc suggests that infection occurred but was probably modified by immunoprophylaxis and that immunity is likely to be prolonged. The presence of anti-HBs alone is indicative of vaccine-induced immunity.
- Susceptible sexual partners of individuals with HBV and those with needlestick injury should receive HBIg (0.04 to 0.07 mL/kg) and the first dose of HBV vaccine at different sites as soon as possible (preferably within 48 hours but no more than 7 days after exposure). A second dose of HBIg should be administered 30 days after exposure, and the vaccination schedule be completed.
- Postexposure prophylaxis with HBIg plus a nucleotide or nucleoside analog should be used initially after liver transplantation to prevent HBV recurrence.

Surgical Management

Liver transplantation is indicated for patients with advanced liver disease and/or HCC due to infection with HBV.

OUTCOME/PROGNOSIS

- Depending on the age at infection, people may have spontaneous resolution or progression to chronicity.
  - Children younger than 5 years old: 90% may develop chronic HBV infection.
  - Adults: 5% to 10% may develop chronic HBV.
- Chronic hepatitis B
  - Morbidity and mortality in chronic HBV are linked to level and persistence of viral replication. Spontaneous clearance of HBsAg occurs in 0.5% of patients annually.
  - Once the diagnosis of chronic HBV is established, the 5-year cumulative incidence of developing cirrhosis ranges from 8% to 20%.
  - Of patients with chronic HBV, 5% to 10% progress to HCC **with or without preceding cirrhosis**.

Hepatitis C

GENERAL PRINCIPLES

Classification

- HCV is an RNA virus that belongs to the **flavivirus** family.
- There are six HCV genotypes with multiple subtypes.

Epidemiology

- **HCV** is a global health problem with approximately **180 million carriers worldwide**.
- The incidence of hepatitis C has declined in the last 30 years. In the United States, about 4.1 million are infected with HCV, and 50% to 75% of these people are unaware of their infection (*Ann Intern Med 2012;156:263*).
- HCV infection is the most common chronic blood-borne infection (see Risk Factors).
- Transmission by transfusion of blood products (and their derivatives) and organ transplantation has been reduced to near zero in developed countries due to sensitive screening methods.
- In the United States, HCV mortality is increasing as the infected population ages and is anticipated to reach 35,000 deaths per year by 2030 (*Ann Intern Med 2012;156:263*).
- Genotype 1 accounts for 75% and genotypes 2 and 3 account for 20% of HCV infections in the United States.
- In industrialized countries, HCV accounts for 20% of cases of acute hepatitis, 70% of cases of chronic hepatitis, 40% of cases of ESLD, 60% of cases of HCC, and 40% of liver transplantations.

Pathophysiology

- The liver damage that ensues after HCV infection is immune mediated.
- Modes of transmission include:
  - **Parenteral** (e.g., transfusion, injection drug use, body piercing, needlestick injury)
  - **Sexual (high-risk sexual practices)** and **from mother to offspring (vertical transmission)**, although at a much lower frequency than HBV

Risk Factors

Risk factors for HCV infection include a history of blood transfusions or clotting factors before the institution of modern screening methodology (1992), hemodialysis, injection drug use, multiple sexual partners, and occupational exposure with blood and blood-derived products. Other risk factors may include tattooing, body piercing, sharing "straws" for intranasal cocaine use, sharing razors, and military service, homelessness, and incarceration (*Gastroenterology 2002;123:2082*).

Prevention

No preexposure prophylaxis or vaccine exists. Prevention of high-risk behaviors and lifestyle modifications should be encouraged.

Associated Conditions

Extrahepatic manifestations include mixed cryoglobulinemia (10% to 25% of patients with HCV), glomerulonephritis, porphyria cutanea tarda, cutaneous necrotizing vasculitis, lichen planus, lymphoma, diabetes mellitus, and other autoimmune disorders.

DIAGNOSIS

Clinical Presentation

- The incubation period varies from 15 to 150 days.
- **Acute hepatitis** can be silent, especially in children and young adults. Symptoms may also vary from mild illness to ALF. Malaise, fatigue, pruritus, headache,

abdominal pain, myalgias, arthralgias, nausea, vomiting, anorexia, and fever are common but nonspecific symptoms.
- **Chronic hepatitis** runs an indolent course, sometimes for decades. Fatigue is a common symptom. The disease may only become clinically apparent late in the natural course, when symptoms are associated with advanced liver disease.

Diagnostic Testing
- **Antibodies against HCV (anti-HCV)** may be undetectable for the first 8 weeks after infection. These antibodies are detected by enzyme immunoassay (EIA). **Antibodies do not confer immunity.** The test has a sensitivity of 95% to 99% and a lower specificity. A false-positive test (anti-HCV positive with HCV RNA negative) may be detected in the setting of autoimmune hepatitis (AIH) or hyper-gammaglobulinemia. A false-negative test (anti-HCV negative with HCV RNA positive) may be seen in immunosuppressed individuals and in patients on hemodialysis.
- **HCV RNA** can be detected by **PCR** in serum as early as **1 to 2 weeks after infection** (qualitative and quantitative assays). It is expressed in international units per milliliter (IU/mL), with lower limits of detection approaching 10 IU/mL. HCV RNA determination is useful for both diagnosis and treatment purposes.
- **HCV genotypes and subtypes** can be detected by commercially available serologic and molecular assays. HCV genotype influences the duration, dosage, and response to treatment.
- **Liver biopsy** is useful to score the degree of inflammation (grade) and fibrosis (stage) in the liver of chronically infected patients. It is useful to grade the amount of liver steatosis and guides treatment decisions.

TREATMENT

- Therapeutic **goals for treatment** of HCV include:
  ○ Eradication of the virus
  ○ Decrease disease progression
  ○ Histologic improvement
  ○ Decrease HCC frequency
- Treatment outcome in HCV is determined by a number of pretreatment and on-treatment factors
  ○ **Pretreatment factors**
    Viral genotype, IL-28B genotype (CC allele), viral load, treatment naïve or previous treatment failure, advanced liver disease (amount of liver fibrosis), metabolism (obesity, steatosis, and insulin resistance), race/ethnicity
  ○ **On-treatment factors**
    ▪ Adherence to the prescribed regimen, dose and duration of ribavirin, pIFN-α, and protease inhibitors boceprevir and telaprevir
    ▪ Rapidity of viral clearance

Medications
Acute infection
IFN-α (standard or pegylated) for 6 months has been associated with a high rate (98%) of sustained HCV RNA clearance (*N Engl J Med 2001;345:1452*).

Chronic infection

- In patients with genotype 1 (all subtypes), the standard of care is to use triple therapy including pIFN, ribavirin, and a direct antiviral agent (DAA). DAAs currently approved are boceprevir and telaprevir. The chosen treatment regimen takes into consideration prior exposure and response to pIFN and ribavirin, presence of cirrhosis, and selected DAA (Figures 19-1 and 19-2, and Table 19-4).
- Side effects of IFN-based therapy include flu-like symptoms, neuropsychiatric disorders, endocrine dysfunction, and bone marrow suppression.

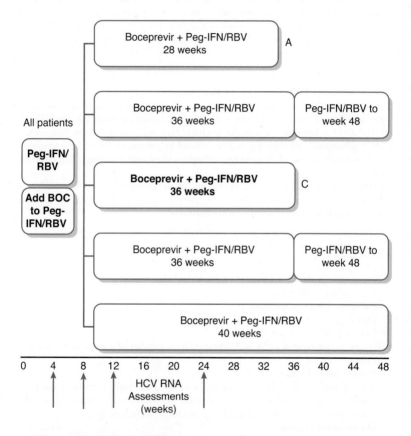

A: Naïve, undetectable HCV RNA at weeks 8 and 24.
B: Naïve, detectable HCV RNA at week 8 and undetectable HCV RNA at week 24.
C: Experienced, undetectable HCV RNA at weeks 8 and 24.
D: Experienced, detectable HCV RNA at week 8 and undetectable HCV RNA at week 24.
E: Cirrhotic, null responder.

Figure 19-1. Response-guided treatment algorithm for boceprevir. HCV, hepatitis C virus; Peg-IFN/RBV, pegylated interferon/ribavirin.

A: Naïve, undetectable HCV RNA at weeks 4 and 12.
B: Naïve, detectable HCV RNA at weeks 4 *and/or* 12; all experienced patients; naïve, cirrhotic, undetectable HCV RNA at weeks 4 and 12.

Figure 19-2. Response-guided treatment algorithm for telaprevir. HCV, hepatitis C virus; Peg-IFN/RBV, pegylated interferon/ribavirin.

- Side effects of ribavirin include teratogenicity, hemolytic anemia, and pulmonary symptoms (dyspnea, cough, and pneumonitis). Contraindications to treatment with ribavirin include pregnancy or unwillingness to practice birth control, chronic renal insufficiency, and the inability to tolerate anemia (15% to 30%).
- Side effects of boceprevir include anemia and dysgeusia. Side effects of telaprevir include rash (maculopapular and eczematous), anemia, pruritis, nausea, and diarrhea. It is important to note that the protease inhibitors can inhibit the hepatic cytochrome P450 enzymes and therefore may interfere with the metabolism of other drugs.
- In patients with genotype 2 or 3, a combination of pIFN (peginterferon alfa-2a 180 μg/wk or peginterferon alfa-2b 1.5 μg/kg/wk, subcutaneous) and oral ribavirin (800 mg daily) is administered for 6 months.

Table 19-4	Futility Rules for Boceprevir and Telaprevir

Triple therapy with boceprevir should be stopped if the patient has:
HCV RNA results $\geq$100 IU/mL at week 12
Confirmed, detectable HCV RNA at week 24

Triple therapy with telaprevir should be stopped if the patient has:
HCV RNA results $\geq$1,000 IU/mL at weeks 4 or 12
Confirmed, detectable HCV RNA at week 24

HCV, hepatitis C virus.

MONITORING/FOLLOW-UP

- Triple therapy with boceprevir should be stopped if the patient has:
  - HCV RNA results ≥100 IU/mL at week 12
  - Confirmed, detectable HCV RNA at week 24
- Triple therapy with telaprevir should be stopped if the patient has:
  - HCV RNA results ≥1,000 IU/mL at weeks 4 or 12
  - Confirmed, detectable HCV RNA at week 24

OUTCOME/PROGNOSIS

HCC develops in approximately **1% to 2% of patients per year**, and rarely occurs in the absence of cirrhosis.

Hepatitis D

GENERAL PRINCIPLES

Classification

HDV is a circular RNA virus and is the only member of the genus *Delta virus*. Originally, it was considered a subviral particle resembling plant pathogens, viroids, and virusoids.

Epidemiology

It is found throughout the world and is endemic to the Mediterranean basin, the Middle East, and portions of South America. Outside these areas, infections occur primarily in individuals who have received transfusions or in injection drug users. **HDV requires the presence of HBV for infection and replication.**

Pathophysiology

HDV infection clinically presents as a **coinfection** (acute hepatitis B and D), as a **superinfection** (chronic hepatitis B with acute hepatitis D) that may progresses to chronic infection and cirrhosis, or as a **latent infection** (i.e., in the liver transplantation setting).

Risk Factors

High-risk groups are similar to HBV (see Epidemiology under Hepatitis B Virus section).

Prevention

Although there is no vaccine to prevent HDV in carriers of HBV, both infections can be prevented by timely administration of the HBV vaccine.

DIAGNOSIS

Clinical Presentation

In patients with coinfection, the course is transient and self-limited. The rate of progression to chronicity is similar to the one reported for acute HBV. In superinfection, the HBV carriers may present with a severe acute hepatitis exacerbation with frequent progression to chronic HDV.

Diagnostic Testing

Diagnosis is made by finding HDV RNA or HDV antigen in serum or liver and by detecting antibody to the HDV antigen in the setting of acute or chronic HBV.

TREATMENT

IFN-α is the **treatment of choice** for chronic hepatitis D.

Hepatitis E

GENERAL PRINCIPLES

Classification

HEV is an **RNA virus** that belongs to the *Hepeviridae* family.

Epidemiology

- It has been implicated in epidemics in India, Southeast Asia, Africa, and Mexico. HEV has also been identified in developed countries, and there have been increasing reports of sporadic cases and food-borne outbreaks within the United States and Western Europe (*Hepatology 2011;54:2218*).
- Acute HEV is now more common than acute HAV in China, France, the United Kingdom, and Japan (*Lancet 2012;379:2477*).
- Pets and consumption of organ meats may play a role in transmission.
- Hepatitis E is considered a zoonotic disease and reservoirs include pigs, wild boar, deer, and potentially, other species (*Virus Res 2007;127:216*).

Pathophysiology

Transmission closely resembles that of HAV (i.e., **fecal–oral route**).

Prevention

- In developing countries, strategies of prevention should include sanitary and hygiene improvements.
- Two hepatitis E vaccines have been investigated in clinical trials. They are highly immunogenic and are 95% to 100% effective. These vaccines are not yet commercially available.

DIAGNOSIS

- Acute hepatitis E is clinically indistinguishable from other acute viral hepatitis and is usually a self-limited illness. In patients with preexisting chronic liver disease, acute hepatitis E may have a more severe course with higher mortality.
- Hepatitis E can cause chronic infection (HEV RNA for >6 months). Most cases have occurred in solid-organ transplant recipients or immunosuppressed individuals (e.g., HIV).

TREATMENT

Treatment is supportive.

OUTCOME/PROGNOSIS

Children under the age of 2 years and pregnant women (third trimester) have high mortality rates when infected with hepatitis E.

DRUG-INDUCED LIVER INJURY

GENERAL PRINCIPLES

New medications and herbal products can cause liver disease. Over 1,000 drugs and herbals have been associated with drug-induced liver injury (DILI).

Classification

- There are three major classifications of DILI that occur as a result of both intrinsic and idiosyncratic hepatotoxicity:
  - ○ Hepatocellular injury refers to injury to the liver cell.
  - ○ Cholestatic injury refers to injury to the biliary system.
  - ○ Mixed hepatocellular and cholestatic injury refers to injury to both the liver cell and the biliary system.
- Other less common types of DILI include chronic hepatitis, chronic cholestasis, granulomatous hepatitis, fibrosis or cirrhosis, and carcinogenesis.

Epidemiology

DILI causes approximately 50% of all the cases of ALF in the United States, with acetaminophen being the most common causative agent.

Pathophysiology

- Intrinsic hepatotoxicity results from the direct hepatotoxic effects of the drug or its metabolites. The mechanism is predictable and dose dependent. Examples include carbon tetrachloride, elemental phosphorus, and supratherapeutic doses of acetaminophen.
- Idiosyncratic hepatotoxicity can be divided into hypersensitivity (allergic) and metabolic (nonallergic). These reactions depend on multiple variables and are not predictable.
- Hypersensitivity responses occur as a result of stimulation of the immune system by a metabolite of a drug alone or after haptenization (covalently binding) to a liver protein (e.g., allopurinol, diclofenac). The latency of the reaction is variable. Repeated challenge with the same agent leads to prompt recurrence of the reaction.
- Metabolic hepatotoxicity occurs in susceptible patients as a result of altered drug clearance or accelerated production of hepatotoxic metabolites (e.g., isoniazid, ketoconazole). The latency of this reaction is variable.

DIAGNOSIS

Clinical Presentation

- The acute presentation can be clinically silent. When symptoms are present, they are nonspecific and include nausea/vomiting, general malaise, fatigue, and abdominal pain.
- In the acute setting, the majority of patients will recover after cessation of the offending drug.
- Fever and rash may also be seen in association with hypersensitivity reactions.

Diagnostic Criteria

- Clinical suspicion
- Temporal relation of liver injury to drug usage
- Resolution of liver injury after the suspected agent has been discontinued

Diagnostic Testing

Laboratories

Biochemical abnormalities

- **Hepatocellular injury:** AST and ALT elevation more than two times the upper limit of normal.
- **Cholestatic injury:** ALP and conjugated bilirubin elevation more than two times the upper limit of normal.
- **Mixed injury** includes increases in all of the mentioned biochemical abnormalities to more than two times the upper limit of normal.

Diagnostic Procedures

Liver biopsy is sometimes needed.

TREATMENT

Nonpharmacologic Therapies

- Treatment includes cessation of offending drug and institution of supportive measures.
- An attempt to remove the agent from the GI tract should be made in most cases of acute toxic ingestion using lavage or cathartics (see Chapter 28, Toxicology).
- Management of acetaminophen overdose is a medical emergency (see Chapter 28, Toxicology).

Surgical Management

Liver transplantation may be an option for patients with drug-induced ALF.

OUTCOME/PROGNOSIS

- Prognosis of DILI is often unique to the offending medication.
- Jaundice portends a poor prognosis and is associated with case-fatality rates in the range of 10% to 50% (*N Engl J Med 2006;354:731*).

ALCOHOLIC LIVER DISEASE

GENERAL PRINCIPLES

Alcohol is a potentially toxic substance to the liver.

Classification

- The spectrum of alcoholic liver disease is broad, and a single patient may be affected by more than one of the following conditions: fatty liver, alcoholic hepatitis, or alcoholic cirrhosis.
- Fatty liver is the most commonly observed abnormality and occurs in up to 90% of alcoholics.
- Alcoholic cirrhosis is a common cause of ESLD and HCC.

Epidemiology

- Alcoholism is a significant medical and socioeconomic problem. Although ethyl alcohol exerts a direct toxic effect on the liver, liver damage develops in 5% to 35% of chronic alcoholics.
- Average alcohol consumption can be measured by units per week. One unit is equal to 7 g of alcohol: one glass of wine, or a can (240 mL) of 3.5% to 4.0% beer. Approximately 30 to 40 units of alcohol per week can induce cirrhosis in 3% to 8% of individuals over a decade.

DIAGNOSIS

Clinical Presentation

- **Fatty liver**
  - Patients are usually asymptomatic.
  - Clinical findings include hepatomegaly and mild liver enzyme abnormalities.
- **Alcoholic hepatitis**
  - Alcoholic hepatitis may be clinically silent or severe enough to lead to rapid development of hepatic failure and death (*Alcohol Alcohol 2008;43:393*).
  - Clinical features include fever, abdominal pain, anorexia, nausea, vomiting, weight loss, and jaundice.
  - In severe cases, patients may have hepatic encephalopathy, ascites, and GI bleeding.
- **Alcoholic cirrhosis**
  The presentation is variable, from clinically silent disease to decompensated cirrhosis.
- Patients frequently give a history of drinking until the onset of symptoms.
- Alcoholics may underestimate or minimize their reported alcohol abuse.

Diagnostic Testing

Laboratories
- In alcoholic fatty liver, laboratory tests may be normal or demonstrate **mild elevation in serum aminotransferases** (AST greater than ALT) and ALP.
- In alcoholic hepatitis, laboratory tests typically demonstrate elevation in serum aminotransferases (AST greater than ALT) and ALP. Hyperbilirubinemia (conjugated) and elevated PT/INR may also be observed.
  - Laboratory abnormalities associated with a poor prognosis include renal failure, leukocytosis, a markedly elevated total bilirubin, and elevation of PT/INR that does not normalize with subcutaneous vitamin K.

Table 19-5	The Glasgow Alcoholic Hepatitis Score		
	Points Given		
Variable	1	2	3
Age	<50	≥50	—
WBC (10^9/L)	<15	≥15	—
Urea (mmol/L)	<5	≥5	—
INR	<1.5	1.5–2.0	>2.0
Bilirubin (μmol/L)	<125	125–250	>250

INR, international normalized ratio; WBC, white blood cell.

- A number of classification systems have been developed to risk stratify patients with alcoholic hepatitis:
  - **A discriminant function (DF)** = 4.6 × ($PT_{patient}$ − $PT_{control}$) + serum bilirubin. A score <32 has 93% and >32 has 68% 1-month survival, respectively.
  - **The Glasgow Alcoholic Hepatitis Score (GAHS)** incorporates patient age, white blood cell count, blood urea, PT/INR, and serum bilirubin (Table 19-5). A score <9 has no difference in survival between untreated and steroid-treated patients. A score >9 has a difference in 1-month survival between untreated (52% 1-month survival) and steroid-treated (78% 1-month survival) patients (*Gut 2007;56:1743*).
- In alcoholic cirrhosis, liver function abnormalities and clinical status vary depending on disease severity.

Diagnostic Procedures
- The typical histopathologic findings in alcoholic liver disease include Mallory hyaline bodies, lobular inflammation, necrosis of hepatocytes, periportal fibrosis, ductal proliferation, and fatty changes.
- The indication of liver biopsy depends on the clinical assessment of the patient. It may be helpful if alternate diagnoses are being considered.

TREATMENT

The cornerstone of treatment is abstinence from alcohol. Nutritional status should be evaluated and corrected accordingly.

Medications
Treatment of acute alcoholic hepatitis with corticosteroids is controversial. However, there is evidence that patients with a DF >32 and GAHS >9 may benefit from steroid therapy. An early decrease in bilirubin levels after 1 week of treatment portends a better prognosis. Response to therapy, as measured by the Lille Model, strongly predicts 6-month survival in patients treated with corticosteroids (*Hepatology 2007;45:1348*).
- **Oral prednisolone** 40 mg/d for 4 weeks, followed by a taper over 2 to 4 weeks has been recommended.
- **Pentoxifylline** is a nonselective phosphodiesterase inhibitor with anti-inflammatory properties and an excellent safety profile that has shown improved survival in severe alcoholic hepatitis at a dose of 400 mg PO tid × 4 weeks. Pentoxifylline may be

considered for individuals with a contraindication to steroids (infection and bleeding).

Surgical Management

Patients with cirrhosis and ESLD can be evaluated for liver transplantation but are required to abstain from alcohol for 6 months prior to evaluation, maintain abstinence, and be part of a rehabilitation program.

Lifestyle Modification

- Rehabilitation (e.g., Alcoholics Anonymous, private counseling) is highly recommended.
- Emphasis must be given to supplemental enteral nutrition to ensure adequate energy and protein intake in patients with severe alcoholic hepatitis (*Clin Nutr 2006;25:285*).

COMPLICATIONS

Potentially dangerous interactions may occur between alcohol and a variety of medications, including sedatives, anticoagulants, and acetaminophen because of shared metabolic pathways.

OUTCOME/PROGNOSIS

- Fatty liver may be reversible with abstinence.
- In alcoholic hepatitis, prognosis depends on the severity of presentation and alcohol abstinence. The in-hospital mortality for severe cases is approximately 50%.
- In cirrhosis induced by alcohol, prognosis is variable and depends on the degree of liver decompensation. Abstinence from alcohol may promote significant liver chemistry improvement even in advanced liver disease.

IMMUNE-MEDIATED LIVER DISEASES

Autoimmune Hepatitis

GENERAL PRINCIPLES

Definition

AIH is a chronic unresolving inflammation of the liver of unknown cause, associated with circulating autoantibodies and hypergammaglobulinemia.

Classification

Two types of AIH have been proposed based on differences in their immunologic markers. They do not have distinctive etiologies and do not vary in response to corticosteroid therapy.

- **Type I AIH** is the most common form of the disease and constitutes 80% of AIH cases. It is associated with antinuclear antibodies (ANAs) and anti–smooth muscle antibodies (SMAs).

- **Type 2 AIH** is characterized by antibodies to liver/kidney microsome type 1 (anti-LKM1) and/or liver cytosol type 1 (anti-LC1). This type is predominately seen in children and young adults (*N Engl J Med 2006;354:54*).
- A less established form of AIH is characterized by the presence of antibodies to soluble liver antigen/liver pancreas (anti-SLA/LP).

Epidemiology

- AIH occurs worldwide and affects all ethnic groups.
- The mean annual incidence of AIH among Caucasian Northern Europeans is 1 per 100,000 and its point prevalence is 11 to 17 per 100,000 (*Hepatology 2010;51:2193*).
- Women are affected more than men (gender ratio, 3.6:1).
- In North America, cirrhosis is present at initial presentation more often in African American patients than Caucasian patients.

Associated Conditions

Extrahepatic manifestations may be found in 30% to 50% and include synovitis, celiac disease, Coombs' positive hemolytic anemia, autoimmune thyroiditis, Graves' disease, rheumatoid arthritis, ulcerative colitis, and other immune-mediated processes.

DIAGNOSIS

Clinical Presentation

In approximately 30% to 40% of cases, the presentation is acute and similar to acute viral hepatitis. Patients may present in ALF or with asymptomatic elevation of serum ALT. It presents with cirrhosis in at least 25% of patients.

History

- The most common symptoms at presentation include fatigue, jaundice, myalgias, anorexia, diarrhea, acne, and right upper quadrant abdominal discomfort.
- Patients with AIH may overlap with clinical and histologic findings consistent with other liver diseases (e.g., PBC, PSC, Wilson's disease [WD], and autoimmune cholangitis).

Physical Examination

AIH is not associated with any specific physical examination findings.

Diagnostic Criteria

Diagnostic criteria have been codified by an international panel and were most recently updated in 1999 (*Hepatology 2002;36(2):479*). This same panel has since put forth simplified diagnostic criteria based on autoantibodies, IgG, histology, and the exclusion of viral hepatitis (*Hepatology 2008;48(1):169*).

Diagnostic Testing

Liver biopsy is essential for the diagnosis.

- **"Piecemeal necrosis" or interface hepatitis** with lobular or panacinar inflammation (lymphocytic and plasmacytic infiltration) are the histologic hallmarks of the disease.
- Histologic changes, such as ductopenia or destructive cholangitis, may indicate overlap syndromes combining characteristics of AIH, PSC, PBC, or autoimmune cholangitis.

TREATMENT

- Treatment should be started in patients with elevated serum aminotransferase levels and hyperglobulinemia.
- Histologic features of interface hepatitis, bridging, or multiacinar necrosis compel therapy.

Medications
First Line
- Therapy is initiated with either prednisone alone (40 to 60 mg/d) or a combination of prednisone (30 mg/d) and azathioprine (1 to 2 mg/kg/d). Azathioprine should be used with caution in patients with pretreatment cytopenias.
- Prednisone is tapered with biochemical and clinical improvement and is eventually discontinued. The average duration of treatment is 18 to 24 months. Some patients require lifelong low-dose therapy.

Second Line
- Budesonide, in combination with azathioprine, has recently been shown to induce and maintain remission in patients with noncirrhotic AIH with fewer steroid-specific side effects (*Gastroenterology 2010;139:1198*).
- **Refractory disease** (remission not achieved with first-line therapy) may require "salvage" therapy with cyclosporine, tacrolimus, or mycophenolate mofetil.

Surgical Management
- Liver transplantation should be considered in patients with ESLD and those with AIH-mediated ALF.
- After transplantation, recurrent AIH is seen in approximately 15% of patients. De novo AIH or immunologically mediated hepatitis, defined as hepatitis with histologic features similar to AIH in patients transplanted for nonautoimmune diseases, has been described in about 5% of transplant recipients.

MONITORING/FOLLOW-UP

- About 90% of adults have improvements in the serum aminotransferase, bilirubin, and γ-globulin levels within 2 weeks of treatment.
- Histologic improvement lags behind clinical and laboratory improvement by 3 to 6 months.

PROGNOSIS

- Remission (normalization of serum bilirubin, Ig levels, AST, ALT; disappearance of symptoms; resolution of histologic changes) is achieved in 65% and 80% of patients within 1.5 and 3.0 years of treatment, respectively.
- Relapses occur in at least 20% to 50% of patients after cessation of therapy, and require retreatment.

Primary Biliary Cirrhosis

GENERAL PRINCIPLES

Definition
PBC is a cholestatic hepatic disorder of unknown etiology with autoimmune features.

Epidemiology
- It most often affects middle-aged women (90% to 95%).
- Although PBC is seen worldwide, it is more commonly described in Caucasians.

Pathophysiology
- PBC is caused by granulomatous destruction of the interlobular bile ducts, which leads to progressive ductopenia.
- Cholestasis is generally slowly progressive and can lead to cirrhosis, and eventual liver failure.

Associated Conditions
Extrahepatic manifestations include keratoconjunctivitis sicca (Sjögren), renal tubular acidosis, gallstones, thyroid disease, scleroderma, Raynaud's phenomenon, CREST syndrome (calcinosis, Raynaud phenomenon, esophageal dysmotility, sclerodactyly, and telangiectasia), and celiac disease.

DIAGNOSIS

Clinical Presentation
The course is highly variable.

History
- Fatigue, jaundice, and pruritus are often the most troublesome symptoms.
- Patients may present de novo with manifestations of ESLD.

Physical Examination
While there are no exam findings that are specific for PBC, xanthomata and xanthelasma can be a clue to underlying cholestasis.

Diagnostic Testing
Laboratories
- Antimitochondrial antibodies are present in >90% of patients.
- Typical features include elevated levels of ALP, total bilirubin, cholesterol, and IgM.

Diagnostic Procedures
Liver biopsy may be helpful for both diagnosis and staging.

TREATMENT

Medications
- No curative therapy is available and treatment aims to slow progression of disease.

- **Ursodeoxycholic acid (UDCA)** (13 to 15 mg/kg/d PO) improves liver function test abnormalities and appears to delay progression of disease when given for long term (>4 years).
  - UDCA increases the rate of transport of intracellular bile acids across the hepatocyte into the canaliculus.
  - UDCA treatment also reduces intracellular hydrophobic bile acid levels providing a cytoprotective effect.

Other Nonpharmacologic Therapies

Symptom-specific therapy for pruritus, steatorrhea, and malabsorption are outlined in the following text.

Surgical Management

- Liver transplantation is an option in advanced disease.
- Recurrent PBC after transplantation has been documented at a rate of 20% to 25% over 10 years.

OUTCOME/PROGNOSIS

- PBC progresses along a path of increasingly severe histologic damage (florid bile duct lesions, ductular proliferation, fibrosis, and cirrhosis).
- Progression to cirrhosis and liver failure may occur years from diagnosis without treatment.

Primary Sclerosing Cholangitis

GENERAL PRINCIPLES

Definition

PSC is a cholestatic liver disorder characterized by inflammation, fibrosis, and eventual obliteration of the extrahepatic and intrahepatic bile ducts.

Classification

- Patients with PSC can be subdivided into those with small duct and large duct involvement. Small duct disease is defined as typical histologic features of PSC with a normal cholangiogram. In classic PSC, characteristic strictures of the biliary tree can be detected by cholangiography.
- Approximately 75% of patients have involvement of both intrahepatic and extrahepatic ducts, 15% have only intrahepatic involvement, and 10% have only extrahepatic disease (*Curr Gastroenterol Rep 2009;11:37*).
- Patients with small duct disease have a more favorable prognosis.

Epidemiology

- Most patients are middle-aged men, and the male to female ratio is 2:1.
- The peak incidence is about age 40 years.
- PSC is frequently associated with inflammatory bowel disease (70% of patients have concomitant ulcerative colitis). The clinical course of these conditions is not correlated.

DIAGNOSIS

Clinical Presentation

- Clinical manifestations include intermittent episodes of jaundice, hepatomegaly, pruritus, weight loss, and fatigue.
- Acute cholangitis is a frequent complication in patients with severe strictures of the biliary ducts.
- Patients slowly progress to cirrhosis.
- Cholangiocarcinoma is the most frequent neoplasm associated with PSC and occurs in 10% to 30% of patients (*Curr Gastroenterol Rep 2012;14:17*).

Diagnostic Testing

Laboratories

- PSC should be considered in individuals with inflammatory bowel disease who have increased levels of ALP even in the absence of symptoms of hepatobiliary disease.
- **ANA** is positive in up to 50% of cases, and perinuclear antineutrophil cytoplasmic antibody (p-ANCA) is positive in 80% of cases.

Imaging

MRCP is a noninvasive study, which can demonstrate abnormalities of the biliary ducts. Liver ultrasound may be useful in establishing the diagnosis if ductal dilation is present.

Diagnostic Procedures

- ERCP can confirm the diagnosis of PSC by demonstrating strictures or irregularities of the intrahepatic or extrahepatic bile ducts. Duct brushings can also be obtained with ERCP to evaluate for associated malignancy. Intraductal endoscopy provides direct visualization of the biliary ducts with the advantage of obtaining biopsies.
- Liver biopsy is helpful in the diagnosis of small-duct PSC, in the exclusion of other diseases, and in staging. Characteristic histologic findings include concentric periductal fibrosis ("onion skinning"), degeneration of bile duct epithelium, ductular proliferation, ductopenia, and cholestasis.
- Fluorescent in situ hybridization (FISH) allows for molecular assessment of malignancy from tissue obtained by brushing or biopsy.

TREATMENT

Medications

- UDCA has been studied for the treatment of PSC. Although UDCA may improve liver chemistries, it is associated with a higher risk of serious adverse events including death and transplantation and is not currently recommended for therapy (*Curr Gastroenterol Rep 2012;14:17*).
- Episodes of cholangitis should be managed with IV antibiotics and endoscopic therapy as outlined in the following text.

Other Nonpharmacologic Therapies

ERCP can be performed to dilate and stent dominant strictures.

Surgical Management

- Colectomy for ulcerative colitis does not affect the course of PSC.
- Patients with decompensated cirrhosis or recurrent cholangitis should be referred for liver transplantation.
- Cholangiocarcinoma may be an indication for liver transplantation in select circumstances.
- Recurrent PSC after liver transplantation has been documented.

COMPLICATIONS OF CHOLESTASIS

Nutritional Deficiencies

GENERAL PRINCIPLES

Any condition that blocks bile excretion (in the liver cells or biliary ducts) is defined as cholestasis. Laboratory manifestations of cholestasis include elevated levels of ALP and bilirubin.

Etiology

- **Nutritional deficiencies** result from fat malabsorption.
- **Fat-soluble vitamin deficiency** (vitamins A, D, E, and K) is often present in advanced cholestatic disease and is particularly common in patients with steatorrhea.

DIAGNOSIS

Clinical Presentation

- Patients may give a history of oily, foul-smelling diarrhea that may stick to the toilet bowl or be difficult to flush.
- Characteristic manifestations of vitamin deficiencies are discussed in Chapter 2, Nutrition Support.

Diagnostic Testing

- Stool can be tested for fecal fat. Both spot tests and 24-hour collections can be done.
- 25-Hydroxyvitamin D serum concentrations reflect the total body stores of vitamin D. Vitamin D deficiency in the setting of malabsorption, and steatorrhea is a good clinical marker for total body concentrations of other fat-soluble vitamins.

TREATMENT

Medications

- Vitamin supplements are available to correct deficiencies.
- Fat-soluble vitamin replacement can be accomplished by water-soluble preparations of vitamin A, 10,000 to 50,000 IU by mouth (PO) daily; vitamin K, 10 mg subcutaneously; and vitamin E, 30 to 100 IU PO daily.
- Vitamin D deficiency can be corrected by 25-hydroxyvitamin D3 (25-cholecalciferol), 50,000 U PO 3 × weekly.
- Zinc deficiency may occur in some patients and is corrected with zinc sulfate, 220 mg PO daily (50 mg elemental zinc) for 4 weeks.

Lifestyle/Risk Modification

In patients with steatorrhea, a low-fat diet (40 to 60 g/d) helps to decrease symptoms.

MONITORING/FOLLOW-UP

Serum levels of the affected vitamins should be monitored to assess the adequacy of replacement therapy and avoid toxicity.

Osteoporosis

GENERAL PRINCIPLES

Definition

Osteoporosis is defined as a decrease in the amount of bone (mainly trabecular bone), leading to a decrease in its structural integrity and, consequently, an increase in the risk of fractures.

Epidemiology

• Osteoporosis is more commonly seen in clinical cholestasis due to PBC.
• The relative risk of osteopenia in cholestatic disease is 4.4 times greater than the general population, matched for age and gender.

Pathophysiology

Both decreased osteoblastic activity and increased osteoclastic activity contribute to the development of osteoporosis.

DIAGNOSIS

Clinical Presentation

Osteoporosis is often insidious and is sometimes diagnosed after development of pathologic fracture.

Diagnostic Testing

Bone mineral density through dual energy X-ray absorptiometry (DEXA) should be measured in all patients at the time of diagnosis and during follow-up (every 1 to 2 years).

TREATMENT

Treatment of bone disease includes weight-bearing exercise, oral calcium supplementation (1.0 to 1.5 g/d), bisphosphonate therapy, and vitamin D supplementation.

Pruritus

GENERAL PRINCIPLES

The pathophysiology is debated and may be due to the accumulation of bile acid compounds or endogenous opioid agonists.

DIAGNOSIS

Patients with cholestasis may present with itching in the setting of a normal or elevated bilirubin level.

TREATMENT

Medications

First Line
- Pruritus is best treated with cholestyramine, a basic anion exchange resin. It binds bile acids and other anionic compounds in the intestine and inhibits their absorption. The dose is 4 g mixed with water before and after the morning meal, with additional doses before lunch and dinner. The maximum recommended dose is 16 g/d. Cholestyramine should be administered apart from other vitamins or medications to prevent impaired absorption.
- Colestipol, another similar resin, is also available.

Second Line
- Antihistamines (hydroxyzine, diphenhydramine, or doxepin, 25 mg PO at bedtime) and petrolatum may provide symptomatic relief.
- Rifampin (300 to 600 mg/d) and naltrexone (25 to 50 mg/d) are reserved for intractable pruritus.

Other Nonpharmacologic Therapies

Plasmapheresis and ultraviolet (UV) light can be administered when medical therapy has failed.

Surgical Management

Liver transplantation is rarely used as a treatment option for intractable pruritus.

METABOLIC LIVER DISEASES

Wilson's Disease

GENERAL PRINCIPLES

Definition

WD is an autosomal recessive disorder (ATP7B gene on chromosome 13) that results in progressive copper overload.

Epidemiology
- Incidence is 1 in 30,000.
- Female to male ratio of 2:1.

Pathophysiology

Absent or reduced function of ATP7B protein leads to decreased hepatocellular excretion of copper into bile. This results in hepatic copper accumulation and injury. Eventually, copper is released into the bloodstream and deposited in other organs, notably the brain, kidneys, and cornea.

Associated Conditions

Other extrahepatic manifestations include Kayser–Fleischer rings on slit-lamp examination (gold to brown rings due to copper deposition in the Descemet's membrane in the periphery of the cornea), Coombs-negative hemolytic anemia, renal tubular acidosis, arthritis, and osteopenia.

DIAGNOSIS

Clinical Presentation

- Liver disease can be highly variable, ranging from asymptomatic with only biochemical abnormalities to ALF.
- The diagnosis of WD should be considered in patients with unexplained liver disease with or without neuropsychiatric symptoms, first-degree relatives with WD, or individuals with ALF (with or without hemolysis).
- The average age at presentation of liver dysfunction is 6 to 20 years, but it can manifest later in life.
- Neuropsychiatric disorders usually occur later, most of the time in association with cirrhosis. The manifestations include asymmetric tremor, dysarthria, ataxia, and psychiatric features.

Diagnostic Testing

Laboratories

- Low serum ceruloplasmin level (<20 mg/dL), elevated serum free copper level (>25 mcg/dL), and elevated 24-hour urinary copper level (>100 μg) are seen in patients with WD.
- Most patients with the ALF presentation of WD have a characteristic pattern of clinical findings including Coombs-negative hemolytic anemia with features of acute intravascular hemolysis, rapid progression to renal failure, modest rise in serum aminotransferases from the beginning of clinical illness (typically <2,000 IU/L), normal or markedly subnormal serum ALP (typically <40 IU/L) (*Hepatology 2008;47:2090*).
- Mutation analysis by whole-gene sequencing is possible and should be performed on individuals in whom the diagnosis is difficult to establish by clinical and biochemical testing. Many patients are compound heterozygotes for mutations in the ATP7B gene, making identification of mutations difficult.

Imaging

Brain imaging (basal ganglia changes) findings are nonspecific.

Diagnostic Procedures

- The liver histology (massive necrosis, steatosis, glycogenated nuclei, chronic hepatitis, fibrosis, cirrhosis) findings are nonspecific and depend on the presentation and stage of the disease.
- Elevated hepatic copper levels of >250 μg/g dry weight (normal <40 μg/g) on biopsy are highly suggestive of WD.

TREATMENT

Medications

Treatment is with the copper-chelating agents penicillamine and trientine. Zinc salts are also used, which block intestinal absorption of copper.

- **Zinc salts** 50 mg tid are indicated in patients with chronic hepatitis and cirrhosis in the absence of hepatic failure. Other than gastric irritation, zinc has an excellent safety profile.
- **Penicillamine** 1 to 2 g/d (in divided doses bid or qid) and pyridoxine 25 mg/d (to avoid vitamin B6 deficiency during treatment) are indicated in patients with hepatic failure. Use may be limited by side effects (e.g., hypersensitivity, bone marrow suppression, proteinuria, systemic lupus erythematosus, Goodpasture syndrome). Penicillamine should never be given as initial treatment to patients with neurologic symptoms.
- **Trientine** 1 to 2 g/d (in divided doses bid or qid) may also be used in hepatic failure. This has similar side effects as penicillamine but at a lower frequency. The risk of neurologic worsening with trientine is less than with penicillamine.

Surgical Management

Liver transplantation is the only therapeutic option in ALF or in progressive dysfunction despite chelation therapy.

Lifestyle/Risk Modification

Patients should avoid intake of foods with high concentrations of copper (shellfish, nuts, chocolate), especially during the first year of treatment.

MONITORING/FOLLOW-UP

- For routine monitoring, serum copper and ceruloplasmin, liver biochemistries, INR, complete blood cell count and urinalysis (especially for those on chelation therapy), and physical examination should be performed regularly, at least twice annually.
- The 24-hour urinary excretion of copper should be measured annually while on medication. More frequent monitoring may be needed if there is suspicion of noncompliance or if dose adjustment is required. The estimated serum free copper may be elevated or low in situations of nonadherence and overtreatment, respectively.
- The American Association for the Study of Liver Diseases (AASLD) recommends that first-degree relatives of any patient newly diagnosed with WD should be screened for WD.

OUTCOME/PROGNOSIS

In the absence of neurologic symptoms, liver transplantation has a good prognosis and requires no further medical treatment.

Hereditary Hemochromatosis

GENERAL PRINCIPLES

Definition

Hereditary hemochromatosis (HH) is an autosomal recessive disorder of iron overload.

Epidemiology

- This is the most common inherited form of iron overload affecting Caucasian populations.
- One in 200 to 400 Caucasian individuals are homozygous for *hemochromatosis* (*HFE*) gene mutations.
- It rarely manifests clinically before middle age (40 to 60 years).

Etiology

- HH is most frequently caused by a missense mutation (C282Y) in the *HFE* gene located on chromosome 6. Approximately 90% of patients with HH are homozygote for the C282Y mutation.
- In one study, however, only 58% of homozygotes for the HH mutation had the full phenotype with iron overload (*N Engl J Med 1999;341:718*).
- Less frequent mutations, which lead to HH, include H63D and S65C and the compound heterozygous C282Y/H63D and C282Y/S65C mutations.

Pathophysiology

HH is a systemic syndrome characterized by increased absorption of iron and toxic deposition of iron into parenchymal cells of various tissues. It can be caused by mutations that affect any of the proteins that limit the entry of iron into the blood. Commonly, increased amounts of iron absorption cause a diminished production of hepcidin, which leads to iron overload (*Gastroenterology 2010;139:393*).

Associated Conditions

Secondary iron overload states include thalassemia major, sideroblastic anemia, chronic hemolytic anemias, iatrogenic parental iron overload, chronic hepatitis B and C, alcohol-induced liver disease, porphyria cutanea tarda, and aceruloplasminemia.

DIAGNOSIS

Clinical Presentation

- Presentation varies from **asymptomatic disease** to **cirrhosis**.
- Clinical findings include slate-colored skin, diabetes, cardiomyopathy, arthritis, hypogonadism, and hepatic dysfunction.

Diagnostic Testing

Diagnosis is based on laboratory testing, imaging, and liver biopsy.

Laboratories
- The diagnosis is suggested by **high fasting transferrin saturation (>45%) (serum iron divided by the total iron binding capacity)**.
- Other nonspecific laboratory tests include serum iron and ferritin levels. **Ferritin level >1,000 ng/mL is an accurate predictor of the degree of fibrosis in patients with HH.**
- Hepatic iron concentration (HIC) can be measured by liver biopsy. The normal content of iron in the liver ranges from 250 to 1,500 μg/g dry weight. In patients with HH, HIC ranges from 2,000 to 30,000 μg/g dry weight.
- In patients with HH (independent of symptoms) and their first-degree relatives, genotype analysis should be performed if transferrin saturation and ferritin are elevated.

- If transferrin saturation >45% and ferritin is elevated, then check for C282Y homozygosity. If patient is a C282Y homozygote, then:
  - Proceed to therapeutic phlebotomy if ferritin <1,000 ng/mL and liver enzymes are normal.
  - Proceed to liver biopsy for histology and HIC if ferritin >1,000 ng/mL or liver enzymes are elevated.
- In patients with elevated transferrin saturation and heterozygosity of the C282Y mutation, exclude other liver or hematologic diseases and consider liver biopsy.

Imaging
MRI is the modality of choice for noninvasive quantification of iron storage in the liver. It allows for repeated measures and minimizes sampling error.

Diagnostic Procedures
In patients with iron overload without typical HFE gene mutations, liver biopsy is still a valuable diagnostic tool. Liver biopsy stages the amount of fibrosis and can be used to quantify the amount of iron (HIC).

TREATMENT

Therapy consists of **phlebotomy** every 7 to 15 days (500 mL blood) until iron depletion is confirmed by a ferritin level of 50 to 100 ng/mL and a transferrin saturation of <40%. Maintenance phlebotomy of one to two units of blood three to four times a year is continued for life with some exceptions. Blood acquired by phlebotomy may be used for blood donation.

Medications
Iron chelation with deferoxamine is an alternative to phlebotomy, but it is often more expensive and has side effects such as GI distress, visual and auditory impairments, and muscle cramps. Deferoxamine binds free iron and facilitates urinary excretion and is recommended only when phlebotomy is contraindicated. Deferoxamine is only given intravenous (IV), intramuscular (IM), or subcutaneous (SC). **Deferasirox** is another alternative in the treatment of iron overload and is given orally (*Curr Opin Gastroenterol 2012;28(3):217*).

Surgical Management
Liver transplantation may be considered in cases of HH with cirrhosis.

SPECIAL CONSIDERATIONS

- Once a diagnosis has been made, the **patient's first-degree relatives** should **undergo screening** for HH by measuring fasting transferrin saturation and ferritin levels.
- Genetic testing may also be performed.

OUTCOME/PROGNOSIS

- The survival rate in appropriately treated noncirrhotic patients is identical to that of the general population.

- Patients with cirrhosis or advanced fibrosis are at increased risk for the development of HCC despite therapy and should be routinely screened for HCC.
- Patients who undergo liver transplantation for hemochromatosis have better survival rates if they are iron depleted via phlebotomy prior to transplantation compared to patients who are iron overloaded prior to transplantation (*Gastroenterology 2010;139:393*).

α_1-Antitrypsin Deficiency

GENERAL PRINCIPLES

Definition

- α_1-Antitrypsin (α_1AT) deficiency is an autosomal recessive disease associated with accumulation of misfolded α_1AT in the endoplasmic reticulum of hepatocytes.
- The gene associated with the disease is located on chromosome 14.
- The most common allele is protease inhibitor M (PiM—normal), followed by PiS and PiZ (deficient variants). African Americans have a lower frequency of these alleles.

Epidemiology

- Severe α_1AT deficiency (PiZZ) is found in approximately 1:3,500 live births. It has been described in all races.
- It is commonly a disease of Caucasians. The most prevalent deficiency alleles Z and S are derived from European ancestry (*Am J Gastroenterol 2008;103:2136*).

Associated Conditions

- α_1AT deficiency can also be associated with emphysema in early adulthood, as well as other extrahepatic manifestations including panniculitis, pancreatic fibrosis, and membranoproliferative glomerulonephritis.
- Patients with α_1AT deficiency and cirrhosis should undergo routine screening for HCC.

DIAGNOSIS

Clinical Presentation

- The disease may present as neonatal cholestasis or later in life as chronic hepatitis, cirrhosis, or HCC.
- The presence of significant pulmonary and hepatic disease in the same patient is rare (1% to 2%).

Diagnostic Testing

Laboratories

- Low serum α_1AT level (10% to 15% of normal)
- Decreased α_1-globulin level on serum electrophoresis
- Deficient α_1AT phenotype (PiSS, PiSZ, and PiZZ)
- Abnormal liver enzymes

Diagnostic Procedures

Liver biopsy shows characteristic periodic acid Schiff–positive diastase-resistant globules in the periportal hepatocytes.

TREATMENT

- Currently, there is no specific medical treatment.
- Gene therapy for α_1AT deficiency is a potential future alternative.

Surgical Management

Liver transplantation is an option for those with cirrhosis.

OUTCOME/PROGNOSIS

- Chronic hepatitis, cirrhosis, or HCC may develop in 10% to 15% of patients with the PiZZ phenotype during the first 20 years of life.
- Controversy exists as to whether liver disease develops in heterozygotes (PiMZ, PiSZ, PiFZ, etc.).
- Liver transplantation is curative, with survival rates of 90% at 1 year and 80% at 5 years.

MISCELLANEOUS LIVER DISORDERS

Nonalcoholic Fatty Liver Disease

GENERAL PRINCIPLES

Definition

- Nonalcoholic fatty liver disease (NALFD) is a clinicopathologic syndrome that encompasses several clinical entities that range from simple steatosis to steatohepatitis, fibrosis, and ESLD in the absence of significant alcohol consumption (*Gastroenterology 2002;123:1705*).
- Nonalcoholic steatohepatitis (NASH) is part of the spectrum of NAFLD and is defined as steatosis with hepatocellular ballooning plus lobular inflammation.

Epidemiology

- NAFLD is a worldwide phenomenon with an estimated prevalence greater than 30% in the general population (10% to 30% of the U.S. population). The prevalence ranges from 3% to 9% with substantial variation among ethnic groups. It affects both children and adults, and the incidence increases with age (*Hepatology 2010;52:913*).
- NAFLD is associated with an increasing prevalence of type II diabetes, obesity, and the metabolic syndrome in the U.S. population.
- Up to 70% of cases of cryptogenic cirrhosis have NASH as the underlying etiology. Cirrhosis due to NASH may also be complicated by HCC (13% of all cases of HCC).

Etiology

Etiologies include metabolic syndrome, drug-induced liver injury (amiodarone, nifedipine, estrogens), surgical procedures (jejuno-ileal bypass, extensive small-bowel resection, biliary and pancreatic diversions), and miscellaneous conditions (total parenteral nutrition, hypobetalipoproteinemia, environmental toxins, etc.).

DIAGNOSIS

Clinical Presentation

The disease may vary from asymptomatic liver fatty infiltration to advanced fibrosis with cirrhosis and HCC.

Diagnostic Testing

- The diagnosis of NAFLD is suspected in patients with abnormal liver chemistries and, in many cases, evidence of metabolic syndrome.
- The distinction between NAFLD and NASH is made with liver biopsy.

Laboratories
- Liver enzyme elevations are mild, up to 80% of patients will have normal liver enzymes.
- Aminotransferases greater than two times normal are predictive of septal bridging and fibrosis across different populations.
- Biochemical abnormalities may reflect the stage of the disease (e.g., cholestasis, hypoalbuminemia, increased INR).

Imaging
- Imaging studies such as ultrasonography, CT scan, and MRI may detect moderate-to-severe steatosis.
- Magnetic resonance spectroscopy offers a quantitative measurement of liver fat content but is not commonly available.

Diagnostic Procedures
- Liver biopsy remains the gold standard by which the diagnosis is made. However, the decision to perform a liver biopsy should take into account the specific clinical questions that are relevant to each case.
- Noninvasive predictive models, serum biomarkers, imaging studies, and breath tests are currently under evaluation as surrogate measures of liver fibrosis, inflammation, and steatosis (*World J Gastroenterol 2010;14:4784*).

TREATMENT

Medications

The effects of metformin, vitamin E, statins, ezetimibe, thiazolidinediones, pentoxifylline, angiotensin-receptor blockers, and UDCA have been studied on patients with NASH. While some of these studies have shown temporary improvements in liver histology and/or liver enzymes, no medication has consistently and safely reversed NASH. There is currently no U.S. Food and Drug Administration (FDA)-approved drug for the treatment of NASH (*Clin Liver Dis 2012;16:397*).

Other Nonpharmacologic Therapies

Therapies to correct or control associated conditions are warranted (weight loss through diet and exercise, tight control of diabetes and insulin resistance, appropriate treatment of hyperlipidemia, and discontinuation of possible offending agents).

Surgical Management

Liver transplantation should be considered in patients with cirrhosis. Recurrence of NASH after transplantation can develop.

OUTCOME/PROGNOSIS

- An unknown proportion of those with simple steatosis will progress to NASH.
- Progression to NASH cirrhosis has been reported at a rate of 11% over a 15-year period (*Clin Liver Dis 2012;16:397*).

Ischemic Hepatitis

GENERAL PRINCIPLES

Definition
Ischemic hepatitis results from liver acute hypoperfusion.

Etiology
Clinical circumstances associated with acute hypotension or hemodynamic instability include severe blood loss, substantial burns, cardiac failure, heat stroke, sepsis, sickle cell crisis, and others.

DIAGNOSIS

Clinical Presentation
Ischemic hepatitis presents as an acute and transient rise of liver enzymes in the thousands during or following an episode of liver hypoperfusion.

Diagnostic Testing
Laboratories
- Laboratory studies show a rapid rise and in levels of serum AST, ALT ($>1,000$ mg/dL), and lactate dehydrogenase (LDH) within 1 to 3 days of the insult.
- Total bilirubin, ALP, and INR may initially be normal but subsequently rise as a result of reperfusion injury.

Diagnostic Procedures
Liver biopsy is not routinely needed, as the diagnosis can usually be made with clinically history. Classic histologic features include variable degrees of zone 3 (centrilobular) necrosis with collapse around the central vein. Coexistent features may include passive congestion, sinusoidal distortion, fatty change, and cholestasis. Inflammatory infiltrates are rare.

TREATMENT

Treatment consists of supportive care and correction of the underlying condition that caused the circulatory collapse.

OUTCOME/PROGNOSIS

Prognosis is dependent upon rapid and effective treatment of the underlying condition.

Hepatic Vein Thrombosis

GENERAL PRINCIPLES

Definition
Hepatic vein thrombosis (HVT; also known as Budd–Chiari syndrome) causes hepatic venous outflow obstruction. It has multiple etiologies and a variety of clinical consequences.

Etiology
- Thrombosis is the main factor leading to obstruction of the hepatic venous system, frequently in association with myeloproliferative disorders, antiphospholipid antibody syndrome, paroxysmal nocturnal hemoglobinuria, factor V Leiden, protein C and S deficiency, Jak-2 mutation, and contraceptive use (*Dig Liver Dis 2011; 43:503*).
- Membranous obstruction of the inferior vena cava (IVC) is an infrequent condition that presents clinically similar to HVT.
- HVT can occur during pregnancy and in the postpartum period.
- Less than 20% of cases are idiopathic.

DIAGNOSIS

Clinical Presentation
- Patients may present with acute, subacute, or chronic illness characterized by ascites, hepatomegaly, and right upper quadrant abdominal pain.
- Other symptoms may include jaundice, encephalopathy, GI bleeding, and lower extremity edema.

Diagnostic Testing
Laboratories
- Serum-to-ascites albumin gradient (SAAG) is >1.1 g/dL. Serum albumin, bilirubin, AST, ALT, and PT/INR are usually abnormal.
- Laboratory evaluation to identify a possible hypercoagulable state should be performed (see Chapter 20, Disorders of Hemostasis and Thrombosis).

Imaging
- Doppler ultrasound can be used as a screening test.
- Definitive diagnosis is made with magnetic resonance venography, hepatic venography, or cavography.

TREATMENT

Medications
Nonsurgical treatment includes anticoagulation, thrombolytics, diuretics, angioplasty, stents, and transjugular intrahepatic portosystemic shunt (TIPS).

Surgical Management
Liver transplantation is an option in selected patients.

Sinusoidal Obstruction Syndrome

GENERAL PRINCIPLES

Definition

Sinusoidal obstruction syndrome (SOS; also known as veno-occlusive disease) refers to alterations in the liver microcirculation that may occur in the absence of large vessel vascular occlusion (*World J Gastroenterol 2007;13:1912*).

Etiology

SOS is seen in bone marrow transplant recipients after therapy with total body irradiation and high-dose cytoreductive chemotherapy, in renal transplant recipients who are immunosuppressed with azathioprine, and with ingestion of pyrrolizidine alkaloids (Jamaican bush teas).

DIAGNOSIS

Clinical Presentation

- Diagnosis is based on the triad of hepatomegaly, weight gain (2% to 5% of baseline body weight), and hyperbilirubinemia (>2 mg/dL), generally occurring within 3 weeks after bone marrow transplantation.
- The severity of SOS ranges from mild-to-moderate to severe disease.
- The clinical presentation depends on the severity of the disease.

Diagnostic Testing

Laboratories

The laboratory findings correlate with the clinical disease, from mild to significant elevations in aminotransferases and bilirubin.

Diagnostic Procedures

- A useful approach to the diagnosis is the transjugular measurement of the hepatic venous pressure. A concomitant liver biopsy can be performed during the same procedure.
- Typical histology shows centrilobular congestion with hepatocellular necrosis and accumulation of hemosiderin-laden macrophages. The terminal hepatic venules exhibit minimal edema without obvious fibrin deposition or thrombosis.

TREATMENT

- Treatment is largely supportive.
- Defibrotide, a single-stranded polydeoxyribonucleotide drug, has demonstrated ability to affect inflammatory, thrombotic, and angiogenic pathways involved in veno-occlusive disease. It has been used in the treatment of cardiovascular disorders and has shown promise in endothelial complications of allogeneic stem cell transplantation (*Expert Opin Biol Ther 2009;9(6):763*).

SPECIAL CONSIDERATIONS

Altering the myeloablative therapy and reducing the dose of radiation may decrease the incidence of SOS.

OUTCOME/PROGNOSIS

Prognosis depends on the severity of disease.

Portal Vein Thrombosis

GENERAL PRINCIPLES

Portal vein thrombosis (PVT) is seen in a variety of clinical settings, including abdominal trauma, cirrhosis, malignancy, hypercoagulable states, intra-abdominal infections, pancreatitis, and after portocaval shunt surgery and splenectomy.

DIAGNOSIS

Clinical Presentation
- PVT can present as an acute or a chronic condition.
- The acute phase may go unrecognized. Symptoms include abdominal pain/distension, nausea, anorexia, weight loss, diarrhea, or features of the underlying disorder.
- Chronic PVT may present with variceal hemorrhage or other manifestations of portal hypertension.

Diagnostic Testing
Laboratories
In patients with no obvious etiology, a hypercoagulable workup should be performed.

Imaging
- **Ultrasonographic Doppler** examination is sensitive and specific for establishing the diagnosis.
- Portal venography, CT, or magnetic resonance venography can also be used.

TREATMENT

Medications
- In patients with acute PVT with or without cirrhosis, anticoagulation is recommended in the absence of any obvious contraindications. Treatment is aimed to prevent further thrombosis and recanalization, to treat complications and concurrent disease, and to identify underlying risk factors (*Neth J Med 2009;67:46*).
- In patients with chronic PVT, anticoagulation is not recommended.

Other Nonpharmacologic Therapies
In the setting of chronic PVT, treatment should focus on the complications of portal hypertension and include nonselective β-blockers, endoscopic banding for varices, and diuretics for ascites.

Surgical Management
Portosystemic derivative surgery carries a high morbidity and mortality, especially in patients with cirrhosis.

Pyogenic Abscess

GENERAL PRINCIPLES

- Pyogenic abscess can result from hematogenous infection, spread from intra-abdominal infection, or ascending cholangitis.
- Approximately 20% of cases are cryptogenic in origin.

DIAGNOSIS

Clinical Presentation
Clinical features include fever, chills, weight loss, jaundice, and tender hepatomegaly.

Diagnostic Testing
Laboratories
- Laboratory studies may demonstrate leukocytosis and elevated ALP.
- Blood cultures are often positive at presentation.

Imaging
Diagnosis is confirmed by CT, MRI, or ultrasonography.

TREATMENT

Treatment consists of a prolonged course of antibiotic therapy and, in some cases, imaging-guided percutaneous drainage or surgery (*World J Gastroenterol 2011; 17:1622*).

MONITORING/FOLLOW-UP

Repeated imaging is recommended to document resolution.

Amebic Abscess

GENERAL PRINCIPLES

Amebic abscess is a diagnostic consideration in patients from and traveling to endemic areas (*Expert Rev Anti Infect Ther 2007;5(5):893*).

DIAGNOSIS

Clinical Presentation
- Diagnosis requires a high index of clinical suspicion.
- Clinical features include fever, chills, and tender hepatomegaly. Concurrent diarrhea is rarely seen. Some patients may give a history of dysentery in the previous few months.

Diagnostic Testing
Specific serologic tests, which detect antibodies for *Entamoeba histolytica*, include enzyme-linked immunosorbent assay (ELISA), EIA, and indirect hemagglutination,

are helpful in establishing the diagnosis in low-prevalence areas. These tests have a high sensitivity as markers of invasive amebiasis (>90%).

TREATMENT

Medications
Amebic abscesses are treated with 5-nitroimidazole (metronidazole, tinidazole, and secnidazole).

Other Nonpharmacologic Therapies
Imaging-guided drainage is reserved for patients with large abscesses, abscesses localized in the left lobe of the liver, bacterial coinfected abscesses, abscesses with extrahepatic involvement, abscesses of uncertain etiology, and those with poor response to 5 to 7 days of antiparastitic treatment with persistent fever and pain.

Granulomatous Hepatitis

GENERAL PRINCIPLES

Definition
Granulomatous hepatitis is the consequence of a nonspecific reaction to a wide spectrum of diverse etiologic stimuli.

Etiology
Etiologies include infections (brucellosis, syphilis, mycobacterial, fungal, and rickettsial diseases), sarcoidosis, AIDS, DILI, lymphoma, and idiopathic causes.

DIAGNOSIS

Clinical Presentation
Patients may present with fever, hepatosplenomegaly, and signs of portal hypertension.

Diagnostic Testing
Laboratories
Laboratory studies show elevated liver enzymes and ALP.

Diagnostic Procedures
Liver biopsy is the most accurate and specific way to diagnose granulomatous hepatitis.

TREATMENT

- Specific therapy is directed at the underlying cause.
- If clinical suspicion for tuberculosis is high, an empiric trial with antituberculous therapy may be warranted despite negative mycobacterial cultures.
- Corticosteroids should be considered in patients with idiopathic granulomatous liver disease in whom tuberculosis is not suspected.

ACUTE LIVER FAILURE

GENERAL PRINCIPLES

Definition

ALF is a condition that includes evidence of coagulation abnormalities (INR >1.5) and any degree of mental alteration (encephalopathy) in a patient without preexisting liver disease and with an illness of <26 weeks' duration.

Classification

Terms used signifying length of illness in ALF such as hyperacute (<7 days), acute (7 to 21 days), and subacute (>21 days to <26 weeks) are not helpful since they do not have prognostic significance distinct from the cause of illness (*Gastroenterol Clin North Am 2011;40:523*).

Epidemiology

Approximately 2,000 cases of ALF occur in the United States each year.

Etiology

- Acetaminophen hepatotoxicity and viral hepatitis are the most common causes of ALF.
- Other causes include AIH, drug and toxin exposure, ischemia, acute fatty liver of pregnancy, WD, and Reye's syndrome.
- In 20% of cases, no clear cause is identified.

Pathophysiology

Acute inflammation with varying degrees of necrosis and collapse of the liver's architectural framework are the typical histologic changes seen in ALF.

DIAGNOSIS

Clinical Presentation

- Patients may present with mild-to-severe mental status changes in the setting of moderate-to-severe acute hepatitis and coagulopathy.
- Jaundice may or may not be initially present.
- Patients may develop cardiovascular collapse, acute renal failure, cerebral edema, and sepsis.

Diagnostic Testing

Laboratories
- Aminotransferases are typically elevated, and in many cases are >1,000 IU/L.
- INR >1.5.
- Initial workup to determine the etiology of ALF should include acute viral hepatitis panel, serum drug screen (including acetaminophen level), ceruloplasmin, AIH serologies, and pregnancy test.

Imaging
- Right upper quadrant ultrasound with Doppler may be obtained to evaluate obstruction of hepatic venous inflow or outflow.

- CT of the head may be obtained to evaluate and track progression of cerebral edema; however, the radiologic findings may lag behind its development and do not substitute for serial bedside assessments of neurologic status.

Diagnostic Procedures

Liver biopsy is seldom used to establish etiology or prognosis. Given the presence of coagulopathy, a transjugular approach to liver biopsy may be attempted if necessary.

TREATMENT

- Supportive therapy in the intensive care unit (ICU) setting of a tertiary center with liver transplant capabilities is essential.
- Precipitating factors should be identified and treated.
- Sedation should be avoided to allow for serial neurologic and mental status exams.
- Blood glucose, electrolytes, acid–base, coagulation parameters, and fluid status should be serially monitored.
- Surveillance for and treatment of infection should be closely monitored.
- Fresh frozen plasma and the use of recombinant activated factor VIIa should be considered in the setting of active bleeding or when invasive procedures are required.
- Cerebral edema and intracranial hypertension are related to severity of encephalopathy. In patients with grade III or IV encephalopathy, intracranial pressure monitoring should be considered (intracranial pressure should be maintained below 20 to 25 mm Hg and cerebral perfusion pressure should be maintained above 50 mm Hg). Therapies to decrease cerebral edema include mannitol (0.5 to 1.0 g/kg IV), hyperventilation (to reduce $PaCO_2$ to 25 to 30 mm Hg), hypothermia (32°C to 34°C), hypernatremia to 145 to 155 mEq/L induced with hypertonic saline, and barbiturates (*Neurocrit Care 2008;9:97*).
- Lactulose is not indicated for encephalopathy in this setting. Its use may result in increased bowel gas that can interfere with the surgical approach for liver transplantation.
- Liver transplantation should be urgently considered in cases of severe ALF.

OUTCOME/PROGNOSIS

- In the United States, 45% of adults with ALF have a spontaneous recovery, 25% undergo liver transplantation, and 30% die without liver transplantation (*Curr Opin Organ Transplant 2011;16:289*).
- Death often results from progressive liver failure, GI bleeding, cerebral edema, sepsis, or arrhythmia.
- Decline in aminotransferases correlates poorly with prognosis and does not always indicate an improved response to therapy.
- Poor prognostic indicators in acetaminophen-induced ALF include arterial pH <7.3, INR >6.5, creatinine >2.3 mg/dL, and encephalopathy grade III through IV.

CHRONIC LIVER DISEASES

Cirrhosis

- Cirrhosis is a chronic condition characterized by diffuse replacement of liver cells by fibrotic tissue, which creates a nodular-appearing distortion of the normal liver architecture. This fibrosis represents the end result of many etiologies of liver injury.
- Cirrhosis affects nearly 5.5 million Americans and in 2009 was the twelfth leading cause of death in the United States.
- The most common etiologies are alcohol-related liver disease, chronic viral infection, and NASH (diagnosis and treatment discussed earlier in respective sections).
- Main complications of cirrhosis include portal hypertension with various clinical manifestations (ascites, esophageal and gastric varices, portal hypertensive gastropathy and colopathy, hypersplenism, gastric antral vascular ectasia, spontaneous bacterial peritonitis [SBP], hepatorenal syndrome [HRS]), hepatic encephalopathy, and HCC. Frequent laboratory abnormalities encountered in a patient with cirrhosis include anemia, leukopenia, thrombocytopenia, hypoalbuminemia, coagulopathy, and hyperbilirubinemia.

Portal Hypertension

GENERAL PRINCIPLES

- Portal hypertension is the main complication of cirrhosis and is characterized by increased resistance to portal flow and increased portal venous inflow. Portal hypertension is established by measuring the pressure gradient between the hepatic vein and the portal vein (normal portosystemic pressure gradient is approximately 3 mm Hg).
- Direct and indirect clinical consequences of portal hypertension appear when the portosystemic pressure gradient exceeds 10 mm Hg (*Dig Liver Dis 2011;43:762*).
- Causes of portal hypertension in patients without cirrhosis include idiopathic portal hypertension, schistosomiasis, congenital hepatic fibrosis, sarcoidosis, cystic fibrosis, arteriovenous fistulas, splenic and portal vein thrombosis, HVT (Budd–Chiari syndrome), myeloproliferative diseases, nodular regenerative hyperplasia, and focal nodular hyperplasia.

DIAGNOSIS

Clinical Presentation

Portal hypertension frequently complicates cirrhosis and presents with ascites, splenomegaly, and GI bleeding from varices (esophageal or gastric), or portal hypertensive gastropathy or colopathy.

Imaging

Ultrasonography, CT, and MRI showing cirrhosis, splenomegaly, collateral venous circulation, and ascites are suggestive of portal hypertension.

Diagnostic Procedures
- Upper endoscopy may show varices (esophageal or gastric), portal hypertensive gastropathy, or gastric antrum vascular ectasia (GAVE).
- Transjugular portal pressure measurements may be performed to calculate the porto-systemic pressure gradient.

TREATMENT

Treatment of GI bleeding due to portal hypertension is covered in Chapter 18, Gastrointestinal Diseases.

Ascites

GENERAL PRINCIPLES

Definition
Ascites is the abnormal (>25 mL) accumulation of fluid within the peritoneal cavity.

Etiology
Causes of ascites besides cirrhosis with portal hypertension include cancer (peritoneal carcinomatosis), heart failure, tuberculosis, myxedema, pancreatic disease, nephrotic syndrome, surgery or trauma to the lymphatic system or ureters, and serositis.

DIAGNOSIS

Clinical Presentation
Presentation ranges from ascites detected only by imaging methods to a distended, bulging, and sometimes tender abdomen. Percussion of the abdomen may reveal shifting dullness.

Diagnostic Testing
Laboratories
- A **serum-to-ascites albumin gradient** ≥1.1 indicates portal hypertension–related ascites (97% specificity).
- A SAAG of <1.1 is found in nephrotic syndrome, peritoneal carcinomatosis, serositis, tuberculosis, and biliary or pancreatic ascites.

Imaging
Ultrasonography, CT, and MRI are sensitive methods to detect ascites.

Diagnostic Procedures
Diagnostic paracentesis (60 mL) should be performed in the setting of new-onset ascites, suspicion of malignant ascites, or to rule-out SBP. **Therapeutic paracentesis** (large volume) should be performed when tense ascites causes significant discomfort or respiratory compromise or when suspecting abdominal compartment syndrome.
- Routine diagnostic testing should include fluid cell and differential counts, albumin, total protein, and culture.
- Amylase and triglyceride measurement, cytology, and mycobacterial smear/culture can be performed to confirm specific diagnoses.

- Bleeding, infection, and intestinal perforation are possible complications.
- Rapid large-volume paracentesis (>7 L) may lead to circulatory collapse, encephalopathy, and renal failure. Concomitant administration of IV albumin (5 to 8 g/L ascites removed) can be used to minimize these complications, especially in the setting of renal insufficiency or the absence of peripheral edema.

TREATMENT

Medications

- **Diuretic therapy** is initiated along with **salt restriction**. The goal of diuretic therapy should be a daily weight loss of no more than 1.0 kg in patients with edema and 0.5 kg in those without edema until ascites is adequately controlled. Diuretics should not be administered to individuals with an increasing serum creatinine level.
- **Spironolactone** 100 mg PO daily is indicated. The daily dose can be increased by 50 to 100 mg every 7 to 10 days to a maximum dose of 400 mg until satisfactory weight loss or side effects occur. Hyperkalemia and gynecomastia are common side effects. Other potassium-sparing diuretics such as amiloride, triamterene, or eplerenone are substitutes that can be used in patients in whom painful gynecomastia develops.
- **Loop diuretics**, such as furosemide (20 to 40 mg, increasing to a maximum dose of 160 mg PO daily) or bumetanide (0.5 to 2.0 mg PO daily), can be added to spironolactone.
- Patients should be observed closely for signs of dehydration, electrolyte disturbances, encephalopathy, muscle cramps, and renal insufficiency. Nonsteroidal anti-inflammatory agents may blunt the effect of diuretics and increase the risk of renal dysfunction.

Other Nonpharmacologic Therapies

- TIPS is effective in the management of refractory ascites (fluid overload that is nonresponsive to a sodium-restricted diet and high-dose diuretic therapy).
- Complications of TIPS include shunt occlusion, bleeding, infection, cardiopulmonary compromise, and hepatic encephalopathy.

Lifestyle/Risk Modification

Dietary salt restriction (2 g sodium or 88 mmol Na^+/d) should be initiated in patients with ascites. In selected cases, it may be necessary to restrict sodium intake further.

- Potassium-containing salt substitutes should not be used with potassium-sparing diuretics.
- Routine water restriction is not necessary in patients with ascites. However, if hyponatremia (serum Na^+ <120 mmol/L) occurs, fluid restriction to 1,000 to 1,500 mL/d is indicated.

Spontaneous Bacterial Peritonitis

GENERAL PRINCIPLES

Definition

- SBP is an infectious complication of portal hypertension–related ascites defined as ascitic fluid containing >250 neutrophils/mm^3 (greatest sensitivity) or >500 neutrophils/mm^3 (greatest specificity).

- Bacterascites is defined as culture positive ascites in the presence of normal ascitic neutrophil counts (<250 neutrophils/mm^3). This condition may be spontaneously reversible, or the first step in the development of SBP. In the presence of signs or symptoms of infection, bacterascites should be treated like SBP.

Risk Factors

Risk factors for SBP include ascitic fluid protein concentration <1 mg/dL, acute GI bleeding, and a prior episode of SBP.

DIAGNOSIS

Clinical Presentation

Clinical manifestations include abdominal pain and distention, fever, decreased bowel sounds, and worsening hepatic encephalopathy. SBP may be asymptomatic. Cirrhotic patients with ascites and evidence of any clinical deterioration should undergo diagnostic paracentesis to exclude SBP.

Diagnostic Testing

The diagnosis is confirmed when the ascitic fluid contains >250 neutrophils/mL. Gram stain reveals the organism in only 10% to 20% of samples.
- Ascitic cultures are more likely to be positive when 10 mL ascitic fluid is inoculated into two blood culture bottles at the bedside.
- The most common organisms are *Escherichia coli*, *Klebsiella*, and *Streptococcus pneumoniae*. Polymicrobial infection is uncommon and should lead to the suspicion of secondary bacterial peritonitis. Checking total protein, LDH, and glucose on ascitic fluid is helpful in distinguishing secondary from spontaneous bacterial peritonitis.

TREATMENT

Medications

- Patients with SBP should receive empiric antibiotic therapy with intravenous third-generation cephalosporins (ceftriaxone, 1 g IV daily; or cefotaxime, 1 to 2 g IV q6–8h, depending on renal function). Therapy should be tailored based upon culture results and antibiotic susceptibility. Paracentesis should be repeated if no clinical improvement occurs in 48 to 72 hours, especially if the initial ascitic fluid culture was negative (*Hepatology 2009;49:2087*).
- Oral quinolones can be considered a substitute for IV third-generation cephalosporins in the absence of vomiting, shock, grade II (or higher) hepatic encephalopathy, or serum creatinine >3 mg/dL (*Hepatology 2009;49:2087*).
- Patients with ascitic fluid polymorphonuclear leukocytes (PMN) counts <250 cells/mm^3 and signs or symptoms of infection (fever or abdominal pain or tenderness) should also receive empiric antibiotic therapy (*Hepatology 2009;49:2087*).
- Concomitant use of albumin 1.5 g/kg body weight at time of diagnosis and 1.0 g/kg body weight on day 3 improves survival and prevents renal failure in SBP (*N Engl J Med 1999;341:403*).

First-Line Prophylaxis
- Patients presenting with acute GI bleed should receive ceftriaxone 1 g IV daily for 5 to 7 days based on severity of liver disease.

- Patients with severe liver disease with ascitic fluid protein <1.5 mg/dL should be treated with long-term norfloxacin 400 mg PO daily.

Second-Line Prophylaxis
Norfloxacin 400 mg PO daily is the treatment of choice for prevention of recurrent SBP (*J Hepatol 2010;53:397*).

Hepatorenal Syndrome

GENERAL PRINCIPLES

HRS is a unique form of functional renal impairment in the setting of acute or, more commonly, chronic liver disease. Common precipitating factors include systemic bacterial infections, SBP, and large-volume paracentesis without volume expansion (*J Gastroenterol 2005;100:460*). HRS is characterized by oliguria, benign urine sediment, low urine sodium excretion, and increasing creatinine. HRS is a diagnosis of exclusion.

DIAGNOSIS

Major and minor diagnostic criteria are summarized in Table 19-6.
- **Type I** HRS is characterized by the acute onset of rapidly progressive (<2 weeks), oliguric renal failure unresponsive to volume expansion. There is a doubling of the initial serum creatinine to a level >2.5 mg/dL.
- **Type II** HRS progresses more slowly but relentlessly and often clinically manifests as diuretic-resistant ascites.

TREATMENT

Medications
No clear or established treatments are available for HRS. Systemic vasoconstrictors including vasopressin analogs (terlipressin), somatostatin analogs (octreotide), and α-adrenergic agonists (midodrine and norepinephrine) with plasma expansion have shown a beneficial role in uncontrolled studies.

Other Nonpharmacologic Therapies
- TIPS is a potential treatment alternative; however, data are limited.
- Hemodialysis may be indicated in patients listed for liver transplantation.

Surgical Management
In suitable candidates, liver transplantation may be curative (type I and II HRS). Patients receiving hemodialysis for more than 12 weeks should be considered for liver and kidney transplantation.

OUTCOME/PROGNOSIS

Without treatment, patients with type I HRS have a poor prognosis, with death occurring within 1 to 3 months of onset. Patients with type II HRS have a longer median survival.

Table 19-6	Diagnostic Criteria of Hepatorenal Syndrome

Major criteria

Low glomerular filtration rate, as indicated by serum creatinine >1.5 mg/dL or 24-hr creatinine clearance <40 mL/min

Absence of shock, ongoing bacterial infection, fluid losses, and current treatment with nephrotoxic drugs

No sustained improvement in renal function (decrease in serum creatinine to 1.5 mg/dL or increase in creatinine clearance to 40 mL/min) after diuretic withdrawal and expansion of plasma volume with 1.5 L of a plasma expander

Proteinuria <500 mg/dL and no ultrasonographic evidence of obstructive uropathy or parenchymal renal disease

Additional criteria

Urine volume <500 mL/d
Urine sodium <10 mEq/L
Urine osmolality greater than plasma osmolality
Urine red blood cells <50 per high-power field
Serum sodium concentration <130 mEq/L

Note: All major criteria must be present for the diagnosis of hepatorenal syndrome. Additional criteria are not necessary for the diagnosis but provide supportive evidence.

Adapted from Arroyo V, Gines P, Gerbes AL, et al. Definition and diagnostic criteria of refractory ascites and hepatorenal syndrome in cirrhosis. International Ascites Club. *Hepatology.* 1996;23:164.

Hepatic Encephalopathy

GENERAL PRINCIPLES

Definition

Hepatic encephalopathy is the syndrome of disordered consciousness and altered neuromuscular activity that is seen in patients with acute or chronic hepatocellular failure or portosystemic shunting.

Classification

The grades of hepatic encephalopathy overlap and can rapidly change.
- Grade I: Sleep reversal pattern, mild confusion, irritability, tremor, asterixis
- Grade II: Lethargy, disorientation, inappropriate behavior, asterixis
- Grade III: Somnolence, severe confusion, aggressive behavior, asterixis
- Grade IV: Coma

Etiology
- The pathogenesis of hepatic encephalopathy is controversial.
- **Precipitating factors** include medication noncompliance to lactulose, azotemia, ALF, opioids or sedative-hypnotic medications, acute GI bleeding, hypokalemia and

alkalosis (diuretics and diarrhea), constipation, infection, high-protein diet, progressive hepatocellular dysfunction, and portosystemic shunts (surgical or TIPS).

DIAGNOSIS

- Presentation varies from subtle mental status changes to coma.
- Asterixis (flapping tremor) is present in stage I through III encephalopathy. This motor disturbance is not specific to hepatic encephalopathy.
- The electroencephalogram shows slow, high-amplitude, and triphasic waves.
- Determination of blood ammonia level is not a sensitive or specific test for hepatic encephalopathy.

TREATMENT

Medications

Medications include nonabsorbable disaccharides (lactulose, lactitol, and lactose in lactase-deficient patients) and antibiotics (neomycin, metronidazole, and rifaximin).

- **Lactulose**, 15 to 45 mL PO (or via nasogastric tube) bid–qid, adjusted to produce three to five soft stools per day is indicated. Oral lactulose should not be given to patients with ileus or possible bowel obstruction. In the acute phase, a starting dose of 30 mL every 2 hours is recommended. This can then be transitioned to every 4, 6, and then 8 hours once the patient starts having bowel movements.
- **Lactulose enemas** (prepared by the addition of 300 mL lactulose to 700 mL distilled water) may also be administered.
- **Rifaximin**, 550 mg PO bid, is used as an alternative to neomycin and metronidazole (*N Engl J Med 2010;362:1071*).
- **Neomycin** can be given by mouth (500 to 1,000 mg q6h) or as a retention enema (1% solution in 100 to 200 mL isotonic saline). Approximately 1% to 3% of the administered dose of neomycin is absorbed with the attendant risk of ototoxicity and nephrotoxicity.
- **Metronidazole** (250 mg PO q8h) is useful for short-term therapy when rifaximin or neomycin is unavailable or poorly tolerated. Long-term metronidazole is not recommended due to its associated toxicities.
- Combination therapy with lactulose and any of the antibiotics mentioned earlier should be considered in cases that are refractory to either agent alone.

Lifestyle Modification

The rationale and benefit of dietary protein restriction is controversial. Once the patient is able to eat, a diet containing 30 to 40 g of protein per day should be initiated. Special diets (vegetable protein or branched-chain amino acid enriched) may be beneficial in patients with encephalopathy that is refractory to the usual measures.

Hepatocellular Carcinoma

GENERAL PRINCIPLES

- HCC frequently occurs in patients with cirrhosis, especially when associated with viral hepatitis (HBV or HCV), alcoholic cirrhosis, $\alpha_1 AT$ deficiency, and hemochromatosis.

- HCC is the fifth most common cancer in men and the seventh most common cancer in women worldwide. Nearly 85% of the cases of HCC occur in developing countries (*Gastroenterology 2012;142:1264*).

DIAGNOSIS

Clinical Presentation

- Clinical presentation is directly proportional to the stage of disease. HCC may present with right upper quadrant abdominal pain, weight loss, and hepatomegaly.
- Suspect HCC in a cirrhotic patient who develops manifestations of liver decompensation.
- Surveillance for HCC should be performed every 6 months with a sensitive imaging study and AFP. In patients with hepatitis B, surveillance should begin after age 40 years even in the absence of cirrhosis.

Diagnostic Testing

Laboratories
- AFP (refer back to section Evaluation of Liver Disease)
- Investigational serum markers for HCC: lens culinaris agglutinin-reactive α-fetoprotein, des-gamma-carboxyprothrombin (DCP), alpha-L-fucosidase, and glypican-3 (GPC3).

Imaging
Liver ultrasound, triple-phase CT, and MRI are sensitive and often used for detection of HCC.

Diagnostic Procedures
Liver biopsy should be considered for patients at risk for HCC with suspicious liver lesions >1 cm with noncharacteristic imaging features (absence of arterial hypervascularity and venous or delayed phase washout).

TREATMENT

Medications

Sorafenib is a small molecule that inhibits tumor cell proliferation and angiogenesis. In patients with advanced HCC, median survival and radiologic progression were 3 months longer for patients treated with sorafenib compared to placebo (*N Engl J Med 2008;359:378*). Currently, there are several new medications being investigated for the treatment of HCC that inhibit angiogenesis, epidermal growth factor receptor, and mammalian target of rapamycin (mTOR).

Nonpharmacologic Therapies

- Transarterial chemoembolization (TACE) improves survival in selected patients. It is recommended as first-line palliative therapy for nonsurgical patients with large or multifocal HCC who do not have vascular invasion or metastatic disease (*Hepatology 2011;53:1020*).
- Selected patients with tumors beyond Milan criteria HCC can be downstaged to meet Milan criteria with TACE, radiofrequency ablation (RFA), and transarterial radioembolization (TARE) prior to liver transplantation.

Surgical Management

- Hepatic resection is the treatment of choice in noncirrhotic patients.
- Liver transplantation is the treatment of choice for select cirrhotic patients that fall into Milan criteria (single HCC <5 cm or up to three nodules <3 cm).
- Milan criteria is utilized by the United Network for Organ Sharing (UNOS) for priority status (exception points) for liver transplantation candidacy in patients with HCC.

OUTCOME/PROGNOSIS

Early diagnosis is essential, as surgical resection and liver transplantation can improve long-term survival with 5-year disease-free survival exceeding 50% (*Hepatology 2011;53:1020*). Advanced HCC has a dismal prognosis with a 5-year survival of 0% to 10%.

LIVER TRANSPLANTATION

GENERAL PRINCIPLES

- Liver transplantation is an effective therapeutic option for irreversible acute and ESLD for which available therapies have failed.
- Whole cadaveric livers and partial livers (split-liver, reduced-size, and living-related) are used in the United States as sources for liver transplantation.
- The prioritization for liver transplantation is determined by the Model for End-Stage Liver Disease (MELD) score. The MELD score is calculated by a formula that takes into account serum bilirubin, serum creatinine, and INR. Regularly patients are evaluated for a liver transplantation when they achieve a MELD of 15. Patients are considered for "exception MELD points" for conditions such as: HCC within Milan criteria, hepatopulmonary syndrome, portopulmonary hypertension, polycystic liver disease, familial amyloidosis, unusual tumors, etc. (*Liver Transpl 2006;12(12 suppl 3):S128*).
- Patients who fulfill criteria for **acute liver failure** are potential candidates for liver transplantation.
- Patients with cirrhosis should be considered for transplant evaluation when they have a decline in hepatic synthetic or excretory functions, ascites, hepatic encephalopathy, or complications such as HRS, HCC, recurrent SBP, or variceal bleeding.
- Candidates for liver transplantation are evaluated by a multidisciplinary team that includes hepatologists, transplant surgeons, transplant nurse coordinators, social workers, psychologists, and financial coordinators.
- General **contraindications** to liver transplant include severe and uncontrolled extrahepatic infection, advanced cardiac or pulmonary disease, extrahepatic malignancy, multiorgan failure, unresolved psychosocial issues, medical noncompliance issues, and ongoing substance abuse (e.g., alcohol and illegal drugs).
- In the United States in the last 5 years, between 15 and 16,000 patients have been actively listed for liver transplantation. The majority of these patients are male and Caucasian. In 2009, there were 5,748 liver transplantations performed. The main etiologies for liver transplantation have included HCV, malignancy, and alcoholic liver disease (*http://www.unos.org/*).

- There continues to be a disparity between supply and demand of suitable livers for transplantation.

TREATMENT

Immunosuppressive, infectious, and long-term complications are discussed in Chapter 17, Solid Organ Transplant Medicine.

20 Disorders of Hemostasis and Thrombosis

Roger Yusen, Charles Eby, Kristen Sanfilippo, and Brian F. Gage

Hemostatic Disorders

GENERAL PRINCIPLES

Normal hemostasis involves a complex sequence of interrelated reactions that lead to platelet aggregation (primary hemostasis) and activation of coagulation factors (secondary hemostasis) to produce a durable vascular seal.

- **Primary hemostasis** is an immediate but temporary response to vessel injury. Platelets and von Willebrand factor (vWF) interact to form a primary plug.
- **Secondary hemostasis (coagulation)** results in formation of a fibrin clot (Figure 20-1). Injury initiates coagulation by exposing extravascular tissue factor to blood, which initiates activation of factors VII, X, and prothrombin. The subsequent activation of factors XI, VIII, and V leads to further generation of thrombin, conversion of fibrinogen to fibrin, and formation of a durable clot (*Semin Thromb Hemost 2009;35:9*).

DIAGNOSIS

Clinical Presentation

History

A detailed history can assess bleeding severity, congenital or acquired status, and primary or secondary hemostatic defects.

- Prolonged bleeding after dental extractions, circumcision, menstruation, labor and delivery, trauma, or surgery may suggest an underlying bleeding disorder.
- Family history may suggest an inherited bleeding disorder.

Physical Examination

- Primary hemostasis defects are suggested by mucosal bleeding and excessive bruising.
  - Petechiae: <2 mm subcutaneous bleeding, do not blanch with pressure, typically present in areas subject to increased hydrostatic force: the lower legs and periorbital area (especially after coughing or vomiting).
  - Ecchymoses: >3 mm black-and-blue (or violaceous) patches due to rupture of small vessels from trauma.
- Secondary hemostasis defects can produce **hematomas** (localized masses of clotted/unclotted blood), hemarthroses, or delayed bleeding after trauma or surgery.

Figure 20-1. Coagulation cascade. *Solid arrows* indicate activation. Solid or dashed lines that run into a vertical line and are associated with drugs represent a point of inhibition. Extrinsic pathway includes the left upper portion of the cascade above FX. Intrinsic pathway includes the right upper portion of the cascade above FX. Common pathway includes the lower portion of the cascade from FX and below. AT, antithrombin; FX, factor X; LMWH, low–molecular-weight heparin; TF, tissue factor.

Diagnostic Testing

Laboratories

The history and physical exam guide test selection. Initial studies should include platelet count, prothrombin time (PT), activated partial thromboplastin time (aPTT), and a blood smear.

- **Primary hemostasis tests**
  - A low **platelet count** requires review of blood smear to rule out platelet clumping artifact (due to the ethylenediaminetetraacetic acid [EDTA] additive, platelet glycoprotein [GP] IIb/IIIa receptor inhibitor drugs), giant platelets.
  - The **PFA-100** (Dade Behring, Deerfield, IL) instrument assesses vWF-dependent platelet activation in flowing citrated whole blood. Most patients with von Willebrand disorder (vWD) and qualitative platelet disorders have prolonged PFA-100 closure times. Anemia (hematocrit [Hct] <30%) and thrombocytopenia (platelet $<100 \times 10^9$/L) can cause prolonged closure times.
  - **In vitro platelet aggregation** studies measure platelet secretion and aggregation in response to platelet agonists (see Qualitative Platelet Disorders section).
  - Laboratory evaluation of suspected vWD begins with measurement of von Willebrand factor antigen (**vWF:Ag**) and performance of at least one **vWF activity assay**:
    - **Ristocetin cofactor (vWF:RCo):** Measures vWF-mediated agglutination of control platelets in the presence of ristocetin.

- **Collagen binding assay:** Measures vWF affinity for collagen.
  - **von Willebrand factor multimer analysis** by agarose gel electrophoresis separates vWF multimers by size to classify vWD type 2 subtypes.
- **Secondary hemostasis** (see Figure 20-1)
  - **PT:** Measures time to form a fibrin clot after adding thromboplastin (tissue factor and phospholipid) and calcium to citrated plasma.
    - Sensitive (i.e., elevated PT) to deficiencies of **extrinsic pathway** (factor VII), **common pathway** (factors X, V, prothrombin), and **fibrinogen**, and to use of vitamin K antagonists and direct factor Xa and thrombin (IIa) inhibitors.
    - Reporting a PT ratio as an international normalized ratio (INR) reduces interlaboratory variation (*Thromb Haemost 1983;49:238*).
    - Most PT reagents contain a heparin-neutralizing additive.
    - Point-of-care instruments measure PT/INR from a drop of whole blood.
  - **aPTT:** Measure the time to form a fibrin clot after activation of citrated plasma by calcium, phospholipid, and negatively charged particles. Besides heparin, low–molecular-weight heparin (LMWH), fondaparinux, and direct anti-Xa and thrombin (IIa) inhibitors, deficiencies and inhibitors of coagulation factors of the **intrinsic pathway** (e.g., high–molecular-weight kininogen, prekallikrein, factor XII, factor XI, factor IX, and factor VIII), **common pathway** (e.g., factor V, factor X, prothrombin), and **fibrinogen prolong the aPTT.**
  - **Thrombin time (TT):** Measures time to form a fibrin clot after addition of thrombin to citrated plasma. Quantitative and qualitative deficiencies of fibrinogen, fibrin degradation products, heparin, LMWH, fondaparinux, and direct thrombin (IIa) inhibitors prolong the TT.
  - **Fibrinogen:** The addition of thrombin to dilute plasma and the measurement of a clotting time determine the level of fibrinogen. Conditions causing hypofibrinogen and potential for bleeding include decreased hepatic synthesis, massive hemorrhage, and disseminated intravascular coagulation (DIC).
  - **D-dimers** result from plasmin digestion of fibrin. Elevated D-dimer concentrations occur in many disease states that include acute venous thromboembolism (VTE), DIC, trauma, and malignancy.
  - **Mixing studies** determine if a factor deficiency or an inhibitor have prolonged the PT or the aPTT. Mixing patient plasma 1:1 with normal pooled plasma (all factor activities = 100%) restores deficient factors sufficiently to normalize or nearly normalize the PT or the aPTT (Table 20-1). If mixing partially corrects

Table 20-1	Factor Deficiencies Cause Prolonged Prothrombin Time and/or Activated Partial Thromboplastin Time that Correct with 50:50 Mix
Abnormal Assay	**Suspected Factor Deficiencies**
aPTT	XII, XI, IX, VIII, HMWK, PK
PT	VII
PT and aPTT	II, V, X, or fibrinogen

aPTT, activated partial thromboplastin time; HMWK, high–molecular-weight kininogen; PK, prekallikrein; PT, prothrombin time.

the prolonged PT or aPTT, a specific factor inhibitor, a nonspecific inhibitor (e.g., lupus anticoagulant [LA]), or an anticoagulant drug may have caused the prolongation.

PLATELET DISORDERS

Thrombocytopenia

GENERAL PRINCIPLES

Thrombocytopenia is defined as a platelet count of $<140 \times 10^9$/L at Barnes-Jewish Hospital. In the absence of qualitative platelet defects or vascular damage, spontaneous bleeding does not typically occur with platelet counts $>30 \times 10^9$/L.

DIAGNOSIS

Thrombocytopenia occurs from decreased production, increased destruction, or sequestration of platelets (Table 20-2). Many infectious diseases have an association with thrombocytopenia through complex or poorly understood mechanisms (*Blood 2009;113:6511*).

Table 20-2	Classification of Thrombocytopenia	
Decreased Platelet Production	**Increased Platelet Clearance**	
Marrow failure syndromes	*Immune-mediated mechanisms*	
Congenital	Immune thrombocytopenic	
Acquired: Aplastic anemia, paroxysmal nocturnal hemoglobinuria	Thrombotic thrombocytopenic purpura/hemolytic uremic syndrome	
Hematologic malignancies	Posttransfusion purpura	
Marrow infiltration: Cancer, granuloma	Heparin-induced thrombocytopenia	
Myelofibrosis: Primary or secondary	*Non–immune-mediated mechanisms*	
Nutritional: Vitamin B_{12} and folate deficiencies	DIC	
Physical damage to the bone marrow: Radiation, alcohol, chemotherapy	Local consumption (aortic aneurysm)	
	Acute hemorrhage	
Increased Splenic Sequestration	**Infections Associated with Thrombocytopenia**	
Portal hypertension		
Felty's syndrome	HIV, HHV-6, ehrlichiosis, rickettsia,	
Lysosomal storage disorders	malaria, hepatitis C, CMV, Epstein–	
Infiltrative hematologic malignancies	Barr, *Helicobacter pylori*, *E. coli*	
Extramedullary hematopoiesis	O157	

CMV, cytomegalovirus; DIC, disseminated intravascular coagulation; HHV-6, human herpesvirus 6.

Immune Thrombocytopenia

GENERAL PRINCIPLES

Immune thrombocytopenia (ITP) is an acquired immune disorder in which antiplatelet antibodies cause shortened platelet survival and suppress megakaryopoiesis leading to thrombocytopenia (platelets $<100 \times 10^9$/L) and increased bleeding risk (*Blood 2009;113:6511*). ITP can be idiopathic (primary), associated with coexisting conditions (secondary), or drug induced.

Epidemiology

Adult primary **ITP** has an incidence of 3.3 cases per 10^5 persons (*Am J Hematol 2010;85:174*).

Etiology

- In **primary ITP**, autoantibodies bind to platelet surface antigens and cause premature clearance by the reticuloendothelial system in addition to immune-mediated suppression of platelet production.
- **Secondary ITP** occurs in the setting of systemic lupus erythematosus (SLE), antiphospholipid antibody (APA) syndrome, HIV, hepatitis C virus (HCV), *Helicobacter pylori*, and lymphoproliferative disorders (*Blood 2009;113:6511*).
- **Drug-dependent ITP** results from drug–platelet interactions prompting antibody binding (*N Engl J Med 2007;357:580*). Medications linked to thrombocytopenia include quinidine and quinine; platelet inhibitors abciximab, eptifibatide, tirofiban, and ticlopidine; antibiotics linezolid, rifampin, sulfonamides, and vancomycin; the anticonvulsants phenytoin, valproic acid, and carbamazepine; the analgesics acetaminophen, naproxen, and diclofenac; cimetidine; and chlorothiazide (*Ann Intern Med 2005;142:474; www.ouhsc.edu/platelets*).

DIAGNOSIS

Clinical Presentation

- **ITP** typically presents as mild mucocutaneous bleeding and petechiae or incidental thrombocytopenia. Occasionally, ITP can present as major bleeding.
- Risk of bleeding is highest with platelet counts $<30 \times 10^9$/L, male gender, and age >40 (*Blood 2010;115:168; Arch Intern Med 2000;160:1630*).

Diagnostic Testing

Normalization of platelet counts with discontinuation of suspected drug, and confirmation if thrombocytopenia recurs when rechallenged supports the diagnosis of **drug-induced thrombocytopenia**.

Laboratories

- Review a peripheral blood smear to confirm automated platelet count, assess for platelet clumping, and platelet, red cell, and white cell morphologies.
- Laboratory tests do not confirm the diagnosis of primary ITP, though they help to exclude secondary causes. Primary **ITP** often has the scenario of isolated thrombocytopenia in the absence of a likely underlying causative disease or medication.

- Test for infection-associated causes: HIV, HCV, *Helicobacter pylori* (*Blood 2011;117:4190*)
- Serologic tests for antiplatelet antibodies generally do not help diagnose **ITP** because of poor sensitivity and low negative predictive value (NPV) (*Am J Hematol 2005;78:193*).

Diagnostic Procedures
Diagnosis of ITP does not typically require bone marrow examination, although it can help to exclude other causes in select patients with additional complete blood cell (CBC) abnormalities, unresponsiveness to immune suppression therapy, or atypical signs or symptoms (*Blood 2011;117:4190*).

TREATMENT

- The decision to treat **primary ITP** depends upon the severity of thrombocytopenia and concerns about bleeding.
- Initial therapy, when indicated, consists of **glucocorticoids** (typically prednisone 1 mg/kg/d orally × 21 days). Nonresponders or patients with active bleeding typically also receive intravenous immunoglobulin **(IVIg**; 1 g/kg × 1) or anti-D immunoglobulin (**WinRho**) if Rh-positive (ineffective postsplenectomy). WinRho works by forming anti–D-coated red blood cell (RBC) complexes, which bind to splenic macrophages saturating the reticuloendothelial system and preventing platelet destruction. This may cause severe hemolysis, and requires postinfusion monitoring for signs and symptoms of hemolysis. Reduce WinRho dose if hemoglobin (Hgb) <10 g/dL and avoid when the Hgb is <8 g/dL. Most primary ITP cases initially respond to therapy within 1 to 3 weeks.
- Nonresponders and 30% to 40% of patients who relapse during a steroid taper have refractory ITP, for whom the therapeutic goal is a safe platelet count to prevent major bleeding (typically ≥30 × 10^9/L), and minimization of treatment-related toxicities. Two-thirds of patients with refractory ITP will obtain a durable complete response following **splenectomy**. Administer pneumococcal, meningococcal, and *Haemophilus influenza* type B vaccines presplenectomy or postsplenectomy.
- Options for patients who do not undergo splenectomy, or those who fail splenectomy, include single or combined therapies with prednisone, IVIg, androgen therapy with danazol, other immunosuppressive agents, or **rituximab** (anti-CD20 monoclonal antibody) (*Blood 2011;117:4190*).
- There are two thrombopoietin receptor (TPO-R) agonists for treatment of refractory primary ITP patients with increased bleeding risk. **Romiplostim** (Nplate), dosed SQ weekly, and **eltrombopag** (Promacta), taken orally once a day, produce durable platelet count improvements in a majority of refractory ITP patients beginning 5 to 7 days after initiation. Potential complications include thromboembolic events and bone marrow fibrosis (*Lancet 2011;377:393; Lancet 2008; 371:395*).
- Management of secondary ITP may include a combination of treating the underlying disease and therapies used for management of primary ITP.
- Platelet transfusion for severe drug-induced thrombocytopenia may decrease risk of bleeding. IVIg, steroids, and plasmapheresis have uncertain benefit.

Thrombotic Thrombocytopenic Purpura and Hemolytic Uremic Syndrome

GENERAL PRINCIPLES

Definition

Thrombotic thrombocytopenic purpura (TTP) and **hemolytic uremic syndrome (HUS)** are thrombotic microangiopathies (TMAs) caused by platelet–vWF aggregates and platelet–fibrin aggregates, respectively, resulting in thrombocytopenia, microangiopathic hemolytic anemia (MAHA), and organ ischemia. Usually, clinical and laboratory features permit differentiation of TTP from HUS. TMA may occur in association with DIC, HIV infection, malignant hypertension, vasculitis, organ and stem cell transplant–related toxicity, adverse drug reactions, and pregnancy-related complications of preeclampsia/eclampsia and HELLP (**H**emolysis, **E**levated **L**iver enzymes, **L**ow **P**latelets) syndrome.

Epidemiology

Sporadic **TTP** has an incidence of approximately 11.3 cases per 10^6 persons, occurring more frequently in women and African Americans (*J Thromb Haemost 2005;3:1432*). **Typical HUS** usually occurs in gastroenteritis outbreaks affecting children. Adults may present with both **typical** and **atypical** (nongastroenteritis-associated) variants of **HUS**.

Etiology

- Autoantibody-mediated removal of plasma vWF-cleaving protease: A disintegrin and metalloproteinase with a thrombospondin type 1 motif, member 13 (ADAMTS13), leading to elevated levels of abnormally large vWF multimers, typically causes **sporadic TTP** (*N Engl J Med 1998;339:1578*). The abnormal vWF multimers spontaneously adhere to platelets and may produce occlusive vWF–platelet aggregates in the microcirculation and subsequent microangiopathy. Second-hit events may involve endothelial dysfunction or injury.
- Severe ADAMTS13 deficiency does not cause HUS and other types of TMA, with the exception of some cases associated with HIV and pregnancy.
- **Typical or enteropathic HUS** has an association with *Escherichia coli* (O157:H7) production of Shiga-like toxins in Shiga toxigenic *Escherichia coli*-hemolytic uremic syndrome (STEC-HUS).
- **HUS** can also be associated with transplantation, endothelial damaging drugs, and pregnancy (*Kidney Int Suppl 2009;112:S8*).
- Inherited or acquired defects in regulation of the alternative complement pathway are present in 30% to 50% of cases atypical HUS cases (*Ann Rev Path Mech Dis 2008;3:249*).

DIAGNOSIS

Clinical Presentation

- The complete clinical pentad of **TTP**, present in <30% of cases, includes consumptive **thrombocytopenia, MAHA, fever, renal dysfunction, and fluctuating neurologic deficits**.
- The findings of thrombocytopenia and MAHA should raise suspicion for **TTP-HUS** in the absence of other identifiable causes.

- Patients with autosomal recessive inherited ADAMTS13 deficiencies have relapsing TTP (Upshaw–Schulman syndrome).
- Diarrhea, usually bloody, and abdominal pain often precede STEC-HUS.
- Marked renal dysfunction usually occurs in HUS.

Diagnostic Testing

- TMAs produce schistocytes (fragmented red cells) and thrombocytopenia on blood smears. The findings of anemia, elevated reticulocyte count, low or undetectable haptoglobin, and elevated lactate dehydrogenase support the presence of hemolysis.
- Sporadic TTP has TMA findings, normal PT and aPTT, mild-to-moderate azotemia, very low or undetectable ADAMTS13 enzyme activity, and sometimes detectable ADAMTS13 inhibitory antibody.
- Typical HUS has TMA and acute renal failure. *E. coli* O157 stool culture has a higher sensitivity than do Shiga toxin assays. However, stool samples obtained after diarrhea has resolved reduce the sensitivity of both tests (*Kidney Int 2009;75:S29*).
- In the absence of precipitating risk factors, testing for **atypical HUS** should include molecular and serologic tests for complement regulator factor H and I mutations or autoantibodies through reference laboratories.

TREATMENT

- The mainstay of therapy for **TTP** consists of rapid treatment with plasma exchange (PEX) of 1.0 to 1.5 plasma volumes daily. PEX is usually continued for several days after normalization of platelet count and lactate dehydrogenase.
  - If PEX is not available or will be delayed, infuse **fresh frozen plasma (FFP)** immediately to replace ADAMTS13.
  - Common practice includes the administration of **glucocorticoids**: Prednisone 1 mg/kg PO/day. Consider a brief course of high-dose corticosteroids (methylprednisolone 0.5 to 1.0 g IV/d) in critically ill or PEX nonresponding patients (*Blood 2010;116:4060*).
  - Platelet transfusion in the absence of severe bleeding is relatively contraindicated due to potential risk of additional microvascular occlusions.
  - About 90% of treated patients have a remission. Relapses may occur within days to year after remission.
  - Therapy with **rituximab** achieves durable remissions following TTP relapses (*Ann Intern Med 2003;138:105*; *Thromb Haemost 2009;101:233*).
  - **Immunosuppression** with cyclophosphamide, azathioprine, or vincristine and splenectomy may have success in the treatment of refractory or relapsing TTP (*Ann Hematol 2002;81:7*; *Blood 2000;96:1223*).
- **STEC-HUS** does not usually improve with PEX and treatment remains supportive. Antibiotic therapy does not hasten recovery or minimize toxicity for STEC-HUS.
- **TMA associated with calcineurin inhibitors** (cyclosporine, tacrolimus) usually responds to drug dose reduction or discontinuation of the offensive agent.
- **Atypical HUS** in the absence of precipitating risk factors often leads to chronic renal failure necessitating dialysis.
  - In 2011, the U.S. Food and Drug Administration (FDA) approved eculizumab for treatment of **non–STEC-HUS**. Eculizumab is a humanized monoclonal antibody that binds to complement protein C5, blocking its cleavage into C5a and the cytotoxic membrane attack complex C5b-9, thus inhibiting complement activation (*Blood 2011;118:3303*).
  - *Neisseria meningitides* vaccination must be performed before starting eculizumab.

Heparin-Induced Thrombocytopenia

GENERAL PRINCIPLES

Definition

Heparin-induced thrombocytopenia (HIT) is an acquired hypercoagulable disorder due to autoantibodies targeting heparin and platelet factor 4 (PF4) complexes. HIT typically presents with a decrease in platelet count by at least 50% from preexposure baseline. Major complications of HITs consist of arterial and venous thromboembolic events.

Epidemiology

The incidence of **HIT** varies with clinical setting, anticoagulant formulation, dose, duration of exposure, and previous exposure. It ranges from 0.1% to 1.0% in medical and obstetric patients receiving prophylactic and therapeutic unfractionated heparin (UFH), to >1% to 5% in patients receiving prophylactic UFH after total hip or knee replacements or cardiothoracic surgery (*Chest 2012;141:e495s*). Patients exposed only to LMWH have a low incidence of HIT (*Thromb Res 2009;124:189*). HIT rarely occurs in association with the synthetic pentasaccharide fondaparinux (*N Engl J Med 2007;356:2653*).

Etiology

Immune-responsive patients produce autoantibodies that bind to PF4/heparin complexes, which can activate platelets, cause thrombocytopenia, and lead to clot formation through increased thrombin generation (*Blood 2003;101:31*).

DIAGNOSIS

Clinical Presentation

- **HIT** usually develops within 5 to 14 days of heparin exposure (**typical-onset HIT**). Exceptions include **delayed-onset HIT**, which occurs after stopping heparin, and **early-onset HIT**, which starts within the first 24 hours of heparin administration in patients with recent exposure to heparin (*Chest 2012;141:e495s*).
- Suspect HIT when thrombocytopenia occurs during heparin exposure by any route in the absence of other causes of thrombocytopenia.
- The **4T scoring system** (Table 20-3) was developed to assist with determining HIT pretest probability (*J Thromb Haemost 2006;4:759*).
- HIT rarely causes severe thrombocytopenia and bleeding.
- **Thromboembolic complications** (i.e., heparin-induced thrombocytopenia and thrombosis [HITT]), venous > arterial, occur in 30% to 75% of HIT patients. Thrombosis can precede, be concurrent with, or follow thrombocytopenia.
- HIT causing venous thrombi at heparin injection sites produces full-thickness skin infarctions, sometimes in the absence of thrombocytopenia.
- HIT can cause systemic allergic responses following an IV bolus of heparin characterized by fever, hypotension, dyspnea, and cardiac arrest.

Diagnostic Testing

- Obtain surveillance platelet counts every 2 to 3 days during heparin exposure in patients with >1% risk of HIT (*Chest 2012;141:e495s*).

Table 20-3	Four T's Scoring System for Pretest Probability of Heparin-Induced Thrombocytopenia		
T	**0 Point**	**1 Point**	**2 Points**
Thrombo-cytopenia	Decrease <30% or nadir <10 k/cumm	Decrease 30%–50% or nadir 10–19 k/cumm	Decrease >50% and nadir ≥20 k/cumm
Timing of thrombo-cytopenia	≤4 d without prior exposure	Likely within 5–10 d, not clear; >10 d; ≤1 d (with exposure 31–100 d)	Within 5–10 d of exposure or ≤1 d (with exposure in last 30 days)
Thrombotic event	No thrombus	Thrombus recurrence or progression; erythematous skin lesion; unproven thrombus	Confirmed thrombus; skin necrosis; acute reaction post-UFH bolus
Other causes for thrombo-cytopenia	Definite alternate explanation	Possible alternate explanation	No other explanation

Sum the points for each of the four categories to determine the clinical probability: High (6–8 points), intermediate (4–5 points), low (0–3 points).
UFH, unfractionated heparin.
Adapted from Lo GK, Juhl D, Warkentin TE, et al. Evaluation of pretest clinical score (4 T's) for the diagnosis of heparin-induced thrombocytopenia in two clinical settings. *J Thromb Haemost* 2006;4:759–765.

- For suspected HIT, laboratory tests for PF4 antibodies improve diagnostic accuracy.
  - Most laboratories use an ELISA method.
  - Detection of IgG, IgM, and IgA PF4 antibodies in patients' serum is a sensitive screening test for seroconversion but lacks specificity for HIT.
  - Specificity improves when only IgG antibodies are detected and a positive enzyme-linked immunosorbent assay (ELISA) is quantified in optical density (OD) units. The higher the OD, the more likely that the patient has HIT.
  - The impact of these refinements on sensitivity is unclear, leading to different criteria for "positive HIT ELISA" (*Blood 2012;119:2209*; *Chest 2012;141 (suppl):e495s*).
- Two functional assays for HIT: serotonin release assay (SRA) and heparin-induced platelet activation (HIPA; more common in Europe).
  - Both tests detect PF4 antibodies in patients' serum capable of activating control platelets in the presence of heparin.
  - They are sensitive and specific for HIT, typically sent to reference laboratories, which delays results for days.
- In a low clinical probability of HIT, testing for HIT antibodies is NOT indicated.
- In a moderate-high clinical probability of HIT, a negative PF4 ELISA effectively rules out HIT.
- In a moderate-high clinical probability of HIT, a functional test (SRA or HIPA) should confirm a positive PF4 ELISA to improve specificity.

TREATMENT

- Since PF4 antibody test results are rarely immediately available, clinical assessment should determine initial management.
- When HIT is strongly suspected, begin treatment by **eliminating all heparin** exposure.
- Patients with and those at high risk for thrombosis require alternative anticoagulation (*Blood 2012;119:2209*) with a parenteral direct thrombin inhibitor (DTI) (**argatroban or lepirudin**; see Medications under Approach to Venous Thromboembolism section). Although it lacks supportive evidence from clinical trials and it does not have FDA approval for the indication of HIT, clinicians could consider using fondaparinux for treatment of HIT if a parenteral DTI is not available/feasible (*J Thromb Haemost 2011;9:2389*). Do not substitute LMWH for UFH due to high rates of cross-reactivity with HIT antibodies.
- Screen (e.g., lower extremity venous compression ultrasound [US]) to assess for asymptomatic venous thromboembolism, which mandates longer duration anticoagulation (*Blood 2003;101:31*).
- Start warfarin only after the platelet count normalizes, at an initial low dose, overlapping with a DTI for 5 days, to reduce the risk of limb gangrene due to ongoing hypercoagulable conditions and depletion of proteins C and S.
- DTIs prolong the INR and require careful monitoring when transitioning from DTI to warfarin (see Medications under Approach to Venous Thromboembolism section for guidelines).
- Oral DTI and anti-Xa inhibitors (dabigatran and rivaroxaban) have not been evaluated for safety and efficacy in HIT patients with or without thromboses.
- The recommended duration of anticoagulation therapy for HIT depends on the clinical scenario: 4 weeks for **isolated HIT** (without thrombosis) and 3 months for **HIT-associated thrombosis** (*Chest 2012;141:e495s*) (see treatment duration in the Approach to Venous Thromboembolism section).

Posttransfusion Purpura

GENERAL PRINCIPLES

Definition

Posttransfusion purpura (PTP), a rare syndrome characterized by the formation of alloantibodies against platelet antigens, most commonly HPA-1a, follows blood component transfusion and causes severe thrombocytopenia.

Epidemiology

PTP has an incidence of 1 in 50,000 to 100,000 blood transfusions, although ~2% of the population has a potential risk for PTP based on the frequency of HPA-1b/1b.

Etiology

GP IIIa has a polymorphic epitope called HPA-1a/b. **PTP** typically occurs in HPA-1b/1b multiparous women or previously transfused patients when reexposed to HPA-1a by transfusion. An amnestic response produces alloantibodies to the HPA-1a epitope, which appear to also recognize the patient's HPA-1a–negative platelets and cause thrombocytopenia. In some cases, alloantibodies recognize different platelet-specific epitopes (HPA-3a/b, HPA-5a/b).

DIAGNOSIS

- In **PTP**, severe thrombocytopenia ($<15 \times 10^9$/L) occurs within approximately 7 to 10 days of transfusion.
- Confirmation of suspected **PTP** requires detection of platelet alloantibodies.

TREATMENT

Although spontaneous platelet recovery eventually occurs, bleeding may require treatment. Effective therapies include IVIg and plasmapheresis. Transfusion with platelets from a donor who lacks the causative epitope (typically HPA-1a) does not clearly have higher efficacy than random platelet transfusion, and most hospitals do not have HPA-1a–negative platelets readily available. Reserve transfusion with platelets of unknown HPA-1 status for patients with PTP and severe bleeding (*Am J Hematol 2004;76:258*).

Gestational Thrombocytopenia

GENERAL PRINCIPLES

Definition

Gestational thrombocytopenia (platelet counts no lower than 70×10^9/L) is a benign, mild thrombocytopenia associated with pregnancy.

Epidemiology

Gestational thrombocytopenia spontaneously occurs in approximately 5% to 7% of otherwise uncomplicated pregnancies (*Clin Obstet Gynecol 1999;42:327*).

Etiology

The mechanism of **gestational thrombocytopenia** remains unknown.

DIAGNOSIS

Clinical Presentation

Gestational thrombocytopenia occurs in the third trimester of pregnancy. The mother has no symptoms and the fetus remains unaffected.

Differential Diagnosis

Other causes of thrombocytopenia during pregnancy include **ITP**, **preeclampsia**, **eclampsia**, **HELLP** syndrome, **TTP**, and **DIC**.

Diagnostic Testing

Diagnostic testing for gestational thrombocytopenia includes a thorough evaluation for evidence of hemolysis, infection, hypertension, and liver dysfunction to distinguish between these syndromes.

OUTCOME/PROGNOSIS

Gestational thrombocytopenia and thrombocytopenia associated with preeclampsia and eclampsia usually resolves promptly after delivery.

Thrombocytosis

GENERAL PRINCIPLES

Definition

Thrombocytosis is defined as a platelet count of $>440 \times 10^9$/L at Barnes-Jewish Hospital.

Classification

Thrombocytosis can be divided into two categories: reactive and clonal (*Thrombosis 2011;2011:536062*).

- **Reactive thrombocytosis** may occur during recovery from thrombocytopenia, after postsplenectomy, or in response to iron deficiency, acute infectious or chronic inflammatory states, trauma, and malignancies and can be extreme ($>1 \times 10^6$/uL). Thrombocytosis should be confirmed by review of a blood smear. Patients with reactive thrombocytosis have very low risks of thrombosis or bleeding. Platelets normalize after improvement of the underlying disorder. Clonal and reactive thrombocytosis may coexist; if accompanied by thrombotic complications, evaluate for an underlying myeloproliferative disorder.
- **Essential thrombocytosis (ET)** is a chronic myeloproliferative disorder. Eventual progression to myelofibrosis, acute myeloid leukemia, or myelodysplastic syndrome occurs in a small minority of ET patients (*Br J Haematol 2005;130:153*).

DIAGNOSIS

Clinical Presentation

History

ET may present as an incidental discovery or present with thrombotic or hemorrhagic symptoms. The risk of thrombosis increases with age, prior thrombosis, duration of disease, and other comorbidities (*Blood 1999;93:417*). Erythromelalgia, due to microvascular occlusive platelet thrombi, presents as intense burning or throbbing of the extremities, typically involving the feet. Cold exposure usually relieves symptoms. Hemorrhage typically occurs with platelet counts $>1,000 \times 10^9$/L, and acquired deficiencies of large vWF multimers often accompany hemorrhage patients with ET (*Blood 1993;82:1749*).

Physical Examination

Approximately 50% of ET patients develop mild splenomegaly. Typical signs of erythromelalgia include erythema and warmth of affected digits.

Diagnostic Criteria

In 2008, the World Health Organization (WHO) revised criteria (requires all 4) included: (*Current Hematologic Malignancy Reports 2007;4:33*)
- Sustained platelet count $>450 \times 10^9$/L.
- Bone marrow biopsy showing increased mature megakaryocytes and no increase in erythropoiesis or granulopoiesis.
- Chronic myelogenous leukemia (CML), polycythemia vera, and primary myelofibrosis not present according to WHO criteria.

- Presence of JAK2V617F mutation or other clonal marker (*Lancet 2005;365:1054*) **or** no evidence for reactive thrombocytosis if clonal marker not present (*Leukemia 2008;22:14*).

TREATMENT

Patients requiring platelet reduction therapy include those with age >60 years, a prior thrombosis or hemorrhage, hypertension, diabetes, smoking, or hyperlipidemia. The majority of thrombotic complications occur at modest platelet count elevations. Treatment typically aims for a platelet count of $\leq 400 \times 10^9/L$. Platelet-lowering drugs include **hydroxyurea** and **anagrelide**, or **interferon-α** in pregnant patients or females in their childbearing years (*Blood 2001;97:863*).
- Limited evidence suggests that long-term hydroxyurea therapy has a very low leukemogenic potential.
- Anagrelide side effects include palpitations, atrial fibrillation, fluid retention, and headache.
- Hydroxyurea and anagrelide provide equivalent platelet count control but anagrelide causes more complications (*N Engl J Med 2005;353:33*).
- Platelet pheresis rapidly lowers platelet counts to manage acute arterial thrombosis.

Qualitative Platelet Disorders

GENERAL PRINCIPLES

Qualitative platelet disorders present with mucocutaneous bleeding and excessive bruising with an adequate platelet count, PT and aPTT, and normal screening tests for vWD. Most potent platelet defects produce prolonged platelet function assay-100 (PFA-100) closure times. However, a high clinical suspicion of a disorder in a patient with normal test results should lead to in vitro platelet aggregation studies.

Classification
- **Inherited disorders** of platelet function include receptor, signal transduction, cyclooxygenase, secretory (e.g., storage pool disease), adhesion, or aggregation defects. In vitro platelet aggregation studies can identify patterns of agonist responses consistent with a particular defect, such as the rare autosomal recessive disorders of adhesion in Bernard–Soulier syndrome (lack of GP IbIX [vWF receptor]) and aggregation in Glanzmann thrombasthenia (lack of GP IIb/IIIa [fibrinogen receptor]).
- **Acquired** platelet defects are more common than hereditary platelet qualitative disorders.
  - Conditions associated with acquired qualitative defects include metabolic disorders (uremia, liver failure), myeloproliferative diseases, myelodysplasia, acute leukemia, monoclonal gammopathy, and cardiopulmonary bypass platelet trauma.
  - **Drug-induced** platelet dysfunction occurs as a side effect of many drugs, including high-dose penicillin, aspirin and other nonsteroidal anti-inflammatory drugs (NSAIDs), and ethanol. Other drug classes, such as β-lactam antibiotics, β-blockers, calcium channel blockers, nitrates, antihistamines, psychotropic drugs, tricyclic antidepressants, and selective serotonin reuptake inhibitors, cause platelet dysfunction in vitro but rarely cause bleeding.

○ Certain **foods and herbal products** may affect platelet function including omega-3 fatty acids, garlic and onion extracts, ginger, gingko, ginseng, and black tree fungus. Patients should stop using herbal medications and dietary supplements in conjunction with anticoagulant therapy and at least 1 week before major surgery (*Thromb Res 2005;117:49*; *Anaesthesia 2002;57:889*).

TREATMENT

• Reserve platelet transfusions for major bleeding episodes. Anecdotal reports have described successful control of severe bleeding with recombinant factor VIIa (rFVIIa).
• Treatment of **uremic platelet dysfunction** includes the following (*Nature Clinical Practice Nephrology 2007;3:138*):
  ○ Dialysis, to improve uremia.
  ○ Increase of Hct to ~30%, by transfusion or erythropoietin.
  ○ Desmopressin (diamino-8-D-arginine vasopressin [DDAVP], 0.3 mcg/kg IV) to stimulate release of vWF from endothelial cells.
  ○ Conjugated estrogens (0.6 mg/kg IV daily for 5 days), which may improve platelet function for up to 2 weeks.
  ○ Platelets transfusions in actively bleeding patients, although transfused platelets rapidly acquire the uremic defect.
• **Reversal of drug-induced platelet dysfunction**
  ○ **Aspirin** irreversibly inhibits cyclooxygenase-1 (COX-1) and cyclooxygenase-2 (COX-2). Its effects diminish over 7 to 10 days due to new platelet production.
  ○ Since other **NSAIDs** reversibly inhibit COX-1 and COX-2, their effect only lasts several days. **COX-2 inhibitors** have antiplatelet activity in large doses, but they have a minimal effect on platelets at therapeutic doses.
  ○ **Thienopyridines** inhibit platelet aggregation by irreversibly (clopidogrel and prasugrel) or reversibly (ticagrelor) blocking platelet ADP receptor P2Y12.
  ○ **Dipyridamole**, alone or in combination with aspirin (Aggrenox), inhibits platelet function by increasing intracellular cyclic adenosine monophosphate (cAMP).
  ○ **Abciximab**, **eptifibatide**, **and tirofiban** block platelet IIb/IIIa–dependent aggregation (see Chapter 4, Ischemic Heart Disease).
  ○ Platelet transfusion compensates for drug-induced platelet dysfunction, except immediately following tirofiban and eptifibatide therapy.
  ○ Withhold irreversible antiplatelet agents for 7 to 10 days before elective invasive procedures.

INHERITED BLEEDING DISORDERS

Hemophilia A

GENERAL PRINCIPLES

Definition
Hemophilia A is an X-linked recessive coagulation disorder due to mutations in the gene encoding factor VIII.

Epidemiology

Hemophilia A affects ~1 in 5,000 live male births. Approximately 40% of cases occur in families with no prior history of hemophilia, reflecting the high rate of spontaneous germline mutations in the factor VIII gene (*N Engl J Med 2001;344:1773*).

DIAGNOSIS

Clinical Presentation

- Patients with severe hemophilia experience frequent spontaneous hemarthroses and hematomas, hematuria, and delayed posttraumatic and postoperative bleeding. Repeated bleeding into a "target" joint causes chronic synovitis and hemophilic arthropathy.
- Moderate hemophiliacs have fewer spontaneous bleeding episodes, and mild hemophiliacs may only bleed excessively after trauma or surgery.

Diagnostic Testing

Factor VIII activity: Severe (<1%), moderate (1% to 5%), and mild (>5% to <40%). Mild hemophiliacs with factor VIII ≥30% may not have a prolonged aPTT.

TREATMENT

Medications

First Line
- Mild-to-moderate hemophilia A with minor bleeding:
  DDAVP (0.3 μg/kg IV in 50 to 100 mL NS infused over 30 minutes, or 300 μg intranasally [Stimate, 1.5 mg/mL] dosed every 12 hours). Increases factor VIII activity threefold to fivefold and has a half-life of 8 to 12 hours. Tachyphylaxis may occur after several doses (*Blood 1997;90:2515*).
- Mild-to-moderate hemophilia A with major bleeding OR severe hemophilia A with any bleeding: **Factor VIII replacement** is the mainstay of therapy.
  - Many hemophiliacs infuse **lyophilized factor VIII concentrates** at home.
  - **Factor VIII concentrate** increases factor VIII activity approximately 2% for every 1 IU/kg infused. A 50 IU/kg IV bolus raises factor VIII activity approximately 100% over baseline. Extended treatment should follow with 25-IU/kg IV bolus q12h to maintain sufficient levels.
  - One to three doses of **factor VIII** concentrates targeting peak plasma activities of 30% to 50% typically stop mild hemorrhages.
  - Major traumas and surgery require maintenance of levels >80%.
  - Adjust doses based on peak and trough factor VIII results to achieve individualized targets based on bleeding risk.
  - Continuous infusion of factor VIII provides an alternative to intermittent infusion in special circumstances (*Hematol Oncol Clin North Am 1998;12:1315*).
  - There are multiple brands of plasma derived **recombinant factor VIII concentrates. Consult with a hematologist or pharmacist for prescribing advice** (*Blood 2012;119:4108*).

Second Line
Second-line factor VIII sources include **cryoprecipitate** and **FFP**.

Hemophilia B

GENERAL PRINCIPLES

Definition

Hemophilia B is an X-linked recessive coagulation disorder secondary to mutations in the gene encoding factor IX.

Epidemiology

Hemophilia B affects ~1 in 30,000 male births.

Diagnostic Testing

Factor IX activity.

TREATMENT

Hemophilia B remains clinically indistinguishable from hemophilia A, but the distinction is important, as the therapy of hemophilia B consists of **factor IX replacement** with either **plasma-derived factor IX** or **recombinant factor IX** (BeneFIX).
- **DDAVP** does not increase factor IX levels.
- Postinfusion peak targets, duration of therapy, and laboratory monitoring for treatment of hemophilia B–related bleeding have guidelines similar to those for hemophilia A.
- Every 1 IU/kg of factor IX replacement typically raises plasma factor IX activity by 1% and has a half-life of 18 to 24 hours.

COMPLICATIONS OF HEMOPHILIA A AND B THERAPY

Inhibitors
- Alloantibodies to factors VIII and IX in response to replacement therapy develop in approximately 20% and 12% of severe hemophilia A and B patients, respectively. These alloantibodies neutralize infused factor VIII or IX and prevent correction of the coagulopathy.
- Determining the titer of a factor VIII or IX inhibitor, using a laboratory assay that reports inhibitor strength in Bethesda units (BUs) predicts inhibitor behavior and guides therapy.
- Treatment options for hemophiliacs with factor VIII or IX inhibitors are as follows (*Lancet 2012;379:1447*):
  - Large doses of factor VIII or IX concentrates sometimes decrease bleeding in hemophiliacs with weak inhibitors (BU <5).
  - rFVIIa (NovoSeven), dosed at 90 µg/kg every 2 hours until achievement of hemostasis (*Semin Hematol 2001;38(4 suppl 12):43*).
  - Activated prothrombin complex concentrate (PCC) and factor eight inhibitor bypassing activity, vapor heated (FEIBA, VH) contains partially activated vitamin K–dependent coagulation factors XI, X, and VII, and thrombin that bypass factors VIII and IX in the coagulation cascade. It is associated with increased risk of thrombosis.

von Willebrand Disease

GENERAL PRINCIPLES

Classification

There are three main types of **vWD** (*J Thromb Haemost 2006;4:2103*) (Table 20-4).
- **Type 1 vWD**, due to a partial deficiency of vWF:Ag and activity and accounts for 70% to 80% of cases.
- **Type 2 vWD includes four qualitative defects.**
- **Type 3 vWD** has a virtual complete deficiency of vWF (*Blood 2001;97:1915*).

Epidemiology

vWD, the most common inherited bleeding disorder, affects an estimated 0.1% of the population.

Etiology

vWD results from an inherited quantitative or qualitative defect of vWF. Most forms of **vWD** have an autosomal dominant inheritance with variable penetrance, although autosomal recessive forms (types 2N and 3) exist (see Table 20-4). vWF circulates as multimers of variable size, and these facilitate adherence of platelets to injured vessel walls and stabilize factor VIII in plasma.

DIAGNOSIS

Clinical Presentation

- The characteristic clinical findings consist of mucocutaneous bleeding (epistaxis, menorrhagia, gastrointestinal [GI] bleeding) and easy bruising.
- Trauma, surgery, or dental extractions may result in life-threatening bleeding in severely affected individuals.
- Patients with mild vWD phenotype may remain undiagnosed into adulthood (*Blood 2001;97:1915*).

Diagnostic Testing

If personal and family bleeding histories support a reasonable pretest likelihood of an inherited primary hemostasis or bleeding disorder, screening for vWD should begin with measurements of vWF:Ag and vWF:RCo and FVIII activity (see Table 20-4). Some laboratories substitute vWF adhesion to collagen for vWF:RCo.
- **vWF:Ag** measures circulating vWF protein by immunoassay and is decreased in vWD caused by quantitative defects (type 1 and 3 vWD) as well as in most type 2A, 2B, and 2M patients.
- **vWF:RCo** measures vWF-mediated adhesion of control platelets in the presence of ristocetin. Both quantitative (types 1 and 3) and qualitative (types 2A, 2B, and 2M) forms will cause decreased vWF:RCo as both lead to decreased adhesion.
- The ratio of vWF:Ag to vWF:RCo can help discriminate between subtypes:
  - Suspect a quantitative vWF defect (type 1 and 3) with vWF:Ag/RCo ratio of ≥0.7.
  - Suspect type 2 (A, B, or M) vWD when vWF:Ag/RCo activity has a ratio of ≤0.7.
- vWF multimer analysis by gel electrophoresis assesses for the presence (2M) or absence (2A and 2B) of large vWF multimers to distinguish between type 2 forms.

Table 20-4	Hemostasis Test Patterns in von Willebrand Disease					
	Normal[a]	Type I	Type 2A	Type 2B	Type 2M	Type 2N	Type 3
aPTT		↑/nl	↑/nl	nl/↑	nl/↑	↑/nl	↑
vWF antigen (IU/dL)	50–200	<30*	↓/nl	↓/nl	↓/nl	50–200	Absent
vWF:RCo (IU/dL)	50–200	<30*	<30*	<30*	<30*	50–200	Absent
Factor VIII:C	50–200	↓/nl	↓/nl	↓/nl	↓/nl	↓↓	↓↓
Multimetric pattern	Normal	Normal	Missing large multimers	Missing large multimers	Normal	Normal	None detected
Inheritance		Dominant	Dominant	Dominant	Dominant	Recessive	Recessive

*Some patients with values of 30%–50% may have bleeding and histories consistent with vWD.
[a]Reference ranges vary between laboratories.
nl, normal; vWF, von Willebrand factor; vWF:RCo, von Willebrand factor ristocetin cofactor.

- **Factor VIII:** A quantitative deficiency of vWF (types 1 and 3) or vWF mutations that reduce FVIII binding to vWF (type 2N) may reduce factor VIII activity.
- Enzyme immunoassays measuring vWF binding affinity for factor VIII can confirm type 2N diagnosis.
- Consider genetic testing for types 2A, 2B, 2M, and 2N when phenotypic testing is difficult to interpret.

TREATMENT

Goal of therapy is to raise vWF:RCo and factor VIII activity to ensure adequate hemostasis. vWF:RCo activities >50% control most hemorrhages.

- **DDAVP** 0.3 μg/kg IV can be used to treat type 1 vWD. Administer test dose to confirm patient responds with expected vWF:RCo and FVIII increase before using to treat bleeding. For **minor invasive procedures**, infuse 1 hour before surgery, followed by q12–24h for 2 to 3 days postoperatively, with or without the oral antifibrinolytic drug aminocaproic acid or tanexamic acid.
  - DDAVP does not effectively treat most type 2A, 2M, and 2N vWD and all type 3 vWD patients.
  - Because of the risk of postinfusion thrombocytopenia, patients with type 2B vWD should not receive DDAVP.
- **vWF plasma-derived concentrate transfusions** (Alphanate, Humate-P, and Wilate) should aim to raise vWF:RCo activity to ~100% and maintain it between 50% and 100% until sufficient hemostasis occurs (typically 5 to 10 days). Cryoprecipitate is a second-line vWF source. Indications for concentrate transfusions:
  - type 1 vWD-DDAVP nonresponders
  - type 1 vWD-major bleeding or surgery
  - all other vWD types requiring hemostasis treatment

ACQUIRED COAGULATION DISORDERS

Vitamin K Deficiency

GENERAL PRINCIPLES

Vitamin K deficiency is usually caused by malabsorption states or poor dietary intake combined with antibiotic-associated loss of intestinal bacterial colonization. Hepatocytes require vitamin K to complete the synthesis (γ-carboxylation) of clotting factors (X, IX, VII, prothrombin) and the natural anticoagulant proteins C and S.

DIAGNOSIS

Vitamin K deficiency is suspected when an at-risk patient has a prolonged PT that corrects after a 1:1 mix with normal pooled plasma.

TREATMENT

- **Vitamin K replacement** (Table 20-5) should be given orally or intravenously. Vitamin K has variable absorption when administered subcutaneously, especially in edematous patients. Intravenous vitamin K carries the risk of anaphylactoid

Table 20-5	Treatment of Elevated International Normalized Ratio >5 (Besides Stopping All Antithrombotic Therapy)	
Bleeding	INR	Action
None	5–9	Evaluate for food and drug interactions and for dosing or laboratory errors Repeat INR in 1–4 d If INR rising or at high risk for bleeding, give vitamin K 1.0–2.5 mg PO
	9	Evaluate for food and drug interactions and for dosing or laboratory errors Repeat INR in 12–24 hr and in 48 hr Vitamin K 2–10 mg PO; repeat vitamin K as needed
Minor	Any	Vitamin K 1–5 mg PO or IVPB INR q8–24h; repeat vitamin K as needed If bleeding not controlled in 24 hr, treat as major bleeding
Major	Any	Vitamin K 10 mg IV over 10–20 min FFP (2–3 U), prothrombin complex concentrate (25–50 U/kg) Repeat INR in 6–12 hr and continue vitamin K and FFP until INR remains normal AND bleeding has stopped Surgical intervention for hemostasis

FFP, fresh frozen plasma; INR, international normalized ratio; IVPB, intravenous piggyback; PO, by mouth.

reactions. With adequate replacement therapy, the PT should begin to normalize within 12 hours and should normalize completely in 24 to 48 hours (*Ann Intern Med 2002;137:251*), but repeated administration may be necessary.

- **FFP** rapidly but temporarily (4 to 6 hours) corrects acquired coagulopathies secondary to vitamin K deficiency. Patients with coagulopathy and actively bleeding or who require immediate invasive procedures should receive FFP or a PCC to replace factors X, IX, II, and VII (some brands have minimal FVII).
  - The usual starting dose of FFP is 2 to 3 U (400 to 600 mL), with measurement of the PT and aPTT after the infusion to determine the need for additional therapy. Up to 10 to 15 mL/kg may be required for severe bleeding with significant PT prolongation.
  - Because factor VII has a half-life of only 6 hours, the PT may again become prolonged and require additional FFP, until adequate production of coagulation factors occurs.
  - Vitamin K replacement should be initiated concomitantly with FFP.

Liver Disease

GENERAL PRINCIPLES

Liver disease can impair hemostasis because the liver produces coagulation factors, with the exception of vWF. Coagulopathy is typically mild with stable liver disease until patients decompensate. Other hemostatic complications include thrombocytopenia due to splenic sequestration, DIC, hyperfibrinolysis, and cholestasis (which impairs vitamin K absorption). While PT and aPTT prolongations imply an increased risk of bleeding, they do not reflect concurrent reductions in protein C and protein S, producing a fragile rebalancing of procoagulant and anticoagulant activities, which can be disrupted by infection, renal insufficiency, and vasomotor dysfunction (*Blood 2010;116:878*).

TREATMENT

- **Vitamin K** replacement may shorten a prolonged PT due to a vitamin K antagonist, dietary deficiency, or cholestasis.
- **FFP** may be indicated for patients who are bleeding or require an invasive procedure and have abnormal coagulation parameters but may cause volume overload. A common threshold is PT >1.5 control despite limited supportive evidence.
- **Cryoprecipitate**, 1.5 U/10 kg body weight, corrects severe hypofibrinogenemia (<100 mg/dL)
- **PCC**, but safety and efficacy are unproven.
- Randomized controlled trials failed to show a hemostasis benefit for **recombinant factor VIIa** in GI bleeding (*Hepatology 2008;47:1604*)
- Reserve **platelet transfusions** for active bleeding or prior to invasive procedures, such as liver biopsy, in patients with thrombocytopenia (<50 × 10^9/L).

Disseminated Intravascular Coagulation

GENERAL PRINCIPLES

Etiology

DIC occurs in a variety of systemic illnesses that include sepsis, trauma, burns, shock, obstetric complications, and malignancies (notably, acute promyelocytic leukemia).

Pathophysiology

Exposure of tissue factor to the circulation generates excess thrombin, leading to platelet activation, consumption of coagulation factors (including fibrinogen) and regulators (antithrombin [AT] and proteins C and S), fibrin generation, generalized microthrombi, and reactive fibrinolysis.

DIAGNOSIS

Clinical Presentation

Consequences of **DIC** include bleeding, organ dysfunction secondary to microvascular thrombi and ischemia, and less often, large arterial and venous thrombosis (*Br J Haematol 2009;145:24*).

Diagnostic Testing

No one test confirms diagnosis of DIC. The International Society for Thrombosis and Hemostasis devised a clinical scoring system for objective detection of DIC (Table 20-6). Serial "DIC panels" help assess clinical management and prognosis.

Table 20-6	International Society for Thrombosis and Haemostasis Disseminated Intravascular Coagulation Scoring System[a]

Use only in patients with an underlying condition known to be associated with DIC

	0 Point	1 Point	2 Points
Thrombocytopenia	>100,000 k/cumm	≤100,000 k/cumm	≤50,000 k/cumm
D-Dimer	Normal	<10 × upper limit of normal	≥10 × upper limit of normal
PT Prolongation	<3 sec	3–6 sec	>6 sec
Fibrinogen	>100 mg/dL	≤100 mg/dL	

Sum the points for each of the four categories to determine the clinical probability: Compatible with overt DIC ≥5 points, and suggestive of nonovert DIC <5 points.
[a]Data from *Thromb Haemost 2001;86:132* and *Crit Care Med 2004;32:24167.*
DIC, disseminated intravascular coagulation.

TREATMENT

DIC treatment consists of supportive care and correction of the underlying disorder if possible. Administer **FFP**, **cryoprecipitate**, and **platelets** to manage bleeding but not based strictly on laboratory parameters. Administer adjusted-dose IV **heparin** to patients with large-vessel venous and arterial thromboses. Nonbleeding patients that have DIC should receive thromboprophylactic dose of with heparin.

Acquired Inhibitors of Coagulation Factors

GENERAL PRINCIPLES

Acquired inhibitors of coagulation factors may occur de novo (autoantibodies) or may develop in hemophiliacs (alloantibodies) following FVIII or IX infusions. The most common acquired inhibitor is directed against factor VIII. De novo cases often arise in patients with underlying lymphoproliferative or autoimmune disorders.

DIAGNOSIS

Patients with factor VIII inhibitors present with an abrupt onset of bleeding, prolonged aPTT that does not correct after 1:1 mixing with normal plasma, markedly decreased FVIII activity, and a normal PT. Very rarely patients develop autoantibodies inhibiting other factors (II, V, X), which can prolong aPTT and PT and do not correct after mixing studies.

TREATMENT

Bleeding complications in patients with factor VIII inhibitors (autoantibodies) are managed in the same manner as for hemophiliacs with alloantibodies to factor VIII (see Inherited Bleeding Disorders section). Long-term therapy consists of immuno-suppression with prednisone ± cyclophosphamide to reduce production of the auto-antibody (*Blood 2002;100:3426*). The role of rituximab in management is controversial (*J Thromb Haemost 2011;9:226*).

VENOUS THROMBOEMBOLIC DISORDERS

Approach to Venous Thromboembolism

GENERAL PRINCIPLES

Definition

- **Thromboses** or blood clots occur in veins, arteries, or chambers of the heart.
- **VTE** refers to the presence of **deep vein thrombosis (DVT)** or **pulmonary embolism (PE)**.
- **Thrombophlebitis** consists of inflammation in a vein due to a blood clot.
- **Superficial thrombophlebitis** may occur in any superficial vein.
- An **APA syndrome** diagnosis requires the presence of at least one clinical and one laboratory criterion (*J Thromb Haemost 2006;4:295*).
  - **Clinical criteria** consist of (a) the occurrence of unprovoked arterial or venous thrombosis in any tissue or organ or (b) pregnancy morbidities (unexplained late fetal death; premature birth complicated by eclampsia, preeclampsia, or placental insufficiency; at least three unexplained consecutive spontaneous abortions).
  - **Laboratory criteria** consist of persistent (two positive tests, at least 12 weeks apart) detection of autoantibodies (LA, anticardiolipin antibody, and β_2-glycoprotein-1 antibodies) that react with negatively charged phospholipids.
  - The APA syndrome may include other features, such as thrombocytopenia, valvular heart disease, livedo reticularis, neurologic manifestations, and nephropathy.

Classification

The anatomic location of DVT/PE, clot burden, and sequelae may affect prognosis and treatment recommendations.

- Thromboses can be classified as **deep** or **superficial** and as **proximal** or **distal**.
  - Avoid using the term **superficial femoral vein** because it really refers to part of the **femoral vein (a deep vein)**.
  - **Proximal** lower extremity DVTs occur in or superior to the popliteal vein (or the confluence of tibial and peroneal veins), whereas **distal** DVTs occur more inferiorly.
- Location in the pulmonary arterial system characterizes **PEs** as **central/proximal** (main pulmonary artery, lobar, or segmental) or **distal** (subsegmental).

Epidemiology

- Symptomatic DVTs most commonly develop in the lower limbs.
- Untreated calf vein DVTs may propagate proximally.
- Without treatment, half of patients with proximal lower extremity DVT develop PE.
- DVTs in the proximal lower extremities and pelvis produce most PEs.
- DVTs that occur in upper extremities, often secondary to an indwelling catheter, may also cause PE.
- DVT may occur concomitantly with superficial thrombophlebitis.

Etiology

- Venous thromboemboli arise under conditions of **blood stasis**, **hypercoagulability** (changes in the soluble and formed elements of the blood), or venous **endothelial dysfunction/injury**.
- Hypercoagulable states may have an inherited or acquired etiology (see Risk Factors section).
- **Superficial thrombophlebitis** occurs in association with varicose veins, trauma, infection, and hypercoagulable disorders.
- Other causes of pulmonary arterial occlusion include in situ thrombi (e.g., sickle cell disease), marrow fat embolism, amniotic fluid embolism, pulmonary artery sarcoma, and fibrosing mediastinitis.

Risk Factors

- A method of classifying VTE risk factors uses the categories of inherited, acquired, or unknown (idiopathic).
- **Inherited thrombophilic disorders** are suggested by a history of spontaneous VTE at a young age (<50 years), recurrent VTE, VTE in first-degree relatives, thrombosis in unusual anatomic locations, and recurrent fetal loss.
- The most common inherited risk factors for VTE include two gene polymorphisms (**factor V Leiden and prothrombin gene G20210A**), deficiencies of the natural anticoagulants **protein C, protein S,** and **antithrombin, dysfibrinogenemia,** and **hyperhomocysteinemia**.
- **Homocystinuria**, a rare autosomal recessive disorder caused by deficiency of cysta-thionine-β-synthase, leads to extremely high plasma homocysteine, and has an association with arterial and venous thromboembolic events that begin in childhood. More commonly, milder homocysteine elevations arise from an interaction between genetic mutations that affect enzymes involved in homocysteine metabolism and acquired factors such as inadequate folate consumption (*N Engl J Med 2001; 344:1222*).
- Spontaneous venous thromboses that occur in unusual locations, such as cavernous sinus mesenteric vein, or portal vein, may be the initial presentation of paroxysmal nocturnal hemoglobinuria (**PNH**) or myeloproliferative disorders.
- **Spontaneous (idiopathic) thrombosis**, despite the absence of an inherited throm-bophilia and detectable autoantibodies, predisposes patients to future thromboses (*N Engl J Med 2001;344:1222*).
- **Acquired hypercoagulable** states may arise secondary to malignancy, immobiliza-tion, infection, trauma, surgery, collagen vascular diseases, nephrotic syndrome, HIT, DIC, medications (e.g., estrogen), and pregnancy.
- Acquired **autoantibodies** associated with HIT and the APA syndrome can cause arterial or venous thrombi (see APA syndrome discussion under Approach to Venous Thromboembolism section; Heparin-Induced Thrombocytopenia section).
- At least 10% of patients with SLE have evidence of LAs; however, most patients with LAs do not have SLE.

Prevention

Identifying patients at high risk and instituting prophylactic measures remains the ideal strategy for dealing with the problem of VTE (see Chapter 1, Patient Care in Internal Medicine).

DIAGNOSIS

Clinical Presentation

- **DVT** may produce pain and edema in an affected extremity, but DVT has neither sensitive nor specific symptoms and signs. Pretest assessment of the probability of a DVT provides useful information when combined with the results of compression US or a D-dimer test, or both, in determining whether to exclude or accept the diagnosis of DVT or perform additional imaging studies (*Lancet 1997; 350:1795*).
- **Superficial thrombophlebitis** presents as a tender, warm, erythematous, and often palpable thrombosed vein. Accompanying DVT may produce additional symptoms and signs.
- **PE** may produce shortness of breath, chest pain (pleuritic), hypoxemia, hemoptysis, pleural rub, new right-sided heart failure, and tachycardia, but these signs and symptoms are neither sensitive nor specific (*Ann Intern Med 1998;129:997*).
  Validated clinical risk factors for a PE in outpatients who present to an emergency department include signs and symptoms of DVT, high suspicion of PE by the clinician, tachycardia, immobility in the past 4 weeks, history of VTE, active cancer, and hemoptysis (*Ann Intern Med 2001;135:98*).
- Clinical **suspicion of DVT or PE should lead to objective testing**.

Differential Diagnosis

- The differential diagnosis for **unilateral lower extremity** symptoms and signs of **DVT**, such as swelling and pain, includes cellulitis, Baker cyst, hematoma, venous insufficiency, postphlebitic syndrome, lymphedema, sarcoma, arterial aneurysm, myositis, rupture of the medial head of the gastrocnemius, and abscess.
  - **Symmetric, bilateral lower extremity edema** suggests the presence of heart, renal, or liver failure much more commonly than a DVT.
  - Additional diseases to consider in association with **lower extremity pain** include musculoskeletal and arteriovascular disorders.
- The **differential diagnosis** of symptoms and signs of **PE** includes dissecting aortic aneurysm, pneumonia, acute bronchitis, pericardial or pleural disease, heart failure, costochondritis, and myocardial ischemia.

Diagnostic Testing

Laboratories

- **D-dimer** and cross-linked fibrin degradation products may increase during VTE but are nonspecific.
  - D-dimer testing for VTE has a low positive predictive value (PPV) and specificity; **patients with a positive test require further evaluation**.
  - D-dimer assays differ in sensitivity and units of measure. Some, but not all, quantitative D-dimer tests are FDA cleared to exclude VTE in patients with low-to-moderate pretest probability scores.
  - The NPV of a sensitive quantitative D-dimer assay is high enough to exclude a **DVT** when the objectively defined clinical probability is low and/or a noninvasive test is negative (*Ann Intern Med 2004;140:589; JAMA 2006;295:199*).
  - A negative D-dimer in combination with low pretest probability can exclude almost all **PEs** (*Ann Intern Med 1998;129:1006*).
  - In the setting of a moderate-to-high clinical pretest probability (e.g., patients with cancer), a negative D-dimer does not have sufficient NPV for excluding

the presence of DVT or PE (*Ann Intern Med 1999;131:417*; *Arch Intern Med 2001;161:567*).

• Guidelines suggest that most patients with idiopathic VTE do not need to undergo **hypercoagulability testing**, although it might make sense to test some individuals that have a high likelihood of having an **inherited thrombophilic disorder**.

• Signs and symptoms of the APA syndrome should lead to laboratory evaluation.
  ○ Serologic tests (IgG and IgM β_2-glycoprotein-1 antibodies, and IgG and IgM cardiolipin antibodies) or clotting assays (LA) detect APAs.
  ○ Performing both serologic and clotting assays improves sensitivity.
  ○ LAs may prolong the aPTT or PT/INR, though they do not predispose to bleeding.

• To assess for **PNH** in the setting of unusual spontaneous venous thromboses, perform flow cytometry to detect missing antigens on red cells and leukocytes.

Imaging
• **DVT-specific testing**
  ○ Initial diagnostic imaging for suspected acute DVT typically consists of **compression ultrasound** (called *duplex examination* when performed with Doppler testing) (*Am J Respir Crit Care Med 1999;160:1043*).
    ▪ In addition to assessing for DVT, compression US, magnetic resonance (MR) venography, and computed tomography (CT) venography may detect other pathology (see Differential Diagnosis section).
    ▪ Compression US has a high sensitivity in **symptomatic** patients, but it has a low sensitivity in **asymptomatic** patients.
    ▪ Compression US has low sensitivity for detecting **calf** DVT and may fail to visualize parts of the deep femoral vein, parts of the upper extremity venous system, and the pelvic veins.
    ▪ Compression US may have difficulty distinguishing between acute and **chronic** DVT.
    ▪ **Lower extremity venous compression ultrasonography** provides useful information in a patient with a suspected PE who has a nondiagnostic ventilation/ perfusion (V/Q) scan and in a patient with a nondiagnostic or negative chest CT scan with high suspicion of disease, because proximal DVT can serve as a surrogate for PE; ultrasonography also serves as a useful surrogate for PE, if positive, in patients who have contraindications to or difficulty completing imaging for PE (see PE-specific testing).
    ▪ **Serial testing** can improve the diagnostic yield. If a patient with a clinically suspected lower extremity DVT has a negative initial noninvasive test result and no satisfactory alternative explanation, one can withhold anticoagulant therapy and repeat testing at least once 3 to 14 days later.
  ○ **Simplified compression US** limited only to the common femoral vein in the groin and the popliteal vein (down to the trifurcation of the calf veins) has reasonable but lower sensitivity than a **complete** proximal lower extremity venous examination. Repeating simplified noninvasive tests within 10 days improves sensitivity.

• **PE-specific testing**
  ○ **Nondefinitive tests** such as electrocardiography (e.g., right-sided strain pattern, with characteristic S wave in lead I, and Q wave in lead III, and T wave inversion in lead III), troponin and brain natriuretic peptide (BNP) levels, blood gases, and chest radiography may help determine the pretest probability, focus the

differential diagnosis, assess the cardiopulmonary reserve, and assist with prognostication, but they do not rule in or rule out PE with acceptable certainty.

Unless an objectively low clinical probability of PE combined with a negative D-dimer test occurs, the suspicion of PE usually requires further evaluation with an imaging test.

○ **Contrast-enhanced spiral (helical) chest CT**
  ▪ PE protocol chest CT requires IV administration of iodinated contrast and exposure to radiation.
  ▪ Contraindications to spiral CT include renal dysfunction and dye allergy.
  ▪ **Multidetector CT** has better sensitivity than single-detector CT for evaluating patients with suspected PE.
  ▪ Used according to standardized protocols in conjunction with expert interpretation, spiral CT has good accuracy for detection of large (proximal) PEs, but it has lower sensitivity for detecting small (distal) emboli (*N Engl J Med 2006;354:2317*).
  ▪ The sensitivity of CT for VTE improves by combining the CT pulmonary angiography (PA) results with objective grading of clinical suspicion.
  ▪ Lower extremity compression US may provide additional useful information, although negative D-dimer and multidetector chest CT tests exclude most PE (*Lancet 2008;371:1343*).
  ▪ **Clinical suspicion discordant with the objective test finding** (e.g., high suspicion with a negative CT scan, or low suspicion with a positive CT scan) **should lead to further testing**.
  ▪ Advantages of CT scan over V/Q scan include more diagnostic results (positive or negative), with fewer indeterminate or inadequate studies, and the detection of alternative or concomitant diagnoses, such as dissecting aortic aneurysm, pneumonia, and malignancy.
○ **V/Q scanning**
  ▪ V/Q scanning requires administration of radioactive material (via both inhaled and IV routes).
  ▪ V/Q scans may be classified as normal, nondiagnostic (i.e., very low probability, low probability, intermediate probability), or high probability for PE.
  ▪ V/Q scanning remains most useful in a patient with a normal chest radiograph, because nondiagnostic V/Q scans commonly occur in the setting of an abnormal chest radiograph.
  ▪ Use of clinical suspicion improves the accuracy of V/Q scanning. In patients with normal or high-probability V/Q scans and matching pretest clinical suspicion, the testing has a PPV of 96% (*JAMA 1990;263:2753*).
○ **Pulmonary angiography**
  ▪ Angiography requires placement of a pulmonary artery catheter, infusion of IV contrast, and exposure to radiation.
  ▪ Similar to venography and PE-protocol CT scanning, contraindications to angiography include renal dysfunction and dye allergy.
  ▪ Less invasive tests (i.e., CT angiography) have mostly replaced PA over the past decade.
○ **Echocardiography** to assess cardiopulmonary reserve and evidence of end-organ damage (right ventricular dysfunction) in patients with PE has a role in decision making regarding the use of thrombolytic therapy (see thrombolytic therapy under Approach to Venous Thromboembolism section).

○ **The search for an associated occult malignancy** in patients with VTE should include a thorough history and physical, routine blood work, standard screening tests done according to recommended schedules (e.g., colonoscopy, mammography, pap smear), and specific cancer screening tests indicated for distinct populations (e.g., chest CT to search for lung cancer in smokers of advanced age).

TREATMENT

- **VTE therapy** should aim to prevent recurrent VTE, consequences of VTE (i.e., postphlebitic syndrome [i.e., pain, edema, and ulceration], pulmonary arterial hypertension, and death), and complications of therapy (e.g., bleeding and HIT).
- Clinicians should perform standard laboratory tests (i.e., CBC, PT/INR, and aPTT) and assess bleeding risk before starting anticoagulants.
- Unless contraindications exist, **initial treatment of VTE should consist of anticoagulation**, either with IV or SC UFH, SC LMWH, SC pentasaccharide (fondaparinux) or a new oral anticoagulant (see next section).

Medications
- **Anticoagulants, oral**
  - **Warfarin, an oral anticoagulant**, inhibits reduction of vitamin K to its active form and leads to depletion of the vitamin K–dependent clotting factors II, VII, IX, and X and proteins C, S, and Z (Figure 20-1).
    - Though warfarin has good oral absorption, it requires 4 to 5 days to achieve the full anticoagulant effect.
    - The initial INR rise primarily reflects warfarin-related depletion of factor VII; the depletion of factor II takes several days due to its relatively long half-life.
    - Because of the rapid depletion of the anticoagulant protein C and a slower onset of anticoagulant effect, patients might develop increased hypercoagulability during the first few days of warfarin therapy if warfarin is not combined with a parenteral anticoagulant (*Thromb Haemost 1997;78:785*).
    - The **starting dose** of warfarin depends on many factors (see *www.WarfarinDosing.org*). The starting dose ranges from ~3 mg in older, or petite patients to 10 mg in young, robust outpatients). Patients with polymorphisms in genes for cytochrome P-450 2C9 (CYP2C9) or vitamin K epoxide reductase (VKORC1) may benefit from cautious warfarin initiation. The INR is used to adjust dosing.
    - **Treatment of DVT/PE with warfarin requires overlap therapy with a parenteral anticoagulant** (UFH, LMWH, or pentasaccharide) for at least 4 to 5 days and until the INR reaches at least 2.0.
      □ For most indications, warfarin has a **target INR** of 2.5 and a therapeutic range of 2 to 3.
      □ Patients with most **mechanical heart valves** require a higher level of anticoagulation (INR target range, 2.5 to 3.5).
    - **INR monitoring should occur frequently during the first month of therapy (e.g., twice weekly for 1 to 2 weeks, then weekly for 2 weeks, then less frequently).**
      □ Patients receiving a stable warfarin dose should have INR monitoring performed monthly, although patients with labile INRs should have more frequent monitoring (e.g., weekly). Typical dose adjustments after the first few weeks of therapy change the weekly dose by 10% to 25%.

▫ The addition or discontinuation of medications, especially amiodarone, certain antibiotics (e.g., rifampin, sulfamethoxazole), or antifungal drugs should trigger more frequent INR monitoring and may require dose adjustments >25%.

▫ In eligible patients, home monitoring can improve INR control, quality of life, and satisfaction with warfarin therapy (*N Engl J Med 2010;363:1608*).

▫ Compliant patients who have unacceptable INR lability, or those with LA and difficulty monitoring due to an elevated baseline INR, may benefit from long-term anticoagulation with an agent other than warfarin.

○ **Oral direct Xa Inhibitors**

▪ As compared to warfarin, the oral Xa inhibitors **rivaroxaban** and **apixaban** have a more rapid onset, shorter half-life, wider therapeutic window, and more predictable pharmacokinetics. These features allow for sole oral therapy without the need for an overlapping parenteral agent, no need for titration or dose adjustments in most patients with normal renal function, and no need for routine monitoring.

▪ Issues of concern regarding oral Xa inhibitors include the inability to accurately monitor the degree of anticoagulation, the limited ability to reverse these agents, risk of thrombosis due to missed doses, and dose reduction in the setting of renal dysfunction.

▪ Several countries, excluding the United States, have approved rivaroxaban (15 mg bid × 3 weeks, then 20 mg qd) for DVT treatment. Presently, rivaroxaban is approved by the FDA for atrial fibrillation stroke prophylaxis and for VTE prophylaxis in orthopedic surgery patients. Apixaban has not been approved for VTE treatment, and a major trial is evaluating efficacy for this indication. Apixaban has been approved outside the United States for VTE prophylaxis in orthopedic surgery patients.

○ **Oral direct thrombin inhibitors**

▪ Compared with warfarin, **dabigatran** has a more rapid onset, shorter half-life, wider therapeutic window, and more predictable pharmacokinetics. Also as compared with warfarin, dabigatran has a lower risk of intracranial (but not gastrointestinal) hemorrhage but a higher risk of myocardial infarction.

▪ Dabigatran is not approved for VTE treatment in the United States, although it is approved in many countries for other indications.

• **Anticoagulants, parenteral**

○ **UFH** comes from porcine intestinal mucosa, and it indirectly inactivates thrombin and factor Xa via AT.

▪ At usual doses, UFH prolongs the TT and aPTT, and it has minimal effect on the PT/INR.

▪ Because the anticoagulant effects of UFH normalize within hours of discontinuation and **protamine sulfate** reverses it even faster, UFH is the anticoagulant of choice during initial therapy for patients with increased risk of bleeding.

▪ Abnormal renal function does not typically affect UFH dosing.

▪ For **DVT prophylaxis**, the typical dosage is 5,000 U SC q8–12h, and aPTT monitoring is not necessary.

▪ For **therapeutic anticoagulation**, UFH is usually administered IV with a bolus followed by continuous infusion (Table 20-7).

▫ **Nomogram**-driven weight-based dosing provides a more rapid and reliable prolongation of the aPTT into the therapeutic range than nonnomogram dosing (see Table 20-7).

Table 20-7	Weight-Based Heparin Dosing for Venous Thromboembolism[a]

Initial Therapy[a]

Bolus[b]	80 U/kg
Infusion[b]	18 U/kg/hr

Adjustments[c]

aPTT <40	80 U/kg bolus; increase infusion by 3 U/kg/hr
aPTT 40–50	40 U/kg bolus; increase infusion by 2 U/kg/hr
aPTT 51–59	Increase infusion by 1 U/kg/hr
aPTT 60–94	No change
aPTT 95–104	Decrease infusion by 1 U/kg/hr
aPTT 105–114	Hold for 0.5 hr; decrease infusion by 2 U/kg/hr
aPTT >115	Hold for 1 hr; decrease infusion by 3 U/kg/hr

Note: Target aPTT can vary among hospitals depending on reagents and instruments used.
[a]For patients with ST-segment elevation myocardial infarction, typical bolus dose is 60 U/kg (maximum 5,000 U) and typical initial infusion dose is 12 U/kg/hr (maximum 1,000 U/hr).
[b]Round all doses to nearest 100 U.
[c]Draw aPTT 6 hours after any bolus or change in infusion rate.
aPTT, activated partial thromboplastin time.
Data from *Ann Intern Med* 1993;119:874.

- □ Bleeding risks lead to use of different-intensity nomograms for different types of patients; patients with VTE often receive larger boluses and higher initial drip rates than patients with unstable angina who also receive antiplatelet therapy.
  - □ **UFH may be administered subcutaneously:** Initial dose of 333 U/kg SC, followed by a fixed dose of 250 U/kg every 12 hours (*JAMA 2006;296:935*), or an aPTT-monitored and dose-adjusted approach.
- ○ **LMWHs** are produced by chemical or enzymatic cleavage of UFH, and they indirectly inactivate thrombin and factor Xa via AT.
  - ▪ Since LMWH inactivates factor Xa to a greater extent than it does thrombin (IIa), LMWH minimally prolongs the aPTT.
  - ▪ Extensive clinical trials have confirmed the efficacy and safety of weight-based SC LMWH for the treatment of VTE.
  - ▪ Factor Xa monitoring is not recommended, except in special circumstances: renal dysfunction, morbid obesity, or pregnancy.
  - ▪ For therapeutic anticoagulation, peak factor Xa levels, measured 4 hours after an SC dose, should be 0.6 to 1.0 IU/mL for q12h dosing and 1 to 2 IU/mL for q24h dosing (*Blood 2002;99:3102*).
  - ▪ Different LMWH preparations have different dosing recommendations (Table 20-8).
  - ▪ Given the renal clearance of LMWHs, they are generally contraindicated in patients with creatinine clearance (CrCl) <10 mL/min, and patients with a CrCl <30 mL/min require dose adjustments (e.g., enoxaparin 1 mg/kg once daily instead of twice daily). Dose adjustments may also be required in patients with cachexia or obesity, or in women who are pregnant.

- Though initial SC LMWH overlap therapy with PO warfarin is typically converted to sole PO warfarin long-term therapy, patients with cancer may have reduced recurrent VTE when treated long term solely with LMWH (*N Engl J Med 2003;349:146*) at a slightly reduced dose.
- Because the anticoagulant effects of LMWHs do not normalize within hours of discontinuation and **protamine sulfate** does not fully reverse the anticoagulant effects, UFH is the anticoagulant of choice during initial therapy for patients with increased risk of bleeding.
- **Because of the SC dosing route, LMWH** facilitates outpatient VTE therapy.
- Patients selected for outpatient DVT therapy should have no other indications for hospitalization (i.e., complications of VTE or concomitant disease), low risk for VTE recurrence and bleeding, adequate cardiopulmonary reserve, adequate instruction and understanding of the warning signs of bleeding and VTE recurrence, access to a telephone and transportation, ability to inject the drug or a responsible caretaker, and adequate outpatient follow-up with a health care provider who can manage frequent lab testing, complications, etc. (*Chest 1999;115:972*).
- **Long-term anticoagulation with SC LMWH** is the first choice in **pregnant** women (without artificial heart valves) with thrombosis, and it is an alternative for patients with **cancer** and patients who have clearly **failed warfarin** (objectively confirmed new DVT/PE despite consistently therapeutic INRs) (*N Engl J Med 2003;349:146*).
- **Fondaparinux**, a synthetic pentasaccharide that is structurally similar to the region of the heparin molecule that binds AT, functions as a selective indirect inhibitor of factor Xa.
  - Because fondaparinux inhibits factor Xa and does not inhibit thrombin, it does not significantly prolong the aPTT.
  - Large clinical trials have confirmed the efficacy and safety of weight-based subcutaneously dosed fondaparinux for the treatment of VTE (*Ann Intern Med 2004;140:867; N Engl J Med 2003;349:1695*).
  - Similar to the LMWHs, factor Xa monitoring is not normally recommended but may be necessary for patients with renal dysfunction, obesity, and cachexia.
  - Fondaparinux may be used for outpatient VTE therapy.
  - The recommended dose for VTE therapy consists of 5.0, 7.5, or 10.0 mg SC daily, and the dose used depends on weight (see Table 20-8).
- **Argatroban** is a synthetic DTI that is used for **HIT** therapy.
  - Argatroban has a half-life of <1 hour, and a reversal agent is not available.
  - Argatroban treatment of HIT uses an IV infusion (without a bolus) rate of ≤2 μg/kg/min. For patients recovering from cardiac surgery and those with heart failure, multiple organ failure, or severe anasarca, guidelines recommend a lower initial infusion rate between 0.5 and 1.2 μg/kg/min (*Chest 2012; 141:e495S*).
  - aPTT monitoring should occur 2 hours after beginning the infusion, and the infusion rate should undergo adjustment (rate not to exceed 10 μg/kg/min) to achieve a steady-state therapeutic aPTT (1.5 to 3.0 times the patient's baseline aPTT, not to exceed 100 seconds).
  - Because of its hepatic clearance, argatroban **requires dose adjustment** (e.g., use an IV infusion rate of 0.5 to 1.0 μg/kg/min) **in patients with hepatic dysfunction**.

Table 20-8	Low–Molecular-Weight Heparin and Pentasaccharide Dosages for Treatment of Venous Thromboembolism

Drug	Dosage
Enoxaparin	Outpatient: 1 mg/kg SC q12h Inpatient: 1 mg/kg SC q12h *or* 1.5 mg/kg SC q24h
Tinzaparin	175 IU/kg SC daily[a]
Dalteparin	200 IU/kg SC daily[b]
Fondaparinux	5.0 mg SC daily for weight <50 kg, 7.5 mg SC daily for weight 50–100 kg, and 10.0 mg SC daily for weight >100 kg

Caution with use of fondaparinux, tinzaparin, dalteparin, or enoxaparin for pregnancy, morbid obesity, or severe renal dysfunction (CrCl <30 mL/min); anti-Xa level monitoring is recommended in these settings.

[a]U.S. Food and Drug Administration (FDA) approved for treatment of pulmonary embolism without deep vein thrombosis.

[b]Not an FDA-approved indication. 200 IU/kg SC daily for month 1, followed by 150 IU/kg SC daily during months 2 to 6 for patients with cancer undergoing prolonged low–molecular-weight heparin therapy.

IU, anti-Xa units; for enoxaparin, 1 mg = 100 anti-Xa units.

- During warfarin coadministration, argatroban should be discontinued when the INR becomes >4, and the INR should undergo repeat measurement within 4 to 6 hours (see Figure 20-1).
  - For monitoring the INR of those that just stopped receiving an argatroban at a dose of ≤2 μg/kg/min, a subtherapeutic INR (<2) should lead to the resumption of argatroban. The warfarin dose should undergo daily measurement and adjustment until a therapeutic INR (e.g., 2 to 3) occurs. Discontinue argatroban after 5 days of overlap therapy with warfarin and when a therapeutic INR is achieved for warfarin.
  - For monitoring an argatroban dose >2 μg/kg/min, reduce the argatroban infusion to 2 μg/kg/min for 4 to 6 hours before assessing the INR as described earlier (*Chest 2008;133(6 suppl):340S*).
- **Bivalirudin (Angiomax)**, a DTI, has an indication for treatment of **HIT** in the setting of percutaneous coronary intervention in patients receiving ASA.
  - Bivalirudin has a half-life of 25 minutes in patients with normal renal function.
  - Because of its renal clearance, bivalirudin requires dose adjustment of the infusion rate (but not the bolus dose) in patients with renal insufficiency.
  - Bivalirudin dosing for HIT uses a bolus of 0.75 mg/kg and then a continuous IV infusion rate of 1.75 mg/kg/hr; for a CrCl of <30 mL/min, reduce the infusion rate to 1 mg/kg/hr, and for those on dialysis, reduce the rate to 0.25 mg/kg/hr.
  - aPTT monitoring during bivalirudin therapy should occur 2 hours after a dose change, and the dose should undergo adjustment to obtain a target range of 1.5 to 2.5 times the patient's baseline or the mean of the laboratory normal aPTT. A lower target aPTT range (1.5 to 2.0 times baseline) may have similar efficacy and less bleeding risk.

- The interpretation of the INRs in patients receiving warfarin must take into account the increased PT/INR caused by bivalirudin.
- **Thrombolytic therapy**
  - **Thrombolytic therapy** (e.g., alteplase or recombinant tissue plasminogen activator as a 100 mg IV infusion over 2 hours) is appropriate for rare patients with VTE (*Chest 2012;141:e419S*).
  - The indications for thrombolytic therapy of **PE** consist of refractory systemic hypotension due to acute PE in patients that do not have a high risk of bleeding.
  - Thrombolytic therapy is uncommonly used for **DVT**. The main indication is DVT leading to venous congestion that compromises the arterial supply to the limb, which is most often seen with massive iliofemoral DVT.
- **Duration of anticoagulation for DVT or PE**
  - **Duration of anticoagulation** decisions require individualization based on patient preferences and assessment of the patient's added risk of recurrent VTE off anticoagulant therapy versus the added risk of bleeding complications from continued anticoagulation (*Chest 2012;141:e419S*).
  - Patients with a **first episode of VTE due to reversible risk factors** (surgery, major trauma) have a low risk of recurrence (<6%/yr), and anticoagulation is recommended for 3 months (*Chest 2012;141:e419S*).
  - Guidelines recommend 3 months of anticoagulant therapy for patients with a **first episode of idiopathic VTE** associated with less compelling and transient risk factors, such as prolonged travel, oral contraceptive pills/hormone replacement therapy, or minor injury (*Chest 2012;141:e419S*).
  - For patients with unprovoked proximal lower extremity DVT, consider anticoagulation longer than 3 months in willing patients with no major risk factors for bleeding and good anticoagulant control.
  - For patients with **unprovoked PE** with no major risk factors for bleeding and good anticoagulant control, we recommend at least 6 months of anticoagulant therapy.
  - Patients with **cancer and VTE** should undergo anticoagulation until cancer resolution or development of a contraindication. In patients with cancer and DVT, VTE recurrence rates are lower with LMWH (e.g., dalteparin 200 IU/kg once daily for 1 month, followed by 150 IU/kg for 5 months) than with standard warfarin therapy (INR of 2 to 3) (*N Engl J Med 2003;349:146*).
  - For patients with a **first VTE and one inherited hypercoagulable risk factor**, consider an extended anticoagulation duration, depending on the type of thrombophilia.
    - Heterozygous factor V Leiden or heterozygous prothrombin 20210A modestly increases the odds of recurrence (relative risk [RR] 1.6 and 1.4, respectively). Deficiency of protein S, protein C, or AT carries a greater risk of recurrence than that of heterozygous factor V Leiden or heterozygous prothrombin 20210A, although these deficiencies less commonly occur (*JAMA 2009;301:2472*).
    - Patients with a **first VTE and APAs or two inherited risk factors** should receive extended-duration anticoagulation (e.g., 12 months) and indefinite therapy should be considered.
  - Patients with **recurrent idiopathic VTE** should receive extended-duration anticoagulation, unless a contraindication develops, or patient preferences or bleeding risk dictate otherwise.
  - Patients with a history of VTE, especially those with ongoing risk factors, should possibly receive temporary prophylactic anticoagulation (e.g., low-dose LMWH

SQ) during **periods of increased VTE risk**, including surgery, trauma, immobilization, prolonged air travel, hospitalization for medical illnesses, and postpartum.

Other Nonpharmacologic Therapies

- **Leg elevation** is useful for the treatment of edema associated with DVT.
- **Ambulation** is encouraged for patients with DVT, especially after improvement of pain and edema, although strenuous lower extremity activity should initially be avoided.
- **Fitted graduated compression stockings** reduce the high incidence of postphlebitic syndrome in patients with lower extremity DVT.
- In patients with **congenital antithrombin (AT) deficiency**, infusion of **AT concentrate** can be used for an acute thrombosis (*Br J Haematol 1982;50:531*).
- **Inferior vena cava (IVC) filters** are mainly indicated for acute DVT situations in which there are **absolute contraindications to anticoagulation** (e.g., active bleeding, severe thrombocytopenia, urgent surgery) or **recurrent thromboemboli despite therapeutic anticoagulation**.
  - Prophylactic IVC filters in patients with acute DVT/PE reduce the risk of recurrent PE; however, a reduction in overall mortality has not been demonstrated, and they do increase DVT recurrence rates (*Circulation 2005;112:416*).
  - In patients who had **IVC filters** placed due to **temporary contraindications to anticoagulation**, anticoagulation therapy should be added when safe to reduce the risk of filter-related thromboses.
  - Several types of removable **IVC filters** exist and can provide a temporary physical barrier against emboli from the lower extremities, but they increase the risk of DVT recurrence. Filter removal requires a second procedure.
- **Catheter embolectomy, often combined with local thrombolytic therapy,** can treat large, proximal, acute PE and DVT, although more clinical trial data are needed to better understand the efficacy and safety of this approach.

Surgical Management

Surgical embolectomy should be considered in patients with life-threatening massive PE that have contraindications to thrombolytic therapy. Predictors of life-threatening massive PE include signs of cardiovascular dysfunction (e.g., elevated plasma BNP, tachycardia, hypotension, right ventricular strain on echocardiogram, and right ventricular enlargement on chest CT) (*Circulation 2004;110:3276*).

SPECIAL CONSIDERATIONS

- **Upper extremity acute DVT** (*N Engl J Med 2011;364:861*) that involves axillary or more proximal veins should receive standard-duration (e.g., 3 months) anticoagulation. If the DVT is associated with a functioning central venous catheter, it does not need to be removed (*Chest 2012;141:e419S*).
- **Isolated calf vein acute DVT** without severe symptoms or risk factors for extension may undergo serial imaging for 2 weeks instead of anticoagulation, although clot extension should lead to full dose anticoagulation.
- **Superficial vein thrombophlebitis (SVT)**
  - SVT associated with IV infusion therapy does not require systemic anticoagulation, and treatment of discomfort may consist of oral NSAIDs.
  - For patients with spontaneous superficial thrombophlebitis, nonextensive disease does not clearly require systemic anticoagulation.

○ Extensive superficial thrombophlebitis (e.g., >5 cm in length) with a short course of prophylactic doses of fondaparinux (2.5 mg SQ daily × 6 weeks) (*N Engl J Med 2010;363:1222*) or LMWH (e.g., enoxaparin 40 mg SQ daily for 8 to 12 days) (*Arch Intern Med 2003;163:1657*) anticoagulation decreases the incidence of SVT recurrence, SVT extension, and VTE (*Chest 2012;141:e419S*).

○ Recurrent superficial thrombophlebitis may be treated with anticoagulation or vein stripping (*Br J Haematol 1982;50:531*).

- **Perioperative management of anticoagulation** requires close coordination with the surgical service (see Perioperative Medicine in Chapter 1, Patient Care in Internal Medicine) to address timing of interventions and therapeutic changes with the aim of thromboembolism prevention and avoidance of bleeding.

- **Chronic PE** occurs in 2% to 4% of patients with PE (*N Engl J Med 2011;364:351*), and patients with this disorder should undergo evaluation by an experienced team for possible pulmonary thromboendarterectomy.

- **Invasive procedures** usually require discontinuation of anticoagulation.
  ○ For patients receiving warfarin, to achieve a preoperative INR ≤1.5, stop the warfarin therapy 4 to 5 days before the invasive procedure.
  ○ In situations where a clinician aims to minimize the patient's time off therapeutic anticoagulation, parenteral anticoagulation should be initiated when the INR becomes subtherapeutic (approximately 3 days after the last warfarin dose), but it should be stopped 6 to 48 hours prior to the procedure (depending on the half-life of the parenteral drug).
  ○ In some instances, intravenous UFH is the preferred choice of therapy (e.g., pregnant woman with a mechanical heart valve undergoing a procedure).
  ○ If an INR around 1.7 is acceptable for the procedure, the warfarin dose can be halved for 4 days preoperatively (*Clin Lab Haematol 2003;25:127*).
  ○ After the procedure, resume warfarin (at the previous dose) and/or parenteral anticoagulation as soon as hemostasis and bleeding risk reach an acceptable level, typically within 24 hours.

COMPLICATIONS

- **Bleeding** is the major complication of anticoagulation.
- Up to 2% of patients who receive short-term UFH, LMWH, or pentasaccharide for VTE therapy experience major bleeding.
- For patients receiving chronic oral warfarin therapy (INR, 2 to 3), the annual incidence of major bleeding is approximately 1% to 3%.
- Concomitant use of **antiplatelet agents** increases the risk of bleeding.
- **Major bleeding in a patient with an acute VTE should lead to the discontinuation of anticoagulation and consideration of IVC filter placement. Reinitiation of standard-duration anticoagulation should occur after the bleeding concerns have resolved.**
- **INR elevation** on warfarin:
  ○ Asymptomatic minor INR elevations <5 should be managed by holding or reducing warfarin dose until the INR returns to the appropriate range and then resuming warfarin at a lower dose (see Table 20-5).
  ○ Moderate (INR ≥5 but <9) elevation of the INR in asymptomatic patients should be treated by holding one or more warfarin doses. Treatment with oral vitamin K_1 1 to 5 mg probably does not reduce the risk of hemorrhage in this setting as compared to warfarin cessation alone (*Ann Intern Med 2009;150:293*).

○ Severe (INR ≥9) should be treated with vitamin K (e.g., oral vitamin K_1 2 to 10 mg) (*Thromb Res 2004;113:205*) unless the INR is likely to be spurious.

- **Bleeding with warfarin**
  ○ Serious hemorrhages should be treated with vitamin K (10 mg) by slow IV infusion and either PCC or FFP. Because of the long half-life of warfarin (~36 hours, depending on genotype), vitamin K should be repeated every 8 or 12 hours to prevent INR rebound.
  ○ Although expensive and potentially thrombogenic (*N Engl J Med 2010;363:1791*), **rFVIIa** may stop life-threatening bleeding (*Br J Haematol 2002;116:178*).
- Bleeding with **parenteral anticoagulants**
  ○ Discontinuation usually sufficiently restores normal hemostasis.
  ○ With moderate-to-severe bleeding, give **FFP**.
- **Bleeding with UFH, LMWH, and pentasaccharide**
  ○ FFP may reduce bleeding associated with UFH, LMWH, and pentasaccharide.
  ○ For patients receiving **UFH** who develop major bleeding, heparin can be completely reversed by infusion of **protamine sulfate** in situations where the potential benefits outweigh the risks (e.g., intracranial bleed, epidural hematoma, retinal bleed).
    - Heparin serum concentrations decline rapidly due to a short half-life after IV administration, and the amount of protamine required decreases over time.
    - Approximately 1 mg protamine sulfate IV neutralizes 100 U of heparin, up to a maximum dose of 250 mg. The dose can be given as a loading dose of 25 to 50 mg by slow intravenous injection over 10 minutes, with the rest of the calculated dose over 8 to 16 hours by intravenous infusion.
    - If 30 minutes to 1 hour has elapsed since a heparin dose, the protamine dose should be reduced to approximately 0.5 mg/100 U heparin.
    - If more than 2 hours has elapsed since a heparin dose, 0.25 mg protamine/100 U heparin should be administered.
    - If heparin was administered subcutaneously, the same reductions in the protamine dose are adequate.
  ○ For major bleeding associated with **LMWH**, protamine sulfate has less efficacy compared to its effect on UFH since it neutralizes only approximately 60% of LMWH (*Reg Anesth Pain Med 2003;28:172*). Protamine does not reverse **pentasaccharide** (e.g., **fondaparinux**).
  ○ For patients with very serious bleeding receiving fondaparinux, concentrated factor VIIa may be used.
- Bleeding with novel oral anticoagulants (NOACs): If NOAC discontinuation is inadequate, then additional treatments can lower NOAC concentrations and hopefully decrease bleeding. FFP does not adequately address bleeding associated with NOACs.
  ○ **Bleeding with apixaban or rivaroxaban:** PCC, especially 4-factor PCC, can reverse direct factor Xa inhibitors (*Circulation 2011;124(14):1573*). The high degree of albumin binding in plasma does not allow dialysis to significantly lower the drug concentration.
  ○ **Bleeding with dabigatran:** Dabigatran does not have an antidote for its anticoagulant effect. Neither Factor VII concentrate nor PCC adequately reverse dabigatran (*Circulation 2011;124(14):1573*). Since the majority of dabigatran remains unbound to plasma proteins, hemodialysis will decrease the drug concentration and lower the thrombin clotting time (TCT).

- **Occult gastrointestinal or genitourinary bleeding** is a relative and not absolute contraindication to anticoagulation, although its presence prior to or during anticoagulation warrants an investigation for underlying disease.
- **Warfarin-induced skin necrosis, associated with** rapid depletion of protein C, occurs during initiation of warfarin therapy.
  - Necrosis occurs most often in areas with a high percentage of adipose tissue, such as breast tissue, and it can be life threatening.
  - Therapeutic anticoagulation with an immediate-acting anticoagulant (UFH, LMWH, etc.) and/or avoidance "loading doses" of warfarin prevents warfarin-induced skin necrosis.
- **Warfarin is absolutely contraindicated in early** (i.e., first trimester) **pregnancy** because of the **risk of teratogenicity**, and it is often avoided during the entire **pregnancy** because of the **risk of fetal bleeding**, although it is safe for infants of nursing mothers.
- **Osteoporosis** may occur with long-term heparin or warfarin use (*Arch Intern Med 2006;166:241*).

MONITORING/FOLLOW-UP

- For a suspicious clinical presentation, **testing for intrinsic hypercoagulable risk factors** ideally should wait until the patient is in stable health and off anticoagulation therapy for at least 2 weeks (e.g., at the end of a standard course of treatment) **to avoid false-positive results** for nongenetic testing.
  - Though uncommon, if reasons exist to screen for hypercoagulable risk factors around the time of diagnosis, collect blood for **factor V Leiden and prothrombin gene mutations and LA.**
  - If done, blood collection for **protein C, protein S, and antithrombin** testing should occur before initiating anticoagulation. Although normal protein C, protein S, and AT tests rule out congenital deficiencies, abnormally low results require confirmation through repeat testing or screening first-degree relatives to rule out a temporary deficiency related to the acute thrombosis.
- Though testing for PE in patients with DVT and testing for DVT in patients with PE will produce many positive findings, such testing rarely affects therapy. However, baseline results may provide useful comparison data for patients who return with symptoms of VTE, though studies have not determined the cost-effectiveness of this practice.
- Decisions regarding the prolongation of anticoagulation duration in patients with residual thrombosis on compression ultrasonography at the end of standard duration anticoagulation for proximal DVT (*Ann Intern Med 2009;150:577*) or in those with a positive D-dimer weeks after completing a standard duration of therapy for VTE (*N Engl J Med 2006;355:1780*) remain controversial, and guidelines do not strongly encourage such testing. Decision making regarding duration of anticoagulation should take into account risk factors for VTE recurrence and bleeding and patient preferences, because prolonged-duration anticoagulation reduces the incidence of VTE recurrence while it increases the incidence of bleeding.

21 Hematologic Disorders and Transfusion Therapy

Ronald Jackups, Kristen Sanfilippo, Tzu-Fei Wang, and Morey Blinder

ANEMIA

GENERAL PRINCIPLES

Definition

Anemia is defined as a decrease in circulating red blood cell (RBC) mass; the usual criteria being hemoglobin (Hb) <12 g/dL or hematocrit (Hct) <36% for women and Hb <14 g/dL or Hct <41% in men.

Classification

Anemia can be broadly classified into three etiologic groups: **blood loss (acute or chronic), decreased RBC production, and increased RBC destruction (hemolysis)**.

DIAGNOSIS

A systematic approach to anemia is best at narrowing down the diagnosis and guiding the subsequent diagnostic workup.

Clinical Presentation

- The history and physical exam play a key role in the evaluation of anemia.
- The clinical presentation of anemia include a variety of signs and symptoms depending on the severity of the anemia, its chronicity, and its pace of development.

History

Based on symptoms, one can often discern timeline (acute, subacute, or chronic), severity, and possibly the underlying etiology.

- Acute anemia. Patients with abrupt onset of anemia tolerate diminished red cell mass poorly. Patients may have symptoms of fatigue, malaise, dizziness, syncope, or angina with relatively mild anemia (i.e., Hct >30%). Acute blood loss most commonly occurs in the gastrointestinal (GI) tract (gastritis due to alcohol or nonsteroidal anti-inflammatory drugs [NSAIDs], diverticulosis, or peptic or gastric ulcer disease) and may be accompanied by epigastric symptoms, nausea and vomiting, diarrhea, hematemesis, and hematochezia.
- Chronic anemia. In contrast to acute anemia, patients with chronic anemia usually have less symptoms, especially if anemia has an insidious onset and/or is present over a prolonged period of time. However, patients usually have symptoms when Hb <7 g/dL.

Physical Examination

Common signs and symptoms of anemia include pallor, tachycardia, hypotension, dizziness, tinnitus, headaches, loss of concentration, fatigue, and weakness. Atrophic glossitis, angular cheilosis, koilonychias (spoon nails), and brittle nails are more common in severe anemia. Patients can also experience reduced exercise tolerance, dyspnea on exertion, and heart failure. High-output heart failure and shock may be seen in the most severe forms.

Diagnostic Testing

Laboratories

- The complete blood cell (CBC) count measures white blood cells (WBC), Hb, Hct, platelets, as well as measures of the red cell indices.
- The Hb level is a measure of the concentration of Hb in blood as expressed in grams per deciliter (g/dL), whereas the Hct level is the percentage of space that the RBC occupies in the blood. Hb and Hct are unreliable indicators of red cell mass in the setting of rapid shifts of intravascular volume (i.e., an acute bleed).
- The most useful red cell indices include the **mean cellular volume (MCV), red cell distribution width (RDW), and mean cellular Hb (MCH).**
  - MCV: Mean volume of the red cells. Normal range: 80 to 100 femtoliters (fL).
    - **Microcytic: MCV <80 fL**
    - **Normocytic: MCV between 80 and 100 fL**
    - **Macrocytic: MCV >100 fL**
  - RDW: A reflection of the variability in the size of the red cells and is proportional to the standard deviation of the MCV. **An elevated RDW indicates an increased variability in RBC size.**
  - MCH: Describes the concentration of Hb in each cell and an elevated level is often indicative of spherocytes or a hemoglobinopathy.
- **The reticulocyte count** measures the percentage of immature red cells in the blood and reflects the bone marrow's (BM's) production of RBCs.
  - A normal RBC has a life span of approximately 120 days; therefore, the normal reticulocyte count is 1% to 2%.
  - In the setting of anemia or blood loss, the BM should increase its production of RBC in proportion to loss of RBC and thus a 1% reticulocyte count in the setting of anemia is inappropriate.
  - **The reticulocyte index** (RI) is calculated as % reticulocytes/maturation correction (Table 21-1) × actual Hct/normal Hct (normally 45) and is important in determining if a patient's BM is responding appropriately to the level of anemia.

Table 21-1	Maturation Correction
Hct (%)	**Maturation Correction**
≥35	1.0
25–34	1.5
20–24	2.0
<20	2.5
Hct, hematocrit.	

- In normal individuals, RI 1 to 2 is expected; however, **RI <2 with anemia indicates decreased production of RBCs (hypoproliferative anemia)**. **RI >2 with anemia may indicate hemolysis or bleeding** leading to increased compensatory production of reticulocytes (hyperproliferative anemia).
- The **peripheral smear** is an essential component of the evaluation of anemia. One should pay special attention to RBC shape, size, the presence of inclusions, and orientation of cells in relation to each other. RBCs can appear in many abnormal forms, such as acanthocytes, schistocytes, spherocytes, or teardrop cells, and abnormal orientation such as Rouleaux formation. Each is associated with several specific disease processes.

Diagnostic Procedures

A **BM biopsy** may be indicated in cases of normocytic anemias with a low reticulocyte count without identifiable causes or anemia associated with other cytopenias. The biopsy may confirm myelophthisic process (i.e., presence of teardrop or fragmented cells, normoblasts, or immature WBCs on peripheral blood smear) in the setting of pancytopenia.

ANEMIAS ASSOCIATED WITH DECREASED RED BLOOD CELL PRODUCTION

Microcytic Anemia

GENERAL PRINCIPLES

- **Iron deficiency** is the most common cause of anemia in the ambulatory setting.
- Menstrual blood loss or pregnancy are the most common etiologies of iron deficiency in premenopausal women.
- In the absence of menstrual bleeding, GI blood loss is the presumed etiology in most patients, and the appropriate radiographic and endoscopic procedures should be pursued to identify a source and exclude occult malignancy.
- Diseases of the stomach and proximal small intestine (e.g., *Helicobacter pylori* infection, achlorhydria, celiac disease, and bariatric surgery) often lead to impaired iron absorption and iron deficiency anemia.
- Other causes of microcytic anemia include sideroblastic anemia, lead poisoning, thalassemia, and anemia of chronic disease (ACD), although it more likely presents as normocytic anemia (please refer to the section Anemia of Chronic Disease).

DIAGNOSIS

Clinical Presentation

Patients may present with fatigue or malaise, which is related to the importance of iron in cellular metabolism and its role in oxygen delivery, as well as pica (consumption of substances such as ice, starch, or clay). Iron deficiency has also been increasingly associated with restless leg syndrome.

History

A careful history of menstrual frequency and duration as well as potential GI blood loss (melena, hematochezia, hematemesis) is essential.

Physical Examination

Splenomegaly, koilonychia ("spoon nail"), and the Plummer-Vinson's syndrome (glossitis, dysphagia, and esophageal webs) are rare findings. The presence of telangiectasias or heme-positive stool may help identify the source of blood loss.

Diagnostic Testing

Laboratories

- **Ferritin** is the primary storage form for iron in the liver and BM and is the best surrogate marker of iron stores.
  - A ferritin level of <10 ng/mL in women or <20 ng/mL in men is a specific marker of low iron stores.
  - Ferritin is an acute-phase reactant, so normal levels may be seen in inflammatory states despite low iron stores. **A serum ferritin level of >200 ng/mL generally excludes an iron deficiency;** however, in renal dialysis patients, a functional iron deficiency may be seen with a ferritin up to 500 ng/mL.
- **Iron, total iron binding capacity (TIBC), transferrin, and transferrin saturation** are often used in combination with ferritin to diagnose iron deficiency anemia and differentiate it from ACD (Table 21-2). Serum iron level alone is often unreliable given its significant fluctuation based on patients' diets.
- With adequate follow-up, a microcytic anemia in a menstruating female needs only a baseline Hb/Hct value to be repeated 2 to 4 months after the initiation of oral iron therapy.
- Postmenopausal women and men require more detailed evaluation, including evaluation of potential RBC losses, commonly via the GI tract (e.g., peptic ulcer disease, colon carcinoma), or rarely, the urinary tract (e.g., paroxysmal nocturnal hemoglobinuria).

Diagnostic Procedures

A **BM biopsy** that shows absent staining for iron is the definitive test to diagnose iron deficiency anemia and is helpful when the serum tests fail to confirm the diagnosis.

Table 21-2	Iron Panel in Iron Deficiency Anemia and Anemia of Chronic Disease				
Disease	**Ferritin**	**TIBC**	**Serum Iron**	**Transferring Saturation**	**Soluble Transferrin Receptor**
Iron deficiency anemia	Decreased	Increased	Decreased	Decreased	Increased
Anemia of chronic disease	Increased (can be normal)	Decreased	Decreased (but can be normal or increased)	Normal or decreased	Normal

TIBC, total iron binding capacity.

Table 21-3	Oral Iron Preparations	
Preparations	**Dose**	**Elemental Iron (mg)**
Ferrous sulfate	325 mg tid	65
Ferrous gluconate	300 mg tid	36
Ferrous fumarate	100 mg tid	33
Iron polysaccharide complex (Niferex)	150 mg bid	150
Carbonyl iron	50 mg bid	50

TREATMENT

- **Oral iron therapy.** Given in stable patients with mild symptoms. Several different preparations are available (Table 21-3).
  - Iron is best absorbed on an empty stomach, and 3 to 10 mg of elemental iron can be absorbed daily.
  - Oral iron ingestion may induce a number of GI side effects, including epigastric distress, bloating, and constipation. As a result, noncompliance is a common problem. These side effects can be decreased by initially administering the drug with meals or once per day and increasing the dosage as tolerated. Concomitant treatment with a stool softener can also alleviate these symptoms.
  - Ferrous gluconate and ferrous fumarate at a similar dose may be better tolerated alternative therapies.
  - Iron polysaccharide complex (Niferex) is as effective as other preparations at a similar cost and seems to have fewer GI side effects.
  - Administration of vitamin C along with iron improves absorption by maintaining the iron in the reduced state.
- **Parenteral iron therapy** (Table 21-4). Indications for parenteral iron over oral iron include:
  - Poor absorption (e.g., inflammatory bowel disease, malabsorption).
  - Very high iron requirements that cannot be met with oral supplementation (e.g., ongoing bleeding).
  - Intolerance to oral preparations.
  - Relative iron deficiency in chronic kidney disease (CKD).
  - **Iron dextran** (INFeD, Dexferrum)
    - Infusion can be complicated by serious side effects including **anaphylaxis**; therefore, an **IV test dose** of 0.5 mL should be administered over 5 to 10 minutes at 30 to 60 minutes prior to the full dose. Methylprednisolone, diphenhydramine, and 1:1,000 epinephrine 1-mg ampule (for subcutaneous administration) should be immediately available at all times during the infusion. For an online dose calculator, go to *www.globalrph.com/irondextran.htm*.
    - Delayed reactions to IV iron, such as arthralgia, myalgia, fever, pruritus, and lymphadenopathy may be seen within 3 days of therapy and usually resolve spontaneously or with NSAIDs.
- Alternatives to iron dextran include sodium ferric gluconate (Ferrlecit) and iron sucrose (Venofer).

Table 21-4	Intravenous Iron Preparations		
Preparations	**IV push**	**Infusion**	**Caution**
Iron dextran (INFeD, Dexferrum)	100 mg over 2 min	Not FDA approved, but the entire dose may be diluted and infused in one setting	A 0.5-mL test dose should be given, and observe patient for at least 1 hr prior to full dose.
Iron sucrose (Venofer)	100 mg over 2–5 min	100 mg/100 mL over 15 min	
	200 mg over 2–5 min	300 mg/250 mL over 1.5 hr	
		400 mg/250 mL over 2.5 hr	
		500 mg/250 mL over 3.5 hr	
Ferric gluconate (Ferrlecit)	125 mg over 10 min	125 mg/100 mL over 1 hr	
Ferumoxytol	510 mg over 17 s	Not FDA approved	Observe patient for at least 30 min after administration.

FDA, U.S. Food and Drug Administration; IV, intravenous.

- These alternative preparations appear to have less hypersensitivity infusion reactions when compared to iron dextran.
- **However, they cannot be used to replenish the entire iron deficit with a single infusion as iron dextran.**

Thalassemia

GENERAL PRINCIPLES

Definition
The **thalassemia syndromes** are inherited disorders characterized by reduced Hb synthesis associated with mutations in either the α- or β-chain of the molecule (Table 21-5).

Epidemiology
Most affected individuals are of Mediterranean, Middle Eastern, Indian, African, or Asian descent.

Etiology
- **β-Thalassemia** results in a decreased production of β-globin and a resultant excess of α-globin, forming insoluble α-tetramers and leading to ineffective erythropoiesis.

Table 21-5	Thalassemias			
	Genotype	Hemoglobin (g/dL)	Mean Cellular Volume (fL)	Transfusion Dependent
α-Thalassemia				
Silent carrier	$\alpha\alpha$ / $\alpha-$	Normal	None	No
Trait	$\alpha-$ / $\alpha-$ or $\alpha\alpha$ /$--$	>10	<80	No
Hemoglobin H	$\alpha-$ / $--$	7−10	<70	+/−
Hydrops fetalis	$--$ / $--$	Incompatible with life		
β-Thalassemia				
Silent carrier	β / β^+	>10	<80	No
β-Thal minor (trait)	β / β^0	>10	<80	No
β-Thal intermedia	β^+ / β^+	7−10	65−75	+/−
β-Thal major	β^0 / β^0	<7	<70	Yes

β^+: β-Thalassemia genes produce some β-globin chains but with impaired synthesis.
β^0: β-Thalassemia genes produce no β-globin chains.

- ○ **β-Thalassemia minor (trait)** occurs with one gene abnormality with underproduction of β-chain globin. Patients are asymptomatic and present with microcytic, hypochromic RBCs, and Hb levels >10 g/dL.
- ○ **β-Thalassemia intermedia** occurs with dysfunction in both β-globin genes so that anemia is more severe (Hb, 7 to 10 g/dL).
- ○ **β-Thalassemia major** (Cooley anemia) is caused by severe abnormalities of both genes that produce no β-globin and requires lifelong transfusion support.
- **α-Thalassemia** occurs with a deletion of one or more of the four α-globin genes, leading to a β-globin excess.
- ○ Mild microcytosis and mild hypochromic anemia (Hb >10 g/dL) is seen with the loss of one or two genes (silent carrier and α-thal trait), whereas Hb H disease (deletion of three α-globin genes) results in splenomegaly and hemolytic anemia.
- ○ In patients with Hb H (β-tetramers) disease, transfusion or splenectomy is often not necessary until after second or third decades of life. In addition, oxidant drugs similar to those that exacerbate glucose-6-phosphate dehydrogenase (G6PD) deficiency should be avoided because increased hemolysis may occur.
- ○ Hydrops fetalis occurs with the loss of all four α-globin genes and is incompatible with life.

DIAGNOSIS

Clinical Presentation

- A family history of microcytic anemia or microcytosis is helpful.
- Splenomegaly may be the only physical manifestation.
- Skeletal deformities and hematopoietic masses from extramedullary hematopoiesis can be especially evident in β-thalassemia major.

Diagnostic Testing

- Microcytic hypochromic RBCs are seen, along with poikilocytosis and nucleated RBCs.
- In thalassemia trait, iron studies are normal, as is the RDW, which help to differentiate from iron-deficiency anemia.
- Hb electrophoresis is diagnostic for β-thalassemia showing an increased percentage of Hb A2 ($\alpha 2\delta 2$) and Hb F ($\alpha 2\gamma 2$).
- Silent carries with a single α-chain loss have an essentially normal electrophoresis. Those with Hb H disease have increased Hb H (β-tetramers). The diagnosis of α-thalassemia is made by α-globin gene analysis.

TREATMENT

- Patients with thalassemia trait require no specific treatment.
- In patients with more severe forms of the disease, RBC transfusions to maintain an Hb level of 9 to 10 g/dL are needed to prevent the skeletal deformities that result from accelerated erythropoiesis.
- In severe forms of thalassemia, repeated transfusions result in tissue iron overload, which may cause congestive heart failure (CHF), hepatic dysfunction, glucose intolerance, and secondary hypogonadism. **Iron chelation therapy** delays or prevents these complications. Once clinical organ deterioration has begun, it may not be reversible.
- **Chelation therapy** is indicated for transfusion-associated iron overload from any cause. It is indicated in patients with iron infusion burden of >20 U of packed RBCs and ferritin consistently >1,000 ng/mL.
  - Deferoxamine, 40 mg/kg subcutaneously (SC) or intravenously (IV) over 8 to 12 hours continuous infusion (*N Engl J Med 2011;364(2):146*).
  - Deferasirox 20 to 30 mg/kg/d (up to 40 mg/kg/d) is another option. Dose can be titrated every 3 to 6 months based on ferritin level. Side effects of deferasirox include mild-to-moderate GI disturbances and skin rash. Efficacy is similar to that of deferoxamine.
  - Chelation therapy should be continued until ferritin levels of <1,000 mg/L is maintained.
- Hydroxyurea (15 to 35 mg/kg/d) to increase Hb F may benefit some patients with β-thalassemia.
- Stem cell transplantation (SCT) is the only curative therapy and should be considered in young patients with thalassemia major who have human leukocyte antigen (HLA)-identical donors.

Surgical Management

Splenectomy should be considered in patients with accelerated (>2 U/mos) transfusion requirements. To decrease the risk of postsplenectomy sepsis, immunization against *Pneumococcus*, *Haemophilus influenzae*, and *Neisseria meningitidis* should be administered at least 2 weeks before surgery if not previously vaccinated (see Appendix A, Immunizations and Postexposure Therapies). Splenectomy is not recommended if the patient is younger than 5 to 6 years because of the risk of sepsis.

Sideroblastic Anemias

GENERAL PRINCIPLES

Definition

Sideroblastic anemias are hereditary or acquired RBC disorders characterized by abnormal iron metabolism associated with the presence of ring sideroblasts in the BM aspirate and normal cytogenetics.

Etiology

- Acquired
  - Primary sideroblastic anemia (myelodysplastic syndrome [MDS])
  - Sideroblastic anemia secondary to drugs (i.e., chloramphenicol, cycloserine, ethanol, isoniazid, pyrazinamide), lead or zinc toxicity, chronic ethanol use, or copper deficiency.
- Hereditary
  - X-linked
  - Autosomal
  - Mitochondrial

DIAGNOSIS

A BM examination including cytogenetics is needed to evaluate for the presence of ring sideroblasts or other abnormal marrow forms.

TREATMENT

- Remove any possible offending agent.
- Pyridoxine 50 to 200 mg daily may be used to treat hereditary sideroblastic anemias.

Macrocytic/Megaloblastic Anemia

GENERAL PRINCIPLES

Definition

Megaloblastic anemia is a term used to describe disorders of impaired DNA synthesis in hematopoietic cells but affects all proliferating cells.

Etiology

- Almost all cases are due to folic acid or vitamin B_{12} deficiency.
- **Folate deficiency** results from a negative folate balance arising from malnutrition, malabsorption, or increased requirement (pregnancy, hemolytic anemia).
  - Patients on slimming diets, alcoholics, the elderly, and psychiatric patients are particularly at risk for nutritional folate deficiency.
  - **Pregnancy and lactation** require threefold to fourfold increased daily folate needs and are commonly associated with megaloblastic changes in maternal hematopoietic cells, leading to a dimorphic (combined folate and iron deficiency) anemia.

- ○ Folate malabsorption can also be seen in celiac disease.
- ○ Drugs that can interfere with folate absorption include ethanol, trimethoprim, pyrimethamine, diphenylhydantoin, barbiturates, and sulfasalazine.
- ○ Dialysis-dependent patients require more folate intake because of increased folate losses.
- ○ Patients with hemolytic anemia, such as sickle cell anemia, require increased folate for accelerated erythropoiesis and can present with aplastic crisis (rapidly falling RBC counts) with folate deficiency.
- **Vitamin B$_{12}$ deficiency** occurs insidiously over 3 or more years because daily vitamin B$_{12}$ requirements are low (6 to 9 μg/d), whereas total body stores are 2 to 5 mg.
  - ○ Because multivitamins, bread, and cereals now contain folic acid, the hematologic manifestations of vitamin B$_{12}$ deficiency may be obscured, and neurologic symptoms may be the sole presentation.
  - ○ Causes of vitamin B$_{12}$ deficiency include partial (up to 20% of patients within 8 years of surgery) or total gastrectomy and pernicious anemia (PA). Older patients with gastric atrophy may develop a food-bound vitamin B$_{12}$ deficiency in which vitamin B$_{12}$ absorption is impaired.
  - ○ PA occurs in individuals who are older than 40 years (mean onset, age 60 years). Up to 30% of patients have a positive family history. PA is associated with other autoimmune disorders (Graves' disease 30%, Hashimoto's thyroiditis 11%, and Addison's disease 5% to 10%). Of patients with PA, 90% have antiparietal cell immunoglobulin (Ig)G antibodies and 60% have anti-intrinsic factor antibodies.
  - ○ Other etiologies include pancreatic insufficiency, bacterial overgrowth, and intestinal parasites (*Diphyllobothrium latum*).

DIAGNOSIS

Clinical Presentation

- Folate-deficient patients present with sleep deprivation, fatigue, and manifestations of depression, irritability, or forgetfulness.
- By the time vitamin B$_{12}$ deficiency anemia is clinically evident, the main manifestations are usually neurologic symptoms, such as peripheral neuropathy, paresthesias, lethargy, hypotonia, and seizures.
- Important physical findings include signs of poor nutrition, pigmentation of skin creases and nail beds, or glossitis. Jaundice or splenomegaly may indicate ineffective and extramedullary hematopoiesis. Vitamin B$_{12}$ deficiency may cause decreased vibratory and positional sense, ataxia, paresthesias, confusion, and dementia. Neurologic complications may occur even in the absence of anemia and may not fully resolve despite adequate treatment. **Folic acid deficiency does not result in neurologic disease.**

Diagnostic Testing

Laboratories

- Macrocytic anemia is usually present, and leukopenia and thrombocytopenia may occur.
- The peripheral smear may show anisocytosis, poikilocytosis, and macro-ovalocytes; hypersegmented neutrophils (containing more than six nuclear lobes) are common.
- Lactate dehydrogenase (LDH) and indirect bilirubin are typically elevated, reflecting ineffective erythropoiesis and premature destruction of RBCs.

- Serum vitamin B_{12} and RBC folate levels should be measured.
- RBC folate is a more accurate indicator of body folate stores than serum folate, particularly if measured after folate therapy or improved nutrition has been initiated.
- **Serum methylmalonic acid (MMA) and homocysteine (HC)** may be useful when the vitamin B_{12} or folate level is equivocal. MMA and HC are elevated in vitamin B_{12} deficiency; only HC is elevated in folate deficiency.
- A **Schilling test** may be useful in the diagnosis of PA due to vitamin B_{12} deficiency but rarely affects the therapeutic approach. Therefore, it is rarely done nowadays.
- Detecting **antibodies to intrinsic factor** is specific for the diagnosis of PA.

Diagnostic Procedures
Bone marrow biopsy may be necessary to rule out MDS or acute leukemia since these disorders may present with findings similar to those of megaloblastic anemia.

TREATMENT

- Treatment is to replace the deficient factors.
- Potassium supplementation may be necessary when treatment is initiated to avoid potentially serious arrhythmias due to hypokalemia induced by enhanced hematopoiesis.
- Reticulocytosis should begin within 1 week of therapy, followed by a rising of Hb over 6 to 8 weeks.
- Coexisting iron deficiency is present in one-third of patients and is a common cause for an incomplete response to therapy.
- Folic acid 1 mg daily is given until the deficiency is corrected. High doses of folic acid (5 mg daily) may be needed in patients with malabsorption syndromes.
- Vitamin B_{12} deficiency is corrected by administering cyanocobalamin. Unless the patient is severely ill (decompensated CHF due to anemia, advanced neurologic dysfunction), treatment with full doses of cyanocobalamin (1 mg/d intramuscular [IM]) should await the laboratory diagnosis.
- After 1 week of daily therapy, 1 mg/wk should be given for 4 weeks and then 1 mg/mo for life.
- Patients who decline or cannot take parenteral therapy can be prescribed oral tablets or syrup at 50 mg/d for life.

Anemia of Chronic Renal Insufficiency

GENERAL PRINCIPLES

Anemia of chronic renal insufficiency is attributed primarily to decreased endogenous erythropoietin (EPO) production and may occur as the creatinine clearance declines to below 50 mL/min. Other causes including iron deficiency may contribute to the etiology (see the previous description).

DIAGNOSIS

- Laboratory evaluation typically reveals a normal MCV.
- Peripheral smear: The RBCs are often hypochromic, with the occasional presence of echinocytes (burr cells).

- If the patient's creatinine level is >1.8 mg/dL, the primary cause of the anemia can be assumed to be EPO deficiency and/or iron deficiency, and an EPO level is unnecessary.
- Iron status should be evaluated in patients who are undergoing dialysis by obtaining levels of ferritin and transferrin saturation. Oral iron supplementation is not effective in CKD, so using parenteral iron to maintain a ferritin level of >500 ng/mL is recommended (*Kidney Int 2005;68:2846*).

TREATMENT

- Treatment has been revolutionized by erythropoiesis-stimulating agents (ESAs) including epoetin alfa and darbepoetin alfa (Table 21-6).
- Therapy is initiated in predialysis patients who are symptomatic.
- Objective benefits of reversing anemia include enhanced exercise capacity, improved cognitive function, elimination of RBC transfusions, and reduction of iron overload. Subjective benefits include increased energy, enhanced appetite, better sleep patterns, and improved sexual activity.
- Administration of ESAs can be IV (hemodialysis patients) or SC (predialysis or peritoneal dialysis patients). In dialysis and predialysis patients with CKD, **the target hemoglobin should be between 11 and 12 g/dL and should not exceed 12 g/dL.** An Hb and Hct should be measured at least monthly while receiving an ESA. Dose adjustments should be made to maintain the target Hb.

Table 21-6	Erythropoietin Dosing	
	Agent and Initial Dose (SC or IV)	
Indication	**Erythropoietin[a]**	**Darbepoetin[b]**
Chemotherapy-induced anemia from nonmyeloid malignancy, multiple myeloma, lymphoma; anemia secondary to malignancy or myelodysplastic syndrome	40,000 U/wk or 150 U/kg three times a week	2.25 μg/kg/wk or 100 μg/wk or 200 μg/2 wk or 500 μg/3 wk
Anemia associated with renal failure	50–150 U/kg three times a week	0.45 μg/kg/wk
Anemia associated with HIV infection	100–200 U/kg three times a week	Not approved
Anemia of chronic disease	150–300 U/kg three times a week	Not approved
Anemia in patients unwilling or unable to receive red blood cells; anemic patients undergoing major surgery	600 U/kg/wk × 3 300 U/kg/d × 1–2 wk	Not recommended

[a]Dose increase after 48 weeks up to 900 U/kg/wk or 60,000 U/wk; discontinue if hematocrit (Hct) is >40%; resume when Hct is <36% at 75% of previous dose.
[b]Dose increase after 6 weeks up to 4.5 mg/kg/wk or 150 mg/wk or 300 mg/2 wk; hold dose if Hct is >36%, then resume when Hct is <36% at 75% of previous dose.
IV, intravenous; SC, subcutaneously.

- Side effects of ESAs: Targeting higher Hb levels and/or exposure to high doses of ESAs is associated with a greater risk of cardiovascular complications and mortality. In addition, a higher Hct level from ESAs increases the risk of stroke, heart failure, hypertension, and deep vein thrombosis (*N Engl J Med 2006;355:2085*).
- **Suboptimal responses to ESA therapy** are a common phenomenon due to iron deficiency, inflammation, bleeding, infection, malignancy, malnutrition, and aluminum toxicity.
  - Because anemia is a powerful determinant of life expectancy in patients on chronic dialysis, IV iron administration has become standard therapy in many individuals who receive ESA therapy and are proven to be iron deficient. It has also been shown to reduce the ESA dosage required to correct anemia.
  - A ferritin and transferrin saturation should be tested at least monthly during the initiation of ESA therapy with a goal ferritin level of >200 ng/mL and a transferrin saturation of >20% in dialysis-dependent patients and a ferritin level of >100 ng/mL and a transferrin saturation of >20% in predialysis or peritoneal dialysis patients.
  - Iron therapy is unlikely to be useful if the ferritin level is >500 ng/mL.
  - Secondary hyperparathyroidism that causes BM fibrosis and relative ESA resistance may also occur.

Anemia of Chronic Disease

GENERAL PRINCIPLES

- ACD often develops in patients with long-standing inflammatory diseases, malignancy, autoimmune disorders, and chronic infection.
- Etiology is multifactorial, including defective iron mobilization during erythropoiesis, inflammatory cytokine-mediated suppression of erythropoiesis, and impaired EPO response to anemia.
- ACD is also a common complication of therapy for the underlying disease (e.g., chemotherapy for malignancy, zidovudine for HIV infection).

DIAGNOSIS

Diagnostic Testing
Laboratories
- **No laboratory tests are diagnostic** for ACD.
- Anemia is normocytic, normochromic in 75% of cases and microcytic, and normochromic in 25% of cases.
- Iron studies may be similar to patients with iron deficiency and are difficult to interpret. **Soluble transferrin receptor** may help distinguish iron-deficiency anemia from ACD (see Table 21-2).
- Clinical responses to iron therapy can be seen in patients with ferritin levels up to 100 ng/mL.

Diagnostic Procedures
A BM evaluation of stored iron may be necessary to rule out iron deficiency anemia accompanying ACD, although rarely indicated.

TREATMENT

- Therapy for ACD is directed toward the underlying disease and eliminating exacerbating factors such as nutritional deficiencies and marrow-suppressive drugs.
- ESA therapy should be considered if the patient is transfusion dependent or has symptomatic anemia.
  - Effective doses of ESA are higher than those reported in anemia from renal insufficiency.
  - If no responses have been observed at 900 U/kg/wk, further dose escalation is unlikely to be effective.
- Transfusion should be considered for patients with Hct levels of <24% or if symptomatic.

Anemia in Cancer Patients

The role of ESAs in patients receiving chemotherapy has been controversial. Recent studies indicate that ESAs may potentiate cancer growth and decrease disease-free survival (*Lancet 2003;362:1255*) and decrease overall survival (*J Clin Oncol 2007; 25:1027*). In addition, ESAs have not shown to significantly reduce the need for RBC transfusions in patients not receiving chemotherapy, nor did they increase quality of life (*J Clin Oncol 2005;23:5960*). Therefore, ESA therapy should only be considered in transfusion-dependent patients with a target Hb level of 11 to 12 g/dL.

Anemia Associated with HIV Infection

GENERAL PRINCIPLES

Epidemiology

Anemia is the most common cytopenia in patients with HIV; the prevalence increases as the disease progresses and the CD4 count drops (*Am J Med 2004;116(suppl 7A):27S*).

Etiology

Similar mechanism as ACD in which inflammatory mediators causes decreased erythropoiesis.

DIAGNOSIS

- CBC: Normochromic, normocytic anemia, although zidovudine and stavudine induce a macrocytic anemia.
- Reticulocyte count: decreased.
- BM exam rarely needed (see Special Considerations section), and dysplasia similar to MDS is common.

TREATMENT

ESA (see Table 21-6) improves the Hb level in patients with an endogenous EPO level of ≤500 mU/mL.

SPECIAL CONSIDERATIONS

- *Mycobacterium avium* complex infections are frequently associated with severe anemia. Diagnosis is established on BM examination or culture. Treatment of *M. avium* complex is described in Chapter 16, Human Immunodeficiency Virus and Acquired Immunodeficiency Syndrome.
- Parvovirus B19 should be considered in HIV-infected patients with transfusion-dependent anemia and a low reticulocyte count.
  - Laboratory studies: Parvovirus by polymerase chain reaction from serum or BM.
  - Treatment with IV immunoglobulin (IVIG) 0.4 g/kg daily for 5 to 10 days results in erythropoietic recovery. Relapses have occurred between 2 and 6 months and can be successfully managed with maintenance IVIG at a dose of 0.4 g/kg IV every 4 weeks (*Ann Intern Med 1990;113(12):926*).

Aplastic Anemia

GENERAL PRINCIPLES

- Aplastic anemia is an acquired abnormality of hematopoietic stem cells that usually presents with pancytopenia.
- Most cases are idiopathic.
- Approximately 20% of cases are associated with drug or chemical exposure.
- Ten percent of cases are associated with viral illnesses (e.g., viral hepatitis, Epstein–Barr virus, cytomegalovirus [CMV]).
- There is a growing body of evidence suggesting that BM failure in aplastic anemia results from immunologic destruction of hematopoietic stem and progenitor cells (*Curr Opin Hematol 2008;15(3):162*).

DIAGNOSIS

Clinical Presentation

Patients usually present with pancytopenia, and symptoms are most commonly due to anemia (fatigue, malaise, dyspnea) or thrombocytopenia (mucosal bleeding, bruising), although some patients present with fever and leukopenia.

Diagnostic Criteria

- Moderate aplastic anemia
  - BM cellularity <30%
  - Absence of criteria for severe aplastic anemia
  - At least two of three blood lines are lower than normal
- Severe aplastic anemia (*Lancet 1987;330(8565):955*)
  - BM cellularity <25% with normal cytogenetics, OR
  - BM cellularity <50% with normal cytogenetics, and <30% are hematopoietic, AND two of three peripheral blood criteria:
    - Absolute neutrophil count (ANC) <500/mm^3
    - Platelet count <20,000/mm^3
    - Absolute reticulocyte count <40,000/mm^3
  - No other hematologic disease

- Very severe aplastic anemia
  - ○ The criteria of severe aplastic anemia are met, AND
  - ○ ANC <200/mm^3

Diagnostic Testing

BM biopsy is required for diagnosis. Morphology of BM may be difficult to distinguish from hypocellular MDS and paroxysmal nocturnal hemoglobinuria.

TREATMENT

- Suspected offending drugs should be discontinued and exacerbating factors corrected.
- Once the diagnosis is established, care should be provided in a center experienced with aplastic anemia.
- Immunosuppressive treatment with cyclosporine, glucocorticoids, and antithymocyte globulin should be considered in patients who do not undergo a SCT (*Ann Intern Med 2002;136(7):534*).
- **SCT.** Early referral to a center that is experienced in managing aplastic anemia is recommended. When feasible, SCT from an HLA-identical sibling is generally recommended and has achieved a long-term survival rate of 60% to 70%.
- **Transfusions in aplastic anemia.** Transfusions with RBCs should be kept to a minimum. Prophylactic platelet transfusions are generally recommended if the platelet count is below 10,000/mm^3. Transfusion with blood products from family members should be avoided while SCT is being considered.

ANEMIAS ASSOCIATED WITH INCREASED RED BLOOD CELL DESTRUCTION

Anemias Associated with Increased Erythropoiesis

GENERAL PRINCIPLES

Definition

Anemias associated with increased erythropoiesis (i.e., an elevated reticulocyte count) are caused by bleeding or destruction of RBCs (hemolysis) and may exceed the capacity of normal BM to correct the Hb. Bleeding is much more common than is hemolysis.

Etiology

- **Blood loss.** If no obvious source, suspect occult loss into GI tract, retroperitoneum, thorax, or deep compartments of thigh depending on history (recent instrumentation, trauma, hip fracture, coagulopathy).
- **Hemolysis** can be categorized into two broad groups based on cause of destruction; intrinsic (caused by deficits inherit to the RBC) and extrinsic (caused by factors external to the RBC).
  - ○ In general, intrinsic causes are inherited where extrinsic causes tend to be acquired. Intrinsic disorders are a result of defects of the red cell membrane (i.e., hereditary spherocytosis), Hb composition (i.e., sickle cell disease), or enzyme deficiency (i.e., G6PD deficiency).

○ Extrinsic disorders can result from antibodies (i.e., cold or warm reactive antibodies), infectious agents (i.e., malaria), trauma, chemical agents (i.e., venom), or liver disease.
○ Hemolytic disorders are also commonly categorized by the location of RBC destruction; intravascular (within the circulation) or extravascular (within the macrophage-monocyte system typically in the liver or spleen).

DIAGNOSIS

Laboratory assessment of patients with suspected hemolysis should include:
• **Decreased Hb** and **Hct**.
• **Elevated reticulocyte count** (occurs within 3 to 5 days of onset).
• **Elevated LDH** and **indirect hyperbilirubinemia** reflect increased RBC turnover.
• **Decreased haptoglobin** due to binding of intravascular Hb.
• The **direct Coombs test** (direct antibody testing [DAT]) is an indicator of the presence of antibodies attached to RBC.
• The **indirect Coombs test** indicates the presence of free antibody in the plasma.
• A peripheral blood smear is essential and can aid in determining the etiology of hemolysis. Intravascular hemolysis may reveal red cell fragmentation (i.e., schistocytes, helmet cells), whereas spherocytes indicate extravascular hemolysis. Polychromasia and nucleated RBCs are indicators of increased erythropoiesis.

Sickle Cell Disease

GENERAL PRINCIPLES

• The sickle cell diseases (SCD) are a group of hereditary Hb disorders in which Hb undergoes a sickle shape transformation under conditions of deoxygenation.
• The most common are homozygous sickle cell anemia (Hb SS) or other heterozygous conditions (Hb SC, Hb S–β thalassemia).
• Hb S results from a substitution of valine for glutamic acid at the sixth position of the β-globin chain.
• Newborn screening programs for hemoglobinopathies identify most patients in infancy.
• In the United States, the incidence of SCD is approximately 1 in 625 births.
• **Sickle cell trait** is present in 8% to 10% of African Americans (*N Engl J Med 1973;288:31*).

DIAGNOSIS

Diagnostic Testing

• Hb electrophoresis can determine the presence of hemoglobinopathies.
• Laboratory study abnormalities are determined by the degree of hemoglobinopathy and include anemia (mean in SCD 8 g/dL), reticulocytosis (3% to 15%), indirect hyperbilirubinemia, elevated LDH, and decreased or absent haptoglobin. Leukocytosis (10,000 to 20,000/mm^3) and thrombocytosis (>450,000/mm^3) are common, due to enhanced stimulation of the marrow compartment and autosplenectomy.
• Peripheral smear shows sickle-shaped RBCs, target cells (particularly in Hb SC and Hb S − β thalassemia), and Howell–Jolly bodies, indicative of functional asplenism.

Clinical Presentation

- Clinical presentation of SCD is heterogeneous and is dependent on type and degree of hemoglobinopathy. The most common clinical manifestations of SCD result from hemolysis and/or vascular occlusions.
- Vascular occlusions include pain crises, avascular necrosis, priapism, and acute chest syndrome, while hemolytic complications include pulmonary hypertension, cholelithiasis, and leg ulcers. Strokes and renal medullary infarctions are complications of both.
- **Vaso-occlusive complications (VOC)** result from polymerization of deoxygenated Hb S. These polymerized RBCs assume the classic sickle shape and develop a marked loss of deformability leading to vaso-occlusion.
  - **Acute painful episodes ("sickle cell pain crisis")**
    - Sickle cell pain crisis is the most common VOC and manifestation of SCD.
    - Pain is typically in the long bones, back, chest, and abdomen.
    - Precipitating factors can include stress, infection, dehydration, alcohol, and weather. However, a majority of cases have no identifiable trigger.
    - Typical duration of the episode is 2 to 6 days.
    - Higher levels of fetal Hb (Hb F) may be protective against VOC.
  - **Acute chest syndrome** is a life-threatening emergency that occurs when decreased oxygen saturation (<90%) leads to increased intravascular sickling and irreversible occlusion of the microvasculature in the pulmonary circulation. It may be precipitated by infection, pulmonary embolism, or fat emboli. Treatment consists of supportive care, treatment of the underlying cause, and may require RBC exchange therapy to decrease the burden of Hb S.
  - **Priapism** often presents in adolescence and may result in eventual impotence.
  - **Retinopathy** is caused by chronic vaso-occlusion of the retina, which causes proliferative retinopathy and may lead to complications including vitreous hemorrhage and retinal detachment.
  - **Functional asplenia** results from recurrent splenic infarcts due to sickling and eventually results in the loss of splenic function. The majority of cases occur before the age of 1 year. Functional asplenia places patients at higher risk of infection, especially with encapsulated organisms.
  - **Avascular necrosis (AVN)** is the result of infarction of bone trabeculae and occurs most commonly in the femoral and humeral heads. Up to 50% of adults affected by SCD can manifest AVN, which is a cause of significant pain.
- **Hemolytic complications**
  - **Cholelithiasis** is present in >80% of patients and is primarily due to bilirubin stones. It may lead to acute cholecystitis or biliary colic.
  - **Leg ulceration** occurring at the ankle is often chronic and recurring.
  - **Pulmonary hypertension (PH)** has been linked to several hemolytic disorders and can occur in up to 60% of patients with SCD (*N Engl J Med 2004;350:857*). The pathophysiology is unclear but may be the result of nitric oxide depletion.
- **Renal medulla infarction** is the result of repeated occlusion of renal medullary capillaries, resulting in CKD in many patients. This can lead to isosthenuria (inability to concentrate urine) and hematuria, predisposing patients to dehydration and thus increasing the risk of VOC.
- **Neurologic complications** occur in up to 25% of patients with SCD by the age of 45 years (*Am J Med 1978;65:461*) and include cerebrovascular accidents (transient ischemic attacks, infarction, cerebral hemorrhage), seizure, and sensory hearing loss.

Ischemic stroke is felt to result from recurrent endothelial injury from hemolysis and vaso-occlusion, resulting in intimal hyperplasia with large-artery arteriopathy (*Stroke 2011;42:227*). High cerebral flow rate (>200 cm/s) detected by transcranial Doppler (TCD) has been associated with increased risk of stroke. This risk is greatly reduced by routine transfusion or exchange therapy (*N Engl J Med 1998;339:5*). Adults are not routinely screened using TCD. Current recommendations for adults include evaluation for known additional stroke risk factors with management accordingly (*Circulation 2006;113:e873*).

- **Infections** typically occur in tissues susceptible to vaso-occlusive infarcts (i.e., lungs, bone, kidney). The most common infectious organisms include *Streptococcus pneumonia, Staphylococcus aureus, Salmonella* spp., *Mycoplasma pneumoniae*, or *H. influenza*. Vaccinations are a key mechanism in prevention.
- **Aplastic "crisis"** occurs when there is a transient halt of erythropoiesis due to an inciting event causing a sudden decrease in Hb. The most common etiology in children with SCD is infection with parvovirus B19. Folate deficiency should also be suspected because of the chronic increased requirements for erythropoiesis.
- **Pregnancy** in a patient with sickle cell anemia should be considered high risk and is associated with increased spontaneous abortions or premature delivery, along with increased occurrence of vaso-occlusive crises.

TREATMENT

- **Acute painful episodes.** Management of **acute painful episodes** consists of rehydration (3 to 4 L/d), evaluation for and management of infections, analgesia, and if needed, antipyretic and empiric antibiotic therapy.
  - The full National Institutes of Health (NIH) guidelines for pain management are available at *http://www.nhlbi.nih.gov/health/prof/blood/sickle/sc_mngt.pdf*.
  - **Opioids** (see Chapter 1, Patient Care in Internal Medicine, the Opioids section) are typically used and are effectively administered by a **patient-controlled analgesia pump**, allowing for the patient to self-administer medication within a set limit of infusions (lockout interval) and basal rate.
    Morphine (2 mg/hr basal rate with boluses of 2 to 10 mg every 6 to 10 minutes) is the drug of choice for moderate or severe pain. If patient-controlled analgesia is not used, morphine (0.1 to 0.2 mg/kg IV q2–3h) or hydromorphone (0.02 to 0.04 mg/kg IV q2–3h) is recommended.
  - Transfusion therapy has no role in the treatment of uncomplicated vaso-occlusive crises.
  - Supplemental oxygen does not benefit acute pain crisis unless hypoxia is present.
- **Acute chest syndrome.** Suspicion of **acute chest syndrome** should prompt aggressive transfusion therapy, including red cell exchange immediately. The presentation of acute chest syndrome is clinically indistinguishable from pneumonia; thus, empiric broad-spectrum antibiotics should also be administered.
- **Priapism** is initially treated with hydration and analgesia. Persistent erections for more than 24 hours may require transfusion therapy or surgical drainage.
- **AVN** management consists of local heat, analgesics, and avoidance of weight bearing. Hip and shoulder arthroplasty may be effective at decreasing symptoms and improving function.
- **Cholelithiasis.** Induced acute cholecystitis should be treated medically with antibiotics followed by cholecystectomy when the attack subsides. Elective cholecystectomy for asymptomatic gallstones is controversial.

- **Leg ulcers** should be treated with rest, leg elevation, and intensive local care. Wet to dry dressings should be applied three to four times per day. A zinc oxide–impregnated bandage (Unna boot), changed weekly for 3 to 4 weeks, can be used for nonhealing or more extensive ulcers.
- There is no standard therapy for treatment of **pulmonary hypertension** in SCD, with clinical trials of sildenafil showing conflicting results (*Br J Haematol 2005;130: 445*; *Blood 2001;118:855*), thus patients should be referred to a clinical specialist.
- **Acute CVA** should be managed based on current standards. Long-term transfusions to maintain the Hb S concentration to $<50\%$ for at least 5 years significantly reduce the incidence of recurrence.
- Patients with suspected **aplastic crisis** require hospitalization. Therapy includes folic acid, 5 mg/d, as well as supportive RBC transfusions.
- **Iron chelation therapy** can be used to prevent or treat iron overload in patients with high transfusion requirements.

Risk Modification

- **Dehydration and hypoxia** should be avoided as they may precipitate or exacerbate irreversible sickling.
- **Folic acid** (1 mg PO daily) is administered to patients with SCD because of chronic hemolysis.
- **Hydroxyurea** (15 to 35 mg/kg PO daily) has been shown to increase levels of Hb F and significantly decreases the frequency of VOC and acute chest syndrome in adults with SCD (*N Engl J Med 1995;332:1317*).
- **Antimicrobial prophylaxis** with penicillin VK, 125 mg PO bid to age 3 years and then 250 mg PO bid until age 5 years, is effective at reducing risk of infection (*N Engl J Med 1986;314:1593*). Patients who are allergic to penicillin should receive erythromycin 10 mg/kg PO bid. Prophylaxis should be stopped at age 5 years to avoid development resistant organisms (*J Pediatr 1995;127:685*).
- **Immunizations** against the usual childhood illnesses should be given to children with SCD, including hepatitis B vaccine. After 2 years of age, a polyvalent pneumo-coccal vaccine should be administered. Yearly influenza vaccine is recommended.
- **Ophthalmologic examinations** are recommended yearly in adults because of the high incidence of proliferative retinopathy.
- Local and regional anesthesia can be used without special precautions. Care should be taken to avoid volume depletion, hypoxia, and hypernatremia. For major surgery, RBC transfusions to increase the Hb to 10 g/dL is as effective as more aggressive thresholds (*N Engl J Med 1995;333:206*).

G6PD Deficiency

GENERAL PRINCIPLES

G6PD deficiency represents the most common disorder of RBC metabolism world-wide. Deficiency of G6PD renders RBCs more susceptible to oxidative damage through decreased glutathione reduction leading to chronic or acute episodic hemoly-sis in the presence of oxidative stress.

Classification

With greater than 400 variants recognized, the severity of hemolysis depends on the degree of deficiency present (*Blood Rev 2007;21:267*).

- Milder forms, such as those seen in men of African heritage in the United States, result in self-limiting acute hemolytic episodes.
- More severe forms, such as the Mediterranean variant, can result in severe hemolysis.
- The most severe type causes a chronic, hereditary, nonspherocytic hemolytic anemia in the absence of an inciting cause.

Epidemiology
- X-linked inheritance, thus degree of involvement in females is dependent on lyonization.
- In the United States, 10% of African American males are affected by a mild form (G6PD A-).
- G6PD is felt to be protective against malaria, thus accounting for its prevalence in malaria-stricken areas.
- Hemolysis is triggered by exposure to mediators of oxidative stress (i.e., drugs [Table 21-7]), infections, and fava beans.

DIAGNOSIS

- Examination of a peripheral blood smear reveals presence of "bite cells" and **Heinz bodies** (represents precipitated Hb within RBCs).
- Diagnosis is determined by showing deficient amounts of reduced nicotinamide adenine dinucleotide phosphate (NADPH) generated from NADP using quantitative spectrophotometric analysis or rapid fluorescent screening test.
- False-negative results may occur in patients with high levels of reticulocytes and young RBCs as these cells have innate higher levels of G6PD.

TREATMENT

- Hemolytic crises tend to be self-limiting; thus, the mainstay of treatment is supportive.
- The underlying cause of oxidative stress should be addressed (i.e., treatment of infection, removal of drug).

Autoimmune Hemolytic Anemia

GENERAL PRINCIPLES

Definition
Autoimmune hemolytic anemia (AIHA) results from autoantibodies targeted to antigens on the patient's own RBCs, resulting in extravascular hemolysis (removal of RBC by tissue macrophages in the liver or spleen.

Classification
There are two main causes of AIHA: warm and cold AIHA. Warm AIHA antibodies interact best with RBCs at 37°C, while cold AIHA antibodies are most active at temperatures below 37°C.

Table 21-7 Drugs that Can Induce Red Blood Cell Disorders

| | | | Immune Hemolytic Anemia | |
| | | | Autoantibody | Hapten | Immune Complex[b] |
Sideroblastic Anemia	Aplastic Anemia[a]	G6PD Deficiency			
Chloramphenicol	Acetazolamide	Dapsone	α-Methyldopa	Ak-Fluor 25%	Amphotericin B
Cycloserine	Antineoplastic drugs	Doxorubicin	Cephalosporins	Cephalosporins	Antazoline
Ethanol	Carbamazepine	Methylene blue	Diclofenac	Penicillins	Cephalosporins
Isoniazid	Chloramphenicol	Nalidixic acid	Ibuprofen	Tetracycline	Chlorpropamide
Pyrazinamide	Gold salts	Nitrofurantoin	Interferon alpha	Tolbutamide	Diclofenac
	Hydantoins	Phenazopyridine	L-Dopa		Diethylstilbestrol
	Penicillamine	Primaquine	Mefenamic acid		Doxepin
	Phenylbutazone	Sulfacetamide	Procainamide		Hydrochlorothiazide
	Quinacrine	Sulfamethoxazole	Teniposide		Isoniazid
		Sulfanilamide	Thioridazine		p-Aminosalicylic acid
		Sulfapyridine	Tolmetin		Probenecid
					Quinidine
					Quinine
					Rifampin
					Sulfonamides
					Thiopental
					Tolmetin

Note: Data compiled from multiple sources. Agents listed are available in the United States.

[a]Drugs with >30 cases reported; many other drugs rarely are associated with aplastic anemia and are considered low risk.

[b]Some sources list mechanisms for many of these drugs as unknown.

G6PD, glucose-6-phosphate dehydrogenase.

Adapted from Cooper DH, Krainik AJ, Lubner SJ, et al., eds. *The Washington Manual of Medical Therapeutics*. 32nd ed. Philadelphia: Lippincott Williams & Wilkins, 2007.

Etiology

- Warm antibody AIHA is usually caused by an IgG autoantibody. It may be idiopathic or secondary to an additional process (i.e., lymphoma, chronic lympho-cytic leukemia [CLL], collagen vascular disorder, or drugs [see Table 21-7]).
- Cold antibody AIHA is typically caused by an IgM autoantibody (in cold aggluti-nin disease).
  - The acute form is often secondary to an infection (*Mycoplasma*, Epstein–Barr virus).
  - The chronic form is usually due to a paraprotein associated with lymphoma, CLL, or Waldenström macroglobulinemia in approximately one-half of cases, and is usually idiopathic in the others.

DIAGNOSIS

Clinical Presentation

- Clinical presentation varies based on the degree of hemolysis and type of AIHA.
- In AIHA, mild cases may be clinically asymptomatic with only lab data suggesting the diagnosis. In fulminant cases, the rapid decrease in Hb can be severe with inadequate compensatory erythropoiesis, leading to fever, chest pain, dyspnea, and hemodynamic instability. Jaundice, scleral icterus, and dark urine can result from indirect hyperbilirubinemia.

Diagnostic Testing

- Basic laboratory data should support the presence of hemolysis with: anemia, reticulo-cytosis, elevated LDH, decreased haptoglobin, and indirect hyperbilirubinemia.
- Peripheral blood smear may show spherocytes, occasional fragmented RBCs, polychromasia, and nucleated RBCs.
- The hallmark of diagnosis is by a positive **DAT (aka direct Coombs)**. The DAT detects the presence of IgG or complement bound to the RBC surface and may be falsely negative in cases of IgM mediated hemolysis.
  - Warm AIHA: IgG and/or C3+
  - Cold AIHA: IgG− and C3+
- The indirect antiglobulin test (indirect Coombs) detects the presence of autoanti-bodies in the serum but can also detect alloantibodies in the serum from alternate causes including those causes from transfusion or maternal–fetal incompatibility.
- An elevated cold agglutinin titer is seen with cold AIHA.
- If secondary AIHA is suspected, a workup for the underlying cause should be performed.

TREATMENT

- Initial therapy should be aimed at correcting complications from the hemolytic anemia. Definitive therapy should include identification and treatment of any underlying cause.
- **RBC transfusions may exacerbate hemolysis** with hemolysis of transfused cells. RBCs should only be transfused when the patient is symptomatic or there is decreased oxygen-carrying capacity (e.g., Hb <6 g/dL). Autoantibodies may con-found plasma antibody screens and conventional cross-matches and, therefore, alloantibodies may go undetected.

- **Warm AIHA**
  - **Glucocorticoids**, such as prednisone 1 mg/kg/d, are the first-line treatment in warm AIHA. They decrease macrophage clearance of antibody coated RBCs. Response is typically seen in 7 to 10 days. When hemolysis has abated, glucocorticoids can be tapered over 2 to 3 months. Rapid steroid taper can result in relapse.
  - **IVIG** is less effective in AIHA than in idiopathic thrombocytopenic purpura (ITP) with a response rate of 40% (*Am J Hematol 1993;44:237*). IgG from the IVIG binds to hepatic and splenic macrophages and prevents binding and clearance of antibody coated RBCs.
  - **Splenectomy** should be considered for steroid-resistant AIHA.
  - Rituximab 375 mg/m^2 weekly for four doses, has shown efficacy in small case series of AIHA (*Br J Haematol 2001;114:244*).
- **Idiopathic cold AIHA**
  - Avoidance of cold exposure can minimize exacerbations. RBC transfusions at 37°C and keeping the room warm can prevent exacerbation of hemolysis.
  - Glucocorticoids and splenectomy have low efficacy in treatment.
  - Plasma exchange removes approximately 80% of IgM thus offer effective control of the disease.
  - Rituximab has been demonstrated as effective in small series (*Blood 2004;103(8): 2925*).

Drug-Induced Hemolytic Anemia

GENERAL PRINCIPLES

- **Drug-induced hemolytic anemia** is anemia resulting from exposure to a medication. Table 21-7 lists common offensive medications. Hemolysis occurs by one of three different mechanisms.
- **Drug-induced autoantibodies** occur with exposure to the offensive agent and act similarly in warm AIHA. Laboratory testing reveals a DAT positive for IgG.
- **Hapten formation** can occur when a drug (usually an antimicrobial) coats RBC membranes, forming a new antigenic determinant. If antibodies against the drug are present and the patient receives the drug (particularly at high doses), a DAT-positive hemolytic anemia may result.
- **Immune complexes** occur in most cases of drug-induced hemolysis. IgM (occasionally IgG) antibodies may develop against a drug and form a drug–antibody complex that adheres to the RBCs. The DAT is positive only for C3.

TREATMENT

Treatment consists of discontinuing the offending agent.

Microangiopathic Hemolytic Anemia

GENERAL PRINCIPLES

Definition

Microangiopathic hemolytic anemia (MAHA) is a syndrome of traumatic (microangiopathic) intravascular hemolysis. MAHA is a morphologic classification in which fragmented RBCs (schistocytes) are seen on peripheral blood smear. It is not a specific diagnosis but suggests a limited differential diagnosis.

Etiology

Possible causes of MAHA include **mechanical heart valve**, **malignant hypertension**, **vasculitis**, **adenocarcinoma**, **preeclampsia/eclampsia**, **disseminated intravascular coagulation (DIC)**, **thrombotic thrombocytopenic purpura (TTP)**, and **hemolytic uremic syndrome (HUS)/atypical HUS** (see Chapter 20, Disorders of Hemostasis and Thrombosis, for a discussion of DIC, TTP, and HUS/atypical HUS).

DIAGNOSIS

MAHA is established by confirming the presence of hemolysis with laboratory data and identifying RBC fragments (schistocytes) on peripheral blood smear.

TREATMENT

The treatment depends on the underlying etiology of microangiopathy.

WHITE BLOOD CELL DISORDERS

Leukocytosis and Leukopenia

GENERAL PRINCIPLES

Definition
- Leukocytosis is an elevation in the absolute WBC count ($>10,000/mm^3$).
- Leukopenia is a reduction in the WBC count ($<3,500$ cells/mm^3).

Etiology
- **Leukocytosis**
  - An elevated WBC can be the normal response of BM to an infectious or inflammatory process, steroid, β-agonist or lithium therapy, splenectomy, or stress and is usually associated with an **absolute neutrophilia**.
  - Occasionally, leukocytosis is due to a primary BM disorder in WBC production, maturation, or death (apoptosis). This may occur in the setting of leukemia or myeloproliferative disorders and can affect any cell in the leukocyte lineage.
  - A "**leukemoid reaction**" is defined as an excessive WBC response (i.e., $>50,000/mm^3$) associated with a cause outside the BM that can be reactive or malignant in origin.
  - Lymphocytosis is less commonly encountered and is typically associated with atypical infections (i.e., viral), medication use, or leukemia/lymphoma.
- **Leukopenia**
  - Leukopenia can occur in response to infection (i.e., HIV), inflammation, primary BM disorders (i.e., malignancy), medications, environmental exposure (i.e., heavy metals or radiation), and vitamin deficiencies.
  - The majority of cases are due to medication induced (i.e., chemotherapeutic or immunosuppressive drugs).

DIAGNOSIS

Clinical Presentation

- Patients can present with a wide variety of nonspecific symptoms, which are typically related to the underlying cause.
- **Leukostasis** is a medical emergency that occurs in settings with extreme elevations of WBC count (i.e., >100,000/mm^3) and results from WBC plugs in the microvasculature leading to tissue hypoperfusion and ischemia. Common symptoms include central nervous system (CNS) symptoms suggestive of stroke, vision changes, dyspnea, renal insufficiency, or even myocardial infarction. The most common disorders associated with leukostasis and their corresponding average WBC counts at onset of leukostasis include acute myelogenous leukemia (AML) (>100,000/mm^3), CLL (>400,000/mm^3), and chronic myeloid leukemia (CML) with blast crisis (>100,000/mm^3).
- A severe neutropenia with an ANC (<500/mm^3) increases the risk of a life-threatening bacterial infection. If patients present with **neutropenic fever**, immediate treatment with broad-spectrum antibiotics should be instituted.

History
A careful history, including the temporal nature of the symptoms, specific infectious symptomatology, and a detailed medication history should be elicited.

Physical Examination
- Splenomegaly and lymphadenopathy may be present depending on underlying cause.
- Associated thrombocytopenia may lead to petechiae and ecchymoses.

Diagnostic Testing

Laboratories
- A CBC with peripheral smear is necessary for the evaluation of WBC disorders.
- The presence of blasts on a peripheral smear is concerning for acute leukemia and warrants emergent evaluation.
- A BCR-abl molecular study may be warranted in cases of unexplained neutrophilia to diagnose CML.
- Additional laboratory abnormalities are related to the underlying disorder and may include elevation in LDH and uric acid from the high cell turnover in acute leukemia.
- An infectious workup should be performed as indicated, including assessment for HIV.

Diagnostic Procedures
A BM biopsy with ancillary studies such as cytogenetics and flow cytometry may be required to establish the diagnosis.

TREATMENT

- The primary goal of therapy is treatment of the underlying cause.
- See Chapter 22, Medical Management of Malignant Disease, for the treatment of acute and chronic leukemia.
- If symptoms are present suggestive of **leukostasis**, emergent leukopheresis should be done to decrease WBC burden and relieve symptoms. If left unattended, leukostasis can result in death.

- Growth factor support should be considered in patients with chronic neutropenia and ongoing infections until the neutropenia resolves (see Oncologic Emergencies in Chapter 22, Medical Management of Malignant Disease).

PLATELET DISORDERS

Discussed in Chapter 20, Disorders of Hemostasis and Thrombosis.

BONE MARROW DISORDERS

Myelodysplastic Syndrome

Discussed in Chapter 22, Medical Management of Malignant Disease.

Myeloproliferative Disorders

GENERAL PRINCIPLES

Myeloproliferative disorders (MPDs) are a group of clonal disorders characterized by clonal expansion of a hematopoietic stem cell resulting in overproduction of mature, largely functional cells. The 2008 World Health Organization (WHO) designated seven conditions as MPDs, including polycythemia vera (PV), essential thrombocytosis (ET) (discussed in Chapter 20, Disorders of Hemostasis and Thrombosis), CML (discussed in Chapter 22, Medical Management of Malignant Disease), primary myelofibrosis (PMF), chronic neutrophilic leukemia, chronic eosinophilic leukemia, and mast cell disease (*Cancer 2009;17:3842*). The most common MPDs include PV, ET, CML, and PMF. This chapter will focus on PV and PMF as ET and CML are discussed elsewhere.

DIAGNOSIS

Clinical Presentation

Presenting symptoms of MPDs are nonspecific and include fatigue, pruritus, drenching night sweats, fever, and weight loss (*Cancer 2007;1:68*). Patients with PV can also present with hemorrhagic or thrombotic symptoms.

Diagnostic Criteria

- **PV**

  Initial diagnostic criteria for PV were established by the Polycythemia Vera Study Group in 1975 (*Semin Hematol 1975;4:339*); however, more recently a modified set of criteria have been proposed (*N Engl J Med 2006;355:2452*). The modified criteria include Hct >52% in males or >48% in females in addition to presence of JAK2 mutation. In the absence of JAK2 mutation, four major criteria or three major and two minor criteria need to be met for diagnosis (Table 21-8).

- **PMF**

  The WHO diagnostic criteria for PMF are listed in Table 21-9 (*Blood 2007;110: 1092*). All three major criteria and at least two minor criteria need to be met for the diagnosis.

Table 21-8	Diagnostic Criteria for Polycythemia Vera	

Presence of JAK2 Mutation	**Absence of JAK2 Mutation** Four Major **or** Three Major + Two Minor	
	Major Criteria	**Minor Criteria**
Hct >52% in males	Hct >60% in males	Platelets >450,000/cumm
Hct >48% in females	Hct >56% in females	Neutrophils >10,000/cumm
	Palpable splenomegaly	Radiographic splenomegaly
	No secondary erythrocytosis	
	Presence of genetic mutations (excludes JAK2)	Low serum erythropoietin

Hct, hematocrit.

Diagnostic Testing

Laboratories

Laboratory data ranges widely depending on the underlying MPD. Patients with PMF may present with cytopenias. Patients with PV typically present with an elevated Hct and platelet count (>400,000), presence of JAK2 V617F mutation (>95%), and decreased EPO levels.

Diagnostic Procedures

A BM biopsy should be included in the diagnostic workup of MPDs and can establish the diagnosis of primary myelofibrosis.

Table 21-9	Diagnostic Criteria for Primary Myelofibrosis

Major Criteria

Presence of megakaryocyte proliferation and atypia, usually accompanied by either reticulin and/or collagen fibrosis.

Not meeting WHO criteria for PV, CML, MDS, or other myeloid neoplasm.

Presence of JAK2 or other clonal marker, or no evidence of bone marrow fibrosis due to underlying inflammatory or neoplastic diseases in the absence of a clonal marker.

Minor Criteria

Leukoerythroblastosis
Increase in serum LDH level
Anemia
Palpable splenomegaly

CML, chronic myelogenous leukemia; LDH, lactate dehydrogenase; MDS, myelodysplastic syndrome; PV, polycythemia vera; WHO, World Health Organization.

TREATMENT

- **PV:** The main treatment options include serial phlebotomy myelosuppressive agents, most commonly hydroxyurea. Aspirin is commonly added for the prevention of thrombosis. Choices depend on the risk for thrombosis.
  - In patients with low risk for thrombosis (age <60 years, no history of thrombosis): serial phlebotomy to keep goal Hct <45% in men and <42% in women.
  - Patients with high risk for thrombosis (age >60 years, prior thrombosis) should be treated with serial phlebotomy and hydroxyurea.
- **PMF:** In the absence of adverse prognostic factors such as anemia and constitutional symptoms, treatments may not be needed. In patients with signs and symptoms of PMF, treatment is recommended.
  - Allogeneic hematopoietic stem cell transplantation (HCT) is the only curative therapy.
  - Other than HCT, multiple supportive modalities can be considered, including:
    - Blood transfusions.
    - Hydroxyurea, to treat splenomegaly, constitutional symptoms, and pruritus.
    - Lenalidomide, to treat symptomatic patients with 5q-.
    - Ruxolitinib, a new JAK inhibitor, approved in 2011 is effective to palliate constitutional symptoms and symptomatic splenomegaly.
    - Splenic irradiation, can treat painful splenomegaly; however, effects are usually transient.
    - Radiation therapy, for symptomatic areas of extramedullary hematopoiesis or cord compression.

OUTCOME/PROGNOSIS

The prognosis of PMF is determined by several scoring systems that can be used at different stage of the disease, which is outside of the scope of this book, but readers can refer to the references for further details.

- IPSS (International Prognostic scoring system): Used upon presentation (*Blood 2009;113(13):2895*).
- DIPSS (Dynamic IPSS): Used over time after diagnosis (*Blood 2010;115(9):1703*).
- DIPSS Plus: Incorporated several IPSS-independent prognostic factors such as unfavorable cytogenetics, red cell transfusion dependence, and thrombocytopenia (*J Clin Oncol 2011;29(4):392*).

MONOCLONAL GAMMOPATHIES

Monoclonal Gammopathy of Unknown Significance

GENERAL PRINCIPLES

Definition

Monoclonal gammopathy of unknown significance (MGUS) is a premalignant condition characterized by the presence of a small (<10%) population of neoplastic, clonal plasma cells in the BM that occurs in the absence of related end organ damage.

Epidemiology

The incidence of MGUS increases with age; with estimates of occurrence in 3.2% of Caucasians >50 years and 7.5% in those ≥85 years (*N Engl J Med 2006;354:1362*).

DIAGNOSIS

- Patients with MGUS are asymptomatic and commonly diagnosed when a small monoclonal protein is detected on serum protein electrophoresis during workup of an elevated protein. Most of the gammopathies are identified as IgG, but gammopathies in all Ig classes occur.
- The Multiple Myeloma International Working Group identified diagnostic criteria for MGUS in 2003. All three criteria are required:
  - Presence of a serum monoclonal protein (M protein) IgG, IgA, or IgM <3 g/dL.
  - Presence of clonal BM plasma cells comprising <10% of the marrow.
  - Absence of end organ damage attributed to the underlying plasma cell disorder, such as hypercalcemia, renal insufficiency, anemia, or lytic bone lesions.

TREATMENT

There is currently no treatment indicated for MGUS. The vast majority of patients will not progress to a malignant disease. Generally, it is accepted practice to follow these patients annually with an evaluation that includes serum protein electropheresis (SPEP), urine protein electrophoresis (UPEP), CBC, and serum creatinine. If patients develop symptoms concerning for a malignant plasma cell disease, they should undergo an extensive evaluation.

PROGNOSIS

MGUS can evolve into multiple myeloma in a small portion of patients with an average rate of 1% per year. Risk of progression is characterized in Table 21-10 (*Blood 2005;106:812*).

Table 21-10	Risk of Monoclonal Gammopathy of Unknown Significance Progression to Multiple Myeloma	
Risk	**Number of Risk Factors**	**Absolute Risk of Progression at 20 Years**
Low	0	5%
Low intermediate	1	21%
Intermediate high	2	37%
High	3	58%

Risk factors: M protein >1.5 g/dL; non-IgG monoclonal gammopathy of unknown significance, abnormal serum free light chain ratio (<0.26 or >1.65).

Multiple Myeloma

Discussed in Chapter 22, Medical Management of Malignant Disease.

Waldenström Macroglobulinemia

GENERAL PRINCIPLES

Waldenström macroglobulinemia is an uncommon IgM monoclonal disorder also known as lymphoplasmacytic lymphoma, characterized by mild hematologic abnormalities, and accompanied by tissue infiltration including lymphadenopathy, splenomegaly, or hepatomegaly. Because of its high molecular weight and concentration, IgM gammopathy can lead to hyperviscosity (CNS, visual, cardiac) manifestations.

TREATMENT

- Treatment with chemotherapy is usually successful in achieving a response (*Am J Hematol 2012;87(4):503*).
- Patients with complications of viscosity often benefit from treatment with plasmapheresis to decrease the IgM concentration.

Amyloidosis

GENERAL PRINCIPLES

Primary (AL) amyloidosis is an infiltrative disorder due to monoclonal, light-chain deposition in various tissues most often involving the kidney (renal failure, nephrotic syndrome), heart (nonischemic cardiomyopathy), peripheral nervous system (neuropathy), and GI tract/liver (macroglossia, diarrhea, nausea, vomiting). Unexplained findings in any of these organ systems should prompt evaluation for amyloidosis.

DIAGNOSIS

- An M protein in urine or serum is found in >90% of patients and helps establish the diagnosis. Biopsy of an affected organ or BM is often done; diagnosis is made by identification of amyloid protein in the biopsy tissue.
- Several effective chemotherapy regimens have been developed during the last decade (*Oncology 2012;26(2):152*). However, treatment of amyloidosis is difficult and progressive organ failure is frequent.

OUTCOME/PROGNOSIS

Cardiac involvement with amyloidosis has a particularly poor prognosis with a median survival of <1 year.

Transfusion Medicine

GENERAL PRINCIPLES

Transfusion is a commonly used therapy for a variety of hematologic and hemostatic disturbances. The benefits and risks must be carefully weighed in each situation because blood products are a limited resource with potentially life-threatening side effects.

TREATMENT

- **Packed red blood cells (pRBCs)**. RBC transfusion is indicated to increase the oxygen-carrying capacity of blood in anemic or bleeding patients.
  - Hb threshold for transfusion (in general):
    - Stable patient, no cardiac risk: 7 g/dL.
    - Coronary artery disease or risk of ischemia: May consider a higher threshold (7 to 10 g/dL), although survival is not improved by higher thresholds (*N Engl J Med 1999;340:409*).
  - One unit of pRBCs increases the Hb level by approximately 1 g/dL or Hct by 3% in the average adult.
  - If the cause of anemia is easily treatable (e.g., iron or folic acid deficiency) and no cerebrovascular or cardiopulmonary compromise is present, it is preferable to avoid transfusion.
- **Fresh frozen plasma (FFP):** Plasma transfusion is used to replace certain plasma proteins, usually coagulation factors, to treat bleeding or as bleeding prophylaxis for patients undergoing invasive procedures.
  - Common indications include:
    - Prolonged prothrombin time (PT) or activated partial thromboplastin time (aPTT) (1.5 times normal) in a bleeding patient.
    - Warfarin overdose with life-threatening bleeding.
    - Factor deficiencies for which specific factor concentrates are unavailable.
  - The usual dose is 10 to 20 mL/kg. One unit of FFP contains approximately 250 mL of plasma and 250 U of factor activity for each factor.
  - Plasma should not be used as a volume expander and is usually not indicated in patients who are not currently bleeding, even those with an abnormal PT or aPTT. In the case of warfarin overdose with a very prolonged PT but no bleeding, vitamin K should be used instead.
- **Platelets:** Platelet transfusion is indicated to prevent or treat bleeding in a thrombocytopenic patient or patients with dysfunctional platelets (e.g., due to aspirin)
  - Platelet count threshold for transfusion (in general):
    - Nonbleeding, stable inpatients: 10×10^9/L.
    - Nonbleeding, stable outpatients: 20×10^9/L.
    - Major invasive procedures or bleeding: 50×10^9/L.
    - High-risk surgery (e.g., neurosurgery) or life-threatening bleeding may require higher thresholds.
  - One unit of platelets increases the platelet count by approximately 30 to 50×10^9/L.
  - Platelets have a short shelf life (<5 days) and are stored at room temperature; they must never be placed on ice or refrigerated, which can cause platelet activation.
  - **Platelet refractoriness** (poor response to transfusion) may be due to immunologic causes (anti-ABO, anti-HLA, or antiplatelet antibodies) or nonimmunologic

causes (e.g., sepsis, DIC, fever, active bleeding, splenic sequestration, certain drugs).

Immunologic causes are likely if a 10- to 60-minute posttransfusion platelet count shows little increment and may be prevented in future transfusions by the use of ABO- and/or HLA-compatible platelets (*Br J Haematol 2008;142:348*).

- **Cryoprecipitate**
  - Cryoprecipitate contains the cold-precipitated portion of plasma and is enriched in the following factors:
    - Fibrinogen
    - von Willebrand factor (VWF)
    - Factor VIII
    - Factor XIII
  - It is most commonly indicated to replace **fibrinogen** in patients with hypofibrinogenemia or DIC, and should not be used to replace VWF or factor VIII, for which specific factor concentrates exist.
  - One unit increases fibrinogen concentration by approximately 7 to 8 mg/dL. Doses are frequently ordered in pools of 5 or 10 U.

SPECIAL CONSIDERATIONS

- **Pretransfusion testing**
  - The **type and screen** procedure tests the recipient's RBCs for the A, B, and D (Rh) antigens and also screens the recipient's serum for antibodies against other RBC antigens.
  - The **cross-match** tests the recipient's serum for antibodies against antigens on the donor's RBCs and is performed before a specific unit of blood is dispensed for a patient. May be omitted and replaced by a virtual "electronic cross-match" when the recipient's type has been confirmed on a repeat typing.
- **Modifications of blood products**
  - **Leukoreduction** is performed by the use of filters to eliminate WBC contamination prestorage or at the bedside. Indicated for all patients to reduce the risk of the following transfusion complications:
    - Nonhemolytic febrile transfusion reactions
    - Transfusion-transmitted CMV infection
    - Formation of HLA alloantibodies
  - **CMV-seronegative** blood products may be indicated for immunocompromised patients who are CMV-seronegative to reduce the risk of CMV transmission. However, prestorage leuko-reduced products are considered equivalently "CMV-reduced-risk" and can be used in place of CMV-seronegative products.
  - **Gamma-irradiation** eliminates immunologically competent lymphocytes in order to prevent transfusion-associated graft-versus-host disease and is indicated for certain immunocompromised patients, BM transplant recipients, or patients who receive directed donations from HLA-matched donors or relatives.
  - **Washing** of blood products is rarely indicated but should be considered for patients in whom plasma proteins may cause a serious reaction (e.g., recipients with IgA deficiency or a history of anaphylactic reactions).
- **Procedures**
  - Patient and blood product identification procedures must be carefully followed to avoid mistransfusion and ABO-incompatible transfusion.
  - The IV catheter should be at least 18 gauge to allow adequate flow.

- All blood products should be administered through a 170- to 260-μm "standard" filter to prevent infusion of macroaggregates, fibrin, and debris.
- Patients should be observed with vital signs for the first 10 to 15 minutes of each transfusion for adverse effects and at regular intervals thereafter.
- Infusion is typically administered over 1 to 2 hours, with a maximum of 4 hours.
- **Emergency transfusion** may be considered in situations in which massive blood loss has resulted in cardiovascular compromise.
  - Volume expansion with normal saline should be attempted initially.
  - Before the patient's ABO type can be confirmed, "emergency release" blood may be used, consisting of uncross-matched group O pRBCs and group AB plasma.
  - If **massive transfusion** (replacement of ≥10 U pRBCs in less than 24 hours) is indicated, hemostatic components (plasma, platelets, and cryoprecipitate) should be included to correct the loss and dilution of hemostatic factors. In addition, care must be taken to manage the potential iatrogenic complications of massive transfusion, such as hypothermia, hypocalcemia (due to the citrated preservative solution), and hyperkalemia.

COMPLICATIONS

- **Transfusion-transmitted infections**
  - Donors and blood products are screened for HIV-1/2, human T-lymphotropic virus I/II (HTLV I/II), hepatitis B, hepatitis C, West Nile virus, syphilis, *Trypanosoma cruzi* (Chagas), and bacteremia.
  - Viral transmission may occur when donors are in the "window period" (i.e., undetectable to testing).
    - The risk of hepatitis B transmission is approximately 1 in 300,000; other tested viruses have a transmission risk of less than 1 in 1,000,000.
    - CMV transmission risk may be reduced in immunocompromised patients by the use of CMV-seronegative or prestorage leuko-reduced products.
  - Bacterial transmission may occur from either a donor infection or a contaminant at the time of collection or processing.
    - Platelet transfusions are more likely than RBCs to have bacterial contamination because they are stored at room temperature.
    - The most common organism identified in RBCs is *Yersinia enterocolitica* and in platelets is *Staphylococcus* spp.
- **Noninfectious hazards of transfusion**
  - **Acute hemolytic transfusion reactions** are usually caused by **preformed antibodies** in the recipient and are characterized by intravascular hemolysis of the transfused RBCs soon after the administration of ABO-incompatible blood.
    - **Fever, chills, back pain, chest pain, nausea, vomiting, anxiety, and hypotension** may develop. Acute renal failure with hemoglobinuria may occur. In the unconscious patient, hypotension or hemoglobinuria may be the only manifestation.
    - If a hemolytic transfusion reaction is suspected, **the transfusion should be stopped immediately and all IV tubing should be replaced**. Samples of the patient's blood should be delivered to the blood bank along with the remainder of the suspected unit for repeat of the cross-match. Direct and indirect Coombs tests should be performed, and the plasma and freshly voided urine should be examined for free Hb.

- Management includes preservation of intravascular volume and protection of renal function. Urine output should be maintained at ≥100 mL/hr with the use of IV fluids and diuretics or mannitol, if necessary. The excretion of free Hb can be aided by alkalinization of the urine. Sodium bicarbonate can be added to IV fluids to increase the urinary pH to ≥7.5 (see Chapter 13, Renal Diseases).

- **Delayed hemolytic transfusion reactions** typically occur 3 to 10 days after transfusion and are caused by either a primary or an anamnestic antibody response to specific RBC antigens on donor RBCs.
  - Hb and Hct levels may fall.
  - The DAT is usually positive, resulting in confusion with AIHA.
  - May at times be severe; these cases should be treated similarly to acute hemolytic reactions.

- **Nonhemolytic febrile transfusion reactions** are characterized by fevers and chills.
  - Cytokines released from white cells are thought to be the cause.
  - Treatment and future prophylaxis may include acetaminophen and prestorage leuko-reduced blood products.

- **Allergic reactions** are characterized by urticaria and, in severe cases, bronchospasm and hypotension.
  - The reactions are due to plasma proteins that elicit an IgE-mediated response. The reaction may be specific to the plasma proteins of a particular donor and therefore may occur infrequently or never again.
  - Treatment and future prophylaxis may include antihistamines such as diphenhydramine.
  - **Anaphylactic reactions** may require the addition of glucocorticoids and washed or plasma-reduced products. Additionally, check serum immunoglobulins because patients with IgA deficiency who receive IgA-containing blood products may experience anaphylaxis with small exposure to donor plasma.

- **Transfusion-associated circulatory overload** (TACO) is a relatively common yet underrecognized complication of blood transfusion. Volume overload with signs of CHF may be seen when patients with cardiovascular compromise are transfused. The clinical and radiographic features may be indistinguishable from that of transfusion-related acute lung injury (TRALI) (see the following text). In critically ill patients, more invasive techniques may be required for a definitive diagnosis (*Crit Care Med 2006;34(5 suppl):S109*). Slowing the rate of transfusion and judicious use of diuretics help prevent this complication.

- **TRALI** is indistinguishable from acute respiratory distress syndrome and occurs within 6 hours of a transfusion.
  - Symptoms include dyspnea, hypoxemia, hypotension, fever, and chills.
  - Anti-HLA or antineutrophil antibodies in the donor's serum directed against the recipient's WBCs are thought to cause the disorder.
  - On recognition, transfusions must be stopped and the blood bank notified so that other products from the donor(s) in question may be quarantined.
  - Hypoxemia resolves rapidly, typically in about 24 hours, but ventilatory assistance may be required.
  - Despite clinical or radiographic findings that suggest pulmonary edema, data indicate that diuretics have no role and may be detrimental (*Blood 2005; 105(6):2266*).

- **Transfusion-associated graft-versus-host disease** is a very rare but serious complication usually seen in immunocompromised patients (and immunocompetent patients receiving blood from a relative) and is thought to result from the infusion of immunocompetent donor T lymphocytes.

- Symptoms include rash, elevated liver function tests, and severe pancytopenia.
- Mortality is >80%.
- **Irradiation** of blood products for at-risk patients prevents this disease.

○ **Posttransfusion purpura** is a rare syndrome of severe thrombocytopenia and purpura or bleeding that starts 7 to 10 days after exposure to blood products. This disorder is described in Chapter 20, Disorders of Hemostasis and Thrombosis, the Platelet Disorders section.

Medical Management of Malignant Disease

Saiama N. Waqar, Janakiraman Subramanian, George Ansstas, and Ramaswamy Govindan

Medical Management of Malignant Disease

Cancer is the leading cause of mortality in developed countries and the second leading cause of death in developing countries (*CA Cancer J Clin 2011;61:69*). The pace of research in oncology has accelerated dramatically over the past decade due to advances in genomics, drug development, and supportive care. Improved understanding of the critical interacting molecular pathways operative in cancer cells has led to the development of molecularly targeted agents that produce meaningful clinical benefit. The successes with trastuzumab in breast cancer, imatinib in gastrointestinal stromal tumors (GISTs) and chronic myeloid leukemia (CML), gefitinib and erlotinib in patients with non–small cell lung cancer (NSCLC) whose tumors carry activating mutations in the tyrosine kinase domain of the epidermal growth factor receptor (EGFR), and vemurafenib in BRAF mutation–positive melanoma illustrate the promise of this approach. This chapter provides an overview of cancer therapy.

Approach to the Cancer Patient

GENERAL PRINCIPLES

Principles of targeted therapy
- The advent of molecularly targeted agents has led to marked advances in the treatment of certain malignancies including CML, breast cancer, and lung cancer. These agents have specific toxicities that can be significant.
- The most common classes of drugs are as follows: (1) monoclonal antibodies, given intravenously, and designed to bind to cell surface molecules (e.g., cetuximab, panitumumab, bevacizumab, trastuzumab) and (2) oral receptor tyrosine kinase inhibitors ([TKIs]; e.g., erlotinib, gefitinib, imatinib, lapatinib, sunitinib, sorafenib) (Table 22-1).
- Most antibodies are used in combination with chemotherapy or radiation, whereas most TKIs are used as single agents.
- The majority of targeted agents have a moderate effect and prolong the time to disease progression. A few of these agents result in a striking benefit, including the following:
  - Imatinib in CML inhibits the bcr-abl tyrosine kinase and leads to prolonged remissions.
  - Imatinib in GISTs inhibits C-Kit and leads to marked disease regression.

Table 22-1   Most Frequently Used Targeted Therapies for Common Malignancies and Typical Side Effects

Target/Agent	Indication										Side effects								
	Gliomas	Lung	Breast	GI stromal tumor	Pancreas/biliary	Colon/rectal	Kidney	Hepatocellular	Chronic myeloid	Head and neck	Acneiform rash	Diarrhea	Pneumonitis	Nausea	Cardiac dysfunction	Hand-foot	Hypertension	Vascular toxicity	Cytopenias
EGFR																			
Erlotinib		■			▨						■	■	▨						
Gefitinib		■									■	▨							
Cetuximab		▨				■				■	■	▨							
Panitumumab						■					▨								
Her2																			
Trastuzumab			■												▨				
Her2 and EGFR																			
Lapatinib			▨											▨					
bcr-abl/c-Kit																			
Imatinib				■					■					▨					▨
Nilotinib									▨					▨					▨
Dasatinib									▨					▨					▨
Antiangiogenics																			
Bevacizumab		■	■			■									▨		▨	■	
Sunitinib				▨			■								▨	▨	▨	▨	
Sorafenib							■	▨							▨	▨	▨	▨	
mTOR																			
Temsirolimus							▨												▨
Everolimus							▨												▨

■ Most frequent   ▨ Common   □ Rare

EGFR, epidermal growth factor receptor; mTOR, mammalian target of rapamycin.

- ○ Gefitinib and erlotinib in lung cancer inhibit EGFR, leading to marked benefits in patients with mutations in EGFR (approximately 10% of lung cancer patients).
- ○ Crizotinib leads to similar benefit in 5% of patients with lung cancer, whose tumors carry EML4-ALK translocations.
- ○ Trastuzumab in resected breast cancer, when used in the adjuvant setting, reduces relapse by 50%.
- Toxicities of targeted therapies are unique to each agent (summarized in Table 22-1), but some helpful generalizations can be made.

Table 22-2	Most Common Cancer Diagnoses and Rates of Death in the United States for 2010				
Sites	New Cases			Deaths		

Sites	Both Sexes	Male	Female	Both Sexes	Male	Female
Lung	222,520	116,750	105,770	157,300	86,220	71,080
Prostate	217,730	217,730	—	32,050	32,050	—
Breast	209,060	1,970	207,090	40,230	390	39,840
Colon	102,900	49,470	53,430	51,370	26,580	24,790
Bladder	70,530	52,760	17,770	14,680	10,410	4,270
Non-Hodgkin's lymphoma	65,540	35,380	30,160	20,210	10,710	9,500

Data from Jemal A, Siegel R, Xu J, Ward W. Cancer Statistics, 2010. *CA Cancer J Clin* 2010;60:277–300.

○ Inhibitors of EGFR frequently cause an acne-like rash on the face and upper chest, which can be severe. Treatment is typically with topical corticosteroids or oral minocycline.
○ Inhibitors of Her2 are associated with a reversible decline in cardiac systolic function and ejection fraction should be monitored.
○ Inhibitors of angiogenesis are associated with endothelial toxicity leading to hypertension, proteinuria, delayed wound healing, mild cardiac toxicity, increased risk of bleeding, thromboembolism, and GI perforation/fistula. All antiangiogenics should be held in the perioperative period.

Epidemiology

• Cancer accounts for 1 in 4 deaths in the United States, with as estimated 1,529,560 new cancer cases, and 569,490 deaths from cancer occurred in the year 2010 (*CA Cancer J Clin 2010;60:277*). Tables 22-2 and 22-3 illustrate the incidence and mortality from the most common malignancies in the United States and worldwide.
• Cancer is associated with aging and has increased as life expectancy has increased. Median age at diagnosis for all cancers in the United States is 67 years (*CA Cancer J Clin 2008;58:71*).
• Tobacco is the most common cause of cancer death and is associated with lung, head and neck, esophageal, gastric, pancreatic, kidney, and bladder cancers.
• Diet, obesity, and inactivity likely contribute to many malignancies.

DIAGNOSIS

• A tissue diagnosis is required prior to any medical or radiation therapy.
• **Cytology** specimens may contain only a few malignant cells and are often the least invasive to obtain. Examples include cervical brushings (Pap smears), endoscopic brushings, and samples of sputum, urine, and pleural, pericardial, or peritoneal fluid. Cytology is not the preferred approach specifically to diagnose and characterize subtypes of lymphoma. Even in other malignancies, the current approach is to get core biopsy with material adequate not just for morphology but also for additional molecular studies. Increasingly, cytology is mainly used either to confirm recurrence of cancer or to confirm the presence of malignancy in an additional site (e.g.,

Table 22-3	Most Common Cancer Diagnoses in Incidence and Mortality Worldwide for 2008		
New Cases		**Deaths**	
Male	Female	Male	Female
Lung (1,095,200)	Breast (1,383,500)	Lung (951,000)	Breast (458,400)
Prostate (903,500)	Colorectal (570,100)	Liver (478,300)	Lung (427,400)
Colorectal (663,600)	Cervix (529,800)	Stomach (464,400)	Colorectal (288,100)
Stomach (640,600)	Lung (513,600)	Colorectal (320,600)	Cervix (275,100)
Liver (522,400)	Stomach (349,000)	Esophagus (276,100)	Stomach (273,600)

Data from Jemal A, Bray F, Center MM, et al. Global cancer statistics. *CA Cancer J Clin* 2011;61:69–90.

cytologic analysis of pleural fluid in a patient with biopsy confirmed lung cancer). **Fine needle aspiration (FNA)** provides a cytology specimen. It is usually validated by a cytopathologist at the bedside and performed with multiple passes of a small-bore needle into a solid lesion. Tissue architecture cannot be observed.

- **Histology** rather than cytology is preferred for most malignancies and is essential for suspected lymphoma. This can be obtained by a large-core needle biopsy, excisional biopsy, or surgical resection.

TREATMENT

- **Staging and treatment planning**
  - Cancer stage is an assessment of the extent of tumor spread and treatment is based on staging.
  - Most malignancies are staged by the tumor, lymph node, and metastasis (TNM) system from stages I to IV. The T classification is based on the size and extent of local invasion. The N classification describes the extent of lymph node involvement, and the M classification is based on the presence or absence of distant metastasis.
  - Appropriate radiologic staging must be performed before therapy, usually including computed tomographic (CT) imaging. Fluorodeoxyglucose-positron emission tomography (FDG-PET) adds to CT in select malignancies. Brain imaging with magnetic resonance imaging (MRI; preferable) or CT with intravenous contrast should be considered in advanced melanoma and lung and kidney cancer. See tumor type discussion for further details.
  - Complete surgical staging provides more accurate extent of the disease than clinical staging and is possible only in patients with resectable disease when surgery is performed with an intent to cure.
  - Tumor grade is an assessment by the pathologist of the tumor's similarity to the cell of origin and the proliferation rate, usually low, moderate, or high grade. Tumor grade is rarely used in treatment decisions, except in certain malignancies (i.e., sarcoma).

Table 22-4	Eastern Cooperative Oncology Group Score

Grade	Description
0	Fully active, able to carry on all predisease performance without restriction.
1	Restricted in physically strenuous activity but ambulatory and able to carry out work of a light or sedentary nature (e.g., light housework, office work).
2	Ambulatory and capable of all self-care but unable to carry out any work activities. Up and about >50% of waking hours.
3	Capable of only limited self-care, confined to bed or chair >50% of waking hours.
4	Completely disabled. Cannot carry on any self-care. Totally confined to bed or chair.
5	Dead.

From Oken MM, Creech RH, Tormey DC, et al. Toxicity and response criteria of the Eastern Cooperative Oncology Group. *Am J Clin Oncol* 1982;5:649.

- Once the staging workup is completed, treatment decisions are made often using a multidisciplinary approach. This process is facilitated by weekly "tumor board" conferences that enable surgeons, radiation oncologists, medical oncologists, radiologists, pathologists, and other support staff collectively plan the treatment approach. Cancer care is truly a **team effort**.
- Presence or absence of comorbidities and performance status guide extent of therapy. The commonly used scale for assessing performance status is the one developed by the Eastern Cooperative Oncology Group (ECOG) (Table 22-4).
- **Principles of radiation**
  - Collaboration with a radiation oncologist is critical for the management of most patients. Radiation planning is designed to deliver a precise dose of ionizing radiation to a tumor while sparing surrounding tissues.
  - External beam radiation is the most common modality, but brachytherapy (radio-active implants) is effective in certain settings.
  - **Curative** intent radiotherapy is used in several settings.
    - **Neoadjuvant:** Preoperative therapy intended to reduce both the extent of surgery and the risk of local relapse.
    - **Adjuvant:** Postoperative intended to reduce the risk of local relapse.
    - **Definitive:** High dose with curative intent, usually not followed by surgery.
    - **Concurrent chemoradiation:** Chemotherapy with definitive radiation significantly increases toxicity but increases efficacy in some settings.
  - **Palliative** radiotherapy is used in lower dosing to reduce symptoms, including bony pain, obstruction (esophageal, bronchial), bleeding (GI, gynecologic, bronchial, cutaneous), and neurologic symptoms (brain metastasis).
- **Principles of chemotherapy**
  - Traditional, cytotoxic chemotherapy targets all dividing cells and has broad toxicities.
  - Chemotherapy is typically given in 2-, 3-, or 4-week "cycles." In most regimens, intravenous treatment is given on the first day of the cycle, with no further treatment until the next cycle. In other regimens, treatments are weekly for 2 or 3 weeks, with 1 week off prior to the next cycle.
  - **Curative** intent chemotherapy includes neoadjuvant, adjuvant, and chemoradiation protocols in solid tumors. Chemotherapy alone is curative in many lymphomas, leukemias, and germ cell tumors (GCT).

- ○ **Palliative** chemotherapy is used in advanced solid tumors and hematologic malignancies, with a focus on prolonging survival without overly affecting quality of life. Should only be used in patients with a good performance status.
- ○ Specific chemotherapy protocols are beyond the scope of this text. Table 22-5 lists the most common malignancies and the chemotherapy agents that are most frequently used in each protocol but is not all inclusive.
- ○ Chemotherapy toxicities are widely variable and potentially life threatening. Table 22-6 lists the most clinically significant toxicities for common chemotherapy agents but should not be considered all inclusive. Toxicities are also entirely dependent on the dose and route of administration. Toxicity management is discussed at the end of this chapter.
- ○ Most agents have a very narrow therapeutic index and dosing is based on body surface area (mg/m^2).

Surgical Management

- Goals of therapy, cure versus palliation, must guide any surgical intervention.
- Surgical resection is often performed only when there is a possibility of cure, although palliative surgery is performed to relieve discomfort (mastectomy for local control in a patient with metastatic disease) in some malignancies.
- Complete lymph node staging provides useful information for postoperative treatment planning (adjuvant therapy).
- Surgical resection of isolated metastatic sites in select patients can improve survival. Examples include solitary brain metastases, pulmonary metastases from colorectal cancer or sarcomas, and liver metastases from colorectal cancer.

OUTCOME/PROGNOSIS

- The goal of therapy (cure vs. palliation) must be clear to the patient. High-risk or highly toxic therapies are not appropriate in a noncurative setting.
- Patients diagnosed with cancer often expect to hear an estimate of life expectancy, and physicians often feel obligated to provide such estimates. However, such temporal estimates are often incorrect and unhelpful, given the variability in disease and response to treatment.
- It is more accurate and easier to describe the likelihood of surviving to a defined time point (i.e., 1-year or 5-year survival rate) rather than giving an individual a specific time frame (i.e., median survival). It is important to underscore the enormous variability in the outcomes even within a seemingly homogenous group (e.g., stage I NSCLC) due to molecular heterogeneity of cancer. It is critical to emphasize the difference between accurately describing a group statistic ("1-year survival of patients with metastatic NSCLC is around 40%") and erroneously attributing the median survival as a true measure of one's individual's life expectancy ("you have 9 months to live").

Lung Cancer

GENERAL PRINCIPLES

Epidemiology

Lung cancer is the most common cause of cancer death in the United States, accounting for 157,300 deaths in 2010. Smoking is the greatest risk factor for lung cancer, with over 90% of cases tobacco related. The risk remains greater even 20 to 30 years after quitting

Table 22-5	Most Frequently Used Chemotherapies for Common Malignancies

Legend: ■ Most frequent ▦ Common ☐ Rare

Agent	Gliomas	Head and neck	Lung	Breast	Esophageal/gastric	Pancreas/biliary	Colon/rectal	Kidney	Bladder	Prostate	Germ cell	Gynecologic	Sarcoma	Lymphoma	Leukemia
Platinum agents															
Cisplatin		■	■		■	▦			■		■	■	■	▦	▦
Carboplatin		■	■	▦							▦	■		▦	
Oxaliplatin					▦		■								
Antimetabolites															
5-FU		■			■	▦	■		■						
Capecitabine				■	▦		■								
Gemcitabine			■	▦		■			■				▦		
Methotrexate		▦							▦					▦	
Pemetrexed			■												
Cytarabine															■
Fludarabine															■
Alkylators															
Cyclophosphamide				■										▦	■
Ifosfamide												▦	■		
Temozolomide	■														
Dacarbazine													▦	▦	
Anthracyclines															
Doxorubicin				■					▦				■	▦	■
Epirubicin				▦	■									▦	
Idarubicin															■
Mitoxantrone										▦					
Microtubule agents															
Vincristine												▦		■	■
Vinorelbine			■	▦											
Paclitaxel		■	■	■	▦							■			
Docetaxel		■	■	■	■					■		▦			
Other															
Etoposide			■								■		■	▦	■
Irinotecan					▦		■								
Topotecan			▦									■			
Bleomycin											■			▦	

■ Most frequent   ▦ Common   ☐ Rare

Am J Clin Oncol 1982;5:649.

Table 22-6 Most Frequent Toxicities for Common Chemotherapy Agents

Legend: ■ Frequent/Severe ▨ Less common/Mild ☐ Uncommon

	Cytopenias	Nausea	Mucositis	Diarrhea	Nephrotoxicity	Cardiac	Neuropathy	Fatigue	Vesicant	Late leukemia	Hair loss	Unique toxicity
Platinum agents												
Cisplatin	▨	■			■	▨	■	■				Hearing loss, low Mg/K
Carboplatin	■	▨			▨			▨				Low Mg/K
Oxaliplatin	▨	▨					■	▨				Cold sensitivity
Antimetabolites												
5-FU	▨		▨	■		▨		▨				Hand–foot syndrome
Capecitabine	▨			■				▨				Hand–foot syndrome
Gemcitabine	▨							▨				TTP/HUS
Methotrexate	■		■	▨	■			▨			▨	Accumulates in effusions
Pemetrexed	▨							▨				
Alkylators												
Cyclophosphamide	▨	■	▨		▨	▨		▨			■	Hemorrhagic cystitis
Ifosfamide	■	■	▨		▨	▨		■			▨	Encephalopathy, cystitis
Temozolomide	▨	▨						▨				
Anthracyclines												
Doxorubicin	■	■	▨			■			▨		■	
Epirubicin	■	■	▨			■			▨	■	▨	
Mitoxantrone	▨	▨	▨			▨		▨		▨	▨	
Microtubule agents												
Vincristine	▨						■	▨			■	Constipation
Vinorelbine	▨						▨	▨				Constipation
Paclitaxel	■			▨			■	▨			■	
Docetaxel	■	▨	▨	▨			▨	■			■	Nail loss, fluid retention
Other												
Etoposide	■	▨						▨		▨	▨	
Irinotecan	■	▨		■				▨			▨	Acute hypercholinergic reaction
Topotecan	■	▨						▨			■	
Bleomycin			▨		▨			▨		■	▨	Pulmonary fibrosis

TTP/HUS, thrombotic thrombocytopenic purpura/hemolytic uremic syndrome.

smoking. Asbestos exposure is strongly linked to mesothelioma (cancer of the pleura) and other lung cancers, particularly in smokers. Another risk factor is radon exposure.

Pathology

NSCLC accounts for over 85% of cases. The most common histologic subtypes are adenocarcinoma and squamous cell carcinoma, with large cell, bronchoalveolar, and other subtypes being less common. Distinction between squamous cell and other histologic subtypes is important and influences treatment options. Small-cell (formerly "oat-cell") carcinoma is of neuroendocrine origin and is treated in a manner different from that of NSCLC.

DIAGNOSIS

Clinical Presentation

- Most common local symptoms are cough, dyspnea, postobstructive pneumonia, hemoptysis, or chest wall pain. Less common symptoms are Pancoast syndrome from superior sulcus tumors (shoulder pain, brachial plexus symptoms, and Horner's syndrome); superior vena cava compression (SVC syndrome) with face and arm plethora or swelling; or voice hoarseness from recurrent laryngeal nerve involvement. Widespread disease presents with fatigue, cachexia, bone pain, or neurologic symptoms from central nervous system (CNS) metastasis.
- **Paraneoplastic syndromes** include hypercalcemia (usually caused by squamous cell), hyponatremia, syndrome of inappropriate antidiuretic hormone secretion (usually caused by small-cell carcinoma), and hypertrophic pulmonary osteoarthropathy (clubbing, joint pain, swelling).

Diagnostic Testing

- Screening for lung cancer is controversial. However, any patient with a smoking history and concerning pulmonary symptoms should undergo a chest CT scan. A normal chest radiograph does not exclude lung cancer. Diagnosis can be made from pleural fluid cytology, bronchoscopy with biopsy, brushings, or washings, or ultrasound/CT-guided needle biopsy. Core needle biopsy is preferable to FNA.
- **Staging evaluation:** In all patients, it should include CT scan of chest and abdomen, bone scan, brain MRI (preferred), or head CT scan. In potentially curable patients, evaluation includes PET scan and mediastinoscopy (Table 22-7).

Table 22-7	Simplified Tumor, Lymph Node, and Metastasis Staging System for Lung Cancer		
Tumor	**Lymph Node Involvement**		
	None	Hilar	Mediastinal
T1–T2: <7 cm, no local invasion	I	II	III
T3: Invasive but resectable	II	III	III
T4: Usually unresectable	III	III	III
Pleural or distant spread	IV	IV	IV

TREATMENT

- **NSCLC**
  General
  - Stage I: Surgery is preferred with no further therapy; 70% chance of cure.
  - Stage II: Surgery followed by adjuvant cisplatin-based chemotherapy; 50% chance of cure (*J Clin Oncol 2008;26:3552*).
  - Stage III: Usually concurrent radiation and chemotherapy; surgery in selected patients; <15% chance of cure.
  - Stage IV: Palliative chemotherapy, not curable; 40% of patients have 1-year survival. Recent advances in the treatment of stage IV NSCLC include the use of targeted agents, such as bevacizumab and erlotinib, and factoring histology and genetic mutations into treatment decisions. Front-line platinum-based doublet chemotherapy provides modest improvement in survival (*N Engl J Med 2002;346:92*). In patients with nonsquamous histology, treatment options include front-line platinum and pemetrexed (a folate antagonist) doublet therapy (*J Clin Oncol 2008;26:3543*) or addition of bevacizumab, a vascular endothelial growth factor (VEGF) inhibitor, to platinum-based doublet chemotherapy (*J Clin Oncol 2009;27:1227*). Epidermal growth factor receptor tyrosine kinase inhibitors (EGFR-TKIs) such as gefitinib and erlotinib can be used as front-line therapy in patients whose tumors carry activating mutations of the EGFR tyrosine kinase domain but not in patients with EGFR wild-type tumors (*N Engl J Med 2009;361:947*). Crizotinib is an anaplastic lymphoma kinase (ALK) inhibitor approved for use in patients with advanced NSCLC whose tumors carry the EML4-ALK fusion gene (*N Engl J Med 363:1693*).
- **Small-Cell Lung Cancer**
  - "Limited stage" (stages I to III): Concurrent chemotherapy (cisplatin and etoposide) and radiation lead to a 10% to 20% chance of cure.
  - "Extensive stage" (stage IV): Combination chemotherapy (cisplatin with etoposide or irinotecan) has very high response rate, but all patients relapse with treatment-resistant disease. One-year survival is 30% from time of diagnosis (*J Clin Oncol 2006;24:2038*).
  - Prophylactic cranial irradiation is used in select patients to prevent brain metastasis.

Breast Cancer

GENERAL PRINCIPLES

Epidemiology

Breast cancer is the most common cause of cancer in women in developed countries. Over 220,000 patients develop breast cancer per year in the United States and less than 1% of cases are reported in men. Approximately 1 in 10 women in the United States eventually develop breast cancer.

Pathophysiology

- Noninvasive: Ductal carcinoma in situ (DCIS) and lobular carcinoma in situ (LCIS).
- Invasive: Ductal carcinoma is more common than lobular carcinoma.

- Estrogen receptor (ER): Positive in 60% of cases; confers a good prognosis and sensitivity to endocrine therapies.
- Progesterone receptor (PR): Usually correlates with ER.
- Her2, measured by immunohistochemistry (IHC) or fluorescent in situ hybridization (FISH): Approximately 20% of all patients have high levels of Her2 expression and it confers not only poor prognosis but sensitivity to targeted therapies (trastuzumab, lapatinib).

Risk Factors
- Risk factors include a family history, early menarche, late menopause, late first pregnancy, obesity, and hormone replacement therapy (*N Engl J Med 2009;360:573*).
- **Genetics:** *BRCA1* and *BRCA2* mutations are associated with approximately 50% lifetime risk of breast cancer. *BRCA1* is also associated with ovarian cancer. Only 5% to 6% of all breast cancers are attributable to mutations involving susceptibility genes.

Prevention
- Prophylactic mastectomy/oophorectomy is recommended for carriers of *BRCA1* or *BRCA2* mutations.
- Chemoprevention with ER modulators tamoxifen and raloxifene is an option in women with high risk for developing breast cancer (family history and LCIS).
- Monthly self-exam starting at age 20 years. Age 20 to 40 years, clinical breast exam every 3 years. Annual mammogram and clinical breast exam at ages 40 to 70 years.

DIAGNOSIS

Clinical Presentation
- Patients present with mass usually found on screening mammography or by examination.
- Premenopausal women: A breast mass can be observed 1 month for change.

Diagnostic Testing
Imaging
- Bilateral mammogram and subsequent biopsy for any clinically concerning mass, even with a normal mammogram.
- Chest radiograph in most patients, CT of chest, abdomen and pelvis if lymph node–positive disease.

TREATMENT

- **Endocrine therapies**
  - Tamoxifen, an estrogen antagonist, in breast cancer treatment (agonist in bone/endometrium).
  - Oophorectomy/ovarian suppression with luteinizing hormone-release hormone (LHRH) agonists (goserelin, leuprolide) for premenopausal women.
  - Aromatase inhibitors (AIs) block androgen to estrogen conversion (letrozole, anastrozole, exemestane) in peripheral tissues for postmenopausal women.
  - Fulvestrant, an ER antagonist, for postmenopausal women

- **Treatment of DCIS:** Lumpectomy with adjuvant radiation. Repeat resections for positive margins are often necessary. Tamoxifen if the tumor is ER positive.
- **Treatment of LCIS:** Usually multifocal disease, no role for multiple resections. Prophylactic mastectomy is an option, otherwise tamoxifen is recommended.
- **Adjuvant medical therapy for resectable breast cancer**
  - Neoadjuvant chemotherapy can be used to facilitate surgery in large tumors.
  - Adjuvant endocrine therapy is recommended for ER/PR+ tumors: With tamoxifen (if premenopausal) or an AI (if postmenopausal). Treatment duration is 5 to 10 years.
  - Adjuvant chemotherapy is generally recommended for lymph node–positive disease, any tumor >2 cm, tumors >1 cm if ER/PR negative, and tumors >0.5 cm if Her2+.
  - AC + T (Adriamycin and cyclophosphamide, followed by paclitaxel) and TC (docetaxel and cyclophosphamide) are some of the most common adjuvant regimens used in the United States. In addition, there are several other chemotherapy regimens that are excellent options.
  - Adjuvant trastuzumab (Herceptin, anti-Her2 antibody) for 1 year improves survival and is used for most Her2+ tumors (*N Engl J Med 2005;353:1673*). Trastuzumab is associated with congestive heart failure (usually reversible), and cardiac function should be monitored.
- **Treatment of metastatic breast cancer**
  - Many patients with ER/PR+ metastatic disease live for >5 years with endocrine therapy alone. The goal of therapy is to prevent symptoms/progressive disease with minimal impact on quality of life.
  - Radiation therapy is preferred for symptomatic bone or brain metastases.
  - Endocrine therapy is recommended in ER/PR+ patients except in the case of symptomatic visceral metastases. Multiple endocrine agents should be tried before chemotherapy.
  - Single agent rather than combination chemotherapy is preferred in most patients.
  - Trastuzumab improves outcomes with endocrine or chemotherapy in Her2+.
  - Lapatinib is an oral inhibitor of EGFR and Her2 and is used in combination with capecitabine (*N Engl J Med 2006;355:2733*).

Surgical Management

- Lumpectomy (breast conservation therapy) with adjuvant radiation is equivalent to mastectomy (*N Engl J Med 1995;332:907*).
- Sentinel lymph node biopsy at the time of surgery, if the result is negative, can substitute for complete axillary lymph node dissection.

Head and Neck Cancer

GENERAL PRINCIPLES

Epidemiology

Head and neck (H&N) cancer includes squamous cell carcinoma of the lip, oral cavity, pharynx, and larynx. In the United States, approximately 40,000 patients were diagnosed with H&N cancer in the year 2012. Tobacco smoking and alcohol consumption are associated with increased risk of developing H&N cancer. Human papillomavirus (HPV) infection is implicated in oropharyngeal squamous cell carcinomas.

DIAGNOSIS

Clinical Presentation

Oral mass/ulcer, dysphagia, voice hoarseness, or neck mass (lymph node involvement).

Diagnostic Testing

- Complete ear, nose, and throat (ENT) evaluation with biopsy of primary lesion and laryngoscopy.
- **Staging evaluation:** Examination under anesthesia. CT of head, neck, and chest. Whole body PET scan in select patients.

TREATMENT

- **Stage Classification:** Stage I to II disease is resectable with no lymph node involvement. Stage III tumors are larger or have isolated lymph node involvement. Local invasion or significant lymph node involvement is stage IVA/B and distant metastasis is stage IVC.
- **Treatment by stage**
  - Early stage (I to II): Either surgery or definitive radiation would be the appropriate choice.
  - Locally advanced (stage III to IVA/B): Treatment approaches include:
    - Definitive surgical resection followed by adjuvant radiation with or without chemotherapy
    - Concurrent chemotherapy with radiation
    - Induction chemotherapy followed by concurrent chemotherapy with radiation
  - Metastatic (IVC): Palliative chemotherapy.
  - **Supportive care:** Dental evaluation is required prior to radiation therapy and in some cases completed dental extraction may be necessary, particularly in patients with poor oral hygiene. Patients undergoing definitive radiation or adjuvant radiation may develop severe mucositis requiring the placement of gastric feeding tube for nutrition.
  - **Chemotherapy:** Cisplatin is the preferred agent in combination with definitive radiation therapy. Induction regimens usually involve taxane and platinum combination followed concurrent chemotherapy with radiation.
  - **Targeted therapy:** Cetuximab, a monoclonal antibody to EGFR, can also be used in combination with definitive radiation (*N Engl J Med 2006;354:567*).
  - **Complications** of treatment can be extensive. Surgery may lead to loss of speech (laryngectomy), permanent tracheostomy, and disfigurement. Swallowing can be impaired and lead to aspiration. Radiation can lead to severe xerostomia.

Sarcoma

GENERAL PRINCIPLES

Epidemiology

In the United States, approximately 14,000 patients were diagnosed with sarcomas in the year 2012. These comprise a minority of adult malignancies but 7% of pediatric malignancies. Risk increases with age and is also associated with prior radiation, chemical, and chemotherapy exposures.

Etiology

Genetics: Neurofibromatosis type I is linked to neurofibrosarcoma. Li-Fraumeni syndrome (loss of p53) has a high rate of osteosarcoma and other sarcomas. Patients with Gardner's syndrome and tuberous sclerosis are also at risk. Several sarcomas have been linked to specific, acquired translocations including Ewing's sarcoma: t(11;22), synovial sarcoma: t(X;18), alveolar rhabdomyosarcoma: t(2;13), and myxoid liposarcoma: t(12;16).

Pathology

The most common sarcomas in adults are "soft tissue sarcomas," with the most common locations being in the extremities or retroperitoneum, and are treated similarly. These include malignant fibrous histiocytoma, liposarcoma, and leiomyosarcoma. GIST, osteosarcoma, and Ewing's sarcoma have unique features and are treated differently.

DIAGNOSIS

Clinical Presentation

Varies according to the site of disease.

Diagnostic Testing

- MRI for sarcomas involving the extremities or pelvis.
- CT for retroperitoneal sarcomas.
- PET/CT not recommended for routine staging but may be helpful in detecting occult metastasis and in distinguishing between malignant peripheral nerve sheath tumor (MPNST) from a neurofibroma.

TREATMENT

- **Soft tissue sarcoma/osteosarcoma:** Resection followed by adjuvant chemotherapy and/or radiation for high-grade tumors. Metastatic sites should be resected if feasible.
- **GIST:** Most common site is stomach, followed by small bowel. Surgery should be performed if feasible. Most GISTs overexpress c-KIT and are highly responsive to imatinib (oral TKI). Adjuvant imatinib can be considered in select patients.
- **Ewing's sarcoma:** Treated similarly to soft tissue sarcoma but more responsive to chemotherapy. Metastatic disease may still be cured with chemotherapy.

GASTROINTESTINAL MALIGNANCIES

Esophageal Cancer

GENERAL PRINCIPLES

Epidemiology

Esophageal cancer accounts for an estimated 14,500 deaths in the United States in 2010. Esophageal cancer is three to four times more common in men than in women.

Risk factors include tobacco, alcohol, obesity, gastroesophageal reflux disease, Barrett's esophagus, achalasia, and caustic injury.

Pathology

Adenocarcinomas are most common in the lower third of the esophagus and at the gastroesophageal junction and have had a sharp increase in incidence over the past few decades in the United States. Squamous cell carcinomas more common in the upper and middle esophagus.

DIAGNOSIS

Clinical Presentation

Usually progressive dysphagia and weight loss. Other symptoms include odynophagia, cough, and hoarseness.

Diagnostic Testing

- CT of the chest and abdomen. If no metastatic disease, endoscopic ultrasound (EUS) for the definition of tumor depth and lymph node status and FDG-PET to rule out regional and distant metastases.
- Upper endoscopy with biopsy.

TREATMENT

- **Early stage disease:** Usually defined as no invasion through the adventitia (T1 to T2) and no nodal or distant metastases. Patients who are medically fit should undergo esophagectomy.
- Locally advanced disease: Patient diagnosed with esophageal cancer with invasion of the adventitia (T3) or lymph node involvement are best considered for potentially curative concurrent chemoradiation, although some prefer to resect these tumors after induction therapy.
- Metastatic disease is usually treated with palliative chemotherapy.

Gastric Cancer

GENERAL PRINCIPLES

Epidemiology

Gastric cancer accounted for an estimated 10,570 deaths in the United States in 2010. Over 70% of new cases are diagnosed in developing countries. The highest incidence rates are in Eastern Asia, Eastern Europe, and South America, while the lowest incidence is in North America and Africa. Risk factors include *Helicobacter pylori* infection, previous partial gastrectomy for benign ulcer, cigarette smoking, and blood group A.

Pathophysiology

More than 90% are adenocarcinomas, subdivided according to Lauren's classification into intestinal or diffuse types. Intestinal type is more common in older patients and has a better prognosis. Diffuse type is more prevalent in younger patients and women, is not associated with dietary patterns, and is the most common subtype in the United States.

DIAGNOSIS

- Most common symptoms are decreased appetite, weight loss, and abdominal discomfort. Dysphagia may occur with gastroesophageal junction tumors and persistent vomiting if there is pyloric obstruction. Physical exam may show metastases to the left supraclavicular node (Virchow's node) or periumbilical node (Sister Mary Joseph's node).
- Diagnosis is established by upper endoscopy. CT of the chest and abdomen in all patients, and CT of the pelvis in women exclude ovarian involvement (Krukenberg tumor). Other tests include *H. pylori* testing, EUS, and PET scan. Staging laparoscopy may be indicated prior to surgery in patients with otherwise resectable tumors.

TREATMENT

Medically fit patients with resectable disease should undergo surgery. Chemotherapy or chemoradiotherapy are commonly used, either before or after the resection, except in patients with very early stage disease. Patients with unresectable disease are treated with palliative chemotherapy. Herceptin should be used in combination with chemotherapy in patients with Her2 gastric cancer (*Lancet 2010;376:687*).

Colorectal Cancer

GENERAL PRINCIPLES

Epidemiology

Colorectal cancer is the third most common malignancy worldwide. The incidence is higher in Western industrialized countries, with 102,900 cases diagnosed in the United States in 2010. Risk factors include age >50 years, physical inactivity, obesity, diet with increased red meat and decreased fiber, personal history of polyps or colorectal cancer, inflammatory bowel disease, and hereditary syndromes (familial adenomatous polyposis and hereditary nonpolyposis colorectal cancer [HNPCC]).

DIAGNOSIS

Clinical Presentation

Most common symptoms include bleeding, abdominal pain, change in bowel habits, and obstruction. Any unexplained iron deficiency anemia should be evaluated with upper and lower endoscopy to evaluate for a GI malignancy. Otherwise, carcinomas are identified from screening colonoscopy.

Diagnostic Testing

- Diagnosis is typically made through colonoscopy with biopsy.
- Imaging studies include CT scan of the chest, abdomen, and pelvis. FDG-PET scan is not routinely indicated.
- Additional studies include serum carcinoembryonic antigen (CEA) levels.

Table 22-8	Simplified Tumor, Lymph Node, and Metastasis Staging System for Colorectal Cancer	
T Status	**Lymph Node Involvement**	
	None	**Present**
T1–T2: No serosal invasion	I	III
T3–T4: Local invasion	II	III
Distant metastases	IV	IV

TREATMENT

- **Treatment of colon cancer**
  - **Localized disease** should be treated with surgical resection. Adjuvant chemotherapy is indicated in patients with stage III disease and may also be beneficial in selected patients with stage II disease (Table 22-8). **Surveillance** after successful therapy includes (1) history, physical exam, and CEA levels every 3 to 6 months for 2 years and then every 6 months for 3 years; (2) CT scan annually for the first 3 years; and (3) colonoscopy within 1 year of resection, at 3 years, and then every 5 years.
  - **Metastatic disease** is treated with combination chemotherapy, usually including fluorouracil (5-FU), leucovorin, oxaliplatin (FOLFOX), or irinotecan (FOLFIRI). The combination of bevacizumab, a VEGF monoclonal antibody, and chemotherapy improves survival compared with chemotherapy alone (*J Clin Oncol 2007;25: 1539*). Cetuximab, an antibody against the EGFR, is also associated with improved outcomes if the *K-ras* gene is not mutated.
  - **Isolated liver metastases** may be treated with surgical resection, preceded or not by neoadjuvant chemotherapy, with curative intention.
- **Treatment of rectal cancer:** Patients without metastatic disease should undergo endorectal ultrasound for the evaluation of T and N status. Adjuvant or neoadjuvant therapy is indicated for patients with stage II or III disease. Concurrent neoadjuvant chemoradiation is commonly used to decrease the risk of local recurrence and downsize the tumor, facilitating sphincter preserving surgery (see Table 22-8). Patients with metastatic disease should be treated similarly to those with colon cancer.

Pancreatic Cancer

GENERAL PRINCIPLES

Epidemiology

Pancreatic adenocarcinoma is the fourth most common cause of cancer-related death in the United States. Incidence increases with age, with median age at diagnosis between 60 and 80 years. Risk factors include cigarette smoking, diabetes mellitus, and inherited syndromes (*BRCA2* mutation, *HNPCC*).

DIAGNOSIS

Clinical Presentation

Common symptoms include jaundice, anorexia, weight loss, and abdominal pain. Pancreatic cancer should be suspected when diabetes mellitus develops suddenly in patients older than 50 years, particularly if associated with abdominal pain, anorexia, or weight loss. Early staged disease is usually found incidentally on abdominal CT.

Diagnostic Testing

Imaging

Diagnosis is usually suspected by the presence of a pancreatic mass or dilated biliary duct on CT scan or ultrasound. Pancreas protocol CT with thin slices is recommended to evaluate for resectability defined as absence of distant metastases, patent superior mesenteric and portal veins, and absence of celiac and superior mesenteric artery involvement.

Diagnostic Procedures

- Those with resectable disease may have a tissue diagnosis by ERCP or EUS-guided FNA.
- In case of metastatic disease, biopsy of the metastatic lesion is preferred.

TREATMENT

- **Treatment of localized disease:** Surgical resection is the only potentially curative therapy. Approximately 20% of patients are candidates for surgery, which is typically a pancreaticoduodenectomy (Whipple procedure). Patients who have adequately recovered from surgery may benefit from adjuvant chemotherapy or chemoradiotherapy. More than 80% of patients suffer relapse even with optimal therapy.
- **Treatment of unresectable disease:** Locally invasive disease may be treated with chemotherapy or chemoradiotherapy, whereas those with metastatic disease are typically treated with chemotherapy. The most frequently used chemotherapy for metastatic pancreatic carcinoma is gemcitabine, either alone or in combination with erlotinib (*J Clin Oncol 2007;25:1960*). FOLFIRINOX, a combination chemotherapy regimen consisting of oxaliplatin, irinotecan, fluorouracil, and leucovorin, is an option for use in patients with good performance status, and is associated with more toxicity than gemcitabine, but improved survival (*N Engl J Med 2011; 364(19):1817*).

Hepatocellular Carcinoma

GENERAL PRINCIPLES

Epidemiology

Hepatocellular carcinoma (HCC) is the fifth most frequently diagnosed cancer in men worldwide, and the second most common cause of cancer death. It is the seventh most commonly diagnosed cancer in women, and the sixth leading cause of cancer-related mortality. An estimated 24,120 patients were diagnosed with liver and intrahepatic bile duct tumors in 2010 in the United States. Risk factors include chronic viral hepatitis B or C, alcohol abuse, autoimmune hepatitis, and hemochromatosis. Approximately 80% to 90% of the patients with HCC have **cirrhosis**.

DIAGNOSIS

Clinical Presentation

Common symptoms include abdominal pain, anorexia with weight loss, jaundice, and vomiting. Invasion of the hepatic veins may cause Budd–Chiari syndrome, characterized by tender hepatomegaly and tense ascites. HCC should be suspected in patients with stable cirrhosis and rapid decompensation, including ascites, encephalopathy, and variceal bleeding. Most common paraneoplastic syndromes include hypoglycemia, hypercalcemia, and erythrocytosis. α-Fetoprotein (AFP) levels are increased in approximately 50% of patients in the United States.

Diagnostic Testing
- The classic feature of HCC in CT or MRI is rapid enhancement during the arterial phase of contrast administration, followed by "washout" during the later venous phases. Patients with liver lesions >2 cm, AFP level >200 ng/mL, and **radiologic features suggestive of HCC on two imaging modalities may be diagnosed without biopsy**. Lesions <1 cm have low probability of being HCC and should be followed with repeated imaging to detect growth suspicious of malignancy (*Hepatology 2005;42:1208*). PET scan may identify extrahepatic metastases.
- Those with lesions between 1 and 2 cm should undergo percutaneous biopsy.

TREATMENT

Other Nonpharmacologic Therapies
- **Local therapy:** Percutaneous ethanol injection, radiofrequency ablation, cryoablation, transarterial chemoembolization, and liver radiation may be used for palliation for nonsurgical candidates or to control tumor growth while waiting for transplant.
- **Chemotherapy** has minimal efficacy in HCC, with doxorubicin being the most common agent used. The small molecule TKI sorafenib is well tolerated and improves survival modestly compared to best supportive care (*N Engl J Med 2008; 359:378*).

Surgical Management
The only potentially curative treatment is surgical resection, which can be considered in lesions <5 cm not involving major vessels. Liver transplant is an option for selected patients with cirrhosis since it addresses both the malignancy and the underlying disease. Indications for liver transplant include the following: (1) absence of distant metastases; (2) not a candidate for liver resection; (3) absence of major vessel involvement; (4) single tumor <5 cm; and (5) three or fewer tumors, not larger than 3 cm.

GENITOURINARY MALIGNANCIES

Renal Cancer

GENERAL PRINCIPLES

Epidemiology
Renal cancer accounts for 60,000 cases per year in the United States, with 13,000 deaths. More commonly diagnosed in men (1.5:1) and the risk increases with age. Other risk factors include tobacco smoking, obesity, and hypertension. Medullary renal carcinoma is associated with sickle cell disease.

Etiology

Genetics: Vast majority of the cases are sporadic. Von Hippel-Lindau syndrome (VHL) carries a high risk of clear cell renal cell carcinoma (RCC). *VHL* gene mutations increase hypoxia-inducible factor, which increases angiogenesis.

Pathology

RCC is a malignancy of the renal parenchyma. Clear cell RCC is the most common (80%), followed by papillary (15%) and chromophobic (5%) RCCs. Transitional cell carcinoma (TCC) of the renal pelvis is similar to bladder cancer and management is also similar to that of bladder cancer.

DIAGNOSIS

Clinical Presentation

Most diagnoses in the United States are incidental findings on CT scan. Most common symptoms are anemia, hematuria, cachexia, and fever. The classic triad of flank pain, hematuria, and a palpable mass is uncommon. Erythrocytosis from erythropoietin production can also be seen but is uncommon.

Diagnostic Testing

Imaging
- Cystic renal lesions (by ultrasound) require no further evaluation. CT is highly sensitive and specific for RCC.
- **Staging evaluation:** Preoperative CT for the evaluation of lymph nodes, metastatic disease, and tumor thrombus is typically sufficient. PET does not have a role.

Diagnostic Procedures
Most lesions can be resected without a biopsy.

TREATMENT

Medical treatment of RCC has changed more in the past 5 years than the treatment of any solid tumor. Cytotoxic chemotherapy is mostly ineffective.
- **Adjuvant therapy** is not currently indicated.
- **Molecularly targeted therapy.** Oral inhibitors of VEGF and other tyrosine kinases have been shown to improve survival outcomes in patients with advanced stage RCC. At present, sunitinib and pazopanib are preferred as the treatment of choice in previously untreated patients. Axitinib and sorafenib are preferred in patients who failed previous treatment. The mammalian target of rapamycin (mTOR) inhibitors temsirolimus and everolimus are also approved for RCC and are typically used in high-risk patients or after the progression of VEGF-targeted therapy (*N Engl J Med 2007;356:2271*; *Lancet 2008;372:449*). Bevacizumab is effective when used in combination with interferon (*Lancet 2007;22:2103*). Metastatic disease can be controlled for more than a year and the median overall survival is >2 years (*N Engl J Med 2007;356:115*).
- **Immunotherapy** was standard for eligible patients prior to targeted therapies. High-dose interleukin (IL)-2 has significant toxicities but has reported complete response rates of 5%. Interferon given subcutaneously can also lead to a response and disease control in some patients.

Surgical Management

Surgical treatment is of primary importance.

- Early disease (stage I/II, no local invasion, no lymph nodes) is treated with radical nephrectomy, or partial nephrectomy in select patients. Increasingly, laparoscopic nephrectomies are being performed in patients with early stage disease.
- Locally invasive tumors should be resected if possible, sometimes requiring partial liver resection or partial resection of the SVC.
- In metastatic disease, resection of the primary tumor should be considered if the overall burden of disease is low.
- Resection of isolated metastases (brain, lung, adrenal) improves survival in select patients.

Bladder Cancer

GENERAL PRINCIPLES

Epidemiology

One of the commonly diagnosed malignancies in the United States (almost 70,000 cases in 2012) but less frequently fatal (one-fifth as many deaths). TCC is the most common histology and is strongly associated with tobacco smoking as well as exposure to benzene and other industrial chemicals. Schistosome infection is linked to squamous cell bladder cancer.

DIAGNOSIS

Clinical Presentation

Ninety percent of patients present with hematuria, often with frequency, urgency, and dysuria.

Diagnostic Testing

- Gross hematuria should be evaluated with urine culture and cytology, imaging (intravenous pyelogram [IVP] or CT), and cystoscopy.
- **Staging:** Based primarily on findings of transurethral resection (TUR), which determines depth of invasion. Lymph node involvement is stage IV.

TREATMENT

Treatment by stage

- **Superficial tumors** (no muscle invasion, stages 0 to I) are treated cystoscopically with TUR, often needing multiple resections and frequent cystoscopy (every 3 months). Intravesical bacillus Calmette-Guérin reduces recurrence. Mitomycin-C and other intravesical chemotherapies may also be used.
- **Muscle invasive disease** (invades bladder muscle or adjacent tissue; stages II to III). Neoadjuvant cisplatin-based chemotherapy followed by surgery is associated with better survival outcomes than surgery alone and should be the preferred approach in eligible patients. Surgery involves radical cystectomy with removal of the bladder, adjacent organs, and regional lymph nodes with urinary diversion by creating an ileal conduit. The ureters are attached to a segment of ileum that is attached to the

abdominal wall. Radiation, often with concurrent chemotherapy, is an alternative to surgery if resection cannot be safely performed.
- **Metastatic disease** (includes node-positive or distant disease) is highly responsive to chemotherapy but inevitably relapses if not resected. The most common regimens are gemcitabine + cisplatin and MVAC (methotrexate, vinblastine, doxorubicin, and cisplatin).

Prostate Cancer

GENERAL PRINCIPLES

Epidemiology
Prostate cancer is the most common cancer in men in the United States, with an estimated 240,000 cases and 28,000 deaths in 2012. Risk factors include African American ethnicity, family history, and a high-fat/low-vegetable diet.

Prevention
Screening with annual prostate-specific antigen (PSA) and digital rectal exam (DRE) has not been definitively shown to improve survival but should be discussed with patients older than 50 years.

DIAGNOSIS

Clinical Presentation
Most common presentation in the United States is asymptomatic elevation in PSA. DRE findings of asymmetric induration or nodules are suggestive. Less common symptoms are obstructive symptoms, new onset erectile dysfunction, hematuria, or hematospermia.

Diagnostic Testing
Specific indications for biopsy are controversial. An abnormal PSA should be repeated for confirmation prior to biopsy. Biopsy should be performed if PSA is >10 ng/mL. For PSA of 4 to 10 ng/mL, biopsy will be positive in approximately 25% and is usually recommended. For PSA levels between 2.6 ng/mL and 4 ng/mL, biopsy is recommended if PSA is increasing by ≥0.75 ng/mL/yr (PSA velocity). Suggestive findings on DRE should lead to biopsy as well.

TREATMENT

- Most important predictors of outcomes are pretreatment PSA levels, Gleason score, and clinical stage.
- Gleason score is determined by transrectal biopsy or resection on a scale of 2 to 10, with most scores being 6 to 7.
- T stage is determined by exam and ultrasound with early-stage disease (T1 to T2), defined as no extension beyond the prostate, and locally advanced disease (T3 to T4), defined as local invasion. Nodal involvement is considered stage IV.
- **Early stage disease:** Outcomes are equivalent with radical prostatectomy, external beam radiation, or brachytherapy. Late toxicities are variable among modalities

but rates of incontinence and erectile dysfunction are 10% to 20%. Robotic-assisted prostatectomy reduces recovery time but does not improve outcomes. Active surveillance is a suitable option for men with low-risk disease.
- **Locally advanced disease:** Can be treated with a combination of surgical, radiation, and hormonal therapy.
- **Metastatic disease** is incurable but can be managed with hormonal therapy for 2 to 10 years. Medical castration with GnRH agonists (leuprolide, goserelin) is the most common first-line therapy. After progression on GnRH agonists, oral androgen receptor blockade (ARB) (bicalutamide or flutamide) is usually effective. Other hormonal treatments include discontinuation of ARB, ketoconazole, and estrogens. Chemotherapy with docetaxel improves survival in hormone refractory disease (*N Engl J Med 2004;351:1502*). Sipuleucel-T, an autologous cell-based vaccine targeting prostatic acid phosphatase, is an alternative option to chemotherapy in patients with hormone refractory disease. In patients who have progressed on docetaxel, treatment with cabazitaxel a semisynthetic taxane, or abiraterone, an irreversible inhibitor of CYP17, are potential second-line options.

Testicular Cancer and Germ Cell Tumors

GENERAL PRINCIPLES

Epidemiology

Testicular cancers are relatively rare tumors (8,000 cases in the United States), but by far the most common tumor in men aged 15 to 35 years. Nonseminomatous tumors are more common in younger men, whereas seminomas are more common after age 30 years. Incidence is higher in Caucasians than in patients of other ethnicities. Other risk factors include cryptorchidism and Klinefelter syndrome.

Pathology

Fifty percent of testicular cancers are seminomas and the remainder are nonseminomas or of mixed histology. Nonseminomas include embryonal carcinoma, teratoma, choriocarcinoma, and yolk sac tumor. Pure seminomas have a better prognosis compared to nonseminomas or mixed histology tumors.

DIAGNOSIS

Clinical Presentation

Most common presentation is that of a painless testicular mass but can also present with testicular pain, hydrocele, or gynecomastia.

Diagnostic Testing
Laboratories

Tumor markers (alpha-fetoprotein [AFP], β human chorionic gonadoropin (β-hCG), and lactate dehydrogenase [LDH]) should be obtained. In patients with pure seminomas, AFP is not elevated and β-hCG may be elevated in only 20% of these patients, whereas AFP and β-hCG are elevated in up to 85% of patients with nonseminomas.

Imaging
- Transillumination or ultrasound can distinguish solid from cystic masses.
- Preoperative CT of the abdomen and pelvis and chest radiograph should be performed.

TREATMENT

- **Staging** is based on TNM status and serum markers. In general, a disease limited to the scrotum is stage I, lymph node involvement is stage II, visceral metastases are stage III, and there is no stage IV. Risk stratification for patients requiring chemotherapy is based on histology, sites of metastasis, and tumor markers.
- Solid masses should be treated with orchiectomy.
- **Treatment by stage**
  ○ Stage I: Orchiectomy followed by adjuvant chemotherapy or radiation to retroperitoneal nodes or active surveillance can result in a very high cure rate of almost 100%.
  ○ Stages II to III: Chemotherapy with BEP (bleomycin, etoposide, and cisplatin) results in high rates of cure, particularly in seminomas. Lymph node dissection is performed for residual tumor (usually in retroperitoneal nodes). Intermediate-risk patients have an 80% cure rate with BEP, and poor risk patients have a 45% chance of cure. High-dose chemotherapy with stem cell rescue (autologous stem cell transplant) is appropriate for treatment refractory patients.

GYNECOLOGIC MALIGNANCIES

Cervical Cancer

GENERAL PRINCIPLES

Epidemiology

Cervical cancer is the third most common cancer in women and is the fourth leading cause of cancer-related death in women worldwide. In countries that lack a cervical cancer screening and prevention program, it is the second most common cancer seen in women. The most important risk factor is persistent HPV infection, detected in over 99% of tumors, usually HPV 16 and 18. Other risk factors include early onset of sexual activity, multiple sexual partners, high-risk partner, history of sexually transmitted disease, and chronic immunosuppression (HIV infection).

Pathophysiology

The most common histologies seen are squamous cell carcinoma (69%), followed by adenocarcinoma (25%).

Prevention

The prophylactic quadrivalent vaccine protects against HPV 6, 11, 16, 18 (Gardasil), whereas the bivalent vaccine protects against HPV 16 and 18. Vaccination can be started as early as 9 years of age and is most effective if given before the initiation of sexual intercourse. Vaccinated women should continue routine Pap smears because the vaccine is not effective against all HPV subtypes (*N Engl J Med 2007;356:1915*). Cervical cancer screening should begin at age 21 years.

DIAGNOSIS

Clinical Presentation

Patients with early-stage lesions are commonly asymptomatic and diagnosed incidentally on Pap smear, which underscores the importance of screening. Symptoms observed at presentation include irregular or heavy vaginal bleeding, or postcoital bleeding. Patients with advanced disease may present with back pain, hematochezia from bowel involvement, or vaginal passage of urine or stool.

Diagnostic Testing

Diagnosis obtained through cervical cytology and biopsy. Cone biopsy is recommended if cervical biopsy is inadequate to define the invasiveness of the lesion.

TREATMENT

Patients with small, early-stage lesions may be treated with radical hysterectomy, whereas locally advanced disease is treated with concurrent chemoradiotherapy. Advanced disseminated disease is treated with chemotherapy alone. The role of angiogenesis inhibitors, such as bevacizumab, in patients with advanced disease is being explored.

Endometrial Cancer

GENERAL PRINCIPLES

Epidemiology

Endometrial cancer is the most common gynecologic cancer in the United States, accounting for 43,470 new cases diagnosed in 2010. Risk factors include obesity, unopposed estrogen, early menarche, late menopause, nulliparity, chronic anovulation, and tamoxifen use. Patients with hereditary cancer syndromes, such as Lynch syndrome, have increased incidence of endometrial cancer.

Pathology

Two distinct subtypes are as follows:
• Type I: More common in younger woman. Associated with unopposed estrogen, endometrioid histology, and slow growth.
• Type II: More common in late postmenopause. Not related to estrogen and shows nonendometrioid histologies (serous, clear cell) and aggressive behavior.

DIAGNOSIS

Clinical Presentation

The most common presentation is abnormal vaginal bleeding. Any vaginal bleeding in a postmenopausal woman, including spotting and staining, should be evaluated.

Diagnostic Testing

Endometrial sampling is most often performed by in-office endometrial biopsy or, less commonly, by dilation and curettage.

TREATMENT

- Surgery is indicated for staging and treatment.
- Patients with cervical extension (stage II) may benefit from adjuvant radiotherapy.
- Patients with extrauterine disease extension and those with distant metastates are treated with chemotherapy.

Ovarian Cancer

GENERAL PRINCIPLES

Epidemiology

Ovarian cancer is the leading cause of gynecologic mortality in the United States. Risk factors include early menarche, late menopause, nulligravidity, family history, and familial syndromes including patients with BRCA1 and BRCA2 mutations and Lynch syndrome.

Pathology

Most tumors are seen in patients between the ages of 40 and 65 years, and 85% of the tumors are epithelial. Nonepithelial ovarian malignancies (germ cell, sex cord-stromal and mixed) are seen in younger patients.

DIAGNOSIS

Clinical Presentation

Patients with early stage disease have vague symptoms including bloating and abdominal discomfort. Patients usually have advanced disease at presentation and may have increasing abdominal girth, ascites, and abdominal pain.

Diagnostic Testing

Laboratories

Cancer antigen 125 (CA-125) is elevated in approximately 80% of patients but is not specific.

Imaging

- Ultrasound may confirm the presence of an adnexal mass.
- CT scan is used to evaluate for metastases.

TREATMENT

- Surgery is usually performed without prior histologic diagnosis and is necessary for tumor debulking.
- Stage I (without pelvic extension): Surgery alone.
- Stage II (extension to uterus, fallopian tubes, or other pelvic tissues): Surgery and adjuvant chemotherapy.
- Stage III (peritoneal or lymph node involvement) and IV (distant metastasis): Debulking/cytoreductive surgery and systemic chemotherapy.
- Poly-ADP-ribose phosphorylase (PARP) inhibitors in combination with platinum-based chemotherapy show promise in patients with recurrent disease.

- **Germ cell ovarian cancers** are rare, typically occur in younger women, and are highly curable with chemotherapy.
- **Stromal tumors** usually present in early stage and are commonly cured with resection alone.

Cancer of Unknown Primary

GENERAL PRINCIPLES

Definition

Cancer of unknown primary site is defined as biopsy-proven malignancy for which the primary site of origin cannot be identified after a thorough history and physical examination, blood tests, and imaging studies.

Pathology

These malignancies are classified using light microscopy into adenocarcinoma (60%), poorly differentiated carcinoma/poorly differentiated adenocarcinoma (29%), squamous carcinoma (5%), poorly differentiated malignant neoplasm (5%), and neuroendocrine carcinoma (1%). Further identification usually requires specialized tests including IHC staining, electron microscopy, and genetic analysis.

TREATMENT

Treatment for favorable subgroups of patients with cancer of unknown primary is tailored based on the likely primary site of origin such as patients with isolated axillary adenopathy are treated as stage II breast cancer, women with peritoneal carcinomatosis are treated as stage III ovarian cancer, and patients with cervical adenopathy are treated as H&N cancer. Most patients have unfavorable disease and are treated with an empiric combination chemotherapy, usually carboplatin and paclitaxel.

OUTCOME/PROGNOSIS

The median survival for patients with cancer of unknown primary is 6 to 9 months. Favorable subsets include women with isolated axillary adenopathy, papillary serous adenocarcinoma of the peritoneal cavity, squamous cell carcinoma of the cervical or inguinal lymph nodes, and single metastatic site.

HEMATOLOGIC MALIGNANCIES

Myelodysplastic Syndrome

GENERAL PRINCIPLES

Epidemiology

- Myelodysplastic syndromes (MDS) comprise a heterogeneous group of malignant stem cell disorders broadly characterized by cytopenias associated with a dysmorphic and usually cellular bone marrow and ineffective blood cell production. Cytopenias are due to clonal abnormalities of marrow cells affecting one or more cell lines.

- The precise incidence of de novo MDS is not known; however, de novo MDS is relatively common form of bone marrow failure with prevalence of 3.5 to >10 per 100,000 persons in the general population. Therapy-related MDS is less common, but as many as 15% of patients within a decade after intensive combination treatment for cancer can develop MDS. Mean age at onset is 68 years for de novo MDS.
- Risk factors are similar to those for acute myeloid leukemia (AML).

Etiology

The exact etiology is unknown; however, chromosome abnormalities occur in up to 80% of cases leading to accumulation of multiple genetic lesions, loss of tumor suppressor genes, and/or activating oncogene mutations causing impaired cell proliferation and differentiation. Most common chromosomal abnormalities include:

- Addition of part or all of chromosome 8 (10%)
- Deletion of part or all of chromosomes 5 (8%), 7 (8%), or both (15%)
- Deletion of Y (7%)
- Abnormal 17p (7%)
- Deletion of 20q (4%)

Pathophysiology

- The French-American-British (FAB) Cooperative Group originally distinguished the following five morphologic groups based on the peripheral blood and bone marrow:
  - Refractory anemia (RA)
  - Refractory anemia with ringed sideroblasts (RARS)
  - Refractory anemia with excess blasts (RAEB)
  - Refractory anemia with excess blasts in transformation (RAEB-t)
  - Chronic myelomonocytic leukemia (CMML)
- The World Health Organization (WHO) classification made changes to the FAB system, including
  - Reducing the threshold for defining AML from 30% to 20% blasts in the marrow and peripheral blood, and eliminating RAEB-t entity.
  - Dividing RA and RARS into five categories, based on presence of single or multilineage dysplasia (MLD) and presence of 5q deletion.
  - Subdividing RAEB into two groups, RAEB-1 and RAEB-2, based on number of blasts in blood and marrow.
  - Movement of CMML to a novel class called myelodysplastic/myeloproliferative.

DIAGNOSIS

Clinical Presentation

- Symptoms usually related to bone marrow failure, including fatigue, fever, bruising, or bleeding.
- At least half of patients are asymptomatic.
- Some patients are discovered incidentally on routine blood counts.
- Leukopenia can lead to frequent infections.
- Splenomegaly is rare except in CMML.
- Autoimmune syndromes can occur in about 14% of patients as cutaneous vasculitis, monoarticular arthritis, fever, and pulmonary infiltrates.

- Cutaneous manifestations such as Sweet's syndrome (acute febrile neutrophilic dermatosis) often herald transformation to AML.
- Acquired α-thalassemia (hemoglobin H disease) is a rare manifestation.

Diagnostic Testing

- Complete blood count usually shows anemia alone or as part of bicytopenia or pancytopenia. Macrocytosis is common. Leukocyte count is usually normal or low (except in CMML). Platelet count is usually normal or low (except in 5q- syndrome).
- Peripheral blood smear can show dimorphic erythrocytes and large platelets. Neutrophils can be hypogranulated, hyposegmented, ringed, or abnormally segmented nuclei (so-called pseudo–Pelger-Huet anomaly).
- Bone marrow aspiration and biopsy show normocellular or hypercellular marrow. Hypocellular marrow is less frequent and only seen in 20% of cases. Morphologically, the cells have dyserythropoietic changes with irregular nuclear contour, ringed sideroblasts in the erythroid lineage, hypogranulation and hyposegmentation in granulocytic precursors with an increase in myeloblasts, and reduced numbers of disorganized nuclei in megakaryocytes.
- Cytogenetic analysis and FISH can identify chromosomal abnormalities, which are essential in disease prognosis and often in therapy approach.

TREATMENT

- Therapy for MDS is generally unsatisfactory, and stem-cell transplantation only offers cure. Specific interventions are influenced by age, performance status, cytogenetics, and International Prognostic Scoring System (IPSS) risk category (Table 22-9). For example, young patients with good performance status and high IPSS are likely to benefit more from allogeneic bone marrow transplant.
- Lenalidomide has 60% response in the erythroids of patients with low/intermediate-1 IPSS score and 83% of those with 5q- syndrome. Hypomethylating agents such as 5- azacytidine improves blood counts and modestly improves survival in about 16% of patients with MDS compared with best supportive care. Antithymocyte

Table 22-9	International Prognostic Scoring System (IPSS) Risk Category for Myelodysplastic Syndromes				
	Score Value				
Prognostic variable	0	0.5	1	1.5	2.0
Marrow blasts (%)	<5	5–10		11–20	21–30
Karyotype*	Good	Inter	Poor		
Cytopenia	0/1	2/3			
Risk groups	Score				
Low	0				
Intermediate 1 (Int-1)	0.5–1.0				
Intermediate 2 (Int-2)	1.5–2.0				
High	2.5–3.5				

*Poor: complex (>2), chromosome 7 abnormalities; good: normal, -Y, 5q-, 20q-; intermediate: other abnormalities.

globulin (ATG) and cyclosporine work better in young patients, hypocellular MDS, overrepresentation of human leukocyte antigen D2, and the presence of paroxysmal nocturnal hemoglobinuria clone.
• Supportive therapy with blood transfusions, hematopoietic growth factors (such as erythropoietin and granulocyte colony-stimulating factor), and antibiotics is still the cornerstone of treatment for many patients.

Acute Myeloid Leukemia

GENERAL PRINCIPLES

Epidemiology

Most common type of acute leukemia in adults. Median age at presentation is 65 years. Risk factors include prior exposure to chemotherapy with alkylating agents or topoisomerase inhibitors, radiotherapy, antecedent hematologic disorder such as MDS or myeloproliferative disorder (MPD), and congenital disorders (Down's syndrome [particularly AML-M7], Turners and Klinefelter syndromes, Fanconi anemia).

Pathophysiology

• Current WHO classification includes the following: (1) AML with recurrent genetic abnormalities; (2) AML with MLD (prior MDS); (3) AML therapy related; and (4) AML not otherwise categorized, which includes the FAB subtypes M0 (AML minimally differentiated), M1 (AML without maturation), M2 (AML with maturation), M4 (acute myelomonocytic leukemia), M5 (acute monocytic leukemia), M6 (acute erythroleukemia), and M7 (acute megakaryoblastic leukemia). M3 (acute promyelocytic anemia) is classified as AML with recurrent genetic abnormalities due to the presence of t(15;17).
• **AML with recurrent genetic abnormalities:** This WHO category contains AML variants that contain genetic abnormalities of prognostic significance (Table 22-10).

Table 22-10	Cytogenetic Abnormalities in Acute Myeloid Leukemia and Associated Prognosis	
Risk Group	**Cytogenetic Findings**	**Preferred Consolidation Strategy**
Favorable	t(15;17), t(8;21), inv(16)	Chemotherapy
Intermediate	Normal or ≤2 nonspecific chromosomal aberrations	Chemotherapy OR allogeneic transplant
Unfavorable	Complex karyotype (defined as ≥3 abnormalities, excluding the favorable-risk cytogenetics) inv(3), t(6;9), t(6;11), t(11;19) del(5q) −5, −7, +8	Allogeneic transplant

Adapted from Mrozek K, Bloomfield CD. Chromosome aberrations, gene mutations and expression changes, and prognosis in adult acute myeloid leukemia. *Hematol Am Soc Hematol Educ Program.* 2006:169–177.

- **AML with t(8;21)(q22;q22); RUNX1-RUNX1T1:** This leukemia may not have 20% blasts but can be identified if the cytogenetic abnormality is present. It typically has associated morphologic features that can suggest its diagnosis. The leukemia is associated with a more favorable prognosis. The presence of c-KIT mutations is an adverse prognostic features in patients with t(8;21). Surprisingly, patients can have transcripts of the RUNX1-RUNX1T1 detected by RT-PCR even in patients who have been in remission for many years.
- **AML with inv(16)(p13.1q22) or t(16;16)(p13.1;q22); CEFB-MYH11** (previously acute myelomonocytic leukemia, AMML, FAB M4Eo): This leukemia occurs in younger patients and can present as an extramedullary myeloid sarcoma. It is associated with a more favorable prognosis, although cases with an additional c-KIT mutation may do more poorly.
- **APL with t(15;17)(q22;q12); PML-RARA:** It is notable that the malignant cells in APL are promyelocytes, making this another AML where the presence of 20% blasts is not required. Outcomes in this variant of AML are generally favorable. It can present with **disseminated intravascular coagulation (DIC)**.
- **AML with t(9;11)(p22;q23); MLLT3-MLL:** This type of leukemia is usually monocytic and more common in children. It can present with DIC and high white cell counts with gingival or skin infiltration. It has an intermediate prognosis.
- **AML with t(6;9)(p23;q34); DEK-NUP214:** This is a rare type of leukemia that is associated with basophilia, pancytopenia, and dysplasia. It has a generally poor prognosis.
- **AML with inv(3)(q21q26.2) or t(3;3)(q21;q26.2); RPN1-EVI1:** This leukemia is also rare, accounting for only 1% or 2% of cases. Patients are anemic but may have normal or elevated platelet counts. It is frequently associated with dysplasia and is associated with aggressive disease and a short survival time.
- **AML (megakaryoblastic) with t(1;22)(p13;q13); RBM15-MKL1:** This type of leukemia is also rare but is typically a megakaryoblastic process occurring in infants, although it is not seen in patients with Down syndrome. Sometimes it can present as a mass and mimic sarcoma.
- Two provisional entities identified at the molecular level include:
  ○ **AML with mutated NPM1:** Leukemias with mutations of NPM1 are considered as a provisional entity. The mutation is seen in about one-third of all cases of AML, making it overlap other types, and thus, it is not a unique group. In almost all cases, the mutation is seen in AML with normal cytogenetics. The presence of the NPM1 mutation confers a better prognosis but only if it is seen alone.
  ○ **AML with mutated CEBPA:** Mutation in CEBPA is seen in about 6% to 15% of AML, commonly in cases with a normal karyotype. Cases with this mutation are associated with a good prognosis.

DIAGNOSIS

Clinical Presentation

Symptoms usually related to bone marrow failure, including fatigue, fever, bruising, or bleeding. Most patients present with pancytopenia and circulating blast forms. Patients with white blood cell count **above 100,000/μL are at risk for leukostasis**, manifested by dyspnea, chest pain, headaches, confusion, and cranial nerve palsies. Extramedullary tissue invasion by leukemic cells (most commonly with AML-M5) may result in hepatomegaly, splenomegaly, lymphadenopathy, rashes (leukemia cutis), gingival hypertrophy, CNS dysfunction and cranial neuropathies, intestinal involvement, lytic bony lesions, or even establishment of infiltrative masses (granulocytic sarcomas or chloromas).

Diagnostic Testing

- Bone marrow specimens should be evaluated for cytochemistry, flow cytometry, and cytogenetics. Markers for AML include positive myeloperoxidase staining, CD33, CD13, CD41, and glycophorin A. AML is classified by cytogenetic findings into three prognostic groups: favorable, intermediate, and unfavorable. Table 22-10 outlines the risk groups.
- In the WHO system, AML is defined by >20% myeloblasts in the bone marrow aspirate. Patients with clonal cytogenetic abnormalities such as t(8;21), inv(16), and t(15;17) have AML regardless of the blast percentage.

TREATMENT

- **Remission induction:** Usually with cytarabine for 7 days and an anthracycline for 3 days (7 + 3 regimen).
- **Consolidation:** Therapy with high-dose cytarabine in patients younger than 60 years who achieved complete remission.
- **Stem cell transplant:** High-dose chemotherapy followed by donor stem cell transplant may be considered in young patients with poor cytogenetic features or antecedent hematologic disorders.
- Acute promyelocytic leukemia (AML-M3) is characterized by the translocation t(15;17), disseminated intravascular coagulopathy, and increased cure rates with the use of all-trans retinoic acid and arsenic trioxide.

Acute Lymphoblastic Leukemia

GENERAL PRINCIPLES

Epidemiology

Most common **childhood** leukemia. Median age at presentation is 35 years. Bimodal distribution with one peak at 4 to 5 years and a second gradual increase after the age of 50 years.

Pathophysiology

- Subdivided into three groups: precursor B cell, mature B cell (Burkitt lymphoma), and T cell. Classification is based on morphologic (FAB system) and immunophenotypic information (Table 22-11). Many different translocations have been reported in B-ALL, three of which are clearly associated with treatment failure or success when using intensive chemotherapy. These include:
  - ○ **The Philadelphia (Ph) chromosome: t(9;22)(a34;q11); BCR/ABL:** Associated with a poor prognosis, this is the most frequent rearrangement in adult ALL. It is present in 25% of adult cases and 3% of childhood cases. The incidence of t(9;22) increases with age and is present in 40% to 50% of patients older than 60 years.
  - ○ **t(v;11q23); MLL rearranged:** Associated with a poor prognosis, seen in infants <1 year and adults.

Table 22-11	Acute Lymphoblastic Leukemia, Immunotype, and French-American-British (FAB) Classification		
Immunotype	Frequency (%)	FAB Subtype	Staining
Pre–B cell	75	L1, L2	+TdT, +CALLA, B-cell markers (CD19, CD20)
T cell	20	L1, L2	+TdT, −CALLA, +acid phosphatase, +T cell markers (CD2, CD7, CD5)
B cell	5	L3	−TdT, +surface IgG

CALLA, common acute lymphoblastic leukemia antigen; TdT, terminal deoxynucleotidyl transferase.

- ○ **t(12;21)(p12;q22) TEL/AML1:** Associated with a good prognosis and hyperdiploidy, this is the most common rearrangement seen in children.
- The t(9;22) and t(v;11q23) are often associated with a pro-B immunophenotype and a poor prognosis, while the t(12;21) is associated with common pre–B-ALL.

DIAGNOSIS

Clinical Presentation

- Symptoms include fatigue, fever, and bleeding. Extremity joint pain may be the only manifestation in children. Leukostasis is uncommon, even with high white blood cell counts.
- Lymphadenopathy and splenomegaly are present in approximately 20% of cases. Much more commonly than in AML, in up to 10% of patients, the CNS may be involved at presentation, manifesting as headache and/or cranial nerve palsies. Hepatosplenomegaly and lymphadenopathy can be seen.
- ALL can be associated with an anterior mediastinal mass (in T-cell subtypes) or large abdominal lymph nodes (in B-cell subtypes).

Diagnostic Testing

- Basic workup is similar to that for AML.
- A peripheral smear will usually demonstrate the presence of circulating blasts. Bone marrow will be hypercellular, with >30% blasts. Cytoplasmic granules and Auer rods should be absent. However, it can be extremely difficult to diagnose ALL on clinical and morphologic grounds alone.
- Immunophenotyping is often necessary to distinguish ALL from AML. Of adult ALL patients, 30% exhibit the Ph chromosome t(9;22), as seen in CML.

TREATMENT

Complex and may be subdivided into induction (initial chemotherapy to achieve a complete remission), consolidation (postremission therapy to destroy clinically occult disease), and maintenance (prolonged low-dose chemotherapy to prevent relapse, given usually for 2 years). Because of the high risk of CNS, relapse prophylactic intrathecal therapy is administered during the induction and consolidation phases. Allogeneic stem cell transplant may be used at relapse or in patients with high-risk disease.

Chronic Myeloid Leukemia

GENERAL PRINCIPLES

Epidemiology

Accounts for 14% of leukemias in the United States. Median age at diagnosis is 65 years.

Pathophysiology

- CML is associated with the fusion of two genes: BCR (on chromosome 22) and ABL1 (on chromosome 9) resulting in the BCR-ABL1 fusion gene. This abnormal fusion typically results from a reciprocal translocation between chromosomes 9 and 22, t(9;22)(q34;q11), that gives rise to an abnormal chromosome 22 called the Philadelphia chromosome. It is this derivative chromosome 22, which harbors the BCR-ABL1 fusion gene. The BCR-ABL1 fusion gene results in the formation of a unique gene product, the BCR-ABL1 fusion protein. This protein product includes an enzymatic domain from the normal ABL1 with tyrosine kinase catalytic activity, but relative to ABL1, whose kinase activity is tightly regulated, the kinase activity of BCR-ABL1 is elevated and constitutive due to fusion with a portion of BCR. It is this deregulated tyrosine kinase that is implicated in the pathogenesis of CML.
- Blast-phase CML is characterized by **cytogenetic evolution** in nearly 70% of patients. The most common chromosomal abnormalities are trisomy 8, additional Ph chromosome, and isochromosome 17.

DIAGNOSIS

Clinical Presentation

Patients can present in any of three phases: chronic, accelerated, and blastic. Approximately 90% present in chronic phase, usually diagnosed incidentally by an abnormal blood cell count. Symptoms are usually related to splenomegaly (pain, left abdominal mass, early satiety) or anemia. Peripheral blood counts show increased white blood cells with all levels of granulocytic differentiation, from myeloblasts to segmented neutrophils. Transformation from chronic phase may be insidious through accelerated phase or abrupt-to-blastic phase.

Diagnostic Testing

- Bone marrow aspirate with cytogenetics, FISH for the bcr-abl rearrangement, and PCR for the *bcr-abl* gene confirm the diagnosis.
- The Ph chromosome is not pathognomonic for CML, as it may also be detected in acute lymphoblastic leukemia (ALL; 15% to 30% adults) and AML (2%).

TREATMENT

Most patients are initially treated with oral TKIs such as imatinib, dasatinib, and nilotinib. Phase III trials comparing dasatinib or nilotinib to imatinib as initial therapy for CML in chronic phase have demonstrated faster and deeper responses with these second generation TKIs. Young patients with HLA-identical siblings or TKI failures may benefit from stem cell transplant.

Chronic Lymphocytic Leukemia

GENERAL PRINCIPLES

Epidemiology

Most common form of leukemia in Western countries. Median age at presentation is 65 years.

Pathophysiology

Chronic lymphocytic leukemia (CLL) is an accumulation of malignant, immunologically incompetent, but mature B-cell lymphocytes. The malignant cells of CLL express high levels of the antiapoptotic protein, bcl-2, and express common B-cell antigens CD19, CD20, and CD23. Of note, CD5 antigen, a T-cell antigen, is found in all cases of CLL. A Coombs-positive, warm antibody, hemolytic anemia occurs in 10% of patients, and an immune thrombocytopenia occurs in ~5% of patients. In 5% of patients, **Richter's syndrome** develops, which is a malignant transformation to diffuse large B-cell lymphoma.

DIAGNOSIS

Staging: Classification of CLL is based on the extent of systemic infiltration of lymphocytes. This helps to determine the prognosis and initiation of treatment (Table 22-12). Molecular and cytogenetic markers have become increasingly useful for prognostication.

Table 22-12	Chronic Lymphocytic Leukemia Staging and Molecular Prognostics
Rai	**Binet**
Stage 0: Lymphocytosis	Stage A: Lymphocytosis
Stage 1: Lymphadenopathy	Stage B: Lymphadenopathy in
Stage 2: Splenomegaly	>3 areas
Stage 3: Hgb <11 g/dL	Stage C: Hgb <10 g/dL or platelets
Stage 4: Platelets <100,000/μL	<100,000/μL
High-risk molecular markers	Good-risk cytogenetics
Elevated β2, LDH, sCD23	Deletion 13q
CD38+ in >30% lymphocytes	High-risk cytogenetics
ZAP70+ in >30% lymphocytes	14q rearrangement
Germline IgVH	11q rearrangement
	Deletion 17p
	Trisomy 12
Low risk: overall survival, 7–10 years	High risk: Overall survival, 2–5 years
Rai 0–1	Rai 3–4
Binet A	Binet C
Deletion 13q	Molecular or cytogenetic changes noted
Doubling time >12 months	Doubling time <12 months

Hgb, hemoglobin; IgVH, immunoglobulin variable heavy chain; LDH, lactate dehydrogenase.

Clinical Presentation

Usually asymptomatic and diagnosed incidentally by routine blood cell counts. Symptoms may include night sweats, weight loss, lymphadenopathy, and splenomegaly. Peripheral blood typically shows absolute lymphocyte count above $5,000/\mu L$ and "**smudge cells**" caused by damage of the fragile lymphocytes during smear preparation. Anemia and thrombocytopenia may also be present from autoimmunity or progressive disease. Infection can result from hypogammaglobulinemia, T-cell dysfunction, and decreased phagocytic function.

Diagnostic Testing

The essential diagnostic criteria for CLL identified by the CLL international working group include an absolute lymphocytosis of $>5000/\mu L$ with a typical morphology, a bone marrow infiltrated with small lymphocytes accounting for $>30\%$ of nucleated cells, and a typical immunophenotype ($CD5^+$, $CD23^+$, $CD10^-$, $CD19^+$, $CD20^{+dim}$, $CyclinD1^-$, $CD43^{\pm}$).

TREATMENT

Many patients do not require treatment. Indications for treatment include bulky disease, cytopenias, recurrent infections, rapid progression, and transformation to large cell lymphoma (Richter's syndrome). Treatment options include oral alkylating agents (chlorambucil, cyclophosphamide, bendamustine), purine analogues (fludarabine, cladribine), and monoclonal antibodies such as rituximab (anti-CD20), ofatumumab (anti-CD20), and alemtuzumab (anti-CD52), either as single agents or in combination.

Hairy Cell Leukemia

GENERAL PRINCIPLES

Epidemiology

Rare disorder, most common in elderly men.

DIAGNOSIS

- Characteristic "hairy" appearing leukocytes on peripheral smear. Flow cytometry is positive for CD20, CD11c, CD103, CD123, cyclin D1, and annexin A1. Also, hairy cells are tartrate-resistant acid phosphatase (TRAP) positive.
- Most patients present with malaise and fatigue. On physical exam, splenomegaly and hepatomegaly are evident in 95% and 40% of cases, respectively. With more advanced disease, pancytopenia develops, and patients may present with bleeding or recurrent infections (bacterial, viral, fungal, or atypical mycobacterial).

TREATMENT

As with other chronic leukemias and lymphomas, early treatment does not improve overall outcome. The decision to treat is based on the development of cytopenias (hemoglobin, $<10\,g/dL$, absolute neutrophil count, $<1,000/\mu L$; platelets, $<100,000/\mu L$)

and recurrent infections. Typically, cladribine or pentostatin is used. However, both of these agents induce significant and prolonged immunosuppression, which may last up to 54 months. Prophylaxis for herpes simplex virus and *Pneumocystis*, especially if concurrent steroids are used, is advised.

Hodgkin's Lymphoma

GENERAL PRINCIPLES

Epidemiology
Bimodal distribution with the first peak at age 25 years and second peak after the age of 50 years.

Pathophysiology
- Hodgkin's lymphoma (HL) is subdivided into nodular lymphocyte predominant (NLPHD) and classical HL (nodular sclerosis, lymphocyte-rich, mixed cellularity, lymphocyte depleted).
- The Reed-Sternberg cells consistently express the CD30 and CD15 antigens. CD30 is a marker of lymphocyte activation that is expressed by reactive and malignant lymphoid cells. CD15 is a marker of late granulocytes, monocytes, and activated T cells that is not normally expressed by cells of B lineage.
- Of note, NLPHD constitutes 5% of cases. In contrast to the other histologic subtypes, the typical Reed-Sternberg cells are either infrequent or absent in NLPHD. Instead, lymphocytic and histiocytic cells, or "popcorn cells," are seen within a background of inflammatory cells, which are predominantly benign lymphocytes.

DIAGNOSIS

Clinical Presentation
Most patients present with painless lymphadenopathy in the cervical or supraclavicular region. Systemic or "B" symptoms (drenching night sweats, fever, and weight loss) are more common in advanced stages.

Diagnostic Testing
- Made with excisional biopsy showing Reed-Sternberg cells within a background of reactive inflammatory cells. FNA is insufficient. Workup includes history and physical, complete blood cell (CBC) count, chemistry, LDH, erythrocyte sedimentation rate, CT, PET, and bone marrow exam.
- **Staging:** The Ann Arbor staging system subdivides the lymphomas into four stages (Table 22-13).

TREATMENT

Chemotherapy with ABVD (Adriamycin, bleomycin, vinblastine, dacarbazine). Radiation may be added in the early-stage or bulky disease. Relapsed disease should be treated with salvage chemotherapy +/− stem cell transplant. Brentuximab vedotin, a CD30-directed antibody-drug conjugate, is recently approved for refractory and relapsed HL (*N Engl J Med 2010;1812:1821*).

Table 22-13	Ann Arbor Staging of Lymphoma[a]

Stage	Description
I	Involvement of a single lymph node region (I) or single extralymphatic organ (IE).
II	Involvement of ≥2 lymph node regions in the same side of the diaphragm.
III	Involvement of lymph node regions in both sides of the diaphragm.
IV	Diffuse or disseminated involvement of one or more extralymphatic organs.

[a]**Modifying features:** A, absence of B features; B, presence of B features; E, involvement of a single extranodal site contiguous or proximal to the involved nodal site; S, spleen involvement; X, bulky disease defined as lymph node ≥10 cm than one-third of mediastinum.

Non-Hodgkin's Lymphoma

GENERAL PRINCIPLES

Epidemiology

Fifth most common malignancy in the United States with over 65,000 new cases in 2010. Risk factors include immunodeficiency, autoimmune disorders, bacterial infections (*H. pylori*, *Borrelia burgdorferi*, and *Chlamydia psittaci*), viral infections (human immunodeficiency virus [HIV], Epstein–Barr virus, human herpesvirus 8, human T-cell leukemia virus-1), and previous transplant, either solid organ or stem cell.

Pathophysiology

Broadly divided into indolent (follicular, marginal, small lymphocytic), aggressive (diffuse large cell, mantle cell, peripheral T cell, anaplastic T cell), and very aggressive (Burkitt lymphoma, lymphoblastic) tumors. Table 22-14 illustrates chromosomal abnormalities in B-cell non-Hodgkin's lymphoma (B-NHL).

DIAGNOSIS

- Clinical manifestations, staging, and therapy depend on the histologic subtype. Essential workup includes history, physical exam, CBC count, chemistry, CT scans ± PET-CT, and bone marrow exam. The cerebrospinal fluid (CSF) evaluation is indicated in patients with high-grade lymphomas, those with HIV-related lymphomas, and those with involvement of the epidural space, nasopharynx, and paranasal sinuses.
- **Staging:** Patients are staged by the Ann Arbor classification. Patient with aggressive lymphoma are usually stratified according to the International Prognostic Index, which uses five adverse prognostic factors: age <60 years; Ann Arbor stage III or IV; abnormal serum LDH; two or more extranodal sites involved; and performance status ECOG 2 or higher. Five-year survival rates for patients with 0–1, 2, 3, or 4–5 risk factors are 73%, 51%, 43%, and 26%, respectively (*N Engl J Med 1993;329:987*).

Table 22-14	Chromosomal Abnormalities in B-Cell Non-Hodgkin's Lymphoma		
Cytogenetic Abnormality	Histology	Antigen Rearrangement	Oncogene Expression
t(14;18)	Follicular, diffuse large cell	IgH	bcl-2
t(11;14)	Mantle cell	IgH	cyclin-D1/bcl-1
t(1;14)	MALT lymphoma	IgH	bcl-10
t(11;18)	MALT lymphoma	IgH	Unknown
t(9;14)	Lymphoplasmacytic lymphoma	IgH	PAX-5
8q24 translocations	Burkitt lymphoma	IgH	c-myc
t(8;14)		Ig-8	
t(2;8)		Ig-6	
t(8;22)			

IgH, Immunoglobulin H; MALT, mucosa-associated lymphoid tissue.

TREATMENT

- **Follicular lymphoma**
  - Second most common NHL and most common indolent lymphoma. Patients are usually older adults with asymptomatic adenopathy and generalized involvement. Bone marrow involvement is common.
  - The cytogenetic hallmark is the t(14;18), which causes overexpression of bcl-2 and protection from apoptosis. Subdivided into three grades according to the microscopic pattern. Grades 1 (0–5 large, noncleaved cells/high-power field [hpf]) and 2 (6–15 large, noncleaved cells/hpf) usually follow an indolent course, whereas grade 3 (>15 large, noncleaved cells/hpf) behaves as an aggressive tumor and is treated like diffuse large cell lymphoma.
  - Prognosis system most commonly used is the Follicular Lymphoma International Prognostic Index, which uses five independent poor prognostic factors including age >60 years, Ann Arbor stage III or IV, hemoglobin <12 g/dL, less than four involved nodal areas, and abnormal serum LDH. Five-year survival for patients with 0–1, 2, or 3–5 risk factors are 90%, 77%, and 52%, respectively (*Blood 2004;104:1258*). Patients with stage I and II lesion are usually treated with radiation therapy and patients with stage III or IV lesion may be observed or treated with chemotherapy.
- **Small lymphocytic lymphoma (SLL)** is a different manifestation of CLL, diagnosed in the absence of lymphocytosis. Treatment of the two disorders is the same.
- **Marginal zone lymphoma** may be subdivided into extranodal marginal zone B-cell lymphoma of the mucosa-associated lymphoid tissue, nodal marginal zone, and splenic marginal zone. Extranodal marginal zone is the most common subtype and most commonly involves the stomach. *H. pylori* is commonly found in these patients and antibiotic therapy for early-stage results in higher rates of cure, particularly in the absence of t(11;18). Advanced stage patients are usually treated similarly to other indolent lymphomas.

- **Diffuse, large B-cell lymphoma** is the most common subtype of NHL. Stage I and II lymphomas are treated with rituximab and CHOP (cyclophosphamide, doxorubicin, vincristine, and prednisone) with or without involved field radiotherapy. Stage III and IV lymphomas are treated with chemotherapy alone. Relapsed tumors should be treated with salvage chemotherapy, followed by autologous stem cell transplant if feasible.
- **Peripheral T-cell lymphomas and anaplastic large cell lymphomas** are treated similarly to diffuse large B-cell lymphoma, with the exception that there is no role for rituximab.
- **Mantle cell lymphoma (MCL)** usually presents as advanced disease in elderly patients. GI tract is frequently involved and the characteristic abnormality is t(11;14), leading to overexpression of cyclin D1. Prognosis system most commonly used is the Mantle Cell Lymphoma International Prognostic Index (MIPI), which uses four independent poor prognostic factors including age, performance status, LDH, and white blood cell count. The MIPI is able to classify patients into three risk groups: low risk (median survival not reached after median 32 months follow-up and 5-year overall survival rate of 60%), intermediate risk (median survival 51 months), and high risk (median survival 29 months). In addition to the four independent prognostic factors included in the model, the cell proliferation index (Ki-67) was also shown to have additional prognostic relevance. MCL exhibits a moderately aggressive course, and it is rarely curable with currently available standard treatment. Standard chemotherapy with CHOP is suboptimal, and fit patients are commonly treated with more aggressive regimens.
- **Burkitt lymphoma** may be subdivided into endemic (young patients, common involvement of the jaw), sporadic, and HIV associated. The typical histologic pattern of benign, clear macrophages in a background of darker malignant cells reveals the "**starry sky**" appearance. The characteristic feature is t(8;14) translocation, leading to overexpression of c-myc. Treated with very aggressive, complex chemotherapy regimens, similar to ALL. Unlike ALL, neither consolidation nor maintenance chemotherapy are required.
- **Lymphoblastic lymphomas** may be of B-cell or T-cell origin, usually present with widespread disease, and are treated with complex regimens. Treated similarly to ALL.
- **Waldenström macroglobulinemia** (see Chapter 21, Hematologic Disorders and Transfusion Therapy).

Multiple Myeloma

GENERAL PRINCIPLES

Epidemiology

Second most frequent hematologic malignancy after NHL. Median age at diagnosis is 68 years.

DIAGNOSIS

- Initial evaluation includes history, physical exam, CBC count, chemistry, β_2-microglobulin, serum protein electrophoresis, urine protein electrophoresis, serum free light chains, bone survey, and bone marrow exam. The diagnosis is confirmed by the presence of 10% of more plasma cells in the bone marrow and monoclonal protein in the serum or urine.

- **Staging:** The International Stage System for multiple myeloma (MM) uses β_2-microglobulin (B2M) and albumin to stratify patients into three stages: stage I (B2M <3.5 mg/dL and albumin >3.5 g/dL), stage II (albumin <3.5 g/dL or B2M 3.5–5.5 mg/dL), and stage III (B2M >5.5 mg/dL). Median survival in months for stages I, II, and III are 62, 44, and 29, respectively. However, it is clear now that the median survival has improved with the introduction of the newer novel agents such as lenalidomide and bortezomib.

Clinical Presentation

Most common presentation is bone pain. Anemia, renal failure, and hypercalcemia are also common.

TREATMENT

Treatment is usually reserved for symptomatic myeloma, including bone lesions, hypercalcemia, renal insufficiency, and anemia. The introduction of novel agents, such as thalidomide, lenalidomide, and bortezomib (usually in combination with dexamethasone), has led to a clear improvement in survival of patients with myeloma. However, much work is needed to determine the best sequence and combinations of therapies, as well as the role of autologous stem transplant in upfront therapy. It is therefore essential that, wherever possible, patients are entered into clinical trials.

Principles of Stem Cell Transplant

GENERAL PRINCIPLES

- **Background:** Hematopoietic stem cell transplant (HSCT) involves the infusion of autologous (patient) or allogenic (donor) stem cells after a "conditioning" regimen of chemotherapy and/or radiation. This allows for an intensification of chemotherapy with the hope of eradicating malignancy (autotransplant and allotransplant), and a graft versus tumor effect (allo only). More than 40,000 HSCTs are performed each year worldwide.
- **Indications:** Transplant can be considered for patients who have progressive or residual disease that is thought to be chemoresponsive (auto) or susceptible to graft versus tumor effect (allo). MM and lymphoma are the most common indications for autotransplant, and MDS and leukemia are the most common indications for allotransplant. Autotransplant is also used for refractory germ cell tumors.
- **Donor selection:** Appropriate allogenic donors are selected on the basis of the following:
  - HLA typing: Major histocompatibility class I and II alleles trigger immune activation. Six to 10 alleles are tested for compatibility and at least a 5 of 6 match is required.
  - Blood group: ABO-incompatible transplants are feasible but complex.
  - Cytomegalovirus (CMV)-negative donors are preferred for CMV-negative patients.
- **Source of stem cells**
  - The observation that the recovery phase after chemotherapy was associated with increased the number of circulating CD34+ cells, the surrogate marker of hematopoietic stem and progenitor cells (HSPCs) in humans, was first described in early 1980s, which led to its use for stem cell collection in preparation for autologous transplantation.

○ For patients undergoing autologous transplant, the number of CD34+ cells collected is a reliable predictor of neutrophils and platelet engraftment after transplantation. Platelet recovery is defined as that day the subject achieves a postnadir platelet count of >20 × 10⁹/L with no platelet transfusion in the prior 7 days; whereas neutrophil engraftment is defined as the first of 3 consecutive days on which the ANC count is >0.5 × 10⁹/L for 24 hours. The engraftment of neutrophils and platelets typically occurs in 8- to 10-day and 12- to 14-day time periods, respectively.

○ Sources of stem cells include:
  ▪ Bone marrow was historically used and is obtained under anesthesia from repeated aspirations from the iliac crest but is becoming less common.
  ▪ Peripheral blood stem cells have become the most common product. Stem cells routinely circulate in low numbers but can be "mobilized" by granulocyte colony-stimulating factor (G-CSF) and then collected by leukopheresis. Stem cells are limited when patients have received multiple cytotoxic agents, and plerixafor (a subcutaneous CXCR4 antagonist) was recently approved to increase stem cell collection in such patients.
  ▪ Umbilical cord blood can be used but is limited by the low volume of cord blood in each cord.

COMPLICATIONS

• **Hematopoietic:** Stem cells may fail to engraft, leading to prolonged cytopenias or failure after engraftment. Prolonged requirements for platelet and red blood cell transfusion are not uncommon. ABO incompatibility may lead to acute or delayed hemolysis.

• **Graft-versus-host disease (GVHD):** Occurs when the donor T cells react with recipient tissues leading to acute and chronic inflammation. Most common tissues affected include skin, cornea, gut, and lungs. Acute, mild GVHD is common but acute, severe GVHD is almost uniformly fatal. Chronic GVHD leads to diarrhea, nausea, sclerodermatous-type skin changes, and corneal irritation. Prophylaxis and treatment of GVHD rely on corticosteroids and a myriad of immunosuppressants.

• **Infectious:** During the immediate transplant period, patients are susceptible to infections associated with neutropenia, including overwhelming gram-negative sepsis, gram-positive infections of indwelling catheters, *Candida* infections, and herpes simplex virus (HSV) reactivation. The postengraftment period is complicated by impaired cell–mediated immunity, with susceptibility to CMV, *Pneumocystis carinii* pneumonia, and *Aspergillus* infections.

ONCOLOGIC EMERGENCIES

Febrile Neutropenia

GENERAL PRINCIPLES

Definition
Febrile neutropenia (FN) is defined as an absolute neutrophil count (ANC) of <500/mm³, with a single core temperature of >38.3°C or a persistent temperature (>1 hour) of >38.0°C.

Risk Factors

Risk of FN is proportional to the duration of neutropenia. Most solid tumor chemotherapy regimens have, if any, a brief (<5 day) duration of neutropenia. The highest risk for FN is with leukemia and transplant regimens in which neutropenia may persist for weeks. Risk is also increased with regimens that cause mucositis (inflammation and ulceration of the oral and GI mucosa).

DIAGNOSIS

- Evaluation should include a complete physical exam, including an assessment for mucositis, of catheter sites, and of the perianal region. DRE should not be performed because of the potential risk of bacterial translocation.
- Cultures of blood and urine in all patients and stool studies and sputum cultures of symptomatic patients should be obtained.
- Chest X-ray should be performed in all patients.

TREATMENT

- Patients should be treated emergently with intravenous antibiotics to prevent life-threatening, gram-negative sepsis.
- **Antimicrobial treatment**
  - Immediate, empiric intravenous antibiotics with coverage of gram-positive cocci and gram-negative bacilli (including *Pseudomonas aeruginosa*) must be included.
  - Empiric coverage of methicillin-resistant *Staphylococcus aureus* (MRSA) with vancomycin is not recommended unless patients are unstable, have active oral mucositis, have evidence of a catheter-related infection, or had a recent infection with MRSA.
  - Antimicrobials should be modified according to the source of infection if one is identified.
  - Persistent fever alone does not warrant a change in antibacterial therapy.
  - Empiric antifungal therapy should be considered if fever persists for >72 hours.
  - Gram-negative coverage should continue until ANC is >500/mm^3.
  - Low-risk patients (afebrile for 24 hours after antibiotics, negative culture results, and expected duration of myelosuppression for <1 week) can be treated as outpatients with oral, broad-spectrum antibiotics such as fluoroquinolone, amoxicillin/clavulanic acid, or trimethoprim-sulfamethoxazole.

SPECIAL CONSIDERATIONS

- Patients should be kept in reverse isolation.
- Consuming raw fruits and vegetables is not associated with excessive risk for infection in neutropenic patients.
- **White cell growth factors**
  - Growth factors may reduce the duration of hospitalization for FN but do not improve survival. Granulocyte colony-stimulating factor (G-CSF) is the most commonly used agent, given subcutaneously in doses of 5 μg/kg/day.

○ Growth factors should not be given within 24 hours after chemotherapy or during radiation because of the potential for increased myelosuppression.
○ Prophylactic G-CSF is used in the curative setting to (1) prevent FN when the risk is >15% and (2) reduce the duration of neutropenia to prevent chemotherapy delays.
○ Use of G-CSF for FN prophylaxis in the palliative setting is controversial since chemotherapy regimens with high rates of FN are usually not appropriate.

Tumor Lysis Syndrome

GENERAL PRINCIPLES

• Tumor lysis syndrome (TLS) is a group of metabolic disturbances resulting from significant tumor breakdown with release of intracellular products into the circulation.
• TLS occurs only in tumors that grow rapidly and are sensitive to cytotoxic chemotherapy. Highest incidence is seen in patients with acute leukemias and high-grade lymphomas.
• Risk is increased in cases of bulky tumors, high leukocyte counts, elevated pretreatment levels of LDH or uric acid, and compromised renal function.

DIAGNOSIS

Manifestations can be divided into laboratory and clinical (Table 22-15) (*Br J Haematol 2004;127:3*).

TREATMENT

• The most important intervention to prevent TLS is aggressive hydration of up to 3 $L/m^2/d$ to maintain a urine output of at least 100 $mL/m^2/hr$. The addition of bicarbonate to intravenous fluids for urine alkalinization remains controversial.
• Hyperuricemia is usually treated with the xanthine oxidase inhibitor, allopurinol. Rasburicase is a recombinant urate oxidase enzyme that degrades uric acid indicated in patients with elevated uric acid prior to treatment and those at high risk for developing hyperuricemia (elevated white blood cell levels, acute leukemias, high-grade lymphomas, and/or high LDH levels).

Table 22-15	Classification of Tumor Lysis Syndrome
Manifestation	**Features**
Laboratory	1. Uric acid ≥8 mg/dL or 25% increase from baseline
	2. Potassium ≥6 mEq/dL or 25% increase from baseline
	3. Phosphorus ≥6.5 mg/dL or 25% increase from baseline
	4. Calcium ≤7 mg/dL or 25% decrease from baseline
Clinical	1. Creatinine ≥1.5 upper normal limit
	2. Cardiac arrhythmia or sudden death
	3. Seizure

- Hyperkalemia is the main immediate threat and should be treated aggressively. Calcium administration should be restricted in patients with symptomatic hypocalcemia or in the treatment of symptomatic hyperkalemia, since it may cause metastatic calcifications in patients with hyperphosphatemia. Hyperphosphatemia should be treated with phosphate binders such as aluminum hydroxide.

Malignant Hypercalcemia

GENERAL PRINCIPLES

- Most common paraneoplastic syndrome, occurring in 10% to 20% of patients with cancer.
- Usually caused by squamous cell lung cancer, breast cancer, MM, and lymphoma.
- The three main mechanisms include focal bone destruction, humoral hypercalcemia due to the production of parathyroid hormone-related protein (PTH-rP), and tumor production of vitamin D analogs.

DIAGNOSIS

Classic symptoms usually develop with total calcium levels above 12 mg/dL and include polyuria, polydipsia, anorexia, constipation, nausea, vomiting, and confusion. Patients usually have severe hypovolemia due to excessive fluid losses and limited intake.

TREATMENT

The most important treatment consists of aggressive fluid replacement with normal saline. Diuretics should not be used unless volume overload is present. Intravenous bisphosphonates, which inhibit bone resorption by osteoclasts, may also be used. The two agents of choice are pamidronate 90 mg and zoledronic acid 4 mg. Refractory cases may be treated with calcitonin. Hypercalcemia caused by tumor production of vitamin D analogs may respond to corticosteroids.

Malignant Spinal Cord Compression

GENERAL PRINCIPLES

- A common problem affecting approximately 5% to 10% of patients with cancer.
- Commonly see in patients with lung cancer, breast cancer, prostate cancer, and lymphoma. When malignant spinal cord compression (MSCC) occurs in patients without a history of previous malignancy, the most common causes are lung cancer, lymphoma, and myeloma.

DIAGNOSIS

- The study of choice for MSCC is MRI of the entire spine. Plain radiography may also be helpful when there are delays in obtaining the MRI, since approximately 80% of the patients with MSCC have abnormal radiographic findings.

- The majority of patients present with back pain and tenderness to palpation in the involved vertebral body. The pain is usually worsened by recumbent position, sneezing, coughing, and Valsalva maneuver. Other symptoms include motor weakness, sensory loss, and dysfunction of the bladder and bowel.

TREATMENT

- Patients with suspected MSCC should be treated immediately with glucocorticoids. If there is a delay in obtaining imaging, treatment should begin even before the diagnostic test. The most commonly used corticosteroid regimen is dexamethasone in a 10- to 16-mg loading dose, followed by 4 mg every 4 hours. Higher doses, up to 100 mg, may be associated with slightly better pain control but are associated with increased toxicity and unclear effect on neurologic recovery.
- Both surgical and radiation consultation should be obtained at time of diagnosis. Surgery should be offered to patients who are candidates, as they are more likely to be ambulatory after treatment than patients with radiation (*Lancet 2005;366: 643*). External beam radiation therapy is the mainstay of treatment for nonsurgical candidates and should begin as soon as the diagnosis is made. Patients with chemosensitive tumors may be treated with systemic chemotherapy alone.

Brain Metastases with Increased Intracranial Pressure

GENERAL PRINCIPLES

- Brain metastases are common in patients with malignancies, with yearly incidence estimated between 90,000 and 170,000 cases. Many patients are asymptomatic and remain undiagnosed until the autopsy.
- Most common causes of brain metastases are lung cancer, breast cancer, and melanoma.
- Most lesions are supratentorial and located at gray–white matter junction, where the change in blood vessel size acts as a trap for emboli.

DIAGNOSIS

Clinical Presentation

Most patients have known cancer, and approximately one-third remain asymptomatic despite the brain metastases. The most common symptoms include headaches, confusion, and focal weakness.

Diagnostic Testing

Brain metastasis should be suspected in patients with cancer who develop neurologic symptoms and is confirmed by brain imaging with either CT scan with intravenous contrast or MRI.

TREATMENT

- Untreated patients usually die because of increasing peritumoral edema causing increased intracranial pressure and cerebral herniation.

- Symptomatic treatment with dexamethasone at the initial dose of 10 mg, followed by 4 mg every 6 hours, usually relieves symptoms.
- Whole-brain radiation is the treatment of choice for patients with multiple lesions. Chemotherapy may have a role in sensitive tumors, particularly in previously radiated patients.
- Anticonvulsants are indicated only in patients with seizures and has no benefit as prophylaxis.
- Selected patients with a solitary lesion in an accessible site and a controlled primary tumor may undergo surgery with curative intent. Stereotactic radiosurgery may also be used in similar patients.

Superior Vena Cava Syndrome

DIAGNOSIS

- Typically diagnosed by history and physical examination with careful evaluation for airway compression. Venous thrombosis should be ruled out, using CT with intravenous contrast.
- It is most commonly associated with primary lung tumors and less commonly with lymphoma, germ cell tumors, or other mediastinal masses and presents as facial and upper extremity erythema, swelling, and venous engorgement. Severe cases are associated with headache and confusion. SVC syndrome is usually a subacute rather than emergent presentation.

TREATMENT

Empiric corticosteroids can reduce swelling and temporarily reduce symptoms. Urgent initiation of radiotherapy is usually indicated for most solid tumors. Chemotherapy is preferable in patients with high grade lymphomas, germ cell tumors, or small cell lung cancer.

MANAGEMENT OF TREATMENT TOXICITIES

Nausea

GENERAL PRINCIPLES

- Historically, nausea was one of the most debilitating side effects of chemotherapy, but with improved antiemetics and newer chemotherapy agents, nausea is less burdensome for patients.
- Incidence of chemotherapy-induced nausea and vomiting (CINV) is widely variable among chemotherapy agents and is dosed dependent (see Table 22-6 for a general summary). With aggressive antiemetics, vomiting is very uncommon for the great majority of chemotherapy regimens.
- CINV is divided into acute (<24 hours) and delayed (>24 hours). Acute CINV is the most important predictor of delayed CINV.
- **Prevention** is by far more effective than treatment when it occurs.
  - Dexamethasone is an active antiemetic and is frequently given intravenously prior to chemotherapy and often continued orally for 2 to 3 days.

- 5HT3 receptor antagonists (ondansetron, granisetron, dolasetron, palonosetron, etc.) are widely used chemotherapy premedications as CINV prophylaxis and are highly effective.
- Aprepitant is a newer agent that is indicated only with regimens with high rates of CINV.

TREATMENT

- Posttreatment nausea should not be immediately assumed to be secondary to chemotherapy, particularly since many agents lead to little or no nausea (see Table 22-6). Secondary causes, including bowel obstruction, brain metastasis with cerebral edema, constipation, narcotics, and gastroenteritis, should all be considered.
- Initial treatment with prochlorperazine is often effective. Lorazepam or other anxiolytics have antiemetic properties. 5HT3 antagonists are less effective in treatment than in prevention but are frequently used. Olanzapine has also been studied and found to be active.

Diarrhea

GENERAL PRINCIPLES

Diarrhea is a common side effect of many chemotherapies (irinotecan, 5-FU, capecitabine) and targeted agents (erlotinib, cetuximab, sunitinib, lapatinib).

TREATMENT

- Empiric and aggressive treatment with loperamide is essential for avoiding volume depletion, particularly with irinotecan.
- When loperamide is ineffective, diphenoxylate, atropine ("Lomotil"), or other agents can be used.

Cytopenias

GENERAL PRINCIPLES

- **Neutropenia** management and prevention are discussed in the previous text with FN.
- **Anemia** is common with many chemotherapy regimens.
  - Evaluation for iron deficiency (ferritin, serum Fe, and total iron-binding capacity) should take place in all patients. Hemolysis or blood loss should be considered if anemia is acute.
  - Red blood cell transfusion should be avoided unless hemoglobin is <8 g/dL or <10 g/dL with cardiac disease or symptoms.
  - Erythropoietin analogs (erythropoietin, darbepoetin) reduce the rate of blood transfusions but should not be used in the absence of significant anemia (<10 mg/dL) and are only reserved for use in patients with incurable malignancies, as there are serious concerns that these agents are associated with increased mortality from disease progression and/or thromboembolism.

- ○ Intravenous iron supplementation may further reduce the need for transfusion and can be considered in patients with a serum ferritin level of <100 ng/mL.
- **Thrombocytopenia** is common with many chemotherapy regimens. Recently, oprelvekin (IL-11, Neumega) is approved for the prevention of severe thrombocytopenia and a reduction in the need for platelet transfusions following myelosuppressive chemotherapy in adult patients with nonmyeloid malignancies who are at high risk of severe thrombocytopenia. Efficacy was demonstrated in patients who had experienced severe thrombocytopenia following the previous chemotherapy cycle. Major side effects include fluid retention with dilutional anemia, peripheral edema, pleural effusions, and atrial arrhythmias. Chemotherapy may need to be held or dose reduced for platelet counts <50,000/mm^3. Patients with hematologic malignancies, particularly after stem cell transplant, may have prolonged thrombocytopenia and require platelet transfusions to keep platelet counts >5,000/mm^3 or to treat bleeding.

Mucositis

GENERAL PRINCIPLES

- Mucositis (inflammation and ulceration of the oral and GI mucosa) is common with many chemotherapy regimens and is worst with chemoradiation and stem cell transplant regimens.
- For **prevention**, oral saline or bicarbonate rinses are minimally effective. Oral cryotherapy has shown to reduce the severity of mucositis with 5-FU by inducing vasoconstriction that leads to less drug exposure. Palifermin, a recombinant keratinocyte growth factor, and calcium phosphate rinse have shown efficacy in patients undergoing high-dose chemotherapy in preparation for HSCT.

DIAGNOSIS

- Presents as oral pain/ulcers, odynophagia/dysphagia, abdominal pain, or diarrhea.
- HSV stomatitis should be ruled out in immunocompromised patients.

TREATMENT

Viscous lidocaine for oral or esophageal pain, with oral or intravenous narcotics for refractory pain. Acid suppression may improve abdominal pain and antimotility agents should be used aggressively for diarrhea.

Pneumonitis

GENERAL PRINCIPLES

Pneumonitis is an uncommon but potentially life-threatening complication of thoracic radiation, EGFR-targeted therapies, carmustine, and bleomycin.

DIAGNOSIS

New cough, shortness of breath, or hypoxia in susceptible patients should be evaluated with a chest radiograph and CT if there is any suspicion for pneumonitis.

TREATMENT

Treatment with corticosteroids (prednisone 50 mg/d) usually improves symptoms but chronic fibrosis may develop.

SUPPORTIVE CARE: COMPLICATIONS OF CANCER

Cancer Pain

GENERAL PRINCIPLES

- Pain is one of the most common manifestations in cancer, with an estimated incidence of 25% at diagnosis and at least 75% in advanced stages.
- The two main mechanisms for pain are nociceptive (somatic or visceral) and neuropathic. Nociceptive pain is caused by stimulation of pain receptors and neuropathic pain by direct injury to the peripheral or central nervous system. Somatic pain typically occurs in bone metastases, musculoskeletal inflammation, or after surgery and is characterized by a well-localized, dull, or aching pain. Visceral pain results from tumor infiltration and compression or distention of viscera and is described as diffuse, deep, squeezing, and pressure-like sensation. Neuropathic pain occurs due to tumor infiltration of peripheral nerves, plexi, roots, or spinal cord, as well as chemical injury caused by chemotherapy, radiotherapy, or surgery. This pain is described as sharp or burning sensation. These three types of pain may occur alone or in combination in the same patient.
- Cancer pain in adults may be classified into three levels on the basis of a 0 to 10 numerical scale: mild pain (1 to 3), moderate pain (4 to 6), and severe pain (7 to 10).

TREATMENT

- The treatment is usually based on the WHO ladder, with a stepwise approach according to the level of pain. Patients with mild pain and not taking opioids may be treated with nonopioid analgesics including nonsteroidal anti-inflammatory drugs (NSAIDs) or acetaminophen (step 1). Patients with no response to nonopioids or moderate pain are treated with weak opioids such as codeine, hydrocodone, and oxycodone, alone or in combination with acetaminophen (step 2). Severe pain is treated with morphine, hydromorphone, methadone, or transdermal fentanyl (step 3). Tramadol, which has weak affinity to μ-opioid receptors and is considered a nonopioid medicine, may be used in patients with mild-to-moderate pain not responding to NSAIDs and who wish to defer opioid treatment. The oral route is usually the most appropriate route because of easier administration and lower costs.

- Patients with mild pain may be reevaluated at the next appointment, whereas those with moderate or severe pain should be reevaluated within 24 to 48 hours. Dose titration should be done aggressively to expedite symptom relief.
- Coanalgesics should be considered in specific cases. Systemic corticosteroids may be useful in pain caused by bone metastases, increased cranial pressure, spinal cord compression, and nerve compression or infiltration. Tricyclic antidepressants, such as nortriptyline, and anticonvulsants, such as gabapentin, are commonly indicated in neuropathic pain, which is usually less responsive to opioids. Bisphosphonates (zoledronic acid and pamidronate) and radiolabeled agents (strontium-89 and samarium-153) may help treat pain resulting from bone metastases.
- Common side effects of opioid therapy include constipation, nausea, respiratory depression, and sedation.
  ○ Constipation should be prevented with the prophylactic use of combined stimulant laxative and stool softener (senna + docusate). If symptoms persist, patients may benefit from the addition of a third agent, including lactulose, magnesium citrate, polyethylene glycol, or enema.
  ○ Nausea may develop during the treatment and should be aggressively treated. Respiratory depression may occur with short-acting agents, but patients usually develop tolerance to repeated administration.
  ○ Sedation and drowsiness may be treated by decreasing the individual dose by increasing the frequency of administration and/or changing to an agent with shorter half-life.
- Patients who experience inadequate pain control despite aggressive opioid therapy or who cannot tolerate opioid titration due to side effects may benefit from interventional therapies, including regional infusion of analgesics and neuroablative or neurostimulatory procedures.

Bone Metastasis

GENERAL PRINCIPLES

Most common in prostate, breast, lung, kidney, and bladder cancers and MM.

DIAGNOSIS

Bone scan (nuclear imaging with technetium-99m) is sensitive for blastic lesions and but will not detect lytic lesions (i.e., MM). Concerning lesions on bone scan should be evaluated with plain X-ray films or CT to identify lesions at risk for pathologic fracture.

TREATMENT

- Pain should be managed aggressively with opioids. NSAIDs may give additional relief.
- Lesions at risk for fracture should be treated with radiation therapy. Bisphosphonates and RANK ligand inhibitors may reduce the risk for fracture and reduce pain.

Pleural Effusion

GENERAL PRINCIPLES

Pleural effusions are common in primary lung cancer and mesothelioma, as well as in advanced breast cancer and lymphoma. Effusions may be malignant (positive fluid cytology or pleural biopsy) or paramalignant (caused by indirect tumor effects). This distinction is critical in lung cancer since patients with malignant effusions are not considered for potentially curative therapies (classified as stage IV disease).

DIAGNOSIS

Routine thoracentesis with cytologic evaluation is typically adequate. However, effusions with negative cytology should be further evaluated with thoracoscopy or open pleural biopsy (see Chapter 10, Pulmonary Diseases).

TREATMENT

- Prompt and complete drainage by therapeutic thoracentesis is necessary to avoid chronic fibrosis and trapped lung. Observation for rate of reaccumulation after initial drainage is appropriate for most patients. Rapidly reaccumulating effusions (<1 month) should be treated aggressively.
- Pleurodesis (obliteration of the pleural space by fibrosis) by complete drainage and instillation of a sclerosant (usually talc) will prevent recurrence of most malignant effusions. Requires hospitalization and chest tube placement causing significant temporary pain.
- Placement of an indwelling pleural catheter for intermittent outpatient drainage is an alternative. Pleural fibrosis and resolution of the effusion occurs over several weeks in most patients.
- Medical therapy may be sufficient in breast cancer or lymphoma but is otherwise ineffective.
- Radiation of the pleural space is not feasible, but treatment of central masses will often alleviate paramalignant effusions.

Venous Thromboembolism

GENERAL PRINCIPLES

- Any malignancy is a hypercoagulable state, which manifests as a spectrum of diseases from migratory superficial thrombophlebitis (Trousseau's syndrome) to life-threatening venous thromboembolism (VTE). VTE is most frequent in hematologic malignancies and adenocarcinomas of the lung and GI tract.
- Empiric **prevention** with warfarin, unfractionated heparin, or low–molecular-weight heparins (LMWHs) is not recommended in patients without known VTE.

TREATMENT

- Anticoagulant treatment in patients with cancer is associated with more recurrent VTE and bleeding complications than in patients without cancer.

- Treatment with LMWH is superior to warfarin in patients with cancer (recurrent VTE in 8% vs. 16%) with no difference in bleeding, but cost and daily injections are prohibitive for many patients. Dalteparin is approved for this indication in the United States (*N Engl J Med 2003;349:146*).
- Treatment with warfarin is complicated by more frequent treatment failures, as well as varying oral intake due to anorexia and chemotherapy, and requires vigilant INR monitoring.
- Treatment should continue indefinitely or until the malignancy resolves.

Fatigue

GENERAL PRINCIPLES

- Common symptom in cancer, occurring in an estimated 80% of patients with advanced disease.
- Underlying depression should be managed appropriately, including antidepressants when indicated.

TREATMENT

First step in the treatment is the identification of treatable contributing factors such as pain, poor nutrition, emotional distress, sleep disturbance, activity level, and comorbidities (anemia, infection, organ dysfunction). Pain management, nutrition support, sleep therapy, exercise, and optimization therapy for comorbidities may improve the fatigue symptoms.

Medications
- Erythropoietin may be helpful in patients with anemia.
- Methylphenidate may provide rapid improvement, and dose escalations may be required over time to maintain benefit.
- Modafinil improves fatigue in multiple sclerosis and may be useful in cancer patients.

Anorexia and Cachexia

GENERAL PRINCIPLES

- Anorexia is defined as loss of appetite in cancer patients with associated weight loss.
- Cachexia is a metabolic syndrome characterized by profound involuntary weight loss.

TREATMENT

- In addition to caloric supplementation, patients may benefit from pharmacologic therapy.
- Megestrol acetate is active, with symptomatic improvement in <1 week. Despite the quick increase in the appetite, it may take several weeks to achieve weight gain. Megestrol is also associated with an increased risk of thromboembolism.
- Dexamethasone provides a short-lived improvement, usually without significant weight gain.
- Dronabinol has limited benefits in anorexia and is associated with sedation.

23 Diabetes Mellitus and Related Disorders

Janet B. McGill

Diabetes Mellitus

GENERAL PRINCIPLES

- **Diabetes mellitus (DM)** is a group of metabolic diseases characterized by hyperglycemia resulting from defects in insulin secretion, insulin action, or both.
- DM is present in 11.3% of persons over the age of 20 years in the United States, and 26.9% of those over the age of 65 years. A substantial percentage of affected persons are not diagnosed. Type 2 diabetes (T2DM) represents 90% to 95% of all cases of diabetes, with type 1 diabetes (T1DM) and other causes representing the remaining 5% to 10% (*http://www.cdc.gov/diabetes/pubs*).
- Persons with diabetes are at risk for microvascular complications, including retinopathy, nephropathy, and neuropathy, and are at increased risk for macrovascular disease.
- T2DM is accompanied by hypertension in about 75% and hyperlipidemia in more than half of adult patients and is considered a "cardiac risk equivalent" because of the excess risk for macrovascular disease, cardiovascular (CV) disease events, and mortality (*Diabetes Care 2012;35(suppl 1):S11*).

Classification

DM is classified into four clinical classes (*Diabetes Care 2012;35(suppl 1):S64*).

- T1DM accounts for <10% of all cases of DM and results from a cellular-mediated autoimmune destruction of the beta (β) cells of the pancreas.
  - The rate of destruction of β cells is rapid in infants and children and slower in adults. Thus, the presentation in young people is often ketoacidosis, whereas older persons may have a longer symptomatic prodrome and may be diagnosed on the basis of hyperglycemia and positive autoantibodies.
  - T1DM is characterized by severe insulin deficiency. Exogenous insulin is required to control blood glucoses (BGs), prevent diabetic ketoacidosis (DKA), and preserve life. When insulin is withheld from a person with T1DM, ketosis will develop in 8 to 16 hours and ketoacidosis in 12 to 24 hours.
  - Early in the course of T1DM, some insulin secretory capacity remains and the insulin requirement may be lower than expected (0.3 to 0.4 U/kg). Tight control of BG level from the onset has been shown to preserve the residual β-cell function and prevent or delay later complications.
  - Latent autoimmune diabetes in adults (LADA) is characterized by mild-to-moderate hyperglycemia at presentation that often responds to noninsulin therapies but progresses over months to years to insulin dependency. Adults with LADA will have one or more β-cell specific autoantibodies and tend to require insulin therapy sooner than patients with classic T2DM.

- T2DM accounts for >90% of all cases of diabetes. T2DM is characterized by insulin resistance followed by reduced insulin secretion from β cells that are unable to compensate for the increased insulin requirements.
  - T2DM is usually diagnosed in adults, with both incidence and prevalence increasing with age; however, T2DM is not uncommon in children and adolescents, and accounts for up to one-third of new cases of diabetes diagnosed between the ages of 5 and 15 years.
  - T2DM is associated with obesity, family history of diabetes, history of gestational diabetes or prediabetes, hypertension, physical inactivity, and race/ethnicity. African Americans, Latinos, Asian Indians, Native Americans, Pacific Islanders, and some groups of Asians have a greater risk of developing T2DM than Caucasians.
  - T2DM may be asymptomatic and therefore remain undiagnosed for months to years in affected individuals.
  - Insulin secretion is usually sufficient to prevent ketosis, but DKA or hyperosmolar nonketotic coma can develop during severe stress. T2DM in patients who present with, or later develop ketosis or DKA, but who do not require insulin between episodes is referred to as ketosis-prone T2DM.
- **Other specific types of DM** include those that result from genetic defects in insulin secretion or action, pancreatic surgery or disease, endocrinopathies (e.g., Cushing syndrome, acromegaly), drugs, and diabetes associated with other syndromes.
- **Gestational DM** (GDM) is defined as any degree of glucose intolerance, with onset or diagnosis during pregnancy. The prevalence of GDM depends on the criteria used for diagnosis, with 2% to 10% of pregnancies affected (old criteria), compared to 18% of pregnancies affected (new criteria). About 60% of women with GDM will develop T2DM in the ensuing 5 to 10 years and all remain at an increased risk for the development of T2DM later in life (*http://www.cdc.gov/diabetes/pubs*).
  - All patients with GDM should undergo diagnostic testing 6 to 12 weeks postpartum and annually thereafter to determine whether abnormal carbohydrate metabolism has persisted or is recurrent.
  - Weight loss and exercise are encouraged to decrease the risk of persistent prediabetes or T2DM after delivery.

DIAGNOSIS

- **The diagnosis of DM** can be established using any of the following criteria (*Diabetes Care 2012;35(suppl 1):S64*):
  - **Hemoglobin A1c (A1C) ≥ 6.5%** using a NGSP-certified method
  - **Fasting plasma glucose (FPG) ≥ 126 mg/dL** (7.0 mmol/L) after an overnight fast. A positive value should be confirmed with a repeat test.
  - **Symptoms of diabetes** (polyuria, polydipsia fatigue, weight loss) and a random plasma glucose level of ≥200 mg/dL (11.1 mmol/L).
  - **Oral glucose tolerance test** (OGTT) that shows a plasma glucose level of ≥200 mg/dL (11.1 mmol/L) at 2 hours after ingestion of 75 g of glucose.
- **Categories of increased risk for diabetes (*prediabetes*).**
  - **Impaired fasting glucose (IFG):** FPG ≥100 and ≤125 mg/dL (5.6 to 6.9 mmol/L).
  - **Impaired glucose tolerance (IGT):** 2-hour glucose 140 to 199 mg/dL (7.8 to 11.0 mmol/L) after ingesting 75 g glucose (OGTT).

- **A1C** in the range 5.7% to 6.4%.
- Progression from IFG or IGT to T2DM occurs at the rate of 2% to 22% (average, about 12%) per year depending on the population studied.
- Lifestyle modification, including a balanced hypocaloric diet to achieve 7% weight loss in overweight patients and regular exercise of $\geq$150 minutes per week, is recommended for persons with prediabetes to prevent progression to T2DM (*Diabetes Care 2012;35(suppl 1):S11*).
- Metformin may be considered in patients with prior GDM, those with BMI >35, or those <60 years of age (*Diabetes Care 2012;35(suppl 1):S11*).

TREATMENT

Principles of Management of Diabetes Mellitus

- **Goals of therapy** are alleviation of symptoms, achievement of glycemic, blood pressure, and lipid targets, and prevention of acute and chronic complications of diabetes.
  - Glycemic control recommendations are the same for type 1 and type 2 diabetes: Fasting and preprandial capillary BG 70 to 130 mg/dL (3.9 to 7.2 mmol/L), postprandial capillary BG <180 mg/dL (<10 mmol/L), and A1C <7% or as close to normal as possible while avoiding significant hypoglycemia (*Diabetes Care 2012;35(suppl 1):S11*). American Association of Clinical Endocrinologists (AACE) and European Association for the Study of Diabetes (EASD) recommend an A1C target of <6.5% (*Endocr Pract 2011;17(suppl 2):1*). This degree of glycemic control has been associated with the lowest risk for microvascular complications in patients with T1DM (*N Engl J Med 1993;329:978*) as well as T2DM (*BMJ 2000;321:405*; *Lancet 1998;352:837*).
  - Tight glycemic control in patients with risk factors for CV disease has been associated with increased mortality (*N Engl J Med 2011;364:818*; *N Engl J Med 2008;359:1577*). Hypoglycemia was implicated as the cause of higher mortality in one, but not all, of the studies (*N Engl J Med 2008;359:1577*). Less tight glycemic goals may be appropriate for patients with a history of CV events or those at high risk for CV events.
  - The blood pressure target for patients with diabetes is <130/80 mm Hg; and the use of either an angiotensin-converting enzyme (ACE) inhibitor or an angiotensin receptor blocker (ARB) is recommended as first-line therapy. For those patients not at goal, a thiazide diuretic should be added if the glomerular filtration rate (GFR) is >30 mL/min/1.73 m^2 and a loop diuretic if the GFR is <30 mL/min/1.73 m^2 (*JAMA 2003;289:2560*).
  - The lipid targets are as follows: low-density lipoprotein (LDL) <100 mg/dL, total cholesterol <150 mg/dL, and high-density lipoprotein (HDL) >40 mg/dL in men and >50 mg/dL in women. In patients with known CV disease or two risk factors in addition to DM, the LDL should be <70 mg/dL, preferably using high-dose statin therapy (*Circulation 2004;110:227*).
  - Aspirin therapy should be advised in patients with diabetes and older than 40 years or who have other risk factors. Low doses (75 to 162 mg) are appropriate for primary prevention (*Diabetes Care 2010;33:1395*).
- **Assessment of glycemic control** consists of the following:
  - **Self-monitoring of blood glucose (SMBG)** is recommended for all patients who take insulin and provides useful information for those on noninsulin therapies. Patients using multiple daily injections or insulin pumps should test

≥3 times daily. Less frequent testing may be appropriate for those on noninsulin therapies. While most SMBG is done before meals and at bedtime, periodic testing 1 to 2 hours after eating may be necessary to achieve postprandial glucose targets (*Diabetes Care 2012;35(suppl 1):S11*).

○ **Continuous glucose monitoring (CGM)** has been shown to reduce A1C in adults older than 25 years on intensive insulin therapy. CGM measures interstitial glucose, which provides a close approximation of BG values. Hypoglycemia and hyperglycemia alarms may help patients with widely fluctuating BG levels or hypoglycemia unawareness. CGM is supplemental to SMBG (*N Engl J Med 2008;359:1464*).

○ **A1C** provides an integrated measure of BG values over the preceding 2 to 3 months. A1C should be obtained every 3 months in patients not at goal or when either diabetes therapy or clinical condition changes, twice yearly in well-controlled patients. A1C should confirm results of SMBG, and discordant values should be investigated. An A1C level that is higher than expected should be evaluated by a diabetes educator to ensure meter accuracy, appropriate technique, and frequency of testing. When the A1C is lower than expected, blood loss, transfusion, hemolysis, and hemoglobin variants should be considered. The correlation between A1C and mean plasma glucose is sufficiently strong that laboratory reports may include both the A1C result and the estimated average glucose (*Diabetes Care 2012;35(suppl 1):S11*).

○ **Ketones** can be detected in a fingerstick blood sample by measuring β-hydroxybutyrate with the handheld glucose/ketone meter, Precision Xtra. Urine ketones can be qualitatively identified, using Ketostix or Acetest tablets. Patients with T1DM should test for ketones, using one of these methods during febrile illness, for persistent elevation of glucose (>300 mg/dL), or if signs of impending DKA (e.g., nausea, vomiting, abdominal pain) develop. Testing for β-hydroxybutyrate is useful in emergency departments to determine whether a patient with hyperglycemia has ketonemia (*Acad Emerg Med 2006;13(6):683*). Hospital laboratories measure serum ketones including acetone, acetoacetate, and β-hydroxybutyrate.

MANAGEMENT

Comprehensive diabetes management includes coordinated diet, exercise, and medication plans. **Patient education** in medical nutrition therapy (MNT), exercise, SMBG, medication use and insulin dosing, and administration is integral to the successful management of diabetes.

Medical Nutrition Therapy

- MNT includes dietary recommendations for a healthy, balanced diet to achieve adequate nutrition and maintain an ideal body weight (*Diabetes Care 2012;35(suppl 1):S11*).
- Caloric restriction is recommended for overweight individuals, with individualized targets that may be as low as 1,000 to 1,500 kcal/d for women and 1,200 to 1,800 kcal/d for men depending on activity level and starting body weight.
- Caloric intake is usually distributed as follows: 45% to 65% of total calories as carbohydrates, 10% to 30% as protein, and <30% as total fat (<7% saturated fat) with <300 mg/d of cholesterol.

- In patients with LDL cholesterol >100 mg/dL (2.6 mmol/L), total fat should be restricted to <25% of total calories, saturated fat to <7%, and <200 mg/d of cholesterol.
- Patients with progressive kidney disease may benefit from restriction of protein intake to 0.8 g/kg/d. Patients with severe chronic kidney disease (CKD) will need additional restrictions of potassium- and phosphorus-containing foods.
- "Carbohydrate counting" is a useful skill for patients on intensified insulin therapy who adjust insulin doses based on carbohydrate content of meals and snacks.

Exercise

Exercise improves insulin sensitivity, reduces fasting and postprandial BG levels, and offers numerous metabolic, CV, and psychological benefits in diabetic patients.

- In general, 150 minutes per week is recommended as part of a healthy lifestyle and has been shown to assist with the prevention and management of T2DM.
- Patients may need individualized guidance regarding exercise, and they are more likely to exercise when counseled by their physician to do so.

Diabetes Mellitus in Hospitalized Patients

GENERAL PRINCIPLES

Diabetes-specific indications for hospitalization

- **DKA** is characterized by a plasma glucose level of >250 mg/dL in association with an arterial pH <7.30 or serum bicarbonate level of <15 mEq/L and moderate ketonemia or ketonuria.
- **Hyperosmolar nonketotic** state includes marked hyperglycemia (≥400 mg/dL) and elevated serum osmolality (>315 mOsm/kg), often accompanied by impaired mental status.
- **Hypoglycemia** is an indication for hospitalization if induced by a sulfonylurea (SFU) medication, is due to a deliberate drug overdose, or results in coma, seizure, injury, or persistent neurologic change.
- **Newly diagnosed T1DM** or newly recognized GDM can be indications for hospitalization, even in the absence of ketoacidosis (see Type 1 Diabetes and Diabetic Ketoacidosis section).
- **Patients with T2DM** are rarely admitted to the hospital for initiation or change in insulin therapy unless hyperglycemia is severe and associated with mental status change or other organ dysfunction.

Management of diabetes in hospitalized patients

Hyperglycemia is a common finding in hospitalized patients and may be due to previously diagnosed diabetes, undiagnosed diabetes, medications, or stress-induced hyperglycemia. Up to 40% of general medical and surgical patients exhibit hyperglycemia, and approximately 80% of intensive care unit (ICU) patients will demonstrate transient or persistent hyperglycemia. Patients with T1DM should be clearly identified as such at the time of admission.

- A1C can help identify previously undiagnosed diabetes in hospitalized patients and may assist with the evaluation of prior glucose control. A1C is not accurate in patients who are severely anemic, bleeding, or hemolyzing or who have been transfused.
- Data are limited to nonexistent regarding use of noninsulin therapies in inpatients.

○ Medication reconciliation on admission should include a careful assessment of home diabetes medications, level of glucose control, kidney function, expected diagnostic studies and treatments, and the possible need for insulin treatment.

○ Patients who are required to fast for diagnostic testing or treatments should have all noninsulin therapies stopped.

○ **Patients hospitalized for reasons other than diabetes and are eating normally** may continue or restart outpatient diabetes treatments, unless specifically contraindicated.

○ Use of noninsulin therapies may be appropriate in psychiatric units, rehabilitation settings, or in stable patients preparing for discharge.

• **Glucose targets for inpatients** have been established to maximize reduction of morbidity and mortality, while minimizing the risk of hypoglycemia (*Endocr Pract 2009;15:353*).

○ In critical care settings, the glucose target is 140 to 180 mg/dL (7.8 to 10.0 mmol/L) with frequent monitoring recommended for scrupulous avoidance of hypoglycemia.

○ In noncritical care settings, the glucose target is 140 mg/dL (7.8 mmol/L) fasting and premeal, <180 mg/dL (10.0 mmol/L) postmeal or on a random glucose check.

Management of hyperglycemia in critical care settings

• Variable intravenous (IV) insulin infusion is recommended for critical illness, emergency surgery, or major surgery (see Perioperative Management on Diabetes Mellitus, Chapter 1, Patient Care in Internal Medicine). Numerous algorithms have been published which direct insulin dose adjustments, based on capillary BG values performed hourly at the bedside.

• An IV infusion of a dextrose-containing solution or other caloric source should be provided to prevent hypoglycemia and ketosis. For fluid restricted patients, 10% dextrose in water (D10W) can be infused at a rate of 10 to 25 mL/hr to provide a steady, consistent source of calories.

• Transition from insulin drip to SC insulin should occur before a meal, preferably before breakfast. The insulin drip should be discontinued 30 minutes to 1 hour after patients have received SC regular insulin and intermediate-acting insulin; however, if a rapid-acting insulin is used, the insulin drip can be discontinued shortly after SC insulin has been administered.

Management of hyperglycemia in noncritical care hospital settings

• BG should be checked on admission in all patients and monitored four times per day in hyperglycemic patients, especially in patients treated with insulin.

• The common practice of using "sliding scale" only has been shown to provide suboptimal glycemic control when compared to a basal/bolus regimen and is inappropriate for a patient with T1DM regardless of the BG on admission or a patient with insulin-requiring T2DM (*Diabetes Care 2007;30:2181*; *Diabetes Care 2011;34:256*). Any patient with a BG level of >150 mg/dL should be considered for basal insulin or basal/bolus therapy, leaving "sliding scale" only to patients with intermittent minor elevations in BG.

• For patients naïve to insulin, a starting dose of basal insulin should equal 0.2 U/kg or 0.1 U/lb. If the presenting BG level is >200 mg/dL, adding premeal insulin is appropriate. The dose should be 0.2 U/kg divided by three meals.
Example: Your patient weighs 80 kg and has a BG level of 250 mg/dL. The starting insulin dose should be 16 units of long-acting insulin plus 5 U of rapid-acting

insulin before each meal. A correction dose of 1 to 2 U per 50 mg/dL of BG, beginning at 150 mg/dL, can be added to the premeal doses.

- Patients with T1DM should continue their home insulin doses and may continue the use of an insulin pump if there is a hospital policy in place to do so. Insulin doses in patients with T2DM should be reduced by 20% to 50% on admission.
- Meal-time insulin doses should be given shortly before or immediately after meals and the correction factor or sliding scale dose should be added to the premeal dose. Correction factor (sliding scale insulin added to basal/bolus regimen) should be reduced or not given at bedtime or during the night; or the glucose scale for intervention should be set higher.
- Adjustments in the next-day basal or premeal insulin doses are indicated if correction doses of insulin are frequently required, or if clinical status or medications change.
- Extreme hyperglycemia (>300 mg/dL, 16.7 mmol/L) on more than one consecutive test should prompt testing for ketoacidosis with electrolytes and ketone measurements.
- Hypoglycemia should be treated promptly with oral or IV glucose and the capillary BG should be repeated every 10 minutes until >100 mg/dL (5.5 mmol/L) stable. Reevaluation of scheduled doses and assessment of risk factors for hypoglycemia (declining renal function, hepatic impairment, poor intake) should be undertaken for any BG <70 mg/dL (3.9 mmol/L) (ACE/ADA Task Force on Inpatient Diabetes) (*Endocr Pract 2006;12:458*).
- **Enteral nutrition** (*Mayo Clin Proc 1996;71:587*). Intermittent tube feeds should be matched by either short-acting (human regular) insulin or intermediate-acting (human NPH) insulin. Patients with baseline hyperglycemia may need a basal insulin dose in addition to the doses given to cover tube feeds. For example, nighttime enteral feeding lasting 6 to 8 hours should be managed with NPH, with or without a basal insulin dose. NPH can be given three to four times daily for continuous tube feeds, allowing a change in insulin dose if the feeding is interrupted.
- **Total parenteral nutrition (TPN).** Patients supported with TPN are likely to develop hyperglycemia, and some require large amounts of insulin. See Chapter 2, Nutrition Support, for insulin management of patients on TPN.

Perioperative guidelines for surgery in patients with diabetes

Comprehensive guidelines have been published by the National Health Service in the United Kingdom for perioperative management of adults with diabetes (*Diabet Med 2012;29:420*).

- Perioperative planning should include risk assessment, minimization of starvation time by scheduling surgery early, use of glucose containing IV solutions and variable insulin infusion for management of hyperglycemia, and resumption of home therapy as soon as possible.
- In general, elective surgery should not be scheduled in patients with poorly controlled diabetes, defined by A1C >8.5%. Efforts should be undertaken to achieve this level of glucose control as an outpatient prior to surgery.
- Preoperative assessment should include glucose, acid–base, electrolyte (potassium, magnesium, and phosphate), and fluid status.
- Recommended glucose targets in the perioperative period and during surgery are 108 to 180 mg/dL (6 to 10 mmol/L). Glucose should be checked hourly in persons with diabetes who have taken insulin or who require insulin perioperatively.
- In emergency situations, DKA and neuropathy complications mimicking surgical emergencies should be excluded. Hyperglycemia or hypoglycemia, acidosis, electrolyte, and volume status should be corrected prior to surgery if possible.

- Patients should continue their basal insulin doses for outpatient surgeries or minor procedures, and resume bolus doses with corrections as soon as possible postoperatively.
- Emergency or major elective surgery may be better handled with a variable IV insulin infusion, supplemented with glucose and potassium as needed to achieve target BG levels. Hourly glucose measurements are mandatory to adjust insulin and glucose infusions. Potassium should be monitored at least every 2 hours and replaced aggressively as required.

TYPE 1 DIABETES AND DIABETIC KETOACIDOSIS

Type 1 Diabetes

GENERAL PRINCIPLES

A comprehensive approach is necessary for successful management of T1DM. A team approach that includes the expertise of physicians, diabetes educators, dietitians, and other members of the diabetes care team offers the best chance of success.

DIAGNOSIS

The diagnosis of T1DM is usually made in childhood or adolescence, often after presenting with DKA or very high BG and ketonuria. T1DM can present at any age, however; and because of the variable prodrome of hyperglycemia, the diagnosis can be challenging in adults.

- T1DM should be suspected when there is a family history of T1DM, thyroid disease, or other autoimmune disease.
- Presentation with ketoacidosis suggests T1DM, but confirmatory tests may be useful to guide therapy.
- Autoantibodies include islet cell autoantibodies (ICA), antibodies to insulin, antibodies to glutamic acid decarboxylase (anti-GAD), and antibodies to tyrosine phosphatases IA-2 and IA-2β. Measuring one or more of these autoantibodies along with a C-peptide can help to confirm the diagnosis of T1DM; however, 20% of insulin deficient adults are antibody negative (*Diabetes Care, 2012;35 (suppl 1):64*).

TREATMENT

Treatment of T1DM requires lifelong insulin replacement, and careful coordination of insulin doses with food intake and activity.

- **Insulin preparations.** After SC injection, there is individual variability in the duration and peak activity of insulin preparations and day-to-day variability in the same subject (Table 23-1).
  - **Rapid-acting insulins** include insulin lispro, insulin aspart, and insulin glulisine. Regular insulin is short acting and can be administered intravenously, intramuscularly, or subcutaneously. An IV bolus of regular insulin exerts maximum effect in 10 to 30 minutes and lasts up to 1 hour.

Table 23-1	Approximate Kinetics of Human Insulin Preparations after Subcutaneous Injection		
Insulin Type	Onset of Action (hr)	Peak Effect (hr)	Duration of Activity (hr)
Rapid acting			
Lispro, aspart, glulisine	0.25–0.50	0.50–1.50	3–5
Regular	0.50–1.00	2–4	6–8
Intermediate acting			
NPH	1–2	6–12	18–24
Lente*	1–2	6–12	18–24
Long acting			
Glargine	4–6	None[a]	20–24
Detemir	3–4		18–24
Ultralente*	3–4	Variable	18–24
PZI*	3–4	Unclear	18–24

*Not available in the United States, possibly generic manufacturers.
[a]Insulin dosage and individual variability in absorption and clearance rates affect pharmacokinetic data. Duration of insulin activity is prolonged in renal failure. After a lag time of approximately 5 hours, insulin glargine has a flat peakless effect over a 24-hour period. PZI, protamine zinc insulin.

○ **Intermediate-acting insulins**, including NPH (isophane) and lente (not available in the United States), are released slowly from SC sites, peak in 6 to 12 hours, and last up to 18 hours.

○ **Long-acting insulins** are absorbed more slowly than the intermediate-acting preparations. Long-acting insulins provide a steady "basal" supply of circulating insulin when administered once or twice a day. Insulin glargine and insulin detemir are "peakless" bioengineered human insulin analogs with an extended duration of activity. These insulins are generally administered once daily as an SC injection at bedtime, in a regimen that includes premeal rapid-acting insulin. Some patients with T1DM have improved control when the basal insulin is given twice a day rather than every day.

○ **Concentration.** The standard insulin concentration is 100 U/mL (U-100), with vials containing 1,000 U in 10 mL. A highly concentrated form of regular insulin containing 500 U/mL (Humulin U-500) is available for the rare patient with severe insulin resistance (usually T2DM). The vial size for U-500 insulin is 20 mL.

○ **Mixed insulin therapy.** Short- and rapid-acting insulins (regular, lispro, aspart, and glulisine) can be mixed with NPH insulin in the same syringe for convenience. The rapid-acting insulin should be drawn first, cross-contamination should be avoided, and the mixed insulin should be injected immediately. Commercial premixed insulin preparations do not allow dose adjustment of individual components but are convenient for patients who are unable or unwilling to do the mixing themselves. Premixed insulins are an option for patients with T2DM who have a regular eating and activity schedule, in general, should not be used in T1DM.

- ○ **SC insulin administration.** The abdomen, thighs, buttocks, and upper arms are the preferred sites for SC insulin injection. Absorption is fastest from the abdomen, followed by the arm, buttocks, and thigh, probably as a result of differences in blood flow. Injection sites should be rotated within the regions, rather than randomly across separate regions, to minimize erratic absorption. Exercise or massage over the injection site may accelerate insulin absorption.
- The **insulin requirement** for optimal glycemic control is approximately 0.5 to 0.8 U/kg/d for the average nonobese patient. A conservative total daily dose (TDD) of 0.4 U/kg/d is given initially to a newly diagnosed patient; the dose is then adjusted, using SMBG values. Higher doses may be required in obese or insulin resistant patients, in adolescents and in the latter part of pregnancy.
- A regimen of **multiple daily insulin injections** that include basal, premeal, and correction doses is preferred to obtain optimal control in both hospitalized patients and outpatients. This regimen implies that capillary glucose monitoring will occur four times daily, 10 to 30 minutes before meals and at bedtime.
  - ○ Basal insulin can be provided by NPH given twice daily, insulin detemir given once or twice daily, or insulin glargine generally dosed once daily. A reasonable starting dose is 0.2 U/kg or 0.1 U/lb for the day, either divided into two parts or given once. Basal insulin should provide 40% to 50% of the TDD of insulin and should be adjusted by 5% to 10% daily until the fasting glucose is consistently <130 mg/dL. In general, basal insulin is given regardless of nothing by mouth (NPO) or dietary status and should not be held without a direct order.
    - ▪ Premeal or bolus doses of insulin are adjusted according to the BG, the anticipated carbohydrate intake and anticipated activity level. Premeal dosing is strongly recommended for inpatients consuming full liquids or regular food. The total premeal complement should roughly equal the total basal dose, with one-third given before or after each meal. Rapid-acting insulin (lispro, aspart, or glulisine) are preferred, but regular human insulin can be used. Orders should be written to hold premeal insulin doses if the patient is NPO, off the medical floor, or not able to eat at least half of the meal provided. Outpatients with T1DM are instructed to check their BG four times daily and administer correction doses if a meal is delayed or missed.
    - ▪ The third component of a comprehensive insulin regimen is "correction factor" insulin, which is similar to sliding scale, adjusted according to the premeal fingerstick glucose testing and the patients estimated insulin sensitivity. In general, thinner patients should use a lower scale than heavier or more insulin-resistant patients. Correction factor and premeal doses should utilize the same insulin and be given together in the same syringe.
  - ○ **Continuous SC insulin infusion** using an insulin pump is widely used for insulin delivery in patients with T1DM, and increasingly in T2DM.
    - ▪ A typical regimen provides 50% of total daily insulin as basal insulin and the remainder as multiple preprandial boluses of insulin, using a programmable insulin pump.
    - ▪ Insulin pumps have advanced features that allow patients to fine tune their basal and bolus doses but require diabetes education in order to utilize the pump to its full potential.
    - ▪ Patients who utilize an insulin pump at home may be allowed to continue this therapy as an inpatient if mental status is not compromised and the regimen can be ordered and supervised by a knowledgeable physician. All doses need to be recorded whether administered by pump or injection. Hospital policies and specific order sets may be needed for these patients.

Diabetic Ketoacidosis

GENERAL PRINCIPLES

Epidemiology

DKA, a potentially fatal complication of diabetes, occurs in up to 5% of patients with T1DM annually and can occur in insulin-deficient patients with T2DM.

Pathophysiology

DKA is a catabolic condition that results from severe insulin deficiency, often in association with stress and activation of counterregulatory hormones (e.g., catecholamines, glucagon).

Risk Factors

Precipitating factors for DKA include inadvertent or deliberate interruption of insulin therapy, sepsis, trauma, myocardial infarction (MI), and pregnancy. DKA may be the first presentation of T1DM and, rarely, T2DM.

Prevention

DKA can be prevented in many cases, and its occurrence suggests a breakdown in education, communication, and problem solving. Diabetes education should therefore be reinforced at every opportunity, with special emphasis on (a) self-management skills during sick days; (b) the body's need for more, rather than less, insulin during such illnesses; (c) testing of blood or urine for ketones; and (d) procedures for obtaining timely and preventive medical advice.

DIAGNOSIS

History

Patients may describe a variety of symptoms including polyuria, polydipsia, weight loss, nausea, vomiting, and vaguely localized abdominal pain generally in the setting of persistent hyperglycemia. A high index of suspicion is warranted because clinical presentation may be nonspecific.

Physical Examination
- Tachycardia; decrease of capillary filling; rapid, deep, and labored breathing (Kussmaul respiration); and fruity breath odor are common physical findings.
- Prominent GI symptoms and abdominal tenderness on exam may give rise to suspicion for intra-abdominal pathology.
- Dehydration is invariable and respiratory distress, shock, and coma can occur.

Diagnostic Testing

Laboratories
- Labs will show an anion gap metabolic acidosis and positive serum β-hydroxybutyrate or ketones (a semiquantitative measurement of acetone, acetoacetate, and β-hydroxybutyrate).
- Plasma glucose level usually is elevated, but the degree of hyperglycemia may be moderate ($\leq$300 mg/dL) in 10% to 15% of patients with DKA. Pregnancy and alcohol ingestion are associated with "euglycemic DKA."

- Urine ketones are generally present in DKA.
- Hyponatremia, hyperkalemia, azotemia, and hyperosmolality are other findings.
- Serum amylase, transaminase, and/or triglyceride levels may be elevated.
- A focused search for a precipitating infection is recommended if clinically indicated.
- An electrocardiogram (ECG) should be obtained to evaluate electrolyte abnormalities and for unsuspected myocardial ischemia.

TREATMENT

Management of DKA should preferably be conducted in an ICU. **If treatment is conducted in a non-ICU setting, close monitoring is mandatory until ketoacidosis resolves and the patient's condition is stabilized.** The therapeutic priorities are fluid replacement, adequate insulin administration, and potassium repletion. Administration of bicarbonate, phosphate, magnesium, or other therapies may be advantageous in selected patients.

- **IV access and supportive measures** should be instituted without delay.
- **Fluid** deficits of several liters are common in DKA patients and can be estimated by subtracting the current weight from a recently known dry weight. The average degree of dehydration for most patients is approximately 7% to 9% of body weight. Hypotension indicates a loss of >10% of body fluids (*Diabetes Care 2004; 27:S94*).
  ○ **Restoration of circulating volume** using isotonic (0.9%) saline should be the initial therapeutic intervention. The first liter should be infused rapidly (if cardiac function is normal) and should be followed by additional fluids at a rate of 0.5 to 1.0 L/hr until vital signs have stabilized and urine output has been established, usually in 2 to 3 hours. The remaining volume deficit can be corrected more slowly. Hypotonic saline (0.45%) can be used in patients with severe hypernatremia (>150 mEq/L) and after stabilization of blood pressure.
  ○ The next goal is to **replenish total body water deficits**; this can be accomplished using a 0.45% saline infusion at 150 to 500 mL/hr if the corrected serum sodium level is normal or elevated; 0.90% NaCl at a similar rate is appropriate if the corrected serum sodium level is low. The rate of the fluid replacement depends on the degree of dehydration and cardiac and renal status. Do not exceed a change in osmolality >3 mOsm/kg/hr. The success of the fluid replacement is judged by improvement in blood pressure, urine output, and clinical examination.
  ○ **Maintenance fluid replacement** is continued until the fluid intake/output records indicate an overall positive balance similar to the estimated fluid deficit. Complete fluid replacement in a typical DKA patient may require 12 to 24 hours to accomplish.
- **Insulin therapy.** Sufficient insulin must be administered to turn off ketogenesis and correct hyperglycemia.
  ○ **An IV bolus of regular insulin**, 10 to 15 U (0.15 U/kg), should be administered immediately. This should be followed by a continuous infusion of regular insulin at an initial rate of 5 to 10 U/hr (or 0.1 U/kg/hr). A solution of regular insulin, 100 U in 100 mL of 0.9% saline, infused at a rate of 10 mL/hr delivers 10 U/hr of insulin.
  ○ **A decrease in BG levels of 50 to 75 mg/dL/hr** is an appropriate response; lesser decrements suggest insulin resistance, inadequate volume repletion, or inadequate insulin dose or delivery. If insulin resistance is suspected, the hourly dose of

regular insulin should be increased progressively by 50% to 100% until an appropriate glycemic response is observed.

- ○ **Excessively rapid correction of hyperglycemia** at rates >100 mg/dL/hr should be avoided to reduce the risk of osmotic encephalopathy.
- ○ **Maintenance insulin infusion rates of 1 to 2 U/hr** can be continued (indefinitely) until the patient is clinically improved, the serum bicarbonate level rises to ≥15 mEq/L, and the anion gap has closed. Once oral intake resumes, insulin can be administered SC and the parenteral route can be discontinued. It is prudent to **give the first SC injection of insulin 30 to 60 minutes before stopping the IV insulin infusion**. Both basal and premeal doses of insulin will need to be restarted, so stopping at a logical time, for example, before breakfast or in the evening, makes sense.
- **Dextrose (5%)** in 0.45% saline should be infused once plasma glucose level decreases to 250 mg/dL and the insulin infusion rate should be decreased to 0.05 U/kg/hr to prevent dangerous hypoglycemia. Consider starting a separate dextrose-containing infusion of 50 to 100 mL/hr and adjusting the fluid replacement accordingly. Rapid rates of dextrose infusion with reduced insulin doses may result in rebound hyperglycemia.
- **Potassium deficit** should always be assumed or anticipated regardless of plasma levels on admission. Insulin administration results in a rapid shift of potassium into the intracellular compartment.
  - ○ The goal is to maintain plasma potassium level in the normal range and thereby prevent the potentially fatal cardiac effects of hypokalemia. Potassium status should be documented from the outset; this includes ECG to rule out rare life-threatening hyperkalemia.
  - ○ Potassium should be added routinely to the IV fluids (consider starting with the second or third liter of fluid replacement) at a rate of 10 to 20 mEq/hr except in patients with hyperkalemia (>6.0 mmol/L and/or ECG evidence), renal failure, or oliguria confirmed by bladder catheterization.
  - ○ Patients who present with hypokalemia should receive higher doses of potassium, ≥40 mEq/hr, depending on severity.
  - ○ Potassium chloride is an appropriate initial choice, but this can later be changed to potassium phosphate to reduce chloride load in patients without severe renal impairment.
- **Monitoring of therapy**
  - ○ BG levels should be monitored hourly, serum electrolyte levels every 1 to 2 hours, and arterial blood gas values as often as necessary for a severely acidotic or hypoxic patient.
  - ○ Serum sodium tends to rise as hyperglycemia is corrected; failure to observe this trend suggests that the patient is being overhydrated with free water.
  - ○ Serial serum ketone measurements are not necessary because ketonemia may persist after clinical recovery and because the most commonly used assays measure all ketones, not just β-hydroxybutyrate. Restoration of renal buffering capacity by normalization of the serum bicarbonate level and closure of the anion gap are more reliable indices of metabolic recovery.
  - ○ Use of a flowchart is an efficient method of tracking clinical data (e.g., weight, fluid balance, mental status) and laboratory results during the management of DKA.
  - ○ Continuous ECG monitoring may be required for proper management of potassium in patients with oliguria or renal failure.

- **Bicarbonate therapy** is not routinely necessary and may be deleterious in certain situations.
  - Bicarbonate therapy may be considered for DKA patients who develop (a) shock or coma, (b) severe acidosis (pH <6.9), (c) severe depletion of buffering reserve (plasma bicarbonate <5 mEq/L), (d) acidosis-induced cardiac or respiratory dysfunction, or (e) severe hyperkalemia.
  - Sodium bicarbonate, 50 to 100 mEq in 1 L of 0.45% saline infused over 30 to 60 minutes, can be given in these situations. Bicarbonate treatment should be guided by arterial pH measurement and continued until the indications are no longer present.
  - Care should be taken to avoid hypokalemia; an additional dose of potassium, 10 mEq, should be included with each infusion of bicarbonate unless hyperkalemia is present.
- **Phosphate and magnesium** stores are reduced in DKA patients, and plasma levels (particularly phosphate) decline further during insulin therapy. The clinical significance of these changes is unclear, and routine replacement of phosphate or magnesium is not necessary, especially if the patient is able to resume usual caloric intake.
  - In hypophosphatemic patients with compromised oral intake, the use of potassium phosphate in maintenance IV fluids can be considered (see Chapter 12, Fluid and Electrolyte Management).
  - Magnesium therapy is indicated in patients with ventricular arrhythmia and can be administered as magnesium sulfate (50%) in doses of 2.5 to 5.0 mL (10 to 20 mEq of magnesium) IV.
- **IV antimicrobial therapy** should be started promptly for documented or suspected bacterial, fungal, and other treatable infections. Empiric broad-spectrum antibiotics can be started in septic patients, pending results of blood cultures. Note that DKA is not typically accompanied by fever, so infection must be considered in a febrile patient.

COMPLICATIONS

Complications of DKA include life-threatening conditions that must be recognized and treated promptly.
- **Lactic acidosis** may result from prolonged dehydration, shock, infection, and tissue hypoxia in DKA patients. Lactic acidosis should be suspected in patients with refractory metabolic acidosis and a persistent anion gap despite optimal therapy for DKA. Adequate volume replacement, control of sepsis, and judicious use of bicarbonate constitute the approach to management.
- **Arterial thrombosis** manifesting as stroke, MI, or an ischemic limb occurs with increased frequency in DKA. However, routine anticoagulation is not indicated except as part of the specific therapy for a thrombotic event.
- **Cerebral edema**, a dire complication of DKA, is observed more frequently in children than in adults.
  - Symptoms of increased intracranial pressure (e.g., headache, altered mental status, papilledema) or a sudden deterioration in mental status after initial improvement in a patient with DKA should raise suspicion for cerebral edema.
  - Overhydration with free water and excessively rapid correction of hyperglycemia are known risk factors.

○ A fall in serum sodium level or failure to rise during therapy for DKA is a clue to imminent or established overhydration with free water. Neuroimaging with a computed tomography (CT) scan can establish the diagnosis. Prompt recognition and treatment with IV mannitol is essential and may prevent neurologic sequelae in patients who survive cerebral edema.

• **Rebound ketoacidosis** can occur due to premature cessation of IV insulin infusion or inadequate doses of SC insulin after the insulin infusion has been discontinued. All patients T1DM and patients with T2DM who develop DKA (indicating severe insulin deficiency) require both basal and premeal insulin in adequate doses to avoid recurrence of metabolic decompensation.

TYPE 2 DIABETES AND NONKETOTIC HYPEROSMOLAR SYNDROME

Type 2 Diabetes

GENERAL PRINCIPLES

• T2DM results from defective insulin secretion followed by loss of β-cell mass in response to increased demand as a result of insulin resistance (*Diabetes 1988; 37:667*).
• The loss of pancreatic β cells is progressive; however, insulin secretion is usually sufficient to prevent ketosis under basal conditions. T2DM patients can develop DKA when hyperglycemia is severe or prolonged or when exposed to severe stress.
• The mechanisms underlying the β-cell loss in T2DM are unknown, but programmed cell death in response to genetic and environmental factors has been demonstrated in animal models (*Diabetes 2003;52:2304*).

TREATMENT

Medications

• The recommended glycemic goals for patients with T2DM are the same as in T1DM, A1C <7% or as low as can be achieved safely. Near normalization of glucose values may be safely achievable in many patients with T2DM.
• The achievement of these goals requires individualized therapy and a comprehensive approach that incorporates lifestyle and pharmacologic interventions. Guidelines have been published by several professional organizations regarding the choice and sequence of antidiabetic therapy (*Endocr Pract 2011;17(suppl 2):1*; *Diabetes Care 2009;32:1903*). Considerations for selecting noninsulin therapy (Table 23-2) in patients with T2DM include:
  ○ Oral therapy should be initiated early in conjunction with diet and exercise.
  ○ Metformin is the recommended first-line therapy if tolerated.
  ○ Monotherapy with maximum doses of insulin secretagogues, metformin, or thiazolidinediones (TZDs) yields comparable glucose-lowering effects.
  ○ The glucose-lowering effects of metformin, insulin secretagogues, and DPP-IV inhibitors and glucagon-like peptide-1 (GLP-1) analogs are observed within days to weeks, while the maximum effects of thiazolidinediones (TZDs) may not be observed for several weeks to months.

Table 23-2 Noninsulin Medications for Diabetes

	Daily Dosage Range	Doses Per Day	Duration of Action (hr)	Main Adverse Effects
Oral antidiabetic medications for type 2 diabetes				
Insulin secretagogues				
SFUs (second generation)				
Glyburide (glibenclamide)	1.25–20 mg	qd or bid	12–24	Hypoglycemia, weight gain
Glipizide	2.5–40 mg	qd or bid	12–24	
Glimepiride	1–8 mg	qd or bid	24	
Gliclazide (not available in the United States)	40–320 mg	bid	12	
Non-SFU secretagogues				
Nateglinide	180–320 mg	tid before meals	4	Hypoglycemia, weight gain; not as severe as SFUs
Repaglinide	1.5–16 mg	tid before meals	4–6	Same
Mitiglinide*	5–20 mg	tid before meals	4–6	Same
Biguanide				
Metformin (available in liquid and long-acting formulations)	500 mg–2.5 g	bid or tid	12–18	Diarrhea, nausea, abdominal pain or cramping, lactic acidosis
α-Glucosidase inhibitors				
Acarbose	75–300 mg	tid before meals	2–3	Gas, bloating, diarrhea, abdominal pain
Miglitol	75–300 mg	tid before meals	2–3	

Voglibose*	600–900 µg	tid before meals	2–3	
Thiazolidinediones				
Pioglitazone	15, 30, 45 mg	qd	24+	Edema, heart failure, fractures in women, increased risk of bladder cancer
Dipeptidyl peptidase-4 inhibitors (DPP-IV)				
Sitagliptin (dose adjustment for CKD: use 50 mg if CrCl ≤50 mL/min; use 25 mg if CrCl ≤30 mL/min)	25, 50, 100	qd	24	Angioedema, Stevens-Johnson syndrome, URI
Saxagliptin (dose adjustment for CKD, use 2.5 mg if CrCl ≤50 mL/min)	2.5 or 5 mg	qd		Urticaria, facial edema, URI
Vildagliptin (not available in the United States and not indicated in severe renal or hepatic impairment, LFT ≥3× upper limit of normal)	50–100 mg	qd or bid	24	Blistering skin lesions in animals, increased LFTs
Linagliptin	5 mg	qd		Safe for use in CKD, fecal route of excretion
Bile acid sequestrant				
Colesevelam hydrochloride (contraindicated in bowel obstruction or GI motility disorders)	3.8 g (each tablet is 625 mg)	3 tablets bid	12	Constipation, reduced absorption of some medications
Dopamine receptor agonist				
Bromocriptine mesylate (do not use with other dopamine agonists or antagonists)	0.8–4.8 mg	1–6 tablets qd	24	Nausea, asthenia, dizziness, headache, constipation, diarrhea

(continued)

| Table 23-2 | Noninsulin Medications for Diabetes (Continued) |

	Daily Dosage Range	Doses Per Day	Duration of Action (hr)	Main Adverse Effects
Injectable medications for type 2 diabetes				
GLP agonists				
Exenatide	5–10 µg	bid	9	Nausea, vomiting, GI distress, reported cases of pancreatitis
Exenatide extended release Liraglutide	2 mg q week 0.6–1.8 mg	qd	24	Nausea, vomiting, GI distress; increased calcitonin and goiter
Injectable medications for type 1 or type 2 diabetes				
Amylin analog				
Pramlintide acetate (given as a separate injection with meals; insulin dose reduction is required when starting)	15–120 µg	tid before meals	2	Nausea, vomiting, diarrhea, headache, hypoglycemia

*Not available in the United States.
CKD, chronic kidney disease; CrCl, creatinine clearance; GI, gastrointestinal; GLP, glucagon-like peptide; LFT, liver function test; SFU, sulfonylurea; URI, upper respiratory infection.

- Combination therapy with two or more oral or injectable agents may be needed at the time of diagnosis to achieve the A1C and glucose targets in patients presenting with significant hyperglycemia and will likely be needed as β-cell function deteriorates over time.
- Insulin therapy should be considered for patients presenting in DKA or with very high glucose levels (A1C >10%). Insulin therapy can sometimes be stopped after glucose toxicity is corrected but may need to be continued in patients with persistent insulin deficiency.
- Because pancreatic β-cell function is required for the glucose-lowering effects of all noninsulin therapies, many patients will require insulin replacement therapy at some point. Insulin therapy can be initiated with basal insulin in addition to other therapies, with premixed insulin or in a basal/bolus regimen.
- The toxicity profile of some oral and injectable antidiabetic agents may preclude their use in patients with preexisting illnesses.

- **Insulin secretagogues**
  - **SFUs** increase insulin secretion by binding to specific receptors in β cells. SFUs are equally effective in controlling hyperglycemia at equivalent doses but have variable pharmacokinetics.
    - These agents should be taken 30 to 60 minutes before food and should never be administered to fasting patients.
    - Glyburide (glibenclamide) has an active metabolite with significant renal excretion and **should be avoided in the setting of impaired renal function and used with caution in elderly patients**.
    - Glipizide has a short duration of action and should be administered two to three times per day or once daily in a modified long-acting formulation.
    - Glimepiride has the longest duration of action and can be administered once per day.
    - Gliclazide is available in either short or longer acting formulations, with a dose range of 40 to 160 mg daily.
    - Therapy should be initiated with the lowest effective dose and increased gradually over several days or weeks to the optimal dose, generally about half of the maximal approved dose.
    - Good responders to SFU include newly diagnosed type 2 diabetics with mild-to-moderate fasting hyperglycemia.
    - Hypoglycemia is seen with all SFUs but is the most common with glyburide.
    - Weight gain is also a notable adverse effect.
  - **Repaglinide** is a meglitinide analog that has a similar mechanism of action as SFUs. Unlike SFUs, however, the meglitinides have a very short onset of action and a short half-life.
    - Repaglinide can be used as a single agent or in a combination with metformin in patients with T2DM.
    - The dose range is 0.5 to 4.0 mg PO with two to four meals daily; the drug should be taken within 30 minutes before meals and skipped if no meal is planned.
    - Adverse effects include hypoglycemia and weight gain.
  - **Nateglinide**, a D-phenylalanine derivative chemically distinct from other insulin secretagogues, acts directly on the pancreatic β cells to stimulate insulin secretion (*Diabetes Care 2000;23:202*).

- It is taken 10 minutes before breakfast, lunch, and dinner and leads to significant insulin secretion within 15 minutes, with a return to baseline in 3 to 4 hours, effectively controlling postprandial hyperglycemia. The maximum effective dosage is 120 mg three times daily.
- Nateglinide is metabolized by the cytochrome P-450 system, so it has potential for drug interactions.
- The drug is well tolerated and the risk of hypoglycemia appears minimal.
  - Meglitinide is a short-acting insulin secretagogue that is available in Europe but not in the United States.
  - **Metformin**, the only biguanide in current clinical use, inhibits hepatic glucose output and stimulates glucose uptake by peripheral tissues. It is the preferred initial agent for most patients with T2DM and particularly those in whom weight gain is not desirable.
    - Metformin should be taken with food and, beginning with a single 500- or 850-mg tablet, the dose is increased every few days to weeks until optimal glycemic effect is achieved or 2,000 mg/d is reached.
    - GI symptoms occur in 20% to 30% of patients and can be managed by dose titration or adjustment; however, about 10% of patients do not tolerate any dose.
    - Lactic acidosis, the most serious adverse effect, has an incidence of approximately 3 per 100,000 patient-years and a significant mortality rate. Risk factors for lactic acidosis include renal dysfunction, hypovolemia, tissue hypoxia, infection, alcoholism, and cardiopulmonary disease.
    - A serum creatinine level of >1.5 mg/dL in men (>1.4 mg/dL in women) or an estimated glomerular filtration rate (eGFR) of <60 mL/min are contraindications to metformin use.
    - Metformin should be discontinued at the time of the radiographic contrast procedure and not restarted for 48 hours.
    - Other situations in which metformin therapy should be avoided include cardiogenic or septic shock, congestive heart failure (CHF) requiring pharmacologic therapy, severe liver disease, pulmonary insufficiency with hypoxemia, and severe tissue hypoperfusion (*N Engl J Med 1996;334:574*).
  - **α-Glucosidase inhibitors** block polysaccharide and disaccharide breakdown and decrease postprandial hyperglycemia when administered with food. Two members of this class, acarbose and miglitol, exert maximal effects at a dosage of approximately 300 mg/d. Voglibose is a similar drug used in Japan.
    - Each drug should be initiated at low doses (25 mg PO daily–tid, with food) and increased slowly in weekly steps of 25 mg to minimize GI intolerance.
    - Monotherapy with these agents provides A1C lowering of 0.4% to 0.7%, which is modest but without risk of hypoglycemia.
    - Dose-related adverse effects are diarrhea, bloating, abdominal cramping, and flatulence in 25% to 50% of individuals.
    - Acarbose has been associated with elevation in liver enzymes, and therefore, periodic monitoring of transaminases is recommended.
    - Hypoglycemia in patients who are receiving regimens that include α-glucosidase inhibitors should be treated with glucose, not sucrose.
  - **TZDs** increase insulin sensitivity in muscle, adipose tissue, and liver. Therefore, patients with considerable endogenous insulin secretion respond better to these agents. Pioglitazone is the only TZD currently available for use.
    - **Pioglitazone** can be used as a single agent (as an adjunct to diet and exercise) or in combination with SFU, metformin, sitagliptin, exenatide, or insulin. The

initial dosage is 15 or 30 mg PO daily, taken with or without food; this can be increased after several weeks to 45 mg PO daily for optimal effect. The maximal dose approved for use with insulin is 30 mg daily.

- Edema is the most common adverse effect and may range from none to mild peripheral edema to precipitation of CHF. Therapy with these agents is not recommended in patients with compromised cardiac function (New York Heart Association class III and IV cardiac status). Before starting TZDs, the physician should determine the existence of cardiac disease, concomitant use of medications associated with fluid retention, edema, and shortness of breath. The risk of CHF is increased in patients with history of heart failure, coronary artery disease (CAD), hypertension, long-standing diabetes, left ventricular hypertrophy, preexisting edema, edema after TZD therapy, insulin therapy, advanced age, renal failure, and aortic and mitral valve disease (*Diabetes Care 2004; 27:256*).
- The risk of drug-induced hepatotoxicity with pioglitazone is considered rare; however, periodic monitoring of liver function is recommended.
- TZDs have been associated with mild decrements in hemoglobin and/or pancytopenia. This has been attributed to increased plasma volume, but there may also be subclinical bone marrow suppression.
- TZDs may increase the risk of fracture in women, particularly smaller bones. The presumed mechanism is inhibition of osteoblast activity.
- Resumption of ovulation may occur during TZD therapy in some premenopausal women with anovulatory cycles. Therefore, contraceptive practice should be reviewed to prevent unintended pregnancy.
- Pioglitazone alters the levels of medications metabolized by cytochrome P-450 isoform CYP 3A4 (carbamazepine, cyclosporine, felodipine, and some oral contraceptives, among others).
- **DPP-IV inhibitors** are orally administered inhibitors of DPP-IV, the enzyme that breaks down endogenous GLP, which is an incretin secreted from the intestinal L cells. Increased levels of GLP reduce BG concentration by inhibiting glucagon secretion from the pancreatic α cells and by stimulating insulin secretion. Pancreatitis has been reported in rare cases in conjunction with DPP-IV inhibitor therapy, and allergic reactions may include angioedema and Stevens-Johnson syndrome.
  - **Sitagliptin** is given once daily at a usual dose of 100 mg. It has been studied for use as monotherapy or in conjunction with metformin, SFUs, TZDs, and insulin. It is well tolerated and without significant adverse effects. Its elimination pathway is predominantly renal, so dose reduction is recommended in patients with reduced renal function (give 50 mg if eGFR is <50 mL/min/1.73 m^2 or 25 mg daily if eGFR is <30 m/min/1.73 m^2).
  - **Vildagliptin** is approved for use in Europe at doses of 50 or 100 mg administered once daily. It has been studied for use as monotherapy and in conjunction with metformin, SFU, TZD, and insulin. It is not indicated in patients with impaired renal function.
  - **Saxagliptin** is administered once daily in doses of 2.5 or 5.0 mg. The lower dose should be used in patients with creatinine clearance <50 mL/min. The main side effects are urticaria and facial edema.
  - **Linagliptin** is given once daily, 5 mg. Because of predominantly fecal route of excretion, no dose adjustment is needed for renal insufficiency.

○ **Colesevelam hydrochloride** is a bile acid sequestrant that has been shown to have glucose-lowering properties. When given at full dose of three (625 mg) tablets bid, it lowers A1C by 0.4% to 0.8% when used as monotherapy or in conjunction with metformin or SFUs. It is also indicated for LDL lowering. The major side effect is constipation, and caution is advised for patients with preexisting GI problems or disease. It should not be used in patients with significant hypertriglyceridemia, as it may raise triglycerides. Colesevelam hydrochloride should be taken on an empty stomach, and before or after other medications so as not to interfere with their absorption. Colesevelam hydrochloride has a pregnancy category B rating and can be used in patients with renal insufficiency and hepatic insufficiency because it is not absorbed. It is also available in powder form for mixing with a liquid.

○ **GLP agonists/mimetics.** These peptides are structurally similar to endogenous GLP1 but resist breakdown by DPP enzymes. Thus, they have a longer half-life than native GLP1 and reach higher blood and tissue levels. GLP1 agonists and mimetics are given by SC injection and, in addition to glucose-lowering properties, may improve satiety and assist with weight loss.

   ▪ Exenatide is a GLP1 mimetic that is given by SC injection in doses of 5 or 10 μg twice daily before meals. Expected A1C lowering is 0.6% to 1.2%, which is accompanied by an average weight loss of 4 kg. Postmarketing cases of pancreatitis and acute renal failure have been reported. An extended release formulation (exenatide extended release, once weekly formulation) is available for once weekly administration at a dose of 2 mg per week.

   ▪ Liraglutide is given by subcutaneous injection once daily at any time in doses of 0.6, 1.2, or 1.8 mg. The main side effects are nausea, vomiting, dizziness, and headache. Increased calcitonin levels and medullary thyroid cancer occurred in rodents.

○ **Pramlintide** is an injectable amylin analog that is used in patients with T1DM or T2DM to improve glucose control by blunting postprandial BG. The dose range is 15 μg to 120 μg before each meal. Side effects are nausea, vomiting, and diarrhea.

○ **Insulin therapy** in T2DM is indicated in the following:

   ▪ Patients in whom oral or injectable agents have failed to achieve or sustain glycemic control.

   ▪ Metabolic decompensation: DKA and nonketotic hyperosmolar crisis

   ▪ Newly diagnosed patients with severe hyperglycemia

   ▪ Pregnancy and other situations in which oral agents are contraindicated

○ **The success of insulin therapy** depends on both the adequacy of the insulin TDD (0.6 to >1.0 U/kg of body weight per day), and the appropriateness of the insulin regimen for a given patient to achieve target glucose and A1C values.

   ▪ A once-daily injection of intermediate- or long-acting insulin at bedtime or before breakfast (basal insulin) added to oral or injectable agents may achieve the target A1C goal.

   ▪ Premeal insulin may be required if basal insulin plus other agents is not adequate. Short- or rapid-acting insulin administered before meals can be added to a basal insulin, or a premixed insulin can be given twice daily before breakfast and dinner. In general, the secretagogues are discontinued when premeal insulin is added, but sensitizing and other agents are continued on the basis of the individual patient needs.

- The TDD of insulin required to achieve glycemic targets varies widely in patients with T2DM and is based on body mass index, the continuation of oral agents, and the presence of comorbid conditions. Large doses of insulin (>100 U/d) may be required for optimal glycemic control. Weight gain with insulin use is a concern.

- Insulin-induced hypoglycemia, the most dangerous side effect, may increase CV event rates and death. Avoidance of hypoglycemia while achieving an A1C as low as can safely be achieved requires close collaboration between physician, patient, and diabetes educators. The frequency of hypoglycemia increases as patients approach normal A1C levels or when deterioration of kidney function occurs.

  o **Combination therapy.** About 60% of patients on monotherapy may have worsening of metabolic control during the first 5 years of therapy, and concurrent use of two or more medications with different mechanisms of action may be necessary (*Am J Med 2010;123(suppl 3):S38*).

  - Dose increases and addition of agents should be performed in a short period of time until glucose control is achieved.
  - Combination therapy first-line therapy in patients with A1C levels of ≥9%. Widely used regimens include an SFU plus metformin (most common), or metformin plus either a DPP-IV inhibitor or GLP analog if weight loss is a goal.
  - The combination of a TZD plus insulin is less accepted because of a higher incidence of CHF exacerbations.
  - Several combination tablets are available: metformin plus a SFU, DPP-IV inhibitors, pioglitazone, or pioglitazone plus an SFU.

Nonketotic Hyperosmolar Syndrome

GENERAL PRINCIPLES

Nonketotic hyperosmolar syndrome (NKHS) is one of the most serious life-threatening complications of T2DM (*J Clin Endocrinol Metab 2008;93:1541*).

Epidemiology

- Hyperosmolar hyperglycemic state (HHS) occurs primarily in patients with T2DM and in 30% to 40% of cases; NKHS is the initial presentation of a patient's diabetes (*Emerg Med Clin North Am 2005;23:629*).
- NKHS is significantly less common than DKA with an incidence of <1 case per 1,000 person-years.

Pathophysiology

- Ketoacidosis is absent because the ambient insulin level may effectively prevent lipolysis and subsequent ketogenesis yet is inadequate to facilitate peripheral glucose uptake and to prevent hepatic residual gluconeogenesis and glucose output.
- Precipitating factors include dehydration, stress, infection, stroke, noncompliance with medications, dietary indiscretion, and alcohol and cocaine abuse. Impaired glucose excretion is a contributory factor in patients with renal insufficiency or prerenal azotemia.

DIAGNOSIS

Clinical Presentation

In contrast to DKA, the onset of NKHS is usually insidious. Several days of deteriorating glycemic control are followed by increasing lethargy. Clinical evidence of severe dehydration is the rule. Some alterations in consciousness and focal neurologic deficits may be found at presentation or may develop during therapy. Therefore, repeated neurologic assessment is recommended.

Differential Diagnosis

The differential diagnosis of NKHS includes any cause of altered level of consciousness, including hypoglycemia, hyponatremia, severe dehydration, uremia, hyperammonemia, drug overdose, and sepsis. Seizures and acute stroke-like syndromes are common presentations.

Diagnostic Testing

Clinical findings include (a) hyperglycemia, often >600 mg/dL; (b) plasma osmolality >320 mOsm/L; (c) absence of ketonemia; and (d) pH >7.3 and serum bicarbonate level of >20 mEq/L. Prerenal azotemia and lactic acidosis can develop. Although some patients will have detectable urine ketones, most patients do not have a metabolic acidosis. Lactic acidosis may develop from an underlying ischemia, infection, or other cause.

TREATMENT

- **The goals of therapy are as follows:**
  - Restoration of hemodynamic stability and intravascular volume by fluid replacement.
  - Correction of electrolyte abnormalities.
  - Gradual correction of hyperglycemia and hyperosmolarity with fluid replacement and insulin therapy.
  - Detection and treatment of underlying disease states and precipitating causes. However, such efforts should not delay fluid replacement and insulin therapy.
- **Initial treatment** can make a difference in the frequency of complications and outcome. Therapy must be individualized on the basis of the degree of dehydration and underlying cause (sepsis and renal and cardiac function). Rapid vein access and urinary catheterization are essential.
  - **Restoring hemodynamic stability** is the first aim. Restoration of intravascular volume should be followed by correction of total body water deficit. Compared to DKA, patients with NKHS may require as much as 10 to 12 L of positive fluid balance over 24 to 72 hours to restore total deficits.
  - **Electrolyte management**
    - Although the potassium level may be initially normal or even high, all patients with NKHS are potassium depleted. Rehydration and insulin therapy usually result in hypokalemia, and this should be corrected.
    - If the initial potassium levels are low, replacement should begin immediately after urine output is ensured. Lactic acidosis requiring bicarbonate therapy may develop as a complication of NKHS or metformin therapy.
  - **Insulin therapy.** Insulin plays a secondary role in the initial management of NKHS, and fluid therapy always should precede insulin administration.

- In patients with marked hyperglycemia (>600 mg/dL), regular insulin, 5 to 10 U IV, should be given immediately, followed by continuous infusion of 0.10 to 0.15 U/kg/hr. Lower doses of a regular insulin bolus can be used for less severe hyperglycemia.
- Once plasma glucose decreases to 250 to 300 mg/dL, insulin infusion can be decreased to 1 to 2 U/hr and 5% dextrose should be added to the IV fluids. After full rehydration and clinical recovery, regular insulin can be given SC and patients can thereafter resume their usual diabetes therapy.

• **Underlying illness.** Detection and treatment of any underlying predisposing illness are critical in the treatment of NKHS. Antibiotics should be administered early, after appropriate cultures, in patients in whom infection is known or suspected as a precipitant to a HHS. A high index of suspicion should be maintained for underlying pancreatitis, GI bleeding, renal failure, and thromboembolic events, especially acute MI.

COMPLICATIONS

Complications of NKHS include thromboembolic events (cerebral and MI, mesenteric thrombosis, pulmonary embolism, and disseminated intravascular coagulation), cerebral edema, adult respiratory distress syndrome, and rhabdomyolysis.

MONITORING/FOLLOW-UP

• **Monitoring of therapy.** Use of a flowchart is helpful for tracking clinical data and laboratory results.
• Initially, BG levels should be monitored every 30 to 60 minutes and serum electrolyte levels every 1 to 2 hours; frequency of monitoring can be decreased during recovery.
• Neurologic status must be reassessed frequently; persistent lethargy or altered mentation indicates inadequate therapy. On the other hand, relapse after initial improvement in mental status suggests too rapid correction of serum osmolarity.

CHRONIC COMPLICATIONS OF DIABETES MELLITUS

Prevention of long-term complications is one of the main goals of diabetes management. Appropriate treatment of established complications may delay their progression and improve quality of life.

Microvascular complications include diabetic retinopathy, nephropathy, and neuropathy. These complications are directly related to hyperglycemia. Tight glycemic control has been shown to reduce the development and progression of these complications.

Diabetic Retinopathy

GENERAL PRINCIPLES

Classification

• Diabetic retinopathy (DR) is classified as background retinopathy (microaneurysms, retinal infarcts, lipid exudates, cotton wool spots, and/or microhemorrhages) with or without macular edema and proliferative retinopathy. Background DR is also known as preproliferative retinopathy.

- Other ocular abnormalities associated with diabetes include cataract formation, dyskinetic pupils, glaucoma, optic neuropathy, extraocular muscle paresis, floaters, and fluctuating visual acuity. The latter may be related to changes in BG levels.
- The presence of floaters may be indicative of preretinal or vitreous hemorrhage; immediate referral for ophthalmologic evaluation is warranted.

Epidemiology
The incidence of DR and vision impairment has dropped significantly with improved management of glycemia, blood pressure, and lipids in patients with both T1DM and T2DM. Early identification and treatment of DR has further reduced vision impairment once it is diagnosed. DR is less frequent in T2DM, but maculopathy may be more severe. DR is still the leading cause of vision loss in adults younger than 65 years (*N Engl J Med 2012;366:1227*).

DIAGNOSIS

Annual examination by an ophthalmologist is recommended at the time of diagnosis of all T2DM patients and at the beginning of puberty or 3 to 5 years after diagnosis for patients with T1DM. Dilated eye examination should be repeated annually by an optometrist or ophthalmologist since progressive DR can be completely asymptomatic until sudden loss of vision occurs. Early detection of DR is critical as therapy is more effective before severe maculopathy or proliferation develops. Any diabetic patient with visual symptoms should be referred for ophthalmologic evaluation (*Diabetes Care 2012;35(suppl 1):S64*).

TREATMENT

The first line of treatment is glycemic control, which has been shown to reduce the incidence and progression of DR in patients with T1DM or T2DM. Blood pressure control was also shown to be effective in the United Kingdom Prospective Diabetes Study (UKPDS), and treatment with either an ACE inhibitor (ACE-I) or ARB have demonstrated additional utility in preventing DR. Fenofibrate, used with simvastatin, reduced the risk of progression of DR in the ACCORD and FIELD clinical trials (*N Engl J Med 2012;366:1227*). Background retinopathy is not usually associated with loss of vision unless macular edema is present (25% of cases). The development of macular edema or proliferative retinopathy (particularly new vessels near the optic disk) requires elective laser photocoagulation therapy to preserve vision. Intraocular injections of vascular endothelial growth factor (VEGF)-neutralizing antibodies or glucocorticoids improve vision outcomes in macular edema but have side effects. Vitrectomy is indicated for patients with vitreous hemorrhage or retinal detachment.

Diabetic Nephropathy

GENERAL PRINCIPLES

Epidemiology
Approximately 25% to 45% of patients with either type of diabetes develop clinically evident diabetic nephropathy during their lifetime. Diabetic nephropathy (DN) is

the leading cause of end-stage renal disease (ESRD) in the United States and a major cause of morbidity and mortality in patients with diabetes (*Med Clin North Am 2004;88:1001*).

Risk Factors

Microalbuminuria precedes overt proteinuria (>300 mg of albumin/d) by several years in T1DM and T2DM. The mean duration from diagnosis of type 1 diabetes to the development of overt proteinuria has increased significantly and is now >25 years. The time from the occurrence of proteinuria to ESRD has also increased and is now >5 years. In T2DM, microalbuminuria can be present at the time of diagnosis. Poor glycemic control is the major risk factor for DN, but hypertension and smoking are contributors. Obesity may contribute to kidney damage in T2DM. Due to the widespread use of ACE-I and ARB agents for the treatment of hypertension, impaired kidney function may occur in the absence of albuminuria (*Diabetes Care 2012; 35(suppl 1):S64*).

Prevention

Prevention of diabetic nephropathy starts at the time of diagnosis with achievement of glycemic, blood pressure, and lipid targets. Smoking cessation is also important. Annual screening for microalbuminuria and measurement of serum creatinine identifies those with early damage who are at risk of progression. Annual screening should be performed in type 1 diabetic patients who have had diabetes for >5 years and all type 2 diabetic patients starting at diagnosis.

Associated Conditions

- Patients with proteinuria (albumin/creatinine >300 mg/g) are at higher risk for anemia due to loss of transferrin and poor production of erythropoietin and should be screened at any stage of CKD and treated.
- **Patients with CKD are at higher risk for CV disease and mortality**, so management of other CV risk factors is particularly important in this group of patients.
- Hypovitaminosis D should be corrected, and secondary hyperparathyroidism prevented or treated as early as possible.
- Diabetic patients with CKD may be at risk for hyperkalemia and metabolic acidosis, which should be identified and managed accordingly.

DIAGNOSIS

Diagnostic Testing

Laboratories

- Measurement of the microalbumin-to-creatinine ratio (normal, <30 mg of albumin/g of creatinine) in a random urine sample is recommended for screening. At least two to three measurements within a 6-month period should be performed to establish the diagnosis of DN (*Diabetes Care 2003;26:S94*).
- Measurement of serum creatinine and serum urea nitrogen should be performed annually, along with calculation of the eGFR. Patients with diabetes may have reduced kidney function without manifesting albumin in their urine. Testing and treatment of associated disorders such as anemia, secondary hyperparathyroidism, hyperkalemia, and acid–base disturbances should begin when the eGFR is <60 mL/min/1.73 m^2, or stage 3 CKD (see Chapter 13, Renal Diseases).

TREATMENT

Intensive control of both diabetes and hypertension is important to reduce the rate of progression of CKD due to diabetes. Achieving the blood pressure target of <130/80 mm Hg is recommended for all patients with diabetes, especially those with evidence of CKD.

Medications

- Antihypertensive treatment with ACE-I or ARB drugs is recommended as first-line therapy for all patients with diabetes and hypertension. These agents have been shown to reduce progression of both retinopathy and nephropathy and may be considered in patients with normal blood pressure or prehypertension.
- Diuretics are considered second line, followed by calcium channel blockers, β-blockers, or centrally acting agents (*Diabetes Care 2004;27:S79*).

Lifestyle/Risk Modification

- Dietary protein restriction may be beneficial in some patients to slow progression.
- Avoidance of renal toxins is important for preservation of kidney function.

Diabetic Neuropathy

GENERAL PRINCIPLES

Classification

Diabetic neuropathy can be classified in (a) subclinical neuropathy, determined by abnormalities in electrodiagnostic and quantitative sensory testing; (b) diffuse symmetrical polyneuropathy with distal symmetric sensorimotor losses ± autonomic syndromes; and (c) focal syndromes.

Epidemiology

Distal symmetric polyneuropathy (DPN) is the most common neuropathy in developed countries and accounts for more hospitalizations than all the other diabetic complications combined. Sensorimotor DPN is a major risk factor for foot trauma, ulceration, and Charcot arthropathy and is responsible for 50% to 75% of nontraumatic amputations (*Med Clin N Am 2004;88:947*).

Prevention

- Sensation in the lower extremities should be documented at least annually, using a combination of modalities such as a light-touch monofilament, tuning fork (frequency of 128 Hz), pinprick, or temperature.
- Foot examination should be conducted at least annually to evaluate the presence of musculoskeletal deformities, skin changes, and pulses, in addition to the sensory examination.

TREATMENT

- **Painful peripheral neuropathy** responds variably to treatment with tricyclic antidepressants (e.g., amitriptyline, 10 to 150 mg PO at bedtime), topical capsaicin (0.075% cream), or anticonvulsants (e.g., carbamazepine 100 to 400 mg PO bid, gabapentin 900 to 3,600 mg/d, or pregabalin 50 to 300 mg should be 150 to 300 mg/d). Patients should be warned about adverse effects, including sedation and anticholinergic symptoms (tricyclics), burning sensation (capsaicin), and blood dyscrasias (carbamazepine). α-Lipoic acid (600 mg bid) and high-dose thiamine (50 to 100 mg tid) have been tested in early DPN.

- **Orthostatic hypotension** is a manifestation of autonomic neuropathy, but other etiologies (e.g., dehydration, anemia, medications) should be excluded. Treatment is symptomatic: Postural maneuvers, use of compressive garments (e.g., Jobst stockings), and intravascular expansion using sodium chloride 1 to 4 g PO qid and fludrocortisone 0.1 to 0.3 mg PO daily. Hypokalemia, supine hypertension, and CHF are some adverse effects of fludrocortisone.

- **Intractable nausea and vomiting** may be manifestations of impaired GI motility from autonomic neuropathy. **DKA** should be ruled out when nausea and vomiting is acute. Other causes of nausea and vomiting, including adrenal insufficiency, should be excluded.
  - ○ **Management of diabetic gastroenteropathy** can be challenging. Frequent, small meals (six to eight per day) of soft consistency that are low in fat and fiber provide intermittent relief. Parenteral nutrition may become necessary in refractory cases.
  - ○ **Pharmacologic therapy** includes the prokinetic agent metoclopramide, 10 to 20 mg PO (or as a suppository) before meals and at bedtime, and erythromycin, 125 to 500 mg PO qid. Extrapyramidal side effects (tremor and tardive dyskinesia) from the antidopaminergic actions of metoclopramide may limit therapy.
  - ○ **Cyclical vomiting** that is unrelated to a GI motility disorder or other clear etiology may also occur in diabetic patients and appears to respond to amitriptyline 25 to 50 mg PO at bedtime.

- **Diabetic cystopathy**, or bladder dysfunction, results from impaired autonomic control of detrusor muscle and sphincteric function. Manifestations include urgency, dribbling, incomplete emptying, overflow incontinence, and urinary retention. Recurrent urinary tract infections are common in patients with residual urine. Treatment with bethanechol 10 mg tid or intermittent self-catheterization may be required to relieve retention.

- **Chronic, persistent diarrhea** in patients with diabetes is probably multifactorial. Celiac disease and inflammatory bowel diseases should be ruled out, particularly in patients with T1DM. Pancreatic mass is reduced with long-standing diabetes, so the possibility of exocrine pancreatic dysfunction should be considered. Bacterial overgrowth has been considered as an etiology but is difficult to diagnose. Empiric treatment with broad-spectrum antibiotics (e.g., azithromycin, tetracycline, cephalosporins) along with metronidazole may be beneficial. Antifungal agents and probiotic replacement can be tried. If diarrhea persists, loperamide or octreotide 50 to 75 mg SC bid can be effective in patients with intractable diarrhea.

MACROVASCULAR COMPLICATIONS OF DIABETES MELLITUS

Coronary Heart Disease

GENERAL PRINCIPLES

- Coronary heart disease (CHD), stroke, and peripheral vascular disease (PVD) are responsible for 80% of deaths in persons with diabetes (*Lancet 1997;350 (suppl 1):SI23*) (see Chapter 4, Ischemic Heart Disease).

- **CAD** occurs at a younger age and may have atypical clinical presentations in patients with diabetes (*Lancet 1997;350(suppl 1):SI23*).
  - MI carries a worse prognosis, and angioplasty gives less satisfactory results in diabetic patients.
  - Persons with diabetes have an increased risk of ischemic and nonischemic heart failure and sudden death.

Risk Factors

Risk factors for macrovascular disease that are common in persons with diabetes include insulin resistance, hyperglycemia, microalbuminuria, hypertension, hyperlipidemia, cigarette smoking, and obesity.

Prevention

- CV risk factors should be assessed at least annually and treated aggressively (see treatment goals in the following text). ECG should be obtained yearly. Stress tests, with or without imaging, should be reserved for those with typical or atypical chest pain or those with abnormalities on ECG (*Diabetes Care 2012;35(suppl 1):S64*).
- Screening asymptomatic persons with cardiac stress test has not been shown to reduce mortality or events in asymptomatic patients with T2DM (*JAMA 2009;301:1547*).
- Aspirin 81 to 325 mg/d is of proven benefit in secondary prevention of MI or stroke in diabetic patients and may be considered for persons over age 40 years with diabetes.

TREATMENT

- Aggressive risk factor reduction lowers the risk of both microvascular and macrovascular complications in patients with diabetes.
  - Glycemic control should be optimized to A1C <7% and as close to normal as possible in the first few years after diagnosis. Patients with long-standing T2DM may have increased risk of mortality with very tight glycemic control (A1C <6.5%), particularly if multiple agents are required and the risk of hypoglycemia increases.
  - Hypertension should be controlled to a target blood pressure of <130/80 mm Hg (or <125/75 mm Hg in patients with proteinuria).
  - Hyperlipidemia should be treated appropriately, with a target LDL cholesterol level of <100 mg/dL, or <70 mg/dL in patients with known CHD. HDL cholesterol levels of >50 mg/dL and triglyceride levels of <150 mg/dL should be achieved.
  - Cigarette smoking should be actively discouraged, and weight loss should be promoted in obese patients.
- **Management of diabetes after acute MI**
  Hyperglycemia (glucose >110 mg/dL), with or without a history of diabetes, is an independent predictor of in-hospital mortality, and CHF in patients admitted for acute MI (*Lancet 2000;355:773*). However, the results of the studies that

investigated tight glucose control with insulin in the setting of acute MI in type 2 diabetic patients are inconclusive (*BMJ 1997;314:1512; J Am Coll Cardiol 1995;26:57; Eur Heart J 2005;26:650*). Nevertheless, given the consistent epidemiologic association, it is reasonable to expect that glucose-lowering effects in acute conditions could lead to clinical benefit.

Peripheral Vascular Disease

GENERAL PRINCIPLES

Diabetes and smoking are the strongest risk factors for PVD. In diabetic patients, the risk of PVD is increased by age, duration of diabetes, and presence of peripheral neuropathy. PVD is a marker for systemic vascular disease involving coronary, cerebral, and renal vessels. Diabetic patients with PVD have increased risk for subsequent MI or stroke regardless of the PVD symptoms.

DIAGNOSIS

Clinical Presentation

Symptoms of PVD include intermittent claudication, rest pain, tissue loss, and gangrene, but patients with diabetes may have fewer symptoms due to concomitant neuropathy.

Physical Examination

Physical examination findings including diminished pulses, dependent rubor, pallor on elevation, absence of hair growth, dystrophic toenails, and cool, dry, fissured skin.

Diagnostic Testing

- The ankle-to-brachial index (ABI) defined as the ratio of the systolic blood pressure in the ankle divided by the systolic blood pressure at the arm is the best initial diagnostic test. An ABI <0.9 by a handheld, 5- to 10-MHz Doppler probe has a 95% sensitivity for detecting angiogram-positive PVD (*Int J Epidemiol 1988;17:248*).
- ABI should be performed in diabetic patients with signs or symptoms of PAD.

TREATMENT

- Risk factors should be controlled, with similar goals described for CAD (see the previous text).
- Antiplatelet agents such clopidogrel (75 mg/d) have additional benefits when compared with aspirin in diabetic patients with PVD (*Diabetes Care 2003;26:3333*).
- Therapy for intermittent claudication could also benefit from exercise rehabilitation and cilostazol (100 mg bid). This medication is contraindicated in patients with CHF.

MISCELLANEOUS COMPLICATIONS

Erectile Dysfunction

GENERAL PRINCIPLES

Epidemiology

It is estimated that 40% to 60% of men with diabetes have erectile dysfunction (ED), and the prevalence varies depending on the age of the patient and duration of diabetes. In addition to increasing age, ED is associated with smoking, poor glycemic control, low HDL, neuropathy, and retinopathy.

Etiology

ED in diabetic patients is multifactorial. It can result from nerve damage, impaired blood flow (vascular insufficiency), adverse drug effects, low testosterone, psychological factors, or a combination of these etiologies.

DIAGNOSIS

Evaluation should include a measurement of total or bioavailable testosterone. If the total testosterone is <300 mg/dL, the test should be repeated in the morning (does not have to be fasting, but a blood draw before 9:00 AM is appropriate) along with a prolactin and prostate-specific antigen (PSA).

TREATMENT

- If testosterone is low, and both PSA and prostate examination are normal, then testosterone replacement can be tried with either testosterone enanthate, 200 mg every 2 to 3 weeks, or a topical gel (AndroGel or Testim).
- A trial of phosphodiesterase type 5 inhibitors (sildenafil, tadalafil, vardenafil) is often warranted in addition to hormonal correction (if indicated). Typical doses include sildenafil 50 to 100 mg or vardenafil 10 mg 1 hour prior to sexual activity and tadalafil 10 mg/d prior to sexual activity. Referral to urology specialist should be considered if the problem persists. CV status should be considered before starting these agents. **This drug class should not be used concurrently with nitrates** to prevent severe and potentially fatal hypotensive reactions. Macular edema should also be ruled out before starting these agents.

Diabetic Foot Ulcers

GENERAL PRINCIPLES

Epidemiology

The prevalence of foot ulcers is 4% to 10% and the lifetime incidence is as high as 25% (*JAMA 2005;293:217*).

Etiology

Causative factors include peripheral sensory neuropathy, excessive plantar pressure, and repetitive trauma. Vascular insufficiency, poor healing, and polymicrobial infection are major contributors to ulcer formation. Poor footwear can add to the risk of ulceration (*Diabetes Care 2008;31:1679*).

Prevention

- **Screening to identify patients at risk for ulcers** includes detection of loss of protective sensation by monofilament (see discussion on peripheral neuropathy) and PVD.
- Patients with prior foot ulcers are at high risk for recurrence and may need ongoing specialized care and footwear.

TREATMENT

- Poorly managed foot ulcers may result in limb loss from amputation. Patient education should emphasize the following prevention: daily foot examination, application of moisturizing lotion, use of proper footwear, and early treatment of tinea and other minor foot infections. Patients should use caution with self-pedicure and seek assistance with nail care if body habitus, limited vision, or thick toenails precludes self-care.
- The exposed feet should be inspected and palpated at every patient encounter; significant findings, such as calluses, hammertoes or other deformities, infections, and soft tissue lesions, should be evaluated.
- Diabetic foot infections should be treated aggressively. Proper management includes a multidisciplinary approach that includes orthopedic surgeons, specialized nursing care, and close monitoring. Evaluation of PVD and referral to a vascular specialist should be considered as an integral part of the management of food ulcers. The presence of deep infection with abscess, cellulitis, gangrene, or osteomyelitis is an indication for hospitalization and prompt surgical drainage. Acute treatment of foot infections is dependent on severity, as outlined in the following text.
- **Mild-to-moderate cellulitis.** Rest, elevation of the affected foot and relief of pressure are essential components of treatment and should be initiated at first presentation. In localized cellulitis and new ulcers, *Staphylococcus aureus* and streptococci are the most frequent pathogens. Therapy with oral dicloxacillin, first-generation cephalosporin, amoxicillin/clavulanate, or clindamycin is recommended. IV antibiotics may be necessary due if the cellulitis does not respond immediately to oral antibiotics.
- **Moderate-to-severe cellulitis.** This type of involvement requires IV therapy and admission to the hospital. Consultation for debridement and aerobic and anaerobic cultures are necessary when necrotic tissue is present. IV oxacillin/nafcillin, a first-generation IV cephalosporin, ampicillin/sulbactam, clindamycin, and vancomycin are options for therapy. Antibiotic coverage should subsequently be tailored according to the clinical response of the patient, culture results, and sensitivity testing.
- **Moderate-to-severe cellulitis with ischemia or significant local necrosis.** It is important to determine the presence of bone involvement and PVD since failure to diagnose osteomyelitis and ischemia often results in failure of wound healing.
  - Bone involvement is present if bone is seen at the base of the ulcer or is easily detected by gentle probing with a blunt sterile probe. Radiographs are not very sensitive for diagnosis and magnetic resonance imaging offers better specificity.
  - Presence of PVD is suspected by the absence of pedal pulses or decreased capillary filling.

- IV antibiotics, bed rest, surgical debridement, culture obtained from the base of the ulcer, and bone culture help direct antibiotic therapy.
- Ampicillin/sulbactam and ticarcillin/clavulanate are first-line agents; piperacillin/tazobactam, clindamycin plus ciprofloxacin, ceftazidime, cefepime, cefotaxime, or ceftriaxone plus metronidazole are good alternatives for initial therapy.
- In the presence of osteomyelitis, 6 to 12 weeks of IV antibiotic therapy is recommended. Ulcers with localized or generalized gangrene require surgical amputation, often limited to a toe or metatarsal head.

Hypoglycemia

GENERAL PRINCIPLES

Classification

Hypoglycemia is uncommon in patients not treated for diabetes. Iatrogenic factors usually account for hypoglycemia in the setting of diabetes, whereas hypoglycemia in the nondiabetic population could be classified as fasting or postprandial hypoglycemia. **Iatrogenic hypoglycemia** complicates therapy with insulin or SFUs and is a limiting factor to achieve glycemic control during intensive therapy in patients with DM (*Diabetes Care 2003;26:1902*).

Risk Factors

Hypoglycemia resulting from too intensive diabetes therapies may increase the risk of mortality in older patients with a long duration of diabetes and should be avoided.

- Risk factors for iatrogenic hypoglycemia include skipped or insufficient meals, unaccustomed physical exertion, misguided therapy, alcohol ingestion, and drug overdose.
- Recurrent episodes of hypoglycemia impair recognition of hypoglycemic symptoms, thereby increasing the risk for severe hypoglycemia (hypoglycemia unawareness).
- Hypoglycemia unawareness results from defective glucose counterregulation with blunting of autonomic symptoms and counterregulatory hormone secretion during hypoglycemia. Seizures or coma may develop in such patients without the usual warning symptoms of hypoglycemia.
- Hypoglycemia unrelated to diabetes therapy is an infrequent problem in general medical practice.

DIAGNOSIS

Clinical Presentation

- Hypoglycemia is a clinical syndrome in which low serum (or plasma) glucose levels lead to symptoms of sympathetic–adrenal activation (sweating, anxiety, tremor, nausea, palpitations, and tachycardia) from increased secretion of counterregulatory hormones (e.g., epinephrine).
- Neuroglycopenia occurs as the glucose levels decrease further (fatigue, dizziness, headache, visual disturbances, drowsiness, difficulty speaking, inability to concentrate, abnormal behavior, confusion, and ultimately loss of consciousness or seizures).

Differential Diagnosis

Plasma or capillary BG values should be obtained, whenever feasible, to confirm hypoglycemia.

- Any patient with a serum glucose concentration of <60 mg/dL should be suspected of having a hypoglycemic disorder, and further evaluation is required if the value is <50 mg/dL.
- Absence of symptoms with these levels of glucose suggests the possibility of artifactual hypoglycemia. These levels are usually accompanied by symptoms of hypoglycemia. Detailed evaluation is usually required in a healthy-appearing patient, whereas hypoglycemia may be readily recognized as part of the underlying illness in a sick patient (*N Engl J Med 1986;315:1245*). Major categories include fasting and postprandial hypoglycemia.
- **Fasting hypoglycemia** can be caused by inappropriate insulin secretion (e.g., insulinoma), alcohol abuse, severe hepatic or renal insufficiency, hypopituitarism, glucocorticoid deficiency, or surreptitious injection of insulin or ingestion of an SFU.
  - These patients present with neuroglycopenic symptoms, but episodic autonomic symptoms may be present. Occasionally, patients with recurrent seizures, dementia, and bizarre behavior are referred for neuropsychiatric evaluation, which may delay timely diagnosis of hypoglycemia.
  - **Definitive diagnosis** of fasting hypoglycemia requires hourly BG monitoring during a supervised fast lasting up to 72 hours and measurement of plasma insulin, C-peptide, and SFU metabolites if hypoglycemia (<50 mg/dL) is documented. Patients who develop hypoglycemia and have measurable plasma insulin and C-peptide levels without SFU metabolites require further evaluation for an insulinoma.
- **Postprandial hypoglycemia** often is suspected, but seldom proven, in patients with vague symptoms that occur 1 or more hours after meals.
  - **Alimentary hypoglycemia** should be considered in patients with a history of partial gastrectomy or intestinal resection in whom recurrent symptoms develop 1 to 2 hours after eating. The mechanism is thought to be related to too rapid glucose absorption, resulting in a robust insulin response. These symptoms should be distinguished from dumping syndrome, which is not associated with hypoglycemia and occurs in the first hour after food intake. Thus, frequent small meals with reduced carbohydrate content may ameliorate symptoms.
  - **Functional hypoglycemia.** Symptoms that are possibly suggestive of hypoglycemia, which may or may not be confirmed by plasma glucose measurement, occur in some patients who have not undergone GI surgery. This condition is referred to as "functional hypoglycemia." The symptoms tend to develop 3 to 5 hours after meals. Current evaluation and management of functional hypoglycemia are imprecise; some patients show evidence of IGT and may respond to dietary therapy.

TREATMENT

Isolated episodes of mild hypoglycemia may not require specific intervention. Recurrent episodes require a review of lifestyle factors; adjustments may be indicated in the content, timing, and distribution of meals, as well as medication dosage and timing. Severe hypoglycemia is an indication for supervised treatment.

- **Readily absorbable carbohydrates** (e.g., glucose and sugar-containing beverages) can be administered orally to conscious patients for rapid effect. Alternatively, milk, candy bars, fruit, cheese, and crackers may be used in some patients with mild hypoglycemia. Hypoglycemia associated with acarbose or miglitol therapy should preferentially be treated with glucose. Glucose tablets and carbohydrate supplies should be readily available to patients with DM at all times.
- **IV dextrose** is indicated for severe hypoglycemia, in patients with altered consciousness, and during restriction of oral intake. An initial bolus, 20 to 50 mL of 50% dextrose, should be given immediately, followed by infusion of D5W (or D10W) to maintain BG levels above 100 mg/dL. Prolonged IV dextrose infusion and close observation is warranted in SFU overdose, in the elderly, and in patients with defective counterregulation.
- **Glucagon**, 1 mg IM (or SC), is an effective initial therapy for severe hypoglycemia in patients unable to receive oral intake or in whom an IV access cannot be secured immediately. Vomiting is a frequent side effect and therefore care should be taken to prevent the risk of aspiration. A glucagon kit should be available to patients with a history of severe hypoglycemia; family members and roommates should be instructed in its proper use.

PATIENT EDUCATION

- **Education** regarding etiologies of hypoglycemia, preventive measures, and appropriate adjustments to medication, diet, and exercise regimens are essential tasks to be addressed during hospitalization for severe hypoglycemia.
- **Hypoglycemia unawareness** can develop in patients who are undergoing intensive diabetes therapy. These patients should be encouraged to monitor their BG levels frequently and take timely measures to correct low values (<60 mg/dL). In patients with very tightly controlled diabetes, slight relaxation in glycemic control and scrupulous avoidance of hypoglycemia may restore the lost warning symptoms.

24 Endocrine Diseases

William E. Clutter

DISORDERS OF THE THYROID GLAND

Evaluation of Thyroid Function

GENERAL PRINCIPLES

The major hormone secreted by the thyroid is **thyroxine (T_4)**, which is converted by deiodinases in many tissues to the more potent **triiodothyronine (T_3)**. Both are bound reversibly to plasma proteins, primarily **thyroxine-binding globulin (TBG)**. Only the free (unbound) fraction enters cells and produces biologic effects. T_4 secretion is stimulated by **thyroid-stimulating hormone (TSH)**. In turn, TSH secretion is inhibited by T_4, forming a negative feedback loop that keeps free T_4 levels within a narrow normal range. Diagnosis of thyroid disease is based on clinical findings, palpation of the thyroid, and measurement of plasma TSH and thyroid hormones.

DIAGNOSIS

Clinical Presentation

Thyroid palpation determines the size and consistency of the thyroid and the presence of nodules, tenderness, or a thrill.

Diagnostic Testing

- **Plasma TSH is the initial test of choice in most patients with suspected thyroid disease**, except when thyroid function is not in a steady state. TSH levels are elevated in very mild primary hypothyroidism and are suppressed to <0.1 microunits/mL in very mild hyperthyroidism. Thus, **a normal plasma TSH level excludes hyperthyroidism and primary hypothyroidism**. Because even slight changes in thyroid hormone levels affect TSH secretion, **abnormal TSH levels are not specific for clinically important thyroid disease**. Changes in plasma TSH lag behind changes in plasma T_4, and TSH levels may be misleading when plasma T_4 levels are changing rapidly, as during treatment of hyperthyroidism.
  - **Plasma TSH is mildly elevated** (up to 20 microunits/mL) in some euthyroid patients with **nonthyroidal illnesses** and in mild (or subclinical) hypothyroidism.
  - **TSH levels may be suppressed to <0.1 microunits/mL in severe nonthyroidal illness**, in mild (or subclinical) hyperthyroidism, and during treatment with dopamine or high doses of glucocorticoids. Also, TSH levels remain <0.1 microunits/mL for some time after hyperthyroidism is corrected.

| Table 24-1 | Effects of Drugs on Thyroid Function Tests |

Effect	Drug
Decreased free and total T$_4$	
True hypothyroidism (TSH elevated)	Iodine (amiodarone, radiographic contrast)
	Lithium
Inhibition of TSH secretion	Glucocorticoids
	Dopamine
Multiple mechanisms (TSH normal)	Phenytoin
Decreased total T$_4$ only	
Decreased TBG (TSH normal)	Androgens
Inhibition of T$_4$ binding to TBG (TSH normal)	Furosemide (high doses)
	Salicylates
Increased free and total T$_4$	
True hyperthyroidism (TSH <0.1 microunits/mL)	Iodine (amiodarone, radiographic contrast)
Inhibited T$_4$ to T$_3$ conversion (TSH normal)	Amiodarone
Increased free T$_4$ only	
Displacement of T$_4$ from TBG in vitro (TSH normal)	Heparin, low–molecular-weight heparin
Increased total T$_4$ only	
Increased TBG (TSH normal)	Estrogens, tamoxifen, raloxifene

T$_3$, triiodothyronine; T$_4$, thyroxine; TBG, thyroxine-binding globulin; TSH, thyroid-stimulating hormone.

- ◦ TSH levels are usually within the reference range in secondary hypothyroidism and are not useful for detection of this rare form of hypothyroidism.
- **Plasma free T$_4$** confirms the diagnosis and assesses the severity of hyperthyroidism when plasma TSH is <0.1 microunits/mL. It is also used to diagnose secondary hypothyroidism and adjust thyroxine therapy in patients with pituitary disease. Most laboratories measure free T$_4$ by immunoassay. Total T$_4$ assays are less reliable and should not be used, except when free T$_4$ is artifactually elevated by heparin treatment (Table 24-1).
  Free T$_4$ measured by equilibrium dialysis is the most reliable measure of unbound T$_4$, but results are seldom rapidly available. It is needed only in rare cases in which the diagnosis is not clear from measurement of plasma TSH and free T$_4$ by analog immunoassay.
- **Effect of nonthyroidal illness on thyroid function tests.** Many illnesses alter thyroid tests without causing true thyroid dysfunction (the nonthyroidal illness or euthyroid sick syndrome). These changes must be recognized to avoid mistaken diagnosis and therapy.
  - ◦ **The low T$_3$ syndrome** occurs in many illnesses, during starvation, and after trauma or surgery. Conversion of T$_4$ to T$_3$ is decreased, and plasma T$_3$ levels are low. Plasma free T$_4$ and TSH levels are normal. This may be an adaptive response to illness, and thyroid hormone therapy is not beneficial.
  - ◦ **The low T$_4$ syndrome** occurs in severe illness. Plasma total T$_4$ levels fall due to decreased levels of TBG and perhaps due to inhibition of T$_4$ binding to TBG. **Plasma free T$_4$ measured by equilibrium dialysis usually remains normal.**

However, when measured by commonly available immunoassays, free T_4 may be low. **TSH levels decrease early in severe illness**, sometimes to <0.1 microunits/mL. **During recovery, they rise, sometimes to levels higher than the normal range** (although rarely >20 microunits/mL).

○ Some drugs affect thyroid function tests (see Table 24-1). Iodine-containing drugs (**amiodarone** and radiographic contrast media) may cause hyperthyroidism or hypothyroidism in susceptible patients. Other drugs alter thyroid function tests, especially plasma total T_4, without causing true thyroid dysfunction. In general, plasma TSH levels are a reliable guide to determine whether true hyperthyroidism or hypothyroidism is present.

Hypothyroidism

GENERAL PRINCIPLES

Etiology

- **Primary hypothyroidism** (due to disease of the thyroid itself) accounts for >90% of cases.
- **Chronic lymphocytic thyroiditis (Hashimoto's disease)** is the most common cause and may be associated with Addison's disease and other endocrine deficits. Its prevalence is greater in women and increases with age.
- **Iatrogenic hypothyroidism** due to thyroidectomy or radioactive iodine (RAI; ^{131}I) therapy is also common.
- Transient hypothyroidism occurs in postpartum thyroiditis and subacute thyroiditis, usually after a period of hyperthyroidism.
- **Drugs that may cause hypothyroidism** include iodine-containing drugs, lithium, interferon (IFN)-α, IFN-β, interleukin-2, thalidomide, bexarotene, and sunitinib.
- Secondary hypothyroidism due to TSH deficiency is uncommon but may occur in any disorder of the pituitary or hypothalamus. However, it rarely occurs without other evidence of pituitary disease.

DIAGNOSIS

Clinical Presentation

History

Most symptoms of hypothyroidism are nonspecific and develop gradually. They include cold intolerance, fatigue, somnolence, poor memory, constipation, menorrhagia, myalgias, and hoarseness. Hypothyroidism is readily treatable and should be suspected in any patient with compatible symptoms, especially in the presence of a diffuse goiter or a history of RAI therapy or thyroid surgery.

Physical Examination

Signs include slow tendon reflex relaxation, bradycardia, facial and periorbital edema, dry skin, and nonpitting edema (myxedema). Mild weight gain may occur, but hypothyroidism does not cause marked obesity. Rare manifestations include hypoventilation, pericardial or pleural effusions, deafness, and carpal tunnel syndrome.

Diagnostic Testing

Laboratories

- Laboratory findings may include hyponatremia and elevated plasma levels of cholesterol, triglycerides, and creatine kinase.

- In suspected primary hypothyroidism, plasma TSH is the best initial test.
  - A normal value excludes primary hypothyroidism, and a markedly elevated value (>20 microunits/mL) confirms the diagnosis.
  - Mild elevation of plasma TSH (<20 microunits/mL) may be due to nonthyroidal illness, but usually indicates **mild (or subclinical) primary hypothyroidism**, in which thyroid function is impaired but increased secretion of TSH maintains plasma free T_4 levels within the reference range. These patients may have nonspecific symptoms that are compatible with hypothyroidism and a mild increase in serum cholesterol and low-density lipoprotein cholesterol. They develop clinical hypothyroidism at a rate of 2.5% per year.
- If secondary hypothyroidism is suspected because of evidence of pituitary disease, plasma free T_4 should be measured. Plasma TSH levels are usually within the reference range in secondary hypothyroidism and cannot be used alone to make this diagnosis. Patients with secondary hypothyroidism should be evaluated for other pituitary hormone deficits and for a mass lesion of the pituitary or hypothalamus (see Disorders of Anterior Pituitary Function section).
- **In severe nonthyroidal illness**, the diagnosis of hypothyroidism may be difficult. Plasma total T_4 and free T_4 measured by routine assays may be low.
  - **Plasma TSH is the best initial diagnostic test.** A normal TSH value is strong evidence that the patient is euthyroid, except when there is evidence of pituitary or hypothalamic disease or in patients treated with dopamine or high doses of glucocorticoids. Marked elevation of plasma TSH (>20 microunits/mL) establishes the diagnosis of primary hypothyroidism.
  - Moderate elevations of plasma TSH (<20 microunits/mL) may occur in euthyroid patients with nonthyroidal illness and are not specific for hypothyroidism. Plasma free T_4 should be measured if TSH is moderately elevated, or if secondary hypothyroidism is suspected, and patients should be treated for hypothyroidism if plasma free T_4 is low. Thyroid function in these patients should be reevaluated after recovery from illness.

Electrocardiography
The electrocardiogram (ECG) may show low voltage and T-wave abnormalities.

TREATMENT

Medications

Thyroxine is the drug of choice. The average replacement dose is 1.6 μg/kg by mouth (PO) daily, and most patients require doses between 75 and 150 μg/d. In elderly patients, the average replacement dose is lower. The need for lifelong treatment should be emphasized. Thyroxine should be taken 30 minutes before a meal, since some foods interfere with its absorption, and should not be taken with medications that affect its absorption (see the following text).
- **Initiation of therapy.** Young and middle-aged adults should be started on 100 μg/d. This regimen gradually corrects hypothyroidism, as several weeks are required to reach steady-state plasma levels of T_4. Symptoms begin to improve within a few weeks. In otherwise healthy elderly patients, the initial dose should be 50 μg/d. Patients with cardiac disease should be started on 25 to 50 μg/d and monitored carefully for exacerbation of cardiac symptoms.

- **Dose adjustment and follow-up.**
  - In primary hypothyroidism, the goal of therapy is to maintain plasma TSH within the normal range. Plasma TSH should be measured 6 to 8 weeks after initiation of therapy. The dose of thyroxine should then be adjusted in 12- to 25-μg increments at intervals of 6 to 8 weeks until plasma TSH is normal. Thereafter, annual TSH measurement is adequate to monitor therapy. TSH should also be measured in the first trimester of pregnancy, since the thyroxine dose requirement often increases at this time (see the following text). Overtreatment, indicated by a subnormal TSH, should be avoided since it increases the risk of osteoporosis and atrial fibrillation.
  - In secondary hypothyroidism, plasma TSH cannot be used to adjust therapy. The goal of therapy is to maintain the **plasma free T_4** near the middle of the reference range. The dose of thyroxine should be adjusted at 6- to 8-week intervals until this goal is achieved. Thereafter, annual measurement of plasma free T_4 is adequate to monitor therapy.
  - **Coronary artery disease** may be exacerbated by the treatment of hypothyroidism. The dose of thyroxine should be increased slowly in patients with coronary artery disease, with careful attention to worsening angina, heart failure, or arrhythmias.

COMPLICATIONS

- **Situations in which thyroxine dose requirements change.** Difficulty in controlling hypothyroidism is most often due to **poor compliance** with therapy. Other causes of increasing thyroxine requirement include
  - Malabsorption due to intestinal disease or drugs that interfere with thyroxine absorption (e.g., calcium carbonate, ferrous sulfate, cholestyramine, sucralfate, aluminum hydroxide)
  - Drug interactions that increase thyroxine clearance (e.g., estrogen, rifampin, carbamazepine, phenytoin) or block conversion of T_4 to T_3 (amiodarone)
  - Pregnancy, in which thyroxine requirements often increase in the first trimester (see the following text)
  - Gradual failure of remaining endogenous thyroid function after RAI treatment of hyperthyroidism
- **Pregnancy. Thyroxine dose increases by an average of 50% in the first half of pregnancy** (*Endocrinol Metab Clin North Am 2011;40:739*). In women with primary hypothyroidism, plasma TSH should be measured as soon as pregnancy is confirmed and monthly thereafter through the second trimester. The thyroxine dose should be increased as needed to maintain plasma TSH within the lower half of the normal range to avoid fetal hypothyroidism.
- **Subclinical hypothyroidism** should be treated with thyroxine if any of the following are present: (a) **symptoms compatible with hypothyroidism**, (b) a **goiter**, (c) **hypercholesterolemia** that warrants treatment, or (d) the **plasma TSH is >10 microunits/mL** (*Endocr Rev 2008;29:76*). Untreated patients should be monitored annually, and thyroxine should be started if symptoms develop or serum TSH increases to >10 microunits/mL.
- **Urgent therapy** for hypothyroidism is rarely necessary. Most patients with hypothyroidism and concomitant illness can be treated in the usual manner. However, hypothyroidism may impair survival in critical illness by contributing to hypoventilation, hypotension, hypothermia, bradycardia, or hyponatremia.

○ Hypoventilation and hypotension should be treated intensively, along with any concomitant diseases. Confirmatory tests (plasma TSH and free T_4) should be obtained before thyroid hormone therapy is started.

○ **Thyroxine, 50 to 100 μg intravenous (IV), can be given q6–8h for 24 hours**, followed by 75 to 100 μg IV daily until oral intake is possible. Replacement therapy should be continued in the usual manner if the diagnosis of hypothyroidism is confirmed. No clinical trials have determined the optimum method of thyroid hormone replacement, but this method rapidly alleviates thyroxine deficiency while minimizing the risk of exacerbating underlying coronary disease or heart failure. **Such rapid correction is warranted only in extremely ill patients. Vital signs and cardiac rhythm should be monitored carefully to detect early signs of exacerbation of heart disease. Hydrocortisone**, 50 mg IV q8h, is recommended during rapid replacement of thyroid hormone, because such therapy may precipitate adrenal crisis in patients with adrenal failure.

Hyperthyroidism

GENERAL PRINCIPLES

Etiology

- **Graves' disease** (*N Engl J Med 2008;358:2594*) causes most cases of hyperthyroidism, especially in young patients. This **autoimmune** disorder may also cause **proptosis** (exophthalmos) and pretibial myxedema, neither of which is found in other causes of hyperthyroidism.
- **Toxic multinodular goiter (MNG)** is a common cause of hyperthyroidism in older patients.
- Unusual causes include **iodine-induced hyperthyroidism** (usually precipitated by drugs such as **amiodarone** or radiographic contrast media), thyroid adenomas, subacute thyroiditis (painful tender goiter with transient hyperthyroidism), painless thyroiditis (nontender goiter with transient hyperthyroidism, most often seen in the postpartum period), and surreptitious ingestion of thyroid hormone. TSH-induced hyperthyroidism is extremely rare.

DIAGNOSIS

Clinical Presentation

History

- Symptoms include heat intolerance, weight loss, weakness, palpitations, oligomenorrhea, and anxiety.
- **In the elderly**, hyperthyroidism may present with only atrial fibrillation, heart failure, weakness, or weight loss, and a high index of suspicion is needed to make the diagnosis.

Physical Examination

- Signs include brisk tendon reflexes, fine tremor, proximal weakness, stare, and eyelid lag. Cardiac abnormalities may be prominent, including sinus tachycardia, atrial fibrillation, and exacerbation of coronary artery disease or heart failure.

Table 24-2	Differential Diagnosis of Hyperthyroidism
Type of Goiter	**Diagnosis**
Diffuse, nontender goiter	Graves' disease or painless thyroiditis
Multiple thyroid nodules	Toxic multinodular goiter
Single thyroid nodule	Thyroid adenoma
Tender painful goiter	Subacute thyroiditis
Normal thyroid gland	Graves' disease, painless thyroiditis, or factitious hyperthyroidism

- Key differentiating physical exam findings include (Table 24-2) the following:
  - The presence of proptosis or pretibial myxedema, seen only in Graves' disease (although many patients with Graves' disease lack these signs)
  - A diffuse nontender goiter, consistent with Graves' disease or painless thyroiditis
  - Recent pregnancy, neck pain, or recent iodine administration, suggesting causes other than Graves' disease

Diagnostic Testing

In rare cases, **24-hour radioactive iodine uptake (RAIU)** is needed to distinguish Graves' disease or toxic MNG (in which RAIU is elevated) from postpartum thyroiditis, iodine-induced hyperthyroidism, or factitious hyperthyroidism (in which RAIU is very low).

Laboratories
In suspected hyperthyroidism, plasma TSH is the best initial diagnostic test.
- A TSH level >0.1 microunits/mL excludes clinical hyperthyroidism. If plasma TSH is <0.1 microunits/mL, **plasma free T_4** should be measured to determine the severity of hyperthyroidism and as a baseline for therapy. If plasma free T_4 is elevated, the diagnosis of clinical hyperthyroidism is established.
- **If plasma TSH is <0.1 microunits/mL but free T_4 is normal**, the patient may have clinical hyperthyroidism due to elevation of plasma T_3 alone; and plasma T_3 should be measured in this case.
- Very **mild (or subclinical) hyperthyroidism** may suppress TSH to <0.1 microunits/mL, and thus suppression of TSH alone does not confirm that symptoms are due to hyperthyroidism.
- TSH may also be suppressed by **severe nonthyroidal illness** (see Evaluation of Thyroid Function section).

TREATMENT

- Some forms of hyperthyroidism (subacute or postpartum thyroiditis) are transient and require only **symptomatic therapy**.
  - A **β-adrenergic antagonist** (such as **atenolol** 25 to 100 mg daily) is used to relieve symptoms of hyperthyroidism, such as palpitations, tremor, and anxiety, until hyperthyroidism is controlled by definitive therapy, or until transient forms of hyperthyroidism subside. The dose is adjusted to alleviate symptoms and tachycardia, then reduced gradually as hyperthyroidism is controlled.

- ○ Verapamil at an initial dose of 40 to 80 mg PO tid can be used to control tachycardia in patients with contraindications to β-adrenergic antagonists.
- Three methods are available for definitive therapy (none of which controls hyperthyroidism rapidly): RAI, thionamides, and subtotal thyroidectomy (*Thyroid 2011;21:593*).
  - ○ **During treatment, patients are followed by clinical evaluation and measurement of plasma free T₄.** Plasma TSH is useless in assessing the initial response to therapy, as it remains suppressed until after the patient becomes euthyroid.
  - ○ Regardless of the therapy used, all patients with Graves' disease require lifelong follow-up for recurrent hyperthyroidism or development of hypothyroidism.
- **Choice of definitive therapy**
  - ○ **In Graves' disease, RAI therapy is the treatment of choice for almost all patients.** It is simple and highly effective but **cannot be used in pregnancy. Propylthiouracil (PTU) should be used to treat hyperthyroidism in pregnancy.** Thionamides achieve long-term control in fewer than half of patients with Graves' disease and they carry a small risk of life-threatening side effects. Thyroidectomy should be used in patients who refuse RAI therapy and who relapse or develop side effects with thionamide therapy.
  - ○ **Other causes of hyperthyroidism.** Toxic MNG and toxic adenoma should be treated with RAI (except in pregnancy). Transient forms of hyperthyroidism due to thyroiditis should be treated symptomatically with atenolol. Iodine-induced hyperthyroidism is treated with thionamides and atenolol until the patient is euthyroid. Although treatment of some patients with amiodarone-induced hyperthyroidism with glucocorticoids has been advocated, **nearly all patients with amiodarone-induced hyperthyroidism respond well to thionamide therapy** (*Circulation 2002;105:1275*).
- **RAI therapy**
  - ○ A single dose permanently controls hyperthyroidism in 90% of patients, and further doses can be given if necessary.
  - ○ A **pregnancy test** is done immediately before therapy in potentially fertile women.
  - ○ A 24-hour RAIU is usually measured and used to calculate the dose.
  - ○ Thionamides interfere with RAI therapy and should be stopped at least 3 days before treatment. If iodine treatment has been given, it should be stopped at least 2 weeks before RAI therapy.
  - ○ Most patients with Graves' disease are treated with 8 to 10 mCi, although treatment of toxic MNG requires higher doses.
  - ○ **Follow-up.** Usually, several months are needed to restore euthyroidism. Patients are evaluated at 4- to 6-week intervals, with assessment of clinical findings and plasma free T₄.
    - ▪ **If thyroid function stabilizes within the normal range**, the interval between follow-up visits is gradually increased to annual intervals.
    - ▪ If symptomatic hypothyroidism develops, thyroxine therapy is started (see Hypothyroidism section).
    - ▪ If symptomatic hyperthyroidism **persists after 6 months, RAI treatment is repeated**.
  - ○ **Side effects**
    - ▪ **Hypothyroidism** occurs in most patients within the first year and continues to develop at a rate of approximately 3% per year thereafter.
    - ▪ Because of the release of stored hormone, a slight rise in plasma T₄ may occur in the first 2 weeks after therapy. This development is important only in

patients with severe cardiac disease, which may worsen as a result. Such patients should be treated with thionamides to restore euthyroidism and to deplete stored hormone before treatment with RAI.

- There is no convincing evidence that RAI has a clinically important effect on the course of Graves' eye disease.
- It does not increase the risk of malignancy or cause congenital abnormalities in the offspring of women who conceive after RAI therapy.

- **Thionamides.** Methimazole and PTU inhibit thyroid hormone synthesis. PTU also inhibits extrathyroidal deiodination of T_4 to T_3. Once thyroid hormone stores are depleted (after several weeks to months), T_4 levels decrease. These drugs have no permanent effect on thyroid function. **In the majority of patients with Graves' disease, hyperthyroidism recurs within 6 months after therapy is stopped.** Spontaneous remission of Graves' disease occurs in approximately one-third of patients during thionamide therapy and, in this minority, no other treatment may be needed. Remission is more likely in mild, recent-onset hyperthyroidism and if the goiter is small. Because of a better safety profile, **methimazole should be used instead of PTU** except in specific situations (see the following text) (*J Clin Endocrinol Metab 2009;94:1881*).
  - **Initiation of therapy.** Before starting therapy, patients must be warned of side effects and precautions. Usual starting doses are methimazole, 10 to 40 mg PO daily, or PTU, 100 to 200 mg PO tid; higher initial doses can be used in severe hyperthyroidism.
  - **Follow-up.** Restoration of euthyroidism takes up to several months.
    - Patients are evaluated at 4-week intervals with assessment of clinical findings and plasma free T_4. If plasma free T_4 levels do not fall after 4 to 8 weeks, the dose should be increased. Doses as high as methimazole, 60 mg PO daily, or PTU, 300 mg PO qid, may be required.
    - Once the plasma free T_4 level falls to normal, the dose is adjusted to maintain plasma free T_4 within the normal range.
    - No consensus exists on the optimal duration of therapy, but periods of 6 months to 2 years are used most commonly. Patients must be monitored carefully for recurrence of hyperthyroidism after the drug is stopped.
- **Side effects** are most likely to occur within the first few months of therapy.
  - Minor side effects include rash, urticaria, fever, arthralgias, and transient leukopenia.
  - **Agranulocytosis** occurs in 0.3% of patients treated with thionamides. Other life-threatening side effects include **hepatitis**, vasculitis, and drug-induced lupus erythematosus. These complications usually resolve if the drug is stopped promptly.
  - **Patients must be warned to stop the drug immediately if jaundice or symptoms suggestive of agranulocytosis develop (e.g., fever, chills, sore throat)** and to contact their physician promptly for evaluation. Routine monitoring of the white blood cell (WBC) is not useful for detecting agranulocytosis, which develops suddenly.
- **Subtotal thyroidectomy.** This procedure provides long-term control of hyperthyroidism in most patients.
  - Surgery may trigger a perioperative exacerbation of hyperthyroidism, and patients should be prepared for surgery by one of two methods.
    - **A thionamide** is given until the patient is nearly euthyroid. **Supersaturated potassium iodide** (**SSKI**), 40 to 80 mg (one to two drops) PO bid, is then added 1 to 2 weeks before surgery. Both drugs are stopped postoperatively.

- **Atenolol** (50 to 100 mg daily) is started 1 to 2 weeks before surgery. The dose of atenolol is increased, if necessary, to reduce the resting heart rate below 90 bpm and is continued for 5 to 7 days postoperatively. SSKI is given as mentioned earlier.
  - **Follow-up.** Clinical findings and plasma free T_4 and TSH should be assessed 4 to 6 weeks after surgery.
    - If thyroid function is normal, the patient is seen at 3 and 6 months, then annually.
    - If symptomatic hypothyroidism develops, thyroxine therapy is started (see Hypothyroidism section).
    - Mild hypothyroidism after subtotal thyroidectomy may be transient, and asymptomatic patients can be observed for further 4 to 6 weeks to determine whether hypothyroidism will resolve spontaneously.
    - Hyperthyroidism persists or recurs in 3% to 7% of patients.
  - **Complications** of thyroidectomy include **hypothyroidism** in 30% to 50% of patients and **hypoparathyroidism** in 3%. Rare complications include permanent vocal cord paralysis, due to recurrent laryngeal nerve injury, and perioperative death. The complication rate appears to depend on the experience of the surgeon.

SPECIAL CONSIDERATIONS

- **Subclinical hyperthyroidism** is present when the plasma TSH is suppressed to <0.1 microunits/mL but the patient has no symptoms that are definitely caused by hyperthyroidism, and plasma levels of free T_4 and T_3 are normal.
  - Subclinical hyperthyroidism increases the risk of **atrial fibrillation** in patients older than 60 years and those with heart disease, and predisposes to **osteoporosis** in postmenopausal women; it should be treated in these patients.
  - Asymptomatic young patients with mild Graves' disease can be observed for spontaneous resolution of hyperthyroidism, or the development of symptoms or increasing free T_4 levels that warrant treatment.
- **Urgent therapy** is warranted when hyperthyroidism exacerbates heart failure or acute coronary syndromes, and in rare patients with severe hyperthyroidism complicated by fever and delirium. Concomitant diseases should be treated intensively, and confirmatory tests (serum TSH and free T_4) should be obtained before therapy is started.
  - **PTU, 300 mg PO q6h,** should be started immediately.
  - **Iodide** (**SSKI**, two drops PO q12h) should be started 1 hour after the first dose of PTU to inhibit thyroid hormone secretion rapidly.
  - **Propranolol**, 40 mg PO q6h (or an equivalent dose IV), should be given to patients with angina or myocardial infarction, and the dose should be adjusted to prevent tachycardia. Propranolol may benefit some patients with heart failure and marked tachycardia but can further impair left ventricular systolic function. In patients with clinical heart failure, it should be given only with careful monitoring of left ventricular function.
  - Plasma free T_4 is measured every 4 to 6 days. When free T_4 approaches the normal range, the doses of PTU and iodine are gradually decreased. RAI therapy should be scheduled 2 weeks after iodine is stopped.
- **Hyperthyroidism in pregnancy.** If hyperthyroidism is suspected, plasma TSH should be measured. Plasma TSH declines in early pregnancy but rarely to <0.1 microunits/mL (*Endocrinol Metab Clin North Am 2011;40:739*).

- If TSH is <0.1 microunits/mL, the diagnosis should be confirmed by measurement of plasma free T_4.
- RAI is contraindicated in pregnancy, and therefore, patients should be treated with PTU. Methimazole is not used because it is associated with certain congenital defects. The dose should be adjusted at 4-week intervals to maintain the plasma free T_4 near the upper limit of the normal range to avoid fetal hypothyroidism. The dose required often decreases in the later stages of pregnancy.
- Atenolol, 25 to 50 mg PO daily, can be used to relieve symptoms while awaiting the effects of PTU.
- The fetus and neonate should be monitored carefully for hyperthyroidism. The maternal plasma level of thyroid-stimulating immunoglobulin should be measured in the third trimester to assess this risk.

Euthyroid Goiter and Thyroid Nodules

GENERAL PRINCIPLES

- The diagnosis of euthyroid goiter is based on palpation of the thyroid and evaluation of thyroid function. If the thyroid is enlarged, the examiner should determine whether the enlargement is **diffuse or multinodular, or whether a single palpable nodule is present**. All three forms of euthyroid goiter are common, especially in women.
- Thyroid scans or ultrasonography (US) provide no useful additional information about goiters that are diffuse or multinodular by palpation and should not be performed in these patients.
- Between 30% and 50% of people have nonpalpable thyroid nodules that are detectable by ultrasound. These nodules rarely have any clinical importance, but their incidental discovery may lead to unnecessary diagnostic testing and treatment (*Clin Endocrinol 2004;60:18*).

Classification

- **Diffuse goiter**
  - Almost all euthyroid diffuse goiters in the United States are due to **chronic lymphocytic thyroiditis (Hashimoto's thyroiditis)**. Since Hashimoto's thyroiditis may also cause hypothyroidism, plasma TSH should be measured even in patients who are clinically euthyroid.
  - Diffuse goiters are usually asymptomatic, and therapy is seldom required. Patients should be monitored regularly for the development of hypothyroidism.
- **Multinodular goiter**
  - MNG is common in older patients, especially women. Most patients are asymptomatic and require no treatment.
  - In a few patients, **hyperthyroidism** (toxic MNG) develops (see Hyperthyroidism section).
  - In rare patients, the gland compresses the trachea or esophagus, causing dyspnea or dysphagia, and treatment is required. Thyroxine treatment has little, if any, effect on the size of MNGs. RAI therapy reduces gland size and relieves symptoms in most patients. Subtotal thyroidectomy can also be used to relieve compressive symptoms.

○ The risk of malignancy in MNG is low, comparable to the frequency of incidental thyroid carcinoma in clinically normal glands. Evaluation for thyroid carcinoma with needle biopsy is warranted if there is a dominant nodule (a nodule that is disproportionately larger than the rest). Some centers have adopted a policy of performing thyroid US in all patients with MNG, and evaluating all nodules larger than 1 cm by needle biopsy. This policy dramatically increases the number of thyroid biopsies and the cost of managing this common condition. There is no evidence that routine thyroid US improves clinical outcomes in patients with MNG, and it is not recommended.

• **Single thyroid nodules**
  ○ **Single palpable thyroid nodules** are usually benign, but about 5% are thyroid carcinomas.
  ○ Clinical findings that increase the likelihood of carcinoma include the presence of cervical lymphadenopathy, a history of radiation to the head or neck in childhood, and a family history of medullary thyroid carcinoma or multiple endocrine neoplasia syndromes types 2A or 2B. A hard, fixed nodule, recent nodule growth, or hoarseness due to vocal cord paralysis also suggests malignancy.
  ○ Most patients with thyroid carcinomas have none of these risk factors, and all **palpable single thyroid nodules should be evaluated with needle aspiration biopsy**. Patients with thyroid carcinoma should be managed in consultation with an endocrinologist.
  ○ Nodules with benign cytology should be reevaluated periodically by palpation. Thyroxine therapy has little or no effect on the size of single thyroid nodules and is not indicated.
  ○ Imaging studies cannot distinguish benign from malignant nodules and are not needed for the evaluation of a palpable thyroid nodule. The management of nonpalpable thyroid nodules discovered incidentally by ultrasound is controversial (*Clin Endocrinol 2004;60:18*).

DISORDERS OF ADRENAL FUNCTION

Adrenal Failure

GENERAL PRINCIPLES

Etiology

• Adrenal failure may be due to disease of the adrenal glands (**primary adrenal failure, Addison's disease**), with deficiency of both cortisol and aldosterone and elevated plasma adrenocorticotropic hormone (ACTH), or due to ACTH deficiency caused by disorders of the pituitary or hypothalamus (**secondary adrenal failure**), with deficiency of cortisol alone.
  ○ **Primary adrenal failure** is most often due to **autoimmune adrenalitis**, which may be associated with other endocrine deficits (e.g., hypothyroidism).
  ○ Infections of the adrenal gland such as **tuberculosis** and **histoplasmosis** may also cause adrenal failure.
  ○ **Hemorrhagic adrenal infarction** may occur in the postoperative period, in coagulation disorders and hypercoagulable states, and in sepsis. Adrenal hemorrhage often causes abdominal or flank pain and fever; computed tomography (CT) scan of the abdomen reveals high-density bilateral adrenal masses.

○ Adrenal failure may develop in patients with AIDS, caused by adrenal lymphoma, disseminated cytomegalovirus, mycobacterial, or fungal infection.

○ Less common etiologies include adrenoleukodystrophy that causes adrenal failure in young males, and drugs such as ketoconazole and etomidate that inhibit steroid hormone synthesis.

• **Secondary adrenal failure** is most often due to **glucocorticoid therapy**; ACTH suppression may persist for a year after therapy is stopped. Any disorder of the pituitary or hypothalamus can cause ACTH deficiency, but other evidence of these disorders is usually obvious.

DIAGNOSIS

Clinical Presentation

• Adrenal failure should be suspected in patients with hypotension, weight loss, persistent nausea, hyponatremia, or hyperkalemia.

• **Clinical findings** in adrenal failure are nonspecific, and without a high index of suspicion, the diagnosis of this potentially lethal but readily treatable disease is easily missed.

○ Symptoms include **anorexia**, **nausea**, **vomiting**, **weight loss**, **weakness**, and **fatigue**. **Orthostatic hypotension** and **hyponatremia** are common.

○ Symptoms are usually chronic, but **shock** may develop suddenly and is fatal unless promptly treated. Often, this adrenal crisis is triggered by illness, injury, or surgery. All these symptoms are due to cortisol deficiency and occur in both primary and secondary adrenal failure.

• **Hyperpigmentation** (due to marked ACTH excess) and **hyperkalemia** and **volume depletion** (due to aldosterone deficiency) occur only in primary adrenal failure.

Diagnostic Testing

Laboratories

• **The cosyntropin (Cortrosyn) stimulation test** is used for diagnosis. Cosyntropin, 250 μg, is given IV or intramuscular (IM), and **plasma cortisol is measured 30 minutes later**. The normal response is a stimulated plasma cortisol >20 μg/dL. This test detects primary and secondary adrenal failure, except within a few weeks of onset of pituitary dysfunction (e.g., shortly after pituitary surgery; see Disorders of Anterior Pituitary Function section).

• **The distinction between primary and secondary adrenal failure** is usually clear.

○ Hyperkalemia, hyperpigmentation, or other autoimmune endocrine deficits indicate primary adrenal failure, whereas deficits of other pituitary hormones, symptoms of a pituitary mass (e.g., headache, visual field loss), or known pituitary or hypothalamic disease indicate secondary adrenal failure.

○ If the cause is unclear, the **plasma ACTH** level distinguishes primary adrenal failure (in which it is markedly elevated) from secondary adrenal failure.

○ Most cases of primary adrenal failure are due to autoimmune adrenalitis, but other causes should be considered. Radiographic evidence of adrenal enlargement or calcification indicates that the cause is infection or hemorrhage.

○ Patients with secondary adrenal failure should be tested for other pituitary hormone deficiencies and should be evaluated for a pituitary or hypothalamic tumor (see Disorders of Anterior Pituitary Function section).

TREATMENT

- **Adrenal crisis** with hypotension must be treated immediately. Patients should be evaluated for an underlying illness that precipitated the crisis.
- **If the diagnosis of adrenal failure is known, hydrocortisone, 100 mg IV q8h**, should be given, and **0.9% saline with 5% dextrose** should be infused rapidly until hypotension is corrected. The dose of hydrocortisone is decreased gradually over several days as symptoms and any precipitating illness resolve, then changed to oral maintenance therapy. Mineralocorticoid replacement is not needed until the dose of hydrocortisone is <100 mg/d.
- **If the diagnosis of adrenal failure has not been established**, a single dose of **dexamethasone**, 10 mg IV, should be given, and a rapid infusion of 0.9% saline with 5% dextrose should be started. A **Cortrosyn stimulation test** should be performed. Dexamethasone is used because it does not interfere with measurement of plasma cortisol. After the 30-minute plasma cortisol measurement, hydrocortisone, 100 mg IV q8h, should be given until the test result is known.
- **Maintenance therapy** in all patients requires cortisol replacement with prednisone. Most patients with primary adrenal failure also require replacement of aldosterone with fludrocortisone.
  ○ **Prednisone**, 5 mg PO every morning, should be started. The dose is then adjusted with the goal being the lowest dose that relieves the patient's symptoms, to prevent osteoporosis and other signs of Cushing's syndrome. Most patients require doses between 4.0 and 7.5 mg PO daily. Concomitant therapy with rifampin, phenytoin, or phenobarbital accelerates glucocorticoid metabolism and increases the dose requirement.
  ○ **During illness, injury, or the perioperative period, the dose of glucocorticoid must be increased.**
    ▪ For minor illnesses, the patient should double the dose of prednisone for 3 days. If the illness resolves, the maintenance dose is resumed.
    ▪ **Vomiting requires immediate medical attention**, with IV glucocorticoid therapy and IV fluid. Patients can be given a 4-mg vial of dexamethasone to be self-administered IM for vomiting or severe illness if medical care is not immediately available.
    ▪ **For severe illness or injury**, hydrocortisone, 50 mg IV q8h, should be given, with the dose tapered as severity of illness wanes. The same regimen is used in **patients undergoing surgery**, with the first dose of hydrocortisone given preoperatively. The dose can be tapered to maintenance therapy by 2 to 3 days after uncomplicated surgery.
- **In primary adrenal failure, fludrocortisone, 0.1 mg PO daily**, should be given. The dose is adjusted to maintain blood pressure (supine and standing) and serum potassium within the normal range; the usual dosage is 0.05 to 0.20 mg PO daily.
- **Patients should be educated in management of their disease**, including adjustment of prednisone dose during illness. They should wear a medical identification tag or bracelet.

Cushing's Syndrome

GENERAL PRINCIPLES

Etiology

- Cushing's syndrome (*J Clin Endocrinol Metab 2008;93:1526*) is most often **iatrogenic**, due to therapy with glucocorticoid drugs.
- **ACTH-secreting pituitary microadenomas (Cushing's disease)** account for 80% of cases of endogenous Cushing's syndrome.
- Adrenal tumors and ectopic ACTH secretion account for the remainder.

DIAGNOSIS

Clinical Presentation

- Findings include truncal obesity, rounded face, fat deposits in the supraclavicular fossae and over the posterior neck, hypertension, hirsutism, amenorrhea, and depression. More specific findings include thin skin, easy bruising, reddish striae, proximal muscle weakness, and osteoporosis.
- Hyperpigmentation or hypokalemic alkalosis suggests Cushing's syndrome due to ectopic ACTH secretion.
- Diabetes mellitus develops in some patients.

Diagnostic Testing

- **Diagnosis** is based on increased cortisol excretion, lack of normal feedback inhibition of ACTH and cortisol secretion, or loss of the normal diurnal rhythm of cortisol secretion.
- The best initial test is the **24-hour urine cortisol** measurement. Alternatively, an **overnight dexamethasone suppression test** (1 mg dexamethasone given PO at 11:00 p.m.; plasma cortisol measured at 8:00 a.m. the next day; normal range: plasma cortisol <2 μg/dL) may be performed; or salivary cortisol may be measured at home during the nadir of normal plasma cortisol at 11:00 p.m. All these tests are very sensitive, and a normal value virtually excludes the diagnosis. If the overnight dexamethasone suppression test or 11:00 p.m. salivary cortisol is abnormal, 24-hour urine cortisol should be measured.
  - If the 24-hour urine cortisol excretion is more than four times the upper limit of the reference range in a patient with compatible clinical findings, the diagnosis of Cushing's syndrome is established.
  - In patients with milder elevations of urine cortisol, a **low-dose dexamethasone suppression test** should be performed. Dexamethasone, 0.5 mg PO q6h, is given for 48 hours, starting at 8:00 a.m. Urine cortisol is measured during the last 24 hours, and plasma cortisol is measured 6 hours after the last dose of dexamethasone. Failure to suppress plasma cortisol to <2 μg/dL and urine cortisol to less than the normal reference range is diagnostic of Cushing's syndrome.
  - Testing should not be done during severe illness or depression, which may cause false-positive results. Phenytoin therapy also causes a false-positive test by accelerating metabolism of dexamethasone.
- Random plasma cortisol levels are not useful for diagnosis, because the wide range of normal values overlaps those of Cushing's syndrome. After the diagnosis of Cushing's syndrome is made, tests to determine the cause are best done in consultation with an endocrinologist.

Incidental Adrenal Nodules

GENERAL PRINCIPLES

- Adrenal nodules are a common incidental finding on abdominal imaging studies.
- Most incidentally discovered nodules are benign adrenocortical tumors that do not secrete excess hormone.

DIAGNOSIS

In patients without a known malignancy elsewhere, the **diagnostic issues are whether a syndrome of hormone excess or an adrenocortical carcinoma is present**.

Clinical Presentation

Patients should be evaluated for hypertension, symptoms suggestive of pheochromocytoma (episodic headache, palpitations, and sweating) and signs of Cushing's syndrome (see Cushing's Syndrome section).

Differential Diagnosis

- The differential diagnosis includes adrenal adenomas causing Cushing's syndrome or primary hyperaldosteronism, pheochromocytoma, adrenocortical carcinoma, and metastatic cancer.
- The imaging characteristics of the nodule may suggest a diagnosis but are not specific enough to obviate further evaluation.

Diagnostic Testing

- **Plasma potassium, metanephrines, and dehydroepiandrosterone sulfate** should be measured, and an **overnight dexamethasone suppression** test should be performed.
- **Patients who have potentially resectable cancer elsewhere** and in whom an adrenal metastasis must be excluded may require positron emission tomography.
- Patients with hypertension and hypokalemia should be evaluated for primary hyperaldosteronism by measuring the ratio of plasma aldosterone (in nanograms per deciliter [ng/dL]) to plasma renin activity (in ng/mL/hr). If the ratio is less than 20, the diagnosis of primary hyperaldosteronism is excluded, while a ratio greater than 50 makes the diagnosis very likely. Patients with an intermediate ratio should be further evaluated in consultation with an endocrinologist.
- An abnormal overnight dexamethasone suppression test should be evaluated further (see Cushing's Syndrome section).
- Elevation of plasma dehydroepiandrosterone sulfate or a large nodule suggests adrenocortical carcinoma.

TREATMENT

- Most incidental nodules are <4 cm in diameter, do not produce excess hormone, and do not require therapy. One **repeat imaging procedure** 3 to 6 months later is recommended to ensure that the nodule is not enlarging rapidly (which would suggest an adrenal carcinoma).
- A policy of resecting all nodules >4 cm in diameter appropriately treats the great majority of adrenal carcinomas while minimizing the number of benign nodules that are removed unnecessarily.

- If clinical or biochemical evidence of a pheochromocytoma is found, the nodule should be resected after appropriate α-adrenergic blockade with phenoxybenzamine.

DISORDERS OF ANTERIOR PITUITARY FUNCTION

GENERAL PRINCIPLES

- The anterior pituitary gland secretes **prolactin**, **growth hormone**, and four **trophic hormones**, including corticotropin (ACTH); thyrotropin (TSH); and the gonado-tropins, luteinizing hormone and follicle-stimulating hormone. Each trophic hormone stimulates a specific target gland.
- Anterior pituitary function is regulated by hypothalamic hormones that reach the pituitary via portal veins in the pituitary stalk. **The predominant effect of hypothalamic regulation is to stimulate secretion of pituitary hormones, except for prolactin**, which is inhibited by hypothalamic dopamine secretion.
- **Secretion of trophic hormones is also regulated by negative feedback** by their target gland hormone, and the normal pituitary response to target hormone deficiency is increased secretion of the appropriate trophic hormone.
- **Anterior pituitary dysfunction** can be caused by disorders of either the pituitary or hypothalamus.

Etiology

- **Pituitary adenomas** are the most common pituitary disorder. They are classified by size and function.
  - **Microadenomas** are <10 mm in diameter and cause clinical manifestations only if they produce excess hormone. They are too small to produce hypopituitarism or mass effects.
  - **Macroadenomas** are >10 mm in diameter and may produce any combination of pituitary hormone excess, hypopituitarism, and mass effects (headache, visual field loss).
  - **Secretory adenomas** produce prolactin, growth hormone, or ACTH.
  - **Nonsecretory macroadenomas** may cause hypopituitarism or mass effects.
  - **Nonsecretory microadenomas** are common incidental radiographic findings, seen in approximately 10% of the normal population, and do not require therapy.
- **Other pituitary or hypothalamic disorders**, such as head trauma, pituitary surgery or radiation, and postpartum pituitary infarction (Sheehan's syndrome) may cause hypopituitarism. Other tumors of the pituitary or hypothalamus (e.g., craniopharyngioma, metastases), inflammatory disorders (e.g., sarcoidosis, histiocytosis X), and infections (e.g., tuberculosis) may cause hypopituitarism or mass effects.

DIAGNOSIS

Clinical Presentation

- In **hypopituitarism** (deficiency of one or more pituitary hormones), gonadotropin deficiency is most common, causing amenorrhea in women and androgen deficiency in men. Secondary hypothyroidism or adrenal failure rarely occurs alone. Secondary adrenal failure causes deficiency of cortisol but not of aldosterone; hyperkalemia and hyperpigmentation do not occur, although life-threatening adrenal crisis may develop.

- **Hormone excess** most commonly results in **hyperprolactinemia**, which can be due to a secretory adenoma or due to nonsecretory lesions that damage the hypothalamus or pituitary stalk. Growth hormone excess (**acromegaly**) and ACTH and cortisol excess (**Cushing's disease**) are caused by secretory adenomas.
- **Mass effects** due to pressure on adjacent structures, such as the optic chiasm, include **headaches** and **loss of visual fields or acuity**. Hyperprolactinemia may also be due to mass effect. **Pituitary apoplexy** is sudden enlargement of a pituitary tumor due to hemorrhagic necrosis.
- **Asymptomatic, incidentally discovered pituitary adenomas on imaging.**

Diagnostic Testing

- **If an incidental microadenoma is found** on imaging done for another purpose, the patient should be evaluated for clinical evidence of hyperprolactinemia, Cushing's disease, or acromegaly.
- Plasma prolactin and **insulin-like growth factor 1** (IGF-1) should be measured, and tests for Cushing's syndrome should be performed if symptoms or signs of this disorder are evident.
- If no pituitary hormone excess exists, therapy is not required. Whether such patients need repeat imaging is not established, but the risk of enlargement is clearly small.
- **Incidental discovery of a macroadenoma** is unusual. Patients should be evaluated for hormone excess and hypopituitarism. Most macroadenomas should be treated since they are likely to grow further.

Hypopituitarism

DIAGNOSIS

Clinical Presentation

Hypopituitarism may be suspected in the presence of clinical signs of target hormone deficiency (e.g., hypothyroidism) or pituitary mass effects.

Diagnostic Testing

Laboratories
- **Laboratory evaluation** for hypopituitarism begins with evaluation of **target hormone function**, including **plasma free T$_4$** and a **Cortrosyn stimulation test** (see Adrenal Failure section).
  - If recent onset of secondary adrenal failure is suspected (within a few weeks of evaluation), the patient should be treated empirically with glucocorticoids and should be tested 4 to 8 weeks later, since the Cortrosyn stimulation test cannot detect secondary adrenal failure of recent onset.
  - In men, **plasma testosterone** should be measured. The best evaluation of gonadal function in women is the **menstrual history**.
- **If a target hormone is deficient**, its trophic hormone is measured to determine whether target gland dysfunction is secondary to hypopituitarism. An elevated trophic hormone level indicates primary target gland dysfunction. In hypopituitarism, trophic hormone levels are not elevated and are usually within (not below)

the reference range. Thus, **pituitary trophic hormone levels can be interpreted only with knowledge of target hormone levels**, and **measurement of trophic hormone levels alone is useless in the diagnosis of hypopituitarism**. If pituitary disease is obvious, target hormone deficiencies may be assumed to be secondary, and trophic hormones need not be measured.

Imaging

Anatomic evaluation of the pituitary gland and hypothalamus is done best by magnetic resonance imaging (MRI). However, hyperprolactinemia and Cushing's disease may be caused by microadenomas too small to be seen with current techniques. The prevalence of incidental microadenomas should be kept in mind when interpreting MRIs. Visual acuity and **visual fields** should be tested when imaging suggests compression of the optic chiasm.

TREATMENT

- Deficient target hormones should be replaced.
- Secondary adrenal failure should be treated immediately, especially if patients are to undergo surgery (see Adrenal Failure section).
- Treatment of secondary hypothyroidism should be monitored by measurement of **plasma free T_4** (see Hypothyroidism section).
- Infertility due to gonadotropin deficiency may be correctable, and patients who wish to conceive should be referred to an endocrinologist.
- Treatment of growth hormone deficiency in adults has been advocated by some, but the long-term benefits, risks, and cost-effectiveness of this therapy are not established.
- Treatment of pituitary macroadenomas generally requires transsphenoidal surgical resection, except for prolactin-secreting tumors.

Hyperprolactinemia

GENERAL PRINCIPLES

- In women, the most common causes of pathologic hyperprolactinemia are prolactin-secreting pituitary **microadenomas** and **idiopathic hyperprolactinemia** (Table 24-3).

Table 24-3	Major Causes of Hyperprolactinemia

Pregnancy and lactation
Prolactin-secreting pituitary adenoma (prolactinoma)
Idiopathic hyperprolactinemia
Drugs (e.g., phenothiazines, metoclopramide, risperidone, verapamil)
Interference with synthesis or transport of hypothalamic dopamine
    Hypothalamic lesions
    Nonsecretory pituitary macroadenomas
Primary hypothyroidism
Chronic renal failure

- In men, the most common cause is a prolactin-secreting **macroadenoma**.
- Hypothalamic or pituitary lesions that cause deficiency of other pituitary hormones often cause hyperprolactinemia.
- **Medications** are an important cause in both men and women (*Pituitary 2008; 11:209*).

DIAGNOSIS

Clinical Presentation

- In women, hyperprolactinemia causes **amenorrhea** or irregular menses and **infertility**. Only approximately half of these women have **galactorrhea**. Prolonged estrogen deficiency increases the risk of **osteoporosis**. Plasma **prolactin should be measured in women with amenorrhea**, whether or not galactorrhea is present. Mild elevations should be confirmed by repeat measurements.
- In men, hyperprolactinemia causes **androgen deficiency** and **infertility** but not gynecomastia; **mass effects and hypopituitarism** are common.

History

The history should include medications and symptoms of pituitary mass effects or hypothyroidism.

Diagnostic Testing

Testing for hypopituitarism is needed only in patients with a macroadenoma or hypothalamic lesion. **Pituitary imaging** should be performed in most cases, as large nonfunctional pituitary or hypothalamic tumors may present with hyperprolactinemia.

TREATMENT

- For **microadenomas and idiopathic hyperprolactinemia** (*J Clin Endocrinol Metab 2011;96:273*), most patients are treated because of **infertility** or to prevent **estrogen deficiency and osteoporosis**.
- Some women may be observed without therapy by periodic follow-up of prolactin levels and symptoms. In most patients, hyperprolactinemia does not worsen, and prolactin levels sometimes return to normal. Enlargement of microadenomas is rare.
- **The dopamine agonists bromocriptine** and **cabergoline** suppress plasma prolactin and restore normal menses and fertility in most women.
  - Initial dosages are bromocriptine, 1.25 to 2.50 mg PO at bedtime with a snack, or cabergoline, 0.25 mg twice a week.
  - Plasma prolactin levels are initially obtained at 2- to 4-week intervals, and doses are adjusted until the lowest dose required to maintain prolactin in the normal range is reached. In general, the maximally effective doses are bromocriptine 2.5 mg tid and cabergoline 1.5 mg twice a week.
  - **Side effects** include **nausea** and **orthostatic hypotension**, which can be minimized by increasing the dose gradually and usually resolve with continued therapy. Side effects are less severe with cabergoline.
  - Initially, patients should use barrier contraception, as fertility may be restored quickly.
    - **Women who want to become pregnant** should be managed in consultation with an endocrinologist.

- **Women who do not want to become pregnant** should be followed with clinical evaluation and plasma prolactin levels every 6 to 12 months. Every 2 years, plasma prolactin should be measured after bromocriptine has been withdrawn for several weeks, to determine whether the drug is still needed. Follow-up imaging studies are not warranted unless prolactin levels increase substantially.
  - Transsphenoidal resection of prolactin-secreting microadenomas is used only in the rare patient who does not respond to or cannot tolerate dopamine agonists. Prolactin levels usually return to normal, but up to one-half of patients experience relapse.
- **Prolactin-secreting macroadenomas** should be treated with a dopamine agonist, which usually suppresses prolactin levels to normal, reduces tumor size, and improves or corrects abnormal visual fields in 90% of cases.
  - If mass effects are present, the dose should be increased to maximally effective levels over a period of several weeks. Visual field tests, if initially abnormal, should be repeated 4 to 6 weeks after therapy is started.
  - Pituitary imaging should be repeated 3 to 6 months after initiation of therapy. If tumor shrinkage and correction of visual abnormalities are satisfactory, therapy can be continued indefinitely, with periodic monitoring of plasma prolactin levels.
  - The full effect on tumor size may take more than 6 months. Further pituitary imaging is probably not warranted unless prolactin levels rise despite therapy.
  - **Transsphenoidal surgery** is indicated to relieve mass effects if the tumor does not shrink or if visual field abnormalities persist during dopamine agonist therapy. However, the likelihood of surgical cure of a prolactin-secreting macroadenoma is low, and most patients require further therapy with a dopamine agonist.
  - **Women with prolactin-secreting macroadenomas should not become pregnant** unless the tumor has been resected surgically or has decreased markedly in size with dopamine agonist therapy, as the risk of symptomatic enlargement during pregnancy is 15% to 35%. Contraception is essential during dopamine agonist treatment.

Acromegaly

GENERAL PRINCIPLES

Acromegaly is the syndrome caused by growth hormone excess in adults and is due to a growth hormone–secreting pituitary adenoma in the vast majority of cases (*J Clin Endocrinol Metab 2009;94:1509*).

DIAGNOSIS

Clinical Presentation

Clinical findings include thickened skin and enlargement of hands, feet, jaw, and forehead. Arthritis or carpal tunnel syndrome may develop, and the pituitary adenoma may cause headaches and vision loss. Mortality from cardiovascular disease is increased.

Diagnostic Testing

- **Plasma IGF-1**, which mediates most effects of growth hormone, is the best diagnostic test. Marked elevations establish the diagnosis.

- If IGF-1 levels are only moderately elevated, the diagnosis can be confirmed by giving 75 mg glucose orally and measuring serum growth hormone q30min for 2 hours. Failure to suppress growth hormone to <1 ng/mL confirms the diagnosis of acromegaly. Once the diagnosis is made, the pituitary should be imaged.

TREATMENT

The treatment of choice is transsphenoidal resection of the pituitary adenoma. Most patients have macroadenomas, and complete tumor resection with cure of acromegaly is often impossible. If IGF-1 levels remain elevated after surgery, radiotherapy is used to prevent regrowth of the tumor and to control acromegaly.

Medications
- The somatostatin analog **octreotide** in depot form can be used to suppress growth hormone secretion while awaiting the effect of radiation. A dose of 10 to 40 mg IM monthly suppresses IGF-1 to normal in about 60% of patients. Side effects include cholelithiasis, diarrhea, and mild abdominal discomfort.
- **Pegvisomant** is a growth hormone antagonist that lowers IGF-1 to normal in almost all patients. The dose is 10 to 30 mg SC daily. Few side effects have been reported, but patients should be monitored for pituitary adenoma enlargement and transaminase elevation.

METABOLIC BONE DISEASE

Osteomalacia

GENERAL PRINCIPLES

- Osteomalacia is characterized by defective mineralization of osteoid. Bone biopsy reveals increased thickness of osteoid seams and decreased mineralization rate, assessed by tetracycline labeling.
- Suboptimal vitamin D nutrition, indicated by plasma 25-hydroxy vitamin D (25[OH]D) levels below 30 ng/mL, is very common and contributes to the development of osteoporosis (*J Clin Endocrinol Metab 2011;96:1911*).

Etiology
- Dietary vitamin D deficiency
- **Malabsorption** of vitamin D and calcium due to intestinal, hepatic, or biliary disease
- Disorders of vitamin D metabolism (e.g., renal disease, vitamin D–dependent rickets)
- Vitamin D resistance
- Chronic hypophosphatemia
- Renal tubular acidosis
- Hypophosphatasia
- Therapy with anticonvulsants, fluoride, etidronate, or aluminum compounds

DIAGNOSIS

Clinical Presentation

- Clinical findings include diffuse skeletal pain, proximal muscle weakness, waddling gait, and propensity to fractures.
- Osteomalacia should be suspected in a patient with osteopenia, elevated serum alkaline phosphatase, and either hypophosphatemia or hypocalcemia.

Diagnostic Testing

Laboratories

- Serum alkaline phosphatase is elevated. Serum phosphorus, calcium, or both may be decreased.
- **Serum 25(OH)D** levels may be low, establishing the diagnosis of vitamin D deficiency or malabsorption.

Imaging

- Radiographic findings include osteopenia and radiolucent bands perpendicular to bone surfaces (pseudofractures or Looser zones).
- Radiography of the chest, pelvis, and hips may reveal characteristic pseudofractures.

TREATMENT

- **Dietary vitamin D deficiency** can initially be treated with ergocalciferol 50,000 international units (IU) PO weekly for 8 weeks to replete body stores, followed by long-term therapy with 600 to 1,000 IU/d.
- **Malabsorption of vitamin D** may require continued therapy with high doses such as 50,000 IU PO per week. The dose should be adjusted to maintain serum 25(OH)D levels above 30 ng/mL. Calcitriol, 0.5 to 2.0 μg PO daily, can also be used. Calcium supplements, 1 g PO daily–tid, may also be required. Serum 25(OH)D and serum calcium should be monitored every 6 to 12 months to avoid hypercalcemia. If the underlying disease responds to therapy, the dose of vitamin D must be reduced accordingly.

Paget's Disease

GENERAL PRINCIPLES

Paget's disease of bone is a focal skeletal disorder characterized by rapid, disorganized bone remodeling. It usually occurs after the age of 40 years and most often affects the pelvis, femur, spine, and skull (*N Engl J Med 2006;355:593*).

DIAGNOSIS

Clinical Presentation

- Clinical manifestations include bone pain and deformity, degenerative arthritis, pathologic fractures, neurologic deficits due to nerve root or cranial nerve compression (including deafness), and rarely, high-output heart failure and osteogenic sarcoma.

- Most patients are asymptomatic, with disease discovered incidentally because of elevated serum alkaline phosphatase or a radiograph taken for other reasons.

Diagnostic Testing

Laboratories

Serum alkaline phosphatase is elevated, reflecting the activity and extent of disease. Serum and urine calcium are usually normal but may increase with immobilization, as after a fracture.

Imaging

The radiographic appearance is usually diagnostic. A bone scan will reveal areas of skeletal involvement, which can be confirmed by radiography.

TREATMENT

Indications for therapy include (a) bone pain due to Paget's disease, (b) nerve compression syndromes, (c) pathologic fracture, (d) elective skeletal surgery, (e) progressive skeletal deformity, (f) immobilization hypercalcemia, and (g) asymptomatic involvement of weight-bearing bones or the skull.

Medications

Bisphosphonates inhibit excessive bone resorption, relieve symptoms, and restore serum alkaline phosphatase to normal in most patients. The effectiveness of therapy is monitored by measuring serum alkaline phosphatase every 3 months. Therapy can be repeated when serum alkaline phosphatase rises above normal. Bisphosphonates may cause esophagitis and are not recommended in patients with renal insufficiency. Typical courses of therapy include the following:
- **Alendronate**, 40 mg/d for 6 months
- **Risedronate**, 30 mg/d for 2 months
- **Pamidronate**, 30 mg IV over 4 hours on 3 consecutive days, or
- **Zoledronic acid**, 5 mg IV by a single infusion

25 Arthritis and Rheumatologic Diseases

Hector Molina and Zarmeena Ali

Basic Approach to the Rheumatic Diseases

GENERAL PRINCIPLES

Definition

Arthritis is any medical process affecting a joint or joints, causing pain, swelling, and stiffness. It has to be distinguished from a periarticular process. The pain from a true articular process is usually present throughout the complete range of motion of a particular joint. The pain from a **periarticular process** is usually evident at a single point in the range of motion, and it is elicited by palpation in a specific area corresponding to a tendon, ligament, or bursa.

Classification

Once it is established that the clinician is dealing with an arthritic process, it can be categorized into an inflammatory versus a noninflammatory process and by the number and type of joints involved (Figure 25-1 and Table 25-1).

DIAGNOSIS

The history and physical exam are essential. In the history, evidence of an inflammatory process includes the presence of morning stiffness lasting more than an hour and worsening of symptoms with inactivity. The review of systems is instrumental in searching for the presence of symptoms related to a particular arthropathy or connective tissue disease (skin rashes, uveitis, iritis, mouth ulcers, and serositis among others). There may be associated swelling, warmth, erythema, or constitutional symptoms. Synovial fluid aspiration helps in the diagnosis. Analysis of the synovial fluid should include a cell count, microscopic examination for crystals, Gram stain, and cultures. Ancillary lab test and imaging techniques are helpful in supporting a diagnosis if their use is directed by the specific findings on the history and physical exam (see Table 25-1).

TREATMENT

The etiology of most rheumatologic disorders is unknown. Therapeutic approaches involve either local or systemic administration of analgesic, anti-inflammatory, immunomodulatory, or immunosuppressive drugs. The initial general therapeutic options will be discussed here. Specific immunomodulatory and immunosuppressive therapies

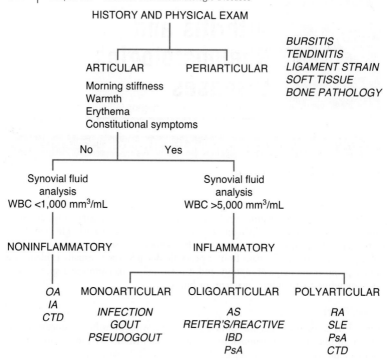

Figure 25-1. Initial general evaluation to a patient with arthritis. AS, ankylosing spondylitis; CTD, connective tissue disease; IA, internal dearrangement; IBD, inflammatory bowel disease; OA, osteoarthritis; PsA, psoriatic arthritis; RA, rheumatoid arthritis; SLE, systemic lupus erythematosus; WBC, white blood cell count.

will be discussed in association with the disease process for which the therapeutic agent is most commonly used.

Medications

- **Nonsteroidal anti-inflammatory drugs (NSAIDs)** exert their effects by inhibiting the constitutive (COX-1) and inducible (COX-2) isoforms of cyclooxygenase, producing a mild-to-moderate anti-inflammatory and analgesic effect. Individual responses to these agents are variable. If one drug is not effective during a 2- to 3-week trial, another should be tried.

  Side effects
  - **Gastrointestinal (GI) toxicity** manifests clinically as dyspepsia, nausea, vomiting, or GI bleeding. Nausea and dyspepsia often respond to the addition of a histamine-2 (H_2)-blocking agent or proton pump inhibitor or to a change in NSAID. Direct GI irritation can be minimized by administration after food, by the use of enteric-coated preparations, and by use of the lowest effective dose. All NSAIDs, however, have a systemic effect on the GI mucosa, resulting in increased permeability to gastric acid. Most serious GI bleeds during NSAID use occur without prior GI symptoms. **Risk factors for GI bleed** include a history of duodenal–gastric ulceration, age, smoking, ethanol use, and concomitant use of corticosteroids,

Table 25-1 General Features of the Most Common Arthritis

Diagnosis	Type	Additional Features	Laboratory and Imaging
Osteoarthritis	Noninflammatory; monoarticular, oligoarticular, or polyarticular	Bone spurs; knees, hips, PIP, DIP, first MTP, first CMC preferentially affected	Normal ESR/CRP, osteophytes, bone sclerosis
Gout	Inflammatory; monoarticular, oligoarticular, or polyarticular	Tophi; acute attacks followed by spontaneous resolution	Elevated uric acid; positive uric acid crystals in joint fluid; elevated ESR/CRP; erosions with overhanging borders
Pseudogout	Inflammatory; monoarticular or polyarticular	Acute attacks or chronic	Elevated ESR/CRP; positive CPPD crystals in joint fluid; chondrocalcinosis
Septic joint	Inflammatory; monoarticular, rarely polyarticular (immunosuppression)	Sepsis, fever	Positive cultures; elevated ESR/CRP; leukocytosis
Rheumatoid arthritis	Inflammatory; polyarticular	Extra-articular manifestations; DIP not affected	Positive RF, CCP; elevated ESR/CRP; erosions; periarticular osteoporosis
Psoriatic arthritis	Inflammatory; oligoarticular; polyarticular	Psoriatic skin rash; asymmetric sacroiliac joint involvement; spondylitis; syndesmophytes	Erosions; ankylosis
Ankylosing spondylitis	Inflammatory	Spondylitis (bamboo spine); syndesmophytes, symmetric sacroiliac involvement	Ankylosis

CCP, citrullinated peptide; CMC, carpometacarpal joint; CPPD, calcium pyrophosphate dehydrate; CRP, C-reactive protein; DIP, distal interphalangeal joint; ESR, erythrocyte sedimentation rate; MTP, metatarsophalangeal joint; PIP, proximal interphalangeal joint; RF, rheumatoid factor.

aspirin, or selective serotonin reuptake inhibitors. The use of proton pump inhibitors such as **omeprazole** 20 mg by mouth (PO) daily decreases the risk of NSAID-induced gastric or duodenal ulceration. **Misoprostol**, a synthetic prostaglandin E analog, is another alternative but may cause diarrhea and is an abortifacient. Consider *Helicobacter pylori* testing prior to beginning NSAIDs, especially in patients with high risk of duodenal–gastric ulceration. If the test is positive, treat accordingly (see Chapter 18, Gastrointestinal Diseases).

○ **Acute renal failure** is the most common form of renal toxicity; however, nephrotic syndrome and acute interstitial nephritis may also occur. **Risk factors** for acute renal failure include preexisting renal dysfunction, congestive heart failure (CHF), cirrhosis with ascites, and a concomitant angiotensin-converting enzyme (ACE) inhibitor or angiotensin-receptor blockers (ARBs). Periodic monitoring of renal function is recommended particularly in elderly patients.

○ **Platelet dysfunction** can be caused by all NSAIDs, particularly aspirin, which is a covalent inhibitor of COX. NSAIDs should be used cautiously or avoided in patients with a bleeding diathesis and those taking warfarin. NSAIDs should be discontinued 5 to 7 days before surgical procedures.

○ **Hypersensitivity reactions** are often seen in patients with a history of asthma, nasal polyps, or atopy. NSAIDs may cause a variety of type I hypersensitivity-like reactions, including urticaria, asthma, and anaphylactoid shock, presumably by increasing leukotriene synthesis. Patients with a hypersensitivity reaction to one NSAID should avoid all NSAIDs and selective COX-2 inhibitors.

○ **Other side effects: Central nervous system** (CNS) toxicity (headaches, dizziness, dysphoria, confusion, aseptic meningitis) is uncommon. Tinnitus and deafness can complicate NSAID use, particularly with high-dose salicylates. **Blood dyscrasias** including aplastic anemia have been observed as isolated case reports with ibuprofen, piroxicam, indomethacin, and phenylbutazone. **Dermatologic reactions** and **elevations in transaminases** have also been described. **Acid–base imbalance** is seen with high doses of salicylates. Nonacetylated salicylates have been reported to have less toxicity but also may be less effective. The use of NSAIDs in general may be associated with an increased risk for **cardiovascular thrombotic events**. NSAIDs might diminish the cardioprotective effect of aspirin.

• **Selective COX-2 inhibitors** exhibit selective inhibition of COX-2, thereby inhibiting inflammation while preserving the homeostatic functions of constitutive COX-1–derived prostaglandins. The anti-inflammatory and analgesic efficacy is similar to that of traditional NSAIDs. Celecoxib is the only selective COX-2 inhibitor approved in the United States.

Side effects

○ Some data demonstrate that **GI symptoms** and **GI ulcerations are reduced** with these agents in comparison to NSAIDs. The potential gastroduodenal-sparing effect of selective COX-2 inhibitors may be eliminated by concurrent warfarin therapy or the use of low-dose aspirin therapy for primary or secondary prevention of cardiovascular or cerebrovascular disease (*JAMA 2000;284:1247*).

○ Acute kidney injury might be precipitated in patients taking selective COX-2 inhibitors.

○ **Platelet function** is not impaired, making selective COX-2 inhibitors a good anti-inflammatory option for patients with thrombocytopenia, hemostatic defects, or chronic anticoagulation. In patients who are taking warfarin, however, the international normalized ratio (INR) should be monitored after the addition of a COX-2 inhibitor (as with any medication change). In addition, there has been controversy as to whether the inhibition of prostacyclin but not thromboxane by these agents may promote clotting.

○ Patients with hypersensitivity reactions to NSAIDs should not use a COX-2 inhibitor. It has been suggested that individuals with a sulfonamide allergy should not use celecoxib, although some studies have found no untoward effect. Celecoxib should be used with caution in patients with sulfonamide allergy.

○ An increase in blood pressure has also been associated with the use of celecoxib. A dose-related **increase in cardiovascular events** has been associated with the use of this medication. These medications might exacerbate CHF.

• **Glucocorticoids** exert a pluripotent anti-inflammatory effect via the inhibition of inflammatory mediator gene transcription.

○ **Preparations, dosages, and routes of administration:** The goal of glucocorticoid therapy is to suppress disease activity with the minimum effective dosage. **Prednisone** (PO) and **methylprednisolone** (intravenous [IV]) are generally the preferred drugs because of cost and half-life considerations. Intramuscular (IM) absorption is variable and therefore is not advised. The dose, route, and frequency of administration are determined by the type of disease and the severity of the disease manifestations. The following are **relative anti-inflammatory potencies** of common glucocorticoid preparations: cortisone, 0.8; hydrocortisone, 1.0; prednisone, 4.0; methylprednisolone, 5.0; dexamethasone, 25.0.

○ **Side effects:** Adverse effects are related to dosage and duration of administration and, except for cataracts and osteoporosis, can be minimized by alternate-day administration once the disease is controlled.

▪ **Adrenal suppression:** Glucocorticoids suppress the hypothalamic–pituitary–adrenal axis. Assume functional suppression in patients receiving more than 20 mg of prednisone (or the equivalent) daily for more than 3 weeks, patients receiving an evening dose for more than a few weeks, or in patients with Cushingoid appearance. Adrenal suppression is unlikely if the patient has received any dose of steroids for less than 3 weeks or if using alternate-day therapy. The degree of adrenal suppression is uncertain in patients receiving 10 to 20 mg of prednisone for more than 3 weeks. Adrenal suppression is minimized by dosing in the morning and using a single daily low dose of a short-acting preparation, such as prednisone, for a short period. In patients who are receiving chronic glucocorticoid therapy, hypoadrenalism (anorexia, weight loss, lethargy, fever, and postural hypotension) may occur at times of severe stress (e.g., infection, major surgery) and should be treated with stress doses of glucocorticoids. These patients should wear a medical-alert bracelet or carry identification.

▪ **Immunosuppression:** Glucocorticoid therapy reduces resistance to infections. **Bacterial infections** in particular are related to the dosage of glucocorticoids and are a major cause of morbidity and mortality. Thus, minor infections may become systemic, quiescent infections may be activated, and organisms that usually are nonpathogenic may cause disease. Local and systemic signs of infection may be partially masked, although fever associated with infection generally is not suppressed completely by glucocorticoids. When possible, a skin test for tuberculosis should be placed before glucocorticoid therapy is instituted, and if it is positive, appropriate prophylaxis is indicated. Prophylaxis with trimethoprim/sulfamethoxazole (TMP-SMX) and acyclovir should be considered to prevent *Pneumocystis carinii* and varicella-zoster viral infections in patients on high-dose steroids in whom therapy is anticipated for a prolonged duration.

- **Endocrine abnormalities:** Possible endocrine abnormalities include a cushingoid habitus and hirsutism. Hyperglycemia may be induced or aggravated by glucocorticoids but usually is not a contraindication to therapy. Insulin therapy may be required, although ketoacidosis is rare. Fluid and electrolyte abnormalities include hypokalemia and sodium retention, which may induce or aggravate hypertension.

- **Osteoporosis** with vertebral compression fractures is common among patients who are receiving long-term glucocorticoid therapy. **Supplemental calcium,** 1.0 to 1.5 g/d PO, should be given along with **vitamin D**, 400–800 U daily PO, as soon as steroid therapy is begun. A bisphosphonate may be indicated in postmenopausal women or in men or premenopausal women who are at high risk for osteoporosis, and calcitonin can be considered for those who cannot tolerate a bisphosphonate. **Teriparatide** (recombinant human parathyroid hormone [1–34]) is another alternative (*N Engl J Med 2007;357:2028*). Determination of baseline bone density is appropriate in these patients. A judicious exercise program may be beneficial in stimulating bone formation.

- **Steroid myopathy** generally involves the hip and shoulder girdle musculature. Muscles are weak but not tender and, in contrast to inflammatory myositis, serum creatine kinase, aldolase, and electromyography are normal. The myopathy usually improves with a reduction in glucocorticoid dosage and resolves slowly with discontinuation.

- **Ischemic bone necrosis** (aseptic necrosis, avascular necrosis) caused by glucocorticoid use often is multifocal, most commonly affecting the femoral head, humeral head, and tibial plateau. Early changes can be demonstrated by bone scan or magnetic resonance imaging (MRI).

- **Other adverse effects:** Changes in **mental status** ranging from mild nervousness, euphoria, and insomnia to severe depression or psychosis may occur. **Ocular effects** include increased intraocular pressure (sometimes precipitating glaucoma) and the formation of posterior subcapsular cataracts. **Hyperlipidemia, menstrual irregularities**, increased perspiration with **night sweats**, and **pseudotumor cerebri** also may occur.

- **Immunomodulatory and immunosuppressive drugs** include a number of pharmacologically diverse agents that exert anti-inflammatory or immunosuppressive effects. Often, such agents are referred to as **disease-modifying antirheumatic drugs (DMARDs)**. They are characterized by a delayed onset of action and the potential for serious toxicity. Consequently, they should be prescribed with the guidance of a rheumatologist or other physician who is experienced in their use and given only to well-informed, cooperative patients who are willing to comply with meticulous follow-up. The specific agents will be discussed in relation to the diseases for which they are indicated.

Other Nonpharmacologic Therapies

Joint aspiration should be performed when an effusion is present in a single joint and its etiology is unclear, for symptomatic relief in a patient with a known arthritis diagnosis, and to monitor the response to therapy in patients with infectious arthritis. Intra-articular glucocorticoid therapy can be used to suppress inflammation when only one or a few peripheral joints are inflamed and infection has been excluded. Intra-articular hyaluronic acid derivatives are used for the treatment of knee osteoarthritis (OA). The joint should be aspirated to remove as much fluid as possible before injection. **Glucocorticoid preparations** include methylprednisolone acetate, triamcinolone acetonide, and triamcinolone hexacetonide. The dose used is arbitrary, but the following guidelines based on volume are useful: large joints (knee, ankle, shoulder), 1 to 2 mL, medium joints (wrists, elbows), 0.5 to 1.0 mL, and small joints of the hands and feet, 0.25 to 0.50 mL. **Lidocaine** (or its equivalent), up to 1 mL of a 1% solution, can be mixed in a single syringe with the glucocorticoid to promote immediate relief but is not generally used in the digits.

- **Technique:** The site of aspiration should be cleansed with antimicrobial/antiseptic skin cleanser. Topical ethyl chloride spray can be used as a local anesthetic. The site can also be infiltrated with local anesthetic in preparation for the procedure, particularly if there is little or no joint effusion or if there is notable joint space narrowing.
- **Contraindications:** Infection overlying the site to be injected is an absolute contraindication. Significant hemostatic defects and bacteremia are relative contraindications to joint aspiration and injection.
- **Complications**
  - **Postinjection synovitis** may develop rarely as a result of phagocytosis of glucocorticoid ester crystals. Such reactions usually resolve within 48 to 72 hours. More persistent symptoms suggest the possibility of iatrogenic infection, which occurs rarely (<0.1% of patients).
  - Localized skin depigmentation and atrophy may result after glucocorticoid injection. Accelerated deterioration of bone and cartilage also may occur when frequent injections are administered over an extended period. Therefore, any single joint should be injected no more frequently than every 3 to 6 months.

Infectious Arthritis and Bursitis

GENERAL PRINCIPLES

Classification

Infectious arthritis is generally categorized into gonococcal and nongonococcal disease.

Etiology

- **Nongonococcal infectious arthritis** in adults tends to occur in patients with previous joint damage or compromised host defenses. It is caused most often by *Staphylococcus aureus* (60%) and *Streptococcus* species. Gram-negative organisms are less common and typically seen with IV drug abuse, neutropenia, concomitant urinary tract infection, or postoperative status.
- In contrast **gonococcal arthritis** causes one-half of all septic arthritis in otherwise healthy, sexually active young adults.

DIAGNOSIS

Clinical Presentation

- **Nongonococcal infectious arthritis** usually presents with fever and an acute monoarticular arthritis, although multiple joints may be affected by hematogenous spread of pathogens.

- The clinical spectrum of **gonococcal arthritis** often includes migratory or additive polyarthralgias, followed by tenosynovitis or arthritis of the wrist, ankle, or knee, and vesicopustular skin lesions on the extremities or trunk (disseminated gonococcal infection).

Diagnostic Testing

- **Joint fluid examination**, including Gram stain, a cell count and differential, and cultures are mandatory to make a diagnosis and to guide management. Synovial fluid Gram stain may be positive in 50% to 70% of nongonococcal infectious arthritis. Cultures of blood and other possible extra-articular sites of infection also should be obtained.
- In contrast to nongonococcal infectious arthritis, Gram staining of synovial fluid is positive in **less than 25% of cases** of gonococcal arthritis. Cultures of synovial fluid are positive in 20% to 50% of cases. Bacteriologic assessment of the throat, cervix, urethra, and rectum may aid in establishing the diagnosis.

TREATMENT

- **Initial antimicrobial therapy** is based on the clinical situation.
  - With a positive Gram stain, antibiotic coverage can be focused accordingly.
  - With a nondiagnostic Gram stain, antibiotics should be chosen to cover *S. aureus*, *Streptococcus* species, and *Neisseria gonorrhoeae*. Vancomycin 15 mg/kg IV every 12 hours and ceftriaxone 1 g IV every 24 hours are good initial treatment choices. Cefepime instead of ceftriaxone is preferred if *Pseudomonas* infection is suspected.
  - IV antimicrobials usually are given for at least 2 weeks, followed by 1 to 2 weeks of oral antimicrobials, with the course of therapy tailored to the patient's response.
  - Treatment of gonococcal arthritis is with an IV antibiotic for the first 1 to 3 days, generally ceftriaxone, 1 to 2 g IV daily. After clinical improvement is noted, therapy is continued with an oral antibiotic to complete 7 to 14 days of treatment. Cefixime 400 mg PO bid or amoxicillin, 500 to 850 mg PO bid may be used. **Treatment of coexisting *Chlamydia* infection** with azithromycin or doxycycline should also be considered.
  - Oral or intra-articular antimicrobials are not appropriate as initial therapy.
- An **NSAID** is often useful to reduce pain and increase joint mobility but should not be used until response to antimicrobial therapy has been demonstrated by symptomatic and laboratory improvement.
- **Drainage** of the affected joint is needed to decrease the possibility of permanent joint damage. Although daily closed needle aspiration might be attempted, arthroscopic lavage and drain insertion has largely replaced closed aspiration of the involved joint. **Surgical drainage** or arthroscopic lavage and drainage are indicated for (a) a septic hip; (b) joints in which either the anatomy, large amounts of tissue debris, or loculation of pus prevent adequate needle drainage; (c) septic arthritis with coexistent osteomyelitis; (d) joints that do not respond in 3 to 5 days to appropriate therapy; and (e) prosthetic joint infection.
- **General supportive measures** include splinting of the joint, which may help to relieve pain. However, prolonged immobilization can result in joint stiffness.
- **Hospitalization** is indicated to ensure drug compliance and careful monitoring of the clinical response.

SPECIAL CONSIDERATIONS

Nonbacterial infectious arthritis is common with many viral infections, especially hepatitis B, rubella, mumps, infectious mononucleosis, parvovirus, enterovirus, and adenovirus.

- It is generally self-limiting, lasting for <6 weeks and responds well to a conservative regimen of rest and NSAIDs.
- Arthralgias (often severe) or a reactive arthritis can also be a manifestation of HIV infection.
- Fungi and mycobacterium can cause septic arthritis and should be considered in patients with chronic monoarticular arthritis.

Septic Bursitis

DIAGNOSIS

- Usually involving the olecranon or prepatellar bursa, it can be differentiated from septic arthritis by localized, fluctuant superficial swelling and by **relatively painless joint motion** (particularly extension).
- Most patients have a history of previous trauma to the area or an occupational predisposition (e.g., "housemaid's knee," "writer's elbow").
- *S. aureus* is the most common pathogen of septic bursitis.

TREATMENT

- Septic bursitis should be treated with aspiration, which can be repeated if fluid reaccumulates. Oral antibiotics (guided by Gram stain and culture of bursa fluid) and outpatient management are usually appropriate. Surgical drainage is indicated only if adequate needle drainage is not possible.
- Preventive measures (e.g., knee pads) should be used in patients with occupational predispositions to septic bursitis.

Lyme Disease

GENERAL PRINCIPLES

Lyme disease is caused by the tick-borne spirochete *Borrelia burgdorferi*.

DIAGNOSIS

- Typical manifestations begin with an erythematous annular rash (**erythema migrans**) and flu-like symptoms.
- Arthralgias, myalgias, meningitis, neuropathy, and cardiac conduction defects may follow in weeks to a few months. Months later, an intermittent or chronic arthritis in one or a few joints, characteristically including the knee, may develop in untreated patients.
- The diagnosis is based on the clinical picture and exposure in an endemic area and supported by serology.

- A two-tiered serologic assay with ELISA and immunoglobulin (Ig)G western blot for *B. burgdorferi* is uniformly positive by the time frank arthritis develops. False positives occur, however, and may signify prior infection. *B. burgdorferi* DNA can be detected by PCR in synovial fluid in 85% of cases.

TREATMENT

- Antibiotic therapy is required, generally with doxycycline 100 mg PO bid or amoxicillin 500 mg PO tid for 28 days.
- NSAIDs are a useful adjunct for arthritis.

Crystal-Induced Synovitis

GENERAL PRINCIPLES

Definition

Deposition of microcrystals in joints and periarticular tissues results in **gout, pseudogout**, and **apatite disease**.

Classification

- Clinical phases of gout can be divided into asymptomatic hyperuricemia, acute gouty arthritis, and chronic arthritis.
- **Asymptomatic hyperuricemia** is defined as serum uric acid levels >7 mg/dL.

Epidemiology

Men are much more commonly affected by gouty arthritis than women. Most premenopausal women with gout have a family history of the disease.

Etiology

- **Primary gouty arthritis** is characterized by hyperuricemia that is usually because of underexcretion of uric acid (90% of cases) rather than its overproduction. Urate crystals may be deposited in the joints, subcutaneous tissues (tophi), and kidneys.
- **Secondary gout**, like primary gout, can be caused by either defective renal excretion or overproduction of uric acid. Intrinsic renal disease, diuretic therapy, low-dose aspirin, cyclosporine, and ethanol all interfere with renal excretion of uric acid. Starvation, lactic acidosis, dehydration, preeclampsia, and diabetic ketoacidosis also can induce hyperuricemia. Overproduction of uric acid occurs in myeloproliferative and lymphoproliferative disorders, hemolytic anemia, polycythemia, and cyanotic heart disease.
- **Pseudogout** results when calcium pyrophosphate dihydrate crystals deposited in bone and cartilage are released into synovial fluid and induce acute inflammation. **Risk factors** include older age, advanced OA, neuropathic joint, gout, hyperparathyroidism, hemochromatosis, diabetes mellitus, hypothyroidism, and hypomagnesemia.

DIAGNOSIS

Clinical Presentation

- **Acute gouty arthritis** presents as an excruciating attack of pain, usually in a single joint of the foot or ankle. Occasionally, a polyarticular onset can mimic rheumatoid arthritis (RA).

- **Chronic gouty arthritis:** With time, acute gouty attacks occur more frequently, asymptomatic periods are shorter, and chronic joint deformity may appear.
- **Pseudogout** may present as an **acute monoarthritis or oligoarthritis**, mimicking gout or as a **chronic polyarthritis** resembling RA or OA. Usually the knee or wrist is affected, although any synovial joint can be involved.
- **Apatite/Basic calcium phosphate crystals** may cause periarthritis or tendonitis. A destructive arthritis also may occur.
- Acute gouty arthritis attacks can be precipitated by surgery, dehydration, fasting, binge eating, or heavy ingestion of alcohol. Although the acute gouty attack will subside spontaneously over several days, prompt treatment can abort the attack within hours.

Diagnostic Testing
Laboratories
- A definitive diagnosis of gout or pseudogout is made by finding **intracellular crystals** in joint fluid examined with a compensated polarized light microscope. **Urate crystals** are needle shaped and strongly negatively birefringent. **Calcium pyrophosphate dihydrate crystals** are pleomorphic and weakly positively birefringent. Hydroxyapatite complexes and basic calcium phosphate complexes can be identified only by electron microscopy and mass spectroscopy. In most cases, the arthritis associated with these compounds are suspected clinically but never confirmed.
- The serum uric acid level is normal in 30% of patients with acute gout and, if elevated, should not be manipulated until an attack has resolved.
- **Apatite disease** should be suspected when no crystals are present in the synovial fluid.

Imaging
- Erosive arthritis may be seen.
- If pseudogout is suspected, films of the wrists, knees, and pubic symphysis may be ordered. These are the most common sites for chondrocalcinosis, a finding that is supportive of (but not diagnostic for) pseudogout.
- Hydroxyapatite disease may be suspected by finding poorly defined cloud-like calcific deposits in the periarticular area on imaging.

TREATMENT

- **Asymptomatic hyperuricemia** is not routinely treated because of expense and the potential drug toxicity. However, patients should be monitored closely for the development of complications if the serum uric acid level is at least 12 mg/dL in men or 10 mg/dL in women. In these patients, antihyperuricemic therapy should be considered.
- **Management of secondary gout** includes treatment of the underlying disorder and urate-lowering therapy.
- The treatment of **apatite disease** is similar to that for pseudogout.

Medications
- **Acute gout**
  - **NSAIDs** are the treatment of choice due to ease of administration and low toxicity. Clinical response may require 12 to 24 hours, and initial doses should

be high, followed by rapid tapering over 2 to 8 days. One approach is to use indomethacin, 50 mg PO q8h for 2 days, followed by 25 mg PO q8h for 3 to 7 days. The long-acting NSAIDs generally are not recommended for acute gout.

○ **Glucocorticoids** are useful when NSAIDs are contraindicated. An intra-articular injection of glucocorticoids produces rapid dramatic relief. Alternatively, prednisone, 40 to 60 mg PO daily, can be given until a response is obtained and then should be tapered rapidly.

○ **Colchicine is most effective if given in the first 12 to 24 hours** of an acute attack and usually brings relief in 6 to 12 hours. In view of the efficacy and tolerability of a short course of NSAIDs, colchicine is not commonly used to treat gout but is useful when NSAIDs or glucocorticoids are contraindicated or not tolerated.

  ▪ **Oral administration** is often associated with severe GI toxicity. The dosage varies but is usually 1.2 mg at onset of symptoms and 0.6 mg taken 1 hour after the initial dose (1.8 mg over 1 hour) is effective therapy. The previous high-dose regimen of 0.6 mg q1–2h or 1.0 to 1.2 mg q2h until symptoms abate is not recommended due to toxicity. The lower dose regimen has recently been shown to be equally effective with less toxicity.

  ▪ **IV colchicine** is not recommended for general use and its administration in almost all circumstances is questionable.

• **Chronic gouty arthritis**

○ **Colchicine**, 0.6 mg PO daily or bid, can be used prophylactically for acute attacks. The dosage needs to be adjusted in patients with renal insufficiency. Colchicine 0.6 mg every other day or every 3 days should be considered in patients with a creatinine clearance between 10 and 34 mL/min. Aspirin (uricoretentive), diuretics, high alcohol intake, and foods high in purines (sweetbreads, anchovies, shellfish, sardines, liver, and kidney) should be avoided. Weight loss should be encouraged. Frequent gout attacks, tophi, joint damage, and urate nephropathy are indications for urate-lowering therapy. **Maintenance colchicine, 0.6 mg PO daily or bid, should be given for a few days before manipulation of the uric acid level to prevent precipitation of an acute attack.** In patients without tophi, prophylactic colchicine can be discontinued 6 months after the target serum urate levels have been obtained and no acute attacks have been documented by the patient. In patients with tophi, duration of prophylaxis is uncertain but consider discontinuation 6 months after resolution of tophi.

○ **Allopurinol**, a xanthine oxidase inhibitor, is effective therapy for hyperuricemia in most patients.

  ▪ **Dosage and administration:** The initial dosage varies. Daily doses can be increased by 100 mg every 2 to 4 weeks to achieve the minimum maintenance dosage that will keep the uric acid level below 6 mg/dL, which is below the limit of solubility of monosodium urate in serum. In patients with impaired renal function, the starting daily dose should be reduced by 50 mg for each 20 mL/min decrease in the creatinine clearance. For patients with a creatinine clearance below 20 mL/min, the starting dosage is 100 mg every other or every third day. The daily dose should also be decreased in patients with hepatic impairment. The concomitant use of a uricosuric agent may hasten the mobilization of tophi. **If an acute attack occurs during treatment with allopurinol, it should be continued at the same dosage while other agents are used to treat the attack.**

- **Side effects: Hypersensitivity reactions** from a minor skin rash to a diffuse exfoliative dermatitis associated with fever, eosinophilia, and a combination of renal and hepatic injury occur in up to 5% of patients. Patients who have mild renal insufficiency and are receiving diuretics are at greatest risk. Severe cases are potentially fatal and usually require glucocorticoid therapy. Allopurinol may potentiate the effect of oral anticoagulants and blocks metabolism of azathioprine and 6-mercaptopurine, necessitating a 60% to 75% reduction in dosage of these cytotoxic drugs.
  - **Febuxostat** is a nonpurine selective inhibitor of the xanthine oxidase that has recently been approved in the United States. It is significantly more expensive than allopurinol. The starting dose is 40 mg/d, with titration to 80 mg/d if needed.
  - **Uricase** catabolizes uric acid to the more soluble compound, allantoin. It is available in the United States for the treatment of tumor lysis syndrome in a recombinant form **(Rasburicase)**. IV **pegloticase** is a recombinant polyethylene glycol–conjugated form of uricase given every 2 weeks that has been shown to provide sustained reductions in plasma uric acid levels to less than the therapeutic target of 6 mg/dL in a substantial proportion of patients with chronic gout who are refractory to, or intolerant of, conventional urate-lowering therapy. The drug is discontinued if serum uric acid levels fail to reach target, or is noted to rise above 6 mg/dL on two consecutive times. There is a high risk of anaphylaxis and infusion reactions with this medication and thus is administered in a controlled setting with health care professionals who are familiar with the medication.
  - **Uricosuric drugs** lower serum uric acid levels by blocking renal tubular reabsorption of uric acid. A 24-hour measurement of creatinine clearance and urine uric acid should be obtained before therapy is started, as these drugs are **ineffective with glomerular filtration rates of <50 mL/min**. They are also not recommended for patients who already have high levels of urine uric acid (800 mg/24 hr) because of the risk of urate stone formation. This risk can be minimized by maintaining a high fluid intake and by alkalinizing the urine. If these drugs are being used when an acute gouty attack begins, they should be continued while other drugs are used to treat the acute attack.
    - **Probenecid**
      - Initial dosage is 500 mg PO daily, which can be raised in 500 mg increments every week until serum uric acid levels normalize or urine uric acid levels exceed 800 mg/24 hr. The maximum dose is 3,000 mg/d. Most patients require a total of 1.0 to 1.5 g/d in two to three divided doses.
      - Salicylates and probenecid are antagonistic and should not be used together.
      - Probenecid decreases renal excretion of penicillin, indomethacin, and sulfonylureas.
      - Side effects are minimal.
    - **Sulfinpyrazone** has uricosuric efficacy similar to that of probenecid; however, it also inhibits platelet function. The initial dosage of 50 mg PO bid can be increased in 100-mg increments weekly until serum uric acid levels normalize, to a maximum dose of 800 mg/d. Most patients require 300 to 400 mg/d in three to four divided doses.
- **Pseudogout**
  - As in gout, the therapy of choice for most patients is a brief high-dose course of an **NSAID**.
  - **Oral corticosteroids** can be used and **colchicine** also may relieve symptoms promptly, but toxicity limits its use. Dosage and administration are similar to the ones used in the treatment of gout.

○ Maintenance therapy with colchicine may diminish the number of recurrent attacks. Allopurinol or uricosuric agents have no role in treating pseudogout.

○ **Aspiration** of the inflammatory joint fluid often results in prompt improvement and intra-articular injection of glucocorticoids may hasten the response.

○ Treatment of underlying disease (hyperparathyroidism, hypothyroidism, hemochromatosis) will also help in disease management.

Rheumatoid Arthritis

GENERAL PRINCIPLES

RA is a systemic disease of unknown etiology that is characterized by symmetric inflammatory polyarthritis, extra-articular manifestations (rheumatoid nodules, pulmonary fibrosis, serositis, vasculitis), and serum rheumatoid factor (RF) in up to 80% of patients.

DIAGNOSIS

Clinical Presentation

• Most patients describe the insidious onset of pain, swelling, and morning stiffness in the hands and/or wrists, ankles, or feet.

• Synovitis may be evident upon exam of the metacarpophalangeal, proximal interphalangeal, wrists, or other joints. Rheumatoid nodules may be palpated most commonly on extensor surfaces.

• The course of RA is variable but tends to be chronic and progressive.

• Clinical criteria for the diagnosis of RA are available (*Arthritis Rheum 2010; 62:2569*). Suspect the diagnosis in patients presenting with symmetric arthritis in three or more joints especially involving small joints and associated with morning stiffness lasting more than 30 minutes.

Diagnostic Testing

RF may be positive in 80% of patients. Cyclic citrullinated peptide (CCP) antibodies may be detected in 50% to 60% of patients with early RA.

• CCP antibodies are more specific (>90%) for RA than is the RF, which can also be elevated in the setting of hepatitis C and other chronic infections.

• Hand and wrist X-rays may show early changes of erosions or periarticular osteopenia.

• Musculoskeletal MRI or ultrasonography are more sensitive than plain X-ray and may be used in equivocal cases to demonstrate clinically inapparent synovitis or erosions.

TREATMENT

Most patients can benefit from an early aggressive treatment program that combines medical, rehabilitative, and surgical services designed with three distinct goals: (a) early suppression of inflammation in the joints and other tissues, (b) maintenance of joint and muscle function and prevention of deformities, and (c) repair of joint damage to relieve pain or improve function.

Medications

- **DMARDs** appear to alter the natural history of RA by retarding the progression of bony erosions and cartilage loss. Because RA may lead to substantial long-term disability (and is associated with increased mortality), the standard of care is to initiate therapy with such agents early in the course of RA. Once a clinical response has been achieved, the chosen drug usually is continued indefinitely at the lowest effective dosage to prevent relapse.
  - **An established diagnosis of RA along with any evidence of disease activity is an indication to initiate disease-modifying therapy.** Initial monotherapy with NSAIDs or steroids is no longer considered appropriate under usual circumstances.
  - **DMARD selection** is tailored to the character of the patient's disease, taking into account the potential toxicity of these agents (see the following text). **Methotrexate** typically is the initial choice for moderate-to-severe RA. **Leflunomide** is also an alternative. **Hydroxychloroquine** or **sulfasalazine** can be used as the initial choice in very mild RA. If response to the initial agent is unsatisfactory after an adequate trial (or if limiting toxicity supervenes), other DMARDs or a biologic agent can be added or substituted.
- **Methotrexate**, a purine inhibitor and folic acid antagonist, is useful in treating synovitis, regardless of the underlying disease process. RA is its most common indication. It is also useful for myositis and may improve the leukopenia of Felty's syndrome.
  - **Dosage and administration:** Typically, methotrexate is administered as a single PO dose once a week starting with 7.5 to 10.0 mg. Clinical response is usually noted in 4 to 8 weeks. The dosage can be increased by 2.5- to 5.0-mg increments every 2 to 4 weeks to a maximum of 25 mg/wk or until improvement is observed. Dosages above 20 mg/wk are generally given by SC injection to promote absorption.
  - **Contraindications and side effects:** Methotrexate is **teratogenic** and should not be used during pregnancy. It should also be avoided in patients with significant hepatic or renal impairment. **Folic acid supplementation** at a dosage of 1 to 2 mg daily may reduce toxicity without attenuating efficacy. Concomitant use of TMP-SMX should be avoided. Serologic testing for hepatitis B and C should be included before initiation of therapy.
    - **Minor side effects** include GI intolerance, stomatitis, rash, headache, and alopecia.
    - **Bone marrow suppression** may occur, particularly at higher doses. Blood and platelet counts should be obtained before initiation, every 2 to 4 weeks during the first 3 to 4 months or if the dose is changed, and every 8 weeks thereafter. **Macrocytosis** may herald serious hematologic toxicity and is an indication for folate supplementation, dose reduction, or both.
    - **Cirrhosis** may occur rarely with long-term use. Aspartate transaminase (AST), alanine transaminase (ALT), and serum albumin should be obtained initially at 4 to 8 weeks intervals during the first 3 to 4 months of therapy or if the dose is changed. Patients on a stable dose should be monitored every 8 to 12 weeks after 3 months of therapy and every 12 weeks after 6 months of therapy. Liver biopsy should be considered if the liver function tests are persistently abnormal or if the liver function tests are abnormal in 6 of 12 monthly determinations (five of nine determinations if measured every 6 weeks). Alcohol consumption increases the risk of methotrexate hepatotoxicity.

- **Hypersensitivity pneumonitis** may occur but usually is reversible. Distinction from the insterstitial lung disease (ILD) associated with RA may be difficult. Patients with preexisting pulmonary parenchymal disease may be at increased risk. **New or worsening symptoms of dyspnea or cough in a patient on methotrexate should prompt evaluation for pneumonitis.**
- **Rheumatoid nodules** may develop or worsen, paradoxically, in some patients on methotrexate.

- **Sulfasalazine** is useful for treating synovitis in the setting of RA and seronegative spondyloarthropathies.
  - **Dosage:** The initial dosage is 500 mg PO daily, with increases in 500-mg increments weekly until a total daily dose of 2,000 to 3,000 mg (given in evenly divided doses) is reached. Clinical response usually occurs in 6 to 10 weeks.
  - **Contraindications and side effects: Sulfasalazine should be used with extreme caution in patients with glucose-6-phosphate dehydrogenase deficiency. Sulfasalazine should not be used in patients with sulfa allergy.** Nausea is the principal adverse effect and can be minimized by the use of the enteric-coated preparation of the drug. Hematologic toxicity including a reduction in any cell line and aplastic anemia rarely occurs. Periodic monitoring of blood and platelet counts is, however, recommended.

- **Hydroxychloroquine** is an antimalarial agent that is used to treat dermatitis, alopecia, and synovitis in systemic lupus erythematosus (SLE) and mild synovitis in RA.
  - **Dosage:** Hydroxychloroquine typically is given at a dosage of 4 to 6 mg/kg PO daily (200 to 400 mg) after meals to minimize dyspepsia and nausea.
  - **Contraindications and side effects: Hydroxychloroquine should be used with caution in patients with porphyria, glucose-6-phosphate dehydrogenase deficiency, or significant hepatic or renal impairment.** It is probably safe during pregnancy. The most common side effects are allergic skin eruptions and nausea. Serious ocular toxicity occurs but is rare with currently recommended dosages. Ophthalmologic evaluation should be performed on an annual basis.

- **Leflunomide** is a pyrimidine inhibitor that has been approved for the treatment of RA.
  - **Dosage and administration:** Treatment is begun with 10 or 20 mg PO daily. Clinical response is generally seen within 4 to 8 weeks.
  - **Contraindications and side effects:** Leflunomide is **teratogenic** and has a very long half-life. Women who plan to become pregnant must discontinue the drug and complete a course of elimination therapy with cholestyramine, 8 g PO tid for 11 days. Plasma levels should then be verified to be <0.02 mg/L on two separate tests at least 14 days apart before pregnancy is considered. Leflunomide is **contraindicated in patients with significant hepatic dysfunction** or in those who are receiving rifampin. **GI side effects** are the most common. **Diarrhea** occurs in up to 20% of patients and may require discontinuation of the drug. Dosage reduction to 10 mg/d may provide relief while maintaining efficacy, and loperamide can be used for symptomatic relief. **Elevations in serum transaminase levels** may occur and should be measured at baseline and then monitored periodically. The dosage should be reduced for confirmed twofold elevations, and greater elevations should be treated with cholestyramine and discontinuation of leflunomide. **Rash** and **alopecia** may occur during therapy.

- **Anticytokine therapies** directed at specific cytokines have been developed. These agents may all be considered **biologic DMARDs.**

○ **Tumor necrosis factor (TNF) inhibitors** have been approved for treatment of RA and seronegative spondyloarthropathies. In general, these agents are used in patients with moderate-to-severe RA who have failed a trial of one or more DMARDs as listed earlier. The effect of these agents on synovitis can be dramatic, with responsive patients reporting the onset of symptomatic benefits within 1 to 2 weeks. In addition to their symptomatic benefits, these agents appear to retard joint damage significantly. Several preparations are currently available, with similar efficacy and toxicity profiles.

■ **Etanercept** is a fusion protein that consists of the ligand-binding portion of the human TNF receptor linked to the Fc portion of human IgG. It binds to TNF, blocking its interaction with cell surface receptors, thus inhibiting the inflammatory and immunoregulatory properties of TNF. This preparation is given in a dosage of 25 mg SC twice a week or 50 mg SC weekly.

■ **Infliximab** is a chimeric monoclonal antibody that binds specifically to human TNF-α, blocking its proinflammatory and immunomodulatory effects. It is given by IV infusion in conjunction with methotrexate to reduce production of neutralizing antibodies against infliximab. The recommended treatment regimen includes infliximab infusions of 3 mg/kg at initiation, at 2 and 6 weeks, and every 8 weeks thereafter, along with methotrexate at a dose of at least 7.5 mg/wk.

■ **Adalimumab** is a recombinant human IgG-1 monoclonal antibody that is specific to human TNF-α. It can be given in a dosage of 40 mg SC every other week.

■ **Golimumab** is a human monoclonal antibody that binds to human TNF-α. It is administered monthly.

■ **Certolizumab pegol** is a pegylated humanized Fab′ fragment of an anti– TNF-α monoclonal antibody. It is given monthly after an initial loading dose.

○ **Contraindications and side effects**

■ **Serious infections and sepsis**, including fatalities, have been reported during the use of TNF-blocking agents. These drugs are contraindicated in patients with acute or chronic infections, and if serious infection or sepsis occurs, the drug should be stopped. Those with a history of recurrent infections and those with underlying conditions that may predispose to infection should be treated with caution and counseled to be vigilant for signs and symptoms of infection. Upper respiratory and sinus infections are most common. Tuberculosis has also been noted, and **a tuberculin skin test and chest radiograph should be obtained before beginning therapy**. These agents are also contraindicated in patients with CHF (usually with a left ventricular ejection fraction less than 30%). Patients who are undergoing elective surgical procedures can omit the last dose of the drug that is scheduled to be given before surgery, as well as the next dose scheduled to follow the surgery.

■ **Local injection site reactions** are common with subcutaneous administration, particularly during the first month of therapy. These reactions are generally self-limited and do not require discontinuation of therapy. Serious systemic allergic reactions are rare but may occur with infliximab infusions.

■ **Other adverse effects** may include induction of antinuclear antibodies and, rarely, a lupus-like illness. A demyelinating disorder has been described as well as exacerbations of preexisting multiple sclerosis. It is unclear whether the frequency of occurrence of lymphoma is increased in patients who receive these agents. A black box warning, however, has been placed on the package insert of these agents.

- **Interleukin inhibitors**
  - **Anakinra** is a recombinant interleukin (IL)-1 receptor antagonist that is approved for use in RA. It blocks binding of IL-1 to its receptor, thus inhibiting the proinflammatory and immunomodulatory actions of IL-1.
    - It is given in a dosage of 100 mg SC daily. Like the TNF blockers, it should not be prescribed to patients with ongoing or recurrent infections.
    - **Adverse effects** include an increased frequency of bacterial infections and injection site reactions.
  - **Tocilizumab** is an antagonist of soluble and membrane bound IL-6 receptors. It is given as an IV infusion. Side effects include increased infections, neutropenia, and elevations in cholesterol.
- **B-cell–directed therapy:** One biologic agent targeting B cells, rituximab, is currently available. **Rituximab** is a monoclonal antibody directed against CD20, a cell surface receptor found on B cells. CD20-positive B cells in peripheral blood are rapidly depleted after two infusions of 1 g of rituximab 2 weeks apart. Methotrexate is generally used as background therapy. The infusion can be repeated in 6 to 12 month intervals, based on patient symptoms.
  - **Contraindications and side effects:** Rituximab has rarely been reported to cause reactivation of JC virus, leading to the clinical syndrome of progressive multifocal leukoencephalopathy (PML), which is uniformly fatal.
  - **Infusion reactions** are more common with the first dose and have rarely been fatal. Antihistamines, IV steroids, and acetaminophen are routinely given prior to infusion.
  - **Infectious complications** are a concern as with all biologics but appear to be less frequent than in TNF-treated patients.
- **Abatacept** is a fusion protein comprising the CTLA-4 molecule and the Fc portion of IgG1. It blocks selective costimulation of T cells. It is given as an IV infusion of 500 to 1,000 mg every 4 weeks. It is also available as a subcutaneous formulation that can be given 125 mg SC weekly with or without an initial loading dose. It is approved in patients with an inadequate response to biologic or nonbiologic DMARDs.
  - **Infections** occur slightly more often than in placebo-treated patients. Opportunistic infections have not been observed. **Infusion reactions** are much less common than with rituximab.
  - **Chronic obstructive pulmonary disease (COPD) exacerbations and respiratory infections** are more common in patients with obstructive lung disease when treated with abatacept.
- **Combinations of DMARDs** can be used if the patient has a partial response to the initial agent.
  - Common combination therapies include methotrexate with either hydroxychloroquine, sulfasalazine, or both. Methotrexate is commonly combined with TNF antagonists as there is evidence for additive efficacy and for a decrease in the formation of human antichimeric antibodies (HACAs) against the TNF blocker. Methotrexate is often used in combination with rituximab or abatacept. Methotrexate and leflunomide may have additive hepatotoxicity, and this combination should be used cautiously.
  - **Combination therapy with two biologic agents is contraindicated because of increased infectious complications.**

- **NSAIDs or selective COX-2 inhibitors** may be used as an adjunct to DMARD therapy. A longer acting NSAID may facilitate patient compliance.
- **Glucocorticoids** are not curative but may delay the formation of erosions with other DMARDs and are among the most potent anti-inflammatory drugs available (see General Principles under Basic Approach to the Rheumatic Diseases section).
  - **Indications** for glucocorticoids include: (a) symptomatic relief while waiting for a response to a slow-acting immunosuppressive or immunomodulatory agent, (b) persistent synovitis despite adequate trials of DMARDs and NSAIDs, and (c) severe constitutional symptoms (e.g., fever and weight loss) or extra-articular disease (vasculitis, episcleritis, or pleurisy).
  - **Oral administration** of prednisone 5 to 20 mg daily usually is sufficient for the treatment of synovitis, whereas severe constitutional symptoms or extra-articular disease may require up to 1 mg/kg PO daily. Although alternate-day glucocorticoid therapy reduces the incidence of undesirable side effects, some patients do not tolerate the increase in symptoms that may occur on the off day.
  - **Intra-articular administration** may provide temporary symptomatic relief when only a few joints are inflamed. The beneficial effects of intra-articular steroids may persist for days to months and may delay or negate the need for systemic glucocorticoid therapy.

Other Nonpharmacologic Therapies

- **Acute care** of inflammatory arthritides involves joint protection and pain relief. Proper joint positioning and splints are important elements in joint protection. Heat is a useful analgesic.
- **Subacute disease** therapy should include a gradual increase in passive and active joint movement.
- **Chronic care** encompasses instruction in joint protection, work simplification, and performance of activities of daily living. Adaptive equipment, splints, orthotics, and mobility aids may be useful. Specific exercises designed to promote normal joint mechanics and to strengthen affected muscle groups are useful. Overall cardiac conditioning also improves functional status.

Surgical Management

- **Corrective surgical procedures** including synovectomy, total joint replacement, and joint fusion, may be indicated in patients with RA to reduce pain and to improve function.
- **Carpal tunnel syndrome** is common, and surgical repair may be curative if local injection therapy is unsuccessful.
- **Synovectomy** may be helpful if major involvement is limited to one or two joints and if a 6-month trial of medical therapy has failed, but usually it is only of temporary benefit.
- Other procedures that may be beneficial include **total joint replacement** of the hip and knee joints, resection of metatarsal heads in patients with bunion deformities, and subluxation of the toes.
- **Surgical fusion of joints** usually results in freedom from pain but also in total loss of motion; this is tolerated well in the wrist and thumb.

- **Cervical spine fusion** of C1 and C2 is indicated for significant cervical subluxation (>5 mm) with associated neurologic deficits.

  Patients with long-standing RA undergoing elective surgical procedures should have a lateral cervical spine radiograph in flexion and extensions performed to screen for subluxation.

Immunizations

- It is recognized that the immune response to influenza and pneumococcal vaccinations in patients receiving methotrexate and biologic therapies may be attenuated, although usually adequate. Therefore, it is recommended that **influenza** vaccinations be given to patients prior to starting therapy with all nonbiologic DMARDs and **pneumococcal** vaccinations to patients starting leflunomide, methotrexate, or sulfasalazine if the patient's vaccinations were not current. In addition, periodic pneumococcal vaccinations and annual influenza vaccinations should be considered for all patients receiving biologic agents, in accordance with the Centers for Disease Control and Prevention (CDC) recommendations for appropriate use and timing of these vaccinations.
- Hepatitis B vaccination is recommended if risk factors for this disease existed and if hepatitis B vaccination had not previously been administered.
- Live vaccines (e.g., varicella-zoster vaccine, oral polio, rabies) are contraindicated during biologic therapy but should be considered before initiation of biologic therapy or high-dose steroids.

COMPLICATIONS

- **Patients with RA and a single joint inflamed out of proportion to the rest of the joints must be evaluated for coexistent septic arthritis.** This complication occurs with increased frequency in RA and carries 20% to 30% mortality.
- **Sjögren syndrome**, characterized by failure of exocrine glands, occurs in a subset of patients with RA, producing sicca symptoms (dry eyes and mouth), parotid gland enlargement, dental caries, and recurrent tracheobronchitis. **Treatment** is symptomatic with artificial tears and saliva, or with pilocarpine up to 5 mg PO qid. Cevimeline, 30 mg tid, can also be considered. Assiduous dental and ophthalmologic care is recommended, and drugs that suppress lacrimal–salivary secretion further should be avoided.
- **Felty syndrome**, the triad of RA, splenomegaly, and granulocytopenia, also occurs in a small subset of patients, and these patients are at risk for recurrent bacterial infections and nonhealing leg ulcers.
- Approximately 70% of patients show irreversible joint damage on radiography within the first 3 years of disease. Work disability is common and life span may be shortened.

REFERRAL

Rehabilitative therapy should be managed by a team of physicians, physical and occupational therapists, nurses, social workers, and psychologists. This approach may benefit patients with any form of arthritis.

PATIENT EDUCATION

Patient education, including pamphlets and support groups, is available in many communities through local chapters of the Arthritis Foundation.

Osteoarthritis

GENERAL PRINCIPLES

Definition

OA, or **degenerative joint disease (DJD)**, is characterized by deterioration of articular cartilage with subsequent formation of reactive new bone at the articular surface. The joints affected most commonly are the distal and proximal interphalangeal joints of the hands, hips, knees, and cervical and lumbar spine.

Epidemiology

The disease is more common in the elderly but may occur at any age, especially as sequelae to joint trauma, chronic inflammatory arthritis, or congenital malformation. OA of the spine may lead to spinal stenosis (neurogenic claudication), with aching or pain in the legs or buttocks on standing or walking.

TREATMENT

- **Acetaminophen** in a dosage of up to 1,000 mg qid is the initial pharmacologic treatment.
- **Low-dose NSAIDs or selective COX-2 inhibitors** are the next step, followed by full-dose treatment (see Treatment under Basic Approach to Rheumatic Diseases section). Because this patient population is often elderly and may have concomitant renal or cardiopulmonary disease, NSAIDs should be used with caution. NSAID-induced GI bleeding also is increased in the elderly population.
- The data for **glucosamine sulfate and chondroitin sulfate** are contradictory. Some studies suggest it may reduce symptoms as well as the rate of cartilage deterioration. Other studies have shown that these agents have little benefit in patients with OA. Glucosamine should not be administered to patients who are allergic to shellfish.
- **Intra-articular glucocorticoid injections** often are beneficial but probably should not be given more than every 3 to 6 months (see General Principles under Basic Approach to the Rheumatic Diseases section).
- Systemic steroids should be avoided. The μ-opioid agonist **tramadol** may be useful as an alternative analgesic agent. Narcotic agents should be avoided for long-term use. Narcotics may be useful for short-term pain relief and in patients in which other therapeutic modalities are contraindicated or have failed.
- **Topical NSAIDs, lidocaine, or capsaicin** may provide symptomatic relief with minimal toxicity.
- Synthetic and naturally occurring hyaluronic acid derivatives can be administered intra-articularly. They may reduce pain and improve mobility in select patients. Commercially, hyaluronan preparations currently available in the United States include sodium hyaluronate (**Hyalgan, Supartz, and Euflexxa**) and hylan G-F 20 (**Synvisc**).

- **Gabapentin** has also been used to help with neural pain modification in patients with severe symptoms of arthritis who are unresponsive to the mentioned modalities.
- **Duloxetine** was also recently approved by the U.S. Food and Drug Administration (FDA) for treatment of OA and chronic lower back pain.

Other Nonpharmacologic Therapies

- **Nonpharmacologic approaches** may complement drug treatment of arthritis. Activities that involve excessive use of the joint should be identified and avoided. Brief periods of rest for the involved joint can relieve pain. Poor body mechanics should be corrected and misalignments such as pronated feet may be aided by orthotics. An exercise program to prevent or correct muscle atrophy can also provide pain relief. When weight-bearing joints are affected, support in the form of a cane, crutches, or a walker can be helpful. Weight reduction may be of benefit, even for non–weight-bearing joints. Thumb splints may be useful for OA of the first carpometacarpal joint. Consultation with occupational and physical therapists may be helpful.
- **OA of the spine** may cause radicular symptoms from pressure on nerve roots and often produces pain and spasm in the paraspinal soft tissues. Physical supports (cervical collar, lumbar corset), local heat, and exercises to strengthen cervical, paravertebral, and abdominal muscles may provide relief in some patients.
- **Epidural steroid injections** may reduce radicular symptoms.

Surgical Management

- **Surgery** can be considered when patients suffer from disabling pain or deformity. Joint replacement surgery usually relieves pain and increases function in selected patients.
- **Laminectomy and spinal fusion** should be reserved for patients who have severe disease with intractable pain or neurologic complications. Lumbar spinal stenosis may require extensive decompressive laminectomy for relief of symptoms.

Spondyloarthropathies

The **spondyloarthropathies** are an interrelated group of disorders characterized by one or more of the following features: spondylitis, sacroiliitis, enthesopathy (inflammation at sites of tendon insertion), and asymmetric oligoarthritis. Extra-articular features of this group of disorders may include inflammatory eye disease, urethritis, and mucocutaneous lesions. The spondyloarthropathies aggregate in families, where they are associated with HLA-B27 antigen.

Ankylosing Spondylitis

DIAGNOSIS

Ankylosing spondylitis (AS) clinically presents as inflammation and ossification of the joints and ligaments of the spine and of the sacroiliac joints.

- Patients are usually young men who classically describe low back pain and morning stiffness, which improve with exercise.

- Hips and shoulders are the peripheral joints that are most commonly involved. Progressive fusion of the apophyseal joints of the spine occurs in many patients and cannot be predicted or prevented.

TREATMENT

Behavioral
- **Physical therapy** emphasizing extension exercises and posture is recommended to minimize possible late postural defects and respiratory compromise.
- Patients should be instructed to sleep supine on a firm bed without a pillow and to practice postural and deep-breathing exercises regularly.
- Cigarette smoking should be discouraged strongly.

Medications
- **Nonsalicylate NSAIDs**, such as indomethacin, are used to provide symptomatic relief, and **selective COX-2 inhibitors** are also effective (see General Principles under Basic Approach to the Rheumatic Diseases section).
- **Methotrexate and sulfasalazine** provide benefit for peripheral disease in some patients (see Treatment under Rheumatoid Arthritis section).
- **TNF blockade** has been shown to be of benefit even in some patients with apparent fixed deformities.
- **Pamidronate**, a bisphosphonate, may provide modest clinical benefits. Systemic glucocorticoids are not commonly used and can worsen osteopenia.

Surgical Management
Many patients develop osteoporosis in the fused spondylitic spine and are at risk of spinal fracture. Surgical procedures to correct some spine and hip deformities may result in significant rehabilitation in carefully selected patients.

REFERRAL

Acute anterior uveitis occurs in up to 25% of patients with AS and should be managed by an ophthalmologist. Generally, this problem is self-limited, although glaucoma and blindness are unusual secondary complications.

Arthritis of Inflammatory Bowel Disease

GENERAL PRINCIPLES

Arthritis of inflammatory bowel disease occurs in 10% to 20% of patients with either Crohn's disease or ulcerative colitis. It may also occur in some patients with intestinal bypass and diverticular disease.

DIAGNOSIS

Clinical features include **spondylitis**, **sacroiliitis**, and **peripheral arthritis**, particularly in the knee and ankle. Although peripheral joint disease may correlate with the activity of the colitis, spinal disease does not.

TREATMENT

- **NSAIDs** relieve joint pain and inflammation in patients with arthritis due to inflammatory bowel disease (IBD). However, GI intolerance due to NSAIDs may be increased among this group of patients. NSAIDs may exacerbate underlying IBD. Since some patients are not able to tolerate NSAIDs, judicious use with careful monitoring is necessary if these agents are to be used.
- **Sulfasalazine, methotrexate, azathioprine, and systemic glucocorticoids** also may be beneficial for this form of arthritis (see Treatment under Rheumatoid Arthritis section).
- **TNF antagonists** may benefit both the colitis and arthritis.
- Local **injection of glucocorticoids** and **physical therapy** are useful adjunctive measures.

Reactive Arthritis

GENERAL PRINCIPLES

- Reactive arthritis refers to the inflammatory arthritis, which occasionally follows certain GI or genitourinary infections. The triad of arthritis, conjunctivitis, and urethritis has classically been referred to as **Reiter syndrome**.
- *Chlamydia trachomatis* is the most commonly implicated genitourinary infection. *Shigella flexneri*, *Salmonella* species, *Yersinia enterocolitica*, or *Campylobacter jejuni* are the most commonly implicated GI infections. *Clostridium difficile* can also trigger the arthritis.
- Of patients, 50% to 80% are HLA-B27 positive. Males and females are equally affected after GI infections, though males more commonly develop the classical Reiter syndrome after *Chlamydia* infection.

DIAGNOSIS

Clinical Presentation

The clinical syndrome may include **asymmetric oligoarthritis**, **urethritis**, **conjunctivitis**, and characteristic **skin and mucous membrane lesions**. The syndrome is usually transient, lasting from 1 to several months, but chronic arthritis may develop in 4% to 19% of patients.

Diagnostic Testing

The triggering infection may have been asymptomatic. Testing for stool pathogens is low yield if the diarrheal illness has resolved, but urine testing for *Chlamydia* may be helpful if the clinical syndrome is consistent with reactive arthritis.

TREATMENT

- Conservative therapy is indicated for control of pain and inflammation in these diseases.
- Spontaneous remissions are common, making evaluation of therapy difficult.
- **NSAIDs** (especially indomethacin) are often useful, and **selective COX-2 inhibitors** also provide relief (see General Principles under Basic Approach to the Rheumatic Diseases section).

- **Sulfasalazine** or **methotrexate** may be of benefit for arthritis that does not resolve after several months (see Treatment under Rheumatoid Arthritis section).
- Trial of an **anti–TNF-α** agent might be considered in patients who do not respond to sulfasalazine or methotrexate.
- In unusually severe cases, **glucocorticoid therapy** may be required to prevent rapid joint destruction (see General Principles under Basic Approach to the Rheumatic Diseases section).
- Appropriate treatment for chlamydia infection, if detected, is appropriate. Prolonged empiric antibiotic therapy has not been shown to be beneficial.

REFERRAL

Conjunctivitis is usually transient and benign, but ophthalmologic referral and treatment with topical or systemic glucocorticoids are indicated for **iritis**.

Psoriatic Arthritis

GENERAL PRINCIPLES

Classification

Five major patterns of joint disease occur: (a) asymmetric oligoarticular arthritis, (b) distal interphalangeal joint involvement in association with nail disease, (c) symmetric rheumatoid-like polyarthritis, (d) spondylitis and sacroiliitis, and (e) arthritis mutilans.

Epidemiology

Approximately 10% of patients with psoriasis have some form of inflammatory arthritis.

TREATMENT

- **NSAIDs**, particularly indomethacin, are used to treat the arthritic manifestations of psoriasis, in conjunction with appropriate measures for the skin disease.
- **Intra-articular glucocorticoids** may be useful in the oligoarticular form of the disease, but injection through a psoriatic plaque should be avoided. Severe skin and joint diseases generally respond well to **methotrexate** (see Treatment under Rheumatoid Arthritis section).
- **Sulfasalazine and leflunomide** may also have disease-modifying effects in polyarthritis.
- **TNF-α blockers** may produce dramatic improvement in both skin and joint disease.

COMPLICATIONS

Colonization of psoriatic skin with *S. aureus* increases the risk of wound infection after reconstructive joint surgery.

Systemic Lupus Erythematosus

GENERAL PRINCIPLES

Definition

SLE is a multisystem disease of unknown etiology that primarily affects women of childbearing age. The usual female to male ratio is 9:1. It is most common in the second and third decade of life and more common in African Americans.

Pathophysiology

Pathophysiology is multifactorial and incompletely understood, with interplay of genetic predisposition and environmental factors. The genetic predisposition is complex and likely involves multiple genes.

DIAGNOSIS

- The course of this disease is highly variable and unpredictable.
- Disease manifestations are protean, ranging in severity from fatigue, malaise, weight loss, arthritis or arthralgias, fever, photosensitivity, rashes, and serositis to potentially life-threatening thrombocytopenia, hemolytic anemia, nephritis, cerebritis, vasculitis, pneumonitis, myositis, and myocarditis.
- Current American College of Rheumatology diagnostic criteria is used primarily in clinical studies and for research purposes but are helpful to review if suspicion arises. They include the following manifestations (4 or more of these 11 criteria establish the diagnosis in clinical studies):
  - Malar rash
  - Discoid rash
  - Photosensitivity
  - Oral and nasopharyngeal ulcers
  - Nonerosive arthritis and arthralgias
  - Serositis
  - Proteinuria and cellular casts
  - Seizures and psychosis
  - Autoimmune hemolytic anemia, leukopenia or lymphopenia, and thrombocytopenia
- They also include positive serologic tests such as:
  - Antinuclear antibodies (ANA) (nonspecific)
  - Anti–double-stranded DNA antibodies (highly specific, increased renal disease)
  - Anti-Smith (SM) antibodies (highly specific) and antiphospholipid antibodies
- Commonly associated positive serology includes anti-SSA (Ro) and SSB (La) antibodies in around 30% of patients, and anti-RNP in 40% of patients. Complement reduction (C3 and C4) is nonspecific but is common in lupus flares, and low levels are more commonly associated with renal disease.
- Patients with lupus have accelerated coronary and peripheral vascular disease, especially with high disease activity and chronic steroid use, and cardiovascular risk factors should be managed aggressively.

TREATMENT

Medications

- **NSAIDs** usually control SLE-associated arthritis, arthralgias, fever, and mild serositis but not fatigue, malaise, or major organ system involvement. The response to

selective COX-2 inhibitors is similar. Hepatic and renal toxicities of the NSAIDs appear to be increased in SLE. NSAIDs should be avoided in patients with active nephritis.

- **Hydroxychloroquine** 200 mg bid may be effective in the treatment of rash, photosensitivity, arthralgias, arthritis, alopecia, and malaise associated with SLE and in the treatment of **discoid and subacute cutaneous lupus erythematosus**. Skin lesions may begin to improve within a few days, but joint symptoms may require 6 to 10 weeks to subside. The drug is not effective for treating fever or renal, CNS, and hematologic problems, but long-term usage may decrease incidence of flares and renal and CNS involvement. Complications are rare, but for potential ophthalmologic complications, patients need annual eye examination.
- **Glucocorticoid therapy**
  - **Indications** for systemic glucocorticoids include life-threatening manifestations of SLE, such as glomerulonephritis, CNS involvement, thrombocytopenia, and hemolytic anemia and debilitating manifestations of SLE (fatigue, rash) that are unresponsive to conservative therapy.
  - **Dosage:** Patients with severe or potentially life-threatening complications of SLE should be treated with prednisone, 1 to 2 mg/kg PO daily, which can be given in divided doses. After disease is controlled, prednisone should be tapered slowly, the dosage being reduced by no more than 10% every 7 to 10 days. More rapid reduction may result in relapse. Alternate-day therapy may reduce many of the adverse effects of long-term glucocorticoid therapy. **IV pulse therapy** in the form of methylprednisolone, 500 to 1,000 mg IV daily for 3 to 5 days, has been used in SLE in such life-threatening situations as rapidly progressive renal failure, active CNS disease, and severe thrombocytopenia. Patients who do not show improvement with this regimen probably are unresponsive to steroids, and other therapeutic alternatives must be considered. A course of oral prednisone should follow completion of pulse therapy.
- **Immunosuppressive therapy**
  - **Indications** for immunosuppressive therapy in SLE include life-threatening manifestations of SLE such as glomerulonephritis, CNS involvement, thrombocytopenia, and hemolytic anemia, and the inability to reduce corticosteroid dosage or severe corticosteroid side effects.
  - **Choice of an immunosuppressive therapy** is individualized to the clinical situation. Often, **cyclophosphamide** is used for life-threatening manifestations of SLE. High-dose monthly IV pulse cyclophosphamide (0.5 to 1.0 g/m^2) may be less toxic but is also less immunosuppressive than low-dose daily oral cyclophosphamide (1.0 to 1.5 mg/kg/d). **Azathioprine** (1 to 3 mg/kg/d) and **mycophenolate mofetil** (500 to 1,500 mg bid) are also used as steroid-sparing agents for serious lupus manifestations. There is increasing evidence that mycophenolate mofetil may be as effective as cyclophosphamide in certain classes of lupus nephritis with fewer side effects, and mycophenolate is particularly preferred in the younger population where fertility maintenance is a concern. Methotrexate (7.5 to 20.0 mg weekly) is often used for musculoskeletal and skin manifestations. **Rituximab**, a monoclonal antibody directed against the B-cell surface molecule CD20, causes depletion of B cells and has been shown in uncontrolled observational studies to be effective in cases of severe SLE not responding to conventional treatment; however, placebo-controlled studies to date have been disappointing. **Belimumab** inhibits B-lymphocytic stimulator (BLyS) binding to B cells inhibiting B cell survival,

including autoreactive B cells, and decreasing B cell differentiation into immunoglobulin-producing plasma cells. This has been shown in trials to reduce SLE disease activity and flares. It was recently approved by the FDA for the treatment of adult autoantibody-positive lupus patients who are receiving standard therapy. The efficacy of belimumab has not been evaluated in patients with severe active lupus nephritis or severe active CNS lupus and has not been studied in combination with other biologics or IV cyclophosphamide. Use of belimumab is therefore not recommended in these situations.

Other Nonpharmacologic Therapies

- **Conservative therapy** alone is warranted if the patient's manifestations are mild.
- **General supportive measures** include adequate sleep and fatigue avoidance, as mild disease exacerbations may subside after a few days of bed rest.
- All patients, especially those with photosensitive rashes, are advised on sunscreens with SPF 30 or greater, protective clothing such as a hat and long sleeves, and sun avoidance. Isolated skin lesions may respond to topical steroids.
- Consider prophylaxis against *Pneumocystis* pneumonia in patients treated with cyclophosphamide. Also consider adding prophylaxis for the prevention of bladder and gonadal toxicity. Appropriate immunizations should be considered prior to initiation of immunosuppressive therapy, especially against influenza and pneumococcus. Immunization with live vaccines is contraindicated in immunosuppressed patients, but varicella-zoster vaccine may be recommended prior to initiation of therapy.

SPECIAL CONSIDERATIONS

- **Transplantation and chronic hemodialysis** have been used successfully in SLE patients with renal failure. Clinical and serologic evidence of disease activity often disappears when renal failure ensues. The survival rate in these patients is equivalent to that of patients with other forms of chronic renal disease. Recurrence of nephritis in the allograft rarely occurs.
- **Pregnancy in SLE:** An increased incidence of second-trimester spontaneous miscarriages and stillbirths has been reported in women with antibodies to cardiolipin or the lupus anticoagulant. Neonatal lupus may occur in offspring of anti-Ro/SSA positive mothers, with skin rash and heart block as the most common manifestations. SLE patients may experience flares during pregnancy if the lupus is active at the time of conception. Differentiation between active SLE and preeclampsia is often difficult. Women in whom SLE is well controlled are less likely to have a flare of disease during pregnancy.
- **Drug-induced lupus** is usually of sudden onset with an equal male to female ratio. It is associated with serositis and musculoskeletal manifestations. Renal and CNS manifestations are rare. Drug-induced lupus is commonly seen with positive ANA and **antihistone antibodies**, negative anti-SM and anti–double-stranded DNA antibodies, and normal complement levels. The disease usually resolves with drug discontinuation, typically in a few weeks. Offending drugs include procainamide, hydralazine, minocycline, diltiazem, penicillamine, isoniazid (INH), chlorpromazine, quinidine, methyldopa, anti-TNF, and interferon (IFN)-α.

Systemic Sclerosis

GENERAL PRINCIPLES

Definition

Systemic sclerosis (scleroderma) is a systemic illness of unknown etiology characterized by thickening and hardening of the skin and visceral organs. Most of the manifestations of scleroderma have a vascular basis (Raynaud's phenomenon, telangiectasias, nail fold capillary changes, early edematous skin changes, nephrosclerosis).

Classification

Scleroderma can be subdivided based on anatomic skin distribution into **localized scleroderma** (morphea and linear scleroderma) and **systemic sclerosis** (diffuse cutaneous, limited cutaneous and systemic sclerosis sine scleroderma). The limited cutaneous form involves extremities distal to the knees and elbows and the face (limited scleroderma was formerly known as the **CREST syndrome**: **c**alcinosis, **R**aynaud's phenomenon, **e**sophageal dysmotility, **s**clerodactyly, **t**elangiectasias). Diffuse cutaneous scleroderma involves the skin of the proximal extremities and the trunk. It is associated with internal organ involvement. Systemic sclerosis *sine* scleroderma affects the internal organs without skin involvement.

DIAGNOSIS

Clinical Presentation

- Nearly all patients with systemic sclerosis have **Raynaud's phenomenon**.
- **Diffuse scleroderma** is characterized by extensive skin disease, the potential for hypertensive "renal crisis," and shortened survival. Multiple internal organs are affected.
  - **GI involvement:** Decreased motility of bowel segments can occur, leading to bacterial overgrowth, malabsorption, diarrhea, and weight loss. Classic endoscopic findings include colonic wide mouth diverticula, patulous esophagus, esophageal strictures, and gastric antral vascular ectasia (GAVE) also known as watermelon stomach.
  - **Renal involvement:** The appearance of sudden hypertension and renal insufficiency indicate potential scleroderma renal crisis. This phenomenon occurs in approximately 10% of systemic sclerosis patients. It is associated with a microangiopathic hemolytic anemia and carries a poor prognosis.
  - **Cardiopulmonary involvement:** Patchy myocardial fibrosis can result in CHF or arrhythmias. Pulmonary involvement includes pleurisy with effusion, inflammatory alveolitis (radiographically seen as ground glass infiltrates) leading to interstitial fibrosis, pulmonary hypertension, and cor pulmonale.
  - **Other organ systems: Skin** involvement appears initially with edematous and erythematous "salt and pepper" pigmentation changes, progressing to skin tightening and thickening. **Musculoskeletal** manifestations range from arthralgias to frank nonerosive arthritis with joint contractures due to the regional skin involvement.
- **Limited scleroderma** may be associated with primary pulmonary hypertension (in the absence of ILD) or biliary cirrhosis and is distinguished by skin thickening that is limited to the face and the distal forearms and hands.

- **Nephrogenic systemic sclerosis** is a recently recognized complication of MRI with gadolinium contrast in the presence of renal failure (acute, chronic and end-stage renal disease). It is associated with skin thickening and internal organ fibrosis resembling scleroderma, without Raynaud's phenomenon or ANA positivity.

Diagnostic Testing

More than 95% of scleroderma patients are ANA positive, 20% to 40% are anti–Scl-70 positive (associated with diffuse disease). Up to 40% of patients with limited scleroderma have anticentromere antibody, which is rarely seen in individuals with diffuse scleroderma.

TREATMENT

No curative therapy for scleroderma exists. Treatment focuses on organ involvement and symptoms.

- **Skin and periarticular changes:** No therapeutic agent is clearly effective for these cutaneous manifestations. **Physical therapy** is important to retard and reduce joint contractures.
- **GI involvement**
  - Reflux esophagitis generally responds to standard therapy (e.g., **H₂-receptor antagonists**, **proton pump inhibitors**, and **promotility agents**).
  - Treatment with broad-spectrum antimicrobials in a rotating sequence including **metronidazole** often improves the malabsorption. Metoclopramide may reduce bloating and distention.
  - Occasionally, esophageal strictures require mechanical esophageal dilation.
  - Rarely, severe constipation or intestinal pseudo-obstruction may occur.
- **Renal involvement:** Aggressive blood pressure control with **ACE inhibitors** may delay, prevent, or even reverse the onset of uremia in patients with suspected scleroderma renal crisis. ARBs do not appear to be as effective.
- **Cardiopulmonary involvement:** Coronary artery vasospasm can cause angina pectoris and may respond to calcium channel antagonists. Pulmonary involvement includes pleurisy with effusion, interstitial fibrosis, pulmonary hypertension, and cor pulmonale. Standard therapies for these conditions are used (see Chapter 10, Pulmonary Diseases). Patients with rapidly progressive pulmonary parenchymal disease may benefit from a course of glucocorticoids and cyclophosphamide.
- Immunomodulatory and antifibrotic therapeutic modalities have yet to be shown effective in scleroderma. The use of penicillamine to arrest the progressive fibrosis is controversial. Most experts consider this an ineffective treatment option.

Raynaud's Phenomenon

GENERAL PRINCIPLES

Raynaud's phenomenon is a reversible vasospasm of the digital arteries that can result in ischemia of the digits. It is characterized by repeated episodes of color changes of the skin of digits on cold exposure or emotional stress. Primary Raynaud's disease has no predisposing factors and is milder, causing fewer complications. Secondary Raynaud's disease occurs in individuals with a predisposing factor, usually a form of collagen vascular disease.

TREATMENT

Medications

Most pharmacologic approaches have had limited success.

- **Calcium channel antagonists** (especially of the dihydropyridine group) are the preferred initial agents, although they may exacerbate gastroesophageal reflux and constipation in these patients.
- Alternative vasodilators such as prazosin are occasionally helpful, but significant side effects, including orthostatic hypotension, may preclude their use.
- Other agents that might improve the vasospasm include topical nitroglycerin applied to the dorsum of the hands, the phosphodiesterase inhibitor sildenafil and the endothelin-1 receptor antagonist bosentan.
- Daily low-dose aspirin therapy is often prescribed for its antiplatelet effects.
- Patients with severe ischemic digits should be hospitalized and conditions such as macrovascular disease, vasculitis, or a hypercoagulable state should be ruled out. An IV infusion of a prostaglandin or prostaglandin analog may also be considered.
- **Sympathetic ganglion blockade** with a long-acting anesthetic agent may be useful when a patient has progressive digital ulceration that fails to improve with conservative therapy.

Surgical Management

Surgical digital sympathectomy may be beneficial.

PATIENT EDUCATION

Patients must be instructed to avoid exposure of the entire body to cold, protect the hands and feet from cold and trauma, and discontinue cigarette smoking.

Necrotizing Vasculitis

GENERAL PRINCIPLES

Definition

Necrotizing vasculitis is characterized by inflammation and necrosis of blood vessels, leading to tissue damage. This diagnosis includes a broad spectrum of disorders that have various causes and involve vessels of different types, sizes, and locations.

Etiology

Although in most cases the inciting antigen has not been identified, some have been associated with chronic hepatitis B and C.

Pathophysiology

The immunopathologic process often involves immune complexes.

DIAGNOSIS

Clinical Presentation

Table 25-2 summarizes clinical features and diagnostic and treatment approaches to the most common forms of vasculitis. **Clinical features** are diverse and depend in

Table 25-2 Clinical Features and Diagnostic and Treatment Approaches to Vasculitis

Vasculitic Syndrome	Clinical Features	Diagnostic Approach	Treatment
Large-vessel involvement			
Temporal arteritis	Headache Jaw claudication	Temporal artery biopsy	Prednisone, 60–80 mg/d
Takayasu arteritis	Finger ischemia Arm claudication	Aortic arch arteriogram	Prednisone, 60–80 mg/d
Medium-vessel involvement			
Polyarteritis nodosa	Skin ulcers Nephritis Mononeuritis Mesenteric ischemia	Skin biopsy Renal biopsy Sural nerve biopsy Mesenteric angiogram Hepatitis B, C testing	Prednisone 60–100 mg/d Cyclophosphamide, 1–2 mg/kg/d can be added
Kawasaki disease	Seen in children Fever Conjunctivitis Lymphadenopathy Mucocutaneous erythema Coronary aneurysms	Clinical Coronary angiogram	Intravenous immunoglobulin Aspirin Anticoagulation
Small-vessel involvement			
Granulomatosis with polyangiitis (c-ANCA vasculitis)	Sinusitis Pulmonary infiltrates Nephritis	c-ANCA, sinus biopsy Lung biopsy Renal biopsy	Prednisone, 60–100 mg/d *and* cyclophosphamide, 1–2 mg/kg/d Rituximab Plasmapheresis

Condition	Clinical features	Diagnostic findings	Treatment
Microscopic polyangiitis	Pulmonary infiltrates Nephritis	p-ANCA Renal biopsy	Prednisone, 60–100 mg/d Cyclophosphamide, 1–2 mg/kg/d can be added
Churg–Strauss syndrome	Asthma, allergic rhinitis Fleeting pulmonary Infiltrates Mononeuritis multiplex	p-ANCA Peripheral eosinophilia Elevated IgE levels Biopsy (sural nerve/skin) with eosinophilic granulomas	Prednisone, 60–100 mg/d Cyclophosphamide if renal, GI, CNS, or cardiac involvement
Vasculitis in SLE or RA	Skin ulcers Polyneuropathy	Skin or sural nerve biopsy	Prednisone, 60–80 mg/d Cyclophosphamide, 1–2 mg/kg/d, can be added
Cutaneous leukocytoclastic vasculitis	Palpable purpura	Skin biopsy	NSAIDs, antihistamine, colchicines, dapsone Low-dose prednisone Discontinue inciting drug
Henoch-Schönlein purpura	Palpable purpura Nephritis Mesenteric ischemia	Skin biopsy Renal biopsy IgA immune complexes deposition	Supportive treatment Prednisone, 20–60 mg/d, may be needed

c-ANCA, cytoplasmic antineutrophil cytoplasmic antibodies; CNS, central nervous system; GI, gastrointestinal; Ig, immunoglobulin; NSAID, nonsteroidal anti-inflammatory drug; p-ANCA, perinuclear antineutrophil cytoplasmic antibodies; RA, rheumatoid arthritis; SLE, systemic lupus erythematosus.

part on the size of the vessel involved. Systemic manifestations including fever and weight loss are common. The response to therapy and long-term prognosis of these disorders are highly variable.

Differential Diagnosis

Vasculitis "mimics" should be considered, including bacterial endocarditis, HIV infection, atrial myxoma, paraneoplastic syndromes, cholesterol emboli, and cocaine and amphetamine use.

TREATMENT

- **Glucocorticoids** are the usual initial therapy. Although vasculitis that is limited to the skin may respond to lower doses of corticosteroids, the initial dosage for visceral involvement should be high (prednisone, 1 to 2 mg/kg/d). **If life-threatening manifestations are present**, a brief course of high-dose pulse therapy with methyl-prednisolone, 500 mg IV q12h for 3 to 5 days, should be considered.
- **Immunosuppressives**, in particular oral **cyclophosphamide**, often are used in the initial management of necrotizing vasculitis, especially when major organ system involvement (e.g., lung, kidney, or nerve) is present. Methotrexate, azathioprine, and mycophenolate mofetil are often used for maintenance therapy and as initial therapy in less severe presentations.
- **TMP-SMX** has been used in variants of granulomatosis with polyangiitis (previously Wegener's granulomatosis) limited to the upper airway and may also be useful in preventing relapse. This drug is not sufficient treatment for systemic disease.
- **Rituximab** combined with glucocorticoids has been approved for the treatment of adult patients with granulomatosis with polyangiitis and microscopic polyangiitis. It is an alternative for remission induction of severe disease especially in patients who cannot take or who refuse cyclophosphamide.

REFERRAL

Management should include consultation with a physician experienced in the treatment of these disorders. Treatment should be tailored to the severity of organ system involvement.

Polymyalgia Rheumatica

DIAGNOSIS

Clinical Presentation

Polymyalgia rheumatica (PMR) presents in elderly patients as proximal limb girdle pain, morning stiffness, and constitutional symptoms. It is associated with **temporal arteritis (TA) in up to 40% of patients**. Patients with TA present with headache, scalp tenderness, jaw or tongue claudication, vision disturbances (including blindness), and stroke (see Table 25-2). Patients who are suspected of having TA should be treated promptly with high-dose steroids, and rheumatology should be consulted immediately.

Diagnostic Testing

- PMR: Elevated erythrocyte sedimentation rate (ESR)
- TA: Elevated ESR (often >100 mm/Hr)

TREATMENT

If PMR is present without evidence of TA, **prednisone**, 10 to 15 mg PO daily, usually produces dramatic clinical improvement within a few days.

- The ESR should return to normal during initial treatment, but subsequent therapeutic decisions should be based on ESR and clinical status.
- Glucocorticoid therapy can be tapered gradually to a maintenance dosage of 5 to 10 mg PO daily but should be continued for at least 1 year to minimize the risk of relapse.
- NSAIDs may facilitate reduction in prednisone dosage.

Cryoglobulin Syndromes

GENERAL PRINCIPLES

Definition

Cryoglobulins are serum immunoglobulins that reversibly precipitate in the cold.

Classification

Cryoglobulinemia is traditionally categorized as monoclonal (formerly type 1) or polyclonal (mixed; formerly types 2 and 3).

Etiology

- Patients with **monoclonal cryoglobulinemia type 1** usually have an underlying lymphoproliferative disorder such as myeloma, lymphoma, or Waldenström macroglobulinemia.
- **Type II cryoglobulinemia** are monoclonal RFs that are associated with small vessel vasculitis. Approximately 80% to 90% of patients have hepatitis C virus infection, although only 5% of patients with hepatitis C and cryoglobulins develop vasculitis.
- **Type III cryoglobulinemia** are polyclonal RFs that are present in patients with chronic inflammatory diseases such as hepatitis B and C virus infection, endocarditis, SLE, and RA.

DIAGNOSIS

- Symptoms in monoclonal (formerly type 1) cryoglobulinemia are related to hyperviscosity (blurring of vision, digital ischemia, headache, lethargy) and respond to treatment of the underlying disorder, although plasmapheresis can be used in the acute setting.
- Clinical manifestations of mixed cryoglobulinemia are mediated by immune complex deposition (arthralgias, palpable purpura, glomerulonephritis, and neuropathy).

TREATMENT

- Therapy for secondary cryoglobulinemia is directed at the underlying disease.
- Treatment of hepatitis C with IFN-α and ribavirin effectively reduces cryoglobulins, although they may recur when treatment is stopped.
- Aggressive therapy is indicated for patients with acute severe disease. Patients with progressive renal failure, distal necroses requiring amputation, or advanced neuropathy should be treated with prednisone and immunosuppression.
- **Plasmapheresis** can be used in addition to immunosuppression in severe disease.

Polymyositis and Dermatomyositis

GENERAL PRINCIPLES

Definition

- **Polymyositis (PM)** is an inflammatory myopathy that presents as weakness and occasionally tenderness of the proximal musculature.
- **Dermatomyositis (DM)** is another inflammatory myopathy associated with a characteristic skin rash.

Classification

PM and DM can occur in three forms: (a) alone, (b) in association with any of the other autoimmune diseases, or (c) with a variety of neoplasms.

Risk Factors

Risk factors for malignancy in the setting of myositis include the presence of DM, cutaneous vasculitis, male sex, and advanced age.

DIAGNOSIS

Diagnostic Testing

Laboratories

- Elevated muscle enzyme levels (creatine kinase, aldolase, aspartate aminotransferase [AST], lactate dehydrogenase [LDH]).
- Certain subsets of disease are associated with myositis-specific antibodies such as Jo-1 (one of the antisynthetase antibodies) and signal recognition particle. These antibodies have therapeutic and prognostic implications, and levels should therefore be measured in all patients.
- Associated with an abnormal electromyogram.

Imaging

An MRI is useful for the localization of inflammation and necrosis.

Diagnostic Procedures

A muscle biopsy is important to establish a diagnosis.

TREATMENT

Medications

- **Prednisone**
  - When PM or DM occurs without associated disease, it usually responds well to prednisone, 1 to 2 mg/kg PO daily.

- Systemic complaints, such as fever and malaise, respond to therapy first, followed by muscle enzymes, and finally, muscle strength.
- Once serum enzyme levels normalize, the prednisone dosage should be reduced slowly to maintenance levels of 10 to 20 mg PO daily or 20 to 40 mg PO every other day.
- Appearance of steroid-induced myopathy and hypokalemia may complicate therapeutic assessment.
- IV infusion of **immunoglobulin** may hasten improvement of severe dysphagia.
- PM or DM associated with neoplasia tends to be less responsive to glucocorticoid therapy but may improve after removal of the malignant tumor.
- Patients who do not respond or cannot tolerate the side effects of glucocorticoids may respond to methotrexate or azathioprine.
- Severe resistant cases may be treated with rituximab, mycophenolate mofetil, and other immunosuppressive agents.

Other Nonpharmacologic Therapies

Physical therapy is essential in the management of myositis. Bed rest with active assisted range of motion is appropriate during very active disease, with more active exercise prescribed to improve strength once inflammation has been controlled.

SPECIAL CONSIDERATIONS

Screening for common neoplasms, such as colon, lung, breast, and prostate cancer, should be considered in these patients as well as individual risk-based assessment.

26 Neurologic Disorders

Robert C. Bucelli and Beau Ances

Alterations in Consciousness

GENERAL PRINCIPLES

Definition

- **Coma** is a state of complete behavioral unresponsiveness to external stimulation. Because some etiologies can lead to irreversible brain damage, evaluation and treatment should be performed concurrently and expeditiously. The need for neurosurgical intervention must be determined promptly.
- **Delirium** is an acute confusional state that can result from diffuse or multifocal cerebral dysfunction and is characterized by relatively rapid reduction in the ability to focus, sustain, or shift attention. Changes in cognition, fluctuations in consciousness, disorientation, and even hallucinations are common.

Epidemiology

- About 30% of older patients (>60 years old) experience delirium during hospitalization.
- Delirious patients often have prolonged hospitalizations and are at greater risk for subsequent cognitive decline.

Etiology

- Coma results from diffuse or multifocal dysfunction involving both cerebral hemispheres or the reticular activating system in the brainstem.
- Etiologies of altered mental status are listed in Table 26-1.
- Mild systemic illness (e.g., urinary tract infections [UTIs]), introduction of new medications, fever, and/or sleep deprivation are common causes of delirium in the elderly and in patients with chronic central nervous system (CNS) dysfunction of any cause.

DIAGNOSIS

- Initial assessment should focus on recognizing the development and progression of altered consciousness. Examiner should query for history of trauma, seizures, stroke, medication changes, and alcohol or drug use as possible etiologies. A collateral source can be extremely helpful and is often necessary.
- If trauma has or may have occurred, **immobilize the spine immediately** and then proceed with imaging to identify or exclude fracture or instability.

Clinical Presentation

Physical Examination

- Search for signs of systemic illness associated with coma (e.g., cirrhosis, hemodialysis shunt, rash of meningococcemia) or signs of head trauma (e.g., lacerations,

| Table 26-1 | Causes of Altered Mental Status |

Metabolic derangements/diffuse etiologies
- Hypernatremia/hyponatremia
- Hypercalcemia
- Hyperglycemia/hypoglycemia
- Hyperthyroidism/hypothyroidism
- Acute intermittent porphyria
- Hypertensive encephalopathy
- Hypoxia/hypercapnia
- Global cerebral ischemia from hypotension

Infections
- Meningitis/encephalitis
- Sepsis
- Systemic infectious with spread to CNS

Drugs/toxins/poisons
- Prescription medications and side effects of medications
- Drugs of abuse
- Withdrawal situations
- Medication side effects
- Inhaled toxins

Inborn errors of metabolism

Nutritional deficiency (i.e., thiamine)

Seizures
- Subclinical seizures
- Postictal state

Head trauma

Structural
- Ischemic stroke (only certain stroke locations cause altered mental status)
- Hemorrhage
- Hydrocephalus
- Tumor

Systemic organ failure
- Hepatic failure
- Renal failure

Psychiatric

CNS, central nervous system.

periorbital or mastoid ecchymosis, hemotympanum). The physical and neurologic examination may reveal systemic illness (e.g., pneumonia) or neurologic signs (meningismus or paralysis) to narrow the differential diagnosis.

- **Herniation** occurs when mass lesions or edema cause shifts in brain tissue. The diagnosis of brain herniation **requires immediate recognition and treatment**. If a risk of herniation is present, the patient should be monitored in a neurosurgical/neurological critical care unit and frequent neurochecks should be performed to evaluate for signs of impending herniation.
  - **Nonspecific signs and symptoms of increased intracranial pressure** include headache, nausea, vomiting, hypertension, bradycardia, papilledema, sixth nerve palsy, transient visual obscurations, and alterations in consciousness.

- ○ **Uncal herniation** is caused by unilateral supratentorial lesions. The earliest sign is a dilated pupil ipsilateral to the mass, diminished consciousness, and hemiparesis, first contralateral to the mass and later ipsilateral to the mass (Kernohan notch syndrome).
- ○ **Central herniation** is caused by medial or bilateral supratentorial lesions. Signs include progressive alteration of consciousness, Cheyne–Stokes or normal respirations followed later by central hyperventilation, midposition and unreactive pupils, loss of upward gaze, and posturing of the extremities.
- ○ **Tonsillar herniation** occurs when pressure in the posterior fossa forces the cerebellar tonsils through the foramen magnum, compressing the medulla. Signs include altered level of consciousness and respiratory irregularity or apnea.
- In general, the neurologic assessment should be to ascertain the patient's ability to focus, sustain, and shift attention appropriately. Due to fluctuations, repeated exams are often necessary.
- **Level of consciousness** can be semi-quantitatively assessed and followed by using the Glasgow coma scale (GCS). Scores range from 3 (unresponsive) to 15 (normal).
- **Respiratory rate and pattern**
  - ○ Cheyne–Stokes respirations (rhythmic crescendo–decrescendo hyperapnea alternating with periods of apnea) occur in metabolic coma and supratentorial lesions, as well as in chronic pulmonary disease and congestive heart failure (CHF).
  - ○ Hyperventilation is commonly seen in the setting of metabolic acidosis, hypoxemia, pneumonia, or other pulmonary disease but can also occur with an upper brainstem injury.
  - ○ Apneustic breathing (long pauses after inspiration), cluster breathing (breathing in short bursts), and ataxic breathing (irregular breaths without pattern) are signs of brainstem injury and are commonly associated with impending respiratory arrest.
- **Pupil size and light reactivity**
  - ○ Anisocoria (asymmetric pupils) in a patient with altered mental status requires immediate diagnosis (i.e., stat head computed tomography [CT]) or exclusion and treatment of possible herniation. Anisocoria may be physiologic or produced by mydriatics (e.g., scopolamine, atropine), and therefore requires well-documented serial examinations.
  - ○ Small but reactive pupils are seen in narcotic overdose, metabolic encephalopathy, and pontine lesions.
  - ○ Fixed mid-position pupils imply midbrain lesions or transtentorial herniation.
  - ○ Bilaterally fixed and dilated pupils occur with severe anoxic encephalopathy or drug intoxication (scopolamine, atropine, glutethimide, or methanol).
- **Eye movements**
  - ○ The oculocephalic (doll's eyes) test is performed (if no cervical injury is present) by quickly turning the head laterally or vertically. Intact brainstem oculomotor function, in the setting of coma, will result in eye movements conjugately opposite to the direction of head movement.
  - ○ The oculovestibular (cold caloric) test is used if cervical trauma is suspected or if eye movements are absent with the oculocephalic test. Brainstem oculomotor function is intact if the eyes move conjugately toward the ear lavaged with ice cold water. Vertical gaze can be assessed with simultaneous lavage of both ears (cold water → eyes depress, warm water → eyes elevate).
  - ○ In the absence of a history to suggest a drug-induced cause (e.g., barbiturates, phenytoin, paralytics) or a preexisting disorder such as progressive external ophthalmoplegia, absence of all eye movements indicates a bilateral pontine lesion.

○ Dysconjugate gaze suggests a brainstem lesion.
○ A gaze preference conjugately to one side suggests a unilateral pontine or frontal lobe lesion. An associated hemiparesis and oculocephalic and oculovestibular tests can help localize the lesion. In pontine lesions, gaze preference is toward the paretic side, and eyes may move toward but do not cross midline. In frontal lobe lesions, gaze preference is away from the paresis, and eyes can move conjugately across midline to both sides.
○ Impaired vertical eye movement occurs in midbrain lesions and central herniation. Conjugate depression and impaired elevation suggests a tectal lesion (e.g., pinealoma) or hydrocephalus.
• **Motor responses** also help with localization. Asymmetric motor responses (spontaneous or stimulus induced, including noxious stimuli if necessary) also have localizing value.

Diagnostic Testing

Laboratories
Obtain serum electrolytes, creatinine, glucose, calcium, complete blood count (CBC), and urinalysis. Drug levels should be ordered if appropriate. An accurate medication list and any history to suggest intoxication are critical features of the evaluation. Toxicology screen of blood and urine should be considered.

Imaging
A head CT should be obtained to evaluate for structural abnormalities. Brain magnetic resonance imaging (MRI) can be useful if head CT is nondiagnostic and there is suspicion for an ischemic or parenchymal lesion (especially of the posterior fossa).

Diagnostic Procedures
• Lumbar puncture (LP) should be considered in patients with fever and/or new headache or those with high risk of infection. Absence of herniation should be confirmed prior to performing an LP.
• Electroencephalography (EEG) can be considered to rule out seizures. Interictal abnormalities can be suggestive of specific etiologies (e.g., periodic lateralized epileptiform discharges [PLEDs] in herpes simplex virus [HSV] encephalitis, triphasic waves in hepatic or uremic encephalopathy, and β activity or voltage suppression in barbiturate or other sedative intoxications).

TREATMENT

Coma
• Ensure adequate airway and ventilation, administer oxygen as needed, and maintain normal body temperature.
• Establish secure intravenous (IV) access and adequate circulation.
• Neurosurgical consult may need to be obtained for arterial, central venous, and intracranial pressures monitoring and treatment, if applicable.

Delirium
• Repeated attempts should be made to reorient the patient and possibly have a sitter present if necessary.
• A quiet room with close observation is necessary. Patients should have a well-lit environment with familiar objects during the day and dark environments at night.

- Physical and pharmacologic restraints should be used only as a last resort and with appropriate documentation in the medical record. If restraints are needed, they should be carefully adjusted and checked periodically to prevent excessive constriction.

Medications

- IV thiamine (100 mg), followed by dextrose (50 mL of 50% dextrose in water = 25 g dextrose), should be administered. Thiamine is administered first as dextrose administration in thiamine-deficient patients may precipitate Wernicke's encephalopathy.
- IV naloxone (opiate antagonist), 0.01 mg/kg, should be administered if opiate intoxication is suspected (coma, respiratory depression, small reactive pupils). Naloxone may provoke opiate withdrawal syndrome in patients on opioids chronically.
- Flumazenil (benzodiazepine antagonist), 0.2 mg IV, may reverse benzodiazepine intoxication, but its duration of action is short, and additional doses may be needed. Flumazenil should be used with caution in certain patient populations (e.g., epileptics) as it reduces the seizure threshold.
- In delirious patients, sedatives should be avoided if possible. If necessary low doses of quetiapine (12.5 to 25.0 mg), lorazepam (1 mg), or chlordiazepoxide (25 mg) can be used. Remember to always consider comorbidities before administering these medications.

Other Nonpharmacologic Therapies

If herniation is identified or suspected, treatment consists of measures to lower intracranial pressure while surgically treatable etiologies are identified or excluded. All of the listed measures are only **temporizing methods**. Consultation with neurosurgery should be performed concurrently.

- Elevate the head of the bed to at least 30 degrees.
- Endotracheal intubation is usually performed to enable hyperventilation to a PCO_2 of 25 to 30 mm Hg. This reduces intracranial pressure within minutes by cerebral vasoconstriction. Bag-mask ventilation can be performed if manipulation of the neck is precluded by possible or established spinal instability. Reduction of PCO_2 below 25 mm Hg is not recommended because it may reduce cerebral blood flow.
- Administration of IV mannitol (1 to 2 g/kg over 10 to 20 minutes), osmotically reduces free water in the brain via elimination by the kidneys and does not require a central line for administration. This effect peaks at 90 minutes. Remember that, given its potent diuretic effect, mannitol can precipitate renal failure if volume is not adequately replaced. Hypertonic saline (23.4% saline) is an alternative option that also carries its own set of side effects and requires central venous access.
- Dexamethasone, 10 mg IV, followed by 4 mg IV q6h, reduces the edema surrounding a tumor or an abscess but is not indicated for diffuse cerebral edema or the mass effect associated with malignant cerebral infarcts.
- Coagulopathy should be corrected if intracranial hemorrhage is diagnosed and before surgical treatment or invasive procedures (e.g., LP) are performed. Each patient's circumstances should be carefully assessed before therapeutic anticoagulation is reversed.

Surgical Management

Surgical evacuation of epidural, subdural, or intraparenchymal (e.g., cerebellar) hemorrhage, and shunting for acute hydrocephalus should be considered in the appropriate clinical circumstances. However, some structural lesions are not amenable to surgical treatment.

SPECIAL CONSIDERATIONS

- **Brain death** occurs from irreversible brain injury sufficient to permanently eliminate all cortical and brainstem functions. Because the vital centers in the brainstem sustain cardiovascular and respiratory functions, brain death is incompatible with survival despite mechanical ventilation and cardiovascular and nutritional supportive measures. Brain death is distinguished from persistent vegetative state in which the absence of higher cortical function is accompanied by intact brainstem function. Patients in a persistent vegetative state are unable to think, speak, understand, or meaningfully respond to visual, verbal, or auditory stimuli, yet with nutritional and supportive care their cardiovascular and respiratory functions can sustain viability for many years.
- Brain death criteria vary somewhat by institution. Refer to your institution's policy for details.
- **Alcohol withdrawal** typically occurs when illness or hospitalization interrupts continued alcohol intake.
  - Tremulousness, irritability, anorexia, and nausea characterize minor alcohol withdrawal. Symptoms usually appear within a few hours after reduction or cessation of alcohol consumption and resolve within 48 hours. Treatment includes a well-lit room, reassurance, and the presence of family or friends. **Thiamine**, 100 mg intramuscular (IM)/IV, followed by 100 mg PO daily; multivitamins containing **folic acid**; and a balanced diet as tolerated should be administered. Serial evaluation for signs of major alcohol withdrawal is essential.
  - Alcohol withdrawal seizures, typically one or a few brief generalized convulsions, occur 12 to 48 hours after cessation of ethanol intake. **Antiepileptic drugs (AEDs) are not indicated for typical alcohol withdrawal seizures.** Other causes for seizures (see Seizures section) must be excluded. If hypoglycemia is present, thiamine should be administered before glucose.
  - Severe withdrawal or delirium tremens consists of tremulousness, hallucinations, agitation, confusion, disorientation, and autonomic hyperactivity (fever, tachycardia, diaphoresis), typically occurring 72 to 96 hours after cessation of drinking. Symptoms generally resolve within 3 to 5 days. Delirium tremens complicates 5% to 10% of cases of alcohol withdrawal, with mortality up to 15%. Other causes of delirium must be considered in the differential diagnosis (see Table 26-1). One should administer supportive management as follows:
    - Chlordiazepoxide is an effective sedative for delirium tremens, 100 mg IV or PO q2–6h as needed (maximum dose, 500 mg in the first 24 hours). One-half the initial 24-hour dose can be administered over the next 24 hours; the dosage can be reduced by 25 to 50 mg/d each day thereafter. Longer lasting benzodiazepines facilitate smoother tapering, but shorter acting agents (i.e., lorazepam, 1 to 2 mg PO or IV q6–8h as needed) may be desirable in older patients and those with reduced drug clearance. In patients with severe hepatic failure, oxazepam (15 to 30 mg PO, q6–8h as needed), which is excreted by the kidney, can be used instead of chlordiazepoxide.
    - Maintenance of fluid and electrolyte balance is important. Alcoholic patients are susceptible to hypomagnesemia, hypokalemia, hypoglycemia, and fluid losses, which may be considerable due to fever, diaphoresis, and vomiting.

Alzheimer's Disease

GENERAL PRINCIPLES

The most common neurodegenerative disorder in older individuals (>60 years old), typically characterized by memory problems and dementia.

Epidemiology

- Prevalence is <1% before age 65, 5% to 10% at age 65, and ~45% by age 85.
- Inherited forms of Alzheimer's disease (AD) manifest typically before age 65 years and are associated with mutations in amyloid precursor protein (APP) gene on chromosome 21, presenilin-1 gene on chromosome 14, and presenilin-2 gene on chromosome 1.
- Lifetime risk doubles if a sibling or parent is diagnosed with AD.

Pathophysiology

Neurofibrillary tangles due to tau with neuritic plaques composed of amyloid.

DIAGNOSIS

Clinical Presentation

- Memory impairment is required for diagnosis of AD.
- Episodic memory for newly acquired information is impaired while memory for more remote events is not affected.
- Declarative memory for facts and events is affected while procedural memory and motor learning are spared at earlier stages of the disease.
- With progression of disease, language, visuospatial skills, abstract reasoning, and executive function deteriorate. Some patients will also develop apraxia, alexia, and delusions.

Differential Diagnosis

See Table 26-2.

Table 26-2	Differential Diagnosis of Alzheimer's Dementia
Frontotemporal dementia Changes in personality, behavior, and executive functioning	
Vascular dementia Stepwise course due to repeated stroke-like events	
Dementia with Lewy bodies Visual hallucinations, cognitive fluctuations, parkinsonism, sensitivity to neuroleptics	
Normal pressure hydrocephalus Triad of dementia, urinary incontinence, and gait instability	
Vitamin B$_{12}$ deficiency **Neurosyphilis** **Thyroid dysfunction** **HIV**	

Diagnostic Testing

Progression of disease can be assessed by the Mini-Mental State Examination (MMSE), the Montreal Cognitive Assessment (MOCA), and the Clinical Dementia Rating Scale (CDR).

Laboratories
- Definitive diagnosis of AD requires histopathologic examination.
- Reversible causes of dementia such as B_{12} deficiency, neurosyphilis, and thyroid abnormalities should be ruled out.

Imaging
- Brain MRI can suggest potential alternative diagnoses.
- MRI may show diffuse atrophy with hippocampal atrophy that is seen with AD.
- [^{18}F] Fluorodeoxyglucose positron emission tomography (FDG-PET) or perfusion single-photon emission computed tomography (SPECT) may demonstrate hypo-metabolism and hypoperfusion, respectively, within the parietotemporal cortex.
- Amyloid PET tracers (florbetapir) can measure amyloid deposition in the brain and are now U.S. Food and Drug Administration (FDA) approved for clinical use.

Diagnostic Procedures
- Neuropsychological testing can establish a baseline. This testing can sometimes differentiate dementia from depression.
- Both structural imaging and PET imaging may assist in early diagnosis.
- Cerebral spinal fluid (CSF) measures of reduced AB_{42} and increased tau may be diagnostic for AD in the research setting.

TREATMENT

- Cholinesterase inhibitors including donepezil, rivastigmine, and galantamine can be considered for early AD.
- Memantine, a noncompetitive *N*-methyl-D-aspartate (NMDA) receptor antagonist, can be considered for moderate to severe dementia.

Seizures

GENERAL PRINCIPLES

Definition
- Seizure: Uncontrolled excessive electrical discharges in the brain that may produce a sudden change in brain function causing physical convulsion, minor physical signs, thought disturbances, or a combination of symptoms.
- Epilepsy is defined as a state of recurrent seizures.
- Status epilepticus is defined by greater than 30 minutes of continuous seizure activity or recurrent seizures without full recovery between episodes. However, in practice, a seizure lasting >5 minutes should be treated as status epilepticus.
- Nonconvulsive status epilepticus is defined by electrographic seizures with clinically absent or subtle motor activity, and impairment or loss of consciousness.
- An aura is a simple partial seizure manifesting as sensory, autonomic, or psychic symptoms.
- A prodrome is a sensation or feeling that a seizure will soon occur.

Classification

- Partial seizures begin focally.
  - **Simple partial:** Consciousness is not impaired. The symptoms can be motor (hand jerking), sensory (focal tingling), autonomic (sensation of epigastric rising), or psychic (déjà vu).
  - **Complex partial:** Consciousness is impaired. The symptoms vary based on whether they involve the temporal (automatisms such as lip smacking or picking at clothes, staring, behavior arrest), frontal (hypermotor behaviors, bicycling, pelvic thrusting, and automatisms), or occipital lobes (unformed images, visual hallucinations). Frontal seizures are often misdiagnosed as nonepileptic seizures (i.e., pseudoseizures) due to their often complex and sometimes bizarre semiology.
- Generalized seizures originate from bilateral hemispheres and, by definition, consciousness is lost.
  - May begin as generalized or as partial seizures with secondary generalization.
  - Include tonic, clonic, tonic–clonic, atonic, myoclonic, and absence.

Epidemiology

- Epilepsy is estimated to affect ~70 million people worldwide with the prevalence being twice as high in low income countries relative to high income countries.
- The median worldwide incidence of epilepsy is ~50/100,000 per year (*Neurology 2011;77(10):1005*).

Etiology

Etiologies for seizures include those listed in Table 26-3. For patients with a known seizure disorder presenting with an increase in seizure frequency, the most common causes are anticonvulsive medication noncompliance, subtherapeutic anticonvulsant levels, or infection.

Table 26-3	Etiologies of Seizures

- CNS infections
- Fever
- Hypoxic brain injury
- Stroke (ischemic or hemorrhagic)
- Tumors
- Head injury
- Eclampsia
- Hyperthyroidism
- Congenital brain malformations
- Genetics (phenylketonuria, Sturge–Weber, tuberous sclerosis, etc.)
- Toxic metabolic (porphyria, uremia, liver failure)
- Drug withdrawal (alcohol, barbiturates, benzodiazepine, AEDS)
- Drug intoxication (TCAs, cocaine, amphetamine)
- Electrolyte abnormalities
  - Hyponatremia
  - Hypocalcemia
  - Hypomagnesemia
  - Hypoglycemia/hyperglycemia

AEDs, antiepileptic drugs; CNS, central nervous system; TCAs, tricyclic antidepressants.

DIAGNOSIS

Clinical Presentation

History

- Query for family history of epilepsy, developmental delay, trauma, medical historical information including preexisting medical conditions, current and recently discontinued medications, drug allergies, recreational drug use, and possible precipitating events.
- Ask the patient about any prodrome/aura. An eyewitness account of the event is also important and a video is even better! Inquire about **incontinence**, **tongue biting**, and how the patient behaved after the event ended (e.g., confused?, if so, for how long?).

Physical Examination

- Convulsive seizures are usually easily identified.
- Carefully observe for subtle signs of nonconvulsive seizures, such as automatisms, facial or extremity twitching, eye deviation, and periods of relatively preserved mental status alternating with periods of impaired consciousness.
- Patients may present during the postictal period, defined as the time between the end of the seizure and the return to baseline mental status. During this time, patients may act confused, obtunded, and have amnesia for events since the seizure. This period can typically last from minutes to hours (rarely, days in the elderly and those with prior CNS injury).
- Postictal paresis (also called Todd's paralysis) is a transient neurologic deficit that lasts for hours or, rarely, days after an epileptic seizure.

Differential Diagnosis

Alternate diagnoses that may mimic seizures include:

- Syncope, especially convulsive syncope in which seizure-like motor activity is observed (*J Am Coll Cardiol 2002;40(1):142*)
- Nonepileptic seizures ("pseudoseizures") (see the following text)
- Toxic-metabolic encephalopathy
- Tremors, dyskinesias
- Nonepileptic myoclonus following a hypoxic event
- Rigors

Diagnostic Testing

Laboratories

Initial laboratory studies should include electrolytes, calcium, magnesium, CBC, urinalysis, urine drug screen, and AED levels if indicated.

Imaging

Neuroimaging is usually indicated to identify structural etiologies.

- Start with a head CT in the acute setting. The administration of contrast can assist in diagnosis of possible tumors.
- Brain MRI with and without contrast, protocolled to evaluate for an ictal focus, is almost always indicated in the evaluation of new onset seizures.

Diagnostic Procedures

- LP should be done if there is concern for CNS infection. Send for routine CSF studies as well as HSV polymerase chain reaction (HSV-PCR). Save extra CSF for any additional testing, if later indicated.

- EEG is not required for initial diagnosis and management of generalized convulsive status epilepticus. If mental status is not improving as expected after convulsive seizures stop, EEG may be necessary to exclude conversion to nonconvulsive status epilepticus.
- Routine EEG is indicated for all new-onset seizures.
- Video EEG is the gold standard test for the evaluation of suspected nonepileptic seizures. A significant (30% to 50% in some studies) number of patients with nonepileptic seizures ("pseudoseizures") will also have epileptic seizures.

TREATMENT

- **Initiation of AED therapy is usually not indicated after a single unprovoked seizure** as about two-thirds of patients who had a single seizure will not have seizure recurrence (*N Engl J Med 1998;338(7):429*). Nonetheless, therapy is not required if a first seizure is provoked by factors that resolve.
- A diagnosis of epilepsy is made after two or more unprovoked seizures. AED treatment is generally started after the second seizure as the patient has a substantially increased risk for repeated seizures after two events.
- Treatment of status epilepticus must be prompt as efficacy of treatment decreases with increased seizure duration (*Semin Neurol 2008;28(3):342*). (See Figure 26-1 for treatment of status epilepticus.) Persistent seizures probably produce permanent brain injury, and definitely result in cardiovascular and respiratory insufficiency, as well as other life-threatening complications.

Medications

- The selection of a specific AED for a patient must be individualized according to the drug effectiveness for seizure type(s), potential adverse effects of the drug, interactions with other possible medications, cost, and mechanism of drug action (*Epilepsia 2006;47:1094*).
- About half of all patients with a new diagnosis of epilepsy will become seizure free with the first AED prescribed (*Epilepsia 2001;42:1255*).
- Treatment should be started with a single drug that can be titrated until adequate control or until side effects are experienced.
- **Combination therapy (polytherapy) should be attempted only after at least two adequate sequential trials of single agents have failed.** Failure to control epilepsy with adequate trials of two drugs meets criteria for treatment-resistant epilepsy and a referral for presurgical evaluation should be considered (*Epilepsia 2010;51(6):1069*).

Lifestyle Modifications

- Patients should not start other medications (i.e., over-the-counter medications, or herbal remedies) without contacting their physician as there may be drug interactions.
- Patients should keep a seizure calendar to identify possible seizure triggers. Screen patients for poor sleep hygiene. Females may have catamenial (perimenstrual) seizures.
- Patients should reduce alcohol intake as heavy consumption (three or more drinks per day) is associated with an increased risk of seizures.

Step 1

Give oxygen, get vital signs, obtain IV access, begin ECG and pulse oximetry monitoring, draw blood, ABG, fingerstick glucose, vital signs

- Lorazepam 2 mg IV over 1 minute, repeat after 1 minute until max dose 0.1 mg/kg
- Fosphenytoin 20 mg/kg PE (phenytoin equivalents) IV at max rate 150 mg/min^

If seizures continue, the patient is in refractory status epilepticus.

Step 2

Additional 10 mg/kg IV Fosphenytoin
or
Valproate 30 mg/kg IV over 15 min
or
Proceed directly to Step 3

Step 3

Intubate, start EEG monitoring,

- Midazolam 0.2 mg/kg IV bolus, followed by continuous IV infusion 0.1 mg/kg/hr
  or
- Propofol 1–2 mg/kg IV load, followed by IV infusion 2 mg/kg/hr*
  or
- Pentobarbital 5 mg/kg load at 50 mg/min, followed by infusion of 1 mg/kg/hr

Titrate above medications to seizure suppression or EEG background suppression

^Check phenytoin level 2 hours post load. Level should be 20–25.
*Using propofol at high doses for >2 days may result in the potentially fatal propofol toxicity.

Figure 26-1. Treatment of status epilepticus. ABG, arterial blood gas; ECG, electrocardiogram; EEG, electroencephalogram; IV, intravenous. (Modified from Arif H, Hirsch LJ. Treatment of status epilepticus. *Semin Neurol 2008;28(3):342*)

REFERRAL

Neurologic consultation may be helpful for managing status epilepticus, and for evaluation and management of new-onset seizures.

PATIENT EDUCATION

Patients with epilepsy, especially those left untreated, have a small risk of sudden death in epilepsy (SUDEP) (*Lancet Neurology 2011;10(11):961*). Patients with epilepsy should not swim unsupervised, bathe in a bathtub of standing water, use motorized tools, or be in position to fall from heights during a seizure (i.e., patients should avoid situations in which they could harm themselves or others if they were to have a seizure). Driver licensing requirements for patients with epilepsy vary from state to state. A complete listing of state laws can be found at *http://www.epilepsy foundation.org/resources/drivingandtravel.cfm*.

MONITORING/FOLLOW-UP

- Regular follow-up visits should be scheduled to check drug concentrations, blood counts, and hepatic and renal function. Side effects after initiating AED should be monitored.
- Correctable causes for seizures (e.g., hyponatremia, drug toxicity, alcohol withdrawal) do not require long-term anticonvulsant therapy.

Cerebrovascular Disease

GENERAL PRINCIPLES

- Stroke is a medical emergency that requires rapid diagnosis and treatment. Remember that "TIME IS BRAIN."
- The hallmark of stroke is the abrupt interruption of cerebral blood flow to a specific brain region resulting in neurologic deficits.
- Fluctuation of functional deficits after stroke onset or a brief deficit known as transient ischemic attack (TIA) suggests tissue at risk for infarction that may be rescued by reestablishing perfusion.

Epidemiology

More than 750,000 strokes occur per year in the United States and it is the fourth leading cause of death in the United States.

Etiology

- **Ischemic stroke** can be subclassified into atherothrombotic, embolic, hypoperfusion, or hypercoagulable state (though relatively rare).
  - **Atherothrombosis** results from reduced flow within an artery or embolism of thrombus into the distal segment of an artery.
    - Atherosclerosis is the most common etiology of thrombus formation in large vessels.

- Less common etiologies include dissection, fibromuscular dysplasia, Moyamoya, giant cell arteritis.
- Lipohyalinosis, usually due to hypertension, is the most common etiology of small-vessel disease.
  - **Cardioembolic** strokes account for about 20% of all ischemic strokes. High-risk cardiac sources include atrial fibrillation, sustained atrial flutter, rheumatic valve disease, atrial or ventricular thrombus, dilated cardiomyopathy, prosthetic valve, bacterial endocarditis, nonbacterial endocarditis (antiphospholipid antibody syndrome, marantic endocarditis, Libman–Sachs endocarditis), sick sinus syndrome, and coronary artery bypass graft (CABG) surgery.
  - **Hypoperfusion** occurs due to general circulatory problems and often results in bilateral symptoms. Infarction commonly occurs in border zones between large vessels, resulting in watershed infarcts.
  - Hypercoagulable states may predispose to arterial thrombosis. These include sickle cell disease, polycythemia vera, essential thrombocythemia, thrombotic thrombocytopenic purpura (TTP), antiphospholipid antibody syndrome, hyperhomocysteinemia, etc.
  - Factor V Leiden, protein C and S deficiency, and anti-thrombin (AT)-III deficiency typically result in venous, not arterial infarcts.
- **Hemorrhagic stroke** occurs in about 20% of all cases.
  - The location of an **intraparenchymal hemorrhage (IPH)** may suggest its etiology.
    - Hemorrhage in basal ganglia, thalamus, or pons is often due to chronic systemic hypertension.
    - Amyloid angiopathy typically causes lobar hemorrhages and is a common etiology in the elderly.
    - Head trauma, anticoagulants, drugs (cocaine or amphetamines), arteriovenous malformation (AVM), tumor, blood dyscrasia, hemorrhagic conversion of an ischemic stroke, and vasculitis are other possible hemorrhagic stroke etiologies.
  - **Subarachnoid hemorrhage (SAH)** is caused by the rupture of an arterial aneurysm resulting in bleeding into the subarachnoid space (which contains CSF). Hypertension, cigarette smoking, genetic factors, and septic emboli (resulting in mycotic aneurysms) can all contribute to an aneurysm formation.
- **Cerebral venous sinus thrombosis** is the occlusion of a venous sinus(es) by a thrombus. Occurs in hypercoagulable states such as late pregnancy, postpartum, cancer, and thrombophilias, as well as with trauma and adjacent inflammation/infection. May manifest with ischemic infarcts and/or hemorrhage.

Risk Factors

Major significant risk factors for ischemic stroke include hypertension, TIA, prior stroke, carotid stenosis, diabetes mellitus (DM), dyslipidemia, cigarette smoking, alcohol consumption, oral contraceptive use, obesity, genetics, and age.

DIAGNOSIS

Clinical Presentation

History

- Time of onset is critical if thrombolytic therapy is to be administered. Time of onset is when the patient was last seen normal and NOT when the patient was found with their deficit.

- Onset of symptoms is typically sudden. Ask about progression or fluctuation of symptoms and when the patient was **last normal**.
- Prior TIA symptoms (e.g., transient monocular loss of vision, aphasia, dysarthria, paresis, or sensory disturbance) suggest atherosclerotic vascular disease, the most common cause for stroke.
- Inquire about cardiac arrhythmias and atherosclerotic risk factors.
- A history of neck trauma or recent chiropractic maneuvers warrants evaluation for arterial dissection.
- SAH commonly presents with sudden onset of a severe headache (i.e., the "worst headache of my life.") Lethargy or coma, fever, vomiting, seizures, and low back pain may also be present.
- IPH presents with neurologic deficits accompanied by headache, vomiting, and possibly lethargy.
- Venous sinus thrombosis often presents with signs and symptoms of elevated intracranial pressure, such as headache, bilateral sixth nerve palsies, blurred vision, and papilledema.

Physical Examination
- A careful neurologic examination can reliably establish the anatomic location of a stroke in most cases.
- In general, carotid artery distribution (anterior circulation) strokes produce combinations of functional deficits (hemiparesis, hemianopsia, cortical sensory loss, often with aphasias or agnosias) contralateral to the affected hemisphere.
- Vertebral-basilar strokes (posterior circulation) produce unilateral or bilateral motor/sensory deficits, usually accompanied by cranial nerve and brainstem signs (vertigo, diplopia, ataxia).
- Horner's syndrome (ptosis, miosis, anhidrosis) contralateral to an acute hemiparesis suggests carotid dissection. A Horner's syndrome with nystagmus and ipsilateral loss of facial pain and temperature sensation with contralateral loss of body pain and temperature sensation is diagnostic of a lateral medullary (posterior inferior cerebellar artery [PICA]) infarct (i.e., Wallenberg syndrome).
- General physical exam should be focused on possible etiologic factors. Examine for abnormal pulses, arrhythmias, murmurs, carotid bruits, and embolic phenomena.

Differential Diagnosis
Mimics of stroke include postseizure paralysis (Todd's paralysis), migraine with neurologic deficit, and hypoglycemia or hyperglycemia.

Diagnostic Testing
Laboratories
- In the acute setting (e.g., acute evaluation for thrombolytic therapy), these should include CBC with platelets, prothrombim time (PT), international normalized ratio (INR), activated partial thromboplastin time (aPTT), and blood glucose.
- The following are indicated but not emergent: basic metabolic panel (BMP), troponin, lipid profile, hemoglobin A1c (HgbA1C). Tests such as erythrocyte sedimentation rate (ESR) and blood cultures (if suspect endocarditis), rapid plasma reagin (RPR), antinuclear antibody, anticardiolipin antibody, drug toxicology screen, and human immunodeficiency virus (HIV) are not part of a "standard screen" but may be indicated in the appropriate clinical contexts.

Electrocardiography

Electrocardiogram (ECG) should be done to look for atrial fibrillation or ischemic changes.

Imaging

- **Noncontrast head CT** scan should be obtained acutely to rapidly differentiate hemorrhagic from ischemic strokes. It can identify acute hemorrhages in most cases. It is insensitive for acute ischemic strokes. It is often the rate limiting step in making decisions on thrombolytic therapy. Head CT scan is diagnostic of SAH in 90% of SAH patients in the first 24 hours.
- **MRI** scan is the most sensitive imaging study for stroke diagnosis. Diffusion-weighted images detect stroke the earliest. If a diagnosis of stroke is clear from clinical exam, MRI is not always necessary as it is unlikely to affect management in a great majority of cases.
- MR angiography (MRA) and venograms are useful noninvasive tests to evaluate large arteries and veins, respectively. MRA of the neck with contrast can serve as a screen for carotid stenosis.
- **Carotid Doppler** studies enable noninvasive estimation of carotid stenosis and should be done for anterior circulation strokes.
- **Two-dimensional transthoracic echocardiography (2D TTE)** is helpful to demonstrate intracardiac thrombi, valve vegetations, valvular stenosis or insufficiency, and right-to-left shunt (bubble study). In some patients, transesophageal echocardiography (TEE) may be necessary to evaluate the left atrium for thrombi.

Diagnostic Procedures

- **Cerebral angiography** is the definitive study for vascular malformations but may miss small aneurysms. Some surgeons prefer having this procedure performed before proceeding with carotid endarterectomy (CEA).
- If suspicion for SAH is high and head CT is negative, **lumbar puncture** is necessary to confirm the diagnosis.
  - Tubes 1 and 4 should be sent for cell count. If the number of red blood cells (RBCs) decreases dramatically from tube 1 to tube 4, a traumatic LP is more likely than SAH.
  - Bloody CSF should be centrifuged and examined for xanthochromia (yellow color). Xanthochromia results from RBC lysis and takes several hours to develop, indicating SAH rather than a traumatic LP.

TREATMENT

- Vital signs, including oximetry and continuous telemetry, should be monitored.
- Hypertension management after ischemic stroke:
  - Perfusion pressure in areas of the brain distal to the arterial occlusion may be low. Cerebral perfusion depends in part on mean systemic arterial pressure. Thus, a degree of hypertension may be necessary to maintain adequate perfusion pressure to injured areas.
  - Aggressive lowering of blood pressure (BP) has been associated with neurologic deterioration (*Neurology 2003;61(8):1047*), although there exists an ongoing debate in the field on this topic (see the following text).
  - Patients with acute stroke often present hypertensive. BP tends to fall on its own over several days following a stroke.
  - While management of hypertension in the setting of acute stroke remains controversial, BP should not be lowered acutely unless necessary for treatment of acute

coronary syndrome (ACS), CHF, hypertensive crisis with end-organ involvement or systolic BP >220 or diastolic BP >120 (*Stroke 2007;38(5):1655*). BP lowering should proceed cautiously, with 15% during the first 24 hours being a reasonable goal.

- Treatment of intracranial hemorrhage consists of supportive care, gradual reduction in BP, and elevation of head of bed by 15 degrees.
- Treatment of SAH depends on etiology (surgical clipping versus intravascular coiling)
  - Supportive measures include bed rest, sedation, analgesia, and laxatives to prevent sudden increases in intracranial pressure.
  - Volume expansion, induced hypertension, and balloon dilation can occasionally be used to reverse neurologic deterioration due to vasospasm.

Medications

- Recombinant tissue plasminogen activator (rt-PA) remains the only FDA-approved pharmacologic therapy for acute ischemic stroke, with additional therapies likely to follow in the near future.
  - Administration of rt-PA must commence within 4.5 hours of stroke onset (*N Engl J Med 2008;359(13):1317*) but should be started as close to onset as possible (i.e., do not delay if early in 4.5-hour window to see if the patient "gets better" on their own).
  - rt-PA treatment increases risk for symptomatic brain hemorrhage, compared to placebo, but without any significant impact on 3- and 12-month mortality rates.
  - Exclusion criteria for the 0- to 3-hour and 3- to 4.5-hour windows are available in Tables 26-4 and 26-5. However, the acute stroke team should be contacted emergently to evaluate ALL acute strokes, as some patients with exclusion for IV t-PA may be eligible for other interventions, such as intra-arterial t-PA or intra-arterial catheter-based interventions.
  - Aspirin, heparin, and warfarin should be held for the first 24 hours post rt-PA.
- Other treatments, including intra-arterial thrombolysis and clot retrieval, which are only available at some centers.
- Aspirin reduces atherosclerotic stroke morbidity and mortality and is typically given at an initial dose of 325 mg within 24 to 48 hours of stroke onset. The dose may be reduced to 81 mg in the post–acute stroke period.
- Other antiplatelet-aggregating drugs (clopidogrel, aspirin/dipyridamole) are available and may be of benefit for certain patients. Both of these drugs have a significant advantage over aspirin in secondary stroke prevention. However, there is no evidence to suggest any benefit to dual antiplatelet therapy for secondary stroke prevention.
- Heparin, low–molecular-weight heparin (LMWH), or warfarin anticoagulation are NOT recommended for acute ischemic stroke.
- Anticoagulation with warfarin, dabigatran, rivaroxaban, or apixaban are indicated to prevent recurrent embolic strokes due to atrial fibrillation. Target INR with Coumadin therapy is 2 to 3 (*Stroke 2007;38(5):1655*).
- Nimodipine, a calcium channel blocker, improves outcome in SAH patients and may reduce the incidence of associated cerebral infarction with few side effects.
- Anticoagulation with heparin/LMWH followed by warfarin is indicated for venous sinus thrombosis both with and without hemorrhagic infarcts. Boluses of heparin to correct the aPTT should be avoided in the setting of hemorrhage. aPTTs should be closely monitored and maintained between 60 and 80 seconds.

Table 26-4	Inclusion/Exclusion Criteria for 0 to 3 Hr Intravenous tPA for Acute Stroke

tPA Eligibility

1. Age ≥18 yr
2. Clinical diagnosis of ischemic stroke causing measurable neurologic deficit and noncontrast head CT showing no hemorrhage.
3. Onset of stroke symptoms well established to be less than 180 min (3 hr) before treatment would begin.

Contraindications

1. Symptoms minor or rapidly improving.
2. Other stroke or serious head trauma within past 3 mo.
3. Major surgery within last 14 d.
4. Known history of intracranial hemorrhage.
5. Sustained systolic blood pressure >185 mm Hg.
6. Sustained diastolic blood pressure >110 mm Hg.
7. Aggressive treatment necessary to lower blood pressure.
8. Symptoms suggestive of subarachnoid hemorrhage
9. Received heparin within 48 hr and has elevated PTT[**]
10. Patient has received treatment (not prophylactic) doses of injectable anticoagulants (e.g., enoxaparin) in the past 48 hr.[**]
11. Patient has taken dabigatran in the last 48 hr (regardless of PTT).[**]
12. Patient has taken dabigatran in >48 hr AND has an elevated PTT.[**]
13. Arterial puncture at noncompressible site within 7 d.
14. GI or GU hemorrhage within 21 d.
15. International normalized ratio (INR) >1.7.[**]
16. Platelet count <100,000/mL.
17. Seizure at onset of stroke (with deficits thought to be related to ictal or post-ictal state and not new stroke).
18. Serum glucose <50 mg/dL. (If glucose is >400 mg/dL, consider other etiology such as unmasking of old deficits vs. new stroke.)

[**]Because time is critical, thrombolytic therapy should not be delayed while waiting for the results of the PT, PTT, or platelet count unless a bleeding abnormality or thrombocytopenia is suspected, the patient has been taking warfarin, heparin, or dabigatran, or anticoagulation use is uncertain.

CT, computed tomography; GI, gastrointestinal; GU, genitourinary; PT, prothrombin time; PTT, partial thromboplastin time; t-PA, tissue plasminogen activator.

Data from AHA Acute Stroke Treatment Guidelines 2007. *Stroke* 2007;38(5):1655.

Other Nonpharmacologic Therapies

- Physical, occupational, and speech therapy can aid in stroke rehabilitation.
- Stroke patients with obvious dysphagia, dysarthria, or a facial droop should be kept nothing by mouth (NPO) until an experienced individual can assess their swallowing abilities.

Surgical Management

- CEA decreases the risk of stroke and death in patients with recent TIAs or nondisabling strokes and ipsilateral high-grade (70% to 99%) carotid stenosis (*N Engl J Med* 1991;325(7):445).

Table 26-5	Inclusion/Exclusion Criteria for 3.0 to 4.5 Hr Intravenous tPA for Acute Stroke

tPA Eligibility

1. Age 18–**80 yr**.
2. Clinical diagnosis of ischemic stroke causing measurable neurologic deficit and noncontrast head CT showing no hemorrhage.
3. Onset of stroke symptoms well established to be between **3.0 and 4.5 hr** before treatment would begin.

Contraindications

1. Symptoms minor or rapidly improving.
2. Seizure at onset of stroke.
3. Major surgery or significant trauma **in past 3 mo**.
4. Blood glucose <50 or **>400 mg/dL**.
5. Prior stroke within the last 3 mo.
6. Known history of or suspected ICH.
7. Systolic blood pressure >185 mm Hg or diastolic blood pressure >110 mm Hg, or aggressive management (**more than a single dose of IV medication**) necessary to reduce BP to these limits.
8. Symptoms suggestive of SAH.
9. Recent (**<10 d**) puncture of a noncompressible blood vessel, external heart massage, or obstetrical delivery.
10. Received heparin within previous 48 hr and an elevated PTT.
11. **Patients receiving Coumadin even with normal PT/INR.**
12. **History of CNS damage** (e.g., neoplasm, aneurysm, intracranial or spinal surgery).
13. Patient has received treatment (not prophylactic) doses of injectable anticoagulants (e.g., enoxaparin) in the past 48 hr.
14. Patient has taken dabigatran in the last 48 hr (regardless of PTT).
15. Patient has taken dabigatran in >48 hr AND has an elevated PTT.
16. Platelet count of below 100,000/mL.
17. Severe stroke assessed clinically (**NIHSS >25**) or by imaging (**>1/3 involvement MCA**).
18. History of prior **disabling** stroke (**MRS 2 or more) and diabetes requiring treatment**.
19. Known hemorrhagic diathesis.
20. Recent severe/dangerous bleeding.
21. **Hemorrhagic retinopathy** (e.g., in diabetes, vision disturbance may indicate hemorrhagic retinopathy).
22. **Acute pancreatitis, documented ulcerative GI disease during last 3 mo, esophageal varices, arterial-aneurysm, or AVM.**
23. **Other major disorders associated with a risk of bleeding** such known bacterial endocarditis, pericarditis, or severe liver disease.

(**BOLD** is different from 0–3 hr criteria.)
AVM, arteriovenous malformation; BP, blood pressure; CNS, central nervous system; CT, computed tomography; GI, gastrointestinal; ICH, intracranial hemorrhage; IV, intravenous; MCA, middle cerebral artery; MRS, modified Rankin Scale; NIHSS, National Institute of Health stroke scale; PT/INR, prothrombin time/international normalized ratio; PTT, partial thromboplastin time; SAH, subarachnoid hemorrhage; tPA, tissue plasminogen activator.

Table 26-6	Secondary Stroke Prevention ("BLASTED")

- **B**lood pressure
- **L**DL
- **A**SA (**a**ntiplatelet), **A**1c
- **S**troke management and rehabilitation team (varies from facility to facility)
  ○ PT, OT, ST, stroke educator, diabetes educator, smoking cessation counseling
- **T**elemetry
- **E**chocardiography
- **D**opplers, **d**iabetes (A1c, educator, etc.)

ASA, acetylsalicylic acid; LDL, low-density lipoprotein; OT, occupational therapy; PT, physical therapy; ST, speech therapy.

- ○ The CREST (Carotid Revascularization Endarterectomy Versus Stenting) trial provides evidence to suggest that carotid stenting is of equal efficacy to CEA (*N Engl J Med 2010;363:11*).
  - ○ Recommendations from a neurologist should be solicited before deciding on which of the two approaches is indicated.
- CEA for asymptomatic high-grade carotid stenosis (≥60%) reduces the 5-year risk of ipsilateral stroke in men, provided that the operator's surgical/angiography complication rate is <3% (*JAMA 1995;273(18):1421; Stroke 2004;35(10):2425*).
- Hemicraniectomy may increase survival in certain patients with large hemispheric infarcts and severe edema. Neurosurgical consultation should be obtained early in these cases.
- Cerebellar infarction or hematomas may result in brainstem compression or obstructive hydrocephalus, which warrant urgent neurosurgical intervention.

Lifestyle/Risk Modification

Modifiable risk factors (see Table 26-6) include
- BP reduction even in normotensive stroke patients is beneficial (*Lancet 2001; 358(9287):1033*).
- Diabetes control is important with care taken to avoid hypoglycemia and hyperglycemia.
- Smoking cessation.
- Cholesterol (serum lipids): Low-density lipoprotein (LDL) <100 mg/dL with some evidence from the SPARCL trial to suggest a more aggressive target of <70 mg/dL (*N Engl J Med 2006;355:549*).
- Treat obstructive sleep apnea (OSA).
- Oral contraceptives may need to be discontinued in women with stroke.

COMPLICATIONS

- Cerebral edema following ischemic stroke peaks at 48 to 72 hours post stroke and patients need to be watched closely during this time.

- Hemorrhagic conversion of an ischemic stroke is more likely in patients who are receiving anticoagulation or in patients with large strokes, particularly those with embolic ischemic infarcts.

Headache

GENERAL PRINCIPLES

Classification

- **Primary headache syndromes** include migraines with (classic) or without (common) aura, the hemicranias and indomethacin-responsive headaches, tension headaches, chronic daily headaches, and cluster headaches.
- **Secondary headaches** have specific etiologies, and symptomatic features vary depending on the underlying pathology (i.e., SAH, tumor, hypertension, posterior reversible encephalopathy syndrome [PRES], analgesic overuse, iatrogenic).
- **Migraine without aura (common):** At least five attacks that last 4 to 72 hours. Symptoms should include at least two of the following: unilateral location, pulsating or throbbing, moderate to severe in intensity, aggravated by activity, and at least one of these associated features: nausea/vomiting, photophobia, and/or phonophobia.
- **Migraine with aura (classic):** Same as the aforementioned, except at least two attacks with an associated aura that lasts from 4 minutes to 1 hour (longer than 60 minutes is a red flag). The aura should have a gradual onset, be fully reversible, and can occur before, with, or after headache onset.
- **Cluster headache:** Unilateral orbital or temporal pain with lacrimation, conjunctival injection, nasal congestion, rhinorrhea, facial swelling, miosis, ptosis, and eyelid edema.
- **Rebound headache** (analgesic overuse headache) occurs in the setting of chronic use of analgesics or narcotics.
- **Trigeminal neuralgia** presents as episodic sharp stabbing pain that is unilateral. Rule out multiple sclerosis.
- **Temporal arteritis** presents as a dull unilateral headache with a thick tortuous artery over temporal region. The disease is almost exclusively limited to individuals over 60 years of age with jaw claudication, low-grade fever, and an elevated ESR and C-reactive protein (CRP).

Etiology

Secondary headache etiologies include:

- Subdural hematoma (SDH), intracerebral hematoma, SAH, AVM, brain abscess, meningitis, encephalitis, vasculitis, obstructive hydrocephalus, and cerebral ischemia or infarction.
- Idiopathic intracranial hypertension (pseudotumor cerebri) presents with headache, papilledema, diplopia, and elevated CSF pressure (>20 cm H_2O in relaxed lateral decubitus position).
- Extracranial causes include giant cell arteritis, sinusitis, glaucoma, optic neuritis, dental disease (including temporomandibular joint syndrome), and disorders of the cervical spine.
- Systemic causes include fever, viremia, hypoxia, carbon monoxide poisoning, hypercapnia, systemic hypertension, allergy, anemia, caffeine withdrawal, and vasoactive or toxic chemicals (nitrites).

- Depression is a common cause of long-standing, treatment-resistant headaches. Specific inquiry about vegetative signs of depression and exclusion of other causes help support this diagnosis.

DIAGNOSIS

Clinical Presentation

History
- The sudden onset of severe headache (**worst headache of my life**) or a severe persistent headache that reaches maximal intensity within a few seconds/minutes warrants immediate investigation for possible SAH.
- History should focus on:
  - Age at onset
  - Frequency, intensity, and duration of attacks
  - Triggers, associations (menstrual cycle), associated symptoms (photophobia, phonophobia, nausea, vomiting, etc.), and alleviating factors
  - Location and quality of pain (sharp, dull, etc.)
  - Number of headaches per month, including number of disabling headaches
  - Family history of migraines
  - Sleep and diet hygiene (caffeine intake)
  - Use of pain medications, including over-the-counter medications

Physical Examination
- On general examination check BP and pulse, listen for possible bruits, palpate head and neck muscles, and check temporal arteries.
- If neck stiffness and meningismus (resistance to passive neck flexion) present on exam then consider meningitis.
- If papilledema observed on exam consider an intracranial mass, meningitis, or idiopathic intracranial hypertension.

Diagnostic Testing

Imaging
Neuroimaging is generally not indicated for known primary headache syndromes, but may be required to exclude secondary etiologies in cases that have not been previously diagnosed or in patients presenting with new headaches, especially those that present with atypical features or abnormal findings.

Diagnostic Procedures
LP is indicated in a patient with severe headache with suspicion of SAH even if the head CT scan is negative.

TREATMENT

- **Acute treatment of migraine**, the most common primary headache syndrome, is directed at aborting the headache. This is easier at onset and often very difficult when the attack is well established. Accordingly, the threshold for treating at the first sign of a headache should be low. Patients have often used nonprescription analgesics (acetylsalicylic acid [ASA], acetaminophen, nonsteroidal anti-inflammatory drugs [NSAIDs]) and oral prescription medications (butalbital with aspirin or acetaminophen), which are the first-line treatments and are most effective early in the course of an attack. Emergent treatments include serotonin agonists and other parenteral medications.

- **Triptans** (serotonin receptor $5HT_{1B}$ and $5HT_{1D}$ agonists) are effective abortive medications available in multiple formulations and may be effective even in a protracted attack. Triptans should not be used in patients with coronary artery disease, cerebrovascular disease, uncontrolled hypertension, hemiplegic migraine, or vertebrobasilar migraine.
- **Dihydroergotamine** (DHE) is a potent venoconstrictor with minimal peripheral arterial constriction. Cardiac precautions are indicated in those with a history of angina, peripheral vascular disease, or elderly patients.
- **Ergotamine** is a vasoconstrictive agent effective for aborting migraine headaches, particularly if administered during the prodromal phase. Ergotamine should be taken at symptom onset in the maximum dose tolerated by the patient; nausea often limits the dose. Rectal preparations are better absorbed than oral agents.
- Chronic daily headaches should not be treated with narcotic analgesics so as to prevent addiction, rebound headaches, and tachyphylaxis.
- Treatment of secondary headaches is directed at the primary etiology, such as surgical treatment of cerebral aneurysm causing SAH, evacuation of subdural hematoma, or shunting obstructive hydrocephalus.
- **Prophylactic medications** should be considered if a patient has at least three disabling migraines per month.
  - It is important to review a patient's use of all medications and comorbidities as they may influence choice of medication and offer additional factors contributing to the headache syndrome.
  - Possible prophylactic medications include propranolol, topiramate, tricyclic anti-depressants (TCAs) (amitriptyline, nortriptyline), and now less commonly, val-proic acid. Second-line agents include verapamil, selective serotonin reuptake inhibitors (SSRIs), and serotonin-norepinephrine reuptake inhibitors (SNRIs).

Lifestyle Modifications

- Patients should keep a headache calendar to identify possible triggers.
- Patients should reduce alcohol, caffeine, and other triggers that may increase risk of migraines.

REFERRAL

Neurosurgical consultation is indicated for managing SAH, SDH, vascular malformations, tumors, and other space occupying lesions resulting in mass effect. Neurologic consultation is indicated if a patient is not well controlled on a first-line prophylactic agent with appropriate use of an abortive therapy.

Head Trauma

GENERAL PRINCIPLES

Definition

- **Traumatic brain injury (TBI)** can occur with head injury due to contact and/or acceleration/deceleration forces.

- **Concussion:** Trauma-induced alteration in mental status with normal radiographic studies that may or may not involve loss of consciousness.
- **Contusion:** Trauma-induced lesion consisting of punctate hemorrhages and surrounding edema.

Classification

- Closed head injuries may produce axonal injury.
- Contusion or hemorrhage can occur at site of initial impact "coup injury" or, opposite to the side of impact, "countercoup injury."
- Penetrating injuries (including depressed skull fracture) or foreign objects cause brain injury directly.
- Secondary increases in intracranial pressure may compromise cerebral perfusion.

Epidemiology

- The overall incidence of TBI in the United States is estimated at ~550 per 100,000 population.
- Rates of TBI are highest in the very young, adolescents, and the elderly.

DIAGNOSIS

Clinical Presentation

- Patients will often present with confusion and amnesia, including loss of memory for the traumatic event as well as inability to recall events both immediately before and after trauma.
- Patients may complain of nonspecific signs including headache, vertigo, nausea, vomiting, and personality changes.
- Intracerebral hematomas may be present initially or develop after a contusion.
- Epidural hematoma is usually associated with skull fractures across a meningeal artery and may cause precipitous deterioration after a **lucid interval**.
- Subdural hematoma is most common in aged, debilitated, and alcoholic individuals and in anticoagulated patients. Antecedent trauma may be minimal or absent.

Physical Examination

- Careful examination for penetrating wounds and other injuries.
- Hemotympanum, mastoid ecchymosis (Battle's sign), periorbital ecchymosis ("raccoon eyes"), and CSF otorrhea/rhinorrhea are indicative of a basilar skull fracture.
- Neurologic examination should focus on the level of consciousness, focal deficits, and signs of herniation. The GCS should be used for an assessment. Serial examinations must be performed and documented to identify neurologic deterioration.
- Degree of impairment due to trauma can be classified using injury severity scores; with GCS being the most common.
- Treatment and diagnostic assessment of patients with severe head injury at admission is done according to the Advanced Trauma Life Support (ATLS) protocol.
- The Standardized Assessment of Concussion (SAC) is a standardized tool for the sideline evaluation of athletes who suffer a head injury.

Diagnostic Testing

Imaging

- Head CT should be considered for patients with GCS <15 two hours after trauma, suspected skull fracture, repeated episodes of vomiting after trauma, >65 years old, dangerous mechanism (e.g., pedestrian struck by motor vehicle, occupant ejected from motor vehicle, fall from ≥3 ft or ≥ five stairs), drug or alcohol intoxication, or persistent anterograde amnesia.
- Noncontrast head CT scan in the emergency room (ER) can rapidly identify intracranial hemorrhage and contusion.
  - A lenticular-shaped extra-axial hematoma is characteristic of epidural hematoma.
  - Bone window views may help to locate fractures, if present.
- Cervical radiographs ± CT of the neck must be performed to exclude fracture or dislocation.
- MRI can assist in evaluation of TBI patients with persistent sequelae as it is more sensitive for demonstrating small areas of contusion or petechial hemorrhage, axonal injury, and small extra-axial hematomas.

TREATMENT

- Hospital admission is recommended for patients at risk for immediate complications from head injury. These include patients with GCS <15, abnormal CT scan, intracranial bleeding, cerebral edema, seizures, or abnormal bleeding parameters.
- When admitted, continuously monitor vital signs and oximetry. ECG should be performed. Arterial pressure monitoring in conjunction with intracranial monitoring may be indicated.
- Immobilize the neck in a hard cervical collar to avoid spinal cord injury from manipulating an unstable or fractured cervical spine.
- **Avoid hypotonic fluids** to limit cerebral edema.
- Steroids are not indicated for head injury.
- Avoid hypoventilation and systemic hypotension as they may reduce cerebral perfusion.
- Anticipate and conservatively treat increased intracranial pressure:
  - Head midline and elevated 30 degrees.
  - In the mechanically ventilated patient, modest hyperventilation (PCO_2 ~35 mm Hg) reduces intracranial pressure by cerebral vasoconstriction; excessive hyperventilation may reduce cerebral perfusion. Remember that these are merely temporizing measures and neurosurgical consultation is always warranted if there is concern for increased intracranial pressure due to head injury.
- Neurologic deterioration after head injury of any severity requires an immediate repeat head CT scan to differentiate between an expanding hematoma that necessitates surgery from diffuse cerebral edema that requires monitoring and reduction of intracranial pressure.
- The use of AEDs in the acute management of TBI can reduce the incidence of early seizures but does not prevent development of epilepsy at a later time. Furthermore, certain AEDs can have adverse effects on cognition and so these agents should only be used when clinically indicated, with careful consideration of the specific agent chosen. There is no evidence to support AED use for seizure prophylaxis.

- Because the risk of a second impact may lead to severe complications, guidelines have been proposed for when individuals can return to play (*PM&R 2009;1(5):406*).

Surgical Management

- Neurosurgical consultation is indicated for patients with contusion, intracranial hematoma, cervical fracture, skull fractures, penetrating injuries, or focal neurologic deficits.
- In some cases of closed head injury complicated by increased intracranial pressure, intracranial pressure monitoring assists medical management.
- Evacuation of chronic subdural hematoma is determined by the symptoms and degree of mass effect.

Acute Spinal Cord Dysfunction

GENERAL PRINCIPLES

- Spinal cord dysfunction is demonstrated by a level below which motor, sensory, and autonomic functions are interrupted.
- **Traumatic spinal cord injury** (TSCI) may be obvious from history or exam but should also be considered in unconscious, confused, or inebriated patients with trauma.
- **Spinal cord concussion** refers to posttraumatic spinal cord symptoms and signs that resolve rapidly (hours to days).

Etiology
See Table 26-7.

DIAGNOSIS

Clinical Presentation

- **Spinal cord compression** often presents with back pain at the level of compression, progressive walking difficulties, sensory impairment, urinary retention with overflow incontinence, and diminished rectal tone. Rapid deterioration may occur.
- **Transverse myelitis or myelopathy** present with symptoms and signs similar to cord compression.
- **Spinal shock** with hypotonia and areflexia may be present soon after traumatic event.
- Acute presentations suggest traumatic or vascular insults, while a subacute course suggests an enlarging mass lesion or infectious process.
- **Radicular signs** (lancinating pain, paresthesias, and numbness in the dermatomal distribution of a nerve root, with weakness and decreased tone and reflexes in muscles supplied by the root) imply inflammation or compression of the nerve root. Tenderness to spinal percussion over the lesion may be present.
- **Spinal cord syndromes include**
  - **Complete cord syndrome:** Bilateral flaccid paralysis (quadriplegia or paraplegia) and loss of all sensation (anesthesia) below a dermatomal level, initially with areflexia and sphincter dysfunction (urinary retention/loss of rectal tone). With time hypertonia and hyperreflexia below the lesion, and extensor plantar responses (Babinski signs).

Table 26-7	Causes of Acute Spinal Cord Dysfunction

Structural

- Tumor (primary or metastatic)
- Herniated disk
- Epidural abscess or hematoma
- Trauma ± fracture of bony elements
- Atlantoaxial instability (e.g., rheumatoid arthritis)
- Fibrocartilaginous

Ischemia/infarction (particularly after aortic surgery)

- Aortic dissection or surgery
- Embolic (cardiogenic, gaseous embolus)
- Prolonged hypotension with underlying vascular disease

Vascular malformations (e.g., AVM)
Inflammatory/infectious (transverse myelitis)

- Multiple sclerosis
- Neuromyelitis optica (longitudinally extensive, > three spinal segments)
- Parainfectious processes (e.g., postmycoplasma pneumoniae)
- Sarcoidosis
- Paraneoplastic
- Systemic lupus erythematosus
- Sjögren syndrome
- Behcet's disease
- Viruses (e.g., entero, HSV, HIV, VZV)
- Tuberculosis
- Syphilis
- HIV

AVM, arteriovenous malformation; HSV, herpes simplex virus; VZV, varicella-zoster virus.

○ **Brown-Séquard syndrome:** Unilateral cord lesion resulting in contralateral pain and temperature loss, with ipsilateral weakness and proprioceptive loss.
○ **Anterior cord syndrome** often results from anterior spinal artery lesion and produces bilateral pain and temperature loss and weakness below the site of the lesion with preserved proprioception and vibratory sensation.
○ **Cauda equina syndrome** from compression of the lower lumbar and sacral roots produces sensory loss in a saddle distribution, flaccid leg weakness, decreased reflexes, and urinary/bowel incontinence.
○ **Central cord syndrome** is often characterized by motor impairment in upper extremities more than lower extremities, bladder dysfunction, and variable degree of sensory loss at the site of the lesion.

Diagnostic Testing

Imaging

- The presence and extent of spinal cord injuries should be confirmed with neuroimaging.

- Plain radiographs of the spine may reveal metastatic disease, osteomyelitis, discitis, fractures, or dislocation.
- Emergent MRI scan of the entire cord can confirm exact level and extent of the lesion(s). Myelography is rarely used but may be necessary in individuals unable to undergo MRI.

Diagnostic Procedures
- Lumbar puncture: Inflammatory and infectious etiologies often require CSF analysis for pleocytosis, malignant cells, abnormal protein/glucose, oligoclonal bands, and immunoglobulin (Ig)G index; if indicated, tests for specific pathogens and cytology/flow cytometry can be considered. Imaging should be performed prior to cautiously attempting a LP. Remember to always check an opening pressure if possible and always save CSF.
- Spinal angiogram is the gold standard diagnostic test to evaluate for a spinal AVM. However, in the setting of a good quality normal MRI, there is low likelihood of finding an abnormality on spinal angiography.

TREATMENT

- Vital signs should be continuously monitored, and adequate oxygenation and perfusion ensured.
- Respiratory insufficiency from high cervical cord injuries requires immediate airway control and ventilatory assistance, without manipulation of the neck.
- Immobilization, especially of the neck, is essential to prevent further injury while the patient's condition is stabilized and radiographic and neurosurgical assessment of the injuries is performed.
- Autonomic dysfunction may occur leading to fluctuating vital signs and BP. Bladder distension can cause sympathetic overactivity (headache, tachycardia, diaphoresis, and hypertension) as a result of autonomic dysreflexia.
  - Management of autonomic dysreflexia should incorporate the help of a spinal cord rehab specialist. These patients require strict attention to bowel and bladder functions (e.g., manual disimpaction, promotility agents, straight catheterization) as a means to prevent an autonomic crisis.
  - Do not treat fluctuations in vital signs blindly, as changes can occur precipitously with potential for iatrogenic injury. Always look first for a cause and treat fluctuations in heart rate or BP with caution.

Medications
- Treatable infections require appropriate antibiotics (i.e., acyclovir for herpes simplex).
- **Dexamethasone**, 10 to 20 mg IV bolus followed by 2 to 4 mg IV q6–8 h, is often administered for compressive lesions, tumors, or spinal cord infarction, although benefit has not been proven for all etiologies.
- For TSCI, **methylprednisolone**, 30 mg/kg IV bolus, followed by an infusion of 5.4 mg/kg/hr for 24 hours when initiated within 3 hours of injury, and infusion for 48 hours when initiated within 3 to 8 hours of injury, may improve neurologic recovery.
- LMWH can be considered to reduce chance of venous thromboembolism and pulmonary embolism.

Surgical Management

Neurosurgical consultation should be obtained because in many cases, spinal cord compression can be decompressed and stabilized. Penetrating injury, foreign bodies, comminuted fractures, misalignment, and hematoma may require surgical treatment.

SPECIAL CONSIDERATIONS

Emergent radiation therapy combined with high-dose steroids is usually indicated for cord compression due to malignancy and generally requires a histologic diagnosis.

MONITORING/FOLLOW-UP

Long-term supportive care is important for patients with spinal cord dysfunction. Pulmonary and urinary infections, skin breakdown, joint contractures, spasticity, and irregular bowel and bladder elimination are common long-term problems.

Parkinson's Disease

GENERAL PRINCIPLES

- Parkinson's disease (PD) is a chronic, progressive neurodegenerative disease characterized by at least two of three cardinal features: resting tremor, bradykinesia, and rigidity. Often, postural instability is seen later in the disease.
- The neurologic exam remains the gold standard diagnostic test for the PD.
- Cognitive dysfunction and dementia are common in PD (one-third of patients in most studies, six times higher than age matched controls).
  - One-third of PD patients are depressed.
  - Olfactory dysfunction and sleep disorders are also common in PD and have a significant impact on quality of life.

Epidemiology

Over 1 million people in the United States have been diagnosed with PD. Usually, the onset of diagnosis is after 50 years of age. Approximately 1% of the population over 50 years of age has the disorder.

DIAGNOSIS

Clinical Presentation

- The parkinsonian tremor is a resting pill rolling tremor (3 to 7 Hz) that is often asymmetric (*Lancet Neurol 2006;5(1):75*).
- Bradykinesia is characterized by generalized slowness of movement, especially in finger movement dexterity and gait (often shuffling).
- Cogwheel rigidity is often observed with a ratchety pattern of resistance and relaxation as examiner moves limbs ("cog wheeling" is due to the rigidity with a superimposed tremor).
- Postural instability can be assessed by the "pull" test, where the examiner pulls the patient by the shoulders while standing behind them.

| Table 26-8 | Differential Diagnosis of Parkinson's Disease |

- Essential tremor
  - Action tremor
- Dementia with Lewy bodies (DLB)
  - Visual hallucinations, fluctuating cognition, sensitivity to neuroleptics
- Alzheimer's disease (AD)
- Frontotemporal dementia (FTD)
  - Changes in personality
- Corticobasal degeneration
- Huntington's disease
- Wilson's disease and other neurodegenerative disorders with metal accumulation
- Toxic/iatrogenic
  - Carbon monoxide, manganese, neuroleptics, other dopamine receptor antagonists

- Other signs that are often associated but not required for diagnosis include masked-like facies, decreased eye blink, increased salivation, hypokinetic dysarthria, micrographia, and sleep disorders (rapid eye movement [REM] sleep behavior disorder).
- Dementia seen with PD is typically subcortical with psychomotor retardation, memory difficulty, and altered personality. Accordingly, an assessment like MOCA is a better screen than the more commonly used MMSE.

Differential Diagnosis
See Table 26-8.

Diagnostic Testing
MRI of the brain should be performed to exclude specific structural abnormalities.

TREATMENT

Medications
- **Parkinson's patients should not be given neuroleptics or any dopamine-blocking medications** (prochlorperazine, metoclopramide) as this may lead to worsening and prolongation of Parkinson's symptoms (*Expert Opin Drug Saf 2006;5(6):759*). If a neuroleptic is absolutely necessary, quetiapine and clozapine are the safest, but the risk/benefit profile needs to be considered.
- Treatment of PD can be divided into neuroprotective and symptomatic therapy.
- Initiation of symptomatic treatment for a PD patient is determined by the degree to which the patient is functionally impaired.

First Line
- Sinemet is the most effective symptomatic therapy for PD and is often considered when both the patient and the physician decide that quality of life of the patient is being affected by PD.
- Dopamine agonists (pramipexole, ropinirole) can be used as monotherapy or in combination with other antiparkinsonian drugs. They are ineffective in patients who show no response to levodopa. They may possibly delay initiation of Sinemet-induced dyskinesia and motor fluctuations but are less efficacious and have increased adverse effects.

Second Line
- Amantadine and catechol-O-methyl transferase (COMT) inhibitors can help supplement the effects of dopamine replacement therapy and are respectively beneficial with regards to the dyskinesias and fluctuations commonly experienced by patients.
- Anticholinergic drugs are used only in younger patients in whom tremor is the predominant symptom.

Third Line
Deep brain stimulation (DBS) has had a remarkable benefit in PD patients who eventually develop motor fluctuations and dyskinesias unresponsive to oral medications. It is important to note that DBS is not a cure for PD and patients will continue to progress.

COMPLICATIONS

- Patients can develop neuroleptic malignant syndrome (NMS) after sudden withdrawal of levodopa or dopamine agonists.
- Serotonin syndrome can occur when monoamine oxidase inhibitors (MAOIs) are combined with TCAs or SSRIs.

NEUROMUSCULAR DISEASE

Guillain–Barré Syndrome

GENERAL PRINCIPLES

Definition
Guillain–Barré syndrome (GBS) or acute immune demyelinating polyneuropathy (AIDP) is an acute immune mediated polyneuropathy/radiculopathy characterized by weakness and areflexia. Classically, GBS follows a viral infection, vaccination, or surgery, but in many instances no prodrome is identified.

Classification
- Classic GBS is a **demyelinating polyneuropathy/radiculopathy** and is the most common acute immune mediated polyneuropathy.
- Acute axonal neuropathies are characterized by axonal degeneration, rather than demyelination, and is much more common in Japan, China, and third world countries than it is in the United States. It includes:
  ○ Acute motor axonal neuropathy (AMAN; affecting only motor axons) and
  ○ Acute motor–sensory axonal neuropathy (AMSAN; affecting both sensory and motor axons affected).
- Miller–Fisher variant consists of ophthalmoparesis, ataxia, and areflexia. It is thought to be associated with presence of GQ1b antibody in serum.

Pathophysiology
- Infections such as *Campylobacter jejuni*, Cytomegalovirus (CMV), Epstein–Barr virus (EBV), or *Mycoplasma pneumonia* often precede GBS by days to weeks.
- GBS is thought to result from an antibody-mediated attack on these infections. These antibodies cross-react with the myelin or axon components of nerves, most likely due to molecular mimicry.

DIAGNOSIS

Clinical Presentation

- Classic GBS typically presents with progressive, symmetric ascending paralysis.
- Mild asymmetries are common, but major asymmetries are a red flag suggestive of an alternative diagnosis.
- Reflexes are almost always hypoactive or absent. Exceptions exist, especially with the axonal variants.
- Sensory symptoms, such as paresthesias in the hands and feet, are often present, but objective sensory loss is uncommon.
- Facial and/or oropharyngeal weakness occurs in about 70% of affected patients.
- Respiratory failure, necessitating intubation, occurs in 25% to 30% of patients (*Lancet Neurol 2008;7(10):939*).
- Pain in the back, hips, and thighs is common. Pain is among the most common presenting symptoms of GBS in the pediatric population.
- Autonomic instability is common (~60%) and potentially life threatening. Includes tachycardia/bradycardia, hypotension alternating with hypertension, and ileus.

Differential Diagnosis

See Table 26-9.

Table 26-9	Differential Diagnosis of Acute Immune Demyelinating Polyneuropathy

- Acute/initial presentation of chronic inflammatory demyelinating polyneuropathy (CIDP)
- Paraproteinemic/paraneoplastic neuropathy
- Diabetic/nondiabetic lumbosacral radiculoplexopathies
- Sarcoidosis
- Mononeuritis multiplex
- West Nile and polioviruses (usually has fever, CSF pleocytosis, and often asymmetric paralysis)
- HIV
- Lyme disease (if in endemic area)
- Postdiphtheric paralysis
- Tick paralysis
- Botulism
- Arsenic
- Lead
- Chemotherapy
- Acute intermittent porphyria
- Myeloradiculopathy
- Carcinomatous meningitis with root involvement

See *http://neuromuscular.wustl.edu/time/nmacute.htm* for further information.

CSF, cerebral spinal fluid; HIV, human immunodeficiency virus.

Diagnostic Testing

Imaging

MRI of the spine is indicated in atypical cases or in those with concern for one of the differentials listed earlier that could result in a myeloradiculopathy. Nerve root gadolinium enhancement and/or thickening can be seen with GBS.

Diagnostic Procedures

- **LP should be performed to narrow the differential and evaluated for cytoalbuminemic dissociation.**
- CSF protein is usually elevated about 1 week after symptoms onset. It may be normal if checked earlier (e.g., 85% of patients with normal CSF within first 2 days).
- CSF leukocytosis is uncommon and, if present (especially greater than 50 cells/mm^3), an alternative diagnosis should be considered.
- Nerve conduction studies (NCS) and electromyography (EMG) are a very important part of the evaluation but should not delay initiation of treatment, particularly in severe cases. NCS should include evaluation of the proximal nerve segments. It is not uncommon to see normal NCSs early on and subsequently abnormal on repeat studies, which can be extremely useful for comparison purposes.

TREATMENT

- Follow **respiratory function closely**, including oximetry, frequent bedside vital capacity (VC), and negative inspiratory force (NIF). Declining VC (<10 to 15 mL/kg, <1 L) and NIF (<25 cm H_2O) are indications for ventilatory assistance and often occur before hypoxia, dyspnea, and acidosis. The threshold for elective intubation should be low. If NIF/forced vital capacity (FVC) testing are not available at the bedside a quick and indirect measure is to ask the patient to count to as high a number as possible on one breath. Each number = 100 mL of VC (i.e., "10" = 1 L).
- Paroxysmal hypertension should not be treated with antihypertensive medications unless absolutely necessary (e.g., signs of end-organ injury or comorbid coronary artery disease). If necessary, extremely low doses of titratable short-acting agents are preferred.
- Hypotension is usually caused by decreased venous return and peripheral vasodilation. Mechanically ventilated patients are particularly prone to hypotension. Treatment consists of intravascular volume expansion; occasionally, vasopressors may be required (see Chapter 8, Critical Care).
- Continuous telemetry monitoring is necessary to monitor for cardiac arrhythmias.
- Prevention of exposure keratitis of the eye, venous thrombosis, and vigilance for hyponatremia (including syndrome of inappropriate diuretic hormone [SIADH]) should be priorities.

Medications

- **Plasma exchange (PLEX) and IV immunoglobulin (IVIG)** are comparably effective in improving outcomes and shortening duration when administered early to patients who cannot walk or have respiratory failure (*Brain 2007;130(pt 9):2245*). The decision between the two depends on the individual patient's comorbidities and medical history.
- Corticosteroids are not indicated.
- Neuropathic pain medications may be needed.

Other Nonpharmacologic Therapies

Physical therapy to prevent contractures and improve strength and function should be started early.

COMPLICATIONS

Complications from prolonged hospitalization and ventilation may occur. These include aspiration pneumonia, sepsis, pressure ulcers, and pulmonary embolism.

PROGNOSIS

- Disease typically progresses over 2 to 4 weeks, with almost all patients reaching their nadir by 4 weeks.
- This is followed by a plateau of several weeks duration.
- Recovery takes place over months.
  - Overall, about 80% of patients recover completely or have only minor deficits (*Lancet 2005;366(9497):1653*).
  - Of patients, 5% to 10% (usually elderly patients and those with more severe disease) have disabling deficits and 3% remain wheelchair bound.
- About 5% of the patients die due to respiratory or autonomic complications despite optimal medical therapy.
- By definition, GBS is a monophasic disease and a recurrence of symptoms should lead you to revisit the original diagnosis (e.g., consider chronic inflammatory demyelinating polyneuropathy [CIDP]). Repeat electrodiagnostic studies are critical in determining the etiology of an apparent "recurrent GBS."

Myasthenia Gravis

GENERAL PRINCIPLES

Definition

Myasthenia gravis (MG) is an autoimmune disorder that involves antibody-mediated postsynaptic dysfunction of the neuromuscular junction of skeletal muscle resulting in fatigable weakness.

Classification

- Generalized disease is most common and affects a variable combination of ocular, bulbar, respiratory, and appendicular muscles.
- Ocular MG is confined to eyelid and oculomotor function. Accounts for 10% to 40% of all MG cases. The longer a patient with ocular MG goes without evidence of generalization, the less likely they are to develop generalized MG (<5% will advance to generalized MG if no symptoms by 2 years).

Epidemiology

Bimodal distribution with peak incidence in women in the second and the third decades and in men in the sixth and seventh decades.

Pathophysiology

MG is an acquired autoimmune disorder resulting from the production of autoantibodies against the postsynaptic acetylcholine receptor (AChR) or less commonly against the receptor-associated proteins, muscle-specific tyrosine kinase (MuSK) or LRP4. However, "antibody-negative" forms account for up to 10% of MG patients. One must be careful to rule out hereditary/congenital forms of MG and avoid mistakenly lumping anti-LRP4 or anti-MuSK patients into this group.

Associated Conditions

- MG is often associated with thymus hyperplasia; 10% may have a malignant thymoma. Hyperplasia is more common in those under 40 years of age. Thymoma is more common in MG patients over age 30 years. Thymectomy is generally recommended in all MG patients with onset of disease under age 55 years, regardless of the presence of thymic hyperplasia or thymoma.
- Autoimmune thyroiditis (hyper more common than hypo) is present in ~15% of patients with MG. MG patients also have an increased risk of other autoimmune diseases including lupus, rheumatoid arthritis, polymyositis, and pernicious anemia.

DIAGNOSIS

Clinical Presentation

History
- The cardinal feature of MG is fluctuating weakness that is worse after exercise or prolonged activity and improves after rest.
- More than 50% of patients present with ptosis, this may be asymmetric.
- Other common complaints include blurred vision or diplopia, trouble smiling, and difficulties with chewing, swallowing, and speaking (e.g., winded at end of sentences, nasal speech, or weak voice).
- Limb weakness is common, especially proximal arms are more prominently affected.
- **Myasthenic crisis** consists of respiratory failure or the need for airway protection and occurs in approximately 15% to 20% of MG patients (*Neurology 2009; 72:1548*). Patients with bulbar and respiratory muscle weakness are particularly prone to respiratory failure, which may develop rapidly and unexpectedly. They require as much vigilance and monitoring as do patients with GBS.
- Respiratory infection, surgery (e.g., thymectomy), medications (e.g., aminoglycosides, quinine, quinolones, β-blockers, lithium, magnesium sulfate), pregnancy, and thyroid dysfunction can precipitate crisis or exacerbate symptoms. However, it is important to note that none of these medications should be withheld if required to treat a concurrent illness. Anticholinergic medications are a notable exception to this rule for obvious reasons, and in the absence of a life-threatening indication, their use should be avoided.

Physical Examination
- Presenting signs include ptosis, diplopia, dysarthria, hypophonia (or nasal quality to speech), dysphagia, extremity weakness, and respiratory difficulty.
- Fatigability on examination is a useful diagnostic feature.
- Ptosis may worsen after prolonged upward gaze (usually by 60 seconds). Patients may also begin to develop diplopia after sustained gaze in one direction.
- Carefully evaluate the airway, handling of secretions, ventilation, and the work of breathing.

- NIF and FVC are useful at the bedside to assess for respiratory muscle weakness. The breath count test described earlier in the GBS section is also useful in this population. The same general rules for ventilatory support (inability to protect airway or ventilate adequately) apply.

Differential Diagnosis

- Lambert–Eaton myasthenic syndrome (LEMS) is an autoimmune disease affecting the presynaptic voltage-gated calcium channels in the neuromuscular junction. It is frequently associated with malignancy (small-cell lung cancer). LEMS also presents with fluctuating weakness, but the weakness improves for a brief period of time after exercise. A quick bedside check is to look at reflexes that are absent before but present after 10 seconds of isometric exercise.
- Amyotrophic lateral sclerosis (ALS) may present with bulbar weakness. However, ALS can be differentiated from MG by presence of upper motor neuron signs in the former. Electrodiagnostic studies are also very useful in distinguishing the two.
- The differential also includes congenital forms of myasthenia, mitochondrial disorders (e.g., Chronic progressive external ophthalmoplegia [CPEO]), as well as acquired and hereditary myopathies or other motor neuronopathies (other than ALS).

Diagnostic Testing

A good rule of thumb is to have two lines of diagnostic evidence (usually serologic and electrodiagnostic) in the appropriate clinical context to make a diagnosis of autoimmune MG.

Laboratories

- Serum **AChR antibodies** are detected in 85% to 90% of adult generalized MG patients and in 50% to 70% of ocular MG cases.
- **MuSK antibodies** are detected in about 30% to 70% of AChR (−) MG patients.
- Thyroid function should be checked to evaluate for autoimmune thyroiditis.

Imaging

Chest CT is indicated to identify **thymoma**.

Diagnostic Procedures

Electrodiagnostic studies are an important step in diagnosing MG.

- Repetitive nerve stimulation (RNS) at 2 to 5 Hz typically shows >10% decrement in the amplitude of the compound muscle action potential (CMAP) in MG. If the patient is taking pyridostigmine, it should be held (if possible) as it could mask a decrement. RNS has a higher yield when it is performed on **weak** proximal muscles. Accordingly, it is only positive in 50% of patients with ocular MG. It should be noted that a decrement on slow RNS is not 100% specific for MG and can also be seen in LEMS, motor neuronopathies/neuropathies, and myopathies. In the Lambert–Eaton syndrome, the response is incremental with fast RNS (20 to 50 Hz). As fast RNS is extremely painful, an adequate supplement is to look for an increment in CMAP amplitude after 10 seconds of tetanic exercise.
- Single fiber EMG has a sensitivity of >95% for both generalized and ocular MG when performed on facial muscles. However, the specificity is much lower (abnormalities also seen in LEMS, motor neuronopathies/neuropathies, and myopa-

thies). It is usually reserved for those with suspected disease (based on clinical symptoms) but negative antibody and RNS testing.
- Edrophonium testing is no longer routinely used.
- Myasthenic weakness is often improved by cold. The "ice pack test" is an easy and safe "bedside" test that can be used in the evaluation of ocular MG symptoms.

TREATMENT

- Treatment of MG is individualized and depends on the severity of the disease, age, comorbidities, and response to therapy.
- **Myasthenic crisis** requires prompt recognition and aggressive support.
  - ○ Consider intensive care unit (ICU) level care and elective intubation for NIF <30 cm H_2O or FVC <15 mL/kg (similar parameters to those used for GBS).
  - ○ Treat superimposed infections and metabolic derangements.
  - ○ **Plasmapheresis** is used to treat acute exacerbations of MG. **IVIG** is less commonly used (*Neurotherapeutics 2008;5(4):535*).
  - ○ Since the effects of PLEX or IVIG are relatively rapid in onset but short lived, corticosteroids are typically started soon after initiating PLEX, usually at a dose of 10 to 20 mg/d and slowly titrated to a dose of 50 mg/d.
  - ○ Anticholinesterases should be temporarily withdrawn from patients who are receiving ventilation support; this avoids uncertainties about overdosage ("cholinergic crisis") and avoids cholinergic stimulation of pulmonary secretions.
  - ○ Neuromuscular blocking agents should be avoided whenever possible.

Medications

First Line
Anticholinesterase drugs can produce symptomatic improvement in all forms of MG. **Pyridostigmine** should be started at 30 to 60 mg PO tid–qid and titrated for symptom relief.

Second Line
- Immunosuppressive drugs are typically used when additional benefit is needed beyond cholinesterase inhibitors.
- High doses of **prednisone** can be used to achieve rapid improvement. **However, up to 50% of patients experience a transient worsening of weakness on initiation of prednisone therapy.** Hence, it is important to start low and increase slow, especially if the patient has not or is not being plasma exchanged.
- Azathioprine, mycophenolate mofetil, cyclosporine A, tacrolimus, and cyclophosphamide are steroid-sparing immunomodulatory agents used to treat MG.
- There is growing evidence that rituximab has great efficacy in treating anti-MuSK MG and can also have some utility in anti-AChR patients that have been medically refractory to the other forms of immunomodulatory therapy listed earlier.

Surgical Management

- Thymectomy may induce remission or reduce medication dependence (*Neurology 2000;55(1):7*).
- Thymectomy in MG patients is indicated in the presence of thymoma and typically in patients younger than 55 years with or without thymoma.

Other Neuromuscular Disorders

GENERAL PRINCIPLES

- **Myopathies:** Rapidly progressive proximal muscle weakness can be caused by many drugs including but not limited to ethanol, steroids, and cholesterol-lowering drugs (particularly in combination). Other common causes include HIV or HIV therapies, particularly zidovudine, and hypothyroidism.
  - **Critical illness myopathy** is increasingly recognized in patients with critical illness and is commonly associated with the use of steroids and neuromuscular blocking agents.
  - **Polymyositis (PM) and dermatomyositis (DM)** fall into a class of diseases now referred to as the idiopathic inflammatory myopathies. Most forms respond well to immunomodulatory therapy with a notable exception being the inclusion body myopathies (IBMs). DM and PM can also be a component of a syndrome affecting multiple different organ systems. Perhaps the best examples are antisynthetase syndromes, like Jo-1 myositis, which involves skin, joint, lung, and muscle. Patients suspected of having DM or PM should have myositis-specific and myositis-associated autoantibodies checked and should be screened for interstitial lung disease, which has a high degree of morbidity if left untreated (see Chapter 25, Arthritis and Rheumatologic Diseases).
- **Rhabdomyolysis** may produce rapid muscle weakness leading to hyperkalemia, myoglobinuria (by definition true rhabdomyolysis causes myoglobinuria), and renal failure (for management, see Chapter 12, Fluid and Electrolyte Management, and Chapter 13, Renal Diseases). The potential etiologies includes **M**etabolic (deficits of lipid or carbohydrate metabolism), **E**xcessive exercise/exertion (including seizures/dystonia), **D**rugs (abuse and Rx), **I**schemic, **C**ompression/crush (trauma), **I**nfection/**I**nflammatory, **N**oxious (toxins), **E**lectrolyte abnormalities (diabetic ketoacidosis [DKA], hyperosmolar hyperglycemic nonketotic syndrome [HHNS], hypokalemia) (**"MEDICINE"**).
- **Botulism** is a disorder of the **neuromuscular junction** caused by ingestion of an exotoxin produced by *Clostridium botulinum*, acquired through a wound, or via an iatrogenic route.
  - The exotoxin interferes with release of acetylcholine from presynaptic terminals at the neuromuscular junction.
  - In infants, it is commonly attributed to gastrointestinal (GI) colonization in the first 6 months of life when normal gut flora is not yet present. Classically, it is associated with ingestion of raw honey but inhalation/ingestion of soil-based spores is probably a more common cause.
  - Symptoms begin within 12 to 36 hours of ingestion in food-borne botulism and within 10 days in wound botulism.
  - Symptoms include **autonomic dysfunction** (xerostomia, blurred vision, urinary retention, and constipation), followed by **cranial nerve palsies**, **descending weakness**, and **possibly respiratory distress**.
  - **Serum assays for botulinum toxin** may be helpful in diagnosis in adults.
  - Management includes removing nonabsorbed toxin with **cathartics**, **supportive care**, and neutralizing absorbed toxin with **equine trivalent (A, B, E) antitoxin** (more immunogenic because it contains both the Fab and Fc portions) or **heptavalent (A, B, C, D, E, F, G) antitoxin** (less immunogenic as Fc portion is cleaved off and has F(ab)$_2$ portions). Penicillin G is often administered but no formal

clinical trials have been performed. There is some evidence that botulism immune globulin can shorten hospital stay by ~2 weeks (*N Engl J Med 2006;354:462*). Recovery is slow and occurs spontaneously, but with appropriate ventilatory and supportive care most make a full recovery.

Neuromuscular Disorders with Rigidity

GENERAL PRINCIPLES

- **NMS** is associated with the use of neuroleptic drugs, certain antiemetic drugs (e.g., metoclopramide, promethazine), or sudden withdrawal of dopamine agonists (L-dopa in PD).
  - Features include hyperthermia, altered mental status, muscular rigidity, and dysautonomia.
  - Laboratory abnormalities include a markedly elevated creatine kinase with myoglobinuria and leukocytosis.
  - Treatment includes discontinuing precipitating drug(s), cooling, monitoring and supporting vital functions (arrhythmias, shock, hyperkalemia, acidosis, renal failure), and administering dantrolene and/or bromocriptine. Treatment is essentially identical to that used for malignant hyperthermia (see the following text).
- **Serotonin syndrome** results from excessive serotonergic activity, especially following recent dosage changes of SSRIs, MAOIs, and TCAs.
  - It presents as a **triad of mental status change**, **autonomic overactivity**, and **neuromuscular abnormalities**. Distinguishing features of serotonin syndrome from NMS include the degree of mental status change, seizures, and the marked hyperreflexia. However, in certain circumstances, the two can be difficult to distinguish from one another.
  - Hyperthermia, tremor, nausea, vomiting, and clonus are common signs.
  - Treatment includes removal of offending drugs, aggressive supportive care, cyproheptadine, and benzodiazepines (*N Engl J Med 2005;352(11):1112*).
- **Malignant hyperthermia** is the acute development of high fever, obtundation, and muscular rigidity following triggering factors (e.g., halothane anesthesia, succinylcholine).
  - The most common etiology is an autosomal dominant mutation in the ryanodine receptor (RyR1) making a screen of the family history a critical part of the preop evaluation. Abnormalities in this calcium channel predispose patients to an elevation in intracytoplasmic calcium triggered by certain anesthetics. Other ion channels have also been identified, and children with dystrophinopathies are also at an increased risk.
  - **Serum creatine kinase is markedly elevated.** Renal failure from myoglobinuria and cardiac arrhythmias from electrolyte imbalance can be life threatening.
  - Successful management requires prompt recognition of early indicators of the syndrome (increased end tidal CO_2, tachycardia, acidosis, and/or muscle rigidity; note, hyperthermia comes later if at all) discontinuation of the offending anesthetic agent, aggressive supportive care that focuses on oxygenation/ventilation, circulation, correction of acid–base and electrolyte derangements, and administration of **dantrolene sodium**, 1 to 10 mg/kg/d for at least 48 to 96 hours to reduce muscular rigidity.
- **Tetanus** typically presents with generalized muscle spasm (especially trismus) caused by the exotoxin (tetanospasmin) from *Clostridium tetani*, a gram-positive bacilli commonly found in intestinal flora and soil.

○ The organism usually enters the body through wounds. Onset typically occurs within 7 to 21 days of an injury (*Expert Rev Anti Infect Ther 2008;6(3):327*).

○ Patients who are **unvaccinated or have reduced immunity** are at risk, underscoring the importance of prevention by tetanus toxoid boosters following wounds. Tetanus may occur in **drug abusers who inject subcutaneously**.

○ Management consists of supportive care, particularly airway control (laryngospasm) and treatment of muscle spasms (benzodiazepines, barbiturates, analgesics, and sometimes neuromuscular blockade). Cardiac arrhythmias and fluctuations in BP can occur. Recovery takes months. Shorter incubation periods (≤7 days) portend more severe courses and a worse prognosis.

○ The patient should be kept in quiet isolation, sedated but arousable.

○ Specific measures include wound debridement, **penicillin G or metronidazole and human tetanus immunoglobulin** (3,000 to 6,000 U IM).

○ **Active immunization** is needed after recovery (total of three doses of tetanus and diphtheria toxoid spaced at least 2 weeks apart).

AIRWAY EMERGENCIES

Acute Upper Airway Obstruction

GENERAL PRINCIPLES

- Airway obstruction must be recognized and addressed quickly as failure to do so can result in dire consequences.
- In awake patients without ventilation, airway obstruction is commonly due to the presence of a foreign body (usually food) or rarely angioedema.
- In unconscious patients without intact ventilation, airway obstruction can be caused by obstruction due to the tongue, foreign body, trauma, infection, or angioedema.

DIAGNOSIS

Clinical Presentation

History

A history is commonly unavailable. In awake patients with adequate ventilation, take a rapid history focused on the causes listed.

Physical Examination

- Manifestations in the **conscious patient** include stridor, impaired phonation, sternal or suprasternal retractions, display of the universal choking sign, and respiratory distress.
- Manifestations in the **unconscious patient** vary from labored breathing to apnea. Suspect airway obstruction if a nonbreathing patient is difficult to ventilate.
- In all patients, look for urticaria, angioedema, fever, and evidence of trauma.
- Partial obstruction in the awake patient with adequate ventilation:
  - Perform a directed physical examination, looking for airway swelling, trismus, pharyngeal obstruction, respiratory retractions, angioedema, stridor, wheezing, grossly swollen lymph nodes, and neck masses.
  - Observe the patient closely and be prepared to intervene to maintain an airway.
- Airway obstruction in an unconscious patient without intact ventilation: Examine the upper airway visually for evidence of obstruction as part of the resuscitative effort.

Differential Diagnosis

Trauma to the face and neck, foreign body, infection (croup, epiglottitis, Ludwig's angina, retropharyngeal abscess, and diphtheria), tumor, angioedema, laryngospasm, anaphylaxis, retained secretions, or blockage of the upper airway by the tongue (in the unconscious patient).

Diagnostic Testing

Imaging

Partial obstruction in the awake patient with adequate ventilation:

- **Soft tissue radiography** of the neck, while sometimes valuable (posteroanterior [PA] and lateral views), is less sensitive and specific than direct examination. Such radiography should be performed in the emergency department or intensive care unit (ICU) as a portable study, as the patient should not be left unattended.
- **Helical computed tomography (CT)** with contrast of the neck (with constant attendance) is a much more sensitive and specific imaging modality for upper airway obstruction. Unless a CT scanner is in close proximity to the clinical environment it may not be possible to safely obtain a CT scan. If you choose to travel to obtain a CT, it is critical that you take emergency airway devices with you and include a 6.0 endotracheal tube (ETT) for nasal intubation and a cricothyrotomy kit.

Diagnostic Procedures

Partial obstruction in the awake patient with adequate ventilation: If the patient's condition is stable, perform indirect **laryngoscopy** or **fiber optic nasopharyngo-laryngoscopy**. A careful examination is unlikely to cause acute airway obstruction in an adult.

TREATMENT

Therapy is directed at **rapid relief of obstruction** to prevent cardiopulmonary arrest and anoxic brain damage.

- **Airway obstruction in the awake patient without ventilation:**
  Perform the **Heimlich maneuver** (subdiaphragmatic abdominal thrust) repeatedly until the object is expelled from the airway or patient becomes unconscious. Up to half of patients may require a second technique (i.e., back slaps, chest thrusts) for success (*Circulation 2005;112(suppl 24):IV19*).
- **Airway obstruction in an unconscious patient without intact ventilation:**
  - If cervical spine trauma is not suspected, perform the head tilt–chin lift maneuver. Perform a jaw thrust if cervical spine trauma is suspected.
  - If these maneuvers are effective, place an oral or nasal airway. If ineffective, attempt to ventilate the patient with a bag-valve-mask (BVM) apparatus. If these attempts are also unsuccessful, rapidly examine the oropharynx and hypopharynx. Avoid a blind finger sweep if it is possible to examine the airway directly using a laryngoscope and McGill forceps (if necessary) to remove a foreign body.
  - If laryngoscopy cannot be performed immediately and a foreign body is suspected, perform **the supine Heimlich maneuver** (straddling the supine patient and applying repeated subdiaphragmatic thrusts). Chest thrusts may generate higher airway pressures and may be successful when abdominal thrusts have failed.
  - Substitute chest thrusts if the patient is very obese or is in late pregnancy.

Surgical Management

Airway obstruction in an unconscious patient without intact ventilation:
- Failure of the supine Heimlich maneuver should prompt an attempt at direct laryngoscopy and endotracheal intubation.
- Establish a surgical airway if the patient cannot be intubated.

- If a surgeon is not immediately available, perform needle cricothyrotomy using a 12- to 14-gauge over-the-needle catheter with high-flow oxygen (15 L/min from a 50-psi wall source). There are commercial devices designed for jet ventilation but you may quickly construct a substitute with a 3 mL syringe with the plunger removed and a 7.5 mm ETT cut off. You may then attach a BVM to the end of the ETT and bag the patient. Keep in mind that this is offering oxygenation only and not ventilation. That said, tracheal jet ventilation can buy you valuable minutes when airway obstruction is suspected.
- **Cricothyrotomy** is a preferred alternative.

Emergent Airway Adjuncts

- **Gum elastic bougie** is a flexible rubbery stick with a hockey stick tip. The bougie can be used blindly but is better suited for direct laryngoscopy where the intubator cannot visualize the cords. The goal is to obtain the best view possible and for the coude tip of bougie to be distal and anterior. When the bougie is in the trachea, you can often feel the clicks of the tracheal rings as you slide the bougie back and forth. Alternatively, you can push the bougie down the oropharynx as deep as possible without losing control of it. If in the esophagus, the bougie will slide all the way down past the stomach with minimal resistance. If in the trachea, the bougie will quickly hit a bronchus and meet resistance. Once you are in the trachea you can simply slide an ETT over the bougie and verify placement as you normally would.
- **Laryngeal mask airway (LMA)** is an easy-to-use rescue device for nearly all airway events. It is an ETT with balloon at the end that is inflated to cup the trachea while occluding the esophagus. Note that it should not be used in patients with upper airway obstruction that cannot be cleared or patients with excessive airway pressures such as with chronic obstructive pulmonary disease (COPD), asthma, or pregnancy. There are models of LMAs (which are preferred) that allow an ETT to be passed through them when a definitive airway is desired. Be cautious with excessive bagging as this can lead to emesis.
- **Supraglottic airway devices** are placed blindly in the oropharynx and inflated with air. An upper balloon obstructs the oropharynx while a lower balloon obstructs the esophagus, allowing ventilation in a similar fashion to an LMA with the same limitations.
- **Fiber optic/digital airway devices** are increasingly common. These devices allow the intubator to get a view of the vocal cords via a camera or fiber optic scope without having to view it through the mouth, making intubation much easier. Excessive secretions or blood can obstruct the camera.

Pneumothorax

GENERAL PRINCIPLES

- Pneumothorax may occur spontaneously or as a result of trauma.
- **Primary spontaneous pneumothorax** occurs without obvious underlying lung disease.
- **Secondary spontaneous pneumothorax** results from underlying parenchymal lung disease including COPD and emphysema, interstitial lung disease, necrotizing lung infections, *Pneumocystis jiroveci* pneumonia, tuberculosis, and cystic fibrosis.

- **Traumatic pneumothoraces** may occur as a result of penetrating or blunt chest wounds.
- **Iatrogenic pneumothorax** occurs after thoracentesis, central line placement, transbronchial biopsy, transthoracic needle biopsy, and barotrauma from mechanical ventilation and resuscitation.
- **Tension pneumothorax** results from continued accumulation of air in the chest that is sufficient to shift mediastinal structures and impede venous return to the heart. This results in hypotension, abnormal gas exchange, and ultimately, cardiovascular collapse.
  ○ It can occur as a result of barotrauma due to mechanical ventilation, a chest wound that allows ingress but not egress of air, or a defect in the visceral pleura that behaves in the same way ("ball-valve" effect).
  ○ Suspect tension pneumothorax when a patient experiences hypotension and respiratory distress on mechanical ventilation or after any procedure in which the thorax is pierced by a needle.

DIAGNOSIS

Clinical Presentation

History
- Patients commonly complain of ipsilateral chest or shoulder pain, usually of acute onset. A history of recent chest trauma or medical procedure can suggest the diagnosis.
- Dyspnea is usually present.

Physical Examination
- Although examination of the patient with a small pneumothorax may be normal, classic findings include decreased breath sounds, decreased vocal fremitus, and a more resonant percussion note on ipsilateral side.
- With a larger pneumothorax or with underlying lung disease, there may be tachypnea and respiratory distress. The affected hemithorax may be noticeably larger (due to decreased elastic recoil of the collapsed lung) and relatively immobile during respiration.
- If the pneumothorax is very large, and particularly if it is under tension, the patient may exhibit severe distress, diaphoresis, cyanosis, and hypotension. In addition, the patient's trachea may be shifted to the contralateral side.
- If the pneumothorax is the result of penetrating trauma or pneumomediastinum, subcutaneous emphysema may be felt.
- Clinical features alone do not predict the relative size of a pneumothorax, and in a stable patient, further diagnostic studies must be used in order to guide treatment strategy. However, tension pneumothorax remains a clinical diagnosis and, if suspected in the appropriate clinical scenario, immediate intervention should be undertaken prior to further testing.

Diagnostic Testing

Electrocardiography
An **electrocardiogram (ECG)** may reveal diminished anterior QRS amplitude and an anterior axis shift. In extreme cases, tension pneumothorax may cause electromechanical dissociation.

Imaging

- A **chest radiograph** will reveal a separation of the pleural shadow from the chest wall. If the PA radiograph is normal and pneumothorax is suspected, a lateral or decubitus film may aid in diagnosis (*Thorax 2003;58(suppl II):ii39*). Air travels to the highest point in a body cavity; thus, a pneumothorax in a supine patient may be detected as an unusually deep costophrenic sulcus and excessive lucency over the upper abdomen caused by the anterior thoracic air. This observation is particularly important in the critical care unit, where radiographs of the mechanically ventilated patient are often obtained with the patient in supine position.
- Although tension pneumothorax is a clinical diagnosis, radiographic correlates include mediastinal and tracheal shift toward contralateral side and depression of the ipsilateral diaphragm.
- **Ultrasonography** is a useful tool for bedside diagnosis of pneumothorax, especially on patients who must remain supine or who are too unstable to undergo CT scanning. Placement of the probe in the intercostal spaces provides information regarding the pleura and underlying lung parenchyma. During normal inspiration, the visceral and parietal pleura move along one another and produce a "sliding sign" phenomenon. In addition, the air-filled lung parenchyma below the pleura produces a ray-like opacity known as "comet tails." Presence of the sliding sign and comet tails on ultrasound during inspiration rule out a pneumothorax with high reliability at the point of probe placement. Conversely, absence of these signs is a highly reliable predictor for the presence of pneumothorax. Several places on the chest should be evaluated, including places that air is most likely to accumulate such as the anterior and lateral chest (*Chest 2012;141:1099*).
- Chest CT is the gold standard for diagnosis and determining the size of pneumothorax. Although not always necessary, it may be particularly useful for differentiating pneumothorax from bullous disease in patients with underlying lung conditions (*Thorax 2003;58(suppl II):ii42*).

TREATMENT

Treatment depends on cause, size, and degree of physiologic derangement.
- **Primary pneumothorax**
  - A small, primary, spontaneous pneumothorax without a continued pleural air leak may resolve spontaneously. Air is resorbed from the pleural space at roughly 1.5% daily, and therefore, a small (~15%) pneumothorax is expected to resolve without intervention in approximately 10 days.
  - Confirm that the pneumothorax is **not increasing in size** (repeat the chest radiograph in 6 hours if there is no change in symptoms) and send the patient home if he or she is asymptomatic (apart from mild pleurisy). Obtain follow-up radiographs to confirm resolution of the pneumothorax in 7 to 10 days. Air travel is discouraged during the follow-up period, as a decrease in ambient barometric pressure results in a larger pneumothorax.
  - If the pneumothorax is **small but the patient is mildly symptomatic**, far from home, or unlikely to cooperate with follow-up, admit the patient and administer high-flow oxygen; the resulting nitrogen gradient will speed resorption.
  - If the patient is **more than mildly symptomatic or has a larger pneumothorax**, simple aspiration is a reasonable initial management strategy. However, aspiration may not be successful for very large pneumothoraces. In patients where

aspiration fails, proceed with thoracostomy tube insertion (*Thorax 2003; 58(suppl II):ii39*).

○ **Pleural sclerosis** to prevent recurrence is recommended by some experts but, in most cases, is not used after a first episode unless a persistent air leak is present.

• **Secondary pneumothorax**
  ○ Individuals with a secondary spontaneous pneumothorax are usually symptomatic and require lung reexpansion.
  ○ Often, a bronchopleural fistula persists and a larger thoracostomy tube and suction are required.
  ○ **Consult a pulmonologist** about pleural sclerosis for persistent air leak and to prevent recurrence.
  ○ **Surgery** may be required for persistent air leak and should be considered for high-risk patients for prevention of recurrence.

• **Iatrogenic pneumothorax**
  ○ Iatrogenic pneumothorax is generally caused either by introducing air into the pleural space through the parietal pleura (e.g., thoracentesis, central line placement) or by allowing intrapulmonary air to escape through breach of the visceral pleura (e.g., transbronchial biopsy). Often, no further air leak occurs after the initial event.
  ○ If the pneumothorax is small and the patient is minimally symptomatic, he or she can be managed conservatively. If the procedure that caused the pneumothorax required sedation, admit the patient, administer oxygen, and repeat the chest radiograph in 6 hours to ensure the patient's stability. If the patient is completely alert and the chest radiograph shows no change, the patient can be discharged.
  ○ If the patient is symptomatic or if the pneumothorax is too large for expectant care, a pneumothorax catheter with aspiration or a one-way valve is usually adequate and can often be removed the following day.
  ○ Iatrogenic pneumothorax due to barotrauma from mechanical ventilation almost always has a persistent air leak and should be managed with a chest tube and suction.

• **Tension pneumothorax**
  When the clinical situation and physical examination strongly suggest this diagnosis, decompress the affected hemithorax immediately with a 14-gauge needle. Place the needle in the second intercostal space, midclavicular line, just superior to the rib. Release of air with clinical improvement confirms the diagnosis. Recognize that an obese patient or a patient with a large amount of breast tissue may require a longer needle than a standard angiocatheter in order to reach the intrathoracic space for decompression. Seal any chest wound with an occlusive dressing and arrange for placement of a thoracostomy tube.

Drowning

GENERAL PRINCIPLES

Definition

• Drowning is defined as the process of experiencing respiratory impairment from submersion/immersion in liquid (*Final Recommendations of the World Congress on Drowning, 2002*).

- Risk factors include youth, inability to swim, alcohol and drug use, barotrauma (in scuba diving), head and neck trauma, and loss of consciousness associated with epilepsy, diabetes, syncope, or dysrhythmias.
- Much has been made of the differences in pathophysiology between fresh- and salt-water drownings. However, the **major insults** (i.e., hypoxemia and tissue hypoxia related to ventilation–perfusion [V/Q] mismatch, acidosis, and hypoxic brain injury with cerebral edema) are common to both.
- Hypothermia, pneumonia, and rarely, disseminated intravascular coagulation (DIC), acute renal failure, and hemolysis may also occur.

DIAGNOSIS

Diagnostic Testing
Laboratories
Obtain serum electrolytes, complete blood cell count (CBC), and arterial blood gases (ABGs). Monitor the cardiac rhythm continuously. Obtain blood alcohol level and drug screen if the mental status is not normal.

Electrocardiography
Obtain ECG.

TREATMENT

Resuscitation
- **Immobilize the cervical spine**, as trauma may be present.
- Begin with resuscitation, focusing on airway management and ventilation with 100% oxygen. The patient may require intubation.
- Establish an intravenous (IV) line with 0.9% saline or lactated Ringer solution.
- **Treat hypothermia** vigorously (see Cold-Induced Illness section).

Medications
Reserve antibiotics for patients who were exposed to grossly contaminated water or sewage.

Disposition
- Admit patients who have survived severe episodes of drowning to an ICU. Noncardiogenic pulmonary edema may still develop in those individuals with less severe immersions.
- Admit any patient with pulmonary signs or symptoms, including cough, bronchospasm, abnormal ABGs or oxygen saturation as measured by pulse oximetry (SpO$_2$), or abnormal chest radiograph.
- Observe the asymptomatic patient with a questionable or brief water immersion for 6 to 8 hours and discharge the patient if the chest radiograph and ABGs are normal (*Ann Emerg Med 1986;15:1048*). However, if a documented long submersion, unconsciousness, initial cyanosis or apnea, or even a brief requirement for resuscitation has occurred, the patient must be admitted for at least 24 hours.

COMPLICATIONS

- **Cerebral edema**
  - Cerebral edema may occur suddenly within the first 24 hours and is a major cause of death. Treatment of cerebral edema does not appear to increase survival, and intracranial pressure monitoring does not appear to be effective (*Crit Care Med 1986;14:529*). Nevertheless, if cerebral edema occurs, hyperventilate the patient to a PCO_2 not lower than 25 mm Hg (to avoid excessive vasoconstriction) and administer mannitol (1 to 2 g/kg q3–4h) or furosemide (1 mg/kg IV q4–6h).
  - Treat seizures aggressively with phenytoin.
  - The routine administration of glucocorticoids is not recommended.
  - It may be necessary to sedate and paralyze the patient to reduce oxygen consumption and facilitate intracranial pressure management.
- **Pulmonary complications**
  - Administer 100% oxygen initially, titrating thereafter by ABGs.
  - Intubate the patient endotracheally and begin mechanical ventilation with positive end-expiratory pressure (PEEP) if the patient is apneic, is in severe respiratory distress, or has oxygen-resistant hypoxemia.
  - Administer bronchodilators if bronchospasm is present.
  - Artificial surfactant has not been shown to be useful (*Acad Emerg Med 1995;2:204*; *Pediatr Emerg Care 1995;11:153*).
- **Metabolic complications:** Manage metabolic acidosis with mechanical ventilation, sodium bicarbonate (if the pH is persistently <7.2), and blood pressure (BP) support.

HEAT-INDUCED INJURY

Heat Exhaustion

GENERAL PRINCIPLES

Heat exhaustion occurs through water or sodium depletion but is often a combination of both. Water depletion heat exhaustion often occurs in the elderly or persons working in hot environments with limited water replacement. Salt depletion occurs in unacclimatized individuals who replace fluid losses with large amounts of hypotonic solution.

DIAGNOSIS

- The patient presents with headache, nausea, vomiting, dizziness, weakness, irritability, and/or cramps.
- The patient may have postural hypotension, diaphoresis, and normal or minimally increased core temperature.

TREATMENT

- Treatment consists of resting the patient in a cool environment, accelerating heat loss by fan evaporation, and repleting fluids with salt-containing solutions.

- If the patient is not vomiting and has stable BP, an oral, commercial, balanced salt solution is adequate.
- If the patient is vomiting or hemodynamically unstable, check electrolytes and give 1 to 2 L 0.9% saline IV.

Lifestyle Modifications

The patient should avoid exercise in a hot environment for 2 to 3 additional days.

Heat Syncope

GENERAL PRINCIPLES

- Heat syncope is a variant of postural hypotension.
- Exercise in a hot environment results in peripheral vasodilation and pooling of blood, with subsequent loss of consciousness. The affected individual has normal body temperature and regains consciousness promptly when supine. These factors separate this syndrome from heat stroke.

TREATMENT

Treatment consists of resting in a cool environment and fluid repletion.

Heat Stroke

GENERAL PRINCIPLES

- Heat stroke occurs in two varieties, classic and exertional. Both varieties present with high core temperatures that result in direct thermal tissue injury. Secondary effects include acute renal failure from rhabdomyolysis. Even with rapid therapy, mortality rates can be very high for body temperatures above 41.1°C (106°F). The distinction between classic and exertional heat stroke is not important because the therapeutics goals are similar in both and a delay in cooling increases mortality rate.
- The cardinal features of heat stroke are **hyperthermia (>40°C, 104°F) and altered mental status**. Although patients presenting with classic heat stroke may have anhidrosis, this is not considered a diagnostic criteria, because 50% of patients are still diaphoretic at presentation.
- The central nervous system (CNS) is very vulnerable to heat stroke with the cerebellum being highly sensitive. Ataxia may be an early sign. Seizures are common. Neurologic injury is a function of maximum temperature and duration of exposure (*N Engl J Med 2002;346:1978*).

DIAGNOSIS

Diagnosis is based on the history of exposure or exercise, a core temperature usually of 40.6°C (105°F) or higher, and changes in mental status ranging from confusion to delirium and coma.

Differential Diagnosis

- Malignant hyperthermia after exposure to anesthetic agents
- Neuroleptic malignant syndrome (NMS) associated with antipsychotic drugs. It is worth noting that NMS and malignant hyperthermia are both accompanied by severe muscle rigidity.
- Anticholinergic poisoning
- Sympathomimetic toxicity (including cocaine)
- Severe hyperthyroidism
- Sepsis
- Meningitis
- Cerebral malaria
- Encephalitis
- Hypothalamic dysfunction due to stroke or hemorrhage
- Brain abscess

Diagnostic Testing

Laboratories

- Laboratory studies should include CBC, partial thromboplastin time (PTT), prothrombin time (PT), fibrin degradation products, electrolytes, blood urea nitrogen (BUN), creatinine, glucose, calcium, and creatine kinase levels, liver function tests (LFTs), ABGs, urinalysis, and ECG.
- If an infectious etiology is suspected, obtain appropriate cultures.

Imaging

If a CNS etiology is considered likely, CT imaging followed by spinal fluid examination is appropriate.

TREATMENT

- **Immediate cooling** is necessary.
  - The best method of cooling is controversial. No study has directly compared ice water application with tepid spray. However, ice water lowers body temperature twice as quickly and is the procedure chosen when exertional heat stroke is anticipated (long-distance races, military training) (*Int J Sports Med 1998;19(suppl 2):S150*; *Ann Intern Med 2000;132:678*).
  - Wrap the patient in sheets that are continuously wetted with ice water.
  - If response is insufficiently rapid, submerge the patient in ice water, recognizing that this may interfere with resuscitative efforts (*Am J Emerg Med 1996;14:355*).
  - Most emergency facilities that do not care for large numbers of heat illness cases are not equipped for this treatment. In this case, mist the patient continuously with tepid water (20°C to 25°C [68°F to 77°F]). Cool the patient with a large electric fan with maximum body surface exposure.
  - Ice packs should be placed at points of major heat transfer, such as the groin, axillae, and chest, to further speed cooling.
  - Antipyretics have no indication.
- **Dantrolene sodium** does not appear to be effective for the treatment of heat stroke (*Crit Care Med 1991;19:176*).

- Monitor core temperatures continuously by rectal probe as oral and tympanic membrane temperature may be inaccurate.
- Discontinue cooling measures when the core temperature reaches 39°C (102.2°F), which should ideally be achieved within 30 minutes. A temperature rebound may occur in 3 to 6 hours and should be retreated.
- **For hypotension, administer crystalloids:** If refractory, treat with vasopressors and monitor hemodynamics. Avoid pure α-adrenergic agents, as they cause vasoconstriction and impair cooling. Administer crystalloids cautiously to normotensive patients.

COMPLICATIONS

- **Treat rhabdomyolysis** or urine output of <30 mL/hr with adequate volume replacement, mannitol (12.5 to 25.0 g IV), and bicarbonate (44 to 100 mEq/L in 0.45% normal saline) to promote osmotic diuresis and urine alkalinization. Despite these measures, **renal failure** may still complicate cases of heat stroke (Chapter 13, Renal Diseases).
- **Hypoxemia and acute respiratory distress syndrome (ARDS)** may occur. Treat as described in Chapter 8, Critical Care.
- Treat seizures with diazepam and phenytoin.

MONITORING/FOLLOW-UP

Patients should be placed on telemetry.

COLD-INDUCED ILLNESS

Exposure to the cold may result in several different forms of injury. Risk factor is accelerated heat loss, which is promoted by exposure to high wind or by immersion. Extended cold exposure may result from alcohol or drug abuse, injury or immobilization, and mental impairment.

Chilblains

GENERAL PRINCIPLES

- Chilblains are among the mildest form of cold injury and result from exposure of bare skin to a cold, windy environment (0.6°C to 15.6°C [33°F to 60°F]).
- The ears, fingers, and tip of the nose typically are injured, with itchy, painful erythema on rewarming.

TREATMENT

Treatment involves rapid rewarming (see Frostnip section), moisturizing lotions, analgesics, and instructing the patient to avoid reexposure.

Immersion Injury (Trench Foot)

GENERAL PRINCIPLES

Immersion injury is caused by prolonged immersion (longer than 10 to 12 hours) at a temperature <10°C (<50°F).

TREATMENT

Treat by rewarming followed by dry dressings. Treat secondary infections with antibiotics.

Frostnip (Superficial Frostbite)

GENERAL PRINCIPLES

Superficial frostbite involves the skin and subcutaneous tissues.

DIAGNOSIS

Areas with first-degree involvement are white, waxy, and anesthetic; have poor capillary refill; and are painful on thawing. Second-degree involvement is manifested by clear or milky bullae.

TREATMENT

The **treatment of choice** is rapid rewarming. Immerse the affected body part for 15 to 30 minutes; hexachlorophene or povidone-iodine can be added to the water bath. Narcotic analgesics may be necessary for rewarming pain. Typically, no deep injury ensues and healing occurs in 3 to 4 weeks.

Deep Frostbite

GENERAL PRINCIPLES

- Deep frostbite involves death of skin, subcutaneous tissue, and muscle (third degree) or deep tendons and bones (fourth degree).
- Diabetes mellitus, peripheral vascular disease (PVD), an outdoor lifestyle, and high altitude are the additional **risk factors**.

DIAGNOSIS

- The tissue appears frozen and hard.
- On rewarming, there is no capillary filling.
- Hemorrhagic blisters form, followed by eschars. Healing is very slow, and demarcation of tissue with autoamputation may occur.
- The majority of deep frostbite occurs at temperatures <6.7°C (44°F) with exposures longer than 7 to 10 hours.

TREATMENT

- The treatment is rapid rewarming as described earlier. **Rewarming should not be started until there is no chance of refreezing.**
- Administer analgesics (IV opioids) as needed.
- Early surgical intervention is not indicated.
- **Elevate** the affected extremity, prevent weight bearing, separate the affected digits with cotton wool, prevent tissue maceration by using a blanket cradle, and prohibit smoking.
- Update tetanus immunization.
- Intra-arterial vasodilators, heparin, dextran, prostaglandin inhibitors, thrombolytics, and sympathectomy are not routinely justified.
- Role of antibiotics is unclear (*Tintinalli's Emergency Medicine Manual. 7th ed. New York: McGraw-Hill, 2010: Chapter 202: Frostbite and Other Localized Cold Injuries*)
- Amputation is undertaken only after full demarcation has occurred.

Hypothermia

GENERAL PRINCIPLES

Definition
Hypothermia is defined as a core temperature of <35°C (95°F).

Classification
Classification of severity by temperature is not universal. One scheme defines hypothermia as mild at 34°C to 35°C (93.2°F to 95°F), moderate at 30°C to 34°C (86°F to 93.2°F), and severe at <30°C (86°F).

Etiology
- The most common cause of hypothermia in the United States is cold exposure due to alcohol intoxication.
- Another common cause is cold water immersion.

DIAGNOSIS

Clinical Presentation
Presentation varies with the temperature of the patient on arrival. All organ systems can be involved.
- **CNS effects**
  - At temperatures **below 32°C (89.6°F)**, mental processes are slowed and the affect is flattened.
  - At **32.2°C (90°F)**, the ability to shiver is lost, and deep tendon reflexes are diminished.
  - At **28°C (82.4°F)**, coma often supervenes.
  - **Below 18°C (64.4°F)**, the electroencephalogram (EEG) is flat. On rewarming from severe hypothermia, central pontine myelinolysis may develop.
- **Cardiovascular effects**
  - After an initial increased release of catecholamines, there is a decrease in cardiac output and heart rate with relatively preserved mean arterial pressure. ECG

changes, manifest initially as sinus bradycardia with T-wave inversion and QT-interval prolongation, and may manifest as atrial fibrillation at temperatures of <32°C (<89.6°F).

- ○ Osborne waves (J-point elevation) may be visible, particularly in leads II and V_6.
- ○ An increased susceptibility to ventricular arrhythmias occurs at temperatures **below 32°C (89.6°F)**.
- ○ At temperatures of **30°C (86°F)**, the susceptibility to ventricular fibrillation is increased significantly, and unnecessary manipulation or jostling of the patient should be avoided.
- ○ A decrease in mean arterial pressure may also occur, and at temperatures of **28°C (82.4°F)**, progressive bradycardia supervenes.
- **Respiratory effects**
  - ○ After an initial increase in minute ventilation, respiratory rate and tidal volume decrease progressively with decreasing temperature.
  - ○ ABGs measured with the machine set at 37°C (98.6°F) should serve as the basis for therapy without correction of pH and carbon dioxide tension (PCO_2) (*Ann Emerg Med 1989;18:72*; *Arch Intern Med 1998;148:1643*).
- **Renal manifestations:** Cold-induced diuresis and tubular concentrating defects may be seen.

Differential Diagnosis

- Cerebrovascular accident
- Drug overdose
- Diabetic ketoacidosis
- Hypoglycemia
- Uremia
- Adrenal insufficiency
- Myxedema

Diagnostic Testing

Laboratories

- Basic laboratory studies should include CBC, coagulation studies, LFTs, BUN, electrolytes, creatinine, glucose, creatine kinase, calcium, magnesium, amylase levels, urinalysis, ABGs, and ECG.
- Obtain toxicology screen if mental status alteration is more profound than expected for temperature decrease.
- Serum potassium is often increased.
- Elevated serum amylase may reflect underlying pancreatitis.
- Hyperglycemia may be noted but should not be treated as rebound hypoglycemia may occur with rewarming.
- DIC may also occur.

Imaging

Obtain chest, abdominal, and cervical spine radiographs to evaluate all patients with a history of trauma or immersion injury.

TREATMENT

Medications

- Administer supplemental oxygen.
- Give **thiamine** to most patients with cold exposure, as exposure due to alcohol intoxication is common.

- Administration of **antibiotics** is a controversial issue; many authorities recommend antibiotic administration for 72 hours, pending cultures. In general, the patients with hypothermia due to exposure and alcohol intoxication are less likely to have a serious underlying infection than those who are elderly or who have an underlying medical illness.

Other Nonpharmacologic Therapies

- **Rewarming:** The patient should be rewarmed with the goal of increasing the temperature by 0.5°C to 2.0°C/hr (32.9°F to 35.6°F/hr), although the rate of rewarming has not been shown to be related to the outcome.
- **Passive external rewarming**
  - This method depends on the patient's ability to shiver.
  - It is effective only at core temperatures of **32°C (89.6°F) or higher**.
  - Remove wet clothing, cover patient with blankets in a warm environment, and monitor.
- **Active external rewarming**
  - Application of heating blankets (40°C to 45°C [104°F to 113°F]) or warm bath immersion may cause paradoxical core acidosis, hyperkalemia, and decreased core temperature, as cold stagnant blood returns to the central vasculature (*J Royal Naval Med Serv 1991;77:139*), although Danish naval research supports arm and leg rewarming as effective and safe (*Aviat Space Environ Med 1999;70:1081*).
  - Pending further investigation, active rewarming is best reserved for young, previously healthy patients with acute hypothermia and minimal pathophysiologic derangement.
- **Active core rewarming is preferred for treatment of severe hypothermia**, although few data are available on outcomes (*Resuscitation 1998;36:101*).
  - **Heated oxygen** is the initial therapy of choice for the patient whose cardiovascular status is stable. This therapeutic maneuver can be expected to raise core temperatures by 0.5°C to 1.2°C/hr (32.9°F to 34.2°F/hr) (*Ann Emerg Med 1980;9:456*). Administration through an ETT results in more rapid rewarming than delivery via face mask. Administer heated oxygen through a cascade humidifier at a temperature of 45°C (113°F) or lower.
  - **IV fluids** can be heated in a microwave oven or delivered through a blood warmer; give fluids only through peripheral IV lines.
  - **Heated nasogastric or bladder lavage** is of limited efficacy because of low-exposed surface area and is reserved for the patient with cardiovascular instability.
  - **Heated peritoneal lavage** with fluid warmed to 40°C to 45°C (104°F to 113°F) is more effective than heated aerosol inhalation, but it should be reserved for patients with cardiovascular instability. Only those who are experienced in its use should perform heated peritoneal lavage, in combination with other modes of rewarming.
  - Closed thoracic lavage with heated fluid by thoracostomy tube has been recommended but is unproved (*Ann Emerg Med 1990;19:204*).
  - **Hemodialysis** can be used for the severely hypothermic, particularly when due to an overdose that is amenable to treatment in this way.
  - **Extracorporeal circulation** (cardiac bypass) is used only in hypothermic individuals who are in cardiac arrest; in these cases, it may be dramatically effective (*N Engl J Med 1997;337:1500*). Extracorporeal circulation may raise the temperature as rapidly as 10°C to 25°C/hr (50°F to 77°F/hr) but must be performed in an ICU or operating room.

Resuscitation

- Maintain airway and administer oxygen.
- If intubation is required, the most experienced operator should perform it (see Airway Management and Tracheal Intubation section in Chapter 8, Critical Care).
- Conduct **cardiopulmonary resuscitation (CPR)** in standard fashion. Perform simultaneous vigorous core rewarming; as long as the core temperature is severely decreased, it should not be assumed that the patient cannot be resuscitated. Reliable defibrillation requires a core temperature of 32°C (89.6°F) or higher; prolonged efforts (to a core temperature of 35°C [95°F]) may be justified because of the neuroprotective effects of hypothermia. **Do not begin CPR if an organized ECG rhythm is present**, as inability to detect peripheral pulses may be due to vasoconstriction, and CPR may precipitate ventricular fibrillation.
- Do not perform Swan–Ganz catheterization, as it may precipitate ventricular fibrillation.
- If ventricular fibrillation occurs, begin CPR as per the advanced cardiac life support (ACLS) protocol (Appendix C). Amiodarone may be administered as per the protocol, although there is no evidence to support its use or guide dosage; some experts suggest reducing the maximum cumulative dose by half. Avoid procainamide because it may precipitate ventricular fibrillation and increase the temperature that is necessary to defibrillate the patient. Rewarming is key.
- Monitor ECG rhythm, urine output, and, possibly, central venous pressure in all patients with an intact circulation.

Disposition

- Admit patients with an underlying disease, physiologic derangement, or core temperature <32°C (<89.6°F), preferably to an ICU.
- Discharge individuals with mild hypothermia (32°C to 35°C [89.6°F to 95°F]) and no predisposing medical conditions or complications when they are normothermic and an adequate home environment can be ensured.

MONITORING/FOLLOW-UP

- Monitor core temperature.
- A standard oral thermometer registers only to a lower limit of 35°C (95°F). Monitor the patient continuously with a rectal probe with a full range of 20°C to 40°C (68°F to 104°F).

28 Toxicology

S. Eliza Halcomb, Evan Schwarz, and
Michael E. Mullins

OVERDOSES

Overdose, General

GENERAL PRINCIPLES

- According to the American Association of Poison Control Centers (AAPCC), there were over 2 million exposures and 1,146 fatalities related to toxins in 2010 (*Clin Toxicol 49(10):910*). Overdoses are common in the emergency department, and although they are rarely fatal, it is important to follow some general guidelines while caring for the poisoned patient.
- Patients who present to the hospital with an overdose can be challenging for the clinician. This section will begin with a review of the general approach to the poisoned patient, followed by a discussion of specific ingestions.
- When managing the poisoned patient, as with all patients, it is vital to make sure the patient has patent airway, intact breathing, and palpable pulses. Beyond the basics of general emergency management, it is important to remember physiologic principles when approaching the poisoned patient. Quite often, patients can be categorized into one of the five toxidromes based on simple clinical examination findings.

Definition

A **toxidrome**, or toxic syndrome, is a constellation of clinical examination findings that assists in the diagnosis and treatment of the patient who presents with an exposure to an unknown agent. The toxicologic physical examination should include documentation of **vital signs**, **pupillary diameter**, **skin findings** (dry, flushed, or diaphoretic), as well as the presence or absence of **bowel sounds**, and **urinary retention**.

Classification

There are **five general toxidromes** that encompass a variety of xenobiotic exposures. They include the following:

- **Sympathomimetic:** This toxidrome is characterized by widespread activation of the sympathetic nervous system. The vital sign abnormalities include **hypertension** due to α-adrenergic stimulation and **tachycardia** due to increased β-adrenergic tone. Patients may also present with pyrexia. Physical examination will reveal **pupillary dilatation**, **diaphoresis**, and occasionally, altered mental status. Drugs that can cause this type of toxidrome include cocaine and amphetamines. Likewise, vasopressors and β-adrenergic agonists can cause a partial syndrome depending on which agent is being used.

- **Cholinergic:** This toxidrome is characterized by the widespread activation of the parasympathetic nervous system. Classically, the vital signs associated with a cholinergic toxidrome include **bradycardia** due to increased vagal tone, **respiratory depression** due to paralysis, and **decreased oxygen saturations** on pulse oximetry, due to **bronchoconstriction** and **bronchorrhea**. Excess acetylcholine (ACh) affects muscarinic receptors leading to the development of pinpoint pupils and the SLUDGE syndrome of **salivation, lacrimation, urination, defecation, gastrointestinal (GI) distress, and emesis**. Excess ACh at the neuromuscular junction (NMJ) results in a depolarizing blockade of the muscles, leading to **fasciculations** and **paralysis**. In the central nervous system (CNS), cholinergic overload is associated with the development of **seizures** and **coma**. Agents linked with the development of this toxidrome all block the function of acetylcholinesterase (AChE), resulting in the accumulation of ACh in the synapse. These agents include organophosphate insecticides and nerve gases, as well as carbamate pesticides. Carbamates are also used therapeutically in anesthesia, myasthenia gravis, and the treatment of anticholinergic toxidromes.
- **Anticholinergic:** This toxidrome should perhaps be more appropriately described as an antimuscarinic syndrome. Its features include **tachycardia** due to vagal blockade and **hyperthermia** (which may be mild to severe). CNS effects include **agitation**, **delirium**, and in severe cases, seizures. Other peripheral effects include **mydriasis**; **dry**, flushed skin; **urinary retention**; and **decreased intestinal motility**. Therapeutic agents that cause this toxidrome include atropine, scopolamine, and antihistamines.
- **Opiate:** The opioids produce a classic vital sign combination of **respiratory depression** and oxygen desaturations in conjunction with **miosis, decreased GI motility**, and **coma**. Opioids produce this toxidrome by binding to one of the four G protein receptors on the cell membrane, leading to analgesia. However, respiratory depression, miosis, and physical dependence are secondary, undesirable effects. Other agents that produce a similar toxidrome include the imidazolines, including clonidine, tetrahydrozoline, and oxymetazoline.
- **Sedative hypnotic:** The benzodiazepines bind to γ-Aminobutyric acid (GABA) receptors in the brain and cause a clinical picture of **sedation or coma** in the setting of **normal** vital signs. A common misconception is that ingested benzodiazepines cause respiratory depression. While this may be true in the setting of intravenously administered benzodiazepines, patients with a **benzodiazepine ingestion generally do not develop respiratory compromise**.

DIAGNOSIS

Diagnostic Testing

If patients do not fall into any of the aforementioned categories, suspect a mixed or undifferentiated exposure, and several diagnostic tests should be ordered.

Laboratories
- **Finger stick blood glucose (FSBG):** This test should be considered one of the vital signs in the patient with altered mental status.
- **Chemistry:** A basic metabolic profile should be ordered on any patient with a toxic exposure. The two important pieces of information gleaned from the basic metabolic panel (BMP) include the presence or absence of a low bicarbonate and the creatinine. If the patient has a low bicarbonate, a metabolic acidosis is present

and the clinician should calculate the **anion gap**. Patients who present with an elevated anion gap acidosis are often subjected to a battery of unnecessary studies because the differential diagnosis is enormous. In order to tailor the diagnosis, the clinician should focus on a mechanistic approach and check serum **ketones** and **lactate**. If these are negative and the **creatinine** is normal, then one should suspect the presence of a toxic alcohol and send the appropriate studies.

- **Blood gas:** In most cases of intoxication, pH rather than oxygenation is of great relevance. Therefore, it is reasonable to send **venous blood gases (VBGs)** rather than arterial blood gases (ABGs) in routine cases of poisoning. However, if adequate oxygenation is a concern (e.g., cyanide, CO poisoning, methemoglobinemia) then an ABG should be sent.

- **Serum drug screen:** In general, the studies included on this panel include acetaminophen, salicylate, and ethanol concentrations. Some laboratories include a tricyclic antidepressant (TCA) screen as well.

  ○ In practice, the piece of information that is critical on this panel is the serum **acetaminophen** (N-acetyl-*para*-aminophenol [APAP]) since patients with this ingestion are often asymptomatic upon presentation and approximately 1/500 overdoses have been found to have an unsuspected and treatable APAP concentration (*Ann Emerg Med 1985;14:562*).

  ○ Acute **salicylate** ingestions, while very serious, produce a clinical syndrome that is readily identifiable at the bedside. Chronic salicylate toxicity should be suspected in elderly patients taking aspirin who present with altered mental status and tachypnea.

  ○ **Ethanol** concentrations are NOT predictive of intoxication, despite the forensic definition of 80 mg/dL as the legal limit for driving. Intoxication is a clinical diagnosis. One of the pitfalls of routinely obtaining ethanol levels is that serious medical conditions may coexist in these often fragile patients. These conditions are frequently missed when the patient is thought to be drunk.

  ○ **TCA** screens are notoriously unreliable and cross-react with many therapeutic agents. In the absence of the characteristic electrocardiogram (ECG) findings and vital sign abnormalities, a positive result is meaningless and is the source of confusion, leading to unnecessary treatment.

- **Urine drug screen:** Rarely contributes to the management of the patient. Many of the assays produce false-positive or false-negative results and may, in fact, cause harm by leading the clinician to attribute a patient's condition to intoxication rather than a medical emergency. Additionally, these tests are expensive to conduct and therefore are of limited value in the management of the poisoned patient. The urine drug screen tends to vary between hospitals but often tests for the following substances:

  ○ **Amphetamines:** The assay for amphetamines commonly cross-reacts with over-the-counter cold medications.

  ○ **Opioids:** This assay frequently misses the presence of the synthetic opioids such as fentanyl, methadone, and meperidine; therefore, it is important to rely on the toxidrome for the diagnosis.

  ○ **Cocaine:** This assay is not directed at the parent compound; rather, it detects the metabolite benzoylecgonine. Since the parent compound is very short lived, this test is very reliable for the identification of recent use, but in no way confirms intoxication.

  ○ **Cannabinoids:** Like cocaine, detection of the tetrahydrocannabinolic acid (THCA) metabolite is a reliable indicator of use; however, its presence does not have any bearing upon the diagnosis of intoxication.

- **Benzodiazepines:** The detection of benzodiazepines most commonly relies upon the detection of oxazepam; however, some commonly used benzodiazepines (such as lorazepam) are therefore often missed by this screening (*Clin Chem 2003; 49:357*). Given that benzodiazepine overdoses tend to be benign, the utility of this component is questionable at best.
- **Phencyclidine (PCP):** Screening assays may cross-react with dextromethorphan, ketamine, and diphenhydramine to produce a false-positive result. Once again, the clinical picture is more important in the diagnosis of PCP intoxication and the presence of PCP on a drug screen does not alter the management of a patient.
- Specific laboratory testing will be further addressed in the following text.

Electrocardiography
- The ECG is a critical part of the toxicologic evaluation, and certain overdoses produce characteristic ECG changes that guide diagnosis and treatment plans.
- In general, the important cardiac toxins tend to prolong the PR interval (reflecting nodal blockade), the QRS (reflecting sodium channel blockade), or the QT interval (potassium channel blockade).
- Electrocardiographic changes specific to certain toxins will be further discussed in the following text.

Imaging
- In general, there is a limited role of diagnostic imaging in toxicology. However, there are a few cases when imaging may be helpful in the diagnosis and management of the poisoned patient. The most useful imaging study in overdose is the abdominal radiograph, which may reveal radiodense material in the stomach or gut in the following ingestions (*Goldfrank's Toxicologic Emergencies. 8th ed. New York: McGraw-Hill, 2006:62*):
  - **C**hloral hydrate
  - **H**eavy metals
  - **I**ron
  - **P**henothiazines
  - **E**nteric-coated preparations
  - **S**ustained-release preparations
- Occasionally, subtle abnormalities on the abdominal film will detect the presence of "rosettes" or elongated packets in the GI tract of body packers. The abdominal film is of limited utility in body stuffers (*Ann Emerg Med 1997;29:596*).

TREATMENT

As with any patient, it is crucial to maintain the airway, check for adequacy of breathing and circulation, and check an FSBG in the patient with altered mental status or coma.
- **Prevention of absorption:** Traditionally, gastric emptying by either inducing **emesis** or **lavage** has been a mainstay in the treatment of the acutely overdosed patient. However, the literature regarding these methods of decontamination suggests that they are of little benefit (*Med J Aust 1995;163:345*). Furthermore, numerous studies have suggested that patients present approximately 3 to 4 hours after ingestion on average, which tends to make it less likely that there will be a large recovery of pills (*Ann Emerg Med 1985;14:562*). Therefore, the routine administration of **ipecac** to children and "stomach pumping" has fallen by the wayside except in very specific circumstances.

- **Activated charcoal (AC)** has largely replaced both of these methods of gastric emptying and has been shown to be effective in the management of acute overdoses (*Ann Emerg Med 2002;39:273*). However, the clinical utility of this method of decontamination is limited if the ingestion occurred more than 1 hour prior to presentation (*J Toxicol Clin Toxicol 1997;35:721*). Certain ingestions benefit from multidose AC as they either bind to concretions in the stomach (aspirin), or they decrease enterohepatic or enteroenteric reabsorption (phenobarbital, phenytoin, theophylline). AC should be dosed at 1 g/kg body weight.
- **Whole-bowel irrigation** is appropriate in patients who have ingested sustained-release medications, body packing, or metals that do not bind to AC. The optimal dose of polyethylene glycol is 1 to 2 L/hr until the rectal effluent is clear. This dose is a large amount of fluid to ingest, so it is often necessary to place a nasogastric tube to achieve this rate of emptying.
- In cases **of life-threatening** ingestions such as colchicine or nondihydropyridine calcium channel blockers (CCBs), it is appropriate to consider **lavage** as well as **AC**.
- **Cathartics** have no role in the management of overdose. They are often present in the premixed AC solutions. If this is the case, only one dose should be administered.
- All of these interventions are **contraindicated** in the presence of airway compromise, persistent vomiting, and the presence of an ileus, bowel obstruction, or GI perforation.
- **Enhanced elimination**
  - **Forced diuresis** with normal saline and Ringer's lactate enhances the elimination of low–molecular-weight agents such as lithium in dehydrated individuals. This should be carefully monitored and diuretics should be avoided in these patients.
  - **Urinary alkalinization** with intravenous sodium bicarbonate enhances the elimination of weak acids and is useful in the setting of salicylate overdose. Typical doses are 1 to 2 mEq/kg, with a goal of maintaining the urinary pH at approximately 7 to 8. Specific recommendations will be further discussed in the following text.
  - There is no role for **urinary acidification** in the management of overdoses.
  - **Hemodialysis and hemoperfusion** are reserved for life-threatening ingestions of substances that have a low volume of distribution, a molecular weight of less than 500 Da, a low endogenous clearance, are water soluble, and have little protein binding. This treatment modality will be further discussed under specific substances.
- **Antidotes** will be discussed under specific toxicities. The regional poison center should be contacted for specific guidelines for treatment.
- **Disposition**
  - Patients who have taken an overdose as a suicidal gesture should all receive a psychiatric evaluation prior to discharge.
  - Most cases of unintentional overdose do not result in significant morbidity, and in cases where the patient is stable and asymptomatic, a brief period of observation may be all that is necessary.
  - In cases where potentially toxic agents have been ingested, patients should be monitored for 4 to 6 hours before discharge.

Acetaminophen

GENERAL PRINCIPLES

APAP is available worldwide as an over-the-counter analgesic and antipyretic and has become the most common pharmacologic agent involved in toxicologic fatalities

(*Am J Emerg Med 2005;23(5):589*). The recommended maximum dose for adults is 4 g/d.

Classification

- An analgesic. Within the United States, APAP is sold under the trade name Tylenol. The most common trade name for APAP outside the United States is Paracetamol.
- Because of its use as an analgesic and antipyretic, APAP has become a common ingredient in various cold and flu remedies. It is also used in the treatment of fevers, headaches, and acute and chronic pain.
- APAP is often sold in combination preparations together with nonsteroidal anti-inflammatory drugs (NSAIDs), opiate analgesics, or sedatives (e.g., Tylenol #3, Percocet, Darvocet, Vicodin, NyQuil, Tylenol PM).

Epidemiology

APAP is the leading cause of toxicologic fatalities per year in the United States, and APAP-induced hepatotoxicity is the most frequent cause of acute liver failure (*Hepatology 2005;42(6):1364*).

Etiology

- APAP is available as tablets, capsules, liquids, and suppositories. In addition to the more common immediate-release form, there is also an extended-release preparation (e.g., Tylenol Arthritis Pain).
- Unintentional overdosing is much more common than intentional ingestion in suicide attempts, especially in elderly patients on chronic pain regimen with several APAP-containing painkillers (*Hepatol Res 2008;38:3*).
- All patients with presumed APAP overdose should be adequately assessed, evaluated, and treated. However, only the minority of poisoned patients require inpatient care (*Acad Emerg Med 1999;6(11):1115*).

Pathophysiology

- **Absorption:** APAP serum levels peak 30 to 60 minutes after oral ingestion; the extended-release preparations peak after 1 to 2 hours. Absorption is often delayed in overdose, and peak levels are usually reached after 2 to 8 hours. The overdose kinetics of extended-release APAP are not yet well established.
- **Overdose:** The hepatic conjugation pathways become saturated in overdose. A cascade of biochemical changes occurs in the liver and centrilobular cell necrosis results (*Clin Pharmacol Ther 1974;16(4):676*).
  - Acetaminophen is metabolized predominantly via glucuronidation (47% to 62%) and sulfation (25% to 36%) by Phase II metabolism in liver as nontoxic conjugate products. However, a small percentage is metabolized via oxidation (5% to 8%) by the cytochrome P450 (2E1) pathway to a toxic metabolite, *N*-acetyl-*p*-benzoquinone imine (NAPQI). NAPQI is conjugated by glutathione to nontoxic cysteine and mercapturic acid conjugates.
  - In cases of acetaminophen toxicity, the Phase II conjugation enzymes are saturated, and a higher fraction of acetaminophen is conjugated via oxidation to NAPQI. The conjugation of NAPQI to glutathione occurs until glutathione is depleted from hepatic reserves, after which the toxic NAPQI accumulates and causes damage to the hepatocytes.

Risk Factors

- Decreased glutathione stores (fasting, malnutrition, anorexia nervosa, chronic alcoholism, febrile illness, chronic disease).

- P450 enzyme inducers (ethanol, Isoniazid [INH], phenytoin and other anticonvulsants, barbiturates, smoking).

DIAGNOSIS

Clinical Presentation
- **First 24 hours**—Asymptomatic stage (stage 1):
  - Early symptoms are very nonspecific and primarily related to the GI tract (nausea, vomiting, anorexia).
  - High-dose APAP can cause pallor or lethargy in some patients.
  - This initial phase is rare in symptoms and patients appear pretty unremarkable. Therefore, always think of other coingestants if a patient exhibits extreme vital sign abnormalities or other significant symptoms during the first 24 hours.
- **24 to 48 hours**—Hepatotoxic stage (stage 2):
  - Right upper quadrant (RUQ) tenderness is the most common symptom.
  - Transaminitis, bilirubinemia, and elevated prothrombin time (PT)/International normalized ratio (INR) are also common findings during the second phase.
- **2 to 4 days**—Fulminant hepatic failure stage (stage 3): Significant hepatic dysfunction develops (i.e., a peak in hepatic enzyme elevation along with jaundice, coagulopathy with high risk of spontaneous bleeding, hypoglycemia, anuria, and cerebral edema with coma or even death).
- **4 to 14 days**—Recovery stage (stage 4): If stage 3 is survived, the hepatic dysfunction usually resolves over the following days/weeks.

History
- In order to predict the risk of hepatotoxicity after acute overdose, a reliable time of ingestion must be obtained from the patient or family/friends.
- Also obtain information about the amount of APAP that has been ingested, in what form (e.g., combination preparations, extended-release form), and over what period of time.
- Inquire about other coingestants (alcohol, other medications, other drugs).

Physical Examination
Assess airway, breathing, and circulation (ABCs) and mental status. The assessment of mental status is crucial, especially in patients who are nauseated or vomiting, to intervene with airway protection in time.

Diagnostic Criteria
- In general, a dose of 150 mg APAP per kilogram is the potentially toxic limit that requires therapeutic intervention. This limit includes an added 25% safety margin that was added by the U.S. Food and Drug Administration (FDA) to adjust for patients with multiple risk factors for increased liver toxicity (*BMJ 1998; 316(7146):1724*).
- If the total amount of ingested APAP is above 150 mg/kg or cannot be obtained from the patient history, it is crucial to predict the risk of toxicity.
- Obtain an APAP serum level at 4 hours or later after ingestion.
- Plot the APAP concentration on the **Rumack–Matthew nomogram** (APAP serum concentration vs. time after ingestion) to assess the possibility of hepatic toxicity. NOTE: The nomogram should only be used for acute ingestions.

- During treatment of APAP overdose, it is important to assess the risk of progressive liver failure. The King's College Hospital (KCH) Criteria provide prognostic markers that help to predict the probability of developing severe liver damage (*Gastroenterology 1989;97(2):439*):
  - pH <7.3, 2 days postingestion.
  - All of the following: PT >100, serum creatinine >3.3 mmol/L, severe hepatic encephalopathy (grade III or IV).
- Elevated serum phosphate levels >1.2 mmol/L (>3.72 mg/dL) on days 2 to 4 (additional criterion, not originally part of KCH criteria) (*Hepatology 2002; 36(3):659*).
- Arterial serum lactate >3.0 mmol/L (>27 mg/dL) after fluid resuscitation (additional criterion, not originally part of KCH criteria) (*Lancet 2002;359(9306): 558*).

Diagnostic Testing

- **APAP serum level at 4 hours** after ingestion or later (see earlier discussion).
- **Liver function tests (LFTs)**—Aspartate aminotransferase (AST) is a relatively sensitive nonprognostic marker for hepatic injury.
- **PT/INR**, **serum bicarbonate**, **blood pH**, serum **lactate**, **renal function panel**, and serum **phosphate** level are the prognostic markers for hepatic injury.
- APAP may interfere with some blood sugar test kits causing measurements higher or lower than actual; always recheck FSBG over the course of hospitalization (*Am J Clin Pathol 2000;113(1):75*).

TREATMENT

Gastric lavage is not useful in APAP overdose; however, it may be indicated in presence of certain other coingestants.

Medications

- **Activated charcoal:** Only indicated in patients with isolated APAP exposure (with no other evidence of mentally altering substances) who present less than 4 hours after ingestion. Give **1 g/kg by mouth (PO)**.
- **N-acetylcysteine (NAC):** NAC is the specific antidote to prevent APAP-related hepatotoxicity (*Toxicol Sci 2004;80(2):343*). NAC replenishes depleted glutathione (GSH) stores. It should be administered early (i.e., within 8 hours after ingestion) to prevent any liver damage. NAC is a nonspecific antioxidant and will still provide some liver protection if given beyond this time window (*J Clin Invest 1983;71(4):980*).
  - **Oral dosing:** Loading dose of 140 mg/kg PO, then 70 mg/kg PO every 4 hours for a total of 17 doses (i.e., 1,330 mg/kg over 72 hours) (*N Engl J Med 1988;319(24):1557*).
  - **Intravenous (IV) dosing:** Prepare the infusion by adding 30 g of a 20% NAC solution (150 mL) to 1 L D_5W. This will result in a final concentration of 30 mg/mL. Load with a dose of 150 mg/kg NAC IV over 1 hour. Thereafter, continue to give 14 mg/kg/hr IV for 20 hours (i.e., 430 mg/kg over 21 hours) (According to IV NAC treatment protocol used by Toxicology Service at Barnes-Jewish Hospital). (See also *Ann Pharmacother 2011;45(6):713*.)
  - **NAC administration** can be safely stopped prior to the completion of the total regimen as soon as the APAP level returns to 0, INR <2.0, and AST normalizes (or reaches less than half of the peak level during acute intoxication).

- **NAC indications:** NAC treatment should be started in the following:
  - Any patient after acute poisoning with a toxic APAP level according to the nomogram.
  - Patients who present beyond 8 hours after acute ingestion. Start NAC therapy while awaiting the initial APAP serum level. Continue treatment if the serum concentration is in the toxic range per nomogram.
  - Patients who present more than 24 hours after acute ingestion and still have a detectable serum APAP level or elevated AST.
  - Patients with chronic APAP exposure (i.e., >4 g/d in adults, >120 mg/kg/d in children) who present with elevated transaminases.
  - Patients with signs of fulminant hepatic failure. NAC treatment should be started immediately and transfer to a transplant center arranged without fail. NAC has been shown to improve survival of patients in fulminant failure (*Lancet 1990;335(8705):1572*; *N Engl J Med 1991;324(26):1852*; *BMJ 1991;303(6809): 1026*).
- **Oral Versus IV NAC:**
  - IV administration of NAC is the preferred route as it is used in all of the studies of patients with fulminant hepatic failure.
  - Oral administration may be slightly safer compared to the IV form; however, NAC has a rather bad odor and taste. Rash, flushing, urticaria, nausea/vomiting, angioedema, bronchospasm, tachycardia, and hypotension have been reported as adverse reactions to IV administration (*BMJ 1984;289(6439):217*).
  - If oral NAC is given, dilute the NAC with juice, provide a drinking straw, give IV antiemetics (e.g., Reglan, Zofran).
  - Consider oral over IV NAC in patients who are prone to anaphylactoid reactions (e.g., severe asthmatics).
  - NAC is effective either way when given within 8 hours after ingestion (*N Engl J Med 1988;319(24):1557*).
  - AC adsorbs oral NAC. Both, PO and IV NAC regimens provide enough excess of the drug to ensure adequate therapeutic effects. Nevertheless, it is advised to administer AC 2 hours apart from NAC when given PO.

COMPLICATIONS

- Overdose with extended-relief APAP (*Ann Emerg Med 1997;30(1):104*):
  - Get APAP serum level 4 hours postingestion.
  - If toxic per nomogram, treat with full NAC course.
  - If below toxic level per nomogram, get repeat APAP at 8 hours postingestion.
  - If now toxic, treat with full course. If remains below toxic level, no therapy necessary.
- Patients with progressing liver failure need to be admitted to an intensive care unit (ICU) bed with close monitoring for hyperglycemia, electrolyte imbalances, GI bleeding, acid–base disturbances, cerebral edema, infections, and renal failure.

REFERRAL

- Involve a clinical toxicologist in all cases where toxic APAP levels are documented. Discuss the initiation of NAC treatment with the toxicology service where possible.
- Inform your regional Poison Control Center (1-800-222-1222).

- Involve the liver or transplant service early in patients presenting with poor prognostic factors for hepatic failure.
- Patients with toxic liver failure should be transferred to a transplant center as early as possible (*BMJ 1991;303(6796):221*; *J R Soc Med 1997;90(7):368*).

Colchicine

GENERAL PRINCIPLES

Definition

Colchicine is the active alkaloid extracted from two plants of the Liliaceae family: *Colchicum autumnale* (autumn crocus) and *Gloriosa superba* or glory lily. It has been used in the therapy of gout for centuries.

Etiology

Colchicine has a very narrow therapeutic index. Severe poisoning and death can result from the ingestion of as little as 0.8 mg/kg of body weight (*Nouv Presse Med 1977;6:1625*).

Pathophysiology

Colchicine is an effective inhibitor of intracellular microtubule formation, leading to impaired leukocyte chemotaxis, and phagocytosis resulting in a decrease in the inflammatory cascade (*JAMA 2003;289:2857*). In overdose, colchicine causes mitotic arrest, leading to cellular dysfunction and death (*J Emerg Med 1994;12:171*).

Prevention

Patients who are started on colchicine for gout symptoms should be explicitly directed to stop taking the medication as soon as symptoms of diarrhea occur. They should also be told that increasing the dose in an acute flare can result in significant toxicity; therefore, if they are unable to control the symptoms at home, they should seek expert care early.

DIAGNOSIS

Clinical Presentation

Patients who present with a colchicine overdose tend to develop a syndrome that progresses through three phases. The initial phase usually begins several hours after the overdose and is characterized by nausea, vomiting, and diarrhea. Over the next 1 to 7 days, patients may develop multiorgan failure requiring intensive support; death is common at this stage. In the final phase, patients develop alopecia and myoneuropathies.

History

Patients with inadvertent overdoses will present with a recent history of an acute gouty flare, followed by the development of nausea, vomiting, and diarrhea within a few hours after the overdose. Intentional overdoses may present late and should be suspected in patients with a GI syndrome followed by multiorgan failure.

Physical Examination

The exam tends to be somewhat unremarkable in these patients. They may exhibit signs of dehydration with tachycardia and dry mucous membranes. They may also have decreased urine output. As the toxicity progresses, patients may develop signs of worsening distress and confusion requiring aggressive resuscitation measures. As the disease evolves, fatal cardiac arrhythmias and refractory cardiovascular collapse may occur, usually within a week of overdose (*J Forensic Sci 1994;39:280*). Reversible alopecia has been reported in survivors (*J Emerg Med 1994;12:171*).

Differential Diagnosis

As with any ingestion, the differential diagnosis is large. However, GI symptoms are common in patients with overdoses of methylxanthines, podophyllin, digoxin and other cardioactive steroids, chemotherapeutic agents, heavy metals, and salicylates.

Diagnostic Testing

There is a very interesting sequence of laboratory findings that should lead one to consider colchicine poisoning in patients.

Laboratories

- **Complete blood cell count (CBC):** In the initial phase of poisoning that lasts for approximately 12 to 24 hours, patients develop a leukocytosis. In the next 48 to 72 hours, signs of bone marrow suppression evolve starting with a profound decline in the leukocyte count and subsequent pancytopenia.
- **BMP:** Colchicine poisoning has also been associated with renal failure and adrenal hemorrhage (*J Anal Toxicol 1991;15:151*); therefore, electrolytes should be monitored.
- **LFTs:** Colchicine overdoses have been reported to cause hepatotoxicity; therefore, LFTs should be monitored.
- **Coagulation studies:** Disseminated intravascular coagulation (DIC) occasionally occurs; therefore, a full panel, including fibrinogen and fibrin split products should be obtained.
- **Colchicine concentrations:** Colchicine has a narrow therapeutic index, and plasma concentrations >3 ng/mL may produce significant toxicity. However, this laboratory test is not readily available and toxicity should be suspected if clinical symptoms and laboratory studies are supportive. This test should be thought of as a confirmatory study.
- **Other studies:** Creatine kinase (CK or creatine phosphokinase [CPK]), troponin, lipase, and other electrolytes should be obtained depending on the clinical scenario.

Electrocardiography

An ECG should be obtained at presentation, given the patient's predilection for developing cardiac arrhythmias, and the patient should be admitted with continuous cardiac monitoring.

Imaging

Colchicine toxicity has been associated with the development of acute respiratory distress syndrome (ARDS). Therefore, a chest X-ray (CXR) should be obtained.

TREATMENT

Colchicine overdoses are often fatal and require aggressive supportive measures. As always, airway protection is of paramount importance followed by adequacy of breathing and support of circulation.

Medications

In cases of severe neutropenia, consider **Granulocyte colony-stimulating factor (G-CSF)** administration.

Other Nonpharmacologic Therapies

- If the patient is **not** vomiting, consider **gastric lavage** and **AC**. If the patient is altered and vomiting, consider early **endotracheal intubation**. **Fluids** and direct acting **vasopressors** should be used in cases of hypotension. **Hemodialysis** is not useful for clearing colchicine, given its large volume of distribution; however, it should be used in the setting of colchicine-induced renal failure.
- All symptomatic patients should be admitted to the ICU. Patients without symptoms should be monitored for 8 to 12 hours prior to discharge.

SPECIAL CONSIDERATIONS

Given its narrow therapeutic window and pharmacokinetics, colchicine should be used cautiously in patients with underlying renal or liver dysfunction. Likewise, colchicine is a P450 drug and is subject to many drug–drug interactions (*Biochem Pharmacol 1997;10:111*). A thorough review of the patient's medication list should be conducted before starting the patient on this agent as toxic concentrations can accumulate rapidly. In this setting, consider using alternative therapies for the management of acute gouty flares.

Nonsteroidal Anti-Inflammatory Drugs

GENERAL PRINCIPLES

- NSAIDs are widely prescribed as analgesics for the management of inflammatory diseases. There are many different classes available; however, the discussion in the following text relates to over-the-counter preparations available in the United States and includes ibuprofen, ketoprofen, and naproxen as well as the selective cyclooxygenase (COX)-2 inhibitors.
- NSAIDs exert their therapeutic effects by inhibiting cyclooxygenase and thereby preventing the formation of prostaglandins. This mechanism accounts for both their therapeutic and toxic side effects, which include ulceration of the GI mucosa and renal dysfunction. In the vast majority of cases, overdose is benign.

DIAGNOSIS

Clinical Presentation

Overdose histories are often unreliable. Consider NSAID overdose in patients who present with **GI distress**. **Massive overdose** with ibuprofen occasionally presents with **coma and seizures**.

Diagnostic Testing

Obtain a **BMP** to evaluate renal function and hydration status. An **APAP** concentration should be obtained as many patients confuse over-the-counter analgesics.

TREATMENT

Usually supportive care is all that is necessary for the management of this overdose. IV fluids (IVF) are beneficial for maintaining hydration in vomiting patients.

Medications
- Consider **AC** 1 g/kg for GI decontamination.
- **Antiemetics and antacids** are beneficial in patients with significant distress.
- **Benzodiazepines** should be used for the management of seizures associated with massive ibuprofen overdose.

Opioids

DIAGNOSIS

Clinical Presentation

Symptoms of opioid overdose are respiratory depression, a depressed level of consciousness, and **miosis**. However, the pupils may be dilated with acidosis or hypoxia or after overdoses with meperidine or diphenoxylate plus atropine. Overdose with fentanyl or derivatives such as α-methyl fentanyl ("China white") may result in negative urine toxicology screens.

Diagnostic Testing

Laboratories

Drug concentrations and other standard laboratory tests are of little use. Pulse oximetry and **ABG**s are useful for monitoring respiratory status. Although less widely available, capnography measuring end-tidal CO_2 is more sensitive in detecting impending respiratory arrest as hypercapnia precedes hypoxemia.

Electrocardiography
- **Methadone** has been reported to cause a **prolonged QT_c**. Obtain an ECG in suspected overdose.
- **Propoxyphene** exhibits type IA antidysrhythmic effects due to sodium channel blockade and may present with a **wide complex QRS** on ECG (*Acta Pharmacol Toxicol 1978;42:171*).

Imaging

A chest radiograph should be obtained if pulmonary symptoms are present.

TREATMENT

- Treatment includes airway maintenance, ventilatory support, and judicious use of opioid antagonist.
- Avoid gastric lavage.
- Limit use of whole-bowel irrigation to body packers. Body packers rarely require surgery, except in cases of intestinal obstruction.
- Endoscopic removal should not be attempted due to the danger of rupture.

Medications
- **Naloxone hydrochloride** specifically reverses opioid-induced respiratory and CNS depression and hypotension.

○ The lowest effective dose should be used. The goal of treatment is adequate spontaneous respiration and not necessarily alertness. The initial dose is 0.04 to 2 mg IV, although the lowest effective dose should be used.

○ Larger doses (up to 10 mg IV) may be required to reverse the effects of propoxyphene, diphenoxylate, buprenorphine, or pentazocine.

○ In the absence of an IV line, naloxone can be administered sublingually (*Ann Emerg Med 1987;16:572*), via endotracheal tube, or intranasally (*Emerg Med J 2006;23:221*). Isolated opioid overdose is unlikely if there is no response to a total of 10 mg naloxone. Repetitive doses may be required (duration of action is 45 minutes), and this should prompt hospitalization despite the patient's return to an alert status.

○ Methadone overdose may require therapy for 24 to 48 hours, whereas levo-α-acetylmethadol may require therapy for 72 hours. A continuous IV drip that provides two-thirds of the initial dose of naloxone hourly, diluted in D_5W, may be necessary to maintain an alert state (*Ann Emerg Med 1986;15:566*).

○ Ventilatory support should be provided for the patient who is unresponsive to naloxone and for pulmonary edema.

• **Disposition**
  ○ If the patient is alert and asymptomatic for 4 to 6 hours after a single dose of naloxone, or for 4 hours after a single treatment for an IV overdose, he or she can be discharged safely.
  ○ Body packers should be admitted to an ICU for close monitoring of the respiratory rate and level of consciousness and remain so until all packets have passed, as documented by computed tomography (CT).

SPECIAL CONSIDERATIONS

• Heroin may be adulterated with scopolamine, cocaine, clenbuterol, or caffeine, complicating the clinical picture. Less common complications include hypotension, bradycardia, and pulmonary edema.

• Be aware of body packers who smuggle heroin in their intestinal tracts. Deterioration of latex or plastic containers may result in drug release and death (*Am J Forensic Med Pathol 1997;18:312*).

Salicylates

GENERAL PRINCIPLES

• Salicylate toxicity may result from **acute or chronic** ingestion of acetylsalicylic acid (aspirin is a generic name in the United States, but a brand name in the rest of the world). Toxicity is usually mild after acute ingestions of <150 mg/kg, moderate after ingestions of 150 to 300 mg/kg, and generally severe with overdoses of 300 to 500 mg/kg.

• Toxicity from chronic ingestion is typically due to intake of >100 mg/kg/d over a period of several days and usually occurs in elderly patients with chronic underlying illness. Diagnosis is often delayed in this group of patients, and mortality is approximately 25%. Significant toxicity due to chronic ingestion may occur with blood concentrations lower than those associated with acute ingestions.

• Topical preparations containing methyl salicylate or oil of wintergreen can cause toxicity with excessive topical use or if ingested.

DIAGNOSIS

Clinical Presentation

- Nausea, vomiting, tinnitus, tachypnea, hyperapnea, and malaise are common. Hyperthermia results in uncoupled mitochondrial oxidative phosphorylation and suggests a poor prognosis.
- Severe intoxications may include lethargy, convulsions, and coma, which may result from cerebral edema and energy depletion in the CNS.
- Noncardiogenic pulmonary edema may occur and is more common with chronic ingestion, cigarette smoking, neurologic symptoms, and older age.
- Severe overdoses of >300 mg/kg may present with tachypnea, dehydration, pulmonary edema, altered mental status, seizures, or coma.

Diagnostic Testing

Laboratories

- Obtain electrolytes, blood urea nitrogen (BUN), creatinine, glucose, and salicylate concentration.
- Obtain either ABGs or VBGs.
- ABGs may reveal an early respiratory alkalosis, followed by metabolic acidosis.
  - Approximately 20% of patients exhibit either respiratory alkalosis or metabolic acidosis alone (*J Crit Illness 1986;1:77*).
  - Most adults with pure salicylate overdose have a primary metabolic acidosis and a primary respiratory alkalosis.
  - After mixed overdoses, respiratory acidosis may become prominent (*Arch Intern Med 1978;138:1481*).
- Serum salicylate concentrations drawn after acute ingestion of salicylates assist in prediction of severity of intoxication and patient disposition. However, **do not rely upon the Done nomogram**.
  - Salicylate concentrations >70 mg/dL at any time represent moderate-to-severe intoxication.
  - Salicylate concentrations >100 mg/dL are very serious and often fatal. This information is useful only for acute overdoses of nonenteric-coated aspirin.
  - Enteric-coated aspirin may have delayed absorption and delayed peak concentration.
  - Chronic ingestion can cause toxicity with lower salicylate concentrations.
  - Bicarbonate concentrations and pH are more useful than salicylate concentrations as prognostic indicators in chronic intoxication.

Imaging

- Repeated blood salicylate concentrations that fail to decline should prompt contrast radiography of the stomach. Salicylate concretions may require endoscopy, multiple-dose AC, or bicarbonate lavage.
- Consider whole-bowel irrigation with polyethylene glycol.

TREATMENT

Medications

- Administer 50 to 100 g **AC** if presentation is within 1 hour of ingestion.
- **Multidose charcoal** may be useful in severe overdose (*Pediatrics 1990;85:594*), or in cases in which salicylate concentrations fail to decline (due to possible gastric bezoar formation).

- **Alkaline diuresis** is indicated for symptomatic patients with salicylate blood concentrations >40 mg/dL.
  - Administer 150 mEq (three ampules) sodium bicarbonate in 1,000 mL D_5W at a rate of 10 to 15 mL/kg/hr if the patient is clinically volume depleted until urine flow is achieved.
  - Maintain alkalinization using the same solution at 2 to 3 mL/kg/hr, and monitor urine output, urine pH (target pH, 7 to 8), and serum potassium. Successful alkaline diuresis requires the simultaneous administration of potassium chloride.
  - Give **40 mEq potassium chloride** intravenous piggyback (IVPB) over 4 to 5 hours. Give additional potassium chloride either orally or intravenously as needed to maintain serum potassium concentration above 4 mEq/L.
  - **Use caution with alkaline diuresis in older patients**, who may have cardiac, renal, or pulmonary comorbidity, as pulmonary edema is more likely to occur in this population.
- **Do not use acetazolamide** (carbonic anhydrase inhibitor). Although acetazolamide alkalinizes the urine, it increases salicylate toxicity because it also alkalinizes the CNS (trapping more salicylate in the brain) and worsens acidemia.
- **Hyperventilate any patient requiring endotracheal intubation.** In salicylate-poisoned patients with tachypnea and hyperapnea, the respiratory alkalosis partially compensates for the metabolic acidosis. Mechanical ventilation with neuromuscular paralysis, sedation, and "normal" ventilator rates will remove the respiratory alkalosis, worsen acidosis, and cause rapid deterioration or death.
- **Treat altered mental status with IV dextrose**, despite normal blood glucose.
- Treat cerebral edema with hyperventilation and osmotic diuresis.
- Treat **seizures** with a **benzodiazepine** (diazepam, 5 to 10 mg IV q15min up to 50 mg) followed by **phenobarbital**, 15 mg/kg IV. Give **dextrose** 25 g IV immediately following seizure control.

Other Nonpharmacologic Therapies

- **Hemodialysis** is indicated for blood concentrations >100 mg/dL after acute intoxication. Hemodialysis rapidly removes salicylate and corrects acidosis. Hemodialysis may be useful with chronic toxicity when salicylate concentrations are as low as 40 mg/dL in patients with any of the following: persistent acidosis, severe CNS symptoms, progressive clinical deterioration, pulmonary edema, or renal failure.
- Treatment of pulmonary edema may also require mechanical ventilation with a high fraction of inspired oxygen concentration and positive end-expiratory pressure (PEEP) (in addition to high respiratory rate).

SPECIAL CONSIDERATIONS

- Patients with minor symptoms (nausea, vomiting, tinnitus), an acute ingestion of <100 mg/kg, and a first blood concentration of <50 mg/dL may be treated in the emergency department. Blood concentrations should be repeated every 2 hours until they show a decline. These patients often are medically stable for discharge, and their disposition can be determined based on psychiatric evaluation.
- Admit moderately symptomatic patients for at least 24 hours. Repeat serum salicylate concentration, electrolytes, BUN, creatinine, and glucose at least every 6 hours to confirm declining salicylate concentration, improving bicarbonate concentration,

and stable potassium concentration. Measure urine pH at least every 6 hours (if patient has urinary bladder catheter) or with each spontaneous void to confirm urinary alkalinization.

• Admit patients with severe overdoses to an ICU. Monitor laboratory studies as with moderately ill patients. Closely monitor ABGs. Arrange for immediate hemodialysis. Use great caution with mechanical ventilation, and hyperventilate any patient who requires mechanical ventilation.

Phenytoin and Fosphenytoin

GENERAL PRINCIPLES

Classification

There are four major mechanisms by which anticonvulsants exert therapeutic activity —sodium channel blockade, GABA agonism, calcium channel antagonism, and inhibition of excitatory amino acids. In overdose, these features are enhanced.

Pathophysiology

• Phenytoin has been a first-line treatment for seizures since its introduction. Fosphenytoin was developed as a response to some of the toxicity associated with intravenous phenytoin administration. Fosphenytoin is a prodrug that is converted to phenytoin after IV or intramuscular (IM) injection and therefore will be referred to as phenytoin in the following text.

• **Neither of these drugs is indicated for the treatment of toxin-induced seizures** (*N Engl J Med 1985;313:145*), **including ethanol withdrawal seizures** (*Ann Emerg Med 1991;20:520*).

• Phenytoin exerts therapeutic activity by binding to sodium channels and inhibiting reactivation (*J Neural Transm 1988;72:173*). Phenytoin exhibits saturable kinetics, and at plasma levels above 20 μg/mL, toxic effects become rapidly apparent.

• Acute toxicity is associated with the development of a **neurologic syndrome** that appears to be cerebellar in origin. **Cardiotoxicity** is **not** associated with phenytoin **ingestion** (*Heart Lung 1997;26:325*); however, it has been **reported with IV administration** of phenytoin. Rapid IV administration slows cardiac conduction and decreases systemic vascular resistance and myocardial contractility. The cardiac toxicity associated with intravenous phenytoin administration is due in part to the presence of propylene glycol and ethanol in the diluent, which are known myocardial depressants and vasodilators (*Am J Cardiol 1966;17:332*). The introduction of fosphenytoin has decreased the incidence of cardiac complications.

Risk Factors

Other than overdose, risk factors for developing phenytoin toxicity are associated with the coadministration of drugs that affect the **cytochrome P450** system.

DIAGNOSIS

There are several classic clinical findings that point to the diagnosis of phenytoin toxicity.

Clinical Presentation

History

Patients exhibiting toxicity from phenytoin will often be brought in by family members who will describe the patient as **ataxic** and increasingly **confused**. There is usually a history of seizure disorder and the medication list will include phenytoin. In intentional overdoses, the patient may be lethargic with slurred speech and an extrapyramidal movement disorder (*Ann Emerg Med 1989;7:61*).

Physical Examination

- At plasma concentrations of >15 μg/mL, patients will exhibit **nystagmus**. **Ataxia** develops at levels of 30 μg/mL. **Confusion** and **frank movement disorders** occur at levels of 50 μg/mL or greater. Chronic phenytoin ingestion is also associated with **gingival hyperplasia**, which is a very useful clinical finding when uncertain of the diagnosis. **Ingestions** are **not** associated with **cardiotoxicity** or vital sign abnormalities (*Ann Emerg Med 1991;20:508*). Rapid **intravenous** administration of phenytoin results in **hypotension** and **bradycardia**. **Death** has been reported (*JAMA 1968;20:2118*).
- **Extravasation** injury is a serious complication of intravenous phenytoin administration and can result in severe tissue injury described as **the purple glove syndrome**. This injury will occasionally require surgical debridement (*Neurology 1998; 51(4):1034*).

Differential Diagnosis

Phenytoin toxicity is similar in presentation to carbamazepine poisoning; however, carbamazepine tends to exhibit cardiotoxicity. Other considerations include a convulsive status epilepticus, meningitis, encephalitis, or other intracerebral lesion.

Diagnostic Testing

Laboratories

- **Serial phenytoin concentrations** (corrected for albumin, as phenytoin is highly protein bound) should be obtained on any patient with a potential history of exposure.
- CBC: Phenytoin has been reported to occasionally cause agranulocytosis.
- LFTs: Phenytoin is associated with the occasional development of hepatotoxicity.

Electrocardiography

ECGs and telemetry are generally not needed in oral overdoses (*Ann Emerg Med 1991;20:508*). However, in IV infusions, it is necessary to have the patient in a monitored setting.

TREATMENT

- Admission is warranted for patients with ataxia, and serial levels should be obtained while in the hospital.
- Supportive care is the mainstay of treatment for acute or chronic phenytoin toxicity. **Multidose activated charcoal** (MDAC) is useful in decreasing the serum half-life; however, given the pharmacokinetic profile of this drug, it is possible to rapidly lower the serum concentration below therapeutic levels and precipitate a seizure.
- **Benzodiazepines** are the mainstay of treatment for seizures.

- Hypotension and bradycardia in the setting of IV administration is usually self-limiting and will resolve with supportive care. In refractory bradycardia or hypotension, advanced cardiac life support (ACLS) principles apply.
- Cases of agranulocytosis are responsive to **G-CSF** administration.
- Hepatotoxicity usually resolves with the discontinuation of the drug.

Surgical Management

In cases of extravasation, it is important to have a surgical evaluation in order to determine the need for operative debridement.

SPECIAL CONSIDERATIONS

Phenytoin is generally of limited use in the treatment of active seizures. Since the mainstay of treatment is benzodiazepine administration and IV phenytoin is associated with significant toxicity, it is better to orally load patients whenever possible.

OUTCOME/PROGNOSIS

Phenytoin overdoses tend to be benign and self-limiting with supportive care. Deaths are exceedingly unusual even in the setting of massive overdose.

Carbamazepine/Oxcarbazepine

GENERAL PRINCIPLES

Definition

Carbamazepine and oxcarbazepine are structurally related to TCAs. Like fosphenytoin, oxcarbazepine is a prodrug that is metabolized to an active metabolite. An anticonvulsant.

Pathophysiology

- The therapeutic efficacy of carbamazepine and oxcarbazepine are due to **sodium channel blockade**, which prevents the propagation of an abnormal focus. The therapeutic serum concentration of carbamazepine is 4 to 12 mg/L. There is no routine laboratory testing for oxcarbazepine; however, the carbamazepine assay will detect the presence of oxcarbazepine.
- The toxicity associated with carbamazepine is likely due to its chemical structure. TCA-like effects include sodium channel blockade, QT prolongation, and anticholinergic features.
- In overdose, carbamazepine is erratically absorbed and may form concretions in the GI tract causing prolonged toxicity.
- Persistently high levels of carbamazepine have been reported to increase antidiuretic hormone secretion leading to syndrome of inappropriate antidiuretic hormone release (SIADH) (*Prog Neuropsychopharmacol Biol Psychiatry 1994;18:211*).

Risk Factors

Carbamazepine toxicity may be enhanced by concomitant use of drugs that are metabolized by the CYP450 system.

DIAGNOSIS

There are several key features of carbamazepine toxicity.

Clinical Presentation

History
Toxicity should be suspected in individuals who present with a history of a seizure disorder and altered mental status. **Delayed toxicity** has been reported after an acute overdose given the variability in GI absorption (*J Toxicol Clin Toxicol 1979;14:263*). Patients may exhibit a relapsing syndrome of coma and altered consciousness due to bezoar formation and enterohepatic recirculation.

Physical Examination
- The predominant clinical findings in carbamazepine toxicity are neurologic and cardiovascular effects. In mild-to-moderate toxicity, patients may present with ataxia, nystagmus, and mydriasis. In serious overdose, patients may develop **coma** and **seizures**, including status epilepticus. Vital sign abnormalities include **tachycardia** due to the anticholinergic effects of the drug as well as **hypotension** and **bradycardia** due to direct myocardial depressant effects.
- The combination of cerebellar findings on exam, in conjunction with an anticholinergic toxidrome, should prompt the clinician to consider carbamazepine as a potential toxicant.

Differential Diagnosis

Mild-to-moderate carbamazepine toxicity resembles phenytoin toxicity. Other considerations include a convulsive status epilepticus, meningitis, encephalitis, or other intracerebral lesion.

Diagnostic Testing

- Serum carbamazepine concentrations should be obtained on any patient who presents with a history of ingestion. The therapeutic range is from 4 to 12 mg/L. Serial levels should be obtained every 4 to 6 hours to evaluate for delayed toxicity or prolonged absorption. Concentrations of >40 mg/L are associated with the development of cardiotoxicity (*J Toxicol Clin Toxicol 1993;31:449*).
- Patients with carbamazepine overdoses will often develop signs of cardiac toxicity. ECG findings include QRS and QT_c prolongation and atrioventricular (AV) conduction delays. Cardiotoxicity will occasionally be delayed, so all patients should be admitted with telemetry.

TREATMENT

Medications

Maintain airway protection at all times, treat seizures with **benzodiazepines**. Although there is a paucity of data regarding the efficacy of **sodium bicarbonate** in this setting, its use should be considered if the QRS duration is >100 milliseconds, given the structural similarity to TCAs.

Other Nonpharmacologic Therapies

Like phenytoin, carbamazepine's half-life is reduced by the administration of **MDAC** by decreasing enterohepatic recirculation of the drug (*Eur J Clin Pharmacol 1980;17:51*).

Lamotrigine

GENERAL PRINCIPLES

Definition

Lamotrigine, an anticonvulsant, is widely prescribed as a mood stabilizer as well as for the treatment of partial complex seizures.

Pathophysiology

Lamotrigine exerts its therapeutic effects by blocking presynaptic and postsynaptic sodium channels. In overdose, excess sodium channel blockade may result in widening of the QRS on the ECG and conduction blocks. Idiopathic cases of dermatologic pathology including Steven–Johnson syndrome and toxic epidermal necrolysis have been reported with the therapeutic administration of lamotrigine.

DIAGNOSIS

Clinical Presentation

History
Suspect lamotrigine toxicity in patients with a seizure disorder and altered mental status.

Physical Examination
Patients with lamotrigine toxicity present with lethargy, ataxia, and nystagmus. Overdose may present with seizures as well.

Differential Diagnosis

Lamotrigine toxicity is similar to other sodium channel blocking anticonvulsant agents.

Diagnostic Testing

Laboratories
Therapeutic concentrations range from 3 to 14 mg/L; concentrations greater than 15 mg/L are associated with the development of toxicity.

Electrocardiography
Lamotrigine overdose has been associated with the development of conduction delays and QRS widening. Patients should be admitted on telemetry.

TREATMENT

AC should be administered to alert patients with an intact airway. Seizures should be treated with **benzodiazepines**. There are theoretical benefits of administering **sodium bicarbonate**, 150 mEq in 1 L of 5% dextrose, in patients with a QRS >100 milliseconds; however, there is a paucity of experimental data to support this practice. In the setting of bicarbonate administration, close monitoring of **serum potassium** levels is required in order to avoid life-threatening hypokalemia.

Levetiracetam

GENERAL PRINCIPLES

- Levetiracetam, an anticonvulsant, is becoming increasingly used in the management of several of the different subtypes of epilepsy.
- The mechanism by which levetiracetam exerts its therapeutic effect is not well described; however, it does block N-type calcium channels on the presynaptic terminals of neurons.

DIAGNOSIS

Clinical Presentation
Very little data exist on levetiracetam overdoses. Lethargy and respiratory depression have been reported in the setting of overdose.

Differential Diagnosis
In patients with a seizure disorder and lethargy, intoxication, infectious, and metabolic disorders should be considered.

Diagnostic Testing
Although a test is available for measuring serum levels, this assay is not routinely available.

TREATMENT

Generally, **supportive care** is required. In cases where respiratory depression is evident, the patient should be intubated and ventilated. Avoid AC in patients with an altered mental status and an unprotected airway.

Valproic Acid

GENERAL PRINCIPLES

Valproic acid (VPA), an anticonvulsant, is widely used for the management of seizures and mood disorders and exerts its effects by inhibiting the function of voltage-gated sodium and calcium channels as well as enhancing the function of GABA.

Pathophysiology
VPA is metabolized by the hepatocytes through a complicated biochemical process that involves β-oxidation in the mitochondria. This drug may result in fatty infiltrates in the liver and accumulation of ammonia.

Risk Factors
Hepatic dysfunction can occur even at therapeutic levels and therefore should be monitored. The therapeutic range runs from 50 to 100 mg/L. In overdose, the risk of hepatic dysfunction and hyperammonemia increases.

DIAGNOSIS

Clinical Presentation

Patients with valproate overdoses may present with tremor, ataxia, sedation, altered sensorium, or coma. Occasionally, patients will present with abdominal pain.

Diagnostic Testing

- Therapeutic concentrations range from 50 to 100 mg/L. Patients who present with overdoses should have a **BMP** drawn to evaluate for hyponatremia and metabolic acidosis.
- In cases of massive overdose, a **CBC** should be sent as cases of pancytopenia have been reported in the literature (*Scott Med J 1987;32:85*). Hematopoietic disturbances may occur up to 5 days after overdose.
- Chronic VPA therapy has been associated with the development of hepatotoxicity and may result in a fatal hepatitis. In cases of chronic toxicity, **LFTs** should be sent to evaluate for transaminitis. Likewise, any patient with VPA toxicity should have an **ammonia** level sent.
- There have been occasional reports of pancreatitis (*J Toxicol Clin Toxicol 1995;33:279*); therefore in massive overdose, consider sending **lipase** as well.

TREATMENT

- Most cases of toxicity resolve with supportive care. In patients who are awake with adequate airway protection, **AC** is warranted.
- In patients with hyperammonemia >35 mmol/L (>80 μg/dL) L-**carnitine** therapy should be instituted. In awake patients, oral carnitine is the preferred route at 50 to 100 mg/kg/d divided every 6 hours up to 3 g/d. In cases where patients are not able to tolerate PO, intravenous L-carnitine may be administered at 100 mg/kg IV up to 6 g as a loading dose, and then 15 mg/kg every 4 hours. Therapy may be discontinued when the patient's ammonia level declines to <35 mmol/L.

Monoamine Oxidase Inhibitors

GENERAL PRINCIPLES

Although several different classes of monoamine oxidase inhibitors (MAOIs) exist, the drugs most frequently implicated in toxicity are the first-generation antidepressant drugs: **phenelzine**, **isocarboxazid**, and **tranylcypromine**. **Clorgiline**, a later generation drug, is also associated with a similar toxic profile. The third-generation drugs, including **moclobemide**, have a better safety profile.

Pathophysiology

Monoamine oxidase is an enzyme responsible for the inactivation of biogenic amines such as **epinephrine**, **norepinephrine**, **tyramine**, **dopamine**, and **serotonin**. Inhibition of this enzyme results in an increase of synaptic concentrations of biogenic amines. An increase in norepinephrine and serotonin, in particular, is thought to be responsible for mood elevation. MAOIs are structurally similar to amphetamine. In overdose, a significant amount of neurotransmitter is released resulting in a **sympathomimetic** toxidrome. Phenelzine and isocarboxazid are also hydrazine derivatives and in overdose have been associated with the development of **seizure** activity. As neurotransmitters become depleted, patients develop cardiovascular collapse, which is often refractory to therapy. Given the fact that MAOIs affect an enzymatic pathway, there is often a **significant delay** in the development of toxicity after overdose, with most cases occurring in a **24-hour** period postingestion, although there are cases of toxicity occurring **up to 32 hours** after overdose (*Ann Emerg Med 1984;13:1137*). This effect may occur with seemingly small overdoses of five or six pills (*J Clin Psychiatry 1983;44:280*).

Risk Factors

The classic risk factors for developing toxicity include increasing a prescribed dose or eating foods rich in **tyramine**, such as aged cheddar cheese or red wine. Drug–drug interactions occur when a new antidepressant (often a selective serotonin reuptake inhibitor [SSRI]) is introduced without an adequate **washout period** of several weeks after discontinuing the MAOI.

Prevention

Patients should be well educated on the risk associated with these drugs. The **duration of action in these drugs significantly outlasts their half-lives**; therefore, physicians should always use a reference guide or consult a pharmacist prior to prescribing a new drug in addition to or as a replacement for the MAOI.

Associated Conditions

- MAOIs have been associated with severe **hypertensive crises** in the setting of coingestions of **tyramine**-containing foods such as **aged cheddar and red wine**. Likewise, coingestion of **indirect-acting sympathomimetics**, which cause presynaptic release of norepinephrine, may precipitate a hypertensive crisis. Agents included in this category are **amphetamine-based drugs, dopamine, and pseudoephedrine**.
- **Serotonin syndrome** is also associated with the coingestion of **SSRIs, St. John's wort, meperidine**, and **dextromethorphan**.

DIAGNOSIS

Clinical Presentation

MAOI overdose is associated with a considerable risk of mortality and morbidity.

History
- In overdose, there may be a **significant delay** in the development of symptoms. Anyone who presents with normal vital signs and history of MAOI overdose must be **admitted and monitored** for at least 24 hours.
- Overdose should be suspected in patients who are taking MAOIs and present in extremis with a florid **sympathomimetic** toxidrome.

Physical Examination
Patients may initially present with minimal signs of toxicity. Subsequently, they will develop **agitation, diaphoresis, tachycardia, severe hypertension, dilated pupils**, and **headache**. As their illness progresses, they may develop **hyperthermia, rigidity, and seizures**. Ultimately, there is depletion of neurotransmitter stores and the patient develops refractory cardiovascular collapse.

Differential Diagnosis

MAOI overdose produces a clinical picture that is similar to severe serotonin syndrome and severe sympathomimetic toxicity. Serotonin syndrome has a relatively faster onset of action and occurs within minutes to hours of ingestion.

Diagnostic Testing

Laboratories

These include routine labs such as a **BMP**, looking for metabolic acidosis, hyperkalemia, and renal failure; **CK** to look for rhabdomyolysis; and **troponins** should be obtained to evaluate for myocardial infarction in severe cases. **Coagulation studies** are important as these patients may DIC.

Electrocardiography

ECG analysis may reveal a range of disorders from a simple sinus tachycardia to a wide complex dysrhythmia.

Imaging

A **head CT** should be obtained on altered patients and patients complaining of a headache in order to evaluate for intracranial hemorrhage.

TREATMENT

- The management of first-generation MAOI overdose can be very difficult as the patient may have dramatically variable vital signs. Patients with MAOI overdose should be aggressively managed with **orogastric lavage**, even if they are asymptomatic on arrival to the hospital.
- In hyperthermic patients, **rapid cooling measures** should be instituted.

Medications

First Line

- **AC** (1 g/kg) should be administered to the patient after the airway is secured. Many patients will be awake and alert and may not need immediate intubation; however, these patients should receive AC as well.
- Given the propensity for wildly fluctuating blood pressure (BP), titratable and short-acting agents are the mainstay of treatment in these patients. Hypertension should be managed with **nitroglycerin**, **nitroprusside**, **or phentolamine**. If the patient develops hypotension, a direct-acting α-agonist such as **norepinephrine** should be used. **Avoid dopamine** in the setting of MAOI overdose as it often fails to improve BP due to catecholamine depletion.
- **Benzodiazepines** should be used for seizures and agitation. Rigidity that does not respond to benzodiazepine administration may be managed with **nondepolarizing** paralytics. There are case reports describing the resolution of rigidity after the administration of **cyproheptadine** (*J Clin Psychopharmacol 1993;13:312*).

Second Line

In patients with refractory seizures, early administration of **pyridoxine** is warranted. Doses of 70 mg/kg not to exceed 5 g should be administered early as an IV infusion of 0.5 g/min.

SPECIAL CONSIDERATIONS

- Patients with MAOI overdoses require admission with monitoring for at least 24 hours, given the propensity for delayed toxicity. Aggressive decontamination measures should be taken, even if the patient seems to be asymptomatic as decompensation is rapid and frequently fatal.
- The **exception** to this is an overdose of **moclobemide**, which has a much better safety profile and tends to have a benign course because of its short duration of MAO inhibition.

PATIENT EDUCATION

- Patients who are placed on MAOIs should be educated about food and drug interactions and warned about the risk of interactions with herbal supplements, including St. John's wort.
- A washout period of at least 2 weeks after discontinuation of an MAOI should be observed before starting another antidepressant.

Tricyclic Antidepressants

GENERAL PRINCIPLES

- Multiple TCAs are on the market, including amitriptyline, clomipramine, doxepin, imipramine, trimipramine, desipramine, nortriptyline, and amoxapine.
- TCAs interact with a wide variety of receptors with many consequent effects in the setting of an overdose. The primary antidepressant effect is due to the inhibition of serotonin and norepinephrine reuptake. Additionally, TCAs modulate the function of central sympathetic and serotonergic receptors, which is thought to contribute to their antidepressant effects.
- TCAs have antimuscarinic effects, resulting in tachycardia, dry mucous membranes and skin, urinary retention, and decreased GI motility. Patients will also have dilated pupils (*Psychopharmacology 1994;114:559*). Sedation is likely due to antihistamine effects. Furthermore, these agents are potent α_1-antagonists leading to the development of hypotension and a reflex tachycardia. Cardiac toxicity is due to sodium channel blockade, resulting in a wide complex rhythm on the ECG (*Annu Rev Med 1984;35:503*). TCAs also exhibit a complex interaction with the GABA receptor, which in overdose likely contributes to seizure activity (*Life Sci 1988;43:303*).

DIAGNOSIS

TCA overdose exhibits its own toxidrome due to the widespread effects on various receptors as outlined earlier. Patients with an acute overdose may present to the emergency department with a normal mental status and vital signs but then rapidly decompensate.

Clinical Presentation

History

As with any overdose, a history is often unreliable. The clinical picture in serious toxicity is fairly stereotypical and a careful physical examination can help establish the diagnosis.

Physical Examination
- Often present with a rapid onset of **CNS depression**
- **Tachycardia** and **hypotension** due to vasodilatation and antimuscarinic effects
- **Dilated pupils**, **dry mucous membranes**, and **urinary retention** due to the anticholinergic effects
- May present with **seizure** activity, if significant overdose present

Diagnostic Criteria

The TCA toxidrome is a fairly consistent constellation of signs including hypotension, tachycardia, coma, and seizures.

Diagnostic Testing

Laboratories
- **Serum TCA concentrations** have a **limited role** in the management of acute TCA toxicity as they are **not predictive of severity of illness** (*N Engl J Med 1985;313:474*). Qualitative measurements of TCA concentrations in the urine are unreliable as there are many common drugs that cross-react on the assay, including diphenhydramine and cyclobenzaprine.
- Serial **VBG**s should be measured in patients undergoing alkalinization. As bicarbonate treatment can cause profound hypokalemia, serial K^+ should be followed and repleted.
- **Dextrose** should be checked in any patient with an altered mental status.

Electrocardiography
The ECG has proved to be a valuable tool in predicting the degree of morbidity in TCA overdose. In one classic study, one-third patients with a **QRS of ≥100 milliseconds** developed **seizures**. Fifty percent of patients with a QRS of ≥160 milliseconds developed **ventricular dysrhythmias** (*N Engl J Med 1985;313:474*). A terminal 40-millisecond axis of greater than 120 degrees is found in patients who are taking TCAs and may help narrow the diagnosis in patients with an altered mental status of unknown etiology. Simply put, the ECG will show an **R′ in aVR**, and an S wave in leads I and aVL. An R′ in aVR of >3 mm has been demonstrated to be predictive of neurologic and cardiac complications in TCA-poisoned patients (*Ann Emerg Med 1995;26(2):195*).

TREATMENT

- Patients with TCA overdose require early aggressive intervention.
- In patients with altered mental status, early **intubation**, **resuscitation**, and **GI decontamination** are warranted.
- Orogastric lavage may be beneficial in patients who are intubated with large ingestions because of decreased GI motility. Avoid this in small children as they only typically take one to two pills.
- **Hyperventilation** to achieve rapid serum alkalinization may be used as a bridge until bicarbonate therapy is started.

Medications

First Line
- **After the patient's airway is protected**, a dose of **AC** 1 g/kg is warranted even in delayed presentations.

- **Sodium bicarbonate** has been demonstrated to narrow the QRS, decrease the incidence of ventricular arrhythmias, and improve hypotension (*Emerg Med 2001;13:204*). A bolus of 1 to 2 mEq/kg every 3 to 5 minutes should be given with continuous ECG monitoring until the QRS narrows or the BP improves. Serial VBGs should be obtained with a goal of maintaining the blood pH at 7.50 to 7.55.
  - A bicarbonate drip should be titrated to the QRS narrowing and resolution of hypotension. The patient should be monitored in an ICU with serial pH and serum potassium measurements as well as monitoring for fluid overload.
  - Alkalinization should continue for 12 to 24 hours until the clinical picture and the ECG improves.
- **Norepinephrine** is the pressor of choice in hypotensive patients who do not respond to alkalinization because of its direct effects on the vasculature.
- **Lidocaine** may be considered in the presence of ventricular dysrhythmias precipitated by TCA toxicity. However, class **Ia and Ic antidysrhythmics are contraindicated in the management of TCA-poisoned patients**.
- **Benzodiazepines** are the mainstay of treatment for seizures. **Phenytoin should be avoided.**

Second Line
Propofol and **barbiturates** may be beneficial in refractory seizures.

Other Nonpharmacologic Therapies
Cardiopulmonary bypass and extracorporeal membrane oxygenation (ECMO) have been used in critically ill patients with refractory hypotension (*Ann Emerg Med 1994;23:480*; *Am J Emerg Med 1994;12:456*).

Selective Serotonin Reuptake Inhibitors

GENERAL PRINCIPLES

Classification
This class of drugs includes **fluoxetine, fluvoxamine, paroxetine, sertraline, citalopram**, and **escitalopram**. These drugs have a much better safety profile than the earlier drugs marketed for the management of depressive disorders and, as such, have largely supplanted MAOIs and TCAs in the treatment of depression.

Pathophysiology
These drugs enhance serotonergic activity by preventing its reuptake into the presynaptic terminal of the neuron, which may partially explain their antidepressant effects. Unlike other antidepressants, SSRIs have limited effects on other receptors and therefore tend to be less toxic in overdose.

DIAGNOSIS

Clinical Presentation
The vast majority of these overdoses have a benign clinical course. However, patients may present with signs of serotonin excess. Patients who have ingested **citalopram** or **escitalopram** may develop delayed toxicity.

History

Overdose histories are unreliable. Many patients who claim to have taken an overdose yet who look well actually took SSRIs.

Physical Examination

Signs of toxicity are usually absent unless the patient has taken a massive overdose. In these cases, patients may present with nausea, vomiting, and tachycardia. Patients with **citalopram** or **escitalopram** ingestions may present with **seizures**.

Diagnostic Testing

Laboratories

- Obtain **BMP** as SSRIs have been implicated in the development of **SIADH**.
- **FSBG** should be checked in patients with an altered mental status or seizures.
- Check **CK**, **lactate**, and **coagulation profile** in patients with **serotonin syndrome**.

Electrocardiography

Patients will occasionally present with a sinus tachycardia. In patients with citalopram or escitalopram, ingestions may develop QT_c prolongation as late as 24 hours after an overdose (*J Toxicol Clin Toxicol 1997;35:237*).

TREATMENT

The vast majority of overdoses require only 6 hours of observation and supportive care. Patients with intentional **citalopram** and **escitalopram** overdoses should be admitted to the floor with 24 hours of telemetry to monitor for QT_c prolongation.

Medications

- In patients who are awake and alert, 1 g/kg of **AC** may be administered.
- Treat seizures with **benzodiazepines**.
- Treat Torsades de pointes (Tdp) with **magnesium**, correction of electrolytes, **lidocaine**, and **overdrive pacing**.

Serotonin Syndrome

GENERAL PRINCIPLES

Definition

Serotonin syndrome is a disorder that can be precipitated by the introduction of a serotonergic agent and has been reported to occur even after ingestion of a single pill (*Ann Emerg Med 1999;33:457*).

Pathophysiology

Serotonin syndrome is thought to occur secondary to excess stimulation of $5HT_{2A}$ receptors (*J Psychopharmacol 1999;13:100*). This syndrome can result from the coadministration of two or more serotonergic agents including SSRIs, MAOIs, meperidine, amphetamines, cocaine, TCAs, and various other drugs.

DIAGNOSIS

Clinical Presentation

History

Suspect serotonin syndrome in any patient who presents with a rapid onset of tremor and clonus after administration of a serotonergic agent. It is important to avoid the addition of other serotonergic agents in the management of these patients.

Physical Examination

- Patients will present with signs of excess serotonergic activity including restlessness, shivering, diaphoresis, and diarrhea.
- Patients may develop myoclonus, ocular clonus, and muscle rigidity later.
- Vital sign abnormalities include tachycardia and hyperpyrexia.

Diagnostic Criteria

- Serotonin syndrome is diagnosed by the presence of four of the following major criteria: alteration of consciousness, coma, or mood elevation; shivering, myoclonus, rigidity, or hyperreflexia; pyrexia; or diaphoresis.
- Additional minor criteria include restlessness or insomnia; mydriasis or akathisia; tachycardia; diarrhea; and respiratory or BP abnormalities (*Med Hypotheses 2000;55:218*).

Differential Diagnosis

Patients who present with altered mental status, rigidity, and hyperpyrexia may be misdiagnosed with neuroleptic malignant syndrome (NMS). NMS tends to develop over days to weeks, whereas serotonin syndrome has a faster onset, usually manifesting over a 24-hour period.

Diagnostic Testing

Serotonin syndrome is diagnosed by a constellation of symptoms and signs rather than any specific laboratory findings; however, as the disease evolves, laboratory abnormalities develop.

Laboratories

- As with any critical illness, patients may succumb to multiorgan failure, and therefore, laboratory studies should be obtained on the basis of the presentation.
- May have no lab abnormalities if present early with mild form.
- On the other hand, more severe presentations may develop complications from psychomotor agitation and muscle rigidity including elevated **CK**, **metabolic acidosis**, and an **elevated lactate**.
- Check **BMP** as **renal failure** may occur in the presence of rhabdomyolysis.
- Check **coagulation studies** as patients with hyperthermia may develop **coagulopathy**.

Electrocardiography

The typical ECG will show a sinus tachycardia; however, there are no specific diagnostic electrocardiographic criteria associated with serotonin syndrome.

TREATMENT

- The treatment of serotonin syndrome is largely supportive and requires the removal of the offending agent. Aggressive cooling and hydration measures should be taken in the hyperthermic patient.

- **Benzodiazepines** should be used liberally to treat psychomotor agitation and myoclonus. In severe cases, **nondepolarizing paralytics** should be used to limit the degree of rhabdomyolysis.
- In patients with mild-to-moderate symptoms, **cyproheptadine**, an antihistamine with $5HT_{1A}$ and $5HT_{2A}$ antagonism, should be considered. A **4- to 8-mg** initial dose should be given orally, which often results in a rapid reversal of symptoms. If there is no response, the dose may be repeated in 2 hours. Subsequent dosing is 2 to 4 mg orally every 6 hours until the patient improves or a maximum dose of 32 mg/d is reached.

Lithium

GENERAL PRINCIPLES

Classification

Toxicity may be classified as **acute, chronic, or acute on chronic**. Lithium, an antidepressant, has a narrow therapeutic index, and therefore, risk of toxicity is high in patients on chronic therapy. The therapeutic range is approximately 0.6 to 1.2 mmol/L (or mEq/L).

Pathophysiology

- The mechanism by which lithium exerts its antimanic properties is not well understood. There is some evidence that lithium enhances serotonin function, which may contribute to its mood-stabilizing properties (*Science 1981;213:1529*).
- Acute toxicity is associated with the development of a GI illness as lithium is a metal.
- Chronic toxicity is primarily associated with neurologic dysfunction.
- Although serum levels are helpful in the management of these patients, the clinical picture should be the basis for therapy.
  - Generally, in **chronically** exposed patients, levels of less than 2.5 mEq/L are associated with tremulousness, ataxia, and nystagmus.
  - Levels greater than 2.5 mEq/L are associated with a deteriorating neurologic syndrome and are an indication for aggressive intervention including dialysis.
  - A serum concentration of 4.0 mEq/L in an **acute** overdose is also an indication for dialysis (*Q J Med 1978;47:123*).

Risk Factors

Lithium has peripheral effects, which may enhance its toxicity, including the development of nephrogenic diabetes insipidus. This phenomenon is thought to occur through the reduction in the binding of aquaporins in the collecting duct of the kidney (*Annu Rev Physiol 1996;58:619*). This development enhances toxicity by causing dehydration, which leads to an increase in proximal tubular reabsorption of lithium (*J Physiol 1991;437:377*). Other dehydration states may enhance toxicity as well.

Prevention

Patients on chronic lithium therapy should have serum levels monitored and regular follow-up with their psychiatrist, which should include evaluation for the clinical signs of toxicity.

Associated Conditions

Lithium therapy has been associated with the development of chronic tubulointerstitial nephropathy (*J Am Soc Nephrol 2000;11:1439*), thyroid dysfunction (*J Toxicol Clin Toxicol 2000;38:333*), serotonin syndrome (*Medicine 2000;79:201*), and other endocrine effects.

DIAGNOSIS

Clinical Presentation

History

Although the history is often unreliable in overdose patients, acutely intoxicated patients may present complaining of nausea and abdominal discomfort. In chronic toxicity, patients may present with worsening confusion.

Physical Examination

- **Acute overdose** presents with a predominately GI syndrome of nausea, vomiting, diarrhea, and abdominal pain. As the illness progresses, patients may develop signs of volume depletion with tachycardia and hypotension. Severe toxicity is associated with neurologic dysfunction including altered mental status, nystagmus, ataxia, or coma.
- **Chronic toxicity** is associated with tremor, nystagmus, and ataxia. Confusion, dysarthria, fasciculations, and myoclonus are frequent physical findings. Seizures are reported in the literature (*Biol Psychiatry 1987;22:1184*).

Diagnostic Testing

Laboratories

- Obtain serial lithium levels in patients who present with evidence of toxicity.
  - A high initial level may be due to the timing of the last dose; therefore, the clinical picture should guide therapy.
  - **Obtain the serum sample in a lithium-free tube.**
- Other laboratories should include a **BMP** to evaluate electrolyte levels, renal function, and hydration status.
- Lithium induces an elevation in the **white blood cell (WBC) count**.

Electrocardiography

The ECG may show nonspecific T-wave flattening or QT_c prolongation; however, cardiac dysfunction is unusual in this overdose.

TREATMENT

- AC does not bind to lithium and therefore has no role in the management of these overdoses.
- Whole-bowel irrigation with **polyethylene glycol** at a rate of 2 L/hr is indicated for overdoses of sustained-release preparations (*Ann Emerg Med 1991;20:536*).
- The mainstay of therapy is the infusion of **0.9% saline solution** at twice the maintenance rate. Closely monitor fluid status in these patients to avoid overload.

Other Nonpharmacologic Therapies

Consider **dialysis** for patients present with signs of severe toxicity with altered mental status, or other neurologic dysfunction but are unable to tolerate the required fluid load for enhanced elimination. In patients with acute overdose and a serum lithium concentration >4.0 mEq/L or chronic overdose and a serum level >2.5 mEq/L, dialysis should be considered.

Bupropion

GENERAL PRINCIPLES

Bupropion is an atypical antidepressant of the monocyclic aminoketone class and is structurally related to amphetamines. It acts by selectively inhibiting dopamine and norepinephrine reuptake.

DIAGNOSIS

Bupropion has been associated with more severe symptoms than the other atypical agents. Common features of toxicity include tachycardia, drowsiness, hallucinations, and convulsions. **Seizures** have been reported at therapeutic doses (*J Clin Psychiatry 1991;52:450*). **QRS prolongation** has also been described in overdose. Symptoms may be **delayed for up to 10 hours** after ingestion of sustained-release pills.

TREATMENT

Treatment of bupropion overdose includes airway protection. **Whole-bowel irrigation** and **MDAC** should be considered in patients who present early with a normal mental status and ingestion of a sustained-release preparation. This modality is **contraindicated** in seizing patients. Seizures should be treated with **benzodiazepines**. Barbiturates and propofol should be considered in patients with status epilepticus.

Antipsychotics, General

GENERAL PRINCIPLES

Epidemiology

According to the AAPC's 2007 report, antipsychotic/sedative hypnotic agents were the fourth leading cause of fatal overdoses in the United States (*Clin Toxicol 2008;46:927*).

Pathophysiology

Antipsychotic agents exert their therapeutic effect largely by binding to dopamine receptors in the CNS, which tends to mitigate the positive symptoms of schizophrenia. Dopamine receptor blockade is also associated with the development of movement disorders, and the newer neuroleptic agents attempt to address this by modulating serotonergic tone. Most antipsychotics affect multiple receptors in the nervous, endocrine, and cardiovascular system, which accounts for a wide range of toxic symptoms. In general, the older "typical" agents in the phenothiazine class tend to have more cardiac toxicity, with varying degrees of sodium channel blockade (wide QRS) and potassium channel blockade (QT_c prolongation). Furthermore, these agents tend to have more significant extrapyramidal effects. The newer or "atypical" antipsychotics tend to exhibit less cardiac toxicity, but they often have pronounced α_1-antagonism, causing hypotension. The atypicals are also associated with the idiosyncratic development of other medical problems. For example, olanzapine has been associated with the development of fatal diabetic ketoacidosis (DKA) (*Am J Psychiatry 2003;160(12):2241*), and clozapine was briefly withdrawn from the market as a small percentage of patients developed agranulocytosis (*J Clin Psychiatry 2000;61:14*).

Phenothiazines

GENERAL PRINCIPLES

These are the prototypic antipsychotic drugs and include chlorpromazine, thioridazine, prochlorperazine, perphenazine, trifluoperazine, fluphenazine, mesoridazine, haloperidol (a butyrophenone), and thiothixene.

DIAGNOSIS

Clinical Presentation

History
The history is often difficult to obtain in these patients.

Physical Examination
- Overdoses are characterized by agitation or delirium, which may progress rapidly to coma. Pupils may be mydriatic and deep tendon reflexes are depressed. Seizures may occur.
- Vital sign abnormalities may include hyperthermia, hypotension (due to strong α-adrenergic antagonism), tachycardia, arrhythmias (including TdP), and depressed cardiac conduction.

Diagnostic Testing

Laboratories
- Serum concentrations are generally not available or useful.
- FSBG and a BMP should be checked on all patients with altered mentation.

Imaging
Abdominal radiographs may reveal pill concretions.

TREATMENT

- Assess airway and breathing, place an IV, and institute cardiac monitoring.
- Hypotensive patients should receive a 20 mL/kg bolus of normal saline (NS).
- Consider whole-bowel irrigation for ingestion of sustained-release formulations.

Medications

- Treat ventricular arrhythmias with lidocaine. Class Ia agents (e.g., procainamide, quinidine, disopyramide) are contraindicated; avoid sotalol.
- Treat hypotension with IV fluid administration and α-adrenergic vasopressors (norepinephrine or phenylephrine). **Avoid epinephrine** as vasodilation may occur because of unopposed β-adrenergic response in the setting of strong α-adrenergic antagonism.

- TdP may require magnesium, isoproterenol, or overdrive pacing (see Chapter 7, Cardiac Arrhythmias).
- Treat seizures with benzodiazepines.
- Treat dystonic reactions with benztropine, 1 to 4 mg, or diphenhydramine, 25 to 50 mg, IM or IV.
- Treat hyperthermia with cooling.

SPECIAL CONSIDERATIONS

- NMS, which may complicate use of these agents, is characterized by rigidity, hyperthermia, altered mental status, and elevated CK. NMS should be treated with aggressive cooling measures, benzodiazepines, and bromocriptine 2.5 to 10 mg IV tid until the patient improves, then taper the dose over several days to avoid recrudescence of symptoms.
- Admit those patients who have ingested a significant overdose for cardiac monitoring for at least 48 hours.

Clozapine

GENERAL PRINCIPLES

An atypical neuroleptic.

DIAGNOSIS

Clinical Presentation
- Overdose is characterized by altered mental status, ranging from somnolence to coma.
- Anticholinergic effects occur, including blurred vision, dry mouth (although hypersalivation may occur in overdose), lethargy, delirium, and constipation. Seizures occur in a minority of overdoses. Coma may occur.
- Vital sign abnormalities include hypotension, tachycardia, fasciculations, tremor, and myoclonus.

Diagnostic Testing
- Obtain CBC and LFTs; follow the WBC counts weekly for 4 weeks.
- Clozapine levels are not useful.

TREATMENT

- As always, support ABCs. Place an IV and institute cardiac monitoring.
- Consider AC 1 g/kg if the patient presents within an hour of ingestion.
- Treat hypotension with 20 mL/kg of IVF; if resistant, treat with norepinephrine or dopamine.
- Treat seizures with benzodiazepines.
- Consider filgrastim for agranulocytosis.

- Forced diuresis, hemodialysis, or hemoperfusion are not beneficial.
- Admit and monitor patients with severely symptomatic overdoses for 24 hours or more.

Olanzapine

GENERAL PRINCIPLES

Definition

An atypical neuroleptic.

DIAGNOSIS

Clinical Presentation

- Overdose is characterized by somnolence, slurred speech, ataxia, vertigo, nausea, and vomiting (*Ann Emerg Med 1999;34:279*).
- Anticholinergic effects occur, including blurred vision, dry mouth, and tachycardia.
- Seizures are uncommon. Coma may occur.
- Vital sign abnormalities include hypotension and tachycardia. Serious dysrhythmias rarely occur.
- **Pinpoint pupils are unresponsive to naloxone.**

TREATMENT

- Pay attention to ABCs, place an IV, and institute cardiac monitoring.
- Give AC if presentation is within 1 hour of ingestion.
- Treat hypotension with fluids and, if ineffective, norepinephrine.
- Give benzodiazepines for seizures.
- Treat DKA aggressively, if present.

Risperidone, Ziprasidone, and Quetiapine

GENERAL PRINCIPLES

These are newer neuroleptic agents and reports of overdoses have increased significantly. Quetiapine overdose is associated with more adverse outcomes than other neuroleptic agents (*Ann Emerg Med 2008;52:541*) and requires aggressive therapy.

DIAGNOSIS

Clinical Presentation

- Clinical effects include CNS depression, tachycardia, hypotension, and electrolyte abnormalities.
- Clinically significant ventricular dysrhythmias are uncommon.
- Quetiapine overdose is associated with respiratory depression (*Ann Emerg Med 2008;52:541*).
- Miosis is a common finding.

Diagnostic Testing

QRS and QT_c prolongation have been reported (*Ann Emerg Med 2003;42:751*).

TREATMENT

- Scrupulous attention should be paid to ventilatory and circulatory support.
- Treat hypotension with 20 mL/kg fluid boluses and, if severe and persistent, consider a direct-acting pressor such as norepinephrine.
- Replete electrolytes as needed.
- Diuresis, hemodialysis, and hemoperfusion do not appear to be useful.

β-Adrenergic Antagonists

GENERAL PRINCIPLES

Definition

Of all of the agents available, propranolol tends to exhibit the most toxicity because it is lipophilic and widely distributed throughout the body and possesses significant membrane-stabilizing activity. Sotalol, which is classically thought of as a class III antiarrhythmic, also has some β-adrenergic antagonist activity and in toxic doses can result in a prolonged QT_c and TdP.

Classification

Cardiovascular agents are a frequent cause of serious poisonings, and according to the 2007 annual report of the National Poison Data System, were the fifth leading cause of fatal drug exposures (*Clin Toxicol 2008;46:927*). Patients with these over-doses require aggressive intervention and close monitoring.

Pathophysiology

The toxicity associated with an overdose of β-blockers is largely due to the effects of antagonism at catecholamine receptors. In general, selectivity is lost in overdose, so bronchospasm may occur in the setting of $β_1$-selective antagonists.

DIAGNOSIS

Clinical Presentation

- Patients with a significant ingestion of an immediate-release product will exhibit signs of toxicity within 6 hours. The exception to this rule is sotalol, which in overdose can have delayed toxicity and prolonged effects with one report of QT_c prolongation persisting up to 100 hours postingestion (*Eur Clin J Pharmacol 1981;20:85*).
- With the exception of propranolol and sotalol, β-blocker overdose in healthy people tends to be benign, with significant number of patients remaining asymptomatic after ingestion (*J Toxicol Clin Toxicol 1993;31:531*).

History

Suspect β-antagonist overdose in patients with altered mental status, bradycardia, and hypotension.

Physical Examination

Patients with significant ingestions present with bradycardia and congestive heart failure (CHF). Patients with propranolol ingestions may develop coma, seizures, and hypotension. Propranolol overdoses have a high mortality (*J Toxicol Clin Toxicol 1997;35:353*).

Differential Diagnosis

In patients with symptomatic bradycardia, also consider overdose of CCB, clonidine, or digoxin.

Diagnostic Testing

Laboratories

Patients with β-antagonist overdoses occasionally become hypoglycemic; therefore, a **FSBG** should be obtained. Likewise, any patient with an altered mental status should have a **BMP** sent. Consider obtaining a **lactate** as patients with profound hypotension may develop mesenteric ischemia.

Electrocardiography

The ECG may reveal sinus bradycardia or AV block. In propranolol ingestions, a wide QRS manifesting sodium channel blockade may be present. With sotalol, QT_c prolongation may appear as a delayed presentation and TdP may develop.

TREATMENT

The treatment of β-blocker overdose is largely supportive in mild-to-moderate cases. The patient should have an IV placed, and continuous cardiac monitoring should be instituted. **Hypoglycemia** should be treated with 50 mL of 50% **dextrose (D_{50})**. Consider **AC** if patients present within 1 hour of ingestion. Intubation and ventilation should be instituted in patients with altered mental status. Likewise, consider **oro-gastric lavage** in patients with potential for severe toxicity such as propranolol overdoses.

Medications

- Patients with significant toxicity, propranolol, or sotalol ingestions should be treated more aggressively.
- **Atropine** 1 mg IV may be given up to 3 mg for symptomatic bradycardia; however, this is usually ineffective as the bradycardia is not vagally mediated.
- **A fluid bolus** of 20 mL/kg should be given and may be repeated; monitor for the development of fluid overload.
- **Glucagon** 2 to 4 mg IV may be given over 1 to 2 minutes. Then start infusion of 2 to 5 mg/hr, not to exceed 10 mg/hr. One of the significant side effects of glucagon administration is nausea and vomiting; monitor for vagally mediated bradycardia.
- **Calcium gluconate** 3 to 9 g IV may be given through a peripheral line in patients with hypotension. Alternatively, consider **calcium chloride** 1 to 3 g through a central line slow IV push over 10 minutes. Calcium chloride is sclerosing and can cause severe extravasation injury.

- Any patient with hypotension is a candidate for **high-dose insulin euglycemia therapy**. Although the mechanism for improvement is unclear, this is routinely used in the management of severe CCB overdose (*J Toxicol Clin Toxicol 1999;37:463*). Animal studies of severe propranolol overdose have shown a survival benefit (*Ann Emerg Med 1997;29:748*). This involves a bolus of **1 U/kg of regular insulin, followed by an infusion of 0.5 to 1.0 U/kg/hr of regular insulin**. This should be accompanied by a dose of **50 mL of D$_{50}$ and a dextrose drip at 1 g/kg/hr of dextrose**. That calculates to 10 mL/kg/hr of D$_{10}$ or 2 mL/kg/hr of D$_{50}$ (*Goldfrank's Toxicologic Emergencies. 8th ed. New York: McGraw-Hill, 2006:933*). FSBG should be obtained every 30 minutes, and potassium levels should be followed every 2 hours with repletion as **profound hypokalemia** may complicate this treatment modality. The BP response tends to be delayed by 15 to 30 minutes.

- **Lipid therapy** is emerging as a promising treatment modality in these often fatal poisonings. Theoretically, lipid administration causes lipophilic drugs to partition into the plasma and away from the heart. The current protocol, which can be found at *http://www.lipidrescue.org*, starts with **1.5 mL/kg of 20% intralipid administration over 1 minute, followed by an infusion rate of 0.25 mL/kg/min**. If there is no response, the patient may have repeat boluses every 3 to 5 minutes until a **3 mL/kg** total dose, and the infusion rate may be increased to **0.5 mL/kg/min**. **The maximum total dose recommended is 8 mL/kg** (*J Med Toxicol 2011;7(2):151*).

- **Catecholamines** should be approached with caution in these patients because α-stimulation in conjunction with β-blockade may precipitate acute heart failure. Therefore, **hemodynamic monitoring** should be instituted with careful titration of **epinephrine at 0.02 μg/kg/min or norepinephrine at 0.10 μg/kg/min**. **Isoproterenol at 0.10 μg/kg/min** may be useful as well; however, monitor closely for the development of hypotension. It is important to note that high doses of these agents may be required.

Other Nonpharmacologic Therapies

- In cases of refractory hypotension and bradycardia, it is reasonable to consider intra-aortic balloon pump (IABP) (*Ann Emerg Med 1987;16:1381*) and ECMO (*Arch Mal Coeur Vaiss 2001;94:1386*).

- Transvenous pacing may be attempted, but it is generally difficult to achieve capture, given the degree of myocardial depression.

Calcium Channel Blockers

GENERAL PRINCIPLES

Definition

CCBs are widely used for the management of tachyarrhythmias and hypertension. Generally speaking, the overdoses of dihydropyridines, such as amlodipine, nimodipine, nicardipine, and nifedipine, tend to be more benign; although in massive overdose, selectivity may be lost and may result in significant symptoms. Nondihydropyridines, verapamil and diltiazem, can produce severe toxicity, even in the setting of a small overdose.

Pathophysiology

CCBs exert their effects by blocking L-type calcium channels on the smooth muscle of the vasculature and the myocardium. This decreases inotropy and chronotropy and results in a decrement of BP and heart rate. In overdose, these effects are accentuated. L-type calcium channels are also involved in the release of insulin from the β-islet cells of the pancreas. In CCB overdose, patients will often present with elevated blood sugars.

DIAGNOSIS

Clinical Presentation

Patients with diltiazem or verapamil overdoses should be considered critically ill and require aggressive intervention.

History
Patients will often present with an unintentional ingestion where they missed a dose and attempt to "catch up" by doubling their next dose. Intentional ingestions will often not be accurately reported.

Physical Examination
Patients with verapamil or diltiazem overdoses will present with profound **hypoten-sion, bradycardia, and generally have a normal mental status until they arrest**. It is thought that CCBs have somewhat of a neuroprotective effect that may explain the preservation of mentation. In the setting of dihydropyridine overdoses, patients usually present with hypotension and a reflex tachycardia.

Differential Diagnosis

CCB toxicity may resemble β-antagonist or clonidine overdoses.

Diagnostic Testing

This is a clinical diagnosis; serum concentrations are not useful in the management of CCB overdose.

Laboratories
- **FSBG** should be checked and is elevated in the setting of CCB toxicity. This is part of the toxidrome associated with this particular overdose.
- A **BMP** should be obtained as well to follow serum calcium levels. In patients on a calcium drip, ionized calcium should be followed.

Electrocardiography
The ECG may show sinus bradycardia, conduction delays, or even complete heart block. With dihydropyridine overdose, a sinus tachycardia may be present.

TREATMENT

The treatment of dihydropyridine CCB overdose is largely supportive in mild-to-moderate cases. The patient should have an IV placed, and continuous cardiac monitoring should be instituted. Consider **AC** if patients present within 1 hour of ingestion. Intubation and ventilation should be instituted in unstable patients. Likewise, consider **orogastric lavage** in patients with potential for severe toxicity. **Whole-bowel**

irrigation with polyethylene glycol should be instituted for sustained-release preparations.

Medications

Patients with significant toxicity, such as verapamil or diltiazem ingestions, should be treated more aggressively.

- **Atropine** 1 mg IV may be given up to 3 mg for symptomatic bradycardia; however, this is usually ineffective as the bradycardia is not vagally mediated.
- **A fluid bolus** of 20 mL/kg should be given and may be repeated; monitor for the development of fluid overload.
- **Calcium gluconate** or **calcium chloride** may be given as described in the treatment section of β-blocker overdose. In addition, a calcium gluconate drip may be started and run up to 2 g/hr. Close monitoring of calcium is required.
- Any patient with hypotension is a candidate for **high-dose insulin euglycemia therapy**. See discussion of this topic under treatment of β-blocker overdose.
- **Lipid therapy** as described in the treatment section of β-blocker overdose should be initiated early.
- **Catecholamines** should be approached with caution in these patients because α stimulation may precipitate acute heart failure. Therefore, **hemodynamic monitoring** should be instituted with careful titration of **epinephrine starting at 0.02 μg/kg/min or norepinephrine at 0.10 μg/kg/min**.

Other Nonpharmacologic Therapies

- In cases of refractory hypotension and bradycardia, it is reasonable to consider IABP (*Clin Cardiol 1991;14:933*) and cardiopulmonary bypass (*Ann Emerg Med 1989;18:984*).
- Transvenous pacing may be attempted but it is generally difficult to achieve capture, given the degree of myocardial depression.

SPECIAL CONSIDERATIONS

Patients with ingestions of a sustained-release preparation should be monitored in an intensive care setting. Immediate-release preparations should be monitored for 6 to 8 hours prior to discharge or psychiatric evaluation.

Clonidine

GENERAL PRINCIPLES

- Clonidine is an orally administered agent used in the management of hypertension.
- Clonidine is an imidazoline drug with centrally acting antihypertensive effects related to α_2-agonism, which decreases sympathetic outflow from the CNS (*N Engl J Med 1975;293:1179*). Other drugs in this family include oxymetazoline and tetrahydrozoline, nasal decongestants that exhibit similar toxicity when orally administered. In overdose, peripheral effects include an initial release of norepinephrine with a **transient increase** in BP, followed by hypotension (*Clin Pharmacol Ther 1976;21:593*).

DIAGNOSIS

Clinical Presentation

Although the clinical presentation of these overdoses can be quite concerning, most patients recover with supportive care. Patients tend to develop symptoms within 30 minutes to an hour after their overdose.

History

The history is unreliable in these patients as they are often somnolent or comatose on arrival to the hospital.

Physical Examination

Suspect clonidine overdose in patients with hypotension, bradycardia, and CNS depression. Occasionally, patients may develop hypoventilation, which is usually responsive to vocal or tactile stimulation (*Ann Emerg Med 1981;10:107*). Pupillary examination reveals miosis, and this finding in the setting of hypotension and bradycardia is highly suggestive of clonidine overdose.

Differential Diagnosis

β-Antagonists, digoxin, and CCB overdose should be included in the differential.

Diagnostic Testing

Laboratories

Serum clonidine concentrations are not routinely used in the management of these patients. An **FSBG** and **BMP** should be obtained on any patient with altered mental status.

Electrocardiography

The ECG generally shows a sinus bradycardia.

TREATMENT

- Patients generally respond with supportive care. In severely poisoned patients, consider intubation and ventilation; however, this is rarely needed.
- **Avoid GI decontamination and AC in these patients as they tend to develop altered mental status quickly.**
- **Atropine** 1 mg IV may be given up to 3 mg for symptomatic bradycardia; however, this is usually not necessary as the bradycardia tends to resolve on its own.
- **A fluid bolus** of 20 mL/kg should be given and may be repeated; monitor for the development of fluid overload.
- An initial dose of 0.4 mg of **naloxone** may be useful in reversing the hypotension and bradycardia associated with clonidine overdose (*Hypertension 1984;69:461*). Occasionally, high doses may be required with redosing every 2 to 3 hours as naloxone has a shorter duration of action than clonidine.

SPECIAL CONSIDERATIONS

Withdrawal syndromes have been reported in patients who have stopped taking clonidine. It is usually manifested as rebound severe hypertension, agitation, and palpitations. Treatment is to administer clonidine, and taper the dose gradually. Benzodiazepines are also useful in this situation.

Other Antihypertensives

GENERAL PRINCIPLES

- These agents include **diuretics, α_1-antagonists, angiotensin converting enzyme (ACE) inhibitors, and angiotensin II receptor blockers (ARBs).**
- **Diuretics** tend to be benign in overdose. Occasionally, they cause dehydration and electrolyte imbalances. Laboratory studies should include a BMP. Management usually only requires gentle fluid hydration.
- α_1-**Antagonists** cause peripheral vasodilation, which usually responds to hydration. Occasionally, they cause enough hypotension to require vasopressors. In these cases, norepinephrine should be administered.
- **ACE inhibitors** rarely cause significant toxicity, although there are case reports of fatal overdoses. Treatment is supportive. In patients with hypotension, naloxone may be useful (*Clin Pharmacol Ther 1985;38:560*).
- **ARBs** may cause hypotension in overdose. Treatment is supportive.

Parasympathetic Agents

GENERAL PRINCIPLES

ACh is a common neurotransmitter of the peripheral and central nervous systems, acting on nicotinic and muscarinic receptors.

Anticholinergics

GENERAL PRINCIPLES

Anticholinergic effects are primarily due to blockade of muscarinic receptors (i.e., antimuscarinic effects), and therefore mainly affect parasympathetic functions.

Epidemiology
Anticholinergic poisoning occurs either from intentional ingestion of certain plants or over-the-counter medications (e.g., Jimson weed, diphenhydramine) (*Can J Emerg Med 2007;9(6):467*), or from accidental overdosing (e.g., medical noncompliance, polypharmaceutical regimens) (*Rev Neurol 2006;43(10):603*).

Etiology
Drugs and medications with anticholinergic effects include the following:
- **Anticholinergics:** Atropine, scopolamine, benztropine, glycopyrrolate, ipratropium
- **Antihistamines:** Diphenhydramine, promethazine, doxylamine
- **Antipsychotics:** Chlorpromazine, clozapine, olanzapine, quetiapine
- **Antidepressants:** Amitriptyline, nortriptyline, imipramine, desipramine
- **Antiparkinson drugs:** Benztropine, trihexyphenidyl
- **Mydriatics:** Cyclopentolate, homatropine, tropicamide
- **Muscle relaxants:** Cyclobenzaprine
- **Plants:** Belladonna, Jimson weed, *Amanita* mushrooms

Pathophysiology

- Blockade of muscarinic receptors (i.e., parasympathetic aurtonomic nervous system [ANS], except for the sympathetically innervated sweat glands) leads to the so-called **anticholinergic toxidrome**.
- **Tachycardia** is one of the main symptoms in anticholinergic poisoning. Vagal blockade of cardiac muscarinic receptors leads to unopposed sympathetic stimulation of the myocardium.
- Some anticholinergic drugs can also cross the blood–brain barrier and interact with muscarinic receptors in the cortex and subcortical regions of the brain causing anticholinergic **CNS manifestations**.

Associated Conditions

- Antihistamines and cyclic antidepressants also block sodium channels and cause additional cardiac symptoms such as dysrhythmias and QRS prolongations.
- Potassium channel blockade may result in QT_c prolongation and TdP.

DIAGNOSIS

Clinical Presentation

Anticholinergic Toxidrome

- **Central effects:** Confusion, agitation, euphoria/dysphoria, hallucinations, incoherent thoughts and speech, lethargy, ataxia, choreoathetoid movements, rarely, seizures or coma
- **Peripheral effects:** Tachycardia, mouth dryness, decreased perspiration with flushed skin and hyperthermia, dilated pupils with photophobia and blurred vision, decreased bowel sounds, urinary retention
- A helpful mnemonic for antimuscarinic effects is "RED as a beet, DRY as a bone, BLIND as a bat, MAD as a hatter, and HOT as a hare."

TREATMENT

- All patients presenting with an anticholinergic toxidrome need **cardiovascular monitoring**. Serial evaluation of vital signs and serial physical exams are essential to address sudden worsening of the patient's condition (dysrhythmia, seizure).
- GI decontamination is only indicated if the patient is fully awake and cooperative due to the high risk of aspiration or loss of airway control in unconscious or combative patients. **Gastric lavage** for GI decontamination may be appropriate, given decreased stomach emptying and slowed GI motility from the anticholinergic effect.
- Patients with hyperthermia may benefit from cooling measures.

Medications

- **Physostigmine** is a reversible **anticholinesterase**, which leads to increased ACh in synapses to overcome receptor blockade. It is useful in the management of severe anticholinergic poisoning with delirium, hallucinations, and seizures (*Int J Clin Pharmacol Ther Toxicol 1980;18(12):523*).

○ In the emergency department setting, the use of physostigmine as a diagnostic tool in patients with high suspicion of anticholinergic agitation or delirium has been found to be relatively safe (*Ann Emerg Med 2003;42(1):14*).

○ **Contraindications:** underlying cardiovascular disease, wide QRS complex or AV block on ECG, asthma, bowel or bladder obstruction, peripheral vascular disease (PVD), or gangrene. Its use is also contraindicated in the setting of cyclic antidepressant overdose.

○ **Adult dosing:** 0.5 mg IV over 5 minutes every 5 minutes up to 2 mg total or until improved level of consciousness.

○ Physostigmine has a short duration of action (20 to 60 minutes) and redosing might be necessary if agitation recurs.

○ NOTE: Always have **atropine** at bedside for reversal if needed, that is, in case of severe bradycardia or asystole from unopposed cholinergic stimulation, or other dysrhythmias from sodium channel blockade (e.g., in TCA overdose) (*J Emerg Med 2003;25(2):185*).

• **Benzodiazepines** should be used as adjuncts to treat anticholinergic agitation or delirium. There is no benefit in benzodiazepine monotherapy in anticholinergic central symptoms (*Ann Emerg Med 2000;35(4):374*).

Cholinesterase Inhibitors

GENERAL PRINCIPLES

Definition

Cholinesterase inhibitors are chemical compounds that inhibit the enzyme cholinesterase. Blockade of **AChE** function leads to excess ACh in synapses of the ANS and sympathetic nervous system (SNS).

Classification

Cholinesterase inhibitors are divided into two classes:
• Organophosphates
• Carbamates

Organophosphates

GENERAL PRINCIPLES

Epidemiology

• Organophosphates (OPs) are commonly used as pesticides and insecticides. Some also have medical indications (e.g., malathion in lice shampoo).

• In the developing world, OP and other pesticide poisonings represent the most common cause of overdose deaths (*QJM 2000;93(11):715*).

• OPs are also potent chemical terrorism and warfare agents ("nerve gas" agents) (e.g., sarin in the Tokyo subway attack, tabun in the Iraq–Iran war) (*Anesthesiology 2002;97(4):989*).

• Although self-inflicted OP poisoning with suicidal intent occurs, exposure is primarily occupational or accidental (*Intern Med 2007;46(13):965*). Since absorption occurs through skin and airways, the handling of OPs requires appropriate protective gear.

Pathophysiology

- Inhibition of AChE leads to accumulation of ACh at nicotinic and muscarinic receptors, resulting in **excessive cholinergic stimulation**.
- The severity of symptoms varies depending on the route of exposure (dermal, inhalation, oral, parenteral), dose, lipid solubility of OP, and enzyme affinity (*Lancet 2008;371(9612):597*).
- Initially, most OPs bind AChE reversibly. Some OPs, however, become permanently bound over time, a phenomenon known as "**aging**." If aging occurs, the only way to overcome the inhibitory effect is for the body to synthesize new enzyme.
- OPs are hepatically metabolized. Some OPs become active toxins after liver metabolism (e.g., Parathion) (*Bull World Health Organ 1971;44(1):289*).
- In severe poisoning, symptoms occur usually within 6 hours after exposure and are unlikely to occur if an exposed person remains free of symptoms for 12 hours or more (*Bull World Health Organ 1971;44(1):289*).

DIAGNOSIS

Clinical Presentation

The cholinergic toxidrome is a result of overstimulation of nicotinic and muscarinic receptors (*Bull World Health Organ 1971;44(1):289; Lancet 2008;371(9612):597*).
- **Muscarinic effects**
  - **SLUDGE syndrome: S**alivation, **L**acrimation, **U**rination, **D**iarrhea, **G**I cramping, **E**mesis.
  - **Bradycardia, bronchorrhea, bronchoconstriction** (NOTE: Asphyxia and cardiovascular collapse are lethal features of OP poisoning).
  - **Other effects:** Miosis, diaphoresis.
  - NOTE: Intoxicated patients may present with tachycardia instead of bradycardia due to hypoxia (bronchoconstriction, bronchorrhea).
- **Nicotinic effects**
  - **Ganglionic:** Tachycardia, hypertension, diaphoresis, mydriasis.
  - **Neuromuscular:** Neuromuscular depolarization, fasciculations, motor weakness, paralysis with respiratory failure (analogous to succinylcholine, which is related to ACh).
  - **Central:** Confusion, agitation, lethargy, seizures, coma.

Diagnostic Testing

- **Cholinesterase levels:** There are two different cholinesterases that are routinely measured in red blood cells and plasma (*Bull World Health Organ 1971;44(1): 289*).
- Both assays are relatively useless in assessing the severity of exposure in acute intoxications because of their wide ranges of normal values.
- They are mostly used as sensitivity markers to compare changes from baseline enzyme activity (e.g., in chronic occupational exposure or after OP elimination) (*Lancet 2008;371(9612):597*).

TREATMENT

- **Protection:** OP-intoxicated patients pose a significant risk for further contamination of others through direct contact. Health care personnel should use special

personal protective equipment (PPE) (gowns, gloves, masks) until the patient is properly externally decontaminated (*Lancet 2008;371(9612):597*). PPE should not consist of latex or vinyl, since OPs are lipophilic and may penetrate such materials.

- **Decontamination:**
  - Remove patient from potential source of poisoning (*Crit Care Med 2002;30(10):2346*). All clothing, especially leather, should be removed from the patient and discarded in a ventilated area (*Crit Care Med 2002;30(10):2346*). Skin and hair decontamination requires thorough irrigation with water and might be enhanced through use of alcohol-based soaps (*Crit Care Med 2002;30(10): 2346*). Ocular decontamination should be irrigated with water only (*Crit Care Med 2002;30(10):2346*).
  - Gastric lavage might be indicated in stable patients who ingested contaminated fluids (*Clin Toxicol 2009;47(3):179*).
  - NOTE: All lavaged/aspirated fluids need to be safely discarded.
- **Stabilization:**
  - ABCs: Have a low threshold for early intubation in order to obtain airway protection.
  - AVOID mouth-to-mouth resuscitation because of contamination risk.
  - Start IV fluids as an initial bolus of 20 mL/kg (*Crit Care 2004;8(6):R391*).
- **Atropine** is an antimuscarinic agent, which competes with ACh for receptor binding.
  - GOAL: **Atropinization** (i.e., drying of bronchial secretions with normalized oxygen saturation [which may require 10 to 100 times the usual atropine doses]), heart rate >80 bpm, and systolic BP >80 mm Hg (*Lancet 2008; 371(9612):597*).
  - The initial **adult dose** is 1 to 3 mg IV bolus. Then titrate according to persistence of bronchorrhea by giving the double of the previously used dose every 5 minutes until atropinization is achieved (*Lancet 2008;371(9612):597*).
  - The initial **pediatric dose** is 0.02 mg/kg IV. Titrate as in adults (*BMJ 2007; 334(7594):629*).
  - Once the patient is stabilized, an infusion of atropine should be started with 10% to 20% of the initial atropinization dose per hour and should be held once anticholinergic effects occur (absent bowel sounds, urinary retention, agitation) (*Lancet 2008;371(9612):597*). Adults and children may develop paradoxical bradycardia through central anticholinergic mechanisms. NOTE: Atropine has no effect on NMJs; therefore, pralidoxime needs to be added as early as possible in order to reverse muscle weakness.
- **Pralidoxime** (2-PAM): Pralidoxime forms a complex with OPs that are bound to AChE. The pralidoxime–OP complex is then released from the enzyme and thus regenerates AChE function.
  - Once the AChE bound OPs start aging, pralidoxime is rendered ineffective. Therefore, it is crucial to start pralidoxime therapy early.
  - Pralidoxime also binds to some degree to free OPs and so prevents further AChE binding.
  - **Adult dosing** used to be administered as boluses given over time. New evidence, however, is favoring an infusion regimen (*Lancet 2006;368(9553):2136*): 1 to 2 g of pralidoxime in 100 mL NS IV over 20 minutes, then infusion of 500 mg/hr (*Lancet 2008;371(9612):597*).
  - NOTE: Pralidoxime use longer than 24 hours might be indicated if unaged OPs are redistributed from fat tissue. In such cases, infusions should be continued

until patient remains symptom free for at least 12 hours without additional atropine doses, or until the patient is extubated (*Lancet 2008;371(9612):597*).

○ Cardiac and respiratory failure have been reported after administration of pralidoxime (*Crit Care Med 2006;34(2):502*).

○ Though pralidoxime might not be effective in all cases of OP poisoning due to the aging effect, it is still recommended to be used routinely in order to decrease the total atropine requirements (*Crit Care Med 2002;30(10):2346*).

• **Benzodiazepines** are the first-line agents for OP-induced seizures (*BMJ 2007;334(7594):629*).

COMPLICATIONS

• **Intermediate syndrome (IMS):**
  ○ This syndrome is a postacute paralysis from persistent ACh excess after the acute cholinergic phase has been controlled.
  ○ Weakness of proximal extremity muscles and muscles supplied by cranial nerves that occurs hours to days after treatment of acute OP poisoning and often leads to respiratory failure if unnoticed (*PLoS Med 2008;5(7):e147*).
• **OP-induced delayed neurotoxicity (OPIDN):**
  ○ Besides AChE some OPs also inhibit other neurotoxic esterases, resulting in polyneuropathy or spinal cord damage due to demyelination of the long nerve fibers.
  ○ OPIDN usually occurs several days to weeks after acute OP poisoning leading to temporary, chronic, or recurrent motor or sensory dysfunctions (*Annu Rev Pharmacol Toxicol 1990;30:405*).

MONITORING/FOLLOW-UP

• All patients with severe or moderate poisoning should be admitted to an ICU after initial stabilization for further monitoring and treatment (*Crit Care 2004; 8(6):R391*).
• Asymptomatic patients presenting with a history of unintentional poisoning or patients with only mild symptoms do not always require hospital admission but should be observed for 6 to 12 hours. In these patients, consider measuring cholinesterase activity 6 hours after ingestion to evaluate for major ingestion (*BMJ 2007;334(7594):629*).

Carbamates

GENERAL PRINCIPLES

Epidemiology

Carbamates are reversible AChE inhibitors that also lead to ACh excess in the synaptic junction. They are occasionally found in pesticides. However, their most common use in this country is medicinal.

• **Physostigmine** is a naturally occurring methyl carbamate found in the Calabar bean. Other common carbamates are pyridostigmine and neostigmine.

• **Pyridostigmine** has been administered to U.S. soldiers while under nerve agent attack to prevent anticholinergic symptoms after possible exposure (*JAMA 1991;266(5):693*).

Pathophysiology

• Inhibition of ACh breakdown through AChE block leads to accumulation of ACh at nicotinic and muscarinic receptors with **excess cholinergic stimulation**.
• Carbamates are reversible enzyme inhibitors; they release AChE spontaneously. There is no "aging" phenomenon with carbamates.

DIAGNOSIS

Clinical Presentation

The clinical picture of the carbamate-induced cholinergic toxidrome is analogous to the one seen in OP poisoning since nicotinic and muscarinic receptors of the ANS and SNS are affected.

• Look for **SLUDGE** syndrome, **bradycardia**, **bronchorrhea**, and **bronchoconstriction** as well as neuromuscular depolarization, and be aware of the risk of cardiovascular or respiratory failure.
• Symptoms from carbamate poisoning are generally milder compared to OP poisoning and of shorter duration.

Diagnostic Testing

Cholinesterase levels are used to compare changes from baseline enzyme activity in mild exposures or to assess treatment success after acute exposure (*Clin Chem 1995;41:1814*).

TREATMENT

• The same measures of **protection** and **decontamination** as with OP poisoning apply to carbamates.
• **Stabilization:**
  ○ ABCs: Have a low threshold for early intubation in order to obtain airway protection.
  ○ Avoid mouth-to-mouth resuscitation because of contamination risk.

Medications

First Line
• **Atropine** is an antimuscarinic agent that competes with ACh for receptor binding.
  ○ GOAL: **Atropinization**. See Treatment under Organophosphates section for dosing guidelines.
  ○ Adults and children may develop paradoxical bradycardia through central anticholinergic mechanisms.

Second Line
Given the reversible action of carbamates, pralidoxime should only be given if more than 2 mg atropine has been required for bronchorrhea control (*Am J Emerg Med 1990;8(1):68*).

- Pralidoxime should be given if there is no clear evidence for isolated carbamate poisoning since additional OP exposure should always be suspected.
- **Benzodiazepines** are the first-line agents for carbamate-induced seizures.

Barbiturates

GENERAL PRINCIPLES

The use of barbiturates has largely fallen by the wayside as safer drugs are now available. Barbiturates are still used as induction agents for anesthesia as well as second-line agents for seizure control.

DIAGNOSIS

Suspect barbiturate overdose in patients who present with CNS and respiratory depression.

Clinical Presentation

History
It is often difficult to elicit a history as these patients are generally comatose on arrival.

Physical Examination
Typical examination findings include **respiratory depression** and **coma**. Other vital sign abnormalities may include hypothermia. Patients may develop cutaneous bullae known as **"barb blisters"** (*Cutis 1990;45:43*). **Miosis** may be present.

Differential Diagnosis

The differential diagnosis includes benzodiazepine overdose, hypoglycemia, ethanol intoxication, CNS, and other metabolic causes of coma.

Diagnostic Testing

Laboratories
This should include routine testing for any presentation of coma: **blood glucose, BMP, LFTs, and thyroid function tests**.

Electroencephalography
In barbiturate overdose, Electroencephalography (EEG) recordings may show no electrical activity.

Imaging
- A **CXR** should be obtained on all of these patients to evaluate for aspiration.
- **Head CT** may help evaluate for the presence of CNS lesions contributing to coma.

Diagnostic Procedures
Consider **lumbar puncture (LP)** in patients with undifferentiated coma to evaluate for meningitis or subarachnoid hemorrhage.

TREATMENT

The most important management strategy in barbiturate overdose is airway and breathing protection. Patients with respiratory depression should be intubated.

Medications

First Line
- Consider **MDAC** in patients with a protected airway and bowel sounds.
- Hypotension should be treated with 20 mL/kg bolus of NS. If this fails, consider a direct-acting vasopressor such as norepinephrine.

Second Line
Urine alkalinization with sodium bicarbonate is reserved for phenobarbital overdoses refractory to MDAC. It is inferior to MDAC (*J Toxicol Clin Toxicol 2004;42:1*).

Other Nonpharmacologic Therapies
Consider **hemoperfusion** in the setting of life-threatening phenobarbital overdose that is refractory to conventional management (*Chest 2003;123:897*). **Hemodialysis** has been reported to be useful as well (*Am J Kidney 2000;36:640*).

Benzodiazepines

GENERAL PRINCIPLES

In general, benzodiazepines have a wide safety margin. Deaths are usually related to the presence of a coingestant or ethanol.

DIAGNOSIS

Clinical Presentation
History
This is often difficult to elicit as patients are frequently comatose.

Physical Examination
The typical presentation of a pure oral benzodiazepine overdose is **coma with normal vital signs**. Respiratory depression is exceedingly unusual in oral overdose of benzodiazepines.

Differential Diagnosis
The differential diagnosis includes barbiturate overdose, hypoglycemia, ethanol intoxication, CNS, and other metabolic causes of coma.

Diagnostic Testing
Laboratories
- This should include routine testing for any presentation of coma: **blood glucose, BMP, LFTs, and thyroid function tests**. Consider **LP** in patients with undifferentiated coma to evaluate for meningitis or subarachnoid hemorrhage.
- **Urine drug screens** are unreliable in the setting of benzodiazepine overdose as the target metabolite, oxazepam or desmethyldiazepam, is not produced by the metabolism of many of the benzodiazepines. Classically, clonazepam, flunitrazepam, alprazolam, and lorazepam are not detected. Therefore, routine screening is not recommended (*Clin Chem 2003;49:357*).

Imaging
- A **CXR** should be obtained on all of these patients to evaluate for aspiration.
- A **head CT** may help evaluate for the presence of CNS lesions contributing to coma.

TREATMENT

Supportive care with observation is the mainstay of therapy. In patients with coingestions and respiratory depression, intubation and ventilation may be required. Since this is a benign overdose, **gastric lavage and AC are not necessary**. These interventions may cause aspiration in an otherwise stable patient.

Medications

- Traditional recommendations include the use of **flumazenil**; however, given the propensity to precipitate seizures and acute benzodiazepine withdrawal in patients on long-term benzodiazepine therapy, this therapy should be **avoided**. Other **contraindications** include a seizure history, coingestion of a cardiotoxic or epileptogenic drug, or ECG evidence of cyclic antidepressant ingestion.
- In **special cases** such as reversal of iatrogenically induced respiratory depression, reversal of sedation, or pediatric benzodiazepine ingestion, flumazenil may be given as a 0.1 mg/min dose intravenously. Repeat injections may be given, as resedation occasionally reoccurs.

Sympathomimetics, General

GENERAL PRINCIPLES

Definition

Patients who overdose on sympathomimetic agents exhibit a syndrome of excess adrenergic tone due to direct stimulation of adrenergic receptors or the effects of norepinephrine and epinephrine. Many of the agents in this category are drugs of abuse; although, several therapeutic agents can produce a similar toxidrome.

Classification

Agents that fall into this category include amphetamines, cocaine, vasopressors, methylxanthines, and β-agonists.

Epidemiology

Stimulants and street drugs were the sixth leading cause of fatal exposures according to the AAPCC in 2007, with 188 fatalities reported (*Clin Toxicol 2007;46(10): 927*).

Pathophysiology

- Agents that stimulate the sympathetic nervous system generally do so by either causing the release or preventing the reuptake of **endogenous catecholamines**, or **directly stimulating α-** and/or **β-receptors**.
- **Methylxanthines** (theophylline, caffeine) and **β-agonists** (albuterol, dobutamine, isoproterenol) enhance chronotropy and inotropy by **facilitating calcium entry into the myocardium**. They also enhance the function of β_2-receptors leading to **bronchodilatation**. Stimulation of the β_2-rich vascular beds to skeletal muscle results in **vasodilatation** as well. Therefore, in a pure β-agonist overdose, **hypotension and tachycardia** predominate.
- **Epinephrine, norepinephrine, cocaine, and amphetamines** have both α- and β- effects resulting in **hypertension and tachycardia**.

- Other α-receptors are found on the **iris**, which when stimulated, results in **pupillary dilatation**.
- Sympathetic stimulation of **sweat glands** is a **cholinergic** effect.

Amphetamines

GENERAL PRINCIPLES

Drugs of abuse in this class include **amphetamine, methamphetamine, and 3,4-methylenedioxymethamphetamine (MDMA)**. MDMA is a potent inducer and/or reuptake inhibitor of presynaptic serotonin, dopamine, and norepinephrine.

DIAGNOSIS

Clinical Presentation

- Suspect amphetamines in any patient presenting with a sympathomimetic toxidrome of **hypertension**, **tachycardia**, **dilated pupils**, and **diaphoresis**.
- Severely intoxicated patients may develop **hyperthermia**, **seizures**, **coma**, and **cardiovascular collapse**.

History
Drug abusers will often deny illicit use; therefore, the history is often unreliable.

Physical Examination
Patients may have **agitation** and **altered mental status** depending on the degree of intoxication.

Differential Diagnosis

The differential includes anything that may result in a sympathomimetic toxidrome including cocaine, ephedrine, pseudoephedrine, and various amphetamine-derived designer drugs.

Diagnostic Testing
Laboratories
Patients with a sympathomimetic toxidrome should be evaluated for end-organ dysfunction.

- A **BMP** is useful to assess the degree of hydration and renal function. MDMA is also associated with the development of hyponatremia due to either SIADH or ingestion of large quantity of water.
- A **CK** should be checked to evaluate for rhabdomyolysis in agitated patients.
- Patients complaining of chest pain should have a **troponin** drawn.
- **Urine drug screens** are often associated with false-negative and false-positive results, are expensive, and **do not contribute to the management of this syndrome**.

Electrocardiography
An ECG should be obtained to evaluate for ischemia and electrolyte disturbances.

Imaging
In select cases, imaging may be useful.
- Obtain a **head CT** in patients complaining of a headache or altered mental status.

- Obtain a **CXR** in patients complaining of chest pain.
- In patients with severe chest pain that radiates to the back or is associated with marked agitation, consider obtaining a **chest CT** to evaluate for aortic dissection.

TREATMENT

Mild-to-moderate cases usually respond to supportive care, including IV hydration. In hyperthermic cases, aggressive cooling measures should be taken. As always, priority should be given to airway protection, breathing, and circulation.

Medications
First Line
- Treat agitation and seizures with **benzodiazepines**. In refractory seizures, consider **barbiturates and propofol**.
- Hypertension and tachycardia may be managed with **CCBs**. **AVOID β-antagonists as they may be associated with the development of a hypertensive crisis.**
- **Nitroglycerin**, **nitroprusside**, and **phentolamine** may be used in the setting of severe hypertension.
- Ventricular arrhythmias should be treated with **lidocaine** or **amiodarone**.

Second Line
- Some data suggest that antipsychotics are useful in the management of agitated delirium in these patients (*N Engl J Med 1968;278:1361*). Consider administration of **haloperidol 5.0 mg IV or droperidol 2.5 mg IV** in patients with hallucinations (*Eur J Emerg Med 1997;4:130*).
- In hyperthermic-agitated patients, consider **paralysis** with a nondepolarizing agent to prevent rhabdomyolysis.

Other Nonpharmacologic Therapies
Patients with renal failure and rhabdomyolysis may require **hemodialysis**.

SPECIAL CONSIDERATIONS

MDMA may cause hyponatremia and serotonin syndrome (see earlier discussion).

REFERRAL

Obtain a chemical dependency consult in patients hospitalized as a result of drug abuse.

Cocaine

GENERAL PRINCIPLES

- Cocaine exerts its effects by inhibiting the reuptake of norepinephrine, serotonin, epinephrine, and dopamine. Excess adrenergic tone in the setting of toxicity is reflected by the development of hypertension and tachycardia. Drug-seeking behavior is likely modulated by dopaminergic effects in the ventral tegmental area of the brain.

- Cocaine has also been implicated in the development of early cardiovascular disease (*Circulation 2001;103:502*), likely due to a combination of vasospastic (*N Engl J Med 1989;321:1557*), prothrombotic (*Heart 2000;83:688*), and atherogenic effects (*J Am Coll Cardiol 2006;47:2120*).

DIAGNOSIS

Clinical Presentation
- Patients with cocaine intoxication often present with complaints of ischemic chest pain.
- Suspect cocaine in any patient presenting with a sympathomimetic toxidrome of **hypertension**, **tachycardia**, **dilated pupils**, and **diaphoresis**.
- Severely intoxicated patients may develop **hyperthermia**, **seizures**, **coma**, and **cardiovascular collapse**.

History
Drug abusers will often deny illicit use; therefore, the history is often unreliable.

Physical Examination
Patients may have **agitation** and **altered mental status** depending on the degree of intoxication.

Differential Diagnosis
The differential includes anything that may result in a sympathomimetic toxidrome, including amphetamines, ephedrine, pseudoephedrine, and various amphetamine-derived designer drugs.

Diagnostic Testing
Laboratories
Patients with a sympathomimetic toxidrome should be evaluated for end-organ dysfunction.
- A **BMP** is useful to assess the degree of hydration and renal function.
- A **CK** should be checked to evaluate for rhabdomyolysis in agitated patients.
- Patients complaining of chest pain should have a **troponin** drawn.
- **Urine drug screens**, although reliable in determining recent use, should not modify the acute management of these patients.

Electrocardiography
- An ECG should be obtained to evaluate for ischemia and electrolyte disturbances.
- Cocaine is a known sodium channel blocker, which may be reflected as a wide complex rhythm on the ECG (*J Pharmacol Exp Ther 1992;261:910*).
- Cocaine has been reported to increase the QT_c (*Emerg Med J 2004;21:252*).

Imaging
In select cases, imaging may be useful:
- Obtain a **head CT** in patients complaining of a headache or altered mental status.
- Obtain a **CXR** in patients complaining of chest pain.
- In patients with severe chest pain that radiates to the back or is associated with marked agitation, consider obtaining a **chest CT** to evaluate for aortic dissection.

TREATMENT

Mild-to-moderate cases usually respond to supportive care, including IV hydration. In hyperthermic cases, aggressive cooling measures should be taken. As always, priority should be given to airway protection, breathing, and circulation.

Medications
First Line
- Treat agitation and seizures with **benzodiazepines**. In refractory seizures, consider **barbiturates and propofol**.
- Hypertension and tachycardia may be managed with **CCBs**.
- **AVOID β-antagonists as they may be associated with the development of a hypertensive crisis.**
- **Nitroglycerin**, **nitroprusside**, and **phentolamine** may be used in the setting of severe hypertension.
- Sodium channel blockade should be treated with **sodium bicarbonate** (*Circulation 1991;83:1799*). Give **1 to 2 mEq/kg** as an IV bolus; may repeat. Monitor for QRS narrowing.
- Ventricular arrhythmias should be treated with **lidocaine**.

Second Line
In hyperthermic-agitated patients, consider **paralysis** with a nondepolarizing agent to prevent rhabdomyolysis.

Other Nonpharmacologic Therapies
Patients with renal failure and rhabdomyolysis may require **hemodialysis**.

SPECIAL CONSIDERATIONS

- Body packers with suspected cocaine toxicity or obstructive symptoms should have emergent surgical intervention.
- Consider whole-bowel irrigation in patients who present without signs of toxicity. Increasingly, cocaine has been found to be adulterated with **levamisole**. This veterinary dewormer has been demonstrated to cause agranulocytosis and vasculitis, which reverse with cessation of cocaine use. Any patient who presents with an unexpected decrease in their WBC or necrotic skin rash should be counseled to stop using cocaine. G-CSF may be used to treat serious neutropenia (*Semin Arthritis Rheum 2011;41(3):445*).

Theophylline

GENERAL PRINCIPLES

Definition
Theophylline is a methylxanthine agent used in the treatment of obstructive pulmonary diseases such as asthma and emphysema. Its use has largely fallen by the wayside as alternative, less toxic medications have been developed. However, patients with refractory pulmonary disease may still be prescribed this drug.

Classification

Toxicity is classified as **acute** or **chronic**. The management strategy is different depending on whether the drug is an **immediate-** or **sustained-release** preparation.

Pathophysiology

Theophylline exerts its therapeutic effects by promoting catecholamine release, which results in enhanced β-agonism (*Circulation 1983;67:162*). Additionally, at high doses, theophylline is a phosphodiesterase inhibitor, which prolongs the effects of β-agonism by preventing the breakdown of cyclic adenosine monophosphate (cAMP). Theophylline is also an adenosine antagonist, which in therapeutic doses, enhances bronchodilatation. However, in toxic doses, adenosine antagonism is associated with the development of tachydysrhythmias and seizures.

DIAGNOSIS

Clinical Presentation

- **Acute toxicity:** Patients with serum concentrations **>20 μg/mL** will present complaining of **nausea** and multiple episodes of **vomiting**. On examination, the patient will be **tremulous** and **tachycardic**. **Hyperventilation** is often present. In more severe cases, **hypotension** and **seizures** occur. **Refractory status epilepticus** is due to adenosine antagonism in the CNS (*Neuroscience 1994;58:245*). These effects are most often present at serum concentrations **>90 μg/mL** in the acutely intoxicated patient.
- **Chronic toxicity** usually occurs in patients with a large body burden of theophylline who develop a concurrent illness or are administered a drug that delays the P450 metabolism and theophylline clearance. Subtle symptoms such as nausea and anorexia may occur; tachycardia is usually present. Severe toxicity may occur at serum levels of **40 to 60 μg/mL**. Patients with these serum concentrations may present with seizures.

Diagnostic Testing

Laboratories

- **Acute toxicity** usually occurs at levels >90 to 100 μg/mL and is associated with the development of **hypokalemia** and **hyperglycemia**. In severe cases, expect a **metabolic acidosis**. Obtain a **BMP and blood glucose**.
- **Serial theophylline** concentrations should be obtained every 1 to 2 hours until a downward trend is present; remember, with sustained-release preparations, a peak may not be evident for 16 hours or later post ingestion.
- **Calcium, magnesium, and CK** should be checked as well.
- **Chronic toxicity** may occur at levels >40 μg/mL and is usually associated with normal laboratory values unless seizures are present. In these cases, obtain the laboratories mentioned earlier. **Serial theophylline** concentrations are also warranted in these patients.

Electrocardiography

Adenosine antagonism and increased catecholamines may result in a sinus tachycardia or supraventricular tachycardia (SVT) on the ECG. In overdose, premature ventricular contractions (PVCs) may be apparent.

TREATMENT

Patients with theophylline toxicity do not require gastric lavage as they tend to vomit. Sustained-release preparations occasionally form bezoars. Severely intoxicated patients require intubation and ventilation. Sustained-release formulations should be treated with **whole-bowel irrigation**. Replete potassium and electrolytes as needed.

Medications

- Administer **AC 1 g/kg**. Consider **MDAC** as theophylline clearance is increased by this modality (*Clin Pharmacol Ther 1983;33:351*). Ensure patients have adequate airway protection as vomiting and aspiration may occur.
- **Vomiting** should be managed with **ondansetron** or **metoclopramide**. **Phenothiazines are contraindicated** as they lower the seizure threshold.
- **Seizures** are often refractory and should initially be treated with **benzodiazepines**. If this modality fails, consider moving to **phenobarbital** as a 10 mg/kg loading dose at a rate of 50 mg/min, followed by up to a total of 30 mg/kg at a rate of 50 mg/min, followed by 1 to 5 mg/kg/d to maintain therapeutic plasma levels. **Propofol** is a reasonable alternative if these fail. Monitor for hypotension.
- **Hypotension** should be treated with 20 mL/kg bolus of IVF, which may be repeated. Direct pressors such as **phenylephrine** and **norepinephrine** may be added if fluid boluses are not sufficient. Since much of the hypotension is mediated by β_2-agonism, **avoid epinephrine**. Consider using short-acting β-antagonists such as **esmolol**, which although counterintuitive, may reverse β_2-mediated vasodilatation. Monitor for bronchospasm.
- **Arrhythmias** should be treated with β-antagonists. Use short-acting agents such as **esmolol** and monitor for bronchospasm.

Other Nonpharmacologic Therapies

Hemoperfusion (charcoal or resin) or **hemodialysis** is indicated for the following:
- Intractable seizures or life-threatening cardiovascular complications, regardless of drug level.
- A theophylline level of ≥ 100 mg/mL after an **acute** overdose.
- A theophylline level >60 mg/mL in acute intoxication, with worsening symptoms, or inability to tolerate oral charcoal administration.
- A theophylline level >60 mg/mL in **chronic** intoxication without life-threatening symptoms.
- A theophylline level >40 mg/mL in a patient with chronic intoxication and CHF, respiratory insufficiency, hepatic failure, or age older than 60 years (*J Emerg Med 1993;11:415*).

Toxic Alcohol, General

GENERAL PRINCIPLES

- High alcohol concentrations increase the measured plasma osmolality and subsequently widen the osmolar gap. A normal gap is <10 mmol/dL and varies from -14 to $+10$ mmol/dL (*N Engl J Med 1984;310(2):102*).

- In presence of a widened gap, the actual serum alcohol level can be estimated if done early after ingestion (*BMC Emerg Med 2008;8:5*) with the following calculation:

$$\text{Osmol gap} \times \frac{\text{Molecular weight of alcohol}}{10} = [\text{Serum alcohol}](\text{mg/dL})$$

- Soon after ingestion, alcohol metabolization begins, the osmolar gap falls, and the anion gap rises (*Clin J Am Soc Nephrol 2008;3(1):208*). Therefore, the osmolar gap should only be used to support the diagnosis of toxic alcohol poisoning and not to draw conclusions about the actual amount of ingested toxin.

$$\text{Calculated osmolarity} = 2\text{Na}^+ + \frac{\text{BUN}}{2.8} + \frac{\text{Glucose}}{18} + \frac{\text{Alcohol/Molecular weight of alcohol}}{10}$$

- The specific molecular weights for each alcohol can be found in the following sections below.

TREATMENT

The general approach to toxic alcohol ingestions is to (*Clin Toxicol 2002;40(4): 415*):
- Prevent the formation of toxic metabolites by inhibiting alcohol dehydrogenase (ADH) (in methanol and ethylene glycol poisoning only).
- Eliminate the toxic alcohol and toxic metabolites from the blood.
- Correct acid–base imbalance.
- Replenish cofactors.

Methanol

GENERAL PRINCIPLES

Definition
Methanol is used in gasoline antifreeze, deicers, windshield washer fluid, paint and varnish removers, fuel, photocopy fluid, embalming fluids; is found in "moonshine" liquor; and is used as a denaturant for ethanol.

Etiology
- Ingestions are mostly intentional as suicide attempts.
- Another common cause of poisoning is the use of methanol as ethanol substitute.

Pathophysiology
Methanol is oxidized to toxic formic acid and this product is responsible for the anion gap metabolic acidosis in methanol poisoning (*Intern Med 2004;43(8): 750*).

DIAGNOSIS

Clinical Presentation

- **Early stage:**
  - Early after ingestion, mild CNS depression or headache evolves, but profound obtundation or inebriation can occur as well.
  - These early symptoms are directly caused by methanol prior to metabolization.
- **Late stage:**
  - After a latent period of about 14 to 18 hours, severe anion gap metabolic acidosis without significant lactate or ketone concentrations develops.
  - Formate accumulation within the retina and optic nerve fibers causes "snow field vision," blurred vision, visual field defects, or blindness (*Arch Ophthalmol 1991;109(7):1012*).
  - Other CNS symptoms during the late phase are lethargy, convulsion, delirium, and coma. Basal ganglia hemorrhage with dyskinesia or hypokinesia has been observed (*Int J Clin Pract 2004;58(11):1042*).
  - Abdominal complaints include nausea, vomiting, pain, and acute pancreatitis (*Clin Toxicol 2000;38(3):297*).

History

Obtain history of what, when, how, and how much of the toxic substance was ingested.

Physical Examination

- Assess mental status and respiratory and cardiovascular stability.
- Kussmaul respirations may indicate underlying metabolic acidosis.
- Visual field testing may reveal central scotoma or other visual field defects. A thorough funduscopic exam may show hyperemia, disk edema, or atrophy (*Med J Aust 1978;2(10):483*).

Diagnostic Testing

Laboratories

- Address possible causes of an anion gap acidosis:
  - BMP: Acidosis, anion gap, renal function
  - Urinalysis (UA): Ketones
  - Serum lactate
- Accu-Cheks.
- Obtain serum osmolality, if toxic alcohol ingestion is suspected. Molecular weight of methanol is 32.04 g/mol.
- ABG or VBG: To assess acid/base status and treatment success.
- Ethanol level: If elevated, toxic methanol manifestations may be delayed; if elevated in presence of acidosis, the acidosis is unlikely to be related to a toxic alcohol ingestion, since ethanol blocks the metabolism of the parent compound (unless the toxic alcohol ingestion occurred hours before ethanol ingestion).
- Serum methanol level: Usually not readily available; therefore, clinically not useful.

TREATMENT

- ABCs and supportive care, monitor urine output.
- GI decontamination: Nasogastric lavage is only indicated in patients who present <30 minutes after ingestion or who ingested large amounts of methanol while maintaining a normal mental status.

- **Do not use AC** since the GI tract rapidly absorbs methanol. AC bears a high risk of aspiration in acutely intoxicated patients.
- Sodium bicarbonate: Give 50 mg IV every 4 hours for arterial pH <7.30 (*N Engl J Med 2009;360(21):2216*).
  - Serum alkalinization limits the amount of undissociated formic acid, which prevents CNS toxicity.
  - Urine alkalinization enhances clearance of formate. CAVEAT: Watch for fluid overload if giving large amounts of bicarbonate.
- Ethanol therapy: EtOH serum levels of 100 mg/dL block ADH sufficiently to inhibit formation of toxic metabolites.
  - Loading dose of **7.6 mL/kg of 10% ethanol** solution IV (correlates with an EtOH serum level of 100 to 200 mg/dL).
  - Maintenance dose of **0.8 mL/kg/hr (nondrinker), or 2.0 mL/kg/hr (drinker), or 2.0 to 3.3 mL/kg/hr (on hemodialysis)** of 10% ethanol solution IV (*Clin J Am Soc Nephrol 2008;3(1):208*).
- **Fomepizole** therapy: 4-Methylpyrazole (Antizol) is an FDA-approved competitive inhibitor of ADH for the treatment of methanol poisoning (*Intensive Care Med 2005;31(2):189*).
  - Loading dose of **15 mg/kg IV**, maintenance dose of **10 mg/kg IV** every 12 hours for 48 hours, then 15 mg/kg IV every 12 hours until methanol level <20 mg/dL.
  - Dose adjustment may be needed for patients on hemodialysis (*N Engl J Med 2009;360(21):2216*).
  - Continue treatment until methanol levels <20 mg/dL and acidosis resolves (*Curr Opin Nephrol Hypertens 2000;9(6):695*).
- Indication: Ethanol or fomepizole therapy should be started early if:
  - Strong evidence of methanol ingestion
  - Methanol serum level >20 mg/dL
  - Osmolar gap >10 mmol/dL
  - Arterial pH <7.3
  - Serum CO_2 <20 mmol/L
  - Or unexplained anion gap metabolic acidosis is present (*N Engl J Med 2009;360(21):2216*)

Other Nonpharmacologic Therapies

- **Hemodialysis** should be used in addition to the aforementioned therapies in order to prevent end-organ toxicity.
- **Hemodialysis** corrects metabolic abnormalities and eliminates nonmetabolized methanol. Indications for hemodialysis are a methanol level >50 mg/dL, severe acidemia (bicarbonate <15 mmol/L, pH <7.30), and/or optic injury from toxicity (*Hum Exp Toxicol 2005;24(2):55*).
- Folic acid 1 mg/kg (up to 50 mg) IV every 4 to 6 hours and folinic acid (leucovorin) 1 mg/kg (up to 50 mg) IV every 4 to 6 hours enhance formate metabolism and should be given until metabolic acidosis resolves (*Alcoholism 1980;4(4):378*).

SPECIAL CONSIDERATIONS

- Coingestion of ethanol might delay the onset of initial symptoms because of ethanol's higher affinity to ADH.
- Ethanol therapy has significant disadvantages; for example, complex dosing regimen, hard to titrate therapeutic levels, intensive care requirements, and severe side-

effect profile. Although very expensive ($500/dose), fomepizole has become the preferred agent in the treatment of methanol intoxication (*Ann Emerg Med 2009;53(4):451*).
- Admit all patients on ethanol infusions to the ICU (risk of hypotension, tachycardia, hypoglycemia, CNS and respiratory depression).
- Stable patients on fomepizole infusion can be safely admitted to the floor. Adverse effects of fomepizole are usually mild and include headache, nausea, dizziness but not sedation (*Alcoholism 1988;12(4):516*; *Lancet 1999;354(9181):831*).
- Report all cases of methanol intoxication to the local poison control center (1-800-222-1222).
- Get a clinical toxicologist involved early.
- Consult ophthalmology or neurology service if signs of optic injury or other neurologic deficits present.

Ethylene Glycol

GENERAL PRINCIPLES

Etiology
- Ingestions are mostly intentional suicide attempts.
- Another common cause of poisoning is the use of ethylene glycol as ethanol substitute.

Pathophysiology
- Ethylene glycol is oxidized to glycolic acid and oxalic acid.
- Glycolate accumulation is responsible for the anion gap metabolic acidosis in ethylene glycol poisoning.
- Oxalate accumulation is responsible for the development of acute renal failure in ethylene glycol poisoning (*Clin Toxicol 1986;24(5):389*).

DIAGNOSIS

Clinical Presentation
- Neurologic stage (30 minutes to 12 hours):
  - CNS depression with altered mental status, hallucinations, ataxia, slurred speech, and cranial nerve palsies are directly caused by ethylene glycol prior to metabolization.
  - Seizures, coma, and respiratory depression can occur in severe intoxications.
- Cardiovascular stage (12 to 24 hours): Glycolate affects the cardiopulmonary system and causes tachycardia, hypotension, heart failure, pulmonary edema, and ARDS.
- Renal stage (24 to 72 hours postingestion):
  - Glycolic acid is further metabolized to oxalic acid. Oxalate is a calcium chelator, and accumulation of oxalate leads to **hypocalcemia**.
  - Calcium oxalate can precipitate in the renal tubules, which subsequently causes acute tubular necrosis with flank pain and acute renal failure (*Acta Clin Belg 1999;54(6):351*).
- Within 4 to 6 hours after ingestion, development of an anion gap metabolic acidosis with absence of significant lactate or ketone concentrations occurs.
- Abdominal complaints (nausea, vomiting, pain) are also common.

History

Obtain history of what, when, how, and how much of the toxic substance was ingested.

Physical Examination
- Assess mental status and respiratory and cardiovascular stability.
- Kussmaul respiration may indicate severe metabolic acidosis.

Diagnostic Testing

Laboratories
- Address causes of a high anion gap metabolic acidosis:
  - BMP: Acidosis, anion gap, renal function.
  - UA: Ketones, oxalate crystals (usually a late sign during intoxication).
  - Serum lactate.
  - **Glycolic acid may also be misinterpreted as a high lactic acid on a point-of-care blood gas analyzer.** Serum levels should be obtained in these cases.
- Obtain serum osmolality if toxic alcohol ingestion is suspected. Molecular weight of ethylene glycol is 62.07 g/mol.
- ABG or VBG to assess acid/base status and treatment success.
- Ethanol level: If elevated, toxic ethylene glycol manifestations may be delayed; if elevated in presence of acidosis, unlikely to be toxic alcohol ingestion (unless toxic alcohol ingestion occurred hours before ethanol ingestion).
- Obtain serum ethylene glycol level: Usually not readily available, therefore clinically often not useful.
- Serum calcium level: Low if increased formation of calcium oxalate.
- Repeated renal function testing: Increased risk of acute kidney injury (AKI).
- Urine microscopy: Calcium oxalate might be visible as envelope-shaped crystals (*Emerg Med J 2007;24(4):310*).
- Wood's lamp examination of urine to detect fluorescence after assumed antifreeze ingestion is not a reliable screening tool (*Am J Emerg Med 2005;23(6):787*).

TREATMENT

- ABCs and supportive care, monitor urine output.
- GI decontamination: Nasogastric lavage is only indicated in patients who present <30 minutes after ingestion or who ingested large amounts of ethylene glycol while maintaining a normal mental status.
- **Do not use AC** since the GI tract rapidly absorbs ethylene glycol. AC bears a high risk of aspiration in acutely intoxicated patients.
- **Thiamine** (Vitamin B$_1$) 100 mg IV every 4 to 6 hours and **pyridoxine** (Vitamin B$_6$) 50 mg IV every 6 to 12 hours enhance glycolate metabolism and should be given until metabolic acidosis resolves (*Eur J Emerg Med 2005;12(2):78*).
- Sodium bicarbonate: Give 50 mg IV every 4 hours for arterial pH <7.30 (*N Engl J Med 2009;360(21):2216*).
  - Serum alkalinization limits the amount of undissociated glycolic acid, which prevents CNS toxicity.
  - Urine alkalinization enhances clearance of glycolate. CAVEAT: Watch for fluid overload if giving large amounts of bicarbonate.

- Ethanol therapy: EtOH serum levels of 100 mg/dL block ADH sufficiently to inhibit formation of toxic metabolites. See discussion of methanol overdose treatment for dosing.
- **Fomepizole** therapy: See discussion of methanol overdose treatment for dosing.
- **Indications:** Ethanol or fomepizole therapy should be started early if:
  - Strong evidence of ethylene glycol ingestion
  - Ethylene glycol serum level >20 mg/dL
  - Osmolar gap >10 mmol/dL
  - Arterial pH <7.3
  - Serum CO_2 <20 mmol/L
  - Unexplained anion gap metabolic acidosis is present (*N Engl J Med 2009;360 (21):2216*)

Other Nonpharmacologic Therapies

- **Hemodialysis** should be used in addition to the aforementioned therapies in order to prevent end-organ toxicity.
- **Hemodialysis** corrects metabolic abnormalities and eliminates nonmetabolized ethylene glycol. Indications for hemodialysis are an ethylene glycol level >50 mg/ dL, severe acidemia (bicarbonate <15 mmol/L, pH <7.30), and/or optic injury from toxicity (*Hum Exp Toxicol 2005;24(2):55*).

Ethanol

GENERAL PRINCIPLES

- Elimination rate: 20 to 25 mg/dL/hr (zero-order kinetics, faster in chronic alcoholics).
- Ethanol is present in all alcoholic beverages, some food extracts, mouthwash, cold syrups, but is also industrially used as a solvent in its denatured form.

Pathophysiology

Ethanol is oxidized to acetic acid (acetate), which is further metabolized to nontoxic intermediates.

DIAGNOSIS

Clinical Presentation

- CNS depression with ataxia, drowsiness, and confusion are common symptoms at blood levels >100 mg/dL. Respiratory depression can occur at higher concentrations (*Emerg Med 1984;2(1):47*).
- Chronic alcohol abuse induces tolerance, and patients appear asymptomatic even with high blood levels (*J Emerg Med 1997;15(5):687*).
- Hypoglycemia is due to an altered NADH/NAD+ ratio with the development of a reduced state. Pyruvate is then shunted off the gluconeogenesis pathway, and lactate production is favored due to increased NADH. Severe hypoglycemia is common in chronic alcoholics and in children.
- Chronic intoxication causes further gluconeogenesis disturbances, an increase in ketogenesis (β-hydroxybutyrate), and eventually the development of alcoholic ketoacidosis (AKA) (*Hum Exp Toxicol 1996;15(6):482*).

Diagnostic Testing

- Obtain glucose levels and BMP (especially in chronic alcoholics).
- Serum ethanol levels are only relevant to rule out poisoning with other alcohols, in presence of coma or altered mental status, or to prove incapacity in an intoxicated patient.
- Serum osmolality (if coingestion with other alcohols is suspected). Molecular weight of ethanol is 46.07 g/mol.
- May also have mild lactic acidosis.

TREATMENT

Treatment is mainly supportive; however, hemodialysis may be indicated in severe poisoning. Administer 100 mg **thiamine** *IV* followed by 50 mL of D_{50} in water IV to any **comatose alcoholic patient**.

SPECIAL CONSIDERATIONS

- Increased morbidity and mortality result from chronic toxicity (liver and GI injuries) and AKA.
- Traumatic injuries and severe hypothermia are frequent findings due to risky behavior or decreased judgment capability during acute intoxication.
- Ethanol withdrawal can lead to life-threatening conditions and requires special attention.
- Patients should be observed until signs of clinical intoxication resolve.

Cyanide

GENERAL PRINCIPLES

Cyanide is one of the most rapidly acting and lethal poisons in existence. Cyanide has an odor of bitter almonds; however, only 50% of the population can detect it (*Clin Toxicol 1981;18(3):367*).

Etiology

- Inhalation of smoke from structural fires is the most common source of cyanide exposure in the United States and Western countries.
- Other etiologies include artificial nail remover, older rodenticides, electroplating solutions, photographic developer solutions, laboratory reagents, laetrile, plants (such aspits from the *Prunus* species), food such as cassava, and from the metabolism of sodium nitroprusside.

Pathophysiology

- Cyanide is a chemical asphyxiant. It induces cellular hypoxia by inhibiting Complex IV (also known as cytochrome c oxidase or cytochrome oxidase aa_3) in the electron transport chain and thus preventing the formation of adenosine triphosphate (ATP).
- Hyperlactemia occurs from inhibition of aerobic metabolism.

DIAGNOSIS

Clinical Presentation

- The dose, duration of exposure, route of exposure, and etiology of the exposure all contribute to the severity of the illness. Signs and symptoms can be nonspecific, so physicians must have a high degree of clinical suspicion to avoid missing the diagnosis (*Hum Exp Toxicol 2007;26:191*).
- Transient increases in heart rate, BP, and respiratory rate can be followed by cardiovascular collapse and respiratory failure. Initially, patients can present with bradycardia and hypertension; this is followed by tachycardia and hypotension before they experience cardiovascular collapse.
- The heart and CNS have high demands for oxygen and are commonly affected. Signs and symptoms include headache, anxiety, lethargy, seizures, coma, respiratory failure, and cardiovascular collapse. Cyanide does not cause cyanosis.
- The cherry-red skin that is classically associated with cyanide toxicity is an uncommon finding. Retinal veins may be bright red.

Laboratories

- Blood and serum levels are available. However due to lengthy delays in obtaining them, they are not clinically useful in treating the acutely ill patient. Smokers may have a slightly elevated baseline level compared to nonsmokers.
- Due to inhibition of aerobic metabolism, patients can have an elevated lactate levels. In smoke inhalation victims, a lactate greater than 10 mmol/L was suggestive of cyanide toxicity (*N Engl J Med 2007;26(3):191*).
- Patients may have an "arterialization" of their venous blood as the venous oxygen saturation may be very elevated due to inhibition of aerobic metabolism. This can be seen when comparing arterial and venous blood gasses that are drawn simultaneously.

TREATMENT

Two antidotes are available for patients with cyanide toxicity.

- The cyanide antidote kit contains **amyl nitrite pearls** and **sodium nitrite**. The pearls can be broken and placed under the patient's nose while IV access is obtained. Sodium nitrite (300 mg) is administered as a 3% solution given over 2 to 4 minutes IV in adults. Nitrites are given to induce a methemoglobinemia so that the cyanide will preferentially bind to them instead of the electron transport chain. However, in patients with smoke inhalation, this can be dangerous as they may already have elevated levels of carboxyhemoglobin and the combination can cause a very severe functional anemia. Nitrites can also cause or exacerbate hypotension. The second part of the antidote is **sodium thiosulfate** administered as 12.5 g IV in adults. Its time of onset is slower than the nitrites; at times, it is given prophylactically to patients on nitroprusside infusions (*Ann Pharmacother 1992;26(4):515*).
- **Hydroxocobalamin** (5 g IV) is another antidote. It combines with cyanide to form cyanocobalamin (vitamin B_{12}). It has few side effects. It turns the urine red and causes skin discoloration, which negatively interferes with co-oximetry. It will also interfere with certain laboratory tests such as bilirubin, creatinine, and serum glucose (*Crit Rev Toxicol 2009;39(7):541*).

- The rest of care is supportive, including adequate volume resuscitation, airway support, and vasopressor and inotropic support as needed (*Hum Exp Toxicol 2007;26:191*).

Carbon Monoxide

GENERAL PRINCIPLES

Carbon monoxide (CO) is a colorless, odorless, and tasteless gas that is produced during incomplete combustion of carbon-containing fuels. It is the leading cause of poisoning morbidity and mortality in the United States (*JAMA 1991;266:659*).

Etiology

Common sources of exposure include smoke inhalation in house fires, malfunctioning heaters and electric generators, automobile exhaust, smoking, forklifts, and chemicals such as methylene chloride (*Emerg Med Clin N Am 2004;22:985*).

Pathophysiology

- CO binds with hemoglobin to form carboxyhemoglobin, which causes a functional anemia and shifts the oxyhemoglobin dissociation curve to the left.
- CO inhibits cellular respiration by binding to mitochondrial cytochrome oxidase and disrupting the electron transport chain (*J Toxicol Clin Toxicol 1989;27(3): 141*).
- Nitric oxide levels, which cause vasodilation, are also increased (likely secondary to activation of nitric oxide synthase) (*Emerg Med Clin N Am 2004;22:985*).

DIAGNOSIS

The diagnosis of CO poisoning is challenging due to its many vague signs and symptoms that can wax and wane depending on the patient's source of exposure.

Clinical Presentation

- Patients may present with flu- or viral-like symptoms, which include headache, myalgias, fatigue, lethargy, nausea, vomiting, and dizziness. If these patients remove themselves from the exposure, such as when they leave their house to seek medical attention, the symptoms may improve before they are evaluated by a physician.
- The heart and CNS have higher oxygen demands and so patients can present with chest pain, myocardial infarctions, cardiac dysrhythmias, syncope, stroke-like symptoms, seizures, coma, and other psychoneurologic symptoms.
- Patients may present with persistent neurologic sequelae (PNS), which occur at the time of exposure or delayed neurologic sequelae (DNS), which can occur anywhere between 2 and 40 days after the exposure (*Ann Emerg Med 1995; 25:474*).

Diagnostic Testing

- Carboxyhemoglobin (CO-Hgb) levels are readily available. They can be obtained on either arterial or venous specimens (*Ann Emerg Med 1995;25:4813*). Levels greater than 5% in nonsmokers and greater than 10% in smokers generally confirm an exogenous exposure. However, levels do not correlate well with a patient's symptoms or prognosis.

- New handheld pulse co-oximeters can be used to noninvasively measure CO-Hgb. Standard pulse oximeters maybe falsely reassuring as they cannot detect a difference between oxyhemoglobin and CO-Hgb. This results in a "gap" between the measured pulse oximetry using a finger probe and the true value found by using co-oximetry.
- Levels need to be interpreted in the context of how long it has been since the exposure and when oxygen therapy was initiated. Both will cause the level to be "falsely low."
- Head CTs may show bilateral lesions in the globus pallidus.
- A lactic acidosis may be present due to the disruption of aerobic respiration.

TREATMENT

- Treatment involves administering oxygen. One hundred percent oxygen administered through a non-rebreather will decrease the half-life of CO to 60 to 90 minutes. Hyperbaric oxygen (HBO) will decrease it to 20 to 30 minutes. Most patients will need to be transported to tertiary centers to receive HBO, hence, improving PNS or preventing DNS and not just decreasing the half-life of CO is the rationale for the use of HBO.
  - Randomized studies have both supported HBO for CO poisoning (*Ann Emerg Med 1995;25:474*; *N Engl J Med 2002;347(14)1057*) and concluded that it was ineffective (*Lancet 1989;334:414*; *Med J Aust 1999;170(5):203*). The studies differed in their inclusion criteria, treatment protocols, and outcome assessment.
  - Indications for and the benefit of HBO are controversial and more research is needed (*Cochrane Database Syst Rev 2011 April 13;(4):CD002041*). Suggested indications include syncope, coma, neurologic deficits, PNS, cardiac ischemia, severe metabolic acidosis, pregnancy, and CO >25%.
  - HBO carries risks including oxygen-induced seizures, barotraumas, claustrophobia, and tympanic membrane rupture. Also, once in the chamber, access to the patient is limited and cardioversion and defibrillation cannot be performed.
- Additional care is supportive including airway and ventilator support, vasopressors for hypotension, and treating any additional concurrent injury such as if the patient has a burn from a house fire.

COMPLICATIONS

- If the patient survives the exposure, DNS and PNS are the most feared long-term complications after CO poisoning.
- The signs and symptoms of DNS are variable and a standard definition does not exist. They can include malaise, fatigue, headache, memory problems, paralysis, dementia, neuropathy, psychosis, and cortical blindness (*Ann Emerg Med 1995; 25:474*).

Appendix A

Immunizations and Postexposure Therapies

Carlos A. Q. Santos and Victoria J. Fraser

- **Active immunization** promotes the development of a durable primary immune response (B-cell proliferation, antibody response, T-cell sensitization) such that subsequent exposure to the pathogen results in a secondary response that protects against the development of disease (Table A-1).
- **Passive immunization** involves the administration of immune globulins that results in transient protection against infection. It is usually utilized in a host with limited capacity to mount a primary immune response after active immunization, in the instance where exposure to a pathogen occurs in a previously unvaccinated host, or to protect against toxin-mediated disease (Tables A-2 and A-3).
- **Postexposure prophylaxis** is required after exposure to blood-borne pathogens in a health care setting (Table A-4) and after exposure to agents of bioterrorism (Table A-5).
- **Health care provider responsibilities** with regard to immunization include
  ○ Following vaccine directives.
  ○ Maintaining records (type of vaccine and dose, site and route of administration, date when vaccine was administered, date when next dose is due, manufacturer and lot number, name and title of person administering the vaccine).
  ○ Reporting adverse events (Vaccine Adverse Events Reporting System [VAERS], *http://vaers.hhs.gov/index*, 1-800-822-7967).
- Additional advice is available from the Division of Immunization at the Centers for Disease Control and Prevention (CDC) (1-404-639-8225).

Table A-1 Adult Immunizations in the United States

Vaccine, Dose	Persons for Whom Indicated	Contraindications	Precautions
Influenza Trivalent inactivated vaccine (TIV): 0.5 mL IM Live attenuated vaccine (LAV) (*FluMist*): 0.2 mL intranasally prior to influenza season **annually.**	**Everyone, prior to influenza season annually.** Persons ≥6 mo of age, including pregnant women, can receive TIV. Healthy, nonpregnant adults <50 yr of age without high-risk medical conditions can receive either LAV or TIV. Health care personnel who care for severely immunocompromised persons (i.e., those who require care in a protected environment) should receive TIV rather than LAV. Other persons should receive TIV.	TIV and LAV: Severe allergic reaction (e.g., anaphylaxis) after previous dose of any influenza vaccine or to a vaccine component, including egg protein. LAV: Immune suppression; certain chronic medical conditions such as asthma, diabetes, heart or kidney disease; pregnancy.	Moderate or severe acute illness with or without fever; history of Guillain–Barre syndrome (GBS) within 6 wk of previous influenza vaccination. LAV: Antivirals (i.e., amantadine, rimantadine, zanamivir or oseltamivir) 48 hr before vaccination; avoid use of these antivirals for 14 d after vaccination.

(continued)

Table A-1	Adult Immunizations in the United States (Continued)		
Vaccine, Dose	Persons for Whom Indicated	Contraindications	Precautions
Tetanus, diphtheria (Td) booster/Tetanus, diphtheria, pertussis (Tdap) booster Td: 0.5 mL IM Tdap: 0.5 mL IM.	**Everyone, every 10 years.** Administer Tdap once to adults who have not received Tdap previously or for whom vaccine status is unknown to replace one of the 10-yr Td boosters. Adults with unknown or incomplete history of completing a three-dose primary vaccination series with Td-containing vaccines should begin or complete a primary vaccination series.	Severe allergic reaction (e.g., anaphylaxis) after a previous dose or to a vaccine component. For Tdap only: Encephalopathy (e.g., coma, decreased level of consciousness or prolonged seizures) not attributable to another identifiable cause within 7 d of administration of a previous dose of Tdap or diphtheria and tetanus toxoids and pertussis (DTP) or diphtheria and tetanus toxoids and acellular pertussis (DTaP) vaccine.	Moderate or severe acute illness with or without fever. GBS within 6 wk after a previous dose of tetanus toxoid-containing vaccine. History of arthus-type hypersensitivity reactions after a previous dose of diphtheria toxoid–containing vaccine For Tdap only: Progressive or unstable neurologic disorder, uncontrolled seizures, or progressive encephalopathy until a treatment regimen has been established and the condition has stabilized.

Vaccine	Indications	Contraindications	Precautions
Varicella 0.5 mL SC, 2 doses 4–8 wk apart.	**Everyone, without evidence of immunity.** Special consideration should be given to those who have close contact with persons at high risk for severe disease (e.g., health care personnel and family contacts of persons with immunocompromising conditions) and are at high risk for exposure or transmission (e.g., teachers, child care employees, residents and staff members of institutional settings, college students, military personnel, adolescents and adults living in households with children, nonpregnant women of childbearing age, and international travelers).	Severe allergic reaction (e.g., anaphylaxis) after a previous dose or to a vaccine component. Known severe immunodeficiency (e.g., from hematologic and solid tumors, receipt of chemotherapy, congenital immunodeficiency, or long-term immunosuppressive therapy or patients with HIV infection who are severely immunocompromised). Pregnancy.	Recent (≤11 mo) receipt of antibody-containing blood product (specific interval depends on product). Moderate or severe acute illness with or without fever. Receipt of specific antivirals 24 hr before vaccination; if possible, delay resumption of antivirals for 14 d after vaccination.
Human papillomavirus (HPV) Quadrivalent HPV vaccine (HPV4): 0.5 mL IM, 3 doses, second and third doses given at 2 and 6 mo after first dose.	**Females:** Administer at 11 or 12 yr of age, and for those 13 through 26 yr of age if not previously vaccinated. **Males:** Administer at 11 or 12 yr of age, and for those 13 through 21 yr of age if not previously vaccinated. Males 22 through 26 yr of age may be vaccinated; HPV4 is recommended for men who have sex with men (MSM) through age 26 yr who did not get any or all doses when they were younger.	Severe allergic reaction (e.g., anaphylaxis) after a previous dose or to a vaccine component.	Moderate or severe acute illness with or without fever. Pregnancy.

(continued)

Table A-1 Adult Immunizations in the United States (Continued)

Vaccine, Dose	Persons for Whom Indicated	Contraindications	Precautions
Zoster 0.65 mg SC once.	**Adults ≥60 yr of age** regardless of whether they report a prior episode of herpes zoster.	Severe allergic reaction (e.g., anaphylaxis) to a vaccine component. Known severe immunodeficiency (e.g., from hematologic and solid tumors, receipt of chemotherapy or long-term immunosuppressive therapy or patients with HIV infection who are severely immunocompromised). Pregnancy.	Moderate or severe acute illness with or without fever. Receipt of specific antivirals 24 hr before vaccination; possible, avoid use of antivirals for 14 d after vaccination.

| Measles, mumps, rubella (MMR)
0.5 mL SC, 1 or 2 doses. | **Adults born after 1957**, unless immune.
Measles/mumps component: Routine second dose of MMR vaccine, administered a minimum of 28 d after the first dose, is recommended for adults who are students in postsecondary educational institutions; work in a health care facility; or plan to travel internationally. Persons who received inactivated (killed) measles vaccine or measles vaccine of unknown type from 1963 to 1967, or persons vaccinated before 1979 with either killed mumps vaccine or mumps vaccine of unknown type who are at high risk for mumps infection (e.g., works at health care facility) should be considered for revaccination with two doses of MMR vaccine.
Rubella component: For women of childbearing age, rubella immunity should be determined. If no immunity, nonpregnant women should be vaccinated. Pregnant women with no immunity should receive MMR vaccine upon completion or termination of pregnancy and before discharge from the health care facility. | Severe allergic reaction (e.g., anaphylaxis) to a vaccine component. Known severe immunodeficiency (e.g., from hematologic and solid tumors, receipt of chemotherapy or long-term immunosuppressive therapy or patients with HIV infection who are severely immunocompromised). Pregnancy. | Moderate or severe acute illness with or without fever.
Recent (within 11 mo) receipt of antibody-containing blood product (specific interval depends on product).
History of thrombocytopenia or thrombocytopenic purpura.
Need for tuberculin skin testing (TST). Measles vaccination might suppress tuberculin reactivity temporarily. Measles-containing vaccine may be administered on same day as TST. If testing indicated after MMR vaccination, test should be postponed ≥4 wk after vaccination.
(continued) |

Table A-1	Adult Immunizations in the United States (Continued)		
Vaccine, Dose	Persons for Whom Indicated	Contraindications	Precautions
Pneumococcal (polysaccharide) (PPSV) 0.5 mL IM, 1 or 2 doses.	**Initial vaccination:** Adults ≥65 yr of age without a history of PPSV vaccination; adults ≤65 yr of age with chronic lung disease, chronic cardiovascular disease, diabetes mellitus, chronic liver disease, alcoholism, cochlear implants, cerebrospinal fluid leaks, immunocompromising conditions, and functional or anatomic asplenia; residents of nursing homes or long-term care facilities; adults who smoke cigarettes; and HIV-infected adults. **Revaccination 5 yr after initial dose:** Persons 19 through 64 yr of age with chronic renal failure or nephritic syndrome, functional or anatomic asplenia, and persons with immunocompromising conditions; and adults ≥65 yr of age.	Severe allergic reaction (e.g., anaphylaxis) after a previous dose or to a vaccine component.	Moderate or severe acute illness with or without fever.

Meningococcal Conjugate vaccine (MCV4) Polysaccharide vaccine (MPSV4) 0.5 mL SC, 1 or more doses.	**One dose:** Microbiologists routinely exposed to isolates of *Neisseria meningitidis*, military recruits, and persons who travel to or live in countries where meningococcal disease is hyperendemic or epidemic, and first-year college students up through 21 yr of age who are living in residence halls if no vaccination on or after their 16th birthday. **Two doses:** HIV-infected persons. **Revaccination every 5 yr:** Adults with functional asplenia or persistent complement component deficiencies. **Note:** MCV4 preferred for adults ≤55 yr of age; MPSV4 preferred for adults ≥56 yr of age.	Severe allergic reaction (e.g., anaphylaxis) after a previous dose or to a vaccine component.	Moderate or severe acute illness with or without fever.
Hepatitis A 1 mL IM, repeated in 6–12 mo (Havrix), or 6–18 mo (Vaqta) If Twinrix used, 1 mL IM at 0, 1, and 6 mo; alternatively, administer on days 0, 7, and 21 to 30, followed by booster dose at month 12.	**Any person seeking protection from hepatitis A virus (HAV) and the following:** MSM; injection drug users; laboratory workers exposed to HAV; persons with chronic liver disease or who receive clotting factor concentrates; travelers to countries with high or intermediate endemicity of HAV; and persons who anticipate close personal contact with an adoptee from a country with high or intermediate endemicity during the first 60 d after arrival.	Severe allergic reaction (e.g., anaphylaxis) after a previous dose or to a vaccine component.	Moderate or severe acute illness with or without fever. Pregnancy.

(continued)

Table A-1   Adult Immunizations in the United States (Continued)

Vaccine, Dose	Persons for Whom Indicated	Contraindications	Precautions
Hepatitis B 1 mL IM (in the deltoid) at 0, 1, and 6 mo (Engerix, Recombivax); If Twinrix used, 1 mL IM at 0, 1, and 6 mo; alternatively, administer on days 0, 7, and 21 to 30, followed by booster dose at month 12. For adults receiving hemodialysis or with other immunocompromising conditions: 1 dose of 40 µg/mL (Recombivax) administered on a 3-dose schedule or 2 doses of 20 µg administered simultaneously on a 4-dose schedule at 0, 1, 2, and 6 mo.	**Any person seeking protection from hepatitis B virus (HBV) and the following:** sexually active persons not in a long-term, mutually monogamous relationship (e.g., persons with more than one sex partner during the previous 6 mo); persons seeking evaluation or treatment for a sexually transmitted disease (STD); injection drug users; MSM; health care personnel; public safety workers; persons with diabetes ≤60 yr of age; persons with diabetes >60 yr of age at discretion of the treating clinician based on increased need for assisted blood glucose monitoring in long-term care facilities, likelihood of acquiring hepatitis B infection and likelihood of immune response to vaccination; persons with end-stage renal disease (ESRD), HIV-infected individuals; persons with chronic liver disease; household contacts and sex partners of persons with chronic HBV infection; travelers to countries with high or intermediate prevalence of HBV; all adults in the following settings: STD and HIV testing and treatment facilities; and facilities providing drug-abuse treatment and prevention services, correctional facilities, ESRD programs, facilities for persons with developmental disabilities.	Severe allergic reaction (e.g., anaphylaxis) after a previous dose or to a vaccine component.	Moderate or severe acute illness with or without fever.

Adapted from Centers for Disease Control and Prevention. Recommended adult immunization schedule—United States, 2012. *MMWR.* 2012;61(4).

Table A-2	Passive Immunization

Disease   **Indications and Dosage**

Diphtheria
Suspected respiratory tract diphtheria: diphtheria antitoxin (DAT–equine source), 20,000–120,000 U IV after cultures taken (given in addition to antibiotics). Must be given early; approximately 10% risk of hypersensitivity and/or serum sickness; prior allergy history should be elicited; scratch test dose of 1:100 dilution should be administered; epinephrine should be immediately available. Not routinely recommended for household contacts given significant risk of anaphylaxis and serum sickness and equivalent efficacy of antimicrobial prophylaxis (benzathine penicillin, 1.2 million U IM once, or erythromycin, 500 mg four times daily for 7–10 d). Not currently commercially available in the United States, but may be obtained from the CDC (404-639-2889).

Hepatitis A
Postexposure: Within 14 d of known exposure in high-risk persons (unvaccinated household and sexual contacts of infected individual; coworkers of infected food handlers; all staff and children at day care centers where ≥1 case has occurred or when cases occur in ≥2 households of center attendees; consider for family members of diapered children who attend such day care centers during outbreaks [cases in ≥3 families])—immune globulin (IG), 0.02 mL/kg IM[1] or HAV vaccine, 1 mL IM. For healthy persons aged 12 mo to 40 yr, HAV vaccine is preferred.

Hepatitis B
Preexposure: Vaccine prophylaxis preferred (see Table A-1).
Postexposure: See Table A-7.

Measles
For nonimmune contacts within 6 d of exposure: IG, 0.25 mL/kg (maximum 15 mL) for normal host; 0.5 mL/kg (maximum 15 mL) for immunocompromised patients. MMR vaccine may provide some protection if given within 72 hr of initial exposure.[2]

Rabies
See Tables A-6 to A-9.

Tetanus
See Table A-3.

Varicella
Vaccine, 0.5 mL SC within 3 d of exposure (possibly effective up to 5 d of postexposure) or varicella zoster IG (VariZIG), 1 vial (125 U) IM for each 10-kg body weight (minimum, 125 U; maximum, 625 U) within 96 hr of exposure.[2,3]

---

[1]Can be ordered from the following distributors; delivery within 24 hr can be arranged: Alternative Site Distributors (1-800-837-5403), BioCare Division, Blood Systems, Inc. (1-800-304-3064), Health Coalition (1-800-456-7283), Chapin Medical (1-800-221-7180), FFF Enterprises (1-800-843-7477), Nationwide (1-800-997-8846), NHS (1-800-344-6087). Anaphylaxis has been reported after injection of IG in immunoglobulin (Ig)A-deficient persons.
[2]Live attenuated vaccines (MMR, varicella zoster virus [VZV]) should be delayed after administration of IG (3 mo for MMR, 5 mo for VZV). Patients who received MMR within 2 wk before IG or VZV within 3 wk before IG should be revaccinated.
[3]Available through expanded access protocol sponsored by Cangene Corporation/FFF Enterprises (1-800-843-7477); delivery within 24 hr can be arranged.
CDC, Centers for Disease Control and Prevention; DAT, direct antiglobulin test; HAV, hepatitis A virus; IM, intramuscular; IV, intravenous; MMR, measles, mumps, rubella.

Table A-3	Tetanus Prophylaxis			
History of Tetanus Immunization (Doses)	Clean, Minor Wounds		Other Wounds	
	Give Td	Give TIG[a]	Give Td	Give TIG
Unknown or <3 doses	Yes	No	Yes	Yes
≥3 doses	Only if last dose given ≥10 yr	No	Only if last dose given ≥5 yr	No

[a]250 U intramuscular (IM), given concurrently with Td at a separate site.
Td, adult tetanus-diphtheria booster; TIG, tetanus immune globulin.

Table A-4	Occupational Blood-Borne Pathogen Postexposure Guidelines[1]
Pathogen	Treatment
HIV[2,3]	For LOW RISK exposures (i.e., solid needle and superficial injury from a low-risk patient,[4] or most exposures of mucous membrane or nonintact skin to blood, visibly bloody fluids or other potentially infectious material such as cerebrospinal fluid or amniotic fluid), two-drug postexposure prophylaxis (PEP) × 4 wk is recommended. Possible regimens include: (i) Truvada (tenofovir 300 mg plus emtricitabine 200 mg) one tablet daily OR (ii) Combivir (zidovudine 300 mg plus lamivudine 150 mg) one tablet twice daily.

For HIGHER RISK exposures (i.e., any contaminated hollow needle, deep puncture, visible blood on device, or needle used in patient's artery or vein; or percutaneous injury from a high-risk patient,[5] or large volume splash or spray exposure from a high-risk patient[5]), a third agent should be added × 4 wk to the two-drug regimen outlined above. Possibilities include: (i) Kaletra (lopinavir 200 mg plus ritonavir 50 mg in each tablet) two tablets twice daily OR (ii) atazanavir 300 mg one capsule daily plus ritonavir 100 mg one capsule daily (Adapted from *MMWR* 2005;54(RR09):1–17).

Assistance with choosing a regimen may be obtained by calling the National Clinicians' Post-Exposure Prophylaxis Hotline (PEPline) at 1-888-448-4911 or an infectious disease expert.

For exposures to other material (e.g., urine), therapy is not recommended unless it is visibly contaminated by blood. |

(continued)

Table A-4	Occupational Blood-Borne Pathogen Postexposure Guidelines[1] (Continued)

Pathogen	Treatment
Hepatitis B	For percutaneous injury with blood or blood-contaminated fluids: Unvaccinated health care worker: Administer hepatitis B immunoglobulin (HBIG), 0.06 mL/kg IM, within 96 hr of exposure AND start hepatitis B vaccine series. Vaccinated health care worker: Known responder: no treatment; Nonresponder after initial vaccination: HBIG × 1 and begin revaccination series; Nonresponder after revaccination: HBIG × 2 doses 1 mo apart; Antibody response unknown: check anti-HBs titer; if ≥10 IU/mL: no therapy; if <10 IU/mL: HBIG × 1 and vaccine booster.
Hepatitis C	Immunoglobulin and PEP not effective. Ensure occupational health follow-up for baseline and subsequent follow-up testing.

[1]All blood and body fluid exposures should be reported to the occupational health department. Source patients should be tested for HIV (with consent), hepatitis B surface antigen (HbsAg), and hepatitis C antibody (anti-HCV).
[2]For exposure to patients with known HIV or at high risk for HIV, postexposure prophylaxis should be started as soon as possible (preferably within 1–2 hr, because there is less evidence for efficacy in preventing transmission after 24–36 hr).
[3]Other antiretrovirals may be indicated if there is a high likelihood that the source patient has drug resistance to components of the standard regimen. If therapy is started for a patient with suspected HIV, it can be stopped if the patient's HIV antibody test is negative unless there is a high suspicion of acute HIV illness.
[4]Asymptomatic HIV or HIV viral load <1,500 copies/mL.
[5]Symptomatic HIV infection, AIDS, acute seroconversion, or known high viral load.

Table A-5	Postexposure Prophylaxis for Centers for Disease Control and Prevention (CDC) Class A Bioterrorism Agents[1]

Pathogen	Treatment
Anthrax	Adults: Ciprofloxacin 500 mg PO bid, or doxycycline 100 mg PO bid, or levofloxacin 500 mg PO daily for 60 d and anthrax vaccine absorbed (AVA) SC series: First dose administered as soon as possible, second and third doses administered 2 and 4 wk after the first dose.[2]
Botulinum toxin	Close observation of exposed person, treat with equine antitoxin or human-derived botulism IG at first sign of illness.
Pneumonic plague	For close contacts (<2 m), doxycycline, 100 mg PO bid (see above for pediatric dosing); alternative is trimethoprim-sulfamethoxazole, DS PO bid for adults, 4 mg/kg of the trimethoprim component bid in children. Watch closely for fever or cough, promptly initiate parenteral therapy with streptomycin, 1 g IM q12h, or gentamicin in symptomatic patients.

(continued)

Table A-5	Postexposure Prophylaxis for Centers for Disease Control and Prevention (CDC) Class A Bioterrorism Agents[1] (*Continued*)

Pathogen	Treatment
Tularemia	If attacks identified during early incubation period: ciprofloxacin or doxycycline PO for 14 d (see earlier section for dosing); if attack unrecognized until multiple people ill, observe exposed persons closely, initiate parenteral therapy at first sign of illness.
Smallpox	Vaccinate[3] ideally within 3 d of exposure; vaccination 4–7 d after exposure may offer some protection.

[1]In the event of a bioterrorism attack, the latest recommendations can be accessed via the CDC Internet site: *http://www.bt.cdc.gov.*

[2]AVA is available from CDC (*http://www.cdc.gov*) and through state and local health departments.

[3]An individualized assessment of risks and benefits of vaccination must be made. In general, vaccination for contacts of smallpox cases is recommended even in the presence of usual contraindications (history of or presence of eczema; atopic dermatitis; other acute, chronic, or exfoliative skin conditions; immunosuppression; pregnancy or intent to become pregnant within 4 wk; breast-feeding; age <1 yr). If an exposed person declines vaccination, the alternative strategy is isolation for 19 d.

DS, double strength; IG, immune globulin; IM, intramuscular; PO, by mouth.

Table A-6	Currently Available Rabies Biologics—United States, 2008

Human Rabies Vaccine	Product Name	Manufacturer	Dose, Route	Indications
Human diploid cell vaccine	Imovax Rabies	Sanofi Pasteur Phone: 800-822-2463 Website: *http:// www.vaccine place.com/ products/*	1 mL IM	Preexposure or postexposure[1]
Purified chick embryo cell vaccine	RabAvert	Novartis Vaccines and Diagnostics Phone: 800-244-7668 Website: *http://www .rabavert.com*	1 mL IM	Preexposure or postexposure[1]

(*continued*)

Table A-6	Currently Available Rabies Biologics—United States, 2008 (*Continued*)			
Human Rabies Vaccine	**Product Name**	**Manufacturer**	**Dose, Route**	**Indications**
Rabies immune globulin	Imogam Rabies-HT	Sanofi Pasteur Phone: 800-822-2463 Website: *http:// www.vaccine place.com/ products/*	20 IU/kg local[2]	Postexposure only
	HyperRab S/D	Talecris Biother-apeutics Bayer Biological Products Phone: 800-243-4153 Website: *http:// www.talecris -pi.info*	20 IU/kg local[2]	Postexposure only

[1]For postexposure prophylaxis, the vaccine is administered on days 0, 3, 7, 14, and 28 in patients who have not been previously vaccinated and on days 0 and 3 in patients who have been previously vaccinated. For preexposure prophylaxis, the vaccine is administered on days 0, 7 and 21 or 28.

[2]As much of the products as is anatomically feasible should be infiltrated into and around the wound. Any remaining product should be administered IM in the deltoid or quadriceps (at a location other than that used for vaccine inoculation to minimize potential interference). IM, intramuscular.

Adapted from Centers for Disease Control and Prevention. Human rabies prevention—United States, 2008. *MMWR Recomm Rep* 2008;57:1.

Table A-7	Rabies Preexposure Prophylaxis Guide—United States, 2008	
Risk Category, Nature of Risk	**Typical Populations**	**Preexposure Recommendations**
Continuous—Virus present continuously, often in high concentrations. Specific exposures likely to go unrecognized. Bite, nonbite, or aerosol exposure.	Rabies research laboratory workers; rabies biologics production workers.	Primary course.[1] Serologic testing every 6 mo; booster vaccination[2] if antibody titer is below acceptable level.[3]
Frequent—Exposure usually episodic, with source recognized, but exposure also might be unrecognized. Bite, nonbite, or aerosol exposure.	Rabies diagnostic laboratory workers, cavers, veterinarians and staff, and animal-control and wildlife workers in areas where rabies is enzootic. All persons who frequently handle bats.	Primary course.[1] Serologic testing every 2 yr; booster vaccination[2] if antibody titer is below acceptable level.[3]
Infrequent (greater than population at large)—Exposure nearly always episodic with source recognized. Bite or nonbite exposure.	Veterinarians and animal control staff working with terrestrial animals in areas where rabies is uncommon to rare. Veterinary students. Travelers visiting areas where rabies is enzootic and immediate access to appropriate medical care including biologics is limited.	Primary course.[1] No serologic testing or booster vaccination.
Rare (population at large)—Exposure always episodic with source recognized. Bite or nonbite exposure.	U.S. population at large, including persons in areas where rabies is epizootic.	No vaccination necessary.

[1]Primary: Human diploid cell vaccine (HDCV) or purified check embryo cell vaccine (PCECV): 1 mL intramuscular (IM) (deltoid area), one each on days 0, 7 and 21 or 28.
[2]Booster: HDCV or PCECV: 1 mL IM (deltoid area), day 0 only.
[3]Minimum acceptable antibody level is complete virus neutralization at a 1:5 serum dilution by the rapid fluorescent focus inhibition test. A booster dose should be administered if the titer falls below this level.
Adapted from Centers for Disease Control and Prevention. Human rabies prevention—United States, 2008. *MMWR Recomm Rep* 2008;57:1.

Table A-8	Rabies Postexposure Prophylaxis Guide—United States, 2008	
Animal Type	**Evaluation and Disposition of Animal**	**Postexposure Prophylaxis Recommendations**
Dogs, cats, and ferrets	Healthy and available for 10 d observation	Persons should not begin prophylaxis unless animal develops clinical signs of rabies.[1]
	Rabid or suspected rabid	Immediately begin prophylaxis.
	Unknown (e.g., escaped)	Consult public health officials.
Skunks, raccoons, foxes, and most other carnivores, bats[2]	Regarded as rabid unless animal proven negative by laboratory tests[3]	Consider immediate prophylaxis.
Livestock, small rodents (rabbits and hares), large rodents (woodchucks and beavers), and other mammals	Consider individually	Consult public health officials. Bites from squirrels, hamsters, guinea pigs, gerbils, chipmunks, rats, mice, other small rodents, rabbits, and hares almost never require antirabies postexposure prophylaxis.

[1]During the 10-day observation period, begin postexposure prophylaxis at the first sign of rabies in a dog, cat, or ferret that has bitten someone. If the animal exhibits clinical signs of rabies, it should be euthanized immediately and tested.

[2]Postexposure prophylaxis should be initiated as soon as possible following exposure to such wildlife unless the animal is available for testing and public health authorities are facilitating expeditious laboratory testing or it is already known that brain material from the animal has tested negative. Other factors that might influence the urgency of decision making regarding initiation of postexposure prophylaxis before diagnostic results are known include the species of the animal, the general appearance and behavior of the animal, whether the encounter was provoked by the presence of a human, and the severity and location of bites. Discontinue vaccine if appropriate laboratory diagnostic test (i.e., the direct fluorescent antibody test) is negative.

[3]The animal should be euthanized and tested as soon as possible. Holding for observation is not recommended.

Adapted from Centers for Disease Control and Prevention. Human rabies prevention—United States, 2008. *MMWR Recomm Rep* 2008;57:1.

Table A-9	Rabies Postexposure Prophylaxis Schedule—United States, 2008	

Vaccination Status	Treatment	Regimen[1]
Not previously vaccinated	Wound cleansing	All postexposure prophylaxis should begin with immediate thorough cleansing of all wounds with soap and water. If available, a virucidal agent such as povidone-iodine solution should be used to irrigate the wounds.
	Rabies immune globulin (RIG)	Administer 20 IU/kg body weight. If anatomically feasible, the full dose should be infiltrated around the wound(s) and any remaining volume should be administered intramuscular (IM) at an anatomical site distant from vaccine administration. Also, RIG should not be administered in the same syringe as vaccine. Because RIG might partially suppress active production of antibody, no more than the recommended dose should be given.
	Vaccine	Human diploid cell vaccine (HDCV) or purified chick embryo cell vaccine (PCECV) 1 mL IM (deltoid area),[3] one each on days 0, 3, 7, 14, and 28.

(continued)

Table A-9	Rabies Postexposure Prophylaxis Schedule—United States, 2008 (*Continued*)	

Vaccination Status	Treatment	Regiment[1]
Previously vaccinated[2]	Wound cleansing	All postexposure prophylaxis should begin with immediate thorough cleansing of all wound with soap and water. If available, a virucidal agent such as povidone-iodine solution should be used to irrigate the wounds.
	RIG	RIG should not be administered.
	Vaccine	HDCV or PCECV 1 mL IM (deltoid area),[3] one each on days 0 and 3.

[1]These regimens are applicable for all age groups, including children.

[2]Any person with a history of a complete preexposure or postexposure vaccination regimen with HDCV, PCECV, or rabies vaccine adsorbed, or previous vaccination with any other type of rabies vaccine and a documented history of antibody response to the prior vaccination.

[3]The deltoid area is the only acceptable site of vaccination for adults and older children. For younger children, the outer aspect of the thigh can be used. Vaccine should never be administered in the gluteal area.

Adapted from Centers for Disease Control and Prevention. Human rabies prevention—United States, 2008. *MMWR Recomm Rep* 2008;57:1.

Appendix B

Infection Control and Isolation Recommendations

Carlos A. Q. Santos and Victoria J. Fraser

- **Standard precautions** should be practiced on **all patients at all times** to minimize the risk of nosocomial infection.
  - **Perform hand hygiene** with an alcohol-based rub or foam before and after patient contact (including **after** gloves are removed), after contact with the environment, and in between caring for different patients. Soap and water should be used for visibly contaminated hands and after contact with patients with confirmed or suspected *Clostridium difficile* infection.
  - **Wear gloves** when direct contact with body secretions or blood is anticipated.
  - **Wear a gown** when clothing may be in contact with body fluids.
  - **Wear a mask** when prolonged procedures including puncture of the spinal canal are performed (e.g., myelography, epidural anesthesia, intrathecal chemotherapy).
  - **Wear a mask and protective eyewear** when splashes of body fluid are possible.
  - **Use proper respiratory hygiene and cough etiquette** (applies to health care workers as well as all patients and visiting family or friends). Mouth and nose must be covered when coughing, and tissues must be disposed of properly. Hand hygiene must be performed after contact with respiratory secretions.
  - **Safely dispose** of sharp instruments, needles, wound dressings, and disposable gowns.
- **Specific isolation** procedures must be performed in addition to standard precautions according to the major mode of microorganism transmission in health care settings.
- **Contact precautions** are used when microorganisms can be transmitted via direct contact between patients and health care workers, or by contact between patients and contaminated objects. **In addition** to standard precautions, the following must be done:
  - **Assign the patient to a private room** if possible. Cohorting is allowed if necessary.
  - **Wear gown and gloves** to enter the room; remove them before leaving the room.
  - **Use a dedicated stethoscope and thermometer.**
  - **Minimize environmental contamination** during patient transport (e.g., patient can be placed in a gown).
- **Droplet precautions** are used when microorganisms can be transmitted by respiratory secretion particles larger than 5 microns. Droplets remain suspended in the air for limited periods, and exposure of less than 3 feet (1 meter) is usually required for human-to-human transmission. **In addition** to standard precautions, the following must be done:
  - **Assign the patient to a private room.** The door must be kept closed as much as possible. Rooms with special air handling systems are NOT required.
  - **Wear a surgical mask** within 6 to 10 feet of patients.
  - **Limit patient transport and activity outside their room.** If transporting the patient outside the room is necessary, the patient must wear a surgical mask.
- **Airborne precautions** must be used when microorganisms can be transmitted by respiratory secretion particles smaller than 5 microns. These airborne particles remain suspended in the air for extended periods. **In addition** to standard precautions, the following must be done:
  - **Assign the patient to a negative-pressure room.** Doors must remain closed.

○ **Wear a tightly fitting respirator that covers the nose and mouth with a filtering capacity of 95%** (e.g., N95 mask) to enter the room. Susceptible individuals should not enter the room of patients with confirmed or suspected measles or chickenpox.

○ **Limit patient transport and activity outside their room.** If transporting the patient outside the room is necessary, the patient must wear a surgical mask. Higher level respirator masks (e.g., N95) are NOT required for the patient.

Table B-1	Isolation for Specific Infections and Duration of Isolation

Infection/Condition	Type	Duration, Comments
Abscess (draining, major)	Contact	Duration of illness
Clostridium difficile	Contact	Duration of illness
Conjunctivitis (acute viral)	Contact	Duration of illness; adenovirus most common
Diphtheria (cutaneous)	Contact	Until off antimicrobial treatment and two cultures taken 24 hr apart negative
Diphtheria (pharyngeal)	Droplet	Same as for cutaneous diphtheria
Hepatitis	Contact	Until 1 wk after onset of symptoms
Herpes simplex (mucocutaneous, disseminated or primary, severe)	Contact	Until lesions dry and crusted
Herpes zoster (disseminated disease in any patient)	Airborne, contact	Duration of illness*
Human metapneumovirus	Contact	Duration of illness
Impetigo	Contact	Until 24 hr after start of therapy
Influenza (human, seasonal)	Droplet	Immunocompetent: 5 d; immunocompromised: duration of illness
Measles (rubeola)	Airborne	Immunocompetent: 4 d after onset of rash; immunocompromised: duration of illness*
Meningitis (*Haemophilus influenzae* type b or *Neisseria meningitides*	Droplet	Until 24 hr after start of therapy

(continued)

Table B-1	Isolation for Specific Infections and Duration of Isolation *(Continued)*

Infection/Condition	Type	Duration, Comments
Meningococcal: sepsis, pneumonia, meningitis	Droplet	Until 24 hr after start of therapy
Monkeypox	Airborne, Contact	Airborne: until monkeypox confirmed and smallpox excluded; contact: until lesions crusted
Multidrug-resistant organisms, infection or colonization (e.g., MRSA, VRE, VISA/VRSA, ESBLs, resistant *S. pneumoniae*)	Contact	Duration of hospitalization and future hospitalizations
Mumps (infectious parotitis)	Droplet	Until 9 d after onset of symptoms*
Mycoplasma pneumonia	Droplet	Duration of illness
Parvovirus B19 (erythema infectiosum)	Droplet	Chronic disease, immunocompromised patient: duration of hospitalization; transient aplastic crisis or red-cell crisis: 7 d
Pediculosis (head lice)	Contact	Until 24 hr after start of therapy
Pertussis (whooping cough)	Droplet	Until 5 d after start of therapy
Plague (pneumonic)	Droplet	Until 48 hr after start of therapy
Pneumonia		
Adenovirus	Droplet, contact	Duration of illness; in immunocompromised hosts, extend duration of precautions
Burkholderia cepacia (in patients with CF, including colonization)	Contact	Unknown; avoid exposure to other persons with CF; private room preferred
Streptococcus, group A	Droplet	Until 24 hr after start of therapy
Poliomyelitis	Contact	Duration of illness
Pressure ulcer (infected)	Contact	Duration of illness
Respiratory syncytial virus	Contact	Duration of illness; in immunocompromised hosts, extend duration of precautions

(continued)

Table B-1	Isolation for Specific Infections and Duration of Isolation (*Continued*)	

Infection/Condition	Type	Duration, Comments
Rhinovirus	Droplet	Duration of illness; add contact precautions if copious moist secretions
Ritter's disease (staphylococcal scalded skin syndrome)	Contact	Duration of illness
Rubella (German measles)	Droplet	Until 7 d after onset of rash*; pregnant women who are not immune should not care for these patients
Scabies	Contact	Until 24 hr after start of therapy For Norwegian scabies: 8 d or 24 hr after the second treatment with scabicide
Severe acute respiratory syndrome (SARS)	Airborne, droplet, contact	Duration of illness plus 10 d after resolution of fever if respiratory symptoms are absent or improving; airborne precautions preferred, droplet if negative pressure room unavailable; eye protection (goggles, face shield)
Smallpox (variola)	Airborne, contact	Duration of illness; until all scabs have crusted and separated (3–4 wk* vaccine within 4 d of exposure protective)
Tuberculosis Extrapulmonary, draining lesion	Airborne, contact	Discontinue precautions only when patient is improving clinically, and drainage has ceased, or there are three consecutive negative cultures of continued drainage; examine for evidence of active pulmonary tuberculosis *(continued)*

Table B-1	Isolation for Specific Infections and Duration of Isolation (*Continued*)

Infection/Condition	Type	Duration, Comments
Pulmonary or laryngeal disease, confirmed	Airborne	Discontinue precautions only when patient on effective therapy is improving clinically and has three consecutive sputum smears negative for acid-fast bacilli collected on separate days
Pulmonary or laryngeal disease, suspected	Airborne	Discontinue precautions only when likelihood of infectious TB disease is deemed negligible, and either there is another diagnosis that explains the clinical syndrome or the results of three sputum smears for AFB are negative; each of the three sputum specimens should be collected 8–24 hr apart, and at least one should be an early morning specimen
Varicella zoster	Airborne, contact	Until lesions dry and crusted*; in immuno-compromised host, prolong duration of precautions for duration of illness
Viral hemorrhagic fevers (Lassa, Ebola, Marburg, Crimean-Congo fever viruses)	Droplet, contact	Duration of illness; single-patient room preferred; emphasize use of sharps safety devices and safe work practices, hand hygiene, barrier protection against blood and body fluids upon entry into room including goggles or face shields and appropriate waste handling; use N95 or higher respirators when performing aerosol-generating procedures

*Susceptible health care workers should not enter room if immune caregivers are available.
AFB, acid-fast bacili; CF, cystic fibrosis; ESBL, extended-spectrum beta-lactamase; TB, tuberculosis; VISA, vancomycin-intermediate *Staphylococcus aureus*; VRE, vancomycin-resistant enterococcus; VRSA, vancomycin-resistant *Staphylococcus aureus*.
Adapted from Sieglel JD, Rhinehart E, Jackson M, Chiarello L; the Healthcare Infection Control Practices Advisory Committee. 2007 Guideline for Isolation Precautions: Preventing Transmission of Infectious Agents in Healthcare Settings. http://www.cdc.gov/ncidod/dhqp/pdf/isolation2007.pdf

Table B-2	Isolation for Centers for Disease Control and Prevention Class A[a] Agents of Bioterrorism	

Infection/Condition	Type	Duration, Comments
Anthrax		
Cutaneous	Standard	Duration of hospitalization; contact precautions if with uncontained copious drainage
Inhalational	Standard	Duration of hospitalization
Gastrointestinal	Standard	Duration of hospitalization
Botulism	Standard	Duration of hospitalization
Ebola hemorrhagic fever (intentional release of bioweapon)	Standard, contact, airborne	Duration of illness; single-patient room preferred
Plague	Standard, droplet	Until 48 hr after start of therapy
Smallpox	Standard, contact, airborne	Until all scabs have separated (3–4 wk); only immune health care workers to care for patients; postexposure vaccine within 4 d
Tularemia	Standard	Duration of hospitalization

[a]Six class A agents have been identified by the Center for Disease Control and Prevention. Criteria for inclusion in class A are easily disseminated or transmitted person to person, high mortality, potential for major public health impact, potential for panic and social disruption, and requirements for special action for public health preparedness.
Adapted from Sieglel JD, Rhinehart E, Jackson M, Chiarello L; The Healthcare Infection Control Practices Advisory Committee. 2007 Guideline for Isolation Precautions: Preventing Transmission of Infectious Agents in Healthcare Settings. http://www.cdc.gov/ncidod/dhqp/pdf/isolation2007.pdf

Appendix C

Advanced Cardiac Life Support Algorithms

1

PULSELESS ARREST
- BLS algorithm: Call for help, give CPR
- Give **oxygen** when available
- Attach monitor/defibrillator when available

2 Check rhythm
Shockable rhythm?

Shockable — **3** **VF/VT**

Not shockable — **9** **Asystole/PEA**

4 *Give 5 cycles of CPR**

Give 1 shock
- Manual biphasic: device specific
  (typically 120 to 200 J)
  Note: If unknown, use 200 J
- AED: device specific
- Monophasic: 360 J
Resume CPR immediately

10 **Resume CPR immediately for 5 cycles**
When IV/IO available, give vasopressor
- **Epinephrine** 1 mg IV/IO
  Repeat every 3 to 5 min
  or
- May give 1 dose of **vasopressin** 40 U IV/IO to
  replace first or second dose of **epinephrine**

5 Check rhythm
Shockable rhythm? — *No*

Shockable

6 Continue CPR while defibrillator is charging
Give 1 shock
- Manual biphasic: device specific
  (same as first shock or higher dose)
  Note: if unknown, use 200 J
- AED: device specific
- Monophasic: 360 J
Resume CPR immediately after the shock
When IV/IO available, give vasopressor during CPR
(before or after the shock)
- **Epinephrine** 1 mg IV/IO
  Repeat every 3 to 5 min
  or
- May give 1 dose of **vasopressin** 40 U IV/IO to
  replace first or second dose of **epinephrine**

11 *Give 5 cycles of CPR** Check rhythm
Shockable rhythm?

12
- If asystole, go to Box 10
- If electrical activity, check
  pulse. If no pulse, go to
  Box 10
- If pulse present, begin
  postresuscitation care

13 Go to
Box 4

Not shockable — *Shockable*

7 *Give 5 cycles of CPR** Check rhythm
Shockable rhythm? — *No*

Shockable

8 Continue CPR while defibrillator is charging
Give 1 shock
- Manual biphasic: device specific
  (same as first shock or higher dose)
  Note: if unknown, use 200 J
- AED: device specific
- Monophasic: 360 J
Resume CPR immediately after the shock
Consider **antiarrhythmics**; give during CPR
(before or after the shock)
  amiodarone (300 mg IV/IO once, then
  consider additional 150 mg IV/IO once) or
  lidocaine (1 to 1.5 mg/kg first dose, then 0.5 to
  0.75 mg/kg IV/IO, maximum 3 doses or 3 mg/kg)
Consider **magnesium**, loading dose
  1 to 2 g IV/IO for torsades de pointes
After 5 cycles of CPR,* go to Box 5 above

During CPR
- **Push hard and fast (100/min)**
- **Ensure full chest recoil**
- **Minimize interruptions in chest compressions**
- One cycle of CPR: 30 compressions
  then 2 breaths; 5 cycles = 2 min
- Avoid hyperventilation
- Secure airway and use waveform
  capnography to confirm and monitor
- * After an advanced airway is placed,
  rescuers no longer deliver "cycles"
  of CPR. Give continous chest com-
  pressions without pauses for breaths.
  Give 8 to 10 breaths/min. Check
  rhythm every 2 min

- Rotate compressions every
  2 minutes with rhythm checks
- Search for and treat possible
  contributing factors:
  – Hypovolemia
  – Hypoxia
  – Hydrogen ion (acidosis)
  – Hypo-/hyperkalemia
  – Hypoglycemia
  – Hypothermia
  – Toxins
  – Tamponade, cardiac
  – Tension pneumothorax
  – Thrombosis (coronary
    or pulmonary)
  – Trauma

1

> **BRADYCARDIA**
> Heart rate <60 bpm and
> inadequate for clinical condition

2

> • Maintain patent **airway**; assist **breathing** as needed
> • Give **oxygen**
> • Monitor ECG (identify rhythm), blood pressure, oximetry
> • Establish IV access

3

> ***Signs or symptoms of poor perfusion caused by the bradycardia?***
> (e.g., acute altered mental status, ongoing chest pain, hypotension or other signs of shock)

4A Adequate Perfusion

> Observe/Monitor

Poor Perfusion **4**

> • **Prepare for transcutaneous pacing;**
>   use without delay for high-degree block
>   (type II second-degree block or third-degree
>   block or third-degree AV block)
> • Consider **atropine** 0.5 mg IV while
>   awaiting pacer. May repeat to a total
>   dose of 3 mg. If ineffective, begin pacing
> • Consider **epinephrine** (2 to 10 μg/min)
>   or **dopamine** (2 to 10 μg/kg/min)
>   infusion while awaiting pacer or if
>   pacing ineffective

> ***Reminders***
>
> • If pulseless arrest develops, go to
>   Pulseless Arrest Algorithm
> • Search for and treat possible contributing factors:
>   – Hypovolemia
>   – Hypoxia
>   – Hydrogen ion (acidosis)
>   – Hypo-/hyperkalemia
>   – Hypoglycemia
>   – Hypothermia
>   – Toxins
>   – Tamponade, cardiac
>   – Tension pneumothorax
>   – Thrombosis (coronary or pulmonary)
>   – Trauma (hypovolemia, increased ICP)

5

> • Prepare for **transvenous pacing**
> • Treat contributing causes
> • Consider expert consultation

Figure C-2. Bradycardia algorithm. AV, atrioventricular; bpm, beats per minute; ECG, electrocardiogram; ICP, intracranial pressure; IV, intravenous. (From *American Heart Association in collaboration with the International Liaison Committee on Resuscitation. Guidelines 2010 for cardiopulmonary resuscitation and emergency cardiovascular care. Circulation 2010;122:S729–S767.*)

Figure C-1. Advanced cardiac life support pulseless arrest algorithm. AED, automated external defibrillator; BLS, basic life support; CPR, cardiopulmonary resuscitation; IO, intraosseous; IV, intravenous; PEA, pulseless electrical activity; VF, ventricular fibrillation; VT, ventricular tachycardia. (From *American Heart Association in collaboration with the International Liaison Committee on Resuscitation. Guidelines 2010 for cardiopulmonary resuscitation and emergency cardiovascular care. Circulation 2010;122:S729–S767.*)

Figure C-3. Advanced cardiac life support tachycardia algorithm. AF, atrial fibrillation; AV, atrioventricular; CHF, congestive heart failure; ECG, electrocardiogram; IV, intravenous; WPW, Wolff–Parkinson–White syndrome. (From *American Heart Association in collaboration with the International Liaison Committee on Resuscitation. Guidelines 2010 for cardiopulmonary resuscitation and emergency cardiovascular care. Circulation 2010;122:S729–S767.*)

Index

Page numbers followed by *f* and *t* denotes figures and tables respectively.